Review for USMLE

United States Medical Licensing Examination *STEP 2 CK*

3rd EDITION

Review for USMLE

United States Medical Licensing Examination STEP 2 CK

3rd EDITION

EDITOR

Kenneth Ibsen, PhD

Emeritus Professor of Biochemistry
College of Medicine
University of California, Irvine
Newport Beach, California
Former Director Academic Development
NMSR/Kaplan Medical
Continuing Medical Education Director
Kaplan Medical, USA

CO-EDITOR

Nandan Bhatt, MBBS, MD, FRCS

Physician and Surgeon
Health Care Services Division
State of California
Faculty, Kaplan Medical

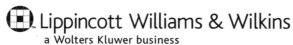 Lippincott Williams & Wilkins
a Wolters Kluwer business
Philadelphia · Baltimore · New York · London
Buenos Aires · Hong Kong · Sydney · Tokyo

Acquisitions Editor: Donna Balado
Managing Editor: Cheryl W. Stringfellow
Marketing Manager: Emilie Linkins
Production Editor: Jennifer P. Ajello
Designer: Holly McLaughlin
Compositor: Circle Graphics
Printer: Courier-Kendallville

Printed in the United States of America

First Edition, 1994
Second Edition, 1999

Library of Congress Cataloging-in-Publication Data

Review for USMLE : United States medical licensing examination step, step 2 CK/editor,
Kenneth Ibsen ; co-editor, Nandan Bhatt.—3rd ed.
    p. cm.
 ISBN 0-7817-6522-6
 1. Medicine—Examinations, questions, etc. I. Ibsen, Kenneth. II. Bhatt, Nandan. III. Title.
R834.5.G78 2006
610.7'6—dc22
                    2005057957

06 07 08 09 10
1 2 3 4 5 6 7 8 9 10

Dedication

To Dr. Victor Gruber, who, while president of National Medical School Review (NMSR), devoted himself to promoting excellence in medical student and physician training; who also made this book possible by sponsoring the first two editions; and to whom I am personally obligated for providing the opportunity to start my second professional career.

To David Hacker, who has dedicated his professional life to the advancement of students and from whom I learned a great deal while working with him for several decades.

And to my wife Marilyn for her love and patience.

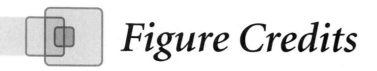

Figure Credits

Test 1 Question 2

From McClatchey KD. *Clinical Laboratory Medicine,* 2nd ed. Philadelphia: Lippincott Williams & Wilkins, 2002.

Test 4 Question 34

Test 7 Question 14

Test 19 Question 1

Adapted from Goldschlager N, Goldman M. *Principles of Clinical Electrocardiography,* 13th ed. Norwalk, CT: Appleton & Lange, 1989. Used with permission from McGraw-Hill.

Test 5 Question 19

Test 15 Question 12

From Fleisher GR, Ludwig S, Baskin MN. *Atlas of Pediatric Emergency Medicine.* Philadelphia: Lippincott Williams & Wilkins, 2004.

Test 7 Question 19

Test 10 Question 23

Test 12 Question 2

Test 17 Question 33

Test 18 Answer 6

Test 20 Question 16

From Rubin E, Farber JL. *Pathology,* 3rd ed. Philadelphia: Lippincott Williams & Wilkins, 1999.

Test 13 Question 16

From Crapo JD, Glassroth J, Karlinsky JB, King TE, Jr. *Baum's Textbook of Pulmonary Diseases,* 7th ed. Philadelphia: Lippincott Williams & Wilkins, 2004.

Test 14, Questions 46, 48–50

Assets provided by Anatomical Chart Company.

Test 15 Question 35

From Smeltzer SC, Bare BG. *Textbook of Medical-Surgical Nursing,* 9th ed. Philadelphia: Lippincott Williams & Wilkins, 2000.

Test 16 Question 29

From Harwood-Nuss A, Wolfson AB, et al. *The Clinical Practice of Emergency Medicine,* 3rd ed. Philadelphia: Lippincott Williams & Wilkins, 2001.

Contents

Contributors... xi

Preface xiii

Examination Preparation Guide xv

Test 1
QUESTIONS 3
ANSWER KEY.. 13
ANSWERS AND EXPLANATIONS.................................. 15

Test 2
QUESTIONS 37
ANSWER KEY.. 47
ANSWERS AND EXPLANATIONS.................................. 49

Test 3
QUESTIONS 69
ANSWER KEY.. 79
ANSWERS AND EXPLANATIONS.................................. 81

Test 4
QUESTIONS 101
ANSWER KEY.. 113
ANSWERS AND EXPLANATIONS.................................. 115

Test 5
QUESTIONS 135
ANSWER KEY.. 145
ANSWERS AND EXPLANATIONS.................................. 147

Test 6
QUESTIONS 165
ANSWER KEY.. 175
ANSWERS AND EXPLANATIONS.................................. 177

Test 7
QUESTIONS 195
ANSWER KEY.. 205
ANSWERS AND EXPLANATIONS.................................. 207

Test 8
QUESTIONS 227
ANSWER KEY.. 235
ANSWERS AND EXPLANATIONS.................................. 237

Test 9
QUESTIONS 255
ANSWER KEY.. 265
ANSWERS AND EXPLANATIONS.................................. 267

Test 10
QUESTIONS 289
ANSWER KEY.. 299
ANSWERS AND EXPLANATIONS.................................. 301

Test 11
QUESTIONS 319
ANSWER KEY.. 329
ANSWERS AND EXPLANATIONS.................................. 331

Test 12
QUESTIONS 351
ANSWER KEY.. 359
ANSWERS AND EXPLANATIONS.................................. 361

Test 13
QUESTIONS 379
ANSWER KEY.. 389
ANSWERS AND EXPLANATIONS.................................. 391

Test 14
QUESTIONS 409
ANSWER KEY.. 419
ANSWERS AND EXPLANATIONS.................................. 421

Test 15
QUESTIONS 441
ANSWER KEY.. 451
ANSWERS AND EXPLANATIONS.................................. 453

Test 16
QUESTIONS 473
ANSWER KEY.. 483
ANSWERS AND EXPLANATIONS.................................. 485

Test 17
QUESTIONS 505
ANSWER KEY.. 515
ANSWERS AND EXPLANATIONS.................................. 517

Test 18

QUESTIONS 535

ANSWER KEY 545

ANSWERS AND EXPLANATIONS.................................... 547

Test 19

QUESTIONS 569

ANSWER KEY 579

ANSWERS AND EXPLANATIONS.................................... 581

Test 20

QUESTIONS 603

ANSWER KEY 613

ANSWERS AND EXPLANATIONS.................................... 615

Discipline Index 633

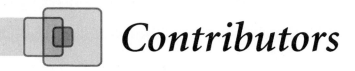

Contributors

Nandan Bhatt, MBBS, MD, FRCS
Physician and Surgeon
Health Care Services Division
State of California
Faculty, Kaplan Medical

Kenneth Ibsen PhD
Emeritus Professor of Biochemistry
College of Medicine
University of California, Irvine
Newport Beach, California
Former Director Academic Development
NMSR/Kaplan Medical
Continuing Medical Education Director
Kaplan Medical, USA

Edward Goljan, MD
Professor and Chairman, Department
    of Pathology
College of Osteopathic Medicine
Oklahoma State University
Tulsa, Oklahoma

Christine E. Koerner, MD, FAAP, FACEP
Associate Professor of Emergency Medicine
University of Texas Health Science Center at
    Houston Medical School
Chief, Division of Pediatric Emergency Medicine
Lyndon B. Johnson General Hospital
Houston, Texas

Elmar P. Sakala, MA, MPH, MD, FACOG
Professor of Gynecology and Obstetrics
Clinical Clerkship Director
School of Medicine
Loma Linda University
Loma Linda, California
Director, Obstetrics and Gynecology
Kaplan Medical, USA

Roderick Shaner, MD
Clinical Professor of Psychiatry
Keck School of Medicine
University of Southern California
Medical Director
Los Angeles County Department of Mental Health
Los Angeles, California

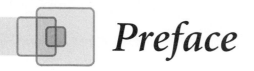

Preface

During the past decade, the first and second editions of the *NMS Review for USMLE Step 2* have served as important adjuncts for students preparing to take the USMLE Step 2 Examination. This, the third edition, is now called *NMS Review for USMLE Step 2 CK* to reflect the fact that it only relates to the CK (clinical knowledge) component of the current two-part Step 2 Examination. In providing this knowledge, it continues the traditions of relevance and excellence established by the previous editions but is also improved as described below:

- All items (an item is defined as a clinical vignette, with distractors, answers, and explanations) have been updated to conform to current clinical practice.
- The number of items has been increased to 1000.
- All distractors, correct and incorrect, are explained.
    - As a consequence, there are more than 5000 explanations, which for the most part, pertain to different clinical conditions.
- The style of the items closely reflects that presently found on the USMLE.
    - Clinical descriptions included in the question stems have been expanded.
    - Some items have more than five distractors.
    - All matching set questions have only one correct answer, and explanations of items not matched are also included.
    - All tests have 50 items.

Of course, the factors that made the second edition so effective have been retained.

- Content is highly relevant to that asked on the examination.
- The questions cover the various clinical disciplines in a random fashion as they do in the USMLE.
- A simplified subject item index is included, making it possible to study each discipline independently. The approximate total percentage of items per disciple is as follows: medicine, 32%: pediatrics, psychiatry, and surgery, 15%; obstetrics and gynecology, 14%; and preventive medicine and public health, 8%.
- Explanations, sometimes detailed, are provided for the incorrect choices as well as for the correct answer, helping the student understand why he or she chose an incorrect distractor and also increasing the breadth of coverage related to a given question.
- A study guide is provided to help students optimize their preparation for the examination and to more effectively use this volume.

We, past and present contributors and publishers, sincerely wish to thank the many past students who benefited from using past editions of this book; nothing made us happier than hearing that this book helped them reach their goal. In the future, we anticipate that the diligent use of this volume will help thousands of additional students to successfully negotiate the road to licensure by helping them obtain a superior score on the Step 2 CK Examination.

Kenneth Ibsen, PhD
Nandan Bhatt, MD

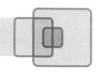

Examination Preparation Guide

I. Steps to Licensure and the Structure of The USMLE Step 2 CK Examination

A. BACKGROUND

During the past decades, the National Board of Medical Examiners (NBME) has transformed the United States Medical Licensing Examination (USMLE) from the multiple choice Steps 1 and 2 of the 1980s and early 1990s to the present four-step process—Step 1, Step 2 CK (Clinical Knowledge), Step 2 CS (Clinical Skills), and Step 3. In doing so, they also changed the process from one that primarily required recall of facts into a process that better tests the application of knowledge and skills to the solution of realistic clinical problems. Of these four steps to licensure, the Step 2 CS examination requires examinee interaction with live simulated patients. In contrast, the Step 1, Step 2 CK, and Step 3 examinations retain a multiple choice format, but the examiners have developed more sophisticated modes of presentation, requiring analytical problem-solving abilities that better simulate those required of practicing physicians. During this period, the examinations also have evolved from pencil-and-paper examinations to the contemporary computerized ones. Although passage of all three multiple choice examination steps requires application of similar types of cognitive skills, each step requires a more sophisticated level of understanding of clinical principles.

- The USMLE Step 1 tests how well the examinee understands the application of the basic sciences to clinical situations at a level expected of a U.S. student who just finished the second year of medical school.
- The USMLE Step 2 CK is designed to test the basic elements of biomedical and clinical knowledge at a level that will permit the student to care for patients under close supervision.
- The USMLE Step 3 is designed to assess the same elements but now at a level permitting safe care of patients under unsupervised conditions and with greater emphasis on management of the ambulatory patient.

Although the steps are designed to be taken in sequence, if you are a student or graduate of a school accredited by the Liaison Committee on Medical Education (LCME) or the American Osteopathic Association (AOA), you may take the Step 1, Step 2 CK, and Step 2 CS examinations in any order. However, if you are an international medical graduate (IMG), you may take the Step 2 CK examination prior to the Step 1 examination, but you must have passed the Step 1 examination before being permitted to register for the Step 2 CS examination. Generally, it is wisest to take these three examinations in the suggested sequence; an exception to this generality may be foreign graduates who had been practicing physicians and who, because of their already developed clinical acumen, may find it easier to slide into the USMLE examinations at the Step 2 CK level. All persons must have passed Step 1 and both parts of Step 2 before being permitted to take Step 3. In general, the Step 3 examination is taken toward the end of the first year of residency. However, several states permit students to take this examination before being admitted into a residency program.

B. STRUCTURE AND CONTENT OF THE STEP 2 CK EXAMINATION

Only the essential highlights will be provided here, since the reader can obtain a detailed and continuously updated description of the examination on the USMLE web site (USMLE.org).

1) Construction. The Step 2 CK Examination is a 9-hour computerized marathon divided into eight 60-minute examination blocks, plus an optional 15-minute tutorial session and 45 minutes of self-scheduled free time. Although the number of questions asked may differ slightly in different examination blocks, the maximum number will be 50, with a probable average number of 46. As long as you work within a given 60-minute examination block, you may review and change your responses as often as you desire. However, once time is up or if you declare you are finished with a block, you cannot return to it, and the next 60-minute examination period will start. On the other hand, if you finish before the 60-minute period ends, you may either start the next one or take a break.

2) Scoring. The score you receive is based upon the total number of correct answers; Incorrect answers are not counted against you, so it behooves you to answer all questions even if you must randomly guess to finish within the allotted time.

3) Score Reporting. Each person takes a different examination, but all examinations are designed to be at an equivalent difficulty level. The 3-digit score you will receive is calculated by a formula that includes your percentage score and your percentile compared with those of recent examinees. You will also be provided with the mean score and the standard deviation of recent examinations, as well as the minimum passing score. The latter may change from year to year and has been raised for the past few years; presently it is set at 182, corresponding to answering 60 to 70% of the questions correctly. A two-digit score is also reported. This score is in reality an anachronism used so that a score of 75 can be reported as the minimal pass as required by some institutions. Students sometimes mistakenly assume that this is a percentage score, but it has no innate meaning, since it is derived from the 3-digit score. Although the two- and three-digit scores report equivalent information, the 3-digit scale provides a better assessment of performance, since scores get condensed in the 2-digit system.

II. Preparation for and Taking the Examination

A. DEVELOPING BASIC KNOWLEDGE

Each of you has a unique set of academic strengths and weaknesses that will affect what and how you should prepare for the examination. In addition, you each are influenced by a set of nonacademic factors including personal relationships and financial resources that influence the time and modes available for study. These factors plus your innate genetic constitution also influence the psychologic and physiologic resources you can make available for preparation as well as for taking the examination itself. This makes it impossible to lay out one set of study rules that will fit everybody. Nonetheless, there are several generalities that fit most students preparing for the USMLE. Each student must decide how to best weigh these generalities and make decisions concerning scheduling study time and selecting topics to study, materials to use, and study and learning modes and how to best care for themselves as they proceed. However, some ideas that will be germane for most students are provided below:

1) Limit Isolated Passive Study. Reading and highlighting textbooks and/or lecture notes is a way to become familiar with basic terminology but continually rereading the same material trying to make the subject matter sink in will almost guarantee failure. Even when studying in isolation, you should make the process more active by asking yourself questions, for example by writing important terms down on flash cards and then testing yourself with them.

2) Use a Study Group to Help Formulate Central Concepts. As your understanding of the basic terminology increases, you will subconsciously be formulating central concepts. These concepts will permit you to extrapolate information derived in a given situation to a different one, a function required to successfully interpret many of the questions on the examination. Concept formulation is even better facilitated by the exchange of ideas that occurs in study groups of four or five persons in which you are exposed to differing opinions. To avoid the fatal error of formulating false concepts, you must be an active participant in your group and not be afraid to freely share your thoughts even if it means you might demonstrate your ignorance. To not share your thoughts is only a half-step up from studying in isolation and will still run the risk of fortifying fallacious central concepts. However, the converse is equally true: you must not try to dominate the group because, in addition to making yourself unpopular, you will not hear what others are saying. How these study groups are best created depends in large part upon your background.

If you attend medical school in the United States or are a U.S. student from an offshore medical school, you probably have such a study group composed of classmates. In addition, you may be able to participate in short review courses provided by your school. Besides highlighting important concepts, such review courses serve as organized study groups.

However, if you are an international medical graduate you probably do not have a preexisting study group available; thus you should seek out like persons with whom you can share information and feelings. Often this is most easily and efficiently done by participating in a commercially available review course in which the material reviewed is presented either via lecture or video. Although these can be expensive, the experience is usually worth the cost. In either case, the opportunity to interact with fellow students can be as important as exposure to the material presented.

Book- or computer-based studies present an effective way to test yourself as your studies progress. Additionally, if a study group of four or five students works in unison using the same study material, they have in effect established a mini-review program; for example, a group can agree beforehand to individually answer *y* questions in test *x* and then subsequently meet as a group to discuss the questions and answers. This way, those who have trouble with a concept can see how those who do not have a problem came up with the correct response. It also provides a chance to discuss ramifications among yourselves and even—rarely, one hopes—decide that the information provided is in error.

B. CONFIRMING YOUR ACADEMIC ABILITY TO TAKE THE EXAMINATION

The study activities described in the preceding paragraphs will increase your familiarity with an ever-increasing number of terms that you will be able to associate with an ever-increasing number of relevant conditions and will help you consolidate some central concepts. However, it will still be necessary to answer simulated USMLE test questions. This will further consolidate your knowledge, increase your test-taking skills, and confirm your readiness to take the examination. To truly test your readiness, you have to take practice examinations that not only probe your knowledge base but also test your ability to apply this knowledge to taking the real examination. Basically there are two ways to obtain realistic testing experiences:

1) Take the Real Examination on a Trial Basis. Since you can repeat the examination without a failure counting against you as far as testing associations are concerned, this may seem to be reasonable option. However, it is not recommended because the attempt will be entered into your record, and if you pass, you will be forever burdened with a score that may not reflect your true potential.

2) Take Commercially Available USMLE-Style Examinations Available in Books or as Computer Programs. Such commercially available examinations are of variable quality. Often they consist of a mix of questions that can be answered by rote along with questions on par with those used in the USMLE. Further value will be obtained if such programs explain both the correct and incorrect responses; this expands the breadth of the question, often clarify why you chose the incorrect response and helps you understand relationships between related conditions, for example, how to distinguish among different diseases to be considered as part of a differential diagnosis.

C. IMPROVING YOUR TEST-TAKING SKILLS

Doing well on multiple choice–type examinations requires development of a set of test-taking skills. Most U.S. students have been exposed to multiple choice examinations since they cut their eyeteeth, while many IMG students have had minimal experience with them. Although this does provide the U.S. student with an advantage, surprisingly the playing field has become more level with the advent of the new type of USMLE examinations, because these require many of the analytical skills used in an oral or essay examination. A practical example of the change is in the advice that can be given concerning the most efficient way to answer questions. The classic response to answering the older single-best-choice question was to simply read the first and last sentences of the stem to determine what the question is about and what is asked and then to look for the most logical distractor. Typically, that minimal effort would put you in a good position to select the best choice among the distractors. However, contemporary Step 2 CK questions usually require that you also understand the significance of the information imparted in the body of the vignette before attempting to answer the question. Consequently, it is recommended that while using USMLE-type practice examinations to test your knowledge, you hone your question-answering skills by using the following approach: (1) look at the last sentence in the vignette and determine what question is asked (i.e., is it a diagnosis, the next best step in management, the pathology, etc.); (2) carefully read the vignette, and in your mind formulate the underlying central concept by asking yourself what of the description is truly relevant to the question asked; and (3) carefully read the distractors, looking for the one that most clearly relates to the central concept you formulated and also answers the question asked. You should be able to identify the one best choice.

Often there will be a second choice that seems as if it too might be correct; perhaps there is a distractor that would be correct under special circumstances or one that relates to a factoid in the vignette not relevant to the central concept. Having read the vignette carefully, you should be able to identify the one that is the best choice, but if you are still in doubt, don't waste time deliberating; make a choice and move on to the next question. Realize that although this might seem like making a guess, because you did think about it, it is an educated guess, and your choice is most likely the correct one. Resist the temptation to brood over a subtlety you may find. This will cause you to waste time, perhaps forcing you to make wild guesses on other questions in the last few seconds before time is up. Moreover, if you do finish before the allotted time is up, you should learn to refrain from going back and changing you first response on the basis of lingering doubts; odds are that your first response was the correct one.

After finishing your practice tests you can go back to look at questions in which you debated between two possible choices and see if whether your instinctive response was correct. It would be surprising if it wasn't more often than not. Furthermore, by analyzing the explanation provided you may be able to understand why you were tempted by the wrong choice. A corollary to this approach is to carefully control the time factor; learn to spend no more than 72 seconds, preferably less, on each question.

The previous paragraphs focus on the one-best-choice type of question. These will constitute some 75 to 80% of the questions on the examination. The remaining ones will be of the matching-set variety, typically presented at the end of an examination block. In these, you are faced with up to 26 optional choices followed by a brief question and a minimum of two relatively brief vignettes asking you to pick the option that best relates to the vignette and also answers the question. Although in the past you may have been asked to select more than one option, the examples and references relating to the 2005 Step 2 CK Examination show only a single choice. Presumably this is the newer format. A suggested approach for efficiently answering such matching item sets is the following: (1) first read the question; (2) glance at the options to get an idea of the type and range of possibilities; (3) read the first questioning vignette; (4) think of an option of the type listed that seems logical; (5) look through the list and choose the one that most closely agrees to the one in your mind. Odds are you will find one close match and this will be the correct choice. However, if you can't come up with a matching choice, attack the problem in the reverse manner and eliminate choices that are obviously wrong; even if this won't necessarily provide one clear choice, it will reduce the number of possibilities, making a correct guess more likely. After completing this cycle by answering the question raised in the first vignette, do the same with the second one, then the third, and so on. Remember that a given option may be used once, more than once, or never, so don't try to eliminate a choice on the basis of its prior use.

Both types of questions may involve a list of clinical values, and as a rule, the only ones relevant to the question are among those that are abnormal. Although you will be able to refer to a table of accepted values to identify abnormal ones, this will take time. Thus, it will behoove you to memorize some of the normal ranges of several of the more common disease states. Although normal values used at various hospitals or clinics may differ to a slight degree from those provided by the USMLE, these differences should be too small to affect an answer. In the real USMLE, the clinical values are readily available via a computerized list. Since this is not possible in a written format, the correct values are provided in the NMS third edition along with the question.

D. IMPROVING YOUR PSYCHOLOGIC AND PHYSIOLOGIC ABILITY TO TAKE THE EXAMINATION

Your psychologic and physiologic status can be as important as your intellectual readiness. There is no escaping the fact that spending almost 9 hours in an intimate relationship with a computer is stressful. Consequently, you need to prepare yourself as well as possible. Some ideas include the following:

- Once you have studied enough to achieve a basic working vocabulary, start answering USMLE-style questions by taking USMLE-style mini-examinations using suitable USMLE-type question-and-answer materials. These mini-examinations serve several purposes. As discussed above, they enhance your examination-taking skills (increase your sense of timing, etc.). They increase your knowledge base directly by exposing you to new information and indirectly by providing feedback to help guide your studies. The consistent improvement you are bound to show will boost your confidence. This can be of critical importance for students who suffer from excessive test anxiety.
- At first these mini-examinations should be composed of a relatively small number of questions because you should still be expanding your knowledge base, and much of your time should be spent analyzing why you missed what you did. If you determine that most of your errors were due to ignorance, you need to go back to your earlier phases of study. If you tend to primarily miss questions in a given area, you should focus on that area. However, more than likely you will find that you more often miss ques-

tions because you misinterpreted the question and/or one or more distractors and consequently jumped to an incorrect assumption. Realizing this and making a conscious effort to reread and interpret this type of question coupled with practice should reduce your tendency to make such erroneous snap judgments, even under the pressure of limited time. Increase the number of questions in your practice sessions as your scheduled time to take the examination draws nearer. At least 2 weeks before the examination you should try simulating a full 9-hour examination. Then about a week later, simulate taking the full examination again, even if you must use the same practice examination. Don't worry, unless you have a photographic memory the improvement you will show will be because you learned something, and this improvement will once again heighten your confidence. As mentioned above, the real examination consists of eight 1-hour examinations. This book has 20 such examinations. Accordingly, it provides enough test material for two full simulated examinations plus four extra tests. It is recommended that four of the 20 tests be used for the initial mini-test before trying to simulate a full examination. These tests can be taken in any order, since they should be approximately equivalent.

- From the beginning you should time yourself. You will have exactly 60 minutes to answer up to 50 questions on the real test. To make the process a bit more challenging, assume only 50 minutes are available. Thus, you should allot 50 minutes for a 50-question test, 25 minutes for 25-question test, etc. You are better off timing the whole group of questions rather than individual ones; not only is this easier to do since you need only set your timing device once, but it will help you develop an intrinsic sense of proper pacing.

- Review the tutorial on the official USMLE CD-ROM, then re-review it until you have memorized the operational key strokes required to navigate from screen to screen and the types and locations of information on the screens. The operational aspects of the program should be second nature for you by the time you take the examination. This again will lead to a feeling of confidence at the start of the test and will also permit you to use most of the 15-minute tutorial session provided to answer questions rather than playing with the computer.

- Establish beneficial sleep habits. About a month before the scheduled examination, start going to bed early and getting up early. This will adjust your circadian rhythm to match that required when the real day comes. It will also improve the odds that you will get a good night's sleep and be able to wake up refreshed and prepared to remain alert during that long examination day that not only will include the 9-hour examination, but also time to eat breakfast, get dressed, travel, etc.

- Plan on getting to the Prometric Center about 30 minutes earlier than your scheduled time. Although this will extend the length of your day, it will provide a margin of safety in case of unexpected travel delays and will give you time to relax and acclimatize yourself.

- Start watching your diet; practice eating a good breakfast that will maintain you into noon. If possible, get into the habit of having a bowel movement after breakfast and before the time you will need to leave to take the examination; you don't want to waste examination time sitting on the toilet. If early hunger becomes a problem, experiment with a power bar or some such supplement that satisfies you, can be readily consumed, and does not stick to your teeth to distract you afterward. Also get into the habit of packing light but nutritious lunches that satisfy, are not messy, are easy to carry around, and sit well on your stomach.

- As much as possible, adjust personal arrangements to reduce stress. Discuss your need for a peaceful interlude with your spouse, significant other, or those in any other close relationships. Get your finances under control; make sure there will be no financial crises arising during the week prior to the examination.

- At least a day before the examination (and ideally earlier if travel is not a major obstacle), go to the Prometric Center where your examination is scheduled. Make sure you know how to get there and how long it will take. Go inside and familiarize yourself with personnel, procedures, and the computer setup.

- If the drive to the Prometric Center from your residence is excessive, make arrangements to spend the night before the examination in a comfortable and quiet place closer to the Center.

- The night before the examination, lay out what you will need the following day, your clothes, lunch, anything you might want as a snack, and any other personal items such as your watch, glasses, and a pen or pencil. You will also want to lay out the items need to be admitted to the examination including your photo identification, scheduling permit, and confirmation ticket and number. Also make arrangements to wake up in time; set an alarm clock or ask for a wake-up call. Not only will that get you started on time, but also it is likely to help you sleep better because you will not subconsciously be worried about waking up. Don't forget transportation. If you are going by public transportation, be sure of the schedule and have the proper change for carfare. If you are going in your own car, make sure it has enough fuel and is otherwise in proper operational order. Also determine ahead of time what parking facilities are available and allow for extra transportation time if it is raining or snowing.

■ On the day before the examination you will be nervous. So rather than trying to do last-minute cramming that is liable to be ineffective at best and will only make you more nervous, try to relax. Go someplace special with a loved one, who very likely has been feeling neglected, or at least take a walk, commune with nature, in short do something peaceful and pleasant, even if part of your day must be spent in travel. Whatever you do, don't use alcohol or drugs as a tool to help you relax; you want to be clear-headed the following morning.

E. TAKING THE EXAMINATION

After having a relaxing day and a good night's sleep, you arrive 30 minutes before your scheduled time at the designated examination site, nervous but bright-eyed and bushy-tailed. After checking in, you then make good use of any free time remaining by taking a brief walk in anticipation of sitting for a long time. Also make a prophylactic trip to the bathroom. The momentous moment arrives; you enter your cubicle and face the computer. Now it is up to you to manage the next 9 hours at maximal efficiency and demonstrate what you really know.

1) Managing Your Scheduled Free Time. You are provided with a total of 9 examination hours, which include eight 1-hour blocks of uninterruptible test time, 45 minutes of free time, and 15 minutes of optional tutorial time. Since you have practiced the tutorial at home ad infinitum, there is no reason for you to do so again. Thus you can use this 15 minutes as extra free time in any manner you like. Remember that the computer will continue to count time even if you depart from your cubicle during an hour scheduled as examination time. This not only shortens the time available for test taking, but the departure will be logged in as a potential irregularity; so use the free time to prevent a need for an interruption, as well as a way to refresh yourself so that you can function well during these intense sessions. We suggest that you use about 30 minutes of the available hour of free time in short 5- to 10-minute breaks between testing blocks to unwind after finishing an intense hour. During these brief intervals, stretch your legs and exercise your arms by doing pushups against the wall. If you are hungry, eat a small bite, if possible go outside and breathe fresh air, and go to the bathroom. Use the remaining 30 minutes of free time after the fourth or fifth examination block as a longer break during which you eat your prepacked light lunch and then relax. Don't try to do last-minute cramming during these breaks. Not only would it be a waste of time but such last-minute cramming is liable to raise your anxiety level and also accelerate the development of fatigue. Above all, remember to keep track of your free time; once you use it up there will be no more breaks, no matter how fatigued you are. Moreover, any nonexamination time you might take in excess of the allotted hour is subtracted from the final hour of examination time. Conversely, by completing an examination block in less than an hour you in effect buy additional free time that may come in handy later in the day.

2) Managing Your Examination Time. Remember that you will have exactly 1 hour in which to finish a question block. When time is up, the computer will switch off. There will be no last seconds to fill in unanswered questions as in the typical paper-and-pencil examination. Consequently, it is best to answer questions one at a time in the order presented, proceeding at a measured pace and always keeping an eye on the clock so that no question will be left unanswered when the program terminates. Should it appear that you will not finish on time, increase the pace, and, as a last resort, guess. An incorrect response is no worse than no response. If there are about 20 minutes remaining and you still have not finished answering the one-best-choice type of questions, quickly glance at them, make your best guess; mark these as questions you may wish to return to, and then start answering the matching questions. Generally, one can answer these faster than the one-best-choice variety. Moreover, the odds of guessing a correct answer is 20% for the typical five-distractor one-best-choice questions and 10% or less for matching questions; thus, guessing is apt to have better returns for the former. If after finishing the matching questions extra time still remains, go back to the first one-best-choice that began the guessing sequence and proceed as if it were the first time you saw it; under these circumstances, changing an answer after making a guess is permissible, since this is not the same as changing an answer on questions that you had time to think about. Make a habit of using the question-marking function but do it very conservatively; use it only on the items for which your guesses were not made on the basis of due deliberation. If you made an "informed" guess, odds are that your first response was the proper one anyway. If you feel a rising sense of panic during an examination time, stop for a moment, take a series of deep breaths, think about the successes you had during your practice sessions, and remember that nobody is asking you to be perfect. Odds are that you will pass even if you miss one of every three questions, and you might be doing better than average if you are answering 25% of the questions incorrectly.

III. Using This Book

A. THE BOOK'S STRUCTURE

The authors of this book have taken great effort to create a product that simulates the questions used in the USMLE Step 2 CK Examination in terms of analytical prowess required and format. However, as whole the difficulty level may be a bit higher than that of the real examination. There are a total of 1000 questions arranged into twenty 50-question examinations in which the subject material is arranged in a random fashion, requiring the test taker to practice the mental gymnastics of rapidly switching from topic to topic as in the real examination. As in the real examination, the initial 75 to 80% of the questions are of the one-best-choice variety, and the remainder are of the matching type. In addition to providing the correct answer, the correct and incorrect distractors and unused matching distractors are explained, often in detail. A subject index at the back of the book describes the subject of each question in terms of the six major clinical disciplines—medicine, obstetrics and gynecology, pediatrics, preventive medicine and public health, psychiatry, and surgery. Most of the many topics included in the USMLE description of the examination are included as belonging to one or another of these six disciplines. For example, dermatology and ophthalmology are considered subdisciplines of medicine and surgery, respectively.

B. SUGGESTED WAYS TO USE THIS BOOK

1) In Preparation for the USMLE. You can use the items in this book as a tool for increasing your knowledge base, for developing the analytical skills that will be required, and as a measure of your readiness to take the examination. It is suggested that during the very early phases of your study, you randomly select 10 to 15 questions for 5 to 10 days, setting aside a period equal to 1 minute per question for the question selected. At the end of each of these mini-tests, you should study both the correct and incorrect responses to try to understand why the correct answer is correct and the others are incorrect. These items can also be used for discussion in your small study group during following days.

After this period, you should be ready to test yourself more seriously. Now set aside an hour and take one of the 50-question examinations. This will give you an average of 72 seconds to answer each question, a time on a par with the real examination. Pace yourself and make sure you answer all the questions even if you have to guess to finish on time; in other words, make believe you are under the same constraints as you will be when the big day arrives. When you finish, study the answers as before but also calculate your overall percentage score and the percentage obtained in each of the six disciplines. Don't worry if you are not getting 100%, remember that correctly answering 60 to 70% of the questions on the real examination should be a passing score, while answering 75 to 80% correctly will result in score that is at or above the mean. However, if your score in one of the disciplines is remarkably below your average, devote extra time for study in that area. For each question, be sure you understand why the correct answer is correct and the incorrect one is not. Once you feel that you have gleaned all the information you can from that examination, repeat the experience using a second 50-question examination. After that, repeat the same process but set aside 2 hours and answer 100 questions found in two examinations. This time it should be easier to finish all the questions in the allotted time and your percentage score should improve as you gain additional knowledge and better hone your test-taking skills.

Ideally, your next step is to simulate taking the full 9-hour examination. Try to arrange your affairs so that you can set aside an uninterrupted 9-hour day in which you take eight 1-hour examinations (400 questions) with 1 hour of free time disbursed in the way you think will be most efficient. In addition to providing further study, this will help you get used to the stress and fatigue factors and serve as a model to guide your future distribution of free time. During this 9-hour period, follow the rules proscribed by the NBME. After finishing, relax and limit your thinking to how you might have better used your free time; for example, were you too tired toward the end and might you have done better if you had saved more free time to refresh yourself? On the following day dissect your performance in more detail; once again make sure you understand why correct answers are correct and wrong ones wrong; determine if your score could be in the passing range or above average; determine if there are topic areas in which you are weaker than average. Then spend time taking appropriate remedial action and finally repeat the process, once again taking advantage of what you learned and using the final 400 questions.

Except for the first 100 to 150 questions taken randomly for the earliest mini-tests, the program outlined does not require using the same question more than once. However, in the unlikely event you still do not feel ready to take the examination you might wish to test yourself further. If so, select a minimum of 50 questions from one of the earlier examinations and repeat the trial test process under timed conditions followed by analysis. You should see further improvement. Don't assume that it is because you have memorized the questions and answers, since there is little chance that a repeated question will be more than vaguely familiar after the passage of a couple of weeks filled with other study materials.

Try hard to set aside the suggested two 9-hour days. However, if for personal reasons this is impossible, set aside an equivalent series of uninterrupted sequences, always making certain that you obey the time restrictions established by the NBME.

2) As a Tool for Study During or for Review of Clerkships. The format of asking clinically relevant questions followed by detailed explanations of the correct and incorrect answers makes this book a potentially valuable tool for study during clerkships for third- and fourth-year students and for review of basic clinical material for physicians who may need to reevaluate their knowledge of basic clinical material (e.g., specialists preparing to take the SPEX). Use of the index at the back of the book will facilitate this process. It will take only minimal effort to select questions in a specific discipline for self-evaluation and/or study.

test **1**

Questions

Single Best Choice Directions: This section consists of numbered statements or questions followed by a list of potential answers; you are to select the ONE BEST answer.

1 A 23-year-old man presents to the emergency department with bizarre delusions, a blunted affect, and tangential thought processes. He has no history of mood episodes and no history of substance abuse. Results of his laboratory studies are unremarkable. Which of the following possible findings from a subsequent, more extensive evaluation would most strongly indicate a favorable prognosis?

(A) An extensive premorbid history of social withdrawal
(B) A family history of schizophrenia
(C) A sudden and dramatic onset of illness
(D) Magnetic resonance imaging (MRI) studies that show gross changes in brain morphology
(E) Catatonic symptomatology

2 A 30-year-old woman has fever and cramping pain in the right upper quadrant, which radiates to the right scapula. Physical examination shows scleral icterus, right upper quadrant tenderness on deep palpation, and splenomegaly. An ultrasonogram of the gallbladder shows gallstones. Laboratory studies reveal a normocytic anemia and an increased reticulocyte count. The photograph shows the morphology of the red blood cells (RBCs) in the peripheral blood smear. Which of the following studies would most likely confirm the cause of the anemia?

(A) Hemoglobin electrophoresis
(B) Osmotic fragility test
(C) Serologic tests for viral hepatitis
(D) Serum ferritin test
(E) Serum transaminase tests

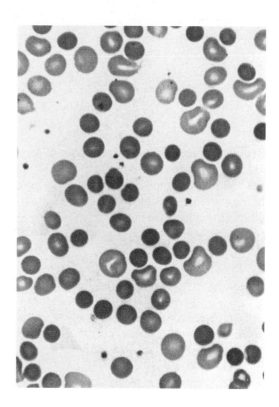

3 A 31-year-old man presents to the emergency department with the sudden onset of weakness in his right hand. Two weeks ago his wife filed a complaint of spousal abuse with the local police, and yesterday he gave several guns to a friend of his because he "didn't trust himself with them." Mental status examination reveals a peculiar calmness and lack of concern about his weakness. Which of the following is the most likely diagnosis?

(A) Conversion disorder
(B) Specific phobia
(C) Obsessive–compulsive disorder
(D) Hypochondriasis
(E) Melancholic depression

4 Morrisville (population 150,000) had 3000 deaths in the year 2003 from all causes, including meningitis. At the beginning of year 2003, 25 patients with meningitis diagnosed the previous year were under treatment. During year 2003, 200 new cases of meningitis were diagnosed. There were 11 deaths from this cohort of newly diagnosed patients; 7 patients died in year 2003, and 4 patients died in 2004. Which of the following represents the meningitis case-fatality rate during year 2003 for Morrisville?

(A) $(7 \div 11) \times 100$

(B) $(7 \div 200) \times 100$

(C) $(200 \div 3000) \times 100$

(D) $[(200 - 11) \div 3000] \times 100$

(E) $[(7 + 11) \div 11] \times 100$

5 After recovering from his third episode of psychosis, a 22-year-old man returns home to live with his parents and his younger siblings. The family asks what they can do to improve his adjustment. Which of the following would be the best advice?

(A) Insist that the patient abstain from social interaction

(B) Keep family stresses and overt conflicts to a minimum

(C) Encourage animated discussions at dinner, with an emphasis on exploring areas of friction among family members

(D) Strongly encourage the patient to return to school or get a job

(E) Keep the patient at home as much as possible

6 A 39-year-old male presented to his physician with a history of back pain that started 2 weeks previously. The patient stated that he had been cleaning the garage for a yard sale when he felt a little pain in his "lower back." He decided to use some hot packs and analgesics that were available over the counter. Unfortunately, over the past few days, he noticed that the pain had gotten worse. He had stiffness of his back and could not sit for long periods. Walking seemed to help. Whenever he coughed or sneezed, the pain would shoot down his right leg. Physical examination revealed that the patient was in moderate distress. He had spasm and tenderness of the paraspinal muscles on the right lumbar region. Straight leg raising test was 50° on the right but full on the left. Additional examination of the right foot revealed weak dorsiflexion and hypesthesia over the first web space. The rest of the neurologic examination was normal. The most likely reason for his symptoms is

(A) Epidural hematoma

(B) Spinal cord astrocytoma

(C) Epidural abscess

(D) Prolapsed intervertebral disk at L4–5 level

(E) Prolapsed intervertebral disk at L5–S1 level

7 An 8-year-old child presents to the physician's office with his mother because of multiple patches of alopecia. The mother states that the child has been in his usual state of good health until approximately 1 month ago. At that time the mother said that she noticed that the patient had small areas of hair loss on the scalp, with associated "black dots." She denies using any new hair products such as gels or shampoos on the patient's scalp. However, she does state that the problem appears to be getting worse. Wood lamp examination of the scalp is negative. A microscopic KOH preparation of an infected hair shows chains of spores within the hair shaft. Which of the following is most likely responsible?

(A) *Epidermophyton floccosum*

(B) *Microsporum canis*

(C) *Candida albicans*

(D) *Trichophyton tonsurans*

(E) Cutaneous *Aspergillus*

(F) Tinea capitis

8 A 55-year-old man presented to his family physician with a history of tiredness, aching, tingling, and cramps in his left leg. These symptoms got progressively worse toward the end of the day, but elevating the leg relieved them. The problem has become worse over the last several weeks, and he is now unable to walk a city block without extreme pain, which lingers even after he sits down and rests for a few minutes. He has tried over-the-counter analgesics, which have given him temporary relief. The patient has noticed that his foot is swollen by the end of the day, when he has to loosen the shoelace to feel comfortable. He is a factory worker and must stand for long hours at his job. Physical examination revealed soft tissue swelling of the left ankle. A reddish brown discoloration of the skin was noted behind the medial malleolus of the left ankle, together with a small area of ulceration in the center. No calf tenderness was elicited, but he did have some scattered areas of venous dilatation under the skin of the leg. No abnormality was noted in the right leg. The femoral, popliteal, and dorsalis pedis pulses were normal and equal in both lower extremities. The most likely condition this patient is suffering from is

(A) Superficial thrombophlebitis
(B) Embolic disease
(C) Arterial insufficiency
(D) Immune vasculitis
(E) Deep venous insufficiency

9 A 31-year-old woman with two living children was seen at the outpatient clinic with a chief complaint of missing her menstrual period. She had been using barrier methods of contraception. Her most recent pregnancy ended in a spontaneous first trimester loss requiring dilation and curettage. Her two previous successful pregnancies were unremarkable, resulting in spontaneous onset labor at term followed by uncomplicated spontaneous vaginal deliveries of healthy neonates who are alive and well. Her last menstrual period was June 10. A qualitative serum β-human chorionic gonadotropin (HCG) test had positive results. Assuming her usual cycle length is 32 days, which of the following is her most likely due date?

(A) March 12
(B) March 17
(C) March 21
(D) November 13
(E) November 17

10 A 65-year-old man was seen by his family physician with a 6-month history of constipation and a recent history of pain in the left lower quadrant of his abdomen. The patient complained of weakness and fever as well. He smoked approximately two packs of cigarettes per month and consumed a six-pack of beer during weekends. Physical examination revealed a moderately obese man. His blood pressure was 138/90, pulse 76/min regular, respirations 16/min and temperature 100°F (37.8°C). His cardiovascular and respiratory systems were normal. Examination of the abdomen revealed tenderness in the left lower quadrant with a positive rebound. In addition, a tender mass was felt on rectal examination. A complete blood count revealed neutrophilic leukocytosis, and the stool guaiac test result was negative. The most likely diagnosis in this patient is

(A) Ulcerative colitis
(B) Irritable bowel syndrome
(C) Acute diverticulitis
(D) Colon cancer
(E) Ischemic colitis

11 A 35-year-old Caucasian man with neurofibromatosis presents to his physician with a complaint of nausea and vomiting, vertigo, nystagmus, tinnitus, and nerve deafness in the right ear. These symptoms had gradually worsened over the past month or so. Upon examination the physician noted hemianesthesia on the right side of the face. Which of the following is the most likely diagnosis?

(A) Mastoiditis
(B) Cerebellar tumor
(C) Vertebrobasilar arterial insufficiency
(D) Glioblastoma multiforme
(E) Acoustic neuroma

12 An 8-year-old child presents with his parents to his physician. His chief complaint is a rash that began on his lower extremities a few hours ago. In addition, his parents state that the patient has had a low-grade fever, arthritis, and colicky abdominal pain. A purpuric rash limited to the lower extremities was observed during physical examination. Laboratory studies are ordered and reveal a guaiac-positive stool, a urinalysis with red blood cell (RBC) casts and mild proteinuria. The platelet count is normal. Which of the following is the most likely diagnosis?

(A) Systemic lupus erythematosus (SLE)
(B) Rocky Mountain spotted fever
(C) Idiopathic thrombocytopenic purpura (ITP)
(D) Henoch-Schönlein vasculitis
(E) Poststreptococcal glomerulonephritis

13 A 50-year-old man with a 35-year history of smoking cigarettes has fatigue, chronic cough, and dyspnea. Physical examination shows jugular neck vein distention, dependent pitting edema, and accentuation of the pulmonic component of the second heart sound. Arterial blood gas analysis shows a chronic respiratory acidosis with severe hypoxemia. Plasma hemoglobin is increased. A chest radiograph shows prominence of the right border of the heart and enlargement of the right and left main pulmonary arteries with tapering of the vessels before they reach the periphery. Which of the following is the most likely diagnosis?

(A) Bronchiectasis
(B) Bronchogenic carcinoma
(C) Cor pulmonale
(D) Left-sided heart failure
(E) Sarcoidosis

14 A 2-year-old boy is brought to the emergency department because of increasing lethargy over the past 4 hours. The past medical history is unremarkable. However, a 7-year-old brother who is a bed wetter has an upper respiratory infection. There have been no other contacts with individuals who are sick. On physical examination, the child's temperature is 37.4°C (99.3°F), and he is noted to be hypotensive. There is no history or evidence of trauma. The cardiac monitor demonstrates a ventricular dysrhythmia, and the child begins to have a seizure. Which of the following is the most likely cause for this child's problem?

- (A) Shaken baby syndrome
- (B) Meningitis
- (C) Imipramine
- (D) Congenital heart disease
- (E) Febrile seizure

15 A 30-year-old man sustains bilateral femoral bone fractures and multiple pelvic fractures after crashing his motorcycle into a tree. About 30 hours after the crash, he suddenly develops acute dyspnea. Physical examination reveals petechial lesions in the upper thoracic area and mental status abnormalities. Laboratory studies show hypoxemia and thrombocytopenia. Which of the following is the most likely diagnosis?

- (A) Air embolism
- (B) Cardiogenic shock
- (C) Fat embolism
- (D) Pulmonary thromboembolism
- (E) Septic shock

16 A 45-year-old male made an appointment to see his family physician because he noted bleeding per rectum. In providing a history, he disclosed that his father had died of cancer of the bowel at age 54 years. He also stated that the bleeding had started about 6 weeks ago and was in small amounts. Although he did not complain of abdominal pain, he did feel somewhat tired and said he had "lost energy." He did not smoke, consumed alcohol in moderation, and avoided red meat. He included a large amount of vegetables and fruits in his diet "for fiber." Anoscopy revealed internal hemorrhoids. Laboratory test results were positive for microcytic hypochromic anemia, and stool samples tested positive for blood. Colonoscopy revealed a moderately large lesion at the splenic flexure of the colon, which was biopsied. The pathology report indicated penetration of the muscle wall and infiltration into serosal fat by sheets of malignant cells without gland or mucin formation. The liver and spleen are of normal size, and a CT scan shows no evidence of distant metastasis, but

3 of 10 lymph nodes contain metastatic tumor. Based on the forgoing data, which of the following choices best describes the most probable prognosis?

- (A) He has an 80% or better chance of surviving for 5 years
- (B) His has a 60% chance of surviving for five more years
- (C) His has a 55% chance of surviving for five more years
- (D) His has a 30% chance of surviving for five more years
- (E) His has a 20% chance of surviving for five more years
- (F) His has less than a 5% chance of surviving for five more years

17 A 65-year-old long-term, heavy smoker has a 9-kg (20-lb) weight loss over the last 3 months that is associated with epigastric pain after eating, diarrhea, and jaundice. Physical examination reveals a palpable, nontender gallbladder and light-colored stools. Laboratory studies show total bilirubin of 8.0 mg/dL (normal, 0.1–1.0 mg/dL), serum alkaline phosphatase of 450 U/L (normal, 20–70 U/L), serum alanine aminotransferase (ALT) of 150 U/L (normal, 8–20 U/L), and urine dipstick test that is positive for bilirubin (normal is negative) and negative for urobilinogen (normal in trace amounts). The primary process, often associated with smoking, most likely responsible for these findings is which of the following?

- (A) Stone in the common bile duct
- (B) Intrahepatic cholestasis
- (C) Carcinoma of the gallbladder
- (D) Carcinoma of the ampulla of Vater
- (E) Carcinoma of the pancreas

18 A 65-year-old woman has an 8-year history of involuntary loss of urine; she leaks small amounts of urine when she coughs, sneezes, and laughs. She comes to the office complaining of pelvic pressure. She denies burning on urination and urinary urgency or frequency. She has no loss of urine at night; however, the symptoms occur frequently enough that she needs to wear a perineal pad. She underwent menopause 12 years ago. For treatment of hot flashes she initially used oral estrogen hormone replacement along with 7 days of medroxyprogesterone acetate 1 week of every month. For the last 8 years she has not used any hormone therapy. Speculum examination reveals an atrophic vagina and cervix without lesions. Bimanual examination reveals a small, symmetrical, midline, mobile, nontender uterus. There are no adnexal masses. With the Valsalva maneuver there is protrusion of her anterior vaginal wall.

Which of the following is the most likely diagnosis for the physical finding?

(A) Cystocele
(B) Urethral diverticulum
(C) Gartner's duct cyst
(D) Rectocele
(E) Enterocele

19 A pediatrician is requested to attend the delivery of a 25-year-old primigravida, with a history of good pre-natal care. The patient tells the pediatrician that she is expecting a full-term single delivery. She denies any history of sexually transmitted diseases, alcohol, or il-licit drug use. Her physical examination is pertinent for a malar rash, alopecia, and polyarticular arthritis. In addition she has a history of renal disease. This pa-tient's newborn will have an increased risk for which of the following disorders?

(A) Complete heart block
(B) Coarctation of the aorta
(C) Open neural tube defects
(D) Microcephaly
(E) Polycystic kidney disease

20 A 75-year-old man develops severe, steady, mid-abdominal pain approximately 30 minutes after eating. He has lost 11 kg (25 lb) over the past few months be-cause he is afraid of the pain after eating. Abdominal examination during an asymptomatic interval is nor-mal. Stool guaiac examination results are negative, as are colonoscopy and barium studies. The complete blood cell count is normal. What is the most likely diagnosis?

(A) Acute sigmoid diverticulitis
(B) Colorectal cancer
(C) Ischemic stricture of large bowel
(D) Meckel's diverticulitis
(E) Mesenteric angina

21 A 55-year-old man who suffered a stroke 6 months ago is administered a Folstein Mini Mental Status Exami-nation. Although he devotes much effort to the task, he is unable to successfully copy intersecting pentagons. Based on this finding, which of the following areas of the brain is most likely to have been affected by the stroke?

(A) Nondominant frontal lobe
(B) Nondominant temporal lobe
(C) Nondominant parietal lobe
(D) Dominant temporal lobe
(E) Dominant frontal lobe

22 A 4-day-old infant born by spontaneous vaginal deliv-ery without complications is brought to the pediatric emergency department. The parents report that the child is vomiting and feeding poorly. Physical exami-nation reveals muscular rigidity with alternating bouts of flaccidity and severe opisthotonos. A bedside glucose determination shows that the infant is hypoglycemic; however, correcting the blood glucose concentration does not improve the patient's clinical condition. The urinalysis does not show evidence of infection, but the urine has a distinct odor. Other routine laboratory studies are unremarkable, except for evidence of se-vere acidosis. Which of the following is the most likely diagnosis?

(A) Sepsis
(B) Neonatal seizure
(C) Maple syrup urine disease (MSUD)
(D) Trauma
(E) Phenylketonuria (PKU)

23 A 65-year-old male with a history of hypertension, di-abetes mellitus, and hypercholesterolemia was admit-ted to the intensive care unit of a university hospital after he sustained a stroke. The patient was obtunded, had a blood pressure of 230/110 mm Hg, heart rate of 68/min regular, and respiratory rate of 24/min. His O_2 saturation was 98% on room air. There was no pa-pilledema or anisocoria, but his eyes were deviated con-jugately to the left. He had right hemiplegia with upper motor neuron signs including a positive Babinski. His cardiovascular examination was positive for a marked left carotid bruit but was otherwise unremarkable. As of January 2006, the leading causes of death in the United States across age groups in descending order are:

(A) Malignancy, heart disease, acquired immune defi-ciency syndrome (AIDS)
(B) Heart disease, AIDS, malignancy, stroke
(C) Stroke, heart disease, malignancy,
(D) Heart disease, malignancy, stroke
(E) Malignancy, stroke, heart disease
(F) Malignancy, heart disease, stroke

24 A 25-year-old man being evaluated for social with-drawal says that he has no friends, is not really inter-ested in other people, and does not feel particularly lonely. A mental status examination reveals no pecu-liar thought processes. Which of the following is the most likely personality diagnosis?

(A) Schizotypal personality disorder
(B) Paranoid personality disorder
(C) Narcissistic personality disorder
(D) Avoidant personality disorder
(E) Schizoid personality disorder

25 A 6-year-old girl who appears healthy is brought to the primary care physician by her mother because of a rash. The mother states that the patient had been in her usual state of good health until 2 days earlier, when she developed a tactile fever and mild upper respiratory symptoms. Yesterday the patient had erythematous facial flushing that spread as a macular red lesion to her proximal extremities and trunk, which now has a lacy appearance. Which of the following is the most likely diagnosis?

(A) Erythema infectiosum
(B) Roseola
(C) German measles
(D) Measles
(E) Scarlet fever

26 A 54-year-old white female presented to her family physician with a recent history of pain in the upper right quadrant of the abdomen associated with nausea, vomiting, and fever. She did have a prior history of discomfort in the stomach, especially after eating a fatty meal, but this lessened after she started eating salads and avoiding butter and fried foods. She had no other medical history. She did not smoke and consumed alcohol only on social or religious occasions. On physical examination, she appeared to be in moderate distress, blood pressure 130/90 mm, pulse 78/min regular, respirations 18/min regular, and temperature 101°F (38.3°C). She was moderately obese. She had minimal guarding and tenderness in the right upper quadrant. Examination of the rest of the abdomen was normal. Examination of the cardiovascular and respiratory systems was noncontributory. A complete blood count showed leukocytosis; chemistry panel showed mildly elevated liver enzymes, but was otherwise unremarkable. X-ray films of the chest and abdomen were normal. Ultrasonography of the abdomen revealed a thickened gallbladder wall with a solitary calculus within. The bile ducts were not dilated. The pancreas and the terminal ducts were normal. Conservative treatment with nasogastric suction, analgesics, and antibiotics failed, and she underwent laparoscopic cholecystectomy. Within 24 hours following surgery, the patient developed a temperature of 102°F (38.9°C); blood pressure 90/60 mm Hg; pulse 100/min regular; respirations 22/min, rapid and shallow; and urine output less than 30 mL/h. Her skin was clammy and cold. She complained about some chest discomfort and pain. The most likely cause for this development is

(A) Hemoperitoneum
(B) Gram-negative sepsis
(C) Acute myocardial infarction
(D) Pulmonary embolus
(E) Pneumothorax

27 Toward the end of her workday a 35-year-old woman complains of tiredness, drooping eyes, and double vision. She also has difficulty swallowing both solids and liquids and states that food seems to "stick near my Adam's apple." The serum antinuclear antibody (ANA) test, complete blood cell count, and serum creatine kinase are negative. Which of the following is the most likely diagnosis?

(A) Multiple sclerosis
(B) Polymyositis
(C) Amyotrophic lateral sclerosis
(D) Myasthenia gravis
(E) Myotonic dystrophy
(F) Achalasia

28 Parents bring their internationally adopted 2-year-old child to the pediatrician's office because he has a temperature of 40°C (104°F) and a morbilliform rash. The parents state that the patient has been in the United States for only 5 days and was scheduled for a well child visit at the end of the week. They report that they thought the child had an upper respiratory infection until the rash began this morning. According to the father, the confluent maculopapular rash started cephalad and spread caudad to include the palms and soles. The mother also notes that prior to developing the rash the child had a dry cough, clear discharge from his nose, and conjunctivitis. The immunization status is unknown. Which of the following complications is most likely to develop in this child?

(A) Acute appendicitis
(B) Subacute sclerosing panencephalitis
(C) Interstitial pneumonia
(D) Myocarditis
(E) Otitis media

29 A 21-year-old woman, gravida 1, para 0, presents at 39 weeks' gestation in active labor. She is 155 cm tall and weighs 75 kg. Her pregnancy weight gain has been 20 kg. On digital vaginal examination the fetus is in cephalic presentation at −1 station. Her cervix is 5 cm dilated, 90% effaced, soft, midposition. Onset of regular uterine contractions was 8 hours ago, and she is now experiencing regular contractions every 3 minutes, lasting 45 seconds, which are firm to palpation. Clinical pelvimetry shows her pelvic dimensions as follows: pelvic sidewalls are straight, ischial spines are not prominent, pubic arch is wide, sacrum is hollow, and sacrosciatic notch is well rounded. Based on general bony architecture, the characteristics of this woman's pelvis identify it as which of the following common female bony shapes?

(A) Gynecoid
(B) Android
(C) Anthropoid
(D) Platypelloid
(E) Obstetroid

30 A 25-year-old man has nodular masses on the Achilles tendons and multiple yellow patches on his eyelids. His father died at 35 years of age of an acute myocardial infarction. His mother is now 52 years old and apparently is in good health. Which of the following biochemical defects is most likely responsible for the physical findings?

(A) Deficiency of apolipoprotein B48
(B) Deficiency of apolipoprotein C-II
(C) Deficiency of apolipoprotein E
(D) Deficiency of capillary lipoprotein lipase
(E) Deficiency of low-density lipoprotein (LDL) receptors

31 A 21-year-old man complains that for the past 4 months he has had morning back pain. The pain improves as the day progresses and when he exercises. Physical examination shows diminished anterior flexion of the lumbar spine, muscle spasms in the lower back, and forward stooping when the patient walks. An x-ray film shows bilateral sclerotic changes in the sacroiliac area. Which of the following tests would provide the most useful information?

(A) Human leukocyte antigen (HLA)-B27
(B) Rheumatoid factor
(C) Serum uric acid
(D) Serum antinuclear antibody test
(E) Erythrocyte sedimentation rate (ESR)

32 A 65-year-old man who recently moved to a new town consulted a family physician concerning a 2-week history of tiredness and weakness. Moreover, he recently noticed blood in the urine, "pain on the right side of the back," fever, and shortness of breath, especially when walking further than 100 yards. In addition, he has a history of chronic headache, which had been attributed to high blood pressure by his previous physician. However, he admitted his compliance was poor, and he seldom remembered to take the prescribed medications regularly. He also provided a history of smoking one pack of cigarettes per week, for more than twenty years and has had long-standing "smoker's cough" with intermittent purulent expectoration. He did have some blood in his sputum a few months previously, and he has also noticed a loss of weight. He consumes alcohol in moderation and has a family history of diabetes mellitus. Vital signs were: blood pressure 170/100

(repeatedly elevated), pulse 78/min regular, respirations 18 breaths/min, and temperature 101°F (38.3°C). He weighed 170 lb and was 6 feet tall. His oxygen saturation was 98% on room air. He had no pallor or cyanosis. Examination of his respiratory system revealed a midline trachea, absence of clubbing or cyanosis, and a few scattered crepitations in both lung fields, but no rales and rhonchi. Cardiovascular examination was normal, except for sinus tachycardia and hypertension. He had no peripheral pitting edema. Examination of the abdomen revealed a tender palpable mass in the right lower quadrant, which could be felt well on ballottement. A complete blood count was normal; a chemistry panel revealed borderline high BUN and creatinine levels but was otherwise unremarkable. Urinalysis revealed a few red and white blood cells per high-power field. The posteroanterior and lateral chest x-ray views revealed multiple well-differentiated masses of homogenous density in both lung fields, changes due to emphysema, and evidence suggesting chronic bronchitis. Which one of the following is the most likely diagnosis?

(A) Renal tuberculosis
(B) Transitional cell carcinoma of the bladder with metastasis to the lung
(C) Primary lung cancer with metastasis to the kidney
(D) Renal adenocarcinoma
(E) Acute pyelonephritis with metastatic abscesses in the lung

33 A 23-year-old man presents to his physician with a complaint of weight loss, dry cough, acute shortness of breath even at rest, and night sweats. On examination he was observed to be in ill health, and he had a low-grade fever, increased respiratory rate, and rales in both lung fields, and his pharynx was coated with a thick white film. In addition, the physician would expect this patient to have which of the following?

(A) A normal skin reaction to intradermal injections of common antigens
(B) An increase in the CD4 helper T-cell/CD8 suppressor T-cell ratio
(C) Hypogammaglobulinemia
(D) An abnormal phytohemagglutinin assay result
(E) Intact cellular immunity

34 A 4-day-old female is brought to the pediatrician because she has a blood-tinged discharge from her vagina. The patient was born at 38 weeks' gestational age to a 22-year-old primigravida. The infant weighed 7 lb 6 oz at birth and had no complications at birth. The infant was discharged home with her mother 24 hours after delivery. The mother reports that since

that time the child has been afebrile and is feeding and sleeping well. At this point, the physician should do which of the following?

(A) Draw blood for a hematocrit (Hct) determination
(B) Notify the Child Protective Services
(C) Reassure the mother that this is normal
(D) Call the endocrinologist
(E) Obtain a urinalysis

35 A 58-year-old man with a widely disseminated small cell carcinoma of the lung has hypotension, decreased serum cortisol levels, and profound electrolyte disturbances. Which set of laboratory data provided below is most closely associated with this patient's clinical abnormality?

	Serum Sodium (136–145 mEq/L)[a]	Serum Potassium (3.5–5.0 mEq/L)	Serum Chloride (95–105 mEq/L)	Serum Bicarbonate (22–28 mEq/L)
(A)	118	3.0	88	21
(B)	152	2.8	110	33
(C)	125	2.9	80	36
(D)	126	5.8	86	18
(E)	140	3.0	110	18

[a]Normal values are indicated in parentheses.

36 A 55-year-old man recently consulted a physician for the first time in several decades because he felt "poorly." The physician determined he had a body mass index (BMI) of 38, a fasting plasma glucose level of 215 mg/dL, and a systolic blood pressure of 185 mm Hg. He immediately recommended a diet and a regimen of drugs that included metformin, hydrochlorothiazide, and acetaminophen; the latter because of mild joint pains associated with incipient osteoarthritis. A series of follow-up appointments were made during which it was determined that the patient was becoming increasingly withdrawn and apathetic. Over a month he has become insomniac, has lost interest in his family, sex, work, eating, and hobbies, and he spends much time brooding about his perceived loss of health. He informs his physician that sometimes he feels as if life is no longer worthwhile. Administration of which of the following is most likely to be prescribed as the initial line of treatment used for his psychiatric symptoms?

(A) A monoamine oxidase inhibitor (MAOI)
(B) A selective serotonin-reuptake inhibitor (SSRI)
(C) A tertiary amine tricyclic antidepressant (TCA)
(D) A secondary amine TCA

(E) A heterocyclic antidepressant
(F) A mixed reuptake inhibitor
(G) Electroconvulsive therapy (ECT)

37 A 67-year-old man consults his physician because of difficulties upon urination. His major concern is that he has difficulty in completely emptying his bladder and that after concluding the act, urine sometimes dribbles down his leg. When asked, he admits that the flow is weaker and slower than it had been and that sometimes it gets interrupted. He is often awakened during the night by an overpowering urge to urinate. He is healthy otherwise. A physical examination was unremarkable, except for findings on a digital rectal examination. This revealed a nontender, smooth but enlarged prostate gland that felt firm but not hard. Routine laboratory workup showed no abnormalities. The prostate-specific antigen (PSA) level was 3.5 ng/dL. Among the following alternatives, which is the best initial treatment to prescribe for this patient?

(A) Transurethral resection of the prostate (TURP)
(B) Trimethoprim-sulfamethiazole (TMP-SMX)
(C) Finasteride (Proscar)
(D) Radical prostatectomy
(E) Interstitial radiotherapy

38 A 28-year-old female, para 0 gravida 1, underwent routine sonography at gestational age 18 weeks. The ultrasound revealed a twin pregnancy, one of which was male, the other female. The fetuses were appropriate for gestational age, and no congenital deformities were detected. The woman did not have a history of bleeding diathesis, but her husband was known to suffer from hemophilia A. The woman's mother is of Scottish descent, and her father, a Ukrainian Jew. Both of her parents are alive and in their 70s. Her mother suffers from hypertension, and the father from diabetes mellitus and hyperlipidemia. Neither suffers from bleeding diathesis. Two of her paternal uncles died at a young age from complications associated with hemophilia A. Which of the following statements about the fetuses she is carrying is factual?

(A) The female fetus has a 50% probability of being a carrier but no possibility of expressing the disease; the male, on the other hand, has no possibility of being a carrier but a 50% probability of expressing the disease
(B) Both the female and the male fetuses have no prospect of either being carriers or expressing the disease
(C) The female fetus has a 75% probability of being a carrier and a 25% probability of expressing the disease; the male cannot be a carrier, but has a 50% possibility of expressing the disease

(D) The female fetus has a 50% likelihood of being a carrier, and a 50% likelihood of expressing the disease; the male on the other hand, has no chance of being a carrier, but a 50% chance of expressing the disease

(E) The female has a 100% chance of being a carrier, but no possibility of expressing the disease; the male has no chance of either being a carrier or of expressing the disease

Directions for Matching Questions (39 through 50): *Each set of matching questions is preceded by a list of 4 to 26 lettered options followed by a brief explanation of the required task and then by a series of numbered statements. For each numbered statement you are to select ONE LETTERED OPTION that best fulfills the task as it relates to that statement. Remember, each of the listed options might be correctly selected once, more than once, or not at all.*

Questions 39–47

(A) Paraovarian cyst of Morgagni

(B) Hydrosalpinx

(C) Tubo-ovarian abscess

(D) Chronic pelvic inflammatory disease (PID)

(E) Pregnancy

(F) Follicular cyst

(G) Corpus luteum cyst

(H) Theca-lutein cyst

(I) Luteoma of pregnancy

(J) Endometrioma

(K) Polycystic ovaries

(L) Mucinous cystadenoma

(M) Benign cystic teratoma

(N) Granulosa cell tumor

(O) Sertoli-Leydig cell tumor

(P) Gonadoblastoma

For each of the following descriptions, select the ONE most appropriate diagnosis in reference to female pelvic masses.

39 A 23-year-old woman, gravida 2, para 1, underwent first-trimester sonography at 10 weeks to rule out twins. A 6-cm, unilateral, fluid-filled, smooth-walled, unilocular pelvic mass was found. The mass is separate from the uterus and is essentially unchanged on serial sonograms. However, it is variable in location, being noted anterior, posterior, and lateral to the uterus.

40 A 34-year-old woman, gravida 1, para 0, at 18 weeks' gestation with severe hyperemesis has a blood pressure of 150/95 mm Hg and 2+ proteinuria. Pelvic examination reveals bilateral adnexal masses that are 8–10 cm in diameter and appear multiloculated on a sonogram.

41 An 18-year-old woman, gravida 1, now para 1, just delivered a 3500-g (7 lb 12 oz) healthy male neonate without complications. At the beginning of this pregnancy, at 8 weeks' gestation, she was noted to have a 5-cm right adnexal cystic mass that spontaneously disappeared and was no longer seen on sonogram at 16 weeks' gestation.

42 A 29-year-old woman experienced her last menses 9 weeks ago. On her first prenatal visit she is noted to have a 9- to 10-cm soft, smooth, symmetrical, midline pelvic mass. The mass is mobile and not tender to palpation. She has experienced morning nausea but no vomiting.

43 A mother brings her 5-year-old daughter to the family physician. The girl shows changes of early breast development and has had vaginal bleeding. Pelvic examination under sedation reveals a normal vagina, but a sonogram shows a 4-cm unilateral, solid pelvic mass.

44 A 55-year-old postmenopausal woman shows evidence of temporal balding, clitoromegaly, and increased facial hair that began 6 months ago. She is noted to have a 5-cm unilateral, solid pelvic mass.

45 A 28-year-old nulligravid woman is found on routine annual examination to have a 6-cm unilateral pelvic mass. On sonogram, the mass is partially solid and partially cystic with foci of calcifications.

46 A 32-year-old infertile, obese nulligravida complains of dysmenorrhea as well as pain with intercourse and bowel movements. Pelvic examination reveals a 7-cm right adnexal mass. She has uterosacral ligament nodularity and a fixed retroverted uterus.

Questions 47 and 48

(A) Altruism

(B) Blocking

(C) Denial

(D) Displacement

(E) Dissociation

(F) Distortion

(G) Humor

(H) Projection

(I) Rationalization

(J) Reaction formation

(K) Regression

(L) Repression

(M) Suppression

(N) Undoing

Match each patient with the ONE associated defense mechanism.

47 A political figure is engaged in a televised debate and comes under increasing pressure from his opponent. As his anxiety mounts, he begins to lose poise, interrupt his opponent, and attack his character. He finally resists an urge to throw down his papers and angrily stalk offstage by telling a self-disparaging joke.

48 A man with a dubious record of compliance with Internal Revenue Service (IRS) regulations faces a tax audit. However he twice missed appointments with the agent after becoming involved with projects at work.

Questions 49 and 50

(A) Polycythemia vera

(B) Chronic obstructive pulmonary disease (COPD)

(C) Relative polycythemia

(D) Renal cell carcinoma

A patient presents with polycythemia. For diagnostic purposes, oxygen saturation, red blood cell (RBC) mass, plasma volume, and plasma erythropoietin levels are obtained. For each set of laboratory results, select the ONE diagnosis it best represents.

49 Decreased oxygen saturation, increased RBC mass, normal plasma volume, and increased erythropoietin

50 Normal oxygen saturation, increased RBC mass, increased plasma volume, and decreased erythropoietin levels

Answer Key

1	C	**11**	E	**21**	C	**31**	A	**41**	G
2	B	**12**	D	**22**	C	**32**	D	**42**	E
3	A	**13**	C	**23**	F	**33**	D	**43**	N
4	B	**14**	C	**24**	E	**34**	C	**44**	O
5	B	**15**	C	**25**	A	**35**	D	**45**	M
6	D	**16**	E	**26**	A	**36**	B	**46**	J
7	D	**17**	E	**27**	D	**37**	C	**47**	G
8	E	**18**	A	**28**	E	**38**	E	**48**	M
9	C	**19**	A	**29**	A	**39**	A	**49**	B
10	C	**20**	E	**30**	E	**40**	H	**50**	A

Answers and Explanations

1 **The answer is C** *Psychiatry*

The symptoms are suggestive of schizophrenia or schizophreniform disorder. In these disorders, the sudden onset of illness (choice **C**), especially with symptoms of agitation and psychosis, has a more favorable prognosis than an insidious onset.

A premorbid history of social withdrawal (choice **A**) is predictive of more severe and long-lasting psychopathology. A family history of schizophrenia (choice **B**) is commonly found in second-degree relatives and has little prognostic significance. Magnetic resonance imaging (MRI) changes (choice **D**) are associated with more severe symptoms and clinical course in schizophrenia. The presence of catatonic symptomatology (choice **E**) is not associated with any particular clinical course.

2 **The answer is B** *Medicine*

The patient has hereditary spherocytosis, an autosomal dominant disorder in which a defect in red blood cell (RBC) membrane spectrin or ankyrin causes macrophages to remove portions of the membrane, leading to the formation of spherocytes. The photograph of the peripheral blood smear shows numerous dense RBCs that lack the central area of pallor typical of the normal biconcave erythrocyte. Spherocytes are phagocytosed by splenic macrophages, resulting in a hemolytic anemia (extravascular type), splenomegaly, and an increase in unconjugated (indirect) bilirubin from macrophage degradation of hemoglobin. Unconjugated bilirubin is converted to conjugated (direct) bilirubin in the liver. Bile becomes saturated with the water-soluble conjugated bilirubin, resulting in the formation of jet black calcium bilirubinate stones. This may precipitate acute cholecystitis, which is the cause of this patient's abdominal pain. The osmotic fragility test (choice **B**) is the confirmatory test for spherocytosis. Spherocytes show increased osmotic fragility. Splenectomy is the treatment of choice. The patient should be given pneumococcal vaccine prior to surgery to prevent *Streptococcus pneumoniae* sepsis.

Hemoglobin electrophoresis (choice **A**) detects changes in the concentration of normal and abnormal forms of hemoglobin, such as hemoglobin S in sickle cell disease. Hemoglobin electrophoresis patterns are normal in spherocytosis. Serologic tests for viral hepatitis (choice **C**) are not indicated because the patient has documented gallstones and an unconjugated hyperbilirubinemia rather than a mixed hyperbilirubinemia with an increase in unconjugated and conjugated bilirubin, which is present in viral hepatitis. Serum ferritin (choice **D**) is used to evaluate iron disorders (e.g., iron deficiency). Iron study results are normal in spherocytosis. Serum transaminase levels (choice **E**) are normal in congenital spherocytosis. Transaminases are increased when there is diffuse liver cell necrosis (e.g., viral hepatitis), which is not present in this patient.

3 **The answer is A** *Psychiatry*

Conversion disorder is suggested by loss of motor control or sensory function that is not fully explained by physiologic mechanisms and is associated with psychologic conflict. Affected individuals often demonstrate an emotional blandness that is sometimes referred to as "la belle indifférence."

Specific phobias (choice **B**), obsessive–compulsive disorder (choice **C**), and hypochondriasis (choice **D**) are often associated with anxiety. Melancholic depression (choice **E**) may be associated with decreased psychomotor activity.

4 **The answer is B** *Preventive Medicine and Public Health*

The case-fatality rate expresses the probability of death from a disease over a specified period of time, i.e.:

$$\text{Case fatality} = \frac{\text{Number of deaths due to a disease during a specified time period}}{\text{Number of new cases diagnosed during that same time period}} \times 100$$

In the situation described, the number of cases of meningitis diagnosed in year 2003 was 200. Even though 11 deaths occurred from this group, the calculation is based only on the 7 deaths that occurred during the year under consideration. Therefore, the answer is $7/200 \times 100$ (choice **B**).

Choice **A**, $(7 \div 11) \times 100$; choice **C**, $(200 \div 3000) \times 100$; choice **D**, $[(200 - 11) \div 3000] \times 100$; and choice **E**, $[(7 + 11) \div 11] \times 100$, do not represent the case-fatality rate.

5 The answer is B *Psychiatry*

This description suggests schizophrenia. Many studies indicate that readjustment to family life is improved if family stress and conflict, sometimes called *expressed emotions,* are kept as low as possible (choice **B**). However, social rehabilitation requires reintegration with others, albeit under conditions of controlled stress.

Shielding the patient from all social interaction (choice **A**) would not promote social rehabilitation. Although it would be inadvisable to put too much pressure on the patient by insisting that he engage in stressful activities, gradual social involvement should be encouraged. Animated and stressful discussions at dinner (choice **C**) or strong pressures to return to school or find a job (choice **D**) would likely increase stress and conflict and would tend to aggravate him. Keeping him home (choice **D**) once again is liable to subvert his social rehabilitation.

6 The answer is D *Surgery*

This patient has a prolapsed intervertebral disk involving the L4–5 level (choice **D**). A herniated disk at this level will typically compress the 5th lumbar nerve root. The distribution of sensory deficit in such cases would be along the medial side of the leg and in the web space between the first and second toes. Since the 5th lumbar nerve root is required for effective dorsiflexion of the foot, weak dorsiflexion is to be expected, and is indeed noted on the vignette. These patients have difficulty standing on their heels. The initial management is conservative, bed rest, nonsteroidal analgesics, muscle relaxants, and physiotherapy.

Choice **A** is incorrect. Epidural hematoma is an acute event. This can result from trauma or in patients who have been on anticoagulants or have bleeding diathesis. The patients usually have sudden localized pain, which could result in cord compression. A computed tomographic (CT) scan will reveal the hemorrhage. Treatment is surgical decompression. Choice **B** is incorrect. A spinal cord astrocytoma is intradural and intramedullary in location. It usually affects people between the ages of 25 and 40. This is a slow-growing tumor that is associated with a long history of slowly progressive backache. The pain is usually localized, and in some cases may be radicular, namely spreading down along the path of a sensory nerve root. The tumor arises from the gray or white matter of the spinal cord. Pain is followed by motor weakness of the lower extremities, and sensory symptoms are usually the last to occur. Treatment is surgical resection. Choice **C** is incorrect. An epidural abscess is an acute event and is rare. The patient would have severe localized pain, and tenderness would be noted over the vertebral spine where the abscess is located. In addition, fever may be present. Radiculopathy is unusual. Treatment is surgical. Choice **E** is incorrect. An L5–S1 prolapsed intervertebral disk compresses the S1 nerve root. The patient has pain along the lateral side of the leg and hypesthesia over this region and along the little toe. These patients have difficulty with plantar flexion and standing on their toes. The ankle jerk is depressed or absent, as the S1 nerve root innervates it. The initial management is the same as that for a prolapsed L4–5 intervertebral disk.

7 The answer is D *Pediatrics*

The three genera generally responsible for dermatophyte infections are *Trichophyton, Microsporum,* and *Epidermophyton.* The most common pathogens are *Trichophyton tonsurans* (choice **D**) followed by *Microsporum canis* (choice **B**). These two pathogens are distinguished by Wood lamp. Hairs infected with *Microsporum* species fluoresce a bright blue-green, whereas those infected by *Trichophyton* species usually do not fluoresce (thus choice **B** is incorrect and choice **D** is correct). In addition, *T. tonsurans* often causes a unique pattern on the scalp known as "black dot ringworm," characterized by circular patches of alopecia with hairs broken off close to the follicle. Microscopic KOH preparations of hair infected with *T. tonsurans* shows chains of spores within the hair shafts, and those infected with *Microsporum* have tiny spores around the hair shaft.

Epidermophyton species usually invade the intertriginous skin, not the scalp. *E. floccosum* (choice **A**) is a cause of tinea cruris, not tinea capitis. Neither *Candida* nor *Aspergillus* species are dermatophytes. *Candida albicans* (choice **C**) is responsible for oral thrush and, in infants, diaper dermatitis. Cutaneous *Aspergillus* species (choice **E**) usually occur in immunocompromised children, resulting from direct inoculation of the skin or hematogenous dissemination. Tinea capitis is a dermatophyte infection of the scalp that may cause multiple patches of alopecia and severe itching. The dermatophytoses are diseases caused by a group of similar filamentous fungi that have a tendency to invade the stratum corneum, hair, and nails. Dermatophyte infections are characterized by the word *tinea,* followed by the Latin name of the site. Thus, tinea capitis is a dermatophyte infection of the head, not a pathogen, and choice **F** is incorrect.

8 The answer is E *Surgery*

The patient has deep venous insufficiency (choice **E**), as indicated by the history of venous symptoms stated in the vignette, stasis dermatitis, and superficial varicosities. Stasis dermatitis is a rusty discoloration of the skin, with or without ulceration, that is located usually behind the medial malleolus. Venous blood from the skin and superficial tissues that lie external to the deep fascia of the leg drains, via perforators (communicating veins), into the deep veins in the calf and is then returned to the right atrium. When the calf muscles contract, valves prevent retrograde flow into the superficial system. Incompetence of the venous valves leads to retrograde flow, increased venous pressure in the dorsal vein of the foot, and ensuing changes to the skin around the ankle. Persistently elevated venous pressure leads to capillary leakage. As a result, blood and fibrin is deposited in surrounding tissues. Breakdown of blood into hemosiderin leads to pigmentation of the skin, while fibrin deposition around capillaries leads to the formation of a barrier. Ischemia predisposes to ulceration of the skin. Finally, the retrograde blood flow from the deep to the superficial venous system causes varicosities as well.

Choice **A** is incorrect. Superficial thrombophlebitis presents with pain and erythema along the course of the superficial saphenous vein. Fever may be present. It is not associated with stasis dermatitis. Superficial thrombophlebitis may occur spontaneously in polycythemia or polyarthritis or may herald the presence of a visceral tumor, such as carcinoma of the pancreas. The condition is known as thrombophlebitis migrans. Choice **B** is incorrect. In embolic disease, the history would suggest an embolus to the lungs and physical findings suggestive of deep venous thrombosis. Deep vein thrombosis may be asymptomatic—presenting as pulmonary embolus—or symptomatic. In the latter case, the patient will have low-grade fever, pain, swelling, redness, and dilated superficial veins. Stasis dermatitis is not a feature. Choice **C** is incorrect. Arterial insufficiency is not associated with stasis dermatitis. However, varicose veins may coexist in patients with arterial insufficiency. The presence of normal arterial pulses and the lack of claudication pain that is characteristic of arterial insufficiency rules out this diagnosis. Choice **D** is incorrect. Rheumatoid arthritis is three times more common in women than in men. Rheumatoid arthritis may be associated with vasculitis. However, varicosities, or stasis dermatitis, are absent. Furthermore, the patient would have evidence of joint involvement, which is absent in the case described.

9 The answer is C *Obstetrics and Gynecology*

A good menstrual history is essential for calculating the estimated due date. Nägele's rule is a convenient method that uses the last menstrual period to calculate an estimated due date. Assuming a 28-day menstrual cycle, 3 months are subtracted from, and 7 days are added to, the date of the last normal menstrual period. This would result in an estimated due date of March 17 (choice **B**). However, adjustments must be made for cycles that are longer or shorter than 28 days. In the question scenario, the cycle length was 4 days over 28 days; therefore, ovulation took place 4 days later than the usual day 14, thus moving the due date 4 days forward. Instead of subtracting 3 months and adding 7 days, in this case one would need to subtract 3 months and add 11 days, thus yielding an estimated due date of March 21 (choice **C**). March 12 (choice **A**), November 13 (choice **D**), and November 17 (choice **E**) are therefore incorrect.

10 The answer is C *Surgery*

The patient has acute diverticulitis (choice **C**). Herniation of the colonic mucosa through the circular muscles of the colon leads to the formation of diverticula. In the United States about 95% of these are located in the sigmoid colon, but among Koreans, Japanese, Chinese, and Malaysians they are twice as likely to form in the ascending colon. In some severely affected individuals the entire colon may be involved; however, diverticula are not found in the rectum because it has a complete circular layer of muscle. Diverticula are usually due to a lack of roughage in the diet. The high fiber content of typical African and Indian diets makes diverticular disease a rarity in these cultures. When one or more diverticula get inflamed, the term *diverticulitis* applies. The clinical presentation in diverticulitis is similar to that of acute appendicitis, except that it is on the left side. Pyrexia, malaise, and leukocytosis are features. Sometimes a tender mass may be palpable on rectal examination.

Presence of urinary symptoms, such as dysuria, may be a forerunner to the formation of a vesicocolic fistula. In such cases, the patient would develop pneumaturia and pass flatus or even fecal material in the urine. The diagnosis is made on clinical grounds. Computed tomography (CT) confirms the diagnosis and also delineates associated pericolic abscesses. Although very mild cases may be treated at home with oral antibiotics and a liquid diet, more commonly acute diverticulitis is treated in a hospital setting with intravenous antibiotics—a combination of cefuroxime and metronidazole. Once the acute attack has resolved, a barium enema and flexible sigmoidoscopy or colonoscopy should be performed. Doing so in the acute phase could result in perforation and peritonitis. Surgery is indicated in approximately 10% of patients. Such surgery is performed in a quiescent period after careful bowel preparation and consists of a one-stage resection and end-to-end anastomosis. If there is bowel obstruction, a Hartmann's procedure is performed. If the patient has fecal peritonitis, the options include primary resection and Hartmann's procedure or, in rare cases, primary resection and anastomosis.

Choice **A** is incorrect. Ulcerative colitis is a nonspecific inflammatory disease that usually affects adults between the ages of 20 and 40. Both sexes are equally affected. In approximately 95% of cases, it commences in the rectum and spreads proximally. In chronic cases, pseudopolyps occur (chronic inflammatory polyps). The sine quo non of this disease is bloody diarrhea and rectal discharge that may be blood stained or foul smelling. Pain is not an early symptom of the disease. The disease is characterized by exacerbations and remissions. In severe cases, mild-grade fever, tachycardia, and hypoalbuminemia could occur. Other complications include toxic megacolon, perforation, and rarely, severe hemorrhage. Carcinoma can occur in those who develop the disease early in life or if the malady involves the whole colon. Colonoscopy and biopsy have an important role to play in the diagnosis of ulcerative colitis. Choice **B** is incorrect. Irritable bowel syndrome (IBS) is the most common gastrointestinal disease seen in clinical practice. It usually begins before the age of 30. Women are twice as likely to suffer from it than are men. Patients with IBS may have psychiatric disorders such as hysteria, obsessive–compulsive disorder, and depression. There are three types of presentation—chronic abdominal pain and constipation (spastic colon), alternating constipation and diarrhea, and finally, chronic painless diarrhea. The patients may also complain of abdominal distention, a feeling of incomplete evacuation, and relief of abdominal pain with evacuation. The diagnosis is based on the Rome criteria and is one of exclusion. Barium enema and colonoscopy are required to exclude inflammatory or neoplastic disease. Treatment includes a high-fiber diet, psyllium extract, and anticholinergics. Psychiatric consultation is indicated in appropriate cases. Choice **D** is incorrect. Carcinoma of the colon is most commonly seen on the left side. It is usually of the stenosing type. Thus, the predominant symptoms are that of progressive intestinal obstruction. In approximately 15% of cases, diverticular disease and colon carcinoma coexist. Loss of weight, positive occult blood test result, and a falling hematocrit should raise concerns about this possibility. Additional features include change in bowel habit such as alternating constipation and diarrhea, colicky pain, and tenesmus (need for evacuation), especially if the tumor is located low in the descending colon. In the latter case, patients may pass blood and mucus, mucus being more common in the morning. If a mass is felt on rectal examination, it will not be tender. Double-contrast barium enema is carried out in patients who have such altered bowel habits, and colonoscopy is indicated in those who have bleeding per rectum. Ultrasonography is used to exclude the presence of hepatic metastases, while CT is indicated in patients who have large palpable masses in the abdomen. Choice **E** is incorrect. Ischemic colitis results from paucity of blood flow to the colon. The most common location is at the splenic flexure. The patient is usually in the sixth decade of life and has degenerative vascular disease. Rectal bleeding and infrequent colicky abdominal pain and vomiting may precede a dramatic onset. Pain may occur several hours after a meal. The onset is usually abrupt with severe lower abdominal pain, vomiting, fever, and bleeding per rectum. Tenderness and guarding of the abdomen will be noted, and bowel sounds may be decreased. An arteriogram confirms the diagnosis. Most cases resolve spontaneously. Treatment is supportive. Some of these patients could develop strictures that would require surgery.

11 **The answer is E** *Medicine*

An acoustic neuroma (choice **E**) is associated with tinnitus, nausea and vomiting, vertigo, nystagmus, and 8th-nerve deafness. It arises in the cerebellopontine angle and may involve the trigeminal nerve, producing ipsilateral sensory changes in the face. It is most commonly a neurilemoma (schwannoma), which is a benign, encapsulated tumor arising from Schwann cells. Patients with neurofibromatosis have an increased incidence of acoustic neuromas.

Untreated mastoiditis (choice **A**) that erodes through bone to produce acoustic nerve damage is rare. Cerebellar tumors (choice **B**) and vertebrobasilar artery insufficiency (choice **C**) produce ataxia. Furthermore, they are not usually associated with 8th-nerve damage. A glioblastoma multiforme (choice **D**) is the most common primary malignancy of the brain in adults and usually involves the frontal lobes. It would not be expected to produce 8th-nerve damage.

12 The answer is D *Pediatrics*

The symptoms of arthritis, gastrointestinal and renal manifestations, and a purpuric rash on the lower extremities and buttocks are characteristic of Henoch-Schönlein vasculitis (choice **D**).

Systemic lupus erythematosus (SLE) (choice **A**), although accompanied by arthritis and fever, usually involves a malar rash. The rash of Rocky Mountain spotted fever (choice **B**) begins peripherally and spreads to the entire body. Idiopathic thrombocytopenic purpura (ITP) (choice **C**) is associated with a petechial rash, primarily on pressure points (e.g., where the elastic band of underwear touches the skin) and a decrease in the platelet count. Poststreptococcal glomerulonephritis (choice **E**) does not typically involve a rash, although hematuria is present.

13 The answer is C *Medicine*

The patient is a smoker who has developed chronic bronchitis (chronic cough) leading to chronic respiratory acidosis and hypoxemia. Respiratory acidosis and hypoxemia produce vasoconstriction of the pulmonary vessels, which eventually produces pulmonary hypertension (tapering of the vessels in the radiograph and accentuation of P_2 upon accommodation) leading to right ventricular hypertrophy. The combination of pulmonary hypertension and right ventricular hypertrophy is called *cor pulmonale* (choice **C**). Patients with cor pulmonale commonly develop right-sided heart failure (jugular neck vein distention and dependent pitting edema). Chronic hypoxemia is a stimulus for the release of erythropoietin, which causes secondary polycythemia (increased plasma hemoglobin).

Smoking cigarettes may cause bronchiectasis (choice **A**). However, the chest radiograph does not show dilation of the bronchi with extension of their lumens to the periphery of the lungs. Cigarette smoking is the most common cause of bronchogenic carcinoma (choice **B**). However, the chest radiograph does not describe a centrally located mass lesion or a lesion at the lung periphery to implicate a primary lung cancer. Left-sided heart failure (choice **D**) is associated with pulmonary edema. The chest radiograph does not show pulmonary edema. Sarcoidosis (choice **E**) is a noninfectious, chronic granulomatous disease that produces restrictive lung disease leading to chronic respiratory alkalosis and hypoxemia. Although cor pulmonale is a potential complication of sarcoidosis, the chest radiograph does not show enlarged hilar lymph nodes or reticulonodular densities in the lungs consistent with interstitial fibrosis.

14 The answer is C *Pediatrics*

The patient is a toddler and at risk for accidental ingestion. Imipramine (choice **C**) is an antidepressant that may be used to treat nocturnal enuresis. Children who have ingested tricyclic antidepressants primarily present with status epilepticus, coma, and dysrhythmias.

Seizures may also be associated with shaken baby syndrome (choice **A**), but retinal hemorrhages are usually noted on physical examination. Congenital heart disease (choice **D**) usually manifests itself earlier than 2 years of age. Febrile seizures (choice **E**) are associated with a rapid rise in temperature and usually develop when the core temperature reaches 39.0°C (102.2°F) or above. This patient is afebrile. Although meningitis (choice **B**) should be included in the differential diagnosis of a lethargic child, it is less likely given the fact that the child presents with symptoms associated with tricyclic antidepressant ingestion, and the child's brother is a bed wetter.

15 The answer is C *Medicine*

The patient has fat embolization (choice **C**). Fat embolization occurs following traumatic fracture of long bones (e.g., femur) and pelvic bones. Microglobules of fat derived from the marrow of the fractured bones and surrounding adipose tissues lodge in the microvasculature throughout the body. Fatty acids damage vessel endothelium, causing formation of platelet thrombi that contribute to occlusion of the microvasculature, and the thrombi consume platelets, causing thrombocytopenia. Symptoms are usually delayed until 24–48 hours after the initial injury. Dyspnea is due to hypoxemia resulting from fat microglobules occluding the pulmonary capillaries. Petechial hemorrhages are due to thrombocytopenia. Neurologic symptoms include restlessness and mental status changes with progression to coma. Treatment includes the use of corticosteroids and administration of oxygen with positive end-expiratory pressure.

Air embolism (choice **A**) occurs during obstetric procedures (e.g., uterine evacuation in abortion), in head and neck surgery, or as a consequence of chest trauma. Suction of air into the venous system mixes with blood in the right side of the heart; this causes a frothy substance to block blood flow into the pulmonary artery. Cardiogenic shock (choice **B**) is most commonly caused by acute myocardial infarction. Cardiac output is decreased, and left ventricular end-diastolic pressure and pulmonary capillary hydrostatic pressure are increased, causing pulmonary edema (left-sided heart failure). The patient's hypoxemia is due to a perfusion defect in the lungs, not pulmonary edema from left-sided heart failure. Pulmonary thromboembolia (choice **D**) most often originate from the femoral vein. The most common cause of deep venous thrombosis in the calf vessels is stasis of blood flow in the lower extremities due to prolonged bed rest. Clots propagate toward the heart and may break off and form an embolus once they enter the femoral vein. Clinically, patients develop a sudden onset of dyspnea and pleuritic-type chest pain due to inflammation of the pleura. Septic (endotoxic) shock (choice **E**) most often occurs in patients with indwelling urinary catheters. Sepsis due to *Escherichia coli* causes the release of endotoxins, which activate the complement system (releasing anaphylatoxins) and damage endothelial cells (releasing vasodilators such as prostacyclin and nitric oxide). Vasodilation of the peripheral resistance arterioles produces warm skin and increases venous return to the heart, causing high-output cardiac failure.

16 **The answer is E** *Surgery*

There are two parameters that are taken into account when dealing with cancers of the colon. The first is the grade, judged histologically: are they well differentiated or not? The less anaplastic the cells, the lower the grade. The second parameter is stage, the depth of penetration and degree of invasion by the tumor; the smaller the depth of penetration and the less the evidence of metastatic activity, the lower the stage. Although both parameters are used to establish treatment and prognosis, staging is the more important factor for patient prognosis, because it describes the size of the tumor and whether it has metastasized to lymph nodes or further on. In the case described, the microscopic appearance described in the pathology report indicates a high-grade colon cancer: the cells are bereft of mucin and glands and appear to be undifferentiated, i.e., anaplastic. Colorectal cancers are commonly staged by use of the modified Dukes' staging system as summarized in the table below.

Dukes' Staging System for Colorectal Cancer

Stage	Description	5-Year Survival Rate
A	Tumor limited to mucosa and submucosa	80%
B1	Tumor into, but not through, muscle wall; no lymph node or distant involvement	60%
B2	Tumor penetrates entire wall; no lymph nodes involved	55%
C1	Tumor into, but not through, muscle wall; lymph node involvement	30%
C2	Tumor penetrates entire wall; lymph node involvement	20%
D	Distant metastasis; any level of invasion; may or may not be lymph node involvement	<5%

Note that the key difference between stages B and C is lymph node involvement and that the key criterion for stage D is distant metastasis.

According to this system, the cancer belongs to modified Dukes' stage C2, because it has penetrated the muscle wall, infiltrated the serosa, and involved the lymph nodes but has not undergone distal metastasis. Accordingly, the most probable prognosis is that the patient has a 20% chance of surviving an additional 5 years (choice **E**). That this tumor is also anaplastic (high grade) does not improve his chances. The overall average 5-year survival rate for colorectal cancer is 35%, obviously the earlier the diagnosis, the better the prognosis.

The tumor was not limited to mucosa and submucosa; as a consequence (choice **A**) is incorrect. The tumor did penetrate the muscle wall and did involve lymph nodes, thus choice **B** is wrong. Choice **C** is incorrect because lymph nodes are involved. Choice **D** is wrong because the cancer did penetrate the wall, and choice **F** is erroneous because there is no evidence of distant metastasis.

17 The answer is E *Medicine*

Carcinoma of the pancreas (choice **E**) is most common in men over 50 years of age. Cigarette smoking and chronic pancreatitis are the most common risk factors. The most common site of the cancer is the head of the pancreas, which causes obstruction of the common bile duct, leading to obstructive jaundice in 65% of cases. Additional findings include weight loss (60% of cases), postprandial epigastric pain (75% of cases), diarrhea owing to malabsorption (decrease in bile salts/acids), and a palpable gallbladder (Courvoisier's sign, in 50% of cases) secondary to distention of the gallbladder by increased pressure in the bile duct. Obstruction to bile flow (cholestasis) produces characteristic laboratory findings. Because bile predominantly contains conjugated (direct) bilirubin, the backflow of bile into the liver eventually results in regurgitation of conjugated bilirubin into the blood, which results in a conjugated hyperbilirubinemia (conjugated fraction > 50% of the total) and bilirubinuria because conjugated bilirubin is water soluble. Absence of bile in the intestine results in light-colored stools. In the intestine, conjugated bilirubin is converted by bacteria into urobilinogen, which is further oxidized to urobilin. Absence of urobilinogen in the stool is associated with its absence in the urine as well, because a small amount is normally reabsorbed via the enterohepatic circulation and recycled back to the liver (90%) and kidneys (10%) for filtration into the urine. Alkaline phosphatase and γ-glutamyltransferase are excellent markers for cholestasis and are preferred over transaminases such as alanine and aspartate amino-transferases (ALT and AST, respectively), which are better indicators of diffuse liver cell necrosis. Computerized tomography (CT) is most useful in identifying pancreatic cancer; however a CT-directed percutaneous biopsy is required to confirm the diagnosis. The tumor antigen CA 19-9 is increased in most cases. In cases that are deemed operative, the Whipple's procedure is performed. It involves an en bloc resection of the pancreatic head/neck, resection of part of the common bile duct, and resection of the antrum with vagotomy in some cases. Radiation and chemotherapy are also used. The average 5-year survival is 5–20% for resectable tumors and less than 1 year with unresectable tumors.

A stone in the common bile duct (choice **A**) is associated with obstructive jaundice; however weight loss and a palpable gallbladder are not present as in this patient. Intrahepatic cholestasis (choice **B**) is most often due to drugs (e.g., oral contraceptives). It is not associated with weight loss and a palpable gallbladder. Carcinoma of the gallbladder (choice **C**) is most often secondary to cholelithiasis and a porcelain gallbladder (gallbladder with dystrophic calcification of the gallbladder wall). It does not cause obstructive jaundice and is not associated with a palpable gallbladder. Carcinoma of the ampulla of Vater (choice **D**) is associated with obstructive jaundice and a palpable gallbladder; however, there is no association with cigarette smoking.

18 The answer is A *Obstetrics and Gynecology*

Urinary stress incontinence is an anatomic problem that develops when the proximal urethra and bladder neck drop below the pelvic floor because of lack of support due to pelvic relaxation. The increase in intra-abdominal pressure is transmitted more to the bladder than to the urethra, resulting in involuntary urine loss with coughing and sneezing. This condition may be associated with a cystocele (choice **A**), the bulging of the bladder into the upper anterior vaginal wall. However, the incontinence is not caused by the cystocele.

A urethral diverticulum (choice **B**) is diagnosed via urethroscopy. Rectocele (choice **D**) is associated with bulging of the posterior vaginal wall. Enterocele (choice **E**) is herniation of the pouch of Douglas into the upper posterior vaginal wall. Gartner's duct cysts (choice **C**) are found in the lateral vaginal wall and are remnants of the embryologic mesonephric duct.

19 The answer is A *Pediatrics*

The mother has systemic lupus erythematosus (SLE). Neonatal lupus syndrome consists of rash, thrombocytopenia, and congenital heart block. Liver disease, hemolytic anemia, and leukopenia occur less frequently. SLE is the most common cause of congenital complete heart block (choice **A**). Injury is caused by maternal immunoglobulin G (IgG). The exact mechanism of damage is unknown. Most infants with congenital heart block have mothers with antibodies to Ro/SSA or La/SSB. The heart damage may be permanent.

Coarctation of the aorta (choice **B**), open neural tube defects (choice **C**), microcephaly (choice **D**), and polycystic kidney disease (choice **E**) have not been associated with SLE.

20 **The answer is E** *Medicine*

The patient has mesenteric angina (choice **E**), which most commonly occurs in elderly men who have evidence of atherosclerotic disease involving the superior mesenteric artery and reduced blood flow to the small and large bowel. Mesenteric angina is characterized by severe midabdominal pain approximately 30 minutes after eating, when splanchnic blood flow is greatest. The pain is so intense that patients are fearful of eating and experience subsequent weight loss. Potential problems include ischemic damage to the large bowel (bloody stools, ischemic colitis), with subsequent development of fibrosis and strictures leading to bowel obstruction. These findings usually occur in the splenic flexure (junction of the transverse colon with the descending colon), where the superior and inferior mesenteric arteries overlap. Ischemic strictures of the colon (choice **C**) produce signs of obstruction, which include colicky pain (pain followed by pain-free intervals), nausea and vomiting, constipation, and obstipation (no passage of gas). Signs of obstruction are not present in the patient.

Acute sigmoid diverticulitis (choice **A**) presents with fever, left lower quadrant pain ("left-sided" appendicitis), rebound tenderness, and neutrophilic leukocytosis. These findings are not present in this patient. Colorectal cancer (choice **B**) does not produce pain following eating. It is usually associated with blood in the stool and alternating bouts of constipation and diarrhea. Meckel's diverticulitis (choice **D**) presents with right lower quadrant pain and rebound tenderness that cannot be clinically differentiated from acute appendicitis.

21 **The answer is C** *Psychiatry*

The construction apraxia seen in this patient is associated with damage to the nondominant parietal lobe (choice **C**).

Damage to the nondominant frontal and temporal lobes (choices **A** and **B**) is associated with problems of mood, orientation, concentration, and memory. Damage to the dominant temporal lobe (choice **D**) is associated with receptive (Wernicke's) aphasia. Damage to the dominant frontal lobe (choice **E**) is associated with expressive (Broca's) aphasia.

22 **The answer is C** *Pediatrics*

The urinary abnormality in maple syrup urine disease (MSUD) (choice **C**) is the presence of high concentrations of branched-chain amino acids—leucine, isoleucine, and valine. The addition of 2, 4-dinitrophenyl-hydrazine (DNPH) will cause the ketoacids of the branched-chain amino acids to precipitate. The urine, skin, or hair has a characteristic smell of maple syrup or caramel. Infants present with symptoms 3 to 5 days after birth, with feeding difficulties, hypoglycemia, seizures, opisthotonos, and muscular rigidity with or without intermittent flaccidity. Cortical atrophy is seen on computed tomography (CT) or magnetic resonance imaging (MRI) scans. Dietary management of intake of branched-chain amino acids is the cornerstone of therapy. However, most patients have already suffered permanent brain damage by the time diagnosis is made and treatment is initiated.

Neonatal seizures (choice **B**) are a disorder of the central nervous system (CNS) that suggests hypoxic ischemic encephalopathy resulting from asphyxia, intracranial hemorrhage, hypoglycemia, infarction, or meningitis. Bruising and retinal hemorrhages might be seen if the patient had been a victim of trauma (choice **D**). Phenylketonuria (PKU) (choice **E**) results from a defect in the metabolism of the amino acid phenylalanine. The infant is normal at birth, but gradually develops mental retardation. Vomiting may be an early symptom of PKU. Children with PKU are fair skinned and have eczematous rash. Some will develop a seizure disorder. A newborn with sepsis (choice **A**) may have vomiting, poor feeding, and hypoglycemia, but the fact that this patient has a distinct odor to the urine, acidosis, no response to glucose, and bouts of flaccidity and opisthotonos makes MSUD the best answer.

23 **The answer is F** *Preventive Medicine and Public Health*

The leading causes of death in the United States across age groups in descending order are malignancy, heart disease, and stroke; in January 2005 the Centers for Disease Control and Prevention (CDC) reported that more deaths now occur from malignancies than from heart disease (choice **F**), reversing the historical order. Women are more likely to have a stroke and men are more likely to die from a heart attack. An increase in the number of women who smoke has led to a rise in lung cancer and subsequent mortality.

Choices **A** and **B** include acquired immune deficiency syndrome (AIDS), which is not one of the three leading causes of death across age groups in the United States. Choices **C, D,** and **E** list the correct three diseases, but in the wrong order.

24 **The answer is E** *Psychiatry*

This case is most consistent with schizoid personality disorder (choice **E**), characterized by emotional aloofness, indifference to praise or criticism, and the absence of any bizarre or idiosyncratic thinking.

Individuals with schizotypal personality disorder (choice **A**) are often withdrawn and aloof, but they also demonstrate peculiar thinking. Paranoid personality disorder (choice **B**) is characterized by unwarranted suspiciousness. Narcissistic personality disorder (choice **C**) involves disdain for most people, but extreme idealization or denigration of a few. Avoidant personality disorder (choice **D**) implies that the individual has a need for human contact and feels lonely.

25 **The answer is A** *Pediatrics*

Erythema infectiosum (choice **A**) (also known as [aka] fifth disease) is a mild exanthematous disease caused by parvovirus B19. Usually there is no prodrome, and fever is low grade or absent. The rash usually starts on the cheeks, which appear to have been slapped. Following the bright-red and confluent rash, an erythematous maculopapular rash appears on the trunk, although it can precede the facial rash. The rash then fades, giving a lacy or reticular appearance. The rash is often pruritic, but does not desquamate, as seen with measles. Other symptoms include headache, rhinitis, and arthralgia, but these symptoms are more common in adults.

In most cases roseola (choice **B**) is caused by herpesvirus 6. Children with roseola present with the differential diagnosis of a fever of unknown origin until the temperature drops precipitously and the rash appears. The rash is maculopapular and nonpruritic, and it blanches on pressure. It first appears on the trunk and spreads to the arms and neck (mild on legs and face). Rubella, aka German measles (choice **C**) or three-day measles, is another viral exanthematous disease of children and adults, with worldwide distribution. The signs and symptoms include adenopathy (posterior auricular), low-grade fever, arthralgias, coryza, and conjunctivitis. The exanthem is descending, beginning on the face or neck and spreading in hours to the trunk and extremities. The lesions are maculopapular and may desquamate. The rash fades in 24–48 hours. Measles (choice **D**) is a highly contagious viral infection transmitted by respiratory droplets. Prodromal symptoms include brassy cough, coryza, conjunctivitis, and fever. Koplik's spots (greyish white spots with a red halo) appear on the buccal mucous membrane 24–48 hours before the rash. The rash begins on the face and ears and spreads to the trunk and extremities in 24–36 hours. The lesion is maculopapular and may become confluent on the face and body (a distinct characteristic of measles). Scarlet fever (choice **E**) is an upper respiratory infection associated with a characteristic diffuse maculopapular "sandpaper"-type rash and group A streptococcal pharyngitis. The face is usually spared, but the cheeks may be erythematous and the area around the mouth spared. Pastia's lines, (prominence of the rash in the creases of the elbow, axillae, and groin) and strawberry tongue (in which the tongue is coated and the papillae may be swollen and reddened) are also associated with scarlet fever.

26 **The answer is A** *Surgery*

This patient has the classic symptoms of hypovolemic shock, namely, hypotension, tachycardia, tachypnea, oliguria, and peripheral vasoconstriction resulting in cold clammy skin. Hemoperitoneum (choice **A**) (i.e., intra-abdominal hemorrhage) is the most common cause of shock in the first 24 hours following abdominal surgery. The most likely cause is a slipped ligature from an artery, for example, the cystic artery. The hematocrit will not fall until several hours after the primary event. Management involves restoration of blood volume and immediate surgical intervention to secure the vessel and arrest the hemorrhage.

Choice **B** is incorrect. Gram-negative sepsis results in endotoxic shock. Toxins released by gram-negative bacteria lead to vasodilatation of blood vessels. As a result, the patient would have a bounding pulse and warm skin. Other features include high fever and hypotension. Choice **C** is incorrect. Myocardial infarction is associated with chest pain. Cardiogenic shock could result from a massive myocardial infarction. In that case, the patient would have hypotension, tachycardia and a weak pulse. The skin would not be warm, and fever, if present, would be low grade. Choice **D** is incorrect. Pulmonary embolus usually presents several days after surgery.

It is seen in patients who have been lying immobile for a few days in bed and then develop deep vein thrombosis. There may be calf swelling and tenderness, but pulmonary embolus without clinical symptoms of deep venous thrombosis has been known to occur. The patient would have sudden chest pain, hemoptysis, hypotension, and tachycardia. Choice **E** is incorrect. A pneumothorax is associated with stabbing chest pain, tachypnea, tachycardia, and, in the case of tension pneumothorax, hypotension. Physical findings will include absent breath sounds, hyperresonance to percussion, and a tracheal shift to the contralateral side. This could follow insertion of a line into the subclavian vein.

27 **The answer is D** *Medicine*

The patient has myasthenia gravis. It is an autoimmune disorder characterized by the presence of IgG antibodies that are directed against acetylcholine receptors in the neuromuscular junction of striated muscle, causing profound weakness (i.e., myasthenia gravis, choice **D**). The most common initial presentation is muscle weakness involving the ocular muscles, causing drooping of the eyelids (ptosis), diplopia (double vision), and generalized fatigue toward the end of the day that improves with rest. In addition, there is dysphagia for solids and liquids in the upper esophagus, since striated muscle is primarily responsible for peristalsis in this location. The IgG antibodies are produced in the thymus, where there are prominent germinal follicles (B-cell hyperplasia). Some patients (15% of cases) develop a thymoma in the anterior mediastinum. The Tensilon (edrophonium) test is used to screen for myasthenia. Edrophonium blocks acetylcholinesterase, which increases the amount of acetylcholine in the synapse, causing reversal of muscle weakness. Autoantibodies against the receptor are present in about 85 to 90% of cases. The treatment of myasthenia involves the use of acetylcholinesterase inhibitors (e.g., pyridostigmine) and corticosteroids. Thymectomy is reserved for very severe cases that do not respond to therapy.

Multiple sclerosis (choice **A**) is an autoimmune disease with destruction of myelin in the central and peripheral nervous systems. Scanning speech, intention tremors, nystagmus, muscle weakness, optic neuritis with blurry vision, and paresthesias are commonly present. None of these findings are present in this patient. Polymyositis (choice **B**) is a female-dominant myositis that occurs primarily in adults. Clinical findings include muscle pain and atrophy (not present in this patient), dysphagia for solids and liquids in the upper esophagus (affects striated muscle). The serum ANA is positive in less than 30% of cases (negative in this patient) and anti Jo-1 and anti PM-1 antibodies are usually present. The serum creatine kinase is increased in all cases (negative in this patient), and a muscle biopsy reveals destruction of muscle tissue and a lymphocytic infiltrate. Amyotrophic lateral sclerosis (choice **C**) is an example of an upper and lower motor neuron disorder. Muscle weakness begins in the hands (ocular weakness in this patient) and progresses throughout the body. It is an uncommon disorder in individuals under 50 years old (patient is 35 years old) and does not present with drooping eyelids and diplopia, as in this patient. Myotonic dystrophy (choice **E**) is an autosomal dominant muscular dystrophy. It is a trinucleotide repeat disorder (repetition of three nucleotide bases) that presents with facial weakness (drooping of the mouth), myotonia (inability to relax muscles), frontal balding, cataract, testicular atrophy, and cardiac muscle weakness. The serum creatine kinase is increased. None of these findings is present in the patient. Achalasia (choice **F**) is a dysphagia caused by a failure of the lower esophageal sphincter (LES) to relax because of lack of inhibitory input from nonadrenogenic, noncholinogenic ganglionic cells. Although it interferes with swallowing both solids and liquids, it is not associated with generalized weakness and fatigue.

28 **The answer is E** *Pediatrics*

The symptoms in this patient clearly describe a case of measles. Otitis media (choice **E**) is the most common complication of measles.

Because of mesenteric node involvement, diffuse lymphadenopathy can cause abdominal pain mimicking appendicitis (choice **A**). Subacute sclerosing panencephalitis (choice **B**) is a rare neurologic complication, with fewer than five new cases per year registered with the U.S. National Sub-Acute Sclerosing Panencephalitis (SSPE) Registry each year since 1982. Interstitial pneumonia (choice **C**) is caused by the measles virus itself and is more common in immunocompromised patients. Bronchopneumonia is more common than interstitial pneumonia and is usually caused by pneumococcus, group A *Streptococcus, Staphylococcus aureus*, or *Haemophilus influenzae* type b. Myocarditis (choice **D**) is a rare but serious complication of measles.

29 **The answer is A** *Obstetrics and Gynecology*

The classification of female bony pelvis types is based on the work of Caldwell and Moloy who examined large numbers of x-ray pelvimetry films. These procedures hark back to the days when radiographs of the pelvis were obtained in cases of protracted labors. The pelvis described in this question is characteristic of the gynecoid shape (choice **A**). It is the most common shape, occurring in approximately 50% of women. The dimensions of the gynecoid shape allow optimal use of the pelvic diameters in obtaining a vaginal delivery.

Android pelves (choice **B**) predispose to arrest of descent, anthropoid pelves (choice **C**) predispose to occiput posterior position at delivery, and platypelloid pelves (choice **D**) predispose to occiput transverse position at delivery. These pelvic shapes occur with frequencies of 30, 20, and 3%, respectively. Some women have combinations of features from more than one pelvic shape. Obstetroid (choice **E**) is not a formally described pelvic shape.

30 **The answer is E** *Medicine*

The patient has familial hypercholesterolemia (type II hyperlipoproteinemia), an autosomal dominant disease with a deficiency of LDL receptors (choice **E**) due to an error in synthesis, processing, or function; this receptor deficiency causes an increase in serum LDL levels. LDL is formed when the very-low-density lipoproteins (VLDLs) and chylomicrons shed much of their triglyceride. This makes the cholesterol content of LDL very high, and its role is to transport this cholesterol to tissues where it should be taken up via its receptors. Obviously when the receptors malfunction this can't happen, and such patients have an extremely high serum LDL cholesterol level, causing deposition of this abnormal excess cholesterol in various tissues. Such anomalous cholesterol deposits commonly occur in the Achilles tendon (tendon xanthomas) and eyelids (xanthelasma). Heterozygous patients like the one described and his father die at an early age of an acute myocardial infarction or stroke. Homozygous individuals usually die before the age of 20. "Statin" drugs that inhibit 3-hydroxy-3-methylglutaryl coenzyme A reductase, the rate-limiting enzyme of cholesterol synthesis, are now given at an early age with the hope of modifying the disease.

Proteins associated with the circulating lipoproteins are called *apolipoproteins* or *apo* for short. These apoproteins serve various functions including structural support, recognition sites for receptor binding, and activators or coenzymes involved in lipid metabolism. Letters from A to H are used to name the major classes, which may be further subdivided into subclasses using various different notations. ApoB-48 is the first of three apoproteins added to chylomicrons as they leave the small intestine; once in the plasma apoE and apo C-II are also added. ApoB-48 and apoE function together as a recognition site for the liver receptor, while apoB-48 and apoC-II act synergistically as activators of capillary lipoprotein lipase (CPL). As a consequence deficiency of apoB-48 (choice **A**) is associated with decreased formation and secretion of chylomicrons from the small intestine.

In the fed state, CPL normally hydrolyzes triglyceride (TG) in chylomicrons and VLDL, causing the release of glycerol and fatty acids into the peripheral circulation where they can be taken up by cells. The lipoprotein fractions that remain after CPL action are respectively called *chylomicron remnants* and *intermediate-density lipoproteins* (IDLs). Consequently, a deficiency of apoC-II (choice **B**) results in accumulation of chylomicrons and VLDLs loaded with triacylglycerides (TGs) as well as an inability to metabolize triglycerides; this condition is known as *type I hyperlipoproteinemia*. Since chylomicrons carry dietary-derived TGs, patients have very high serum TG levels and do not have lipid deposits in tendons or eyelids. A deficiency of apoC-II is a very rare condition that primarily occurs in children. ApoE primarily mediates the uptake of chylomicron remnants and IDLs by hepatocytes. Deficiency of this apolipoprotein (choice **C**) or a mutant form of apoE produces type III hyperlipoproteinemia (dysbetalipoproteinemia or remnant disease). Serum cholesterol and TG levels are increased; however, the lipid deposits are primarily located in the palmar creases. Genetic deficiency of CPL (choice **D**) is another cause of type I hyperlipoproteinemia, which also primarily occurs in children. Chylomicrons are markedly increased. Since chylomicrons carry diet-derived TGs, patients have very high serum TG levels and do not have lipid deposits in tendons or eyelids.

31 **The answer is A** *Medicine*

This man most likely has ankylosing spondylitis, a seronegative, human leukocyte antigen (HLA)-B27-(choice **A**) positive (95% of cases) spondyloarthropathy that occurs primarily in young men between 15 and 30 years of age. Characteristic features include an insidious onset of morning stiffness in the lower back that persists for more than 3 months and improves as the day progresses or when the person exercises. Sclerotic changes in the sacroiliac area are the first radiographic evidence of the disease. Patients have diminished anterior flexion of the spine. Over time, the vertebral column fuses to produce the classic "bamboo spine." Additional complications include restriction of chest movement and subsequent restrictive-type lung disease, iridocyclitis (25% of cases), aortitis with aortic valve insufficiency (3–10% of cases), and reactive (secondary) amyloidosis. Indomethacin and exercise are the treatments of choice.

Ankylosing spondylitis is not a variant of rheumatoid arthritis, and as a consequence, it is not rheumatoid factor positive (choice **B**). Gout does not present with lower back pain; therefore, a uric acid level determination (choice **C**) is not indicated. The serum antinuclear antibody test (choice **D**) result is negative in ankylosing spondylitis, because it is not a collagen vascular disease. The erythrocyte sedimentation rate (ESR) (choice **E**) is a nonspecific indicator of inflammation; therefore, it is not useful in arriving at a specific diagnosis of a rheumatologic disease.

32 The answer is D *Surgery*

The patient has metastatic renal adenocarcinoma (choice **D**) and hypertension secondary to ectopic production of renin by the tumor. Renal adenocarcinoma is the most common neoplasm of the kidney. It affects men twice as often as women, usually in the sixth to seventh decade of life. The neoplasm arises from renal tubular cells. Smoking is a predisposing factor. The tumor affects the poles of the kidney, more commonly the upper. Hematuria is the most consistent sign (90%), sometimes associated with colic due to clot formation, followed by a dragging discomfort in the loin (45%), a palpable mass (30%), and fever (20%). "Cannonball" metastases to the lung occur in 60% of cases. Fever is not related to infection but results from chemicals released by the tumor.

The tumors can ectopically secrete erythropoietin (leading to secondary polycythemia), parathormone-like peptide (leading to hypercalcemia), renin (leading to hypertension as noted in this case), gonadotropins (leading to feminization or masculinization), or cortisol (leading to Cushing's syndrome). Serum levels should be determined to confirm potentially elevated levels. A plain x-ray of the abdomen may show abnormal calcification in the tumor and distortion of the renal outline. An intravenous pyelogram (IVP) will reveal the mass, and the calyces may be stretched and distorted. Ultrasonography will show if the lesion is solid or cystic, and computed tomography (CT) with enhancement will demonstrate the extent of the lesion, including presence of hilar lymphadenopathy or involvement of the renal vein. Needle aspiration of the mass using CT for needle guidance is usually performed to obtain a histologic diagnosis. Angiograms are rarely done, as CT scans with contrast are adequate. Occasionally, an inferior venacavagram is indicated to establish extent of inferior vena caval involvement by the tumor. Radical nephrectomy is the treatment of choice if the tumor is confined to the kidney. The presence or absence of renal vein or capsular invasion affects overall survival—45% of patients without renal vein or capsular invasion achieve a 5-year survival, as opposed to 15 to 30% of those with invasion. Adenocarcinoma of the kidney does not respond well to radiotherapy or conventional chemotherapy.

Choice **A** is incorrect. Although the kidney is the most common extrapulmonary site for tuberculosis (TB); the homogeneous nodular masses in the lung go against this diagnosis. Furthermore, renal tuberculosis usually occurs between the ages of 20 and 40. Other properties of renal TB include that it is 50% more likely to occur in men than in women, urinary frequency is the most common and earliest symptom, and the urine remains negative for bacteria in the early stages. Dysuria sets in when the patient develops cystitis. Hematuria occurs in less than 5% of cases, and it is very uncommon to be able to palpate a renal mass in TB of the kidney. Transitional cell carcinomas of the bladder (choice **B**) usually involve the renal pelvis and produce obstruction. They are not as common as renal cell adenocarcinoma. Primary lung cancer (choice **C**) is not multifocal, and metastasis to the kidney is rare. Choice **E** is incorrect. Acute pyelonephritis is more common in females. The patient may have headache, nausea, and fatigue. Pain is usually sudden in onset and is associated with fever and chills. Soon after onset, the patient develops cystitis, which causes enhanced urinary frequency and urgency as well as dysuria. The patient has tenderness in the loin and in the hypochondrium, but no mass is felt. A midstream specimen of urine will reveal a few pus cells and bacteria. In some cases, the blood urea nitrogen (BUN) and creatinine levels may be elevated. While acute pyelonephritis is usually unilateral, it could be bilateral. Acute pyelonephritis does not produce metastatic abscesses; however, if untreated, it could cause pyonephrosis that could be life threatening.

33 The answer is D *Medicine*

The respiratory symptoms described are characteristic of *Pneumocystis carinii* pneumonia, and the white film on his pharynx is a typical symptom of candidiasis. These opportunistic infections plus his general appearance, his weight loss, and night sweats strongly suggest that he has the acquired immune deficiency syndrome (AIDS). AIDS is the most common acquired immunodeficiency in the United States, where it is usually caused by human immunodeficiency virus-1 (HIV-1), an RNA retrovirus. (HIV-2 infection is common in West Africa but is rarely observed in the United States). The virus attacks and destroys CD4 helper T cells, thus lowering the CD4 helper T-cell count, potentially to fewer than 200 cells/µL in full-blown cases of AIDS. As a consequence of its effect on these T cells, the normal in vitro response to T-cell stimulation by phytohemagglutinin, a potent T-cell mitogen, is also impaired (choice **D**).

Intradermal injections of common antigens do not elicit the expected immune response in patients with AIDS (not a normal response [choice **A**]). This lack of immune response is called *anergy*. By lowering the CD4 helper T-cell count the virus also reverses the CD4 helper T-cell/CD8 suppressor T-cell ratio from a normal ratio of 2:1 to less than 1:2 (not an increase in the ratio [choice **B**]). Opportunistic infections with additional infective agents such as the Epstein-Barr virus (EBV) and cytomegalovirus also are common in AIDS. These agents are potent polyclonal stimulators of B cells, which produce a polyclonal gammopathy (hypergammaglobulinemia, not hypogammaglobulinemia [choice **C**]). However, because patients are unable to mount an antibody response to a new antigen, they are still susceptible to bacterial infections. Because helper T cells are integral to normal cellular immunity (type IV hypersensitivity), tests that evaluate cellular immunity show impaired immunity (not intact immunity [choice **E**]). Defective cellular immunity is responsible for *P. carinii* lung infection, the most common initial presentation in AIDS.

34 The answer is C *Pediatrics*

Vaginal bleeding, or pseudomenses, may occur in a newborn female. In utero, the vaginal epithelium is stimulated by circulating maternal estrogens, which diffuse across the placenta. After birth, these hormone levels rapidly fall, which results in endometrial sloughing. There may be a thick mucoid discharge from the newborn's vagina, which is sometimes bloody. The discharge will usually resolve within 10 days after birth. No testing or treatment is necessary (choices **A** and **E**), only reassurance (choice **C**). Because the vaginal bleeding is not related to abuse, the Child Protective Services need not be informed (choice **B**). It is not necessary to call an endocrinologist (choice **D**) because this is not an endocrinopathy.

35 The answer is D *Medicine*

A patient with small cell carcinoma of the lung with disseminated disease, hypotension, decreased serum cortisol, and electrolyte abnormalities most likely has adrenal insufficiency, or Addison's disease. Metastatic carcinoma must destroy more than 90% of both adrenal glands before symptoms and signs of adrenal insufficiency are manifested. The loss of cortisol, mineralocorticoids, and catecholamines has profound effects on body homeostasis. Hypocortisolism results in hypoglycemia, because cortisol is a gluconeogenic hormone. Hypoaldosteronism affects the distal tubule exchange of sodium for potassium and hydrogen ions. This causes a hypertonic loss of sodium in the urine and subsequent hyponatremia and hypotension from volume depletion. The retention of potassium produces hyperkalemia, which alters cardiac function. Inability to secrete hydrogen ions causes them to combine with chloride ions in the extracellular fluid to form hydrochloric acid (HCl). This produces metabolic acidosis that is manifested by a fall in serum bicarbonate levels. Loss of catecholamines has the potential for affecting heart rate, cardiac contractility, and vascular tone by decreasing β-receptor stimulation. Only choice **D** shows the proper electrolyte changes, namely decreased sodium, chloride, and bicarbonate and elevated potassium levels.

Choice **A** with hyponatremia, hypokalemia, hypochloremia, and a low bicarbonate level is most often due to the inappropriate antidiuretic hormone (ADH) syndrome. Excess release of ADH causes an increase in the reabsorption of free water, which has a dilutional effect on sodium, chloride, potassium, and bicarbonate. A useful rule of thumb is that any serum sodium level below 120 mEq/L is most likely due to inappropriate secretion of ADH. Choice **B** with hypernatremia, hypokalemia, hyperchloremia, and metabolic alkalosis is commonly associated with mineralocorticoid excess states, such as primary aldosteronism. In this disease, autonomous (unregulated) production of aldosterone by the adrenal gland results in excess reabsorption of sodium to produce hypernatremia. The increased exchange of sodium for potassium produces hypokalemia. In addition, the excess exchange of sodium for hydrogen ions leaves bicarbonate behind in the tubules because the hydrogen ions came from the dissociation of carbonic acid into hydrogen ions and bicarbonate. The excess bicarbonate that is left behind produces metabolic alkalosis. Choice **C** with hyponatremia, hypokalemia, hypochloremia, and metabolic alkalosis is commonly seen with diuretic therapy using either loop or thiazide diuretics; as these drugs block sodium reabsorption, the excess delivery of sodium to the distal tubule increases the exchange of sodium for potassium, which produces hypokalemia, and also decreases retention of hydrogen ions. This leaves bicarbonate behind, resulting in metabolic alkalosis. Choice **E** with normal serum sodium, hypokalemia, hyperchloremia, and low bicarbonate commonly occurs in adult diarrhea. The loss of bicarbonate in the stool is counterbalanced by an equal gain in chloride in the plasma, which produces hyperchloremia and normal anion gap metabolic acidosis.

36 The answer is B *Psychiatry*

The symptoms are most strongly suggestive of a depressive episode. Although it may have been precipitated by the realization that he had medical problems, they are not likely to provide a physiologic basis for his depression, nor are any of the drugs listed likely to cause depression. His symptoms, in particular his somewhat oblique references to possible suicide, indicate that antidepressive therapy should be started at once. This would most likely consist of cognitive counseling plus the administration of an antidepressant. The most probable initial choice would be an SSRI (choice **B**) such as fluoxetine (Prozac), sertraline (Zoloft), paroxetine (Paxil) fluvoxamine (Luvox), or escitalopram (Lexapro). These drugs have significantly fewer adverse effects than the other antidepressants, and treatment is effective 70 to 75% of the time. However it usually takes some 4 weeks for the treatment to become fully effective, and doses may have to be adjusted. Combining cognitive therapy with drug treatment will potentially enhance the therapeutic effect and make it longer lasting.

MAOIs (choice **A**) were developed in the 1950s; they have antidepressive activity and still are used to treat resistant cases of depression. However they have lost popularity as a first line of treatment because of adverse effects. A particularly worrisome adverse effect, especially in this already hypertensive patient, is a tendency to provoke a hypertensive crisis. This is most likely to occur when the drug is used in combination with certain foods such as red wine or aged cheese or as a result of interaction with a multitude of different drugs. Other common adverse effects include dizziness, orthostatic hypotension, insomnia (with daytime sleepiness), and sexual malfunction. Tertiary amine tricyclic antidepressants (choice **C**) were among the earliest antidepressants to be developed. Adverse effects include sedation, orthostatic hypotension, and anticholinergic effects. Overdosing readily induces death and consequently they should not be used if there is danger of the patient committing suicide. They are converted to secondary amines in the body, and not surprisingly, secondary amine TCAs (choice **D**) act similarly to the tertiary amine TCAs but are less prone to cause sedation or orthostatic hypotension or to have anticholinergic effects; however they are more likely to exacerbate psychosis. Heterocyclic antidepressants (choice **E**) act on dopamine receptors and may have a tendency to provoke convulsions. Mixed reuptake inhibitors (choice **F**) block the action of norepinehrine, 5-hydroxyytrptamine (5HT), and dopamine. They are sometimes used as a first-line treatment but less often than SSRIs. Bupropion (Wellbutrin) especially may be prescribed if decreased libido is an important primary concern. Electroconvulsive therapy (ECT) (choice **G**) may be used if the patient is resistant to other forms of treatment, cannot tolerate antidepressant drugs, or is in immediate danger of committing suicide. An advantage of ECT is that positive effects are immediately evident. In the hands of an experienced psychiatrist, the current procedure is far less traumatic than it was years ago.

37 The answer is C *Surgery*

The symptoms described in the case history clearly suggest a diagnosis of benign prostatic hypertrophy (BPH). Normally the prostate is a walnut-sized gland situated just below the bladder and is wrapped around the urethra; with age it tends to enlarge and constrict the urethra, making urination more difficult. BPH affects about 50% of men in their 50s and as many as 80% after the age of 70 years. Initially only a nuisance, if left untreated too long BPH can become a serious medical problem; nonvoided urine can lead to infection, and relentless back pressure can irreversibly damage bladder muscles and even the kidney. Normally the first line of treatment is medical. Finasteride (Proscar) (choice **C**) has proved to effectively reduce prostate size by as much as 20% and to relieve mild-to-moderate symptoms effectively over the long term, with few adverse effects. It is an inhibitor of 5α-reductase, the enzyme that converts testosterone to its more active derivative dihydro-testosterone, the hormone that promotes the abnormal growth of the prostate, causing BPH. The major shortcoming of finasteride is that it takes up to a year to become fully effective. As a consequence a selective α_1-blocker such as doxazosin (Cardura), terazosin (Hytrin), or prazosin (Minipress) often is also prescribed. The α_1-blocker acts more rapidly to relax prostatic smooth muscle tone, resulting in reduction of urethral resistance and permitting urine to flow more freely. Thus, the two classes of drugs act synergistically short term; however, it is not clear if that is also true long term.

TURP (choice **A**) remains the "gold standard" of treatment for BPH against which other treatments are compared. It is relatively safe and effective about 80% of the time; however as with any surgical procedure, complications, sometimes severe, may arise, and many patients are left with urinary incontinence and/or impotence, and a smaller fraction with infection and other more serious problems. Therefore it is not usually the first line of treatment and is generally reserved for cases more severe than the one described, for chronic cases, and cases in which medical treatment is ruled out or has proved ineffective. Trimethoprim–sulfamethiazole (TMP-SMX) (choice **B**) is one of the several antibiotics that might be used to treat prostatitis. It has no role in treating BPH unless a secondary infection has set in. Radical prostatectomy (choice **D**), interstitial radiotherapy (choice **E**) or external beam radiotherapy are three of the more common therapies used to treat prostatic cancer. Prostate carcinoma is the most common malignancy in males. The prevalence is estimated to be 30% for men in their 60s, close to 70% for those in their 80s, and approaching 100% for men in their 90s. However because it often is slow growing, older men often die from causes other than problems arising from prostatic carcinoma. Early symptoms of BPH and prostatic cancer are similar. However, the digital rectal examination can often help distinguish between the two, since the cancerous prostate tends to be hard, and nodular, not smooth and firm as in BPH. Although both conditions tend to elevate the PSA, the value in cancer is often above 10 ng/dL. Unfortunately, PSA values for both BPH and cancer can sometimes fall into a gray area, between 4 and 10 ng/dL, adding possible ambiguity to the diagnosis. The ultimate confirmatory test is biopsy.

38 **The answer is E** *Preventive Medicine and Public Health*
Hemophilia A is a sex-linked recessive disease carried on the X chromosome. Normally, males inherit an X chromosome from their mother and a Y chromosome from their father, while females inherit one X chromosome from their mother and the other from their father. Therefore, a male cannot pass an X-linked disease to a son, but has a 100% chance of passing the defective gene to a daughter.

In the genealogy described, there is no reason to suspect that the mother has a defective gene. Despite the fact that her paternal uncles had hemophilia, her father is a healthy male; therefore, the solitary X chromosome that he possesses is normal. In addition, the fact that the woman's mother is of Scottish ancestry and her father is a Ukrainian Jew eliminates consanguinity in that generation. This heritage reduces the chances of the twin's mother carrying a recessive gene even further. On the other hand the father suffered from hemophilia A; as a consequence, his X chromosome carried the mutant gene. Therefore, the female fetus has a 100% chance of being a carrier, but she will not express the disease, and the male fetus will neither be a carrier nor will it express the disease (choice **E**).

If the mother was a carrier and the father did not have the disease, the male fetus would have a 50% chance of expressing the disease, but none of being a carrier. The female fetus on the other hand, would have a 50% chance of being a carrier, but have no chance of expressing the disease (choice **A**). If neither parent had the disease (i.e., both parents carried normal X genes), neither the female nor the male fetus would have a possibility of being a carrier or expressing the disease (choice **B**). Choice **C** is impossible because the mother only has two X chromosomes. If neither is affected, she is normal; if one is affected, she has a 50% chance of passing it on; if both are affected (an unlikely event), she has the disease herself. To have a 75% chance of being a carrier, she would require three X chromosomes, two of which would have to be abnormal. If the father had the disease and the mother was a carrier, the female fetus would have a 50% probability of being a carrier (one normal X gene from the mother and one defective X gene from the father) and a 50% probability of expressing the disease (one defective X gene from each parent). The male fetus would have a 50% likelihood of expressing the disease, but none of being a carrier (choice **D**).

39 **The answer is A** *Obstetrics and Gynecology*
The case scenario describes a hydatid cyst of Morgagni (choice **A**), also known as a paraovarian cyst. They are thin-walled, pedunculated, benign cysts attached to the tubal fimbria. They are of paramesonephric origin and are usually small, but they can grow to 10 cm in size and can be very mobile.

40 **The answer is H** *Obstetrics and Gynecology*

The case scenario describes theca-lutein cysts (choice **H**), which occur as a response of normal ovaries to excessively high β-human chorionic gonadotropin (HCG) titers produced by the trophoblastic tissue of a molar pregnancy. Preeclampsia before 20 weeks' gestation, as is seen in this scenario, is common with a hydatidiform mole. The cysts are bilateral and fluid filled, growing to massive size. They disappear when the source of the increased β-HCG levels is removed by a suction dilation and curettage. Follow-up with serial β-HCG titers is essential for at least a year.

41 **The answer is G** *Obstetrics and Gynecology*

The case scenario describes a classic corpus luteum cyst of pregnancy (choice **G**) that resolved spontaneously when the placenta took over the function of progesterone production. These are unilateral, simple cysts that are an exaggerated response to a normal physiologic event. Management is conservative observation.

42 **The answer is E** *Obstetrics and Gynecology*

The case scenario describes a normal intrauterine pregnancy (choice **E**). This is the most common cause of an enlarged pelvic mass in the reproductive years. Confirmation by sonogram is appropriate if the diagnosis is uncertain. A pelvic mass in the reproductive years is always an indication for a β-HCG test.

43 **The answer is N** *Obstetrics and Gynecology*

The case scenario describes a child undergoing isosexual (in the expected direction for a female), complete (evidence of all pubertal changes) precocious (prior to the age of 8) puberty with the finding of a unilateral pelvic mass. This must be assumed to be a hormonally functional ovarian tumor producing estrogen, such as a granulosa cell tumor (choice **N**), until proved otherwise. Management is surgical removal.

44 **The answer is O** *Obstetrics and Gynecology*

The case scenario describes a postmenopausal woman with virilization and a unilateral pelvic mass. Until proved otherwise, this must be assumed to be a hormonally functional ovarian tumor producing androgens, such as a Sertoli-Leydig cell tumor (choice **O**).

45 **The answer is M** *Obstetrics and Gynecology*

The case scenario describes a benign cystic teratoma (choice **M**). Because these tumors derive from primordial germ cells, they may contain any combination of well-differentiated ectodermal, mesodermal, and endodermal elements. Foci of calcification, even the presence of teeth, are common. Management is surgical removal by laparoscopy.

46 **The answer is J** *Obstetrics and Gynecology*

The case scenario is characteristic for endometriosis (choice **J**). Endometriomas are cysts on the ovary that result from accumulation of menstrual-like detritus from endometriosis. These "chocolate cysts" can enlarge to several centimeters in size.

INCORRECT CHOICES

Hydrosalpinx (choice **B**) is a condition in which the fallopian tube is occluded at both ends, leading to collection of fluid within it. Bacterial or viral infections that are sexually transmitted, lead to inflammation and scarring of the fallopian tubes and their subsequent closure. The patient may have infertility as a result of it. Diagnosis is made by pelvic ultrasonography.

Tubo-ovarian abscess (choice **C**) is an advanced form of pelvic inflammatory disease (PID), which is usually caused by anaerobic bacteria that spread in a retrograde manner from the lower genital tract. Sexually transmitted disease, douching, and multiple sexual partners are risk factors. Women who use IUDs are at increased risk for PID and tubo-ovarian abscess. Patients usually present with pelvic pain. Complications include infertility, a greater risk for ectopic pregnancy, and chronic pelvic pain secondary to adhesions. Diagnosis is made by pelvic ultrasonography.

Chronic pelvic inflammatory disease (PID) (choice **D**) is usually the result of sexually transmitted disease. The most common infection is that caused by *Chlamydia*. The infection is low grade for many years, ultimately leading to chronicity. The patient has crampy or constant pelvic pain. Menorrhagia or intermenstrual irregular bleeding can occur, and infertility is the invariable result. Acute exacerbations could lead to severe pain and fever. Treatment includes antibiotics, steroids (to combat inflammation), and removal of adhesions by surgery. In advanced cases with extensive fallopian tube involvement, the tubes may have to be sacrificed.

Follicular cyst (choice **F**) is usually seen in early pregnancy and resolves during the second trimester. It usually results from failed ovulation. Most cases are asymptomatic. However, if hemorrhage occurs within the cyst, the patient presents with acute pelvic pain, which, if on the right side, could be mistaken for acute appendicitis. Diagnosis is made by ultrasonography.

Luteoma of pregnancy (choice **I**) is a rare nonneoplastic condition usually affecting both ovaries, which show enlargement during pregnancy. It is more common in black multiparous women than in others. The patients are usually asymptomatic, and the condition is usually noted at cesarean section. The characteristic finding is replacement of normal ovarian parenchyma by a solid mass made up of luteinized stromal cells. These cells are under the influence of human chorionic gonadotrophin. However, unlike patients with gestational trophoblastic disease, these patients do not have elevated levels of human chorionic gonadotrophin levels. Virilization of the mother and fetus could occur because stromal cells secrete androgens. No treatment is necessary, as the disorder is self-limiting.

Polycystic ovaries (choice **K**): Polycystic ovarian syndrome is the most common hormonal reproductive disorder in women of childbearing age. Patients usually have pelvic pain, absent or irregular periods (which are usually anovulatory), increased androgen production leading to hirsutism, dandruff, acne and increased body weight, and, in many cases, cysts in their ovaries. Other features include hypertension, hypercholesterolemia, and type 2 diabetes mellitus. Progesterone is essential for the shedding of the endometrium at the end of a menstrual cycle. The absence of menstruation, therefore, leads to thickening of the endometrium over time. As a result, endometrial hyperplasia or carcinoma could occur. Diagnosis is made by ultrasonography. Other tests include measuring serum hormone and blood glucose levels. Treatment includes birth control pills to regularize menstruation for those who do not wish to become pregnant and medications to promote fertility in women who do want to become pregnant. If fertility medications do not work, surgery is an option. Diabetes mellitus should be treated; metformin is a good drug to choose. Not only will it lower blood sugar levels, it will decrease testosterone production too. The latter effect will slow down androgenic effects such as hirsutism.

Mucinous cystadenoma (choice **L**) is a benign ovarian neoplasm that is slow growing and usually affects women between the ages of 30 and 50. The tumor may be bilateral. The patient presents with heaviness and distention of the abdomen, which can grow to a very large size. Ultrasonography usually reveals a multiloculated cyst. Rupture of the cyst leads to pseudomyxoma peritonei. Treatment is surgical.

Gonadoblastoma (choice **P**) is a rare benign tumor that can turn malignant, especially in patients with intersex disorders. Phenotypically, 80% are females, while 20% are males. Gonadoblastomas are usually found within the second decade of life. The usual presentation is primary amenorrhea following puberty. Gonadoblastoma could develop in patients with male pseudohermaphroditism, (46, XY), mixed gonadal dysgenesis, (45, X/46, XY) and Turner's syndrome (45, XO).

47 The answer is G *Psychiatry*

His initial impulses are most suggestive of regression (choice **K**), characterized by a return to less mature levels of functioning. However, he instead lowered his high anxiety levels by using humor (choice **G**) a more mature defense mechanism.

48 The answer is M *Psychiatry*

These behaviors are most suggestive of suppression (choice **M**), a defense mechanism that involves forcing anxiety-provoking feelings into the unconscious by substituting other feelings or thoughts. Denial (choice **C**) differs in that it is simply the failure to acknowledge the disturbing effects of an external reality.

REMAINING INCORRECT CHOICES

Altruism (choice **A**) involves decreasing one's own internal fears or anxiety by caring for others.

Blocking (choice **B**) is defined as the sudden repression of anxiety-provoking thoughts in midsentence. Conversation, if it resumes, is usually about another topic.

Displacement (choice **D**) occurs when the emotions associated with a psychologically unacceptable object, idea, or activity are transferred to another object or situation. The new object or situation is often symbolically related to the original. For example, a patient who was badly injured in an accident becomes angry with his surgeon for leaving a small scar during reconstructive procedures.

Dissociation (choice **E**) involves sealing off disturbing thoughts or emotions from consciousness.

Distortion (choice **F**) is altering the perception of disturbing aspects of external reality to make it more palatable.

Rationalization (choice **I**) is a distortion of reality that makes an undesirable act or event seem more desirable.

Reaction formation (choice **J**) occurs when an unacceptable thought or feeling is transformed into its opposite.

Repression (choice **L**) is the complete separation of aspects of reality (e.g., memories, cognitions, impulses) from conscious awareness.

Sublimation (choice **M**) occurs when unacceptable impulses are channeled into more acceptable activities.

Undoing (choice **N**) involves performing an activity that symbolically reverses a previous behavior or thought.

PROLOGUE

Polycythemia refers to an increase in hemoglobin (Hgb), hematocrit (Hct), and red blood cell (RBC) count. The RBC count is the number of RBCs per μL of blood, while RBC mass is the total absolute number of RBCs in the body in mL/kg. There are two types of polycythemia—relative and absolute. Relative polycythemia refers to an increased RBC count that is due to a decrease in plasma volume (e.g., volume depletion from sweating). The RBC mass, or the absolute number of RBCs in the body, is normal because the bone marrow has not produced more RBCs. Absolute polycythemia refers to an increase in bone marrow RBC production; therefore, there is an increase in the RBC count and RBC mass. Absolute polycythemia is appropriate if there is a hypoxic stimulus for erythropoietin (EPO) release. Examples include primary lung disease (e.g., chronic obstructive lung disease), cyanotic congenital heart disease (e.g., tetralogy of Fallot), or living at high altitude. Absolute polycythemia is inappropriate if there is no hypoxic stimulus for EPO release. Examples include polycythemia vera, and ectopic secretion of EPO (e.g., renal disorders, cysts/cancer; hepatocellular carcinoma). One of the dangers of absolute polycythemia is vessel thrombosis. This underscores the importance of phlebotomy in the treatment of absolute polycythemia due to polycythemia vera.

An arterial blood gas (ABG) determination is the first step in the workup of polycythemia, because it immediately characterizes the polycythemia as appropriate or inappropriate. RBC mass and plasma volume are also useful, because they define whether the polycythemia is absolute or relative. Erythropoietin levels are increased only if the polycythemia is appropriate or ectopically secreted.

49 The answer is B *Medicine*

Decreased oxygen saturation, increased RBC mass, normal plasma volume, and increased erythropoietin indicate an appropriate polycythemia, because the oxygen saturation is decreased. It is also absolute, because the RBC mass is increased. The normal plasma volume and increased erythropoietin levels are expected when hypoxemia is the cause of the secondary polycythemia. Hypoxemia is associated with chronic obstructive pulmonary disease (COPD, choice **B**), restrictive lung diseases, cyanotic congenital heart disease, and high-altitude residence, to name a few.

50 The answer is A *Medicine*

Normal oxygen saturation, increased RBC mass, increased plasma volume, and a decreased erythropoietin level indicate an inappropriate polycythemia because the oxygen saturation is normal. It is an absolute polycythemia, because the RBC mass is increased. Since the EPO is decreased, it cannot be ectopic secretion of EPO; therefore, it must be polycythemia vera (choice **A**). Polycythemia vera is a myeloproliferative disease with unregulated production of RBCs, leukocytes, and platelets in the marrow. The oxygen saturation is normal, RBC mass and plasma volume are both increased, and the erythropoietin is decreased, because the total oxygen content is increased. Oxygen content (oxygen bound to heme groups in Hgb and oxygen dissolved in plasma) is the normal feedback for EPO. A decrease in oxygen content causes an increase in EPO, while an increase in oxygen content causes a decrease in EPO. Note how an increase in plasma volume and a decrease in EPO are unique to polycythemia vera. All other absolute polycythemias have a normal plasma volume and an increase in EPO that is either appropriate (e.g., COPD, tetralogy) or inappropriate (e.g., ectopic secretion).

INCORRECT CHOICES

Relative polycythemia (choice **C**) has a normal oxygen saturation, normal RBC mass, decreased plasma volume, and a normal EPO level. Renal cell carcinoma (choice **D**) and other disorders characterized by ectopic production of erythropoietin (e.g., hepatocellular carcinoma, renal cysts) have normal oxygen saturation, increased RBC mass, normal plasma volume, and increased EPO level.

SUMMARY

The following chart summarizes the different types of polycythemia and the expected laboratory findings.

Condition	RBC Mass	Plasma Volume	SaO$_2$	EPO
Polycythemia vera	↑	↑	Normal	↓
Hypoxemia (COPD)	↑	Normal	↓	↑
Ectopic	↑	Normal	Normal	↑
Relative	Normal	↓	Normal	Normal

EPO, erythropoietin; SaO$_2$, oxygen saturation in arterial blood.

test **2**

Questions

Single Best Choice Directions: This section consists of numbered statements or questions followed by a list of potential answers; you are to select the ONE BEST answer.

1 A 48-year-old female who is a known diabetic and mild hypertensive presents with a 6-week history of tiredness that has come on gradually. She states that her clothes have become tighter and that she has difficulty getting into her shoes. Her voice also seems to have become "hoarse." There are days when she feels that there is no point in getting up in the morning. She has been turning up late for work, and her supervisor has "written her up" for tardiness. In the past few days, she has noticed pain in the right wrist, especially when she uses the computer to send e-mail. She constantly fights with her husband, saying that the bedroom is cold at night, and insists on using several blankets. She even spends more time in the toilet. Her only medications are metformin for diabetes and hydrochlorothiazide for hypertension. Her vital signs are as follows: blood pressure, 130/90 mm Hg; pulse 60/min regular; respirations, 16/min; and a body temperature of 36.50°C (97.70°F). She has rather coarse features, her face and eyelids are puffy, and pretibial nonpitting edema is present. Examination of her neck reveals a diffuse nontender enlargement in the anterior region that moves with swallowing. No other abnormality is noted. Which of the following set of laboratory test values best supports the proper diagnosis?

	Total Serum T_4	Free Serum T_4	Serum TSH
(A)	↑	Normal	Normal
(B)	↑	↑	↓
(C)	↓	Normal	Normal
(D)	↓	↓	↑
(E)	↓	↓	↓

TSH, thyroid-stimulating hormone.

2 A 23-year-old woman, gravida 3, para 1, aborta 1, comes to the maternity unit examination room at 39 weeks' gestation by dates. Onset of prenatal care was at 10 weeks. Gestational age was confirmed by a 12-week sonogram. Her diabetes screening at 26 weeks gestation was within normal limits. She reports uterine contractions that have been regular for the past 3 hours. On examination, you find that the contractions are 3 minutes apart, last 50 seconds each, and are firm to palpation. Her membranes ruptured 1 hour ago, and you note clear Nitrazine-positive fluid leak-ing from her vagina. Digital cervical examination reveals dilation of 5 cm, effacement of 100%, and the presenting vertex at 0 station. Which of the following criteria is most accurate for assessing whether she has entered the active phase of labor?

(A) Cervical effacement over 90%
(B) Contraction duration over 30 seconds
(C) Presenting part below +3 station
(D) Cervical dilation of at least 4 cm
(E) Ruptured membranes

3 A physician sees a 7-year-old girl who has been referred to him by the school nurse, who informs him that the child often has cessation of speech in midconversation, accompanied by a blank stare and flickering of the eyelids. These symptoms last approximately 10 seconds before she resumes regular activity. The physician suspects that the child has a seizure disorder and asks the child to hyperventilate. During hyperventilation, the aforementioned symptoms appear. Which of the following electroencephalogram (EEG) patterns is most characteristic of this disorder?

(A) Hypsarrhythmia
(B) Interictal slow-spike waves
(C) Centrotemporal spikes
(D) Three-per-second spike-and-wave pattern
(E) Four- to six-per-second spike-and-wave pattern

4 A 55-year-old woman comes to see a family physician for the first time since she recently moved to New York City after a job change. She informs the physician that she has had a 10-year history of pain in the joints of her hand. Upon examination, the physician notes the patient has ulnar deviation of both hands, swelling of the metacarpophalangeal (MCP) joints, and nodules on the extensor surface of both forearms. In addition, he finds an ulcer overlying the right lateral malleolus. Which additional finding would you expect the physician to uncover after further examination?

(A) A high rheumatoid factor titer
(B) Monoclonal gammopathy observed on a serum protein electrophoresis
(C) Deep venous insufficiency
(D) Osteophytes at the margins to the joints
(E) Iron deficiency anemia

5 A 38-year-old male was taken to the emergency department after his car skidded on the freeway and struck a pillar. His vital signs were as follows: pulse, 88/min; respirations, 20/min; blood pressure, 100/70 mm Hg. Physical examination revealed nonprominent jugular neck vein, no indication of cyanosis, and breath sounds that were symmetric. A posterior–anterior chest x-ray film revealed a widened mediastinum. Which of the following choices is the most likely diagnosis?

(A) Ruptured aortic aneurysm
(B) Cardiac tamponade
(C) Dissection of the thoracic aorta
(D) Myocardial contusion
(E) Pulmonary contusion

6 An executive was fired 2 years ago and experienced several months of depression. However, he seemed to regain his confidence spontaneously and now states that losing his job has been helpful in that it gives him more time to spend with his family. Which of the following psychodynamic defenses is most strongly suggested by this statement?

(A) Splitting
(B) Compensation
(C) Displacement
(D) Rationalization
(E) Projection

7 A 20-year-old woman who is a business major at a local university sees her physician because she has not had a period for the past 5 months. She knows she is not pregnant because she is not sexually active. She attained menarche at 12 years of age, but her menses always have been irregular. She also expressed concern about being at least 25 pounds overweight and volunteers that her roommate has recently lost weight and was diagnosed with hepatitis A, suggesting that maybe she could do so too. Physical examination revealed that she is 168 cm (66 in) tall and weighs 46 kg (102 lb). Her secondary sex characteristics are normal, but she appears thin and underweight. Her pelvic examination is normal. Findings of laboratory studies of serum prolactin, estradiol, and human chorionic gonadotropin (HCG) measurements are normal. Which of the following is the most likely diagnosis?

(A) Turner's syndrome
(B) Hypogonadotropic hypogonadism
(C) Polycystic ovary syndrome
(D) Asherman's syndrome
(E) Anorexia nervosa

8 A man married a young woman who lost her vision at the age of 28 years. They had three children, two girls and one boy, all of whom started to become blind after the age of 20. All three of these children married sighted persons and had children. One daughter had two boys and a girl all of whom became blind. The other daughter had a boy and girl; both of them lost their vision as well. The son had three boys and a girl, all of whom were sighted and had excellent vision as long as they lived. In the third generation, all the boys who remained sighted and those who lost their vision early married women who remained sighted until they died, and all their offspring also remained sighted well into old age. The daughter of the second generation male who retained her sight married a normally sighted man, and their offspring could see throughout their lives as well. The second generation women who became blind married men who retained their sight but their offspring of either sex lost their sight at an early age. Which of the following inheritance patterns is most likely to be present?

(A) Autosomal dominant
(B) Autosomal recessive
(C) Mitochondrial
(D) X-linked dominant
(E) X-linked recessive

9 A 3-year-old child presents with recurrent right lower lobe pneumonia. His growth parameters are at the 25th percentile, and he is developmentally appropriate for his age. His past medical history is positive for an ear infection at 18 months of age and gastroenteritis at 2 years of age. He has completed two courses of antibiotic therapy with minimal if any improvement. Which of the following conditions is most likely responsible for this patient's disease?

(A) Primary B- or T-cell immunodeficiency disorder
(B) Cystic fibrosis
(C) Chédiak-Higashi syndrome
(D) Congenital lung abnormality
(E) Foreign body aspiration

10 A 65-year-old male jumps off of a bus to catch a train. He immediately feels very severe pain in the front of the knee and hears a snap. He falls to the ground and is unable to rise. The emergency physician determines that the patient is a diabetic whose diabetes is controlled by oral hypoglycemics. He has no allergies and is not on any other medications. He exercises occasionally, and he is overweight. His vital signs are as follows: pulse, 86/min; respirations, 18/min; blood pressure, 150/97 mm Hg. His temperature is normal. The patient complains of pain in the right knee. Clinical examination reveals swelling and tenderness in the anterior aspect of the knee, and a sulcus is palpable proximal to the superior pole of the patella; no fragments can be moved. The patient is unable to extend the knee. Hemarthrosis is absent. Which of the following is the most likely diagnosis?

(A) Tear of the posterior cruciate ligament
(B) Tear of the anterior cruciate ligament
(C) Transverse fracture of the patella
(D) Tear of the quadriceps expansion
(E) Avulsion of the quadriceps tendon from the tibial tuberosity

11 A 35-year-old woman, gravida 5, para 4, aborta 1, is seen for an annual examination and cervical cancer screening. Her four successful pregnancies all ended with term spontaneous vaginal deliveries of neonates weighing between 3000 g (6 lb 10 oz) and 4000 g (8 lb 13 oz). All children are alive and well. She had an uncomplicated elective laparoscopic tubal sterilization procedure performed 2 years ago under general anesthesia. Her 30-year-old sister also comes in for a routine annual examination. She has never been pregnant. She uses combination oral contraceptive pills for birth control. Which of the following physical examination findings of the cervix would be more typical of this 35-year-old woman than of her 30-year-old sister?

(A) Increased bluish hue
(B) Purulent discharge
(C) Retracted squamocolumnar junction
(D) Transverse-appearing external os
(E) Absence of scarring

12 A 25-year old single mother takes her 5-year-old child to see a pediatrician for a rash that started on her trunk and then spread to her face and extremities. According to the mother, the rash occurred in varying stages. It began with crops of small, red papules that progressed to teardrop vesicles on an erythematous base. These vesicles became cloudy, broke open, and then formed scabs. Which of the following is the most common complication of this infection in a normal host?

(A) Reye's syndrome
(B) Pneumonia
(C) Thrombocytopenia
(D) Encephalitis
(E) Secondary bacterial skin infection

13 A very anxious 25-year-old man complains of severe right lower quadrant pain. Physical examination reveals rebound tenderness, and laboratory results include leukocytosis. He experiences much subjective pain relief after normal saline solution is administered. Which of the following is most strongly suggested by this situation?

(A) The pain is psychogenic
(B) He has a histrionic personality disorder
(C) He was volume depleted
(D) He has factitious disorder
(E) He is responding to a placebo

14 A 65-year-old man presents with a 7-kg (15-lb) weight loss over the last 3 months and recent onset of streaks of blood in the sputum. He gives a history of smoking 40 packs of cigarettes per year. Physical examination reveals a thin, afebrile man with clubbing of the fingers, an increased anteroposterior diameter of the chest, scattered coarse rhonchi and wheezes over both lung fields, and distant heart sounds. A chest radiograph exhibits left hilar adenopathy, dilated tubular markings, and flattened diaphragms. Sputum cytology using a Pap stain shows numerous cells with deeply eosinophilic-staining cytoplasm and irregular, hyperchromatic nuclei intermixed with inflammatory cells. Which of the following is the most likely diagnosis?

(A) Small cell carcinoma of the lung
(B) Tuberculosis
(C) Pulmonary embolism with infarction
(D) Bronchiectasis
(E) Squamous cell carcinoma of the lung

15 A 28-year-old woman complains that her mother is selfish, undereducated, devious, and bereft of any redeeming qualities. On the other hand, she idealizes an aunt whom she describes as kind, sage, and the source of strength in her life. Which of the following defense mechanisms is this woman using?

(A) Projection
(B) Idealization
(C) Conversion
(D) Splitting
(E) Symbolization

16 A 74-year old African-American male recently noticed difficulty in swallowing pills and solid foods. The symptoms had started to worsen over the past 4-week period. He was alarmed and decided to consult his primary care physician. In taking a history it was determined that the patient thought that although his problem with solids had progressed rapidly, he had little or no problem with liquids. He had a long-standing history of gastroesophageal reflux disease (GERD) and although omeprazole had been prescribed to treat it, he admitted to not using it regularly. At the present time he did not smoke, but he had started smoking at the age of 14 and quit some 10 years ago. He drank beer on social occasions. Which of the following conditions is the most likely diagnosis?

(A) Diffuse esophageal spasm
(B) Achalasia
(C) Esophageal stricture
(D) Esophageal ring (Schatzki ring)
(E) Esophageal carcinoma
(F) Zenker's diverticulum
(G) Esophageal varices

17 A multicentered retrospective research study, involving 724 women of childbearing age, with pregestational diabetes mellitus investigated the relationship between mean blood glucose values and major fetal malformations. The purpose of the study was to estimate the relative risk of pregestational women with diabetes mellitus to have major fetal malformations during their pregnancy. The presence of malformation was confirmed by sonography and amniocentesis. Of the 724 women, 60 had mean plasma glucose values of 130 mg/dL or above, while 302 women had mean plasma glucose values below 130 mg/dL. The first group had 10 cases of major fetal malformations in their pregnancies, while in the second group; only 2 had major fetal malformations in their pregnancies. Findings from the study are summarized in the table below:

Major Fetal Malformation is	Maternal Mean Plasma Glucose Values		
	Totals	≥130 mg/dL	<130 mg/dL
Present	12	10	2
Absent	350	50	300
Totals	362	60	302

Which of the following equations represents the odds ratio for this study?

(A) $300 \div 50 = 6$
(B) $50 \div 10 = 5$
(C) $60 \div (2 + 10) = 5$
(D) $(300 \div 2) \div (60 \div 10) = 25$
(E) $(10 \div 2) \div (50 \div 300) = 30$

18 A 26-year-old medical student with a history of hepatitis A virus (HAV) is immunized against hepatitis B virus (HBV). Which set of hepatitis serology data is most closely associated with this student's history?

	Anti-HAV IgM	Anti-HAV IgG	Anti-HBc IgM	Anti-HBs	HBsAg	HBeAg
(A)	−	+	+	−	−	−
(B)	−	+	−	+	−	−
(C)	−	+	+	−	+	+
(D)	+	−	−	+	−	−
(E)	+	−	−	−	−	−

c, core antigen; e, e antigen; HAV, hepatitis A virus; HBeAg, e antigen; HBsAg, surface antigen; HBV, hepatitis B virus; Ig, immunoglobulins.

19 A 10-year-old girl is brought to the physician's office because she has a rash on her trunk. The parents state that the child was in her usual good health until 1 week ago when she developed fever; generalized lymphadenopathy; and an expanding, annular, erythematous papular rash on the trunk. In addition, her right knee is painful and slightly swollen. The findings of the physical examination are otherwise unremarkable. The parents deny that the patient had any contacts with others who are ill or any exposure to pets. She had recently returned from visiting with her grandparents. Which of the following is the most likely diagnosis?

(A) Rocky Mountain spotted fever
(B) Babesiosis
(C) Colorado tick fever
(D) Lyme disease
(E) Juvenile rheumatoid arthritis

20 A 73-year-old Scandinavian male was undergoing a routine physical examination when his physician noted a roundish spot about 6 mm (¼ inch) in diameter that was slightly pinker than the remainder of the man's face. When he ran his finger across it he also noted that was dry and rough. The patient informed him that something had been going on with that spot for a year or so; its appearance seemed to wax and wane essentially disappearing once in a while but then returning, sometimes covered with white scales that then dropped off. When asked, the patient admitted that as a boy and a young man he spent countless hours at the beach body surfing and never used sunscreen. The physician cauterized the lesion with liquid nitrogen. Within 2 weeks the area became crusted, shrank and fell off. Two weeks thereafter the rough spot returned, and after a month, the patient developed an open sore at the same location that would not heal. The sore is most likely to be which one of the following?

(A) Actinic keratosis
(B) Basal cell carcinoma
(C) Squamous cell carcinoma
(D) Nodular melanoma
(E) Herpes infection

21 A 62-year-old woman with a 35-year history of treatment with antipsychotic medications for schizophrenia complains of the insidious onset of peculiar writhing movements that she could not control. These include unintended lip smacking, contorted facial expressions, and movements of her tongue and fingers. Her psychotic manifestations had been well controlled for some time, and her physician had begun to taper her medication doses. Moreover, she had been fairly successful in reintegrating herself into a normal social milieu but found these movements so embarrassing that she started to withdraw again. Which of the following is most likely responsible?

(A) Tardive akathisia
(B) Huntington's disease
(C) Parkinsonism
(D) Tardive dyskinesia
(E) Wilson's disease

22 A 60-year-old man, who has smoked two packs of cigarettes daily for 40 years, complains of difficulty with breathing at rest and with exercise. Physical examination reveals a man with an emaciated appearance and pink discoloration of the skin. It is difficult to hear heart and lung sounds. A chest radiograph shows hyperinflation in both lung fields, depression of both diaphragms, an increase in the anteroposterior diameter, and a vertically oriented cardiac silhouette. The pulmonary function test indicative of this condition would be

(A) Decreased functional residual capacity (FRC)
(B) Decreased total lung capacity (TLC)
(C) Increased arterial P_{CO_2} and decreased arterial P_{O_2}
(D) Increased forced expiratory volume 1 second to forced vital capacity ratio (i.e., the FEV_{1sec}/FVC)
(E) Increased residual volume (RV)

23 Fortunesville, USA, population 200,000, has an annual rate of 15 new cases of acute leukemia. A leading pharmaceutical company decided to try an experimental medication for the treatment of the disease. Patients with confirmed acute leukemia were selected from this population. Of the 300 known patients with cases of leukemia, 200 were female and 100 were male. All patients had received treatments earlier with established therapies. The treatment trial was double blinded. Approximately 150 patients received the new treatment, while 130 received a placebo. Twenty patients dropped out of the study due to noncompliance/nonacceptance. The trial clearly showed that it extended the life span of the patients with the disease and increased the length of remission. It did not, however, cure the disease. From this study, one could conclude that with treatment with this new drug

(A) Incidence of acute leukemia will increase
(B) Prevalence of acute leukemia will increase
(C) Incidence of acute leukemia will decrease
(D) Prevalence of acute leukemia will decrease
(E) Both incidence and prevalence of acute leukemia will decrease

24 A first-year pediatric resident is called to the nursery to examine an infant who had a cyanotic and choking episode associated with feeding. The infant was born full term, weighed 3.5 kg (7 lb 14 oz), and no complications occurred during delivery. The mother had no prenatal care but denies use of alcohol, illicit drugs, or tobacco. She also denies any sexually transmitted disease. Physical examination of the infant reveals excessive oral secretions. These oral secretions improve with suctioning of the mouth and pharynx, but recur after a short time. The resident suspects tracheoesophageal fistula. Which of the following additional findings would support her suspicion?

(A) Cyanosis that occurs at rest but is relieved by crying
(B) A history of oligohydramnios during pregnancy
(C) The ability to pass a catheter into the stomach
(D) A stomach filled with air
(E) An associated renal anomaly

25 A 45-year-old man has chronic myelogenous leukemia. He is currently being treated with multiple antileukemic agents. One week into therapy, he develops oliguric renal failure with an increase in serum blood urea nitrogen, creatinine, and uric acid levels. Urinalysis reveals an acid pH, and numerous crystals are present on sediment examination. Which of the following best explains the mechanism for the renal failure?

(A) Drug nephrotoxicity
(B) Increased degradation of purine nucleotides
(C) Increased degradation of pyrimidine nucleotides
(D) Leukemic infiltration of the kidneys

26 An 18-year-old woman, gravida 1, para 0, underwent spontaneous vaginal delivery 10 minutes ago. She gave birth to a 4,030-g (8 lb 14 oz) male neonate with 1- and 5-minute Apgar scores of 8 and 9. Her prenatal course was uncomplicated, and labor began spontaneously. Pain relief in labor was achieved by continuous epidural analgesia. Monitoring of the fetal heart rate and uterine contractions was by external cardiotocography. The second stage of labor lasted 90 minutes. She did not receive an episiotomy. You note only minimal first-degree vaginal lacerations. The umbilical cord begins to lengthen and you observe a gush of blood from the vagina. Which of the following is the most likely cause of these events?

(A) Rapidly falling estrogen levels in maternal circulation

(B) Avulsion of anchoring villi by contracting myometrium

(C) Falling levels of circulating, placentally produced prolactin

(D) A gradual decrease in P_{CO_2} in the umbilical vein

(E) A progesterone-mediated decrease in gap junctions

27 A 25-year-old woman has had to change her prescription for eyeglasses on two separate occasions over the last 4 months because of blurry vision. In addition, she complains of weight loss, increased appetite, increased frequency of urination, and a fruity odor to her breath. Findings from the physical examination are unremarkable. Which of the following laboratory tests is most useful for determining the cause of the blurry vision over the past 2 months?

(A) Hemoglobin A_{1c}

(B) Serum cortisol

(C) Serum thyroid-stimulating hormone

(D) Urine dipstick test for glucose

(E) Urine dipstick test for ketones

28 A 35-year-old woman presents with moderate hypertension, muscle weakness, polyuria, and paresthesias with tetanic manifestations. There is no evidence of pitting edema. A 24-hour urine test for potassium and free cortisol shows increased loss of potassium and normal levels of free cortisol. A computed tomography (CT) scan of the adrenal glands shows a localized, encapsulated mass in the left adrenal gland. Which set of laboratory data would most likely be present in this patient?

	Serum Aldosterone	PRA[a]	Serum Potassium	Serum Bicarbonate
(A)	↑	↑	↓	↑
(B)	Normal	↓	↓	↑
(C)	↑	↓	↓	↑
(D)	↓	↓	↑	↓
(E)	↓	↑	↑	↓

[a]PRA, plasma renin activity.

29 An African-American couple, with no known family history of sickle cell disease, wants to know the probability that their child will have sickle cell disease. To obtain a more precise assessment, a hydrolysate of their red blood cells (RBCs) is subjected to electrophoresis. The male has no HbS, but the female has an obvious HbS band. Given that the carrier rate among African Americans is approximately 8%, or 1 in 12, the likelihood that their child will have sickle cell disease would most likely be:

(A) 0

(B) 1/4

(C) 1/144

(D) 1/576

(E) 1/1936

30 A 22-year-old woman, gravida 2, para 1, presents for a routine prenatal visit. She is 42 and 1/2 weeks' gestation by dates, 170 cm (67 in) tall and weighs 67 kg (147 lb). During her pregnancy she has had a total weight gain of 19 kg (43 lb). This was a planned pregnancy that was complicated in the first trimester by severe nausea and vomiting that ended by 15 weeks gestation. She required intravenous hydration and antiemetic medications. She has a positive history of chronic hypertension treated with methyldopa. She has had five sonograms performed during her pregnancy, at 10, 20, 25, 30, and 40 weeks' gestation. Which of the following five sonograms will have provided the most accurate estimate of the duration of pregnancy?

(A) 10 weeks

(B) 20 weeks

(C) 25 weeks

(D) 30 weeks

(E) 40 weeks

31 A 5-month-old nonimmunized child presents with a 2-week history of paroxysmal coughing, low-grade fever, posttussive emesis, and a viscid nasal discharge. Physical examination reveals bilateral otitis media and conjunctival hemorrhages. Scattered inspiratory rales are present bilaterally. The complete blood count (CBC) shows a white blood cell (WBC) count of 45,000 cells/mm^3, 95% of which represent lymphocytes. Which of the following is the most likely diagnosis?

(A) Acute lymphoblastic leukemia

(B) *Chlamydia trachomatis* pneumonia

(C) Whooping cough

(D) Bronchiolitis

(E) Respiratory syncytial viral pneumonitis

32 A 2-year-old child presents to the physician's office with her mother. The mother states that for the past few days the child has had a low-grade fever, upper respiratory tract symptoms, and has been tugging at her right ear. An examination of the right ear with the pneumatic otoscope reveals a hyperemic, opaque, bulging, tympanic membrane with poor mobility. The patient attends daycare three times a week. There has been no recent travel, and no one else is ill in the household. Which of the following organisms is the most likely causative pathogen?

(A) *Haemophilus influenzae*
(B) *Staphylococcus aureus*
(C) *Moraxella catarrhalis*
(D) *Streptococcus pneumoniae*
(E) Respiratory syncytial virus

33 A 24-year-old male football player fell on his outstretched hand while running with the ball, hoping to make a touchdown. He was writhing in pain and had to be taken to the emergency room of a local hospital. The patient complained of severe pain in his right arm. His vital signs were blood pressure, 140/80; pulse, 98/min regular; temperature 37°C (98.6°F); and respirations 22/min and regular. The right arm was swollen and angulated in the midarm area. It was tender to touch, and movement was painful. The humeral shaft appeared to be fractured. Capillary circulation in the nail beds was normal. However, there was clinical evidence of nerve damage. The arm was splinted, and the patient was given narcotic analgesia to minimize the pain. An x-ray film of the arm confirmed fracture of the humeral shaft, with some angular displacement. Which of the following is the nerve injury associated with this fracture?

(A) Axillary nerve
(B) Median nerve
(C) Ulnar nerve
(D) Radial nerve
(E) Brachial plexus

34 A 16-year-old woman, gravida 1, para 0, presents to the outpatient office for a routine prenatal visit at 34 weeks' gestation. Her blood pressure (BP) is 150/95 mm Hg and remains elevated after 10 minutes of rest in the left-lateral position. Urine dipstick testing reveals 1+ glucose and 2+ albumin. She denies vaginal bleeding, leakage of vaginal fluid, headache, epigastric pain, or visual disturbances. Her BP on her initial prenatal visit at 14 weeks' gestation was 120/75 mm Hg. An obstetric sonogram obtained at 18 weeks gestation confirmed her dates and showed normal fetal anatomy. Her maternal grandfather has adult-onset diabetes.

Her mother and maternal grandmother both have chronic hypertension. Which of the following is the most likely explanation for the findings in this patient?

(A) Blunted angiotensin response
(B) Elevated β-endorphin level
(C) Acute diffuse vasoconstriction
(D) Primary renal disease
(E) Chronic hypertension

35 A 4-year-old child presents with a temperature of 40°C (104°F), which she has had for the past 4 days. Her primary care physician had seen her on the first and third day of fever. He was unable to ascertain the source of the fever. However, he had assured the mother that the fever would go away spontaneously. The mother is very concerned about the fever and brings the child to you for a second opinion. On physical examination the patient is noted to have conjunctivitis, an erythematous rash, cervical adenopathy, and swollen hands and feet. Laboratory findings include an absolute neutrophilic leukocytosis, left shift, normal platelets, and an elevated erythrocyte sedimentation rate (ESR). Which of the following is the most likely diagnosis?

(A) Scarlet fever
(B) Acute rheumatic fever
(C) Juvenile rheumatoid arthritis
(D) Toxic shock syndrome
(E) Kawasaki syndrome

36 A 15-year-old boy presents to his family physician with a history of dysuria, fever, and urethral discharge of 3 days' duration. He confesses to having sex with an older girl a few days earlier. Physical examination reveals a well-nourished boy with no pallor. His blood pressure is 110/76 mm Hg, his pulse 79/minute regular, his respirations 18/min, and he has an oral temperature of 100°F (37.7°C). A yellowish white discharge is noted through the urethra, and he has bilateral tender inguinal lymphadenopathy. Prior to treating this patient, the physician should:

(A) Obtain parental consent
(B) Counsel him on safe sexual practices
(C) Notify state health authorities
(D) Notify his sexual partner
(E) Notify his parents after treating him

37 While riding his bicycle, a 9-year-old boy loses control and falls. During the process, his abdomen strikes the handlebar. His parents bring him to the emergency department because he has vague midabdominal pain and some bruising of the anterior abdominal wall. His vital signs are stable, and he has no other visible injuries. Which of the following is the most likely diagnosis?

(A) Ruptured spleen
(B) Ruptured liver
(C) Ruptured pancreas
(D) Hematoma in the rectus muscle
(E) Ruptured duodenum

38 A patient with the last name Smith, who has O negative blood type, is transfused with a unit of A-negative blood ordered for a different person, whose last name is also Smith. The patient develops fever, hypotension, chills, and severe backache. Blood is noted to ooze out of the multiple venipuncture sites as well. Which of the following is the most appropriate initial step in the management of this patient?

(A) Administer 0.45% normal saline solution to maintain adequate tissue perfusion
(B) Stop infusing the unit of blood and keep the intravenous line open with an isotonic saline solution
(C) Give an intravenous dose of a loop diuretic
(D) Give an intravenous dose of mannitol to begin osmotic diuresis
(E) Administer antipyretics

39 Four hours ago, a 28-year-old woman, gravida 1, para 0, at 38 weeks' gestation was admitted to the labor and delivery suite. On admission she had regular uterine contractions occurring every 2–3 minutes, a dilation of 4 cm on cervical examination, effacement of 80%, and blood pressure of 115/75 mm Hg. The fetus is in longitudinal lie and cephalic presentation with an estimated weight of 3500 g (7 lb 11 oz) by abdominal palpation. Her prenatal course was characterized by first-trimester bleeding that spontaneously resolved. Her blood pressure (BP) has gradually increased over the past 4 hours; it is now sustained at 150/95 mm Hg. Her patella deep tendon reflexes are brisk, but she has no clonus. A urine dipstick test shows 2+ albumin. Administration of which of the following agents is indicated as the next step in management?

(A) Phenobarbital
(B) Diazepam
(C) Magnesium sulfate
(D) Diphenylhydantoin
(E) Magnesium gluconate

Directions for Matching Questions (40 through 50): Each set of matching questions is preceded by a list of 4 to 26 lettered options followed by a brief explanation of the required task and then by a series of numbered statements. For each lettered statement you are to select ONE LETTERED OPTION that best fulfills the task as it relates to that statement. Remember each of the listed options might be correctly selected once, more than once, or not at all.

Questions 40–42

(A) Photophobia
(B) Raccoon sign
(C) Lucid interval
(D) Optic atrophy
(E) Enlarged sella
(F) Cavernous sinus thrombosis

For each patient description, select the ONE most likely finding.

40 A 28-year-old motorcyclist collided with an automobile and was thrown off. His helmet was not secured properly and came off during the event. He sustained a linear fracture to the left temporal bone.

41 A 26-year-old college student was in an automobile accident. She sustained a fracture to the base of the skull.

42 A 75-year-old male was brought to the hospital by his daughter. She stated that he fell and hit his head several weeks ago. Since that time he has had a dull headache, has become uncharacteristically aggressive, and has been unable to concentrate.

Questions 43–48

(A) *Staphylococcus aureus*
(B) *Staphylococcus saprophyticus*
(C) *Bacillus anthracis*
(D) *Bacillus cereus*
(E) *Clostridium perfringens*
(F) *Clostridium tetani*
(G) *Clostridium botulinum*
(H) *Corynebacterium diphtheriae*
(I) *Listeria monocytogenes*
(J) *Actinomyces israelii*

43 A farmer and his wife are brought into an emergency room by their son. Examination reveals diplopia and mydriasis.

44 A 25-year-old man develops nausea, vomiting, and diarrhea 6 hours after eating refried rice. Gram-positive rods are noted in his stool.

45 A 22-year-old man, who is an intravenous drug abuser, develops muscle stiffness in the jaw. Examination reveals a mentally alert male who cannot open his mouth.

46 A 40-year-old woman has a draining sinus underneath her chin that contains a purulent exudate and yellow granular material. She had a dental extraction of an abscessed lower incisor 6 weeks ago.

47 An afebrile 20-year-old sexually active woman complains of dysuria, increased urinary frequency, and suprapubic pain. A urine dipstick test for nitrites is negative, and a dipstick test for leukocyte esterase is positive. A urine culture is pending.

48 A 4-year-old child presents with problems with swallowing and breathing. Examination reveals a gray–tan exudate in the posterior pharynx and prominent, painful cervical lymph node enlargement.

Questions 49–50

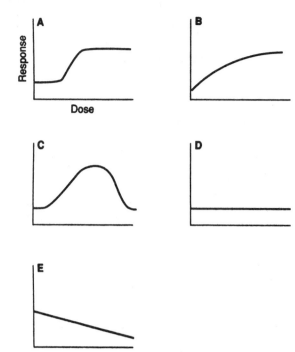

The dose/response curves illustrated above represent the changes in therapeutic response for different medication doses. The ordinate (the vertical axis) represents increasing therapeutic response; the abscissa (the horizontal axis) represents increasing medication dose. Match each drug listed below with the proper graph.

49 Nortriptyline

50 Lithium

Answer Key

1	D	**11**	D	**21**	D	**31**	C	**41**	B
2	D	**12**	E	**22**	E	**32**	D	**42**	A
3	D	**13**	E	**23**	B	**33**	D	**43**	G
4	A	**14**	E	**24**	D	**34**	C	**44**	D
5	C	**15**	D	**25**	B	**35**	E	**45**	F
6	D	**16**	E	**26**	B	**36**	B	**46**	J
7	E	**17**	E	**27**	A	**37**	E	**47**	B
8	C	**18**	B	**28**	C	**38**	B	**48**	H
9	E	**19**	D	**29**	A	**39**	C	**49**	C
10	D	**20**	C	**30**	A	**40**	C	**50**	A

Answers and Explanations

1 **The answer is D** *Medicine*

The clinical vignette describes a patient with hypothyroidism. This diagnosis is confirmed by the laboratory test profile of decreased total T_4, decreased free T_4, and increased TSH levels (choice **D**). The TSH value is the most sensitive test for diagnosing primary hypothyroidism, because it is increased even when the serum T_4 is only on the low side of normal, indicating a gland that is on the verge of failing. The presence of a smooth, non-tender thyroid gland is a typical finding in Hashimoto's thyroiditis, the most common cause of hypothyroidism in the United States in patients older than 6 years of age. Initially, these patients have hyperthyroidism due to leakage of T_3 and T_4 from the cells; after that phase hypothyroidism sets in. Antibodies to thyroglobulin (TBG) and thyroid microsomes are found in the plasma of patients with Hashimoto's thyroiditis, indicating that autoimmunity plays a prominent role in causing the disease. Additional clinical features of hypothyroidism include macroglossia, congestive cardiomyopathy, depression, constipation, slow mentation, menstrual irregularities, and proximal muscle weakness. Elevated serum creatinine kinase should alert one to muscle problems. Levothyroxine is the treatment of choice, with a goal of bringing serum TSH into the normal range.

An analytic pattern of increased total T_4, normal free T_4, and normal TSH values typically is obtained from a person with an increase in TBG levels (choice **A**); for example, a woman taking oral contraceptives. Increased total T_4, increased free T_4, and decreased TSH levels (choice **B**) represent data that might be presented by a patient with hyperthyroidism, most commonly due to Graves' disease. A decreased total T_4, normal free T_4, and normal TSH values (choice **C**) is a pattern that would be obtained from a person with a decrease in TBG levels; for example, an athlete taking anabolic steroids. A decrease in total T_4, decrease in free T_4, and decrease in TSH values (choice **E**) is characteristic of a patient with a problem in either the anterior pituitary (secondary hypothyroidism) or the hypothalamus (tertiary hypothyroidism), with decreased release of thyrotropin-releasing hormone (TRH).

2 **The answer is D** *Obstetrics and Gynecology*

The determination of the stage of labor is important because the normal progress expected varies by which stage and phase of labor the patient is in. The first stage of labor (from onset of true labor to complete cervical dilation) has two phases: a latent phase, during which cervical effacement and early dilation occur, and an active phase, during which more rapid cervical dilation occurs. Cervical dilation of at least 4 cm (choice **D**) marks the active phase.

Cervical effacement over 90% (choice **A**), contraction duration over 30 seconds (choice **B**), and the presenting part below +3 station (choice **C**) are frequently noted in active labor but can also occur in early labor. Membrane rupture (choice **E**) is not essential for active labor diagnosis.

3 **The answer is D** *Pediatrics*

Absence, or petit mal, seizures cease as quickly as they commence. Motor activity stops abruptly, and patients develop a blank stare with fluttering of the eyelids. The seizures are brief (10–30 seconds), but may occur many times throughout the day. They end abruptly and have no postictal stage. Absence seizures can be triggered by hyperventilation. Electroencephalogram (EEG) shows a typical three-per-second spike-and-wave pattern (choice **D**).

Hypsarrhythmia (choice **A**) is seen on EEG in patients with infantile spasms. Interictal slow-spike waves on EEG (choice **B**) are seen with Lennox-Gastaut syndrome. Centrotemporal spikes (choice **C**) is the EEG finding diagnostic of benign partial epilepsy. A four-to six-per-second irregular spike-and-wave pattern (choice **E**) can be found on the EEG of a patient with juvenile myoclonic epilepsy (Janz syndrome).

4 **The answer is A** *Medicine*

The patient has rheumatoid arthritis (RA) involving both hands. There is ulnar deviation of both hands and swelling of the metacarpophalangeal (MCP) and proximal interphalangeal (PIP) joints. Rheumatoid nodules extend in chainlike fashion on the extensor surface of both forearms. The pathogenesis of the joint injury in RA involves synovial tissue production of rheumatoid factor (RF) (choice **A**), which is an immunocomplex composed of IgM autoantibodies against the Fc receptor of IgG. RF activates complement, attracting neutrophils that phagocytize RF and produce inflammation. Chronically inflamed synovial tissue proliferates (forms a pannus) and destroys articular cartilage. Left untreated, reactive fibrosis occurs in the joint, leading to joint fusion (ankylosis). The disease begins with the insidious onset of morning stiffness lasting over an hour. This occurs most commonly in the hands, wrists, and foot joints. In the hands, it produces symmetric involvement of the MCP and PIP joints. In addition, there is ulnar deviation of the hands secondary to the laxity of the surrounding soft tissue. Radiologic findings in the hand include the presence of marginal bone erosions where pannus has destroyed bone, joint space narrowing due to destruction of the articular cartilage, and fusion (ankylosis) of the joint in severe cases. RA in the neck frequently involves the atlantoaxial joint, which can produce subluxation that, in turn, could produce compression of the vertebral artery and vertebrobasilar insufficiency. RA involving the knee is sometimes associated with formation of a synovial cyst in the popliteal fossa. This is called a Baker's cyst. One or more of the so-called disease modifying antirheumatic drugs (DMARDs) are now commonly prescribed during early stages of the disease to halt disease progression before irreversible damage occurs. These DMARDs include methotrexate, injection of gold salts, auranofin (oral gold), antimalarials (e.g., hydroxychloroquine), chlorambucil, cyclophosphamide, cyclosporine, leflunomide, minocycline, sulfasalazine, and penicillamine. A newer group of drugs called biologic response modifiers (BRMs) that inhibit cytokines also have been developed. These may be used in conjunction with a standard DMARD and have proved remarkably effective, sometimes even inducing long-term remissions. Unfortunately they must be administered by injection and are expensive. Corticosteroids and/or nonsteroidal anti-inflammatory drugs (including aspirin) are also used, often in conjunction with a DMARD or a BRM to treat acute inflammation. Physical therapy is extremely important to prevent ankylosis of the involved joints.

A polyclonal gammopathy (benign plasma cell proliferation) is more likely to be present in RA than a monoclonal gammopathy (choice **B**), which is more likely to be due to malignant plasma cell proliferation. The ulcer overlying the right malleolus is not likely caused by a deep venous insufficiency (choice **C**) but more likely represents rheumatoid vasculitis, which is commonly associated with a high titer of rheumatoid factor. Osteophytes at the margins of the joints (choice **D**) represent reactive bone formation and are typically found in osteoarthritis not RA. Anemia of chronic inflammation is more likely to complicate RA than iron deficiency (choice **E**).

5 **The answer is C** *Surgery*

This patient most likely has traumatic dissection of the thoracic aorta (choice **C**) caused by a deceleration injury. Disruption of the aorta can occur at the root (the origin of the ligamentum arteriosum) or at the diaphragm. Prognosis is poor, with 85% of patients dying at the scene of the accident, and only 15% making it to the hospital. These patients have small tears or effective tamponading. The intima and media are fractured, leaving the adventitia intact. Blood collects subjacent to the adventitia, giving rise to a pseudoaneurysm, which is seen as a widened mediastinum on a posterior–anterior chest x-ray film. A widened mediastinum is the most consistent sign associated with traumatic disruption of the thoracic aorta and should immediately make one suspect this lesion. Approximately one third of patients have no presenting clinical symptoms after traumatic disruption of the thoracic aorta.

Ruptured aortic aneurysm (choice **A**) is usually seen in the elderly. The most common cause for this condition is atherosclerosis. There may be a long-standing history of hypertension and associated coronary artery disease. A palpable pulsatile mass is present in the epigastric region. Unlike traumatic disruption of the thoracic aorta, this is a true aneurysm. Cardiac tamponade (choice **B**) most often follows blunt chest injury. It is associated with elevated venous pressure, hypotension, and muffled heart sounds. These three signs compose Beck's triad. Of these, hypotension is the most reliable symptom, because elevated venous pressure may not be seen in the presence of severe hypotension, and the heart sounds are not muffled on many occasions. Tachycardia is present, and the chest radiograph is noncontributory, as acute effusions are not discernible. Two-dimensional echocardiography is the best test to confirm the diagnosis. Treatment involves pericardiocentesis. Myocardial contusion (choice **D**) follows blunt chest trauma. It mainly involves the right ventricle. Patients may not have symptoms at initial presentation. Presence of a new right bundle branch block on electrocardiogram should point to the diagnosis. Radionuclide angiography is the most sensitive test to detect this condition. Pulmonary contusion (choice **E**) may also follow blunt chest trauma. Patients may appear remarkably fit. It is the most common cause of potentially lethal injury in the United States. Chest x-ray films may show a few patchy infiltrates that progress with time. Respiratory failure can develop rapidly. Therefore, one should have a high index of suspicion when confronted with a patient with vague symptoms after blunt chest injury.

6 **The answer is D** *Psychiatry*

Rationalization (choice **D**) refers to the distortion of reality so that an act or event that actually is unpleasant seems to be desirable. This defense mechanism is often used when an individual cannot accept the implications of a particular outcome of events. The other defense mechanism choices do not apply as well to this patient.

Splitting (choice **A**) occurs when an individual psychologically separates positive qualities into one individual or group and negative qualities into another. Compensation (choice **B**) is an effort to use skills or competencies in one area to counterbalance self-perceived deficiencies in other areas. Displacement (choice **C**) occurs when the emotions associated with a psychologically unacceptable object, idea, or activity is transferred to another object or situation. Projection (choice **E**) is the attribution of uncomfortable internal feelings or thoughts, especially anger and guilt, to other individuals.

7 **The answer is E** *Obstetrics and Gynecology*

The patient's height/weight discordance as well as her misconception concerning her weight suggests anorexia nervosa (choice **E**) causing secondary amenorrhea.

Turner's syndrome (choice **A**) is associated with primary amenorrhea, absence of secondary sexual development, and short stature due to aneuploidy (45, X); estradiol levels are low, but FSH levels are high. Hypogonadotropic hypogonadism (choice **B**) is associated with absence of secondary sexual development due to hypothalamic–pituitary insufficiency; an example is Kallmann syndrome. Estradiol levels are low, and FSH levels are also low. Polycystic ovary syndrome (choice **C**) is associated with male-pattern hair, infertility, and irregular menses. Estradiol and FSH levels are within normal limits, but luteinizing hormone (LH) level is increased. Asherman's syndrome (choice **D**) is characterized by secondary amenorrhea, the result of intrauterine synechiae following overzealous curettage. Estradiol and FSH levels are within normal limits.

8 **The answer is C** *Medicine*

In this pedigree all affected females transmit a trait that caused early vision loss to offspring of both sexes. However, affected males and normal individuals of both sexes do not transmit loss of sight to their offspring. This nonMendelian pattern of inheritance is characteristic of conditions caused by a mutation in a mitochondrial gene (choice **C**) due to the fact that only females transmit mitochondria to the ovum. This particular family has Leber's hereditary optic neuropathy. Individuals who inherit this condition suffer precipitous vision loss, usually in their 20s, due to optic nerve degeneration. In different families 11 different missense mutations in three different mitochondrial genes encoding respiratory chain subunits have been described. Although the ultimate phenotype, loss of vision, remains consistent, the rate of vision loss and the age of onset vary considerably, even among members of the same family. Such variability in the phenotypic expression of conditions transmitted by mitochondrial mutations is characteristic of these conditions and is called heteroplasmy. It occurs because each cell carries multiple mitochondria, of which on average only half will be affected, but transmission of mitochondria with normal and mutated genes will occur in a random manner. Because mtDNA-encoded proteins are primarily associated with electron transport and ATP synthesis, tissues that depend upon the electron transport system are affected most.

In an autosomal dominant disorder (choice **A**) either an affected male or female may transmit the mutant gene to a child of either sex and the mutant trait will be expressed.

In an autosomal recessive disorder (choice **B**) both parents must transmit a mutant gene to the gamete for the trait to be expressed. An offspring of either sex who inherits one mutant gene from either parent will be a carrier.

In an X-linked dominant disorder (choice **D**) affected males will carry only one X chromosome, which will bear the mutated gene; this X chromosome will be transmitted to his daughters in whom the trait is expressed since it is dominant. However, characteristically the disease is more severe in hemizygous affected males than in heterozygous affected females. Since his sons will inherit his Y chromosomes they will be neither affected nor carriers. Affected females almost certainly will have one X chromosome with the normal gene and one with the mutated gene; thus they transmit the mutant gene to 50% of their daughters and to 50% of their sons. Since the trait is dominant, the mother as well as offspring of both sexes who inherit the affected chromosome will express the trait.

In an X-linked recessive disorder (choice **E**) males carrying an X chromosome with a mutated gene will express the trait since they only have one X chromosome; females carrying an X chromosome on the other hand will be carriers but will not expresses the trait since the recessive trait will not be expressed in the presence of an X chromosome carrying the normal gene. Sons of affected males will be neither carriers nor affected because they inherit a Y, not an X chromosome; however 100% of the daughters will be carriers because they will receive the affected X chromosome from their father and a normal one from their mother. Fifty percent of the daughters of women who are carriers will become carriers themselves, since there is a 50% chance they will inherit the affected X chromosome. Although there is also a 50% chance that her son will inherit an X chromosome bearing the mutated gene, those who do will express the disease because that will be their only X chromosome.

9 **The answer is E** *Pediatrics*

Foreign body aspiration (choice **E**) is the most common cause of recurrent pneumonia in an otherwise healthy 3-year-old child. Because of the lung's anatomy, right side aspiration is more common. When a child presents with pneumonia, a history of choking can often be elicited.

Immunodeficiency disorders (choice **A**) are characterized by recurrent infections, usually by opportunistic organisms, and failure to thrive. Cystic fibrosis (choice **B**) similarly results in failure to thrive, and malabsorption and clubbing are often seen. In cystic fibrosis, common organisms responsible for pneumonia are *Staphylococcus aureus, Pseudomonas aeruginosa,* and *Haemophilus influenzae.* In addition, *Burkholderia cepacia* is another organism that is increasing in frequency in patients with cystic fibrosis and may be associated with rapid pulmonary deterioration and death. Chédiak-Higashi syndrome (choice **C**) is autosomal recessive and is associated with giant granules in neutrophils and recurrent infections of the skin, mucous membranes, and the respiratory tract. Moreover, the fact that the patient is healthy indicates that this is not Chédiak-Higashi syndrome, in which albinism is a key to diagnosis. Congenital lung abnormalities (choice **D**) generally present at a much earlier stage.

10 **The answer is D** *Surgery*

This patient has a tear of the quadriceps expansion (choice **D**), which may result from direct or indirect injury. It can occur within the muscle, at the tendomuscular junction, within the tendon itself, or at the tendoosseus junction (most common in the elderly). Tears of the quadriceps expansion are most common in older individuals who are overweight and in poor physical condition. The usual history is of missing a step and tripping while descending a staircase or suddenly jumping down from a height. Patients complain of severe pain, often feel or hear a snap, and fall to the ground. Physical examination reveals swelling and tenderness at the site of the tear, and a sulcus or gap is felt at the site of separation, especially if the tear is complete. If the tear is partial, the patient has difficulty extending the knee; if the tear is complete, the patient cannot extend the knee. Tears of the quadriceps expansion can also occur in athletes and young individuals. In athletes, the tears are most often at the insertion of the tendon into the tibial tubercle.

Tears of the posterior cruciate ligament (choice **A**) usually occur because of hyperextension and are associated with a positive sag sign. They are not associated with inability to straight leg raise, swelling of the anterior aspect of the knee, or a gap between the fibers of the quadriceps expansion or tendon. While it is true that a snapping sound is heard in tears of the anterior cruciate ligament (choice **B**), there is hemarthrosis and a positive Lachman's test result. The inability to straight leg raise, a gap felt at the site of the tear, and swelling confined to the anterior aspect of the knee are not features of this condition. Transverse fracture of the patella (choice **C**) is the main differential diagnosis. Fractures of the patella can result from direct or indirect trauma. In older individuals who are obese and in poor physical shape, an indirect injury resulting from tripping down stairs, jumping from a height, or even forcefully squatting can result in fracture of the patella. The patient complains of severe pain and falls to the ground. Difficulty in straight leg raise, swelling over the knee, and hemarthrosis are seen. A gap can be felt in the patella, and the fragments can be moved, which distinguishes it from a pure tear of the quadriceps expansion. Avulsion of the quadriceps tendon from the tibial tuberosity (choice **E**) usually occurs in a younger individual. In teenagers, the epiphysis is weaker than the tendon, and it can be sheared off from its moorings. The gap is felt below the inferior pole of the patella. In the case presented, the gap is felt above the superior pole of the patella.

11 The answer is D   *Obstetrics and Gynecology*

On physical examination the astute observer can identify the irreversible changes that pregnancy brings to the female body, especially in the reproductive tract. A transverse-appearing external os (choice **D**) is more typical of a multiparous than a nulliparous cervix. This is sometimes described as a "fish-mouth"–shaped cervical os.

Increased bluish hue (choice **A**) is true of pregnancy (Chadwick sign) because of the increased vascularity of the cervix but is unrelated to parity. Purulent discharge (choice **B**) is characteristic of cervicitis but is unrelated to parity. A retracted squamocolumnar junction (choice **C**) is found in postmenopausal women but is unrelated to parity. Absence of scarring (choice **E**) is a characteristic of nulliparous, not multiparous, women.

12 The answer is E   *Pediatrics*

The patient has a presentation that is most consistent with varicella (chickenpox). The most common complication of varicella is secondary bacterial infection of skin lesions (choice **E**).

The association of Reye syndrome (choice **A**) with varicella has become rare since salicylates are no longer prescribed as antipyretics for children. Pneumonia (choice **B**) is more common in adolescents and adults than in children. Thrombocytopenia (choice **C**) can result in hemorrhages of skin and mucous membranes and may be associated with transient petechiae. Hemorrhagic vesicles can be seen. Encephalitis (choice **D**) is the most common central nervous system (CNS) complication of varicella but is far less common than secondary bacterial infection of skin lesions.

13 The answer is E   *Psychiatry*

Normal saline solution is unlikely to have corrected the patient's underlying pathology. However, it is common for patients to respond to the placebo effect (choice **E**) inherent in many medical interventions.

Such responses do not suggest that pain or discomfort is psychogenic (choice **A**), exaggerated as in a histrionic personality disorder (choice **B**) or factitious (choice **D**). The response does not suggest that the patient was volume depleted (choice **C**).

14 The answer is E   *Medicine*

Patients with a history of smoking, weight loss, clubbing of the fingers, hemoptysis, and hilar adenopathy are strongly suspect for a primary bronchogenic carcinoma, particularly squamous and small cell carcinoma (oat cell carcinoma). Cough is the most common presenting symptom of lung cancer (75%), followed by weight loss (40%) and hemoptysis (25–30%). The physical findings indicate chronic obstructive lung disease. The bronchitic component consists of productive cough, rhonchi, wheezes, and dilated tubular shadows representing thickened bronchial walls. The emphysematous component is represented by an increased anteroposterior diameter, distant heart sounds and flattened diaphragms. Cytology is the gold standard test for bronchogenic carcinoma and has its highest diagnostic yield in centrally located cancers such as squamous and small cell carcinoma; sputum cytology using a Pap stain reports cells with deeply eosinophilic-staining cytoplasm and irregular, hyperchromatic nuclei. Because keratin becomes bright red with this stain, the patient most likely has a primary squamous cell carcinoma (choice **E**).

Small cell carcinoma of the lung (choice **A**) has small, lymphocyte-sized, basophilic-staining cells in cytology smears. Tuberculosis (choice **B**), pulmonary embolism (choice **C**), and bronchiectasis (choice **D**) are all associated with hemoptysis; however, they have clinical presentations that differ from those described and do not have neoplastic cells in sputum.

15 The answer is D   *Psychiatry*

Splitting (choice **D**) is described as the psychologic separation of all good qualities into one individual and all bad qualities into another. This separation occurs when an individual cannot tolerate ambivalent feelings toward a particular individual. Children and persons with borderline personality disorder often manifest evidence of splitting.

Projection (choice **A**) refers to the attribution of one's feelings or beliefs to another. Idealization (choice **B**) refers to the exaggeration of an individual's qualities by an admirer. Conversion (choice **C**) refers to the transformation of psychologic stressors into physical complaints. Symbolization (choice **E**) refers to the selection of a particular object or event to represent other meanings.

16 The answer is E   *Surgery*

The incidence of esophageal cancer in the United States is some 3–6 cases per 100,000 individuals; it is more common after the sixth decade, seven times more prevalent in males than in females, and also is more common in African Americans than in Caucasians. The factors pointing toward esophageal carcinoma (choice **E**) include dysphagia that is rapidly progressing (even though at this time he has no problems with liquids, if it is carcinoma he soon will) and a long history of acid reflux disease, which apparently was never adequately treated. In addition he is an older African-American male. This diagnosis must be confirmed by endoscopy and biopsy. Almost all esophageal cancers are either squamous cell or basal cell carcinomas. Historically squamous cell carcinoma was the more common form, accounting for 95% of the cases in the United States as recently as the mid-20th century. However, during the past few decades the trend has been for the proportion of basal cell carcinomas to increase, and squamous cell carcinomas to decrease, and by the mid-1990s each accounted for about 50% of cases. Squamous cell carcinomas still predominate in much of the world. They are induced by exposure of the nonkeratinizing stratified epithelial squamous cells lining the esophagus to carcinogens. In the United States the primary source of such carcinogens was tobacco smoke, and the decline in squamous cell carcinomas is likely linked to a decrease in the number of smokers. Other risk factors for squamous cell carcinoma are heavy alcohol consumption, nitrosamine and other nitrosyl compounds found in smoked and pickled foods, and a host of irritants that might be ingested. Most squamous cell carcinomas are located in the middle third of the esophagus. In contrast, adenocarcinomas are primarily found in the lower third of the esophagus. Adenocarcinomas are the end result of a series of transformations started by chronic exposure to gastric acid regurgitated as the result of an incompetent gastroesophageal sphincter. The acid first inflames the stratified squamous epithelial cells, which then undergo metaplasia. These cells eventually transform into specialized epithelial cells called Barrett's epithelium. Barrett's epithelial cells may transform into adenocarcinoma in about 10% of cases. The earliest symptom of esophageal carcinoma, regardless of tissue type, is a mild dysphagia. Patients may state that "food tends to stick in the throat" or they may feel a mild discomfort while eating, which they may very well ignore. As a consequence, by the time the diagnosis is made, the cancer would probably have penetrated the esophageal wall. As the esophagus does not have a serosal layer, and only a mucosal and muscular one, infiltration beyond the confines of the esophagus can occur readily and fairly rapidly. Metastasis to regional lymph nodes and neighboring structures is fairly common. The overall 5-year survival rate for both types of cancer is an abysmal 20% but is much better than the 5% of only a decade ago.

Diffuse esophageal spasm (choice **A**), or "nutcracker esophagus," produces dysphagia and chest pain that is often relieved with nitroglycerin. It is characterized by uncoordinated spasms that occur after a swallow. A barium study reveals a "corkscrew" esophagus, and it is treated with bougienage, calcium channel blockers, or nitrates. Achalasia (choice **B**) is caused by incoordination of the esophageal peristaltic muscles and the failure of the lower esophageal sphincter (LES) to relax because of a lack of inhibitory input from nonadrenergic, noncholinergic, ganglionic cells. It is also associated with dysphagia for solids and liquids, but it is a rare disorder with an incidence in the United States of about 1 per 100,000 and unlike esophageal cancer, does not primarily affect older males and is not progressive. The proximal esophagus is dilated and aperistaltic. It is treated with pneumatic dilatation, drugs that decrease lower esophageal sphincter tone (e.g., nifedipine), or surgery (esophagocardiomyotomy) in 20 to 25% of patients. An esophageal stricture (choice **C**) is a narrowing of the esophageal lumen inhibiting the passage of foods. It usually is caused by scarring, most often by gastric juice due to chronic GERD at the distal end, but stricture formation also can occur in response to other types of trauma, including swallowing caustic solutions, chronic swallowing of pills without water, or residual scarring after surgery. The usual treatment is dilation. A Schatzki ring (choice **D**) is usually characterized by an intermittent, nonprogressive dysphagia for solid foods that occurs while consuming a heavy meal with meat that was "wolfed down"; hence the pseudonym the "steakhouse syndrome." Sometimes the meal is regurgitated, relieving the block, and eating can be resumed. There is no known etiology but such a ring has been observed in 6 to 15% of older patients undergoing a barium swallow. Despite their common occurrence only 0.5% of those with rings have significant symptoms. The presence and severity of symptoms correlate with the diameter of the ring's lumen. Radiographic barium swallow or endoscopy is used to confirm the diagnosis and, if deemed advisable, the ring can be split by dilatation. Zenker's diverticulum (choice **F**) is the most common acquired diverticulum of the esophagus and is treated by surgery. Because of stagnant food collected in the pouch, the patient has halitosis. Esophageal varices (choice **G**) are caused by portal hypertension and do not cause a progressive dysphagia.

17 The answer is E *Preventive Medicine and Public Health*

The odds ratio is a method of estimating relative risk in case-control studies.

$$\text{Odds ratio} = \frac{\text{Odds of exposure among the diseased group}}{\text{Odds of exposure among the disease-free group}}$$

Using the data from the table, the numerator is $(10 \div 2)$ and the denominator is $(50 \div 300)$. Thus (choice **E**) $(10 \div 2) \div (50 \div 300) = 30$

Choices **A**, $300 \div 50 = 6$; **B**, $50 \div 10 = 5$; **C**, $60 \div (2 + 10) = 5$; and **D**, $(300 \div 2) \div (60 \div 10) = 25$ are incorrect.

18 The answer is B *Medicine*

In 90% of cases people who have been immunized against hepatitis B virus (HBV) with Heptavax-B or Recombivax-HB develop protective antibodies only against surface antigen (anti-HBs, choice **B**). Patients who have recovered from hepatitis A virus (HAV) have anti-HAV immunoglobulin G (IgG) antibodies, which offer lifelong protection against HAV (choice **B**). In HAV infections, the first antibody is anti-HAV immunoglobulin M (IgM) (the IgM indicating active infection), which appears after the prodrome and persists for 6 weeks or longer. A switch over to IgG marks recovery. In HBV infections, the first marker is surface antigen (HBsAg), "s" antigen, which is noninfective. This is followed by HBeAg, or "e" antigen, and HBV DNA, which are infective particles. The first antibody to appear is IgM against core antigen (anti-HBc IgM), which persists if the infection becomes chronic (presence of HBsAg beyond 6 months), but switches over to an IgG antibody, only when the last viral particle is eliminated. If the patient is going to recover (90%), HBeAg and HBV DNA disappear first, followed by HBsAg, usually after 4 months. Between the fourth and fifth month (serologic gap, or window), when HBsAg and HBeAg are gone, the only serologic marker for infection is the anti-HBc IgM antibody. In the fifth to sixth month, anti-HBs develops, conferring immunity against future attacks of that particular HBV serotype.

Choice **A** is consistent with someone with a history of HAV (anti-HAV IgG) who is presently recovering from HBV in the serologic gap (anti-HBc IgM only present). Choice **C** is consistent with a patient with a history of HAV (anti-HAV IgG) who now has active HBV in the first 4 months of the disease, because HBsAg, HBeAg, and anti-HBc IgM are present. Choice **D** represents a patient who has active HAV and either had HBV or was immunized against HBV, because anti-HBs is present. Presence of anti-HBc IgG would indicate that the patient had recovered from HBV, whereas a negative result would be consistent with immunization. It is also consistent with a patient who has chronic HBV (HBsAg > 6 months). Chronic carriers are either infective or "healthy." Infective carriers have HBeAg, while those who are healthy carriers do not. Choice **E** represents a patient who has active HAV and no evidence of HBV.

19 The answer is D *Pediatrics*

Lyme disease (choice **D**) is caused by *Borrelia burgdorferi*. It is transmitted by the ticks of the *Ixodes* species, specifically the deer tick *Ixodes dammini* in the United States. It is endemic in the coastal areas of the Northeast, but has been described in 43 states as well as Europe and Australia. Lyme disease is characterized by rash, carditis, arthritis, and meningitis. The rash (erythema chronicum migrans) starts as an erythematous macule or papule at the site of the tick bite. The lesion continues to expand in a ringlike manner, with central clearing. Multiple secondary lesions may develop. Nonspecific symptoms of headache, fever, and chills accompany this stage, which resolves with or without treatment. Disseminated disease occurs in untreated patients after a latent period of weeks to months and can involve the central nervous system (CNS), heart, and musculoskeletal system. Persistent infection can occur. Treatment consists of doxycycline for children above 8 years of age. Amoxicillin should be used for children less than 8 years of age or for those allergic to doxycycline. Cefuroxime is also approved for treatment of Lyme disease as an alternative to doxycycline or amoxicillin.

Rocky Mountain spotted fever (choice **A**) has discrete, pale, rose–red macules or maculopapules. It begins on the extremities and spreads to the entire body, involving the palms and soles. In babesiosis (choice **B**), nausea and vomiting, jaundice, and dark urine occur with hemolysis. Colorado tick fever (choice **C**) occurs periodically among campers and hunters in the western United States. Rash is uncommon. Juvenile rheumatoid arthritis (choice **E**) is a chronic inflammatory disease in children, involving one or more joints. Systemic juvenile rheumatoid arthritis is characterized by a high, spiking fever; a salmon-colored, morbilliform rash; hepatosplenomegaly; arthritis; and leukocytosis.

20 The answer is C *Surgery*

The hallmark of a squamous cell carcinoma (choice **C**) is an open sore that won't heal. It is the second most prevalent form of skin cancer, with a yearly incidence in the United States of about 200,000 cases per year. Most occur in elderly subjects on areas exposed to the sun and are more prevalent in light-skinned individuals with an early history of time spent outdoors as a youth. Most of them are slow growing but if left untreated, will eventually penetrate the dermis and invade underlying tissue. A small fraction may become malignant. As a rule squamous cell carcinomas of the lip are most dangerous; these are most commonly found among habitual pipe smokers.

Actinic keratosis (choice **A**) is a reddening and roughening of the skin found in sun-exposed areas, most commonly in light-skinned elders. It may present as a single spot as in the case described or it may be spread over a wider area, giving the affected person a blotchy appearance. Some 15% will transform into a cancer, almost always a squamous cell carcinoma as in the case described. A basal cell carcinoma (choice **B**) is the most common of all the skin cancers. It has been estimated that some 800,000 Americans are affected at any given time. It too appears to be sun induced and is most commonly found on the exposed areas of skin in lightly pigmented persons. They have several modes of presentation, the most common one being a shiny, pearly translucent nodule. Basal cells carcinomas arise from the basal cells of the epidermis and almost never metastasize. A nodular melanoma (choice **D**) is the most aggressive of all the melanomas. It generally is first recognized as a pigmented, usually dark brown or black, bump or node. Unlike most melanomas, it does not initially spread superficially but rapidly grows into deeper tissues, infiltrating the subcutaneous lymphatics and metastasizing to the nodes. The prognosis is understandably poor. Contrary to common opinion, nodular and other melanomas (with the exception of lentigo melanoma) are not usually induced by exposure to the sun, and most melanomas are more commonly found on the trunk or limbs than on the face or other exposed areas. A herpes infection (choice **E**) may exist as an open sore but rarely as an isolated lesion and is never preceded by a rough, pinkish lesion.

21 The answer is D *Psychiatry*

Tardive dyskinesia (choice **D**) emerges in a substantial number of patients who have had long-term treatment with antipsychotics. This dyskinesia consists of choreoathetoid movements that are often first evident in the fingers and tongue, but later become more generalized, extending to the face, then to the limbs, and eventually even to the trunk in the most severe cases. Unfortunately the symptoms do not necessarily reverse themselves when the drug is withdrawn and are difficult to treat, often creating untenable embarrassment for an indefinite period.

Tardive akathisia (choice **A**) also is sometimes drug induced; it is characterized by motor restlessness caused by painful feelings of inner tension and anxiety. It too is often induced by neuroleptic (antipsychotic) medications. Huntington's disease (choice **B**) is also characterized by choreoathetoid movements, but also by increasingly severe behavioral and cognitive problems, and eventually dementia. It is inherited as an autosomal dominant trait due to a repeat expansion of a CAG trinucleotide sequence at the beginning of the "huntington" gene sequence. Normal individuals have 11 to 34 CAG repeats, Huntington disease-afflicted individuals have 37 to 121; the longer the sequence, the earlier the onset of symptoms. Moreover, the number of repeats increases as the affected gene is passed on from generation to generation. Parkinsonism (choice **C**) (aka pseudoparkinson's) is a catchall phrase used to describe disease conditions that mimic classical idiopathic Parkinson's disease by presenting with tremor, bradykinesia, rigidity, and postural instability or impaired postural reflexes; as is true with Parkinson's disease, these dyskinetic traits result from striatal dopamine deficiencies. There is a very rare X-linked recessive type almost exclusively found among young Filipino men, but nonidiopathic parkinsonism is more often drug induced, commonly by neuroleptics. Wilson's disease (choice **E**) can also present with a dyskinesis mimicking parkinsonism, but is an autosomal recessive condition affecting copper metabolism and usually has an early onset.

22 The answer is E   *Medicine*

The chronic dyspnea, hyperinflated lungs, and depressed diaphragms indicate that the patient has emphysema, no doubt related to a long history of smoking cigarettes. Emphysema is a chronic obstructive pulmonary disease (COPD) that produces permanent enlargement of all or part of the respiratory unit, including respiratory bronchioles, alveolar ducts, and alveoli, as well as destruction of the pulmonary capillary bed. Elastic tissue destruction in small airways causes trapping of air and distention of the distal air space, which increases the RV (choice **E**). (The RV is the volume of air left in the lung after maximal expiration.)

An increase in residual volume RV always increases the TLC (not decreased [choice **B**]). (The TLC is the total amount of air in the lungs after a maximal inspiration.) An increase in TLC causes hyperinflation of the lungs, an increase in the anteroposterior diameter, and depression of the diaphragms, as in this patient. The FRC is the total amount of air in the lungs at the end of a normal expiration. It is the sum of the expiratory reserve volume (amount of air forcibly expelled at the end of a normal expiration) and the RV. In emphysema, the RV is increased, which increases the FRC (not decreased [choice **A**]). In emphysema, lung compliance (ability to fill the lung with air) is increased and elasticity (recoil of the lung) is decreased because of destruction of elastic tissue by elastases and oxidant free radicals released from neutrophils. The FEV_{1sec}, or the amount of air expelled from the lungs in 1 second after a maximal inspiration, is decreased (e.g., 1 L vs. the normal 4 L) because of trapping of air in the distended distal airways. The FVC, or total amount of air expelled after a maximal inspiration, is also decreased (e.g., 3 L vs. the normal 5 L) causing the FEV_{1sec}/FVC ratio to be decreased (not increased [choice **D**]). In emphysema, the arterial PO_2 is decreased late in the disease due to loss of the alveoli and corresponding vascular bed. The arterial PCO_2 is normal to decreased (not increased [choice **C**]), because the patient has a hypoxic stimulus to breathe faster causing increased elimination of CO_2. Unlike emphysema, in chronic bronchitis, there is trapping of CO_2 behind mucous plugs in the terminal bronchioles, causing respiratory acidosis. These relationships are summarized in the table below.

	Emphysema
Total lung capacity	Increased
Residual volume	Increased
Tidal volume	Decreased
Vital capacity	Decreased
FEV_1	Decreased (2+)
FVC	Decreased (3+)
FEV_{1sec}/FVC	Decreased
$PaCO_2$	Normal to decreased
PaO_2	Decreased late in the disease

+ Indicates magnitude of change.

23 The answer is B   *Preventive Medicine and Public Health*

The study clearly demonstrated an extension in the lifespan of patients with acute leukemia. Thus, there will be a larger number of patients with active leukemia at any given point in time. In other words, the *prevalence* will increase (choice **B**). This of course assumes that the rate of new cases of acute leukemia (incidence) remains the same (i.e., 15 new cases per year).

Based on the aforementioned explanation, it is apparent that the other choices, namely, **A, C, D,** and **E,** are incorrect.

24 **The answer is D** *Pediatrics*

Esophageal atresia is an esophageal malformation causing upper intestinal obstruction. In approximately 85% of cases, a fistula between the trachea and distal esophagus is present, usually allowing air to enter the abdomen (choice **D**).

Cyanosis that occurs at rest but is relieved by crying (choice **A**) is characteristic of choanal atresia, which is diagnosed by the inability to pass a catheter through each naris into the nasopharynx. There is an association with polyhydramnios during pregnancy, not oligohydramnios (choice **B**). Often, a catheter used at birth for resuscitation cannot be inserted into the stomach; there is an inability not an ability to pass a catheter into the stomach (choice **C**). Approximately 30% of infants with esophageal atresia have associated anomalies, the most common being cardiac anomalies, not renal (choice **E**).

25 **The answer is B** *Medicine*

Treatment of disseminated malignancies such as chronic myelogenous leukemia or a malignant lymphoma causes the release of purine nucleotides from the nuclei of the killed cancer cells. This markedly increases the synthesis of uric acid, which is the end-product of degradation of purine nucleotides (choice **B**). An acid urine pH causes uric acid to form crystals in the tubules of the nephron, leading to renal failure (urate nephropathy). This complication is prevented by allopurinol, which blocks xanthine oxidase and prevents the conversion of xanthine to uric acid.

Although many chemotherapy drugs are directly nephrotoxic (choice **A**), they do not produce uric acid crystals in the urine, and as a rule, they induce a dyskinesis rather than renal failure. Pyrimidines (choice **C**) are degraded to CO_2, ammonia, and amino acids. Ammonia is metabolized in the urea cycle and converted to urea, which is excreted in the kidneys. Urea does not produce crystals in the urine. Although leukemic cells metastasize to all organ systems including the kidney (choice **D**), the report of crystals in the patient's urine and an increase in uric acid rules out leukemic infiltration as the primary cause of renal failure.

26 **The answer is B** *Obstetrics and Gynecology*

This woman is in the third stage of labor, which starts with delivery of the infant and ends with delivery of the placenta. The upper limit of normal for duration of the third stage of labor is 30 minutes. The factor that contributes most to the mechanism of the third stage of labor is avulsion of anchoring villi by contracting myometrium (choice **B**).

It is true that the estrogen level falls after delivery of the placenta, providing the hormonal stimulus for breast engorgement but this decrease does not contribute to the third stage of labor (choice **A**). The levels of prolactin and umbilical vein P_{CO_2} are not involved in placental separation (choices **C** and **D**). A progesterone-mediated decrease in gap junctions is not relevant to the third stage of labor or placental separation (choice **E**).

27 **The answer is A** *Medicine*

The patient most likely has type 1 diabetes mellitus (weight loss, polyuria, increased appetite). Due to the fruity odor in her breath (acetone), she is currently in diabetic ketoacidosis, a hallmark of uncontrolled type 1 diabetes, rarely found in type 2, which usually is also characterized by obesity rather than weight loss and is more often found in older adults. Although not used to diagnose diabetes mellitus. HbA_{1c} (choice **A**) is an excellent test to evaluate glycemic control over the past 4 to 8 weeks. If the HbA_{1c} value is above 7%, the patient had chronic hyperglycemia, which would account for the blurry vision due to alteration of the refractive index of the lens from conversion of glucose to sorbitol by aldose reductase in the lens. Sorbitol is osmotically active and draws water into the lens, causing changes in the lens that vary with the glucose level in the blood. Cataracts are an eventual complication of osmotic damage.

An increase in serum cortisol (choice **B**) is associated with Cushing's syndrome. Although hypercortisolism can cause hyperglycemia (cortisol stimulates gluconeogenesis) and is a secondary cause of diabetes mellitus, findings of her physical examination are normal. Although weight loss, increased appetite, and eye abnormalities (e.g., lid stare, exophthalmos) are present in Graves' disease, it is not associated with increased frequency of urination and a fruity odor to the breath. Therefore, a serum thyroid-stimulating hormone test (choice **C**) is not indicated. The patient most likely has glucose and ketone bodies in the urine (choices **D** and **E**); however, they are not screening tests for diagnosing diabetes mellitus and do not provide the most relevant information about the cause of the blurry vision over the last 2 months.

28 The answer is C   *Medicine*

Based on the examination and test findings, this patient has primary aldosteronism, which is characterized by autonomous (unregulated) production of aldosterone from an adrenal adenoma and, less frequently, by bilateral adrenal hyperplasia of the zona glomerulosa. Aldosterone normally acts on the distal convoluted tubules and collecting ducts to increase sodium reabsorption in exchange for either potassium or hydrogen ions. Excessive aldosterone would be expected to result in increased reabsorption of sodium to produce hypernatremia and an increase in plasma volume. Increased plasma volume plus the effect of sodium on increasing peripheral vascular resistance leads to hypertension. Furthermore, the increased plasma volume results in increased hydrostatic pressure in the peritubular capillaries; this inhibits the reabsorption of sodium in the proximal tubules, leading to a loss of sodium in the urine. This "escape mechanism" for sodium is enough to prevent clinical evidence of pitting edema. Increased plasma volume also decreases the plasma renin concentration. Hypokalemia also results from the enhanced sodium exchange and loss in the urine. It is associated with proximal muscle weakness and, if chronic, can render the tubules resistant to the action of antidiuretic hormone (ADH) (acquired nephrogenic diabetes insipidus), leading to polyuria. In addition, the excess exchange of sodium for hydrogen ions leaves bicarbonate behind in the tubules because the hydrogen ions come from the dissociation of carbonic acid into hydrogen ions and bicarbonate. The excess bicarbonate produces metabolic alkalosis. Clinical evidence of tetany in this patient is due to the effect of alkalosis (metabolic or respiratory) on ionized calcium levels in the blood. Serum calcium is the sum total of calcium bound to proteins (40%); calcium bound to nonproteins (13%); and free, ionized calcium (47%), which is the metabolically active form of calcium. Alkalosis increases the negative charges on binding proteins, such as albumin, which increases the binding of the divalent ionized calcium to albumin, leading to clinical evidence of tetany, without altering the total serum calcium. In summary, serum aldosterone and bicarbonate levels are increased while plasma renin activity and potassium levels are decreased (choice **C**)

Choice **A** (↑ serum aldosterone, ↑ PRA, ↓ potassium, ↑ bicarbonate) represents either a patient on diuretics or a patient with Bartter's syndrome. Choice **B** (normal aldosterone, ↓ PRA, ↓ potassium ↑ bicarbonate) represents Liddle's syndrome. This syndrome is exactly the same as primary aldosteronism except for the presence of normal serum aldosterone levels. It is thought to be secondary to increased sensitivity of the tubules to normal levels of aldosterone. Choice **D** (↓ serum aldosterone, ↓ PRA, ↑ potassium, ↓ bicarbonate with metabolic acidosis) represents hyporeninemic hypoaldosteronism. This condition is due to destruction of the juxtaglomerular apparatus, which synthesizes renin. Low renin ultimately results in low aldosterone, with subsequent loss of sodium in the urine, hypotension from volume depletion, hyperkalemia, and retention of hydrogen ions, leading to metabolic acidosis. Diabetes mellitus and tubulointerstitial diseases of the kidney (e.g., Legionnaire's disease, leptospirosis) are associated with this disease, otherwise known as type IV renal tubular acidosis (RTA). This disease should offer no confusion with primary aldosteronism. Choice **E** (↓ serum aldosterone, ↑ PRA, ↑ potassium, ↓ bicarbonate with metabolic acidosis) represents Addison's disease. Patients present with hypotension, hyperpigmentation (hypocortisolism increases plasma ACTH), and weakness, none of which are present in this patient.

SUMMARY TABLE

Serum Aldosterone	PRA	Serum K+	Serum HCO₃⁻	
↑	↑	↓	↑	Patient on thiazide/loop diuretic; Bartter's syndrome
Normal	↓	↓	↑	Liddle's syndrome
↑	↓	↓	↑	Primary aldosteronism
↓	↓	↑	↓	Type IV RTAᵃ (hyporeninemic hypoaldosteronism)
↓	↑	↑	↓	Addison's disease

ᵃRTA, renal tubular acidosis.

[29] **The answer is A** *Preventive Medicine and Public Health*

Patients with sickle cell disease are homozygous for HbS. Because in the case described only one potential parent has the HbS allele, the only way their child could inherit two HbS genes is if one of the father's normal Hb genes underwent a new mutation in a sperm cell, an extremely unlikely event. Therefore, their child does not have a reasonable chance of inheriting the disease (choice **A**). However, there is a 1/4 chance that their child would be a carrier. Such heterozygous carriers may have mild symptoms and are said to have the sickle cell trait.

The probability that two heterozygous carriers of the trait will have a child with the disease is 1/4 (choice **B**); that is, 25% of their children will have the disease, while 50% will have the trait and another 25% will be normal.

Assuming there is no knowledge of family histories or hemoglobin (Hb) patterns, choice **C** (1/144) represents the probability that two carriers will meet. That is, the carrier rate among African Americans is approximately 1 in 12, and 1/12 × 1/12 equals 1/144.

Choice **D** (1/576) corresponds to the likelihood of a child having the disease if two African Americans having no knowledge of family histories or Hb patterns had children. As indicated in choice **C** the random chance of two African-American heterozygotes meeting is 1/144. Since only 25% of their children will have the disease (see choice **B** above) those having the disease will equal 1/144 × 1/4, or 1/576.

Choice **E** is not a sensible representation of the probability of a child inheriting sickle cell anemia.

[30] **The answer is A** *Obstetrics and Gynecology*

Determination of gestational age is of crucial importance. The last menstrual period, obtained from patient history, albeit subjective, can be very useful in identifying the number of pregnancy weeks if it is reliable. An objective parameter for estimating the duration of pregnancy is ultrasonic measurement of fetal size. The earlier in pregnancy that the sonogram is performed the more accurate it is, because the proportionate change in fetal growth from week to week is greater earlier in the pregnancy than it is later. As pregnancy progresses, the accuracy of gestational age estimation from sonographic measurement of fetal size is progressively less. Therefore, sonograms performed at 20 (choice **B**), 25 (choice **C**), 30 (choice **D**), and 40 (choice **E**) weeks' gestation would not be as precise as a sonogram performed at 10 weeks' gestation (choice **A**).

[31] **The answer is C** *Pediatrics*

Pertussis (whooping cough) (choice **C**) is an extremely contagious respiratory disease caused by *Bordetella pertussis*. Neither natural disease nor vaccination can provide lifelong immunity against the disease. In the United States approximately 50% of cases occur in children less than 1 year of age, and 25% occur in adolescents or adults. After a 1-week incubation period, children present with three successive stages of the disease. The catarrhal stage consists of symptoms of an upper respiratory infection, thick nasal discharge, and conjunctivitis. The paroxysmal stage is characterized by spasms of forceful coughing ending in an inspiratory whoop. The cough is strong enough to force vomiting, and facial redness and cyanosis are often observed. Often, there is no whoop in infants, but apnea may be manifested. In the convalescent stage, the cough and vomiting gradually subside. Cough can persist for several months. Petechiae and conjunctival hemorrhages are seen. Otitis media is a common complication. Complete blood count (CBC) usually shows leukocytosis, predominantly lymphocytes toward the end of the catarrhal stage and during the paroxysmal stage.

The diagnosis of acute lymphoblastic leukemia (choice **A**) would be suggested by the presence of blast cells on a peripheral blood smear. Patients with *Chlamydia trachomatis* pneumonia (choice **B**) have cough, tachypnea, and lack of fever. Eosinophilia (>400 cells/mm^3) may be present. Patients with bronchiolitis (choice **D**) usually have a normal white blood cell (WBC) count and differential count. The peripheral WBC count of patients with respiratory syncytial viral pneumonitis (choice **E**) tends to be normal or elevated, and the differential count may be normal with a neutrophilic or mononuclear prevalence.

[32] **The answer is D** *Pediatrics*

The presentation of this patient is most consistent with the diagnosis of acute otitis media. The most common causes of acute otitis media are *Streptococcus pneumoniae* (choice **D**), found in approximately 40% of cases; *Haemophilus influenzae* (choice **A**) was found in approximately 25–30% prior to the advent of a vaccine;

and *Moraxella catarrhalis* (choice **C**), in approximately 15%; while *Staphylococcus aureus* (choice **B**), group A *Streptococcus,* and gram-negative organisms (e.g., *Pseudomonas aeruginosa*) are less common causes of acute otitis media, and together account for approximately 5% of cases. Respiratory syncytial virus (RSV) (choice **E**) and other respiratory viruses are also associated with acute otitis media. However, even though otitis media can be a sequela of bronchiolitis caused by RSV, rarely, if ever, is the aspirate from the middle ear solely positive for RSV. These children usually have a bacterial pathogen isolated in their aspirate. It remains to be discovered whether viruses alone can cause acute otitis media or if their presence only enhances the chances for bacterial invasion.

33 The answer is D *Surgery*

Fractures of the shaft of the humerus involve the radial nerve (choice **D**), which winds around its posterior aspect, in the radial groove. As a result, a wrist drop may be present.

Dislocations of the shoulder or fractures involving the surgical neck of the humerus may be associated with trauma to the axillary nerve (choice **A**). In such an event, sensations over the lateral aspect of the shoulder will be impaired. The median nerve (choice **B**) may be traumatized in supracondylar fractures of the humerus. The brachial artery may be compressed as well. The ulnar nerve (choice **C**) can be injured after posterior dislocation of the elbow. The brachial plexus (choice **E**) is not injured in fractures of the upper extremities. Acute lateral flexion of the neck (e.g., after a fall) can damage the lower cord of the brachial plexus.

34 The answer is C *Obstetrics and Gynecology*

The case presentation describes the findings in a patient with preeclampsia associated with acute diffuse vasoconstriction (choice **C**), which typically occurs in primigravidas during the last trimester of pregnancy. This entity is characterized by sustained hypertension (with BP ≥ 140/90) along with significant proteinuria (1–2+ on dipstick testing or ≥300 mg on a 24-hour urine collection).

Preeclampsia is characterized by an enhanced angiotensin response rather than a blunted one (choice **A**) which is the normal physiologic response with pregnancy. This condition is usually unrelated to elevated β-endorphin level (choice **B**), which is a frequent physiologic stress response to the pain of labor. The history provided is not characteristic of primary renal disease (choice **D**) or chronic hypertension (choice **E**), which is diagnosed if the hypertension either was present prior to the pregnancy or had its onset prior to 20 weeks gestation.

35 The answer is E *Pediatrics*

Kawasaki syndrome (mucocutaneous lymph node syndrome [MLNS]) is a febrile vasculitis that affects all blood vessels but primarily affects the medium-sized arteries, with predilection for the coronary arteries. Criteria for diagnosis are unexplained fever of 5 days' duration and four of the following five conditions: bilateral nonpurulent conjunctivitis, changes of the mucosa of the oropharynx (dry, cracked lips; strawberry tongue), changes of the peripheral extremities (edema, erythema), a polymorphous rash, and cervical lymphadenopathy. Desquamation of the palms and soles is a late finding, usually appearing during the second or third week of the disease. Many experts believe that in the presence of classic features, the diagnosis can be made before 5 days of fever. Kawasaki syndrome (choice **E**) occurs generally in children under 5 years of age. Thrombocytosis appears in the second or third week. Leukocytosis, elevated C-reactive protein, and elevated erythrocyte sedimentation rate (ESR) are common laboratory findings.

Scarlet fever (choice **A**) causes a strawberry tongue, maculopapular rash, Pastia's lines, and circumoral pallor. Acute rheumatic fever (choice **B**) is diagnosed using the Jones criteria. The Jones criteria consist of major and minor manifestations. Major criteria include carditis, polyarthritis, erythema marginatum, and subcutaneous nodules. Minor criteria include arthralgia, fever, elevated ESR and C-reactive protein, as well as a prolonged PR interval. Two major criteria, or one major and two minor criteria, plus evidence of a preceding group A streptococcal infection indicate a high probability of rheumatic fever. Juvenile rheumatoid arthritis (choice **C**) includes findings of lymphadenopathy, hepatosplenomegaly, and an evanescent salmon-colored rash. Many features of toxic shock syndrome (TSS) (choice **D**), a multisystem disease, resemble those of Kawasaki disease. Both include findings of strawberry tongue, conjunctival hyperemia, and an erythematous macular rash. However, in TSS other abnormalities such as hypotension, vomiting, diffuse myalgia, azotemia, and shock help to differentiate the two.

36 **The answer is B** *Preventive Medicine and Public Health*

Good medical practice would include counseling the patient about prevention (choice **B**).

Although parents must usually grant consent for medical procedures involving minor children, neither consent nor notifying them is necessary when they demonstrate drug or alcohol dependence, have emergencies, require medical care in pregnancy, or, as in this case, have sexually transmitted disease (choice **A**). In this case, it is not necessary to notify state health authorities (choice **C**) or his sexual partner (choice **D**), nor is it required to notify his parents after treating him (choice **E**). Although true as of January 2006, some of these rulings are under legislative review.

37 **The answer is E** *Surgery*

The presentation of this patient is classic for rupture of the duodenum (choice **E**). Patients have vague symptoms because the duodenum is retroperitoneal. If left untreated, mortality is almost 100%. The best way to diagnose it is to maintain a high index of suspicion and conduct repeated physical examinations. Serum amylase is often elevated but is not diagnostic. X-ray films of the abdomen reveal retroperitoneal air, which is the sine qua non of duodenal rupture. Duodenal rupture in children could also result from the use of the lap belt without shoulder support in motor vehicles. This results from acute hyperflexion of the thoracolumbar spine, which crushes the duodenum. Drivers of motor vehicles can also sustain duodenal rupture as a result of compression against the steering wheel.

This patient does not have a ruptured spleen (choice **A**) or a ruptured liver (choice **B**), because his vital signs are stable. Moreover, neither condition is associated with midabdominal pain. Rather, pain is in the left or right upper quadrant, respectively, and there may be associated fractures of the lower ribs. A diagnostic peritoneal lavage is positive for hemorrhage, and a computed tomography (CT) scan confirms the diagnosis.

Rupture of the pancreas (choice **C**) usually follows blunt trauma. Although this diagnosis is a possibility, the duodenum more usually ruptures in injuries like the one described in the scenario. Pancreatic rupture is associated with hypovolemic shock due to tear of the gastroduodenal artery. The common bile duct may be avulsed as well. Serum amylase is raised, but this alone does not confirm the diagnosis. However, a persistently elevated serum amylase suggests this possibility. The diagnosis is best established by maintaining a high index of suspicion. A CT scan confirms the diagnosis. Hematoma of the rectus muscle (choice **D**) is a benign condition. The pain is confined to the region of injury and is not vaguely defined. Pain increases with contraction of the abdominal muscles. A localized mass may be present. The diagnosis is clinical, and treatment is supportive.

38 **The answer is B** *Medicine*

Most hemolytic transfusion reactions are due to clerical error, such as giving the wrong blood to a patient with the same name, a mislabeled unit, or not checking the patient's blood bank identification tag with the identification number on the unit. Because the patient in question has blood group O, immunoglobulin M (IgM) antibodies against A and B antigens are already present. Anti-A IgM antibodies in the patient will attach to the donor A cells, activate the classic complement pathway, and cause massive intravascular hemolysis (a type II hypersensitivity reaction), with subsequent hypotension and the potential for developing ischemic acute tubular necrosis. Approximately 50% of patients develop disseminated intravascular coagulation (DIC), as did this patient, who has blood oozing out of the venipuncture sites from the consumption of clotting factors (fibrinogen, factor V, prothrombin, factor VIII) and platelets. The initial step in management of a hemolytic transfusion reaction is to stop the transfusion and keep the IV open with isotonic (normal) saline (choice **B**).

Isotonic saline (not 0.45 normal saline [choice **A**]) is important to keep the blood pressure stabilized to prevent acute renal failure due to ischemic tubular necrosis. The unit and a sample of blood and urine should immediately be sent to the blood bank for a transfusion reaction workup. Pink-staining plasma and hemoglobin in the urine are presumptive evidence of intravascular hemolysis. If the urine output is not increasing with the IV fluids or if there is volume overload from congestive heart failure, IV furosemide is given (choice **C**). If the patient's volume status is stable, IV mannitol is used to maintain an osmotic diuresis (choice **D**) to prevent acute tubular necrosis. Antipyretics (choice **E**) are not indicated, because this reaction is not a febrile type of transfusion reaction, in which preexisting anti-HLA antibodies in the patient are reacting against donor leukocytes.

39 **The answer is C**   *Obstetrics and Gynecology*

This patient meets two criteria for mild preeclampsia: sustained BP elevation (≥140/90) developing after 20 weeks gestation along with significant proteinuria. At term, the goal of management with mild preeclampsia is prompt delivery, so induction of labor is appropriate. Patients with preeclampsia, however, are also at risk for progressing to eclampsia, which is characterized by generalized seizures. Prevention of seizures is a crucial aspect of the care of any woman with a hypertensive disorder of pregnancy. In the United States, magnesium sulfate (choice **C**) is the most commonly used preventive agent for this condition.

   Phenobarbital (choice **A**), diazepam (choice **B**), and diphenylhydantoin (choice **D**) are standard anticonvulsant medications, but are not used primarily for seizure prophylaxis in preeclampsia. Randomized controlled head-to-head studies show that magnesium sulfate is superior to these standard anticonvulsants in prevention as well as treatment of eclamptic seizures. Magnesium gluconate (choice **E**) has no anticonvulsant activity.

40 **The answer is C**   *Surgery*

This patient has sustained an epidural hematoma, which usually results from tear of the middle meningeal artery, which enters the middle cranial fossa through the foramen spinosum. Fracture of the thin temporal bone across the groove of the middle meningeal artery results in it tearing. As a consequence the dura is stripped from the inner table of the skull, forming an expanding mass. Failure to intervene results in herniation of the uncus of the temporal lobe, pressure on the brainstem, and death. Fractures of the occipital bone tear the venous sinuses, resulting in a venous epidural hematoma. Patients with epidural hematoma have a lucid interval (choice **C**), which is a hallmark of the condition. The initial period of coma is followed by recovery and then coma again. The pupil on the side of the lesion begins to dilate, and inequality of the pupils (anisocoria) is noted. Hyperventilation should be instituted early to decrease intracranial pressure. A computed tomography (CT) scan shows a bright-white, lens-shaped (lentiform) mass on the side of the hematoma, which represents blood that has collected between the inner table of the skull and the dura. A burr hole is made at the pterion to evacuate the hematoma. A lumbar puncture is contraindicated because it will induce herniation and death.

41 **The answer is B**   *Surgery*

This patient has sustained a basal skull fracture involving the anterior cranial fossa. The fracture occurs across the cribriform plate of the ethmoid bone. Cerebrospinal fluid (CSF) leaks through the nose (CSF rhinorrhea) and may be unilateral or bilateral. Presence of glucose in the discharge is diagnostic of CSF as its source. A CT scan locates the fracture and excludes presence of injury to the frontal lobe and other areas of the brain. Hyperventilation is essential to avoid raising intracranial pressure. In about 24 hours the patient has circumorbital discoloration, which is known as a raccoon sign (choice **B**). Blood leaks into the subcutaneous tissues of the periorbital area. This resolves on its own without treatment. Meningitis can result because of transmission of pneumococci (which are resident flora in the nose) to the intracranial cavity. In such an event, a lumbar puncture can be done, provided there is no clinical evidence of raised intracranial pressure. Performing a spinal puncture in the presence of raised intracranial pressure is fraught with risk of herniation and death. In patients with fractures of the petrous temporal bone, CSF escapes through the external auditory meatus and is associated with discoloration behind the ear (Battle's sign).

42 **The answer is A**   *Surgery*

This patient has a chronic subdural hematoma, which results from tear of the bridging veins. Cortical atrophy in alcoholics and the elderly results in stretching of the bridging veins that connect the cortical veins with the sagittal sinus; this tenuous connection ruptures even after minor trauma. In 20% of cases, the hematoma is bilateral. Symptoms usually begin about 3 weeks after minor head injury and include dull headache, change in personality or mental status, lack of concentration, poor memory, and seizures. Unlike Alzheimer's disease, this condition is associated with fluctuating symptoms. CT scan shows a dark lesion due to collection of blood that contains methemoglobin. Raised intracranial pressure is relatively rare in these patients, because the blood occupies the space vacated by the shrinking brain; thus, hyperventilation is usually not required. A burr hole is required to evacuate the hematoma. Photophobia (choice **A**), retinal hemorrhages, and papilledema (rare) are features of this condition.

INCORRECT CHOICES

Optic atrophy (choice **D**). Optic nerve atrophy results in visual loss that is almost proportional to the degree of atrophy that has occurred. It is a physical sign and not a diagnosis. The etiology could be primary or secondary. In primary optic atrophy, the disk is white, has a sharp margin, and the physiologic cup and lamina cribrosa are clearly visible. The blood vessels are normal. Primary optic atrophy occurs in tabes dorsalis, in pernicious anemia, and as a consequence of chronic raised intracranial pressure, or where the optic nerve is compressed. In secondary optic atrophy, the disc is pale, margins are indistinct; the optic cup and lamina cribrosa cannot be seen. White lines may be seen along the emerging vessels, as a result of perivascular lymph sheathing. Like primary optic atrophy, secondary atrophy can result from increased intracranial pressure secondary to brain tumors.

Enlarged sella (choice **E**). An enlarged sella could result from a tumor such as a pituitary adenoma. These patients will complain of headache and have bitemporal hemianopsia on testing of the visual field.

Cavernous sinus thrombosis (choice **F**). Cavernous sinus thrombosis is a rare disease that results from infection that travels in a retrograde manner via the ophthalmic or facial vein to the cavernous sinus. The patient complains of headaches and difficulty in vision, especially diplopia due to paresis of cranial nerve VI, which lies within the sinus. Oculoparesis, conjunctival edema, and blindness could occur. This is a potentially fatal condition that should be treated early.

43 The answer is G *Medicine*

The farmer and his wife have adult botulism due to *Clostridium botulinum* (choice **G**). The bacteria produce a heat-labile toxin that irreversibly blocks acetylcholine release from cholinergic receptors, leading to descending paralysis (diplopia first sign) and mydriasis followed by generalized muscle paralysis. Adult botulism is usually caused by ingestion of preformed neurotoxin in home-canned vegetables that have not been properly sterilized. On the other hand, infant botulism is more often due to ingestion of spores, which colonize the bowel and then produce the toxin. Honey is a common source of the spores, which is why children should not eat honey for the first 2 years of life. Botulinum toxin is used clinically in the treatment of muscle spasm disorders (e.g., achalasia, blepharospasm torticollis) and by cosmetic plastic surgeons in temporarily treating wrinkles. Treatment for adult botulism is with trivalent antitoxin.

44 The answer is D *Medicine*

The patient has food poisoning due to *Bacillus cereus* (choice **D**), which is a gram-positive rod that produces preformed toxin that stimulates adenylate cyclase, causing gastroenteritis. It is transmitted via reheated fried rice or tacos with rice. The disease is self-limiting and does not require antibiotic treatment.

45 The answer is F *Medicine*

The patient has tetanus due to *Clostridium tetani* (choice **F**), a gram-positive rod that has spores in soil that gain entrance to individuals via closed wounds, "skin popping" among intravenous drug abusers (this patient), or the umbilical cord or circumcision site in newborns. Germination of spores is enhanced by the presence of necrosis and poor blood supply. Wounds have no inflammatory exudate, and organisms are rarely isolated from the wound. Bacterial proliferation in the wound releases a neurotoxin, called *tetanospasmin,* which is carried intraaxonally (retrograde) to the central nervous system where it binds to ganglioside receptors of spinal afferent fibers and inhibits the release of the inhibitory neurotransmitters glycine and γ-aminobenzoic acid within the spinal cord. This causes sustained motor stimulation of all voluntary muscles.

The incubation period is a few days to 2 months. The disease begins with muscle stiffness eventually causing lockjaw (an inability to open the mouth) as in this patient. The contraction of the muscles around the mouth is called *risus sardonicus* (perpetual, sardonic smile on the face). The slightest stimulus causes generalized, painful muscle contractions. Contractions of back muscles produce opisthotonus (painful arching of the back). Patients are mentally alert throughout the course of the disease.

Tetanus toxoid (Td) is given for active immunization. Hyperimmune tetanus immune globulin (TIg) provides passive immunization and must be administered before the neurotoxin is fixed in the central nervous system (part of immune globulin is directly injected into the wound).

Débriding the wound is extremely important, because it removes necrotic tissue, which is the breeding ground of the bacteria. Hyperbaric oxygen therapy is very useful and metronidazole or penicillin G is used to kill proliferating bacteria. Mortality is 10 to 30% in generalized disease. Pneumonia and cardiac failure are the most common causes of death. If the patient survives, no permanent sequelae remain. Protective antibody titers are not high enough to prevent the disease in the future, which is why tetanus toxoid is required every 10 years.

There are established recommendations for prevention of tetanus in clean wounds and dirty wounds in immunized and nonimmunized patients. In an immunized individual with a clean wound, no Td booster is necessary if the last booster was within 10 years. In a nonimmunized patient (no history of immunization or <3 doses of Td), the wound should be cleaned with quaternary ammonium compounds and the patient should receive Td toxoid.

A patient who is immunized and has a dirty wound should first have the wound cleaned.

If the last booster was given within 5 years, no Td booster is necessary; however, if the last booster was given more than 5 years previously, a Td booster is given. A nonimmunized patient with a dirty wound should first have the wound cleaned. Following débriding, one half the dose of tetanus immune globulin (passive immunization) is injected into the wound, and the other half injected into another site. Finally, Td (active immunization) should be administered.

History	Clean Minor Wounds Non–Tetanus-Prone Wound		Dirty Wounds Tetanus-Prone Wound	
	Td	TIg	Td	TIg
Unknown or <3 doses	Yes	No	Yes	Yes
≥3 doses	No (yes if last dose >10 years ago)	No	No (yes if last shot >5 years ago)	No

46 The answer is J *Medicine*

The patient has actinomycosis due to *Actinomyces israelii* (choice **J**), which is an anaerobic, gram-positive filamentous bacterium that is part of the normal flora in the tonsils and crevices around the teeth. Transmission in the oral region is via dental extractions or trauma to the teeth. It presents with a draining sinus in the jaw. The pus contains yellow sulfur granules, which contain the organism. Other infections caused by the pathogen include draining sinuses in the chest and abdomen and endometritis associated with intrauterine devices (now uncommon). Treatment is with penicillin.

47 The answer is B *Medicine*

The patient has a lower urinary tract infection due to *Staphylococcus saprophyticus* (choice **B**), which is coagulase negative and catalase positive. It accounts for 10 to 20% of acute urinary tract infections in young, sexually active women. Since the pathogen is not a nitrate reducer and produces a neutrophilic inflammatory reaction, the dipstick test result for nitrite is negative and that for leukocyte esterase is positive. The treatment of choice is trimethoprim–sulfamethoxazole.

48 The answer is H *Medicine*

The patient has diphtheria due to *Corynebacterium diphtheriae* (choice **H**), which is a gram-positive rod that produces a toxin that inhibits protein synthesis and the β-oxidation of fatty acids. In the oropharynx, larynx, and trachea, the toxin produces an inflammatory reaction causing the development of a pseudomembrane that interferes with swallowing and breathing. There is pronounced cervical lymph node enlargement in response to the inflammation ("bulls-neck" lymphadenopathy). The toxin also damages cardiac muscle (myocarditis) as well as peripheral and cranial nerves, causing paralysis. Heart failure due to myocarditis is the most common cause of death. Diphtheria is treated with horse antitoxin (neutralizes toxin) and erythromycin. The disease is prevented by administration of diphtheria toxoid in combination with tetanus toxoid and acellular pertussis vaccine.

INCORRECT CHOICES

Staphylococcus aureus (choice **A**) is a gram-positive coccus that is the most common cause of skin/breast abscesses, surgical wound infection, scalded skin syndrome (toxin-induced epidermolytic damage to skin in young children), toxic shock syndrome (usually occurs in menstruating women who use tampons), osteomyelitis in children, and acute bacterial endocarditis in intravenous drug abusers. It is also a common cause of food poisoning (preformed enterotoxin), pneumonia in cystic fibrosis, acute conjunctivitis, and nosocomial infections. Oxacillin or nafcillin are recommended for the treatment of methicillin-sensitive strains and vancomycin for methicillin-resistant strains (20% of cases). Mupirocin is used for topical treatment of skin infections.

Bacillus anthracis (choice **C**) is the cause of anthrax. It is a gram-positive rod, whose spores are present in soil. Normally it is transmitted to humans by contact with animal skins or products (most commonly sheep and cattle). Cutaneous anthrax (90%–95% of cases) occurs through direct contact with infected or contaminated animal products. It resembles an insect bite; however, it eventually swells to form a black scab, or eschar, with a central area of necrosis (called a "malignant pustule"). If untreated, death occurs in 20% of patients. Pulmonary anthrax is caused by inhalation of spores, which may potentially be dispersed as a terror weapon, a form of germ warfare. It produces a necrotizing pneumonia and rapidly disseminates throughout the rest of the body. Sterilizing dead animals and animal products prevents soil contamination by the pathogen. A vaccine is available for high-risk patients (e.g., veterinarians, soldiers entering developing countries). Treatment is with ciprofloxacin.

Clostridium perfringens (choice **E**) is the most common cause of gas gangrene (myonecrosis of tissue). It is a gram-positive rod that produces gas bubbles in tissue, causing the tissue to have crepitans when palpated. Gas also is evident in radiographs. Other features of the infection include pain, edema, cellulitis, and a foul-smelling exudate. Complications include hemolytic anemia, jaundice, shock, disseminated intravascular coagulation, and renal failure. Debridement of wound tissue is essential along with antibiotic therapy (penicillin G with or without clindamycin) and hyperbaric oxygen therapy. *C. perfringens* is also a common cause of food poisoning (meat dishes such as beef and turkey), septicemia, intraabdominal infections (e.g., peritonitis, gangrenous cholecystitis), pelvic inflammatory disease, and "back-room abortion" septic endometritis.

Listeria monocytogenes (choice **I**) is a small gram-positive rod that is transmitted to humans via vertical transmission (transplacental or during delivery), by eating contaminated, ready-to-eat foods (e.g., soft cheeses, unpasteurized milk or cheese); or by direct contact (e.g., butchers, veterinarians) or it is a potential complication of immunosuppression. In pregnancy it may cause spontaneous abortion, premature delivery, or peripartum sepsis. It is the third most common cause of neonatal meningitis and produces granulomatous abscesses in disseminated disease (i.e., granulomatis infantisepticum). In immunocompromised patients (e.g., patients with cancer or renal transplants), it produces meningitis. The treatment of choice is ampicillin.

49 The answer is C   *Psychiatry*

Nortriptyline is a tricyclic antidepressant with a "therapeutic window." Dosages that achieve a blood level of 50–100 ng/mL are associated with good patient response. Increasing the dosage diminishes the therapeutic response (graph **C**). This therapeutic window has not been demonstrated for other antidepressants, but may be present with risperidone, an atypical antidepressant that demonstrates greatest therapeutic response at doses of 4–6 mg daily.

50 The answer is A   *Psychiatry*

Lithium has a threshold for responses at a dosage that produces a blood level of approximately 1.0 mEq/L. Lower doses are ineffective. Higher doses do not appreciably increase the response (graph **A**), but are associated with more untoward effects.

Graph **B** represents a gradually increasing response with increasing dosage, as might be seen with many antipsychotic medications. Graph **D** represents a lack of response. Graph **E** represents an increasingly poor response to medication with increasing doses, usually associated with increasing adverse effects.

test **3**

Questions

Single Best Choice Directions: This section consists of numbered statements or questions followed by a list of potential answers; you are to select the ONE BEST answer.

1 A 33-year-old woman, gravida 4, para 3, presents to the obstetric unit at 29 weeks' gestation by dates with painless vaginal bleeding. The bleeding began 2 hours ago and has been accompanied by passage of a significant amount of blood and clots. An intravenous infusion of normal saline is in place. No record of her prenatal obstetric ultrasound examination is available. Her vital signs are as follows: temperature, 37.4°C (99.3°F); pulse, 105/min; respiration, 16/min; blood pressure, 100/70 mm Hg. The fetal heart rate by Doppler stethoscope is 150 beats/min with no audible decelerations. Uterine contractions are absent, and the patient appears very anxious. Her last pregnancy was delivered by emergency cesarean section at 37 weeks' gestation due to double-footling breech presentation in labor. The type of uterine incision is unknown. Which of the following is the best working diagnosis?

(A) Placenta previa
(B) Abruptio placenta
(C) Vasa previa
(D) Bloody show
(E) Uterine rupture

2 Parents present to the emergency department carrying their 4-year-old child, who is lethargic and has excessive oral secretions, miosis, tearing, and "soiled" trousers from urination and defecation. Remnants of emesis are seen on his clothing. Tremors, fasciculations, and hypertension are also present. The parents tell the physician that the child had been in his usual state of good health until that afternoon. The patient's symptoms developed while playing in a field recently sprayed with insecticides. The physician suspects organophosphate poisoning. To treat the nicotinic effects, the physician should use which of the following?

(A) Atropine
(B) British antilewisite (BAL)
(C) Pralidoxime (2-PAM)
(D) Calcium disodium ethylenediaminetetraacetate (CaEDTA)
(E) Naloxone

3 A new blood test, test X, was developed for the detection of colon cancer in patients. As part of the clinical trial, the test was tried on two population groups: those with documented colon cancer and those who did not have the disease. The multicenter trial involved a total of 860 individuals. Of these, 60 dropped out, as they did not wish to participate in the trial. Of the remaining individuals, 400 had colon cancer, and 400 were free of disease. Each cohort had 150 women. The diagram below shows the findings of test X for colon carcinoma in the cohort without colon cancer, and in those with it. Which of the following statements regarding establishing reference intervals (normal range) for this test and interpreting them is true?

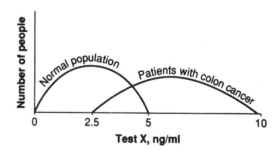

(A) If the reference interval is 0–2.5 ng/mL, the test has 100% specificity
(B) If the reference interval is 0–2.5 ng/mL, a patient with a test result of 4 ng/mL must have colon cancer
(C) If the reference interval is 0–5 ng/mL, the test has 100% sensitivity
(D) If the reference interval is 0–5 ng/mL, a test result of 4 ng/mL may represent a true-negative (TN) or a false-negative (FN) result
(E) If the reference interval is 0–5 ng/mL, the number of FNs and false-positives (FPs) increases

4 A 65-year-old man presents to the emergency room of a small town hospital with a history of crushing substernal chest pain that occurred while he was watching television. This was his first such episode. The patient did give a history of chest pains that came and went, which he had chosen to ignore. He did not smoke, drank alcohol in moderation, and had been retired for 4 years. He had no past history of medical illness or long-term medications. In the emergency room his temperature was 37°C (98.4°F), pulse was 100/min regular, and blood pressure was 140/60 mm Hg. His respirations were 20/min. The patient was diaphoretic and had pallor and a hint of peripheral cyanosis. He was given 100% oxygen by nasal canula at 4 L/min, morphine for pain, sublingual nitroglycerin, and aspirin. An ECG showed an inferior MI based on ST changes in leads II, III, and AVF. As percutaneous coronary intervention was unavailable, and the event was less than 6 hours in duration, thrombolytic therapy was carried out. Thereafter, he was transferred to the coronary intensive care unit. On the fourth day post-MI, he complained of severe substernal pain similar in intensity and character to the one that heralded the first event. Positive physical findings included a third heart sound and bibasilar rales. Pertinent negative findings included the absence of a murmur and friction rub. Laboratory studies revealed the presence of creatine kinase (CK) isoenzyme MB (CK_2) and a lactate dehydrogenase (LDH) isoenzyme study with an LDH_1/LDH_2 flip. Which of the following findings is the most specific indication of reinfarction?

(A) Recurrent pain
(B) A third heart sound
(C) Bibasilar rales
(D) The presence of creatine kinase (CK) isoenzyme MB (CK_2)
(E) A lactate dehydrogenase (LDH) isoenzyme LDH_1/LDH_2 flip

5 A 9-month-old child presents for a well-care examination. The mother states that the child has not been feeding well and seems to be less active than usual. The patient's vital signs are within normal limits, and the patient is afebrile. On physical examination the head circumference is found to be two standard deviations above the norm. The child has frontal bossing, the skin is translucent, and the eyes manifest a "setting sun" sign. The child also has a meningomyelocele. A computed tomography (CT) scan of the head would show which of the following?

(A) Epidural hematoma
(B) Chronic subdural hematoma
(C) Shaken baby syndrome
(D) Noncommunicating hydrocephalus
(E) Leptomeningeal cyst

6 A 19-year-old woman becomes very concerned that a small lump in her left breast is malignant cancer. Workup and biopsy show it to be entirely benign, but she remains excessively worried in spite of reassurance by her physician. Which of the following is the best treatment in this case?

(A) A careful explanation of the benign nature of the physical complaint
(B) Use of benzodiazepine
(C) Skillful physician reassurance and frequent follow-up
(D) Use of placebo medication
(E) Psychotherapy to explore her current life circumstances

7 An 18-year-old female presents to the emergency department with a history of severe retrosternal chest pain that is aggravated by swallowing and deep breathing. The patient appears anxious. She is afebrile, has sinus tachycardia, slightly elevated blood pressure, and tachypnea. Mild pallor is noted, but she seems well hydrated and has no icterus. Examination of the cardiovascular system had normal findings, except for sinus tachycardia. The abdomen is scaphoid, and no tenderness, masses, or organomegaly is noted. Her weight is less than the norm for her age and height. The patient however feels that she is obese and has taken to binge eating followed by self-induced vomiting. Which of the following is the most probable cause of her pain?

(A) Gastroesophageal reflux
(B) Boerhaave's syndrome
(C) Tension pneumothorax
(D) Gastric ulcer disease
(E) Esophageal cancer

8 A 33-year-old woman who underwent a total thyroidectomy for a papillary carcinoma of the thyroid is noted to have both carpal spasm when her blood pressure is taken and facial muscle contraction with tapping over the facial nerve. Which of the following set of laboratory data would most closely represent the expected findings in this patient?

	Serum Calcium	Serum Phosphorus	Serum Parathormone (PTH)
(A)	Increased	Decreased	Increased
(B)	Increased	Decreased	Decreased
(C)	Decreased	Increased	Decreased
(D)	Decreased	Decreased	Increased
(E)	Decreased	Increased	Increased

9 A 29-year-old male presents to the emergency room with a history of pain and swelling in the left side of the scrotum of 4 days' duration. There is no history of trauma. He did have sex recently with a woman whom he had met through the internet and did not use a condom. The patient stated that he had some burning sensation while passing urine, but other than that there was no problem. Physical examination revealed a young man in moderate distress who, as a consequence, walked with a broad-based gait to avoid hurting the scrotum with his thighs. Examination of the genitalia revealed no penile abnormality or discharge through the urethra. Examination of the scrotum revealed dilated veins under the scrotal sac on the left side, which was tender to touch. Which of the following conditions is a possible diagnosis that must be excluded or confirmed?

(A) Torsion of the testis
(B) Incarcerated inguinal hernia
(C) Fournier's gangrene
(D) Epididymitis caused by chlamydia
(E) Renal carcinoma

10 A pediatric intern is called to the newborn nursery to evaluate a 2-day-old who has passed a bloody stool. The patient was born by normal spontaneous vaginal delivery to a 34-year-old prima gravida. The birth weight was 8 lb 3 oz (3.7 kg), and Apgar scores were 8 at 1 minute and 9 at 5 minutes. The mother had good prenatal care throughout the entire pregnancy. She denied using tobacco, alcohol, or drugs during her pregnancy. The patient has been sleeping, feeding, defecating, and urinating well since birth. Vital signs are stable, and the rest of the physical examination findings are within normal limits. Which of the following tests would be most indicated in this patient to determine the cause of the bloody stool?

(A) Apt test on the blood in the stool
(B) Hemoglobin electrophoresis of the blood from the stool
(C) Barium enema
(D) Clinitest examination of the stool
(E) Methylene blue stain of the stool

11 An 18-year-old nulligravid woman complains of painful menses for the past 3 years. These symptoms are associated with cramping located in her lower abdomen and radiating to her lower back and inner thighs. She also has nausea and vomiting. She experienced menarche at age 13. Initially her menses were irregular and not associated with any cramping or pain. She is not sexually active and is not requesting contraception. The only medication she is taking is thyroid hormone replacement for a diagnosis of hypothyroidism that was made 2 years ago. General and pelvic examinations are unremarkable. Her uterus is midline, symmetrical, not enlarged, nontender, and freely mobile. She has no cervical motion tenderness. Which of the following is the most likely mechanism causing this patient's symptoms?

(A) Excessive prostaglandin-induced myometrial contractions
(B) Myometrial irritation from ectopic endometrial glands
(C) Pelvic congestion from dilated spiral arterioles
(D) Excessive endometrial proliferation from unopposed estrogen
(E) Bleeding into proliferated myometrial fibroids

12 A 56-year-old grandmother whose hobby is gardening presents with a red swelling in her right ring finger. She does not remember any specific trauma to the area, but frequently sustains small cuts on her hands while tending to her garden. Physical examination reveals a small red nontender papule on the right ring finger, which shows erythema and swelling, with a small draining pustule on the lateral side. There are ascending erythematous streaks up the right arm with several draining pustules along their course. Bacterial cultures are negative. Which of the following is the least expensive effective medication for this patient?

(A) Dicloxacillin
(B) Erythromycin
(C) Amphotericin B
(D) Saturated solution of potassium iodide (SSKI)
(E) Cephalexin

13 A 2-week-old infant is brought to the emergency department because of diarrhea, poor feeding, abdominal distention, and vomiting for the past 3 days. Physical examination is pertinent for temperature (39°C [102.2°F]), cataracts, hepatomegaly, and jaundice. The patient has poor skin turgor and a capillary refill of 3 seconds. The physician suspects that the infant is septic and has galactosemia. Which of the following would be the most probable pathogen involved in the sepsis?

(A) Group B streptococcus
(B) *Listeria monocytogenes*
(C) *Escherichia coli*
(D) *Staphylococcus aureus*
(E) Pneumococcus (*Streptococcus pneumoniae*)

14 A 35-year-old businessman comes to see his primary care physician for a complete physical. The patient has no medical history suggestive of hypertension, diabetes, seizures, or other chronic disease. He does consume ibuprofen tablets for "tension headaches" at his job. He does not have chest pain, nor does he have a history of shortness of breath. There is no family history of chronic medical illness. Physical examination reveals a well-nourished male, who is afebrile and has normal vital signs. He has no pallor, cyanosis, or icterus. Examination of his cardiovascular and respiratory systems shows normal findings. Findings of his abdominal examination are normal as well. During his interaction with his primary care physician, he stated, rather warily, that he visited a prostitute on one of his travels and did not use protection. Examination of his genitalia did not reveal any abnormal physical findings. He was tested for sexually transmitted disease. His HIV Elisa test result was negative, as were results of the tests for chlamydia and herpes genitalis. His serum rapid plasmin reagin test result (RPR) showed a reaction at 1:10, and the microhemagglutination-*Treponema pallidum* (MHA-TP) showed a reaction as well. Which of the following statements about this patient is true?

(A) He should be treated with procaine penicillin
(B) He must have syphilis because the RPR test is specific
(C) The RPR assay should become nonreactive between 12 and 24 months after treatment
(D) His disease is not communicable, and his sexual partners do not need testing
(E) The MHA-TP should become nonreactive within 6 months after treatment

15 A 2-year-old male child from a Vietnamese immigrant family is brought to the emergency department by a Child Protective Services (CPS) worker for suspected physical abuse. The worker states that earlier that morning she received a call from a daycare facility that the child attends. According to the CPS worker the daycare employee stated that she thought that the child had been physically abused. The physician performs a thorough history and physical examination to determine

evidence of maltreatment. Which of the following would be specific evidence of child abuse in this case?

(A) Bruises on the back in a fir-tree pattern from "coining"
(B) A blue, nontender macular lesion in the presacral area
(C) Weight less than the 5th percentile
(D) Bruised knees
(E) A circular burn restricted to the buttocks

16 A 24-year-old man presents to the emergency room with fever, severe myalgias, and headache. He just returned from a trip to Alaska where he ate a variety of foods, including walrus meat. The patient has a temperature of 39°C (102.2°F), BP of 120/90 mm Hg, pulse of 95/min regular, and a respiratory rate of 20/min regular. The patient is in moderate distress. He has some pallor but no cyanosis. He has periorbital edema and subconjunctival hemorrhages affecting both eyes. There is evidence of blood under the bed of his fingernails. His heart sounds are normal, and he has sinus tachycardia. Findings of an examination of the respiratory system are normal. His abdominal examination also is unremarkable. Laboratory examination reveals a white blood cell (WBC) count of 9.5 cells/µL with 25% eosinophils. Which of the following is the best diagnostic test to first perform on this patient?

(A) Blood culture
(B) Stool examination for ova and parasites
(C) Muscle biopsy for histologic examination
(D) Echocardiogram
(E) Serologic test for febrile agglutinins

17 55-year-old man is being treated for diabetes, hypertension, and degenerative joint disease. His physician prescribed metformin for the diabetes; methyldopa, propranolol, and hydrochlorothiazide for his hypertension; and acetaminophen to treat the pain associated with degenerative joint disease. Over several months, he becomes increasingly withdrawn and apathetic. He loses interest in his family, work, and hobbies, and he spends much time brooding about his loss of health. Which of the following medications has been most consistently associated with his psychiatric symptoms?

(A) Hydrochlorothiazide
(B) Metformin
(C) Acetaminophen
(D) Methyldopa
(E) Propranolol

18 A 25 year-old female comes to the emergency room of a local hospital with severe right-sided headache that has not responded to treatment with ibuprofen or acetaminophen. She states that she has been having these headaches for quite some time and that the stress at her job makes them worse. During the attacks she also gets nausea and vomiting, and she sees bright flashes of light during the attacks. She prefers quiet. The most distressing symptom in this patient is most likely which of the following?

(A) Headache
(B) Nausea
(C) Vomiting
(D) Flashing lights
(E) Increased sensitivity to sound

19 A 13-year-old basketball player presents to the pediatrician with a limp and right knee pain for the last week. He tells the pediatrician that the basketball season has just begun and the training is physically demanding. The patient thinks that he may have pushed himself too hard during workouts. He reports that running, jumping, or climbing stairs exacerbates his knee pain. On physical examination the tibial tuberosity is enlarged. However, there is no synovial effusion or thickening of the knee joint. Which of the following is the most likely diagnosis?

(A) Legg-Calvé-Perthes disease
(B) Slipped capital femoral epiphysis
(C) Osgood-Schlatter disease
(D) Septic arthritis of the knee
(E) Idiopathic adolescent anterior knee pain syndrome

20 A 24-year-old female college student presents to the physician's office with complaints of watery diarrhea, abdominal cramping and bloating, and nausea. She returned from a backpacking trip in the mountains 4 days previously. The patient was in moderate distress, had mild pyrexia, moderate tachycardia, and normal blood pressure and respiratory rate. There was no pallor or cyanosis. She was mildly dehydrated, and showed no signs of icterus. The cardiovascular system was normal except for sinus tachycardia. The respiratory system was normal. The abdomen was soft, and there was diffuse tenderness without guarding. No masses were felt, and there was no organomegaly. Bowel sounds were increased. A complete blood count revealed leukocytosis, and the hematocrit was elevated. Her serum electrolytes revealed moderate hypernatremia but were otherwise unremarkable. Microscopic examination of stool revealed pear-shaped,

dorsally convex, flattened parasites with two nuclei and four pairs of flagella. Which of the following represents the best treatment for this patient?

(A) Reassurance
(B) Penicillin
(C) Tetracycline
(D) Azidothymidine (AZT)
(E) Metronidazole

21 A 29-year-old woman, gravida 2, para 2, had a liquid-based thin-layer cervical Pap smear performed in the office a week ago. A high-grade squamous intraepithelial lesion was reported. Human papilloma virus (HPV) typing was positive for serotypes 16 and 18. She returned to the office and underwent colposcopically directed cervical biopsy. The entire transformation zone was seen with no lesion entering the endocervical canal. A specimen from a biopsy of a lesion at 6 o'clock on the cervix exhibited abnormal vessels and mosaicism. The histologic report showed full-thickness dysplastic epithelial changes with malignant cells that had penetrated the basement membrane and had invaded lymphatics. Which of the following procedures would be considered appropriate in identifying the stage of her disease?

(A) Intravenous pyelogram
(B) Laparoscopy
(C) Exploratory laparotomy
(D) Lymphangiogram
(E) Lymphadenectomy

22 A 25-year-old man presents with complaints of dysuria for the past 6 days. He has had multiple sexual partners in the past 2 months. Physical examination shows a yellowish penile discharge with inguinal adenopathy but no genital ulcers. Gram's stain of the discharge shows intracellular gram-negative diplococci in leukocytes. Which of the following should be used in the treatment of this patient?

(A) Ceftriaxone
(B) Ciprofloxacin
(C) Procaine penicillin
(D) Ceftriaxone plus doxycycline
(E) Doxycycline

23 A 15-year-old boy is brought to the pediatrician for a school physical examination. The mother states that they have just moved to this area from Georgia. According to the mother the child, who is mentally retarded, has been in his usual state of good health. His past medical history is pertinent for a few ear infections and upper respiratory tract infections.

Although the mother did not bring the child's previous medical record with her, she believes that the patient's immunizations are current. Pertinent findings on the physical examination include a prominent jaw, protruding ears, macroorchidism, and developmental delay. Which of the following is the most likely diagnosis?

(A) Klinefelter's syndrome
(B) Trisomy 18
(C) Prader-Willi syndrome
(D) Trisomy 21
(E) Fragile X syndrome

24. A 44-year-old woman presents complaining of lower left leg pain. Three weeks ago, she started intensive training in preparation for an upcoming 10-kilometer race. Her pain becomes more severe while she is running and intermittently occurs while she is walking. On physical examination, there is localized tenderness at the junction of the middle and distal portions of the tibia. Which of the following is the most likely diagnosis?

(A) Stress fracture of the tibia
(B) Chronic exertional compartment syndrome
(C) Overuse myositis
(D) Acute compartment syndrome
(E) Anterior tibialis tendinitis

25. Prostate cancer is a very common malignancy in males, ranking ahead of colon cancer in the annual incidence of new cases and deaths, approximately 230,000 and 29,900 annually, respectively. The risk of developing it increases markedly with age, as indicated in the table below:

Risk of Prostate Cancer with Increasing Age

Age in Years	Percentage Risk Range
50–59	10–42
60–69	17–38
70–79	25–60
80 and over	Up to 90

Modified from the report of the U.S. Preventive Services Task Force: Guide to Clinical Preventive Services. 2nd ed. Williams & Wilkins, 1996;121.

Obviously, if you are male and live long enough there is a good chance you will develop prostate cancer. However, if you are old enough when you first develop the cancer you will probably die of something other than this malignancy, so it behooves men to reduce

their risk of developing or at least delaying the development of prostate cancer. Which of the following statements describes the most practical and effective method available for reducing or delaying the development of prostate cancer?

(A) Orchiectomy
(B) Take finasteride
(C) Eat an appropriate diet
(D) Avoid vasectomy
(E) Supplement a diet with 100 mg or more of zinc daily

26. A 26-year-old man with multiple fractures and soft-tissue injuries from a motorcycle accident has diffuse bleeding from all needle puncture sites and open wounds on the second day of hospitalization. His prothrombin time (PT) is 20 seconds (normal is 11–15 seconds), his partial thromboplastin time (PTT) is 100 seconds (normal is 60–85 seconds), and his platelet count is 45,000 cells/μL (normal is 150,000–400,000 cells/μL). Result of his d-dimer assay is positive. Which of the following is the most likely diagnosis?

(A) Thrombotic thrombocytopenic purpura (TTP)
(B) Disseminated intravascular coagulation (DIC)
(C) Fat embolism syndrome
(D) Primary fibrinolysis
(E) A circulating anticoagulant

27. A mother brings her 3-year-old son to the clinic with a history of recurrent blister formation after minor trauma. An interview with the mother reveals that this is a second marriage for both, and each parent brought two children into the union. The child in question is hers, and the step-father is an alcoholic, a heavy smoker, and has temper tantrums. Which of the following is the most likely diagnosis?

(A) Ehlers-Danlos syndrome
(B) Systemic sclerosis
(C) Epidermolysis bullosa
(D) Osteogenesis imperfecta
(E) Child abuse

28. A large multicenter trial was conducted to test the efficacy of a new screening test to confirm exposure to a viral disease of Asian origin. There were two groups of adults, one group had been exposed to the disease and the other had not. There were 600 adult men and women in each group. The mean age for each group was 35. Given the standardized 2 × 2

table below, which of the following options reflects the study group in a cohort study design?

	Disease Present (D+)	Disease Absent (D−)	Totals
Exposed (E+)	*a*	*b*	*a* + *b*
Nonexposed (E−)	*c*	*d*	*c* + *d*
Totals	*a* + *c*	*b* + *d*	

(A) *a* + *c*
(B) *c* + *b*
(C) *a* + *b*
(D) *c* + *d*
(E) (*a* + *c*) + (*c* + *d*)

29 A 65-year-old man makes an emergency appointment to see his family physician because of sudden loss of vision in the right eye. In presenting a history, the patient states that he first noticed it when he closed his left eye while taking aim at target practice. He further reveals that he has no pain, and other than a history of coronary artery disease, which causes angina, he has no other medical problems. His only medication is nitroglycerin sublingual tablets on an as-needed basis. Physical examination reveals a patient who is not in pain and has normal vital signs. His eyelids are normal. There is no conjunctival or circumcorneal injection. In the affected eye the anterior chamber appears normal and the pupil is moderately dilated and fails to react to direct light, but responds to consensual light reflex. Funduscopy reveals pallor of the optic disc, a cherry-red fovea, and bloodless arterioles. These findings are most consistent with which one of the following choices?

(A) Central retinal vein occlusion
(B) Acute angle-closure glaucoma
(C) Corneal abrasion
(D) Central retinal artery occlusion
(E) Optic neuritis

30 A 20-year-old African-American woman, gravida 3, para 2, has a history of a seizure disorder since 10 years of age. She is currently at 17 weeks' gestation and is being treated with phenytoin orally three times per day. A phenytoin level determined on a sample drawn a week ago is within the therapeutic range. First-trimester bleeding that spontaneously resolved with conservative management complicated her prenatal course. Blood for a maternal serum triple marker screen was drawn 10 days ago, but the results are not yet available. A complete blood count (CBC) was obtained as part of her routine prenatal laboratory tests. On her first prenatal visit she was given a pre-scription for prenatal vitamins. At this time, the following values are noted: hemoglobin (Hgb), 9.3; hematocrit (Hct), 29; mean corpuscular volume (MCV), 150 μm³ (normal is 80–100 μm³). Which of the following is the most likely diagnosis?

(A) Sickle cell trait
(B) Iron deficiency
(C) Physiologic anemia
(D) Folate deficiency
(E) Thalassemia

31 A 17-year-old woman presents to the emergency department with sudden onset of abdominal pain. She was playing in the school band when it began. She describes the pain as starting 30 minutes ago in the left lower quadrant without any radiation. The pain is 7 on a scale of 1 to 10 and not associated with nausea, vomiting, or diarrhea. Onset of menarche was age 13. Although initially her menses were irregular, she has had regular menstrual periods for the past 6 months. She has no fever, and her vital signs are stable. She is sexually active and is on combination oral contraceptive pills. She denies taking other medications. Physical examination reveals a flat abdomen with normal peristalsis. Pelvic examination reveals a normal vagina with a normal-appearing cervix. There is no mucopurulent cervical discharge. Bimanual examination is remarkable with a tender 5-cm mass in the left adnexa. A pregnancy test result is negative. A pelvic sonogram exhibits a 5 × 6 cm complex mass of the left ovary, with focal areas of calcification. Which of the following is the most likely diagnosis?

(A) Follicular cyst
(B) Mucinous cystadenoma
(C) Cystic teratoma
(D) Brenner tumor
(E) Serous cystadenoma

32 A 26-year-old flight attendant presents with a history of palpitations and difficulty breathing. She denies a history of allergies, long-term medications, or previous medical problems. She does not smoke but is a social drinker. Physical examination reveals a tall, medium-build female who appears anxious. Her vital signs are as follows: pulse, 88/min regular; blood pressure, 130/90 mm Hg; temperature, 37°C (98.6°F). Cyanosis, clubbing of the fingers, and pedal edema are absent. Which of the following is the most likely diagnosis?

(A) Aortic stenosis
(B) Mitral stenosis
(C) Aortic regurgitation
(D) Mitral regurgitation
(E) Congestive heart failure

33 A 27-year-old woman presents with a history of two episodes of agitation, pressured speech, grandiose delusions, and disorganized behavior. One episode occurred 4 years ago and lasted several weeks. The current episode has been present for 1 month. Between episodes, the woman is friendly, outgoing, and emotionally stable. Mental status examination reveals increased psychomotor activity and impaired judgment. Which of the following is the most likely diagnosis?

(A) Bipolar disorder, manic phase
(B) Brief psychotic disorder
(C) Delusional disorder, erotomanic type
(D) Major depressive disorder with mood congruent psychosis
(E) Schizophrenia

34 A 75-year-old man presents with puffiness of the face, arms, and shoulders associated with a bluish to purple discoloration of the skin. In addition, he complains of dizziness, shortness of breath, and cough. He has a 35 pack-year history of smoking. Physical examination reveals clubbing of the fingernails, emphysematous chest, and distended neck veins. The pathogenesis for this patient's findings most likely results from which of the following disorders?

(A) Primary lung cancer
(B) Pericardial effusion
(C) Sclerosing mediastinitis
(D) Polycythemia rubra vera
(E) Right ventricular failure

35 A 35-year-old man involved in an automobile accident is rushed to the nearest emergency room. The patient is conscious and in acute pain. He has tachypnea and sinus tachycardia, and his blood pressure is 90/60 mm Hg. He has bruising over the left lower rib cage, and point tenderness is noted here. Air entry is normal in both lungs. These findings are most likely secondary to which of the following?

(A) Pulmonary contusion with hemorrhage into the pleural cavity
(B) Rupture of the spleen
(C) Rupture of the colon
(D) Transection of the abdominal aorta
(E) Rupture of the kidney

36 A 7-month-old infant is brought to the emergency department. The mother states that the patient had been previously well but fell from a sofa onto the carpeted floor while taking a nap. The infant cried immediately according to the mother. However, on physical examination the child is noted to be lethargic. He is also noted to have retinal hemorrhages. Computed tomography of the head is performed and shows a subdural hematoma. After initial stabilization of this patient which of the following is the most appropriate next step in management?

(A) Administer a pain reliever
(B) Notify the patient's primary care provider
(C) Contact the state agency that deals with child abuse
(D) Obtain consent from the mother to admit the infant to the hospital
(E) Tell the parents that you suspect that the child has been abused

37 At a routine prenatal visit, a 28-year-old woman, gravida 5, para 4, at 28 weeks' gestation reports that she has not felt the baby move for 2 days. She first felt fetal movement at 17 weeks' gestation. She denies any vaginal bleeding or fluid leakage. Her pregnancy has been complicated by chronic hypertension for which she is being treated with twice-daily tablets of methyldopa. She is afebrile and her vital signs are stable. On physical examination you measure the fundal height at an appropriate 30 cm. Four weeks ago the fundus measured 26 cm. Leopold's maneuvers reveal the fetus to be in transverse lie. Her blood pressure is 145/85 mm Hg. A urine dipstick test result is negative for albumin. You are unable to obtain fetal heart tones with a Doppler fetoscope. Which of the following is the most appropriate next step in the management of this patient?

(A) Perform a nonstress test
(B) Perform an amniocentesis
(C) Obtain a real-time ultrasound assessment for cardiac motion
(D) Obtain a maternal abdominal x-ray assessment of the fetus
(E) Perform a quantitative β-human chorionic gonadotropin (HCG) assay

38 As a teenager a 46-year-old man secretly set several major fires that caused much property damage. He was never caught and says that he rarely thinks about what he now calls "dead history." Although he is married and works as an accountant, he spends many weekends planting trees in parklands and volunteering as a firefighter. Which of the following defense mechanism is most strongly suggested by this behavior?

(A) Denial
(B) Dissociation
(C) Intellectualization
(D) Sublimation
(E) Undoing

39 A 31-year-old woman seeks medical assessment for an overwhelming number of physical complaints involving practically every organ system. She has seen numerous physicians over the last 10 years and describes them all as "quacks." A complete medical assessment yields unremarkable findings. Which of the following is the most appropriate next step in the management of this patient?

(A) Refusal to see her again
(B) A warning to use medical resources sparingly
(C) Referral to another clinician
(D) Regularly scheduled medical visits
(E) Trials of various medications

40 A 35-year old single female was taking a shower while vacationing in Hawaii. While applying soap onto her body, she felt a lump in her left breast. She was alarmed, as she had never felt the lump before, and it seemed to have crept up on her without causing any pain or discomfort. The patient was nulliparous, had a healthy lifestyle, and exercised regularly. She had no medical illness, did not smoke, and imbibed alcohol sparingly. Physical examination revealed a healthy slim woman who was rather anxious. Apart from a moderate tachycardia brought on by anxiety, her vital signs were normal. The left breast revealed an indrawn nipple. However, no nipple discharge was noted. A nontender hard lump that was immobile and measured approximately 2 × 3 cm was felt in the left breast. Examination of the axilla revealed no palpable lymph nodes. Examination of the right breast and axilla yielded normal findings. Examination of the cardiovascular and respiratory systems also yielded normal findings. Abdominal examination was unremarkable. The most likely location where the lump was discovered would be:

(A) Lower inner quadrant of the breast
(B) Upper inner quadrant of the breast
(C) Lower outer quadrant of the breast
(D) Upper outer quadrant of the breast
(E) Subjacent to the areola.

Directions for Matching Questions (41 through 50): Each set of matching questions is preceded by a list of 4 to 26 lettered options followed by a brief explanation of the required task and then by a series of numbered statements. For each lettered statement you are to select ONE LETTERED OPTION that best fulfills the task as it relates to that statement. Remember each of the listed options might be correctly selected once, more than once, or not at all.

Questions 41–44

(A) Red blood cell (RBC) casts
(B) White blood cell (WBC) casts
(C) Hyaline casts
(D) Renal tubular cell casts
(E) Waxy casts
(F) Fatty casts

Select the ONE urinary finding listed above that best fits the conditions described below.

41 Urinary finding in an 8-year-old boy with anasarca and a 24-hour urine protein level above 3.5 g

42 Urinary finding that distinguishes acute pyelonephritis from acute cystitis

43 Urinary finding that indicates a patient with end stage renal disease

44 Urinary finding that would be expected in a 12-year-old child who develops hypertension, periorbital edema, and pink-colored urine 2 weeks after recovering from scarlet fever

Questions 45–46

(A) Altruism
(B) Blocking
(C) Denial
(D) Displacement
(E) Dissociation
(F) Distortion
(G) Intellectualization
(H) Projection
(I) Rationalization
(J) Reaction formation
(K) Regression
(L) Repression
(M) Sublimation
(N) Undoing

Match each patient with the ONE most closely associated defense mechanism on the previous page.

45 A political figure is engaged in a televised debate and comes under increasing pressure from his opponent. As his anxiety mounts, he begins to lose his poise, interrupt his opponent, and attack his character. He finally throws down his papers and stalks offstage angrily.

46 A man with a dubious record of compliance with Internal Revenue Service (IRS) regulations faces a tax audit. He begins to speak a great deal about "welfare cheats" and other people who do not pay their fair share of the costs of society.

Questions 47–50 Medicine

(A) Acetaminophen with codeine

(B) Rofecoxib

(C) Auranofin

(D) Alendronate

(E) Fluoxetine

(F) Allopurinol

(G) Cyclosporine ophthalmic emulsion

(H) Ibuprofen

Select the ONE most appropriate drug to prescribe for the patient and/or condition described below.

47 Prescribed for a 109-lb 74-year-old woman of Chinese descent who has no obvious medical problems other than a pronounced buffalo hump

48 Drug prescribed for a 35-year-old male by his dentist after performing a root canal procedure

49 A drug prescribed for a 37-year-old woman to stop the ravages of rheumatoid arthritis. Her pain is already adequately controlled.

50 Prescribed for a 55-year-old male who is overweight, has an inflamed big toe on his right foot, and a higher than normal serum uric acid level

Answer Key

1 A		**11** A		**21** A		**31** C		**41** F
2 C		**12** D		**22** D		**32** D		**42** B
3 D		**13** C		**23** E		**33** A		**43** E
4 D		**14** C		**24** A		**34** A		**44** A
5 D		**15** E		**25** C		**35** B		**45** K
6 E		**16** C		**26** B		**36** C		**46** H
7 B		**17** D		**27** C		**37** C		**47** D
8 C		**18** D		**28** C		**38** E		**48** A
9 E		**19** C		**29** D		**39** D		**49** C
10 A		**20** E		**30** D		**40** D		**50** F

Answers and Explanations

1 **The answer is A**   *Obstetrics and Gynecology*

Placenta previa is bleeding arising from a placenta abnormally implanted in the lower uterine segment. The bleeding is typically painless and is mediated by normal stretching of the lower uterine segment, which avulses the anchoring placental villi (choice **A**).

Abruptio placenta (choice **B**) usually involves painful bleeding from a normally implanted placenta. Risk factors include severe preeclampsia, blunt abdominal trauma, and cocaine use. Bleeding from vasa previa (choice **C**) is of fetal origin, mediated by either spontaneous or artificial rupture of a fetal vessel traversing the membranes overlying the cervix. While the mother's vital signs remain stable, the bleeding from the fetoplacental circulation usually results in exsanguination of the fetus. The normal fetal heart rate with no decelerations rules this diagnosis out. A bloody show (choice **D**) is usually blood-tinged mucus from early cervical dilation and would not have significant clots. Uterine rupture (choice **E**) is often a catastrophic event for both mother and fetus and is never painless.

2 **The answer is C**   *Pediatrics*

The specific antidote for nicotinic manifestations of organophosphate toxicity is pralidoxime (2-PAM) (choice **C**). It restores the activity of acetylcholinesterase. Nicotinic effects for organophosphates include fasciculations, twitching, weakness, areflexia, tachycardia, and hypertension.

Atropine (choice **A**) is an antidote for the muscarinic effects of organophosphate toxicity. Some muscarinic effects include salivation, lacrimation, urination, defecation, and abdominal cramps. British antilewisite (BAL) (choice **B**) and calcium disodium ethylenediaminetetraacetate (Ca-EDTA) (choice **D**) are used for the treatment of lead toxicity. These therapies are used in patients with a venous blood lead level concentration of 70μg/dL or above. Ca-EDTA and BAL are used in combination for children with encephalopathy or evidence of encephalopathy. Naloxone (choice **E**) is used as an antidote for opioid poisoning.

3 **The answer is D**   *Preventive Medicine and Public Health*

A laboratory test shows how often the result is positive in patients with a disease; that is, the sensitivity of the test ("positivity in disease") and how often the test result is negative (normal) in persons who do not have the disease; that is, the specificity of the test ("negativity in health"). A test that is performed on persons with a disease can return with a positive or negative test result. A positive test result is called a *true-positive* (TP), whereas a negative test result is called a *false-negative* (FN). An FN misclassifies the patient as normal. Similarly, a test that is performed on a normal person can return with a negative or positive test result. A negative test result is called a *true-negative* (TN), whereas a positive test result is called a *false-positive* (FP). An FP misclassifies the person as having the disease.

The sensitivity of the test is established by testing only patients with known disease, who may have positive (TP) or negative (FN) test results. The formula is as follows: Sensitivity = TP/TP + FN × 100. A test with 100% sensitivity has no FNs; that is, every person in the known disease population has a positive result. Therefore, a negative (normal) test result must be a TN rather than an FN, because the test has no FNs. This test then qualifies as useful in screening for disease because normal test results exclude disease. However, a positive test result may represent a TP or an FP, so another test must be performed. Note that the formula for sensitivity says nothing about the FP rate, because it deals only with the diseased population.

The specificity of a test applies only to normal persons, who can have negative (TN) or positive (FP) test results. The formula is as follows:

$$\text{Specificity} = TN/TN + FP \times 100$$

A test with 100% specificity has no FPs; that is, the result is always normal in normal persons. Therefore, the test result must be a TP. However, a normal test result can represent a TN or an FN, because nothing in the formula relates to findings in the diseased population (e.g., the FN rate). A test with 100% specificity is useful for confirming disease because a positive test result must be a TP and not an FP.

Ideally, a test with 100% sensitivity is first used on a patient who is suspected of having a particular disease. If the test result is negative, that patient does not have that disease. However, if the test result is positive, a test with 100% specificity is used. If that test result is positive, the screening test result is a TP. However, if that test result is negative, the screening test result is an FP. For example, if the physician thinks that a patient is human immunodeficiency virus (HIV)–positive, the first test to order is an enzyme-linked immunosorbent assay (ELISA). If the test result is negative, the patient is not HIV-positive. However, if the test result is positive, a Western blot assay is automatically performed. If this test result is also positive, the ELISA screen is a TP. If the test result is negative (normal), the ELISA screen is an FP. In this example, the ELISA test has a high sensitivity and can screen for HIV, whereas the Western blot assay has a high specificity and can confirm HIV positivity.

The reference interval for the test can be adjusted to create a test with high sensitivity or high specificity. Note that the test illustrated shows an overlap of the normal and cancer populations between 2.5 and 5 ng/mL; this area includes normal persons and persons with disease. Establishing a test with 100% sensitivity (no FNs) means setting the upper limit of the reference interval at that value at the beginning of the disease curve. In this case, the reference interval is 0–2.5 ng/mL. This range has no FNs. However, a positive test result (>2.5 ng/mL) does not necessarily mean that the patient has the disease; i.e., some normal persons are in the overlap area between 2.5 and 5 ng/mL. These patients are considered FPs (choice **B**). Thus, creating a test with 100% sensitivity automatically lowers the specificity of the test because some persons with a positive test result are FPs.

Establishing a test with 100% specificity (no FPs) means setting the value at the end of the normal curve as the upper limit of normal. In this case, it is 0–5 ng/mL (choice **A**). Note that test results above 5 ng/mL are all TPs (choice **E**). However, a normal test result (0–5 ng/mL) does not mean that the patient is normal. The overlap area between 2.5 and 5 ng/mL contains some persons with the disease. These patients are classified as FNs. Thus, creating a test with 100% specificity automatically lowers the sensitivity of the test because the number of FNs is increased.

With this information, if the reference interval is 0–5 ng/mL (100% specificity) and a test result is 4 ng/mL, the test result is either a TN or an FN (choice **D**). The sensitivity of the test is decreased in this interval because there are more FNs, but the specificity of the test is 100% because there are no FPs beyond 5 ng/mL. A reference interval of 0–2.5 ng/mL creates a test with 100% sensitivity (choice **C**). Test results between 2.5 and 5 ng/mL are either TPs or FPs because some normal persons are in the overlap area.

4 | The answer is D *Medicine*

Creatine kinase (CK) is a dimeric protein with two types of subunits, the M-type (CK_3) and the brain BB type (CK_1). The myocardium is the only tissue that expresses the MB hybrid at significant concentration. As a consequence, an increase in the circulating level of the MB isozyme specifically signifies damage to heart muscle. After an MI the MB begins to rise within 4 to 8 hours, peaks in 24 hours, and disappears in 36 to 72 hours. Thus its presence 4 days after the initial infarct signifies reinfarction (choice **D**).

Recurrent pain (choice **A**) could be due to reinfarction, gastroesophageal reflux, or a vivid imagination. A third heart sound (choice **B**) is usually a low-pitched sound that is apical in location. It is physiologic in children. However, after the age of 30, it signifies volume overload or left ventricular failure. Bibasilar rales (choice **C**) usually occur in congestive cardiac failure. The patient would be dyspneic and may have cyanosis and distended jugular veins. In patients with extensive myocardial infarction, bibasilar rales and a third heart sound could result from the reasons elaborated above. Lactate dehydrogenase (LDH) isoenzymes are composed of tetramers of H and M polypeptides. These polypeptides form five distinct isoenzymes, which are numbered from 1 to 5. These isoenzymes are tissue specific. LDH_1 and LDH_2 are primarily located in the red blood cells, cardiac muscle, and the kidneys. LDH_3 is located primarily in the lungs, while LDH_4 and LDH_5 are found in the skeletal muscles, skin, and liver. The wide distribution of these enzymes therefore limits their usefulness. However, in myocardial infarction, they are useful in ruling out other causes of chest pain. The proportion of these polypeptides varies from tissue to tissue. LDH_2 is in greatest concentration and that of LDH_1 exceeds LDH_3. The concentrations of

LDH$_3$ and LDH$_4$, on the other hand, are almost equal to one another. The concentrations of LDH$_1$ and LDH$_2$ in red blood cells and myocardial tissue are as follows:

Location	Activity of LDH$_1$	Activity of LDH$_2$
Red blood cell	Low	High
Cardiac muscle	High	Low

Therefore, in normal situations, the concentration LDH$_1$ in the serum will remain low, and that of LDH$_2$ high, because there is no myocardial damage nor hemolysis. Following myocardial tissue damage, LDH$_1$ will spill into the blood. As a result, the concentration of LDH$_1$ in the serum will exceed that of LDH$_2$, resulting in the flip. The LDH$_1$/LDH$_2$ flip has a sensitivity of 80% and a specificity of 95%. However it is first evident 14 hours post-MI, peaks in 2 to 3 days, and disappears in 7 days. Therefore, in this patient, who is 4 days post-myocardial infarction, one would expect to find an LDH$_1$/LDH$_2$ flip (choice **E**) even in the absence of reinfarction, as the flip remains for up to 7 days. Therefore, in this case it does not contribute to the diagnosis of reinfarction.

5 The answer is D *Pediatrics*

The Arnold-Chiari syndrome type II consists of progressive hydrocephalus and myelomeningocele. The hydrocephalus is a noncommunicating one (choice **D**). The fourth ventricle is elongated, there is kinking of the brainstem, and portions of the brainstem and cerebellum are displaced into the cervical spinal canal, causing obstruction of flow of cerebrospinal fluid (CSF). Skull films show a small posterior fossa and widened cervical canal (platybasia). Type I Chiari malformation is usually not associated with hydrocephalus and is first noted during adolescence or adult life.

A leptomeningeal cyst (choice **E**) is a rare and late complication of a linear skull fracture and appears as an expanding pulsatile mass on the surface of the skull. Chronic subdural hematomas (choice **B**) are characterized by headache, personality change, and loss of consciousness. Classically, patients with epidural hematoma (choice **A**) experience a brief period of unconsciousness followed by a variable lucid interval and are unconsciousness thereafter. Expansion of the hematoma also leads to headache, vomiting, and focal neurologic signs. Children who are victims of shaken baby syndrome have acute subdural hematomas. In addition, retinal hemorrhages are present, and there may be additional clinical evidence to support child abuse (choice **C**).

6 The answer is E *Psychiatry*

This patient's worrying suggests hypochondriasis, which is characterized by misinterpretation of the meaning of a physical symptom. Moreover, this patient does not respond to physician reassurance after an adequate workup. Hypochondriacal symptoms usually become evident during periods of psychologic stress. Resolution of the stressor through brief psychotherapy that includes exploration of current life problems (choice **E**) often results in symptom resolution.

By definition, reassurance (choice **A**) and explanations (choice **C**) are ineffective and suggesting she have frequent follow-ups will only reinforce her fear that there is something wrong. Benzodiazepines (choice **B**) may be used to help reduce anxiety; however, they cannot be considered central to treatment because they will not alleviate the psychologic stressors that presumptively cause the condition, and they carry a risk of creating drug dependency if used over a long period. Placebo (choice **D**) response is usually temporary, at best.

7 The answer is B *Surgery*

Boerhaave's syndrome (choice **B**) refers to a full-thickness rupture of the distal thoracic esophagus or stomach and is associated with vomiting or retching. In most cases, this syndrome is associated with alcoholics who have forceful vomiting or retching. However, it is also the most serious complication of bulimia nervosa, an eating disorder associated with binging on excessive amounts of food followed by self-induced vomiting.

Gastroesophageal reflux (choice **A**), tension pneumothorax (choice **C**), gastric ulcer disease (choice **D**), and esophageal cancer (choice **E**) all may cause retrosternal pain but are not associated with vomiting and bulimia.

8 The answer is C *Medicine*

Hypoparathyroidism is most commonly caused by a total thyroidectomy. Because parathormone (PTH) normally increases calcium reabsorption in the kidney and decreases the reabsorption of phosphate, patients develop hypocalcemia, hyperphosphatemia, and decreased PTH (choice **C**). Hypocalcemia results in clinical evidence of tetany, such as carpal spasm after pumping up a blood pressure cuff (Trousseau's sign) and facial muscle contractions after tapping on the facial nerve (Chvostek's sign).

Hypercalcemia, hypophosphatemia, and increased PTH (choice **A**) are present in primary hyperparathyroidism, which is most commonly (85% of the time) due to a benign parathyroid adenoma. It is the most common cause of hypercalcemia in the ambulatory population. Hypercalcemia, hypophosphatemia, and decreased PTH (choice **B**) are characteristic of malignancy-induced hypercalcemia. This condition is most commonly due to secretion of a PTH-like peptide that acts on the kidney. The result is increased calcium reabsorption (hypercalcemia) and decreased phosphorus reabsorption (hypophosphatemia), but the hypercalcemia suppresses the patient's own PTH production. Other mechanisms for hypercalcemia in malignancy relate to the secretion of osteoclast-activating factor or prostaglandins. Hypocalcemia, hypophosphatemia, and increased PTH (choice **D**) are seen in malabsorption of vitamin D due to celiac disease or other gastrointestinal (GI) diseases. Vitamin D normally increases the reabsorption of both calcium and phosphorus from the gut. Therefore, deficiency results in hypocalcemia and hypophosphatemia, the former serving as a potent stimulus for PTH synthesis and secondary hyperparathyroidism. Hypocalcemia, hyperphosphatemia, and increased PTH (choice **E**) are seen in renal failure. Because PTH normally increases the synthesis of the hydroxylating enzyme located in the renal tubules and is responsible for the second hydroxylation step of vitamin D, renal disease results in functional hypovitaminosis D, with subsequent hypocalcemia and secondary hyperparathyroidism. The kidney is also the excretion route for phosphate; therefore, renal failure results in retention of phosphate. This constellation of findings is also seen in pseudohypoparathyroidism, which is a genetic disease that is associated with resistance of the target tissue to PTH. Therefore, hypocalcemia and hyperphosphatemia are present; but, unlike primary hypoparathyroidism, the PTH is usually increased.

9 The answer is E *Surgery*

This patient has a varicocele involving the pampiniform plexus of veins. The classic description of this is that it feels like a bag of worms. Varicoceles are benign conditions and may be associated with a small hydrocele. However, the main concern on the left side is the presence of a latent renal carcinoma that can herald itself by presenting as a varicocele. This is because the right testicular vein drains directly into the inferior vena cava, the left testicular vein on the other hand, drains into the left renal vein. As a consequence, renal carcinoma (choice **E**), can infiltrate into the left renal vein and block the inflow of blood from the left testicular vein, leading to backup and dilated veins in the scrotum. In such instances, the varicocele will not decompress when the patient is lying supine. Hence, the presence of renal carcinoma should be excluded at the earliest, rather than just dealing with the varicocele itself.

Torsion of the testis (choice **A**) is an unlikely diagnosis. This is usually associated with severe lower abdominal pain, retching, and vomiting, and the testis will be exquisitely tender. Moreover, the testis will be lying in a horizontal position. This man also does not have an incarcerated inguinal hernia (choice **B**). An incarcerated inguinal hernia will usually extrude from the inguinal canal into the scrotum. The scrotum will be swollen and tender. Dilated veins will not be found. The hernia will be distinct from the testis and will fail to reduce. Furthermore, one will not be able to "get above the swelling." Fournier's gangrene, (choice **C**), also known as idiopathic scrotal edema, is a rare condition. Scrotal inflammation occurs suddenly, followed by rapid onset of gangrene. This leads to sloughing of the scrotal skin. Patients usually have severe scrotal pain, fever, prostration, and pallor. Treatment involves antibiotics and analgesics. Epididymitis (choice **D**) in young men most commonly results from sexually transmitted disease. Chlamydia is the leading cause, followed by gonorrhea. The epididymis is tender to palpation; however no dilated veins or scrotal swelling is noted. If it spreads to the testis, the resultant disorder is called epididymo-orchitis.

10 The answer is A *Pediatrics*

The most common cause of blood in the stool of a newborn is swallowed maternal blood. The Apt test (choice **A**) helps distinguish adult hemoglobin (Hb) from fetal Hb. It is easier and less expensive than electrophoresis (choice **B**). If adult Hb is detected, the blood swallowed is maternal blood. If fetal Hb is found, a search begins for the cause of the bleeding.

A barium enema (choice **C**) is both diagnostic and therapeutic for intussusception, which is rare before 3 months of age. The Clinitest (choice **D**) is used to quantify the urinary level of reducing sugars. The presence of leukocytes in the stool is determined by the methylene blue stain (choice **E**).

11 The answer is A *Obstetrics and Gynecology*

The case scenario is characteristic of primary dysmenorrhea, which is classically associated with normal pelvic examination findings. Onset is typically within 2 years of menarche when ovulatory cycles begin. When progesterone withdrawal bleeding occurs, there is prostaglandin-induced spiral arteriolar spasm resulting in excessive myometrial contractions (choice **A**), which cause uterine ischemia and pain.

Myometrial irritation from ectopic endometrial glands (choice **B**) is known as adenomyosis. This is a cause of secondary dysmenorrhea and is associated with an enlarged, soft, tender uterus. Pelvic congestion from dilated spiral arterioles (choice **C**) is also associated with a tender, enlarged uterus. Excessive endometrial proliferation from unopposed estrogen (choice **D**) is found with chronic anovulatory syndromes but does not result in pain. Bleeding into proliferated myometrial fibroids (choice **E**) is known as red or carneous degeneration. This occurs with high-estrogen states such as pregnancy when fibroid proliferation occurs so rapidly the fibroid outgrows its own blood supply resulting in ischemia and severe pain. This is not a cause of primary dysmenorrhea.

12 The answer is D *Medicine*

The disease described is cutaneous sporotrichosis, caused by the fungus *Sporothrix schenckii*. It is found on plants in many areas of the world and can cause infection when minor trauma inoculates the fungus into the subcutaneous tissue.

Spread of the infection along lymphangitic channels is common, but extracutaneous forms of infection are rare. Pain is unusual. Diagnosis is confirmed by culture of a skin biopsy or, when present, pus from a draining pustule. Without treatment, the infection becomes chronic and usually does not heal. Oral administration of a saturated solution of potassium iodide (SSKI) (choice **D**) is the classic and least expensive mode of treatment.

Amphotericin B (choice **C**) is primarily used for extracutaneous forms. The newer azoles (itraconazole and fluconazole) are better tolerated and more effective than SSKI. Dicloxacillin (choice **A**), erythromycin (choice **B**), and cephalexin (choice **E**) are antibiotics used to treat bacterial, not fungal, infections.

13 The answer is C *Pediatrics*

There is a strong association between galactosemia and *Escherichia coli* (choice **C**) sepsis, which may be a presenting feature in infants with galactosemia. Classic galactosemia results from a deficiency of galactose-1-phosphate uridyltransferase. Galactose, derived from lactose (milk sugar), is not metabolized past galactose-1-phosphate, which then accumulates and damages the liver, kidney, and brain. Galactitol, a polyol byproduct of galactose, also can accumulate, causing cataracts. Among other manifestations are jaundice, hepatomegaly, hypoglycemia, vomiting, aminoaciduria, and failure to thrive. Early diagnosis is important, and dietary management contributes to a good prognosis. Although group B streptococcus (choice **A**), *Listeria monocytogenes* (choice **B**), *Staphylococcus aureus* (choice **D**), and pneumococcus *(Streptococcus pneumoniae)* (choice **E**) are also pathogens seen in neonatal sepsis, only *E. coli* has a strong association with galactosemia.

14 The answer is C *Medicine*

This patient has latent syphilis because he has no physical findings to point to the disease, but has a positive result for a screening test that is highly sensitive. The diagnosis of syphilis is usually made by serology. The highly sensitive nontreponemal tests (also known as reagin tests) VDRL and RPR are used for initial screening. They usually become nonreactive after 1 year of treatment (choice **C**). They are called *nontreponemal* because they are directed against a cardiolipin–lecithin–cholesterol antigen and not against the spirochete itself. False-positive VDRL and RPR test results occur in many conditions, but the titers rarely exceed 1:8. In those who are suspected of having the disease titers above 1:8 have a false-positive incidence of 1–3%. Patients with HIV and IV drug users may have concomitant syphilis. Treponemal tests, that target the spirochete, such as the FTA-ABS (fluorescent treponemal antibody absorbed test) and MHA-TP (microhemagglutination-*Treponema pallidum* test) are highly specific. They confirm syphilis when nontreponemal tests are positive, identify false-positive VDRL and RPR results, and, unlike the nontreponemal tests, remain positive even after therapy. Evaluation for neurosyphilis by examining the cerebrospinal fluid obtained by lumbar puncture is recommended for those with neurologic symptoms and signs. Other indications include untreated syphilis, failed therapy, disease for more than 1 year, or a serum VDRL or RPR titer above 1:32. Cerebrospinal fluid examination should also be done in patients with a positive VDRL or RPR result after 1 year of treatment.

Choice **A** is incorrect. Because of the organism's unusually slow rate of multiplication, a long exposure to medication is required. Therefore, short-acting penicillins, such as procaine penicillin, will be ineffectual. The treatment of choice for primary, secondary or early latent syphilis is penicillin G benzathine. For neurosyphilis, the treatment is aqueous penicillin G or aqueous penicillin G procaine with oral probenecid. Tetracycline is approved for treatment of patients who are allergic to penicillin. Treatment should be monitored by determining quantitative VDRL or RPR titers repeated in the first, third, sixth, and twelfth month. If the titer rises or it fails to fall fourfold or if the symptoms recur, the patient should be retreated and cerebrospinal fluid examined to exclude the presence of neurosyphilis. Choice **B** is incorrect because RPR is not a specific test but a sensitive one. Choice **D** is incorrect because the disease is communicable and sexual partners should be tested. Choice **E** is incorrect. Treponemal test results remain positive even after treatment.

15 The answer is E *Pediatrics*

Specific evidence of child abuse includes old healed fractures, belt marks, bruises on the buttocks or lower back (areas where children are unlikely to harm themselves), subdural hematomas, and rupture of internal organs. Hot-water-dunking burns occur when a parent holds the child's thigh against the abdomen and places the buttocks and perineum in scalding water. This causes a circular type of burn restricted to the buttocks (choice **E**). The hands and feet are spared, which is not compatible with falling into a tub. Evidence of sexual abuse includes genital or anal trauma, sexually transmitted disease, and urinary tract infection.

Coin rubbing (choice **A**) is a nonabusive healing practice of the Vietnamese that involves vigorous stroking of the skin of a febrile child, producing a peculiar bruising pattern. A blue, nontender lesion in the presacral area (choice **B**) is a "Mongolian spot" often seen in African-American, Oriental, and East Indian infants. Unlike a bruise, the Mongolian spot does not change color. Although caloric insufficiency from child abuse may explain weight below the 5th percentile for age (choice **C**), it is not the sole reason for failure to thrive. Bruised knees (choice **D**) are commonly seen in children of this age because of falls and are not specific evidence of child abuse.

16 The answer is C *Medicine*

The symptoms of fever, myalgias, periorbital edema, hemorrhages, and eosinophilia are suggestive of trichinosis, especially in a patient with a history of eating potentially infected meat. The most common cause is ingestion of infected, undercooked pork products, but it can also be found in a variety of carnivorous and omnivorous animals including walrus. Diagnosis is made by a muscle biopsy in which histologic examination (choice **C**) shows larvae of *Trichinella spiralis* encysted in the muscle. Currently available antihelminthic drugs are ineffective against the larvae in muscle, and therapy is primarily supportive.

Because the cysts are in muscle, they will not be found in blood (choice **A**) or stool (choice **B**). An echocardiogram (choice **D**) will not identify them in heart muscle. There is no specific serologic test for febrile agglutinins (choice **E**).

17 The answer is D *Psychiatry*

His symptoms of becoming increasingly withdrawn and apathetic are strongly suggestive of a depressive episode. There is a relationship between hypertension and depression. Studies show that hypertensive patients run a higher risk of undergoing a depressive episode than normotensive individuals and vice versa. Several different mechanisms have been postulated. One is that certain drugs used to treat hypertension promote depression, and some drugs used to treat depression affect blood pressure; in the latter case this effect is, not surprisingly, most strongly demonstrated by the monoamine oxidase inhibitors. Although one can still read articles that implicate hypertensive agents in general as potential causes of depression, a high risk appears to be limited to reserpine, and methyldopa (choice **D**). Methyldopa is a centrally acting α_2 agonist, while reserpine depletes the brain of norepinephrine and serotonin (possibly accounting for its action as a depressant) and the peripheral store of norepinephrine in the sympathetic nerve terminal. Although some studies also implicate the β-blocker propranolol as potentially having a risk of causing depression, others do not; in this case competition for cytochrome P450 isozymes is the cited mechanism, implying that this effect is only seen if the patient is already being treated with an antidepressant.

The antihypertensives clonidine, guanethidine, prazosin, and hydralazine, and thiazide diuretics, such as hydrochlorothiazide (choice **A**) all may have some, but if so only low, risk of causing depression. Other agents used to combat hypertension including angiotensin-converting enzyme (ACE) inhibitors, calcium channel blockers, and nonthiazide diuretics have not been implicated in causing depression. Neither have oral hypoglycemic agents such as metformin (choice **B**) or the analgesic acetaminophen (choice **C**).

18 The answer is D *Medicine*

The most distressing symptom is photophobia. Flashing lights (choice **D**) tend to zigzag within the visual field. Patients have a hard time keeping their eyes open, as even the available light tends to distress them. Headache (choice **A**) while severe and throbbing is not as distressing. It can be relieved by medication. Likewise, nausea (choice **B**) and vomiting (choice **C**) can be relieved and are not as distressing as photophobia. While there is certainly increased sensitivity to sound (choice **E**), it is not as distressing as photophobia.

19 The answer is C *Pediatrics*

Osgood-Schlatter disease (choice **C**) is an overuse injury that is more common in physically active boys around puberty. It is characterized by pain and swelling of the tibial tubercle. The treatment is focused on reduction of the activity. Antiinflammatory medications are usually not helpful. The condition is usually self-limiting and resolves in 12–24 months.

Legg-Calvé-Perthes (choice **A**) presents with a gradual limp, stiffness, and pain in the groin, hip, thigh, or knee. This avascular necrosis of the femoral head usually occurs between the ages of 2 and 12 years (mean 7 years). Slipped capital femoral epiphysis (choice **B**) typically occurs in adolescents who are overweight and have delayed skeletal maturity or those who are tall and thin and have had a recent growth spurt. The chronic condition is associated with endocrine abnormalities such as hypothyroidism. Septic arthritis (choice **D**) is an infection within a joint space causing pain and limitation of motion. Analysis of the joint fluid is mandatory for diagnosis. Patients with idiopathic adolescent anterior knee pain syndrome (choice **E**) formally known as chondromalacia patellae develop knee pain of unknown cause in early adolescence. Strenuous physical activity such as running may cause knee pain in these adolescents. However, there are no other associated findings.

20 The answer is E *Medicine*

This patient is suffering from giardiasis, a widespread protozoal disease that causes diarrhea, abdominal pain, bloating, belching, flatus, nausea, and vomiting. Surface waters, such as mountain streams, are at risk for contamination. Treatment with metronidazole (choice **E**) or quinacrine is effective, with cure rates over 80%. Infections are caused by ingestion of the hardy cysts, which exist in the duodenum and live and multiply in the small intestine. Acute giardiasis usually lasts for more than a week, but untreated infections can become chronic and last for years. Therefore, reassurance (choice **A**) is not the appropriate treatment. Humoral responses appear to be important for development of immunity because patients with hypogammaglobulinemia commonly suffer from prolonged, severe infections that are resistant to treatment.

Penicillin (choice **B**) and tetracycline (choice **C**) are effective against bacteria but have no effect on protozoa. Azidothymidine (AZT) (choice **D**) is used to combat human immunodeficiency virus (HIV) infections and has no antiprotozoal activity.

21 The answer is A *Obstetrics and Gynecology*

Cervical cancer is the third most common female reproductive malignancy; it is responsible for 20% of all gynecologic cancers. The prevalence of cervical cancer has been markedly decreased over the past decades because of the widespread use of the Pap smear for cytologic screening. The most common tumor type is squamous cell carcinoma. This is the only gynecologic cancer that is not surgically staged. Although staging is clinical, intravenous pyelogram (choice **A**) can be used.

Laparoscopy (choice **B**) is not used for surgical staging of any gynecologic cancer because adequate visualization can not be achieved. Exploratory laparotomy (choice **C**) is used for staging of ovarian and endometrial carcinoma. Lymphangiogram (choice **D**) and lymphadenectomy (choice **E**) may be helpful in assessing spread of vulvar cancer but are not used for cervical cancer staging.

22 The answer is D *Medicine*

This patient has gonococcal urethritis (GCU), which is caused by *Neisseria gonorrhoeae.* GCU is more common among homosexual men and those of the lower socioeconomic strata. Nongonococcal urethritis (NGU) on the other hand, is more commonly encountered in heterosexual males and those of higher socioeconomic class. NGU is twice as common as gonococcal urethritis in the United States; it is the most common STD in men and is usually due to *Chlamydia trachomatis.* However, *Trichomonas vaginalis* or herpes simplex virus (HSV) can also cause NGU. At one time, the standard treatment would have been penicillin (choice **C**). However, because of increasing resistance, penicillin is no longer recommended for gonorrhea. Ceftriaxone (choice **A**) and cefixime are drugs that inhibit cell wall synthesis but are not susceptible to β-lactase hydrolysis; therefore, they are recommended replacements for penicillin in the treatment of gonorrhea. The quinolones, ciprofloxacin (choice **B**) and ofloxacin inhibit bacterial DNA gyrase and have a relatively broad spectrum of activity. They too are effective against gonorrhea. However, because chlamydial infections so often accompany gonococcal infections, the Centers for Disease Control (CDC) recommends that all patients with suspected or proved gonococcal urethritis also be treated as if they had chlamydial NGU. Although the quinolones have anti-chlamydial activity in vitro, they have not been recommended for clinical infections. *C. trachomatis* is susceptible to tetracyclines such as doxycycline (choice **E**), but strains of tetracycline-resistant *N. gonorrhoeae* have also become too common to recommend its use. Therefore, combined therapy, such as ceftriaxone and doxycycline (choice **D**), is required to treat both infections. Alternatively, because both organisms are still susceptible to the relatively new drug azithromycin, it can be used alone.

23 The answer is E *Pediatrics*

Associated characteristics of fragile X syndrome (choice **E**) include mental deficiency, prominent jaw, large ears with soft cartilage, and macroorchidism in postpubertal males. Fragile X syndrome is the most common form of inherited mental retardation, affecting approximately 1 in 1250 males and 1 in 2000 females. Although inheritance is X-linked, inheritance does not follow classic Mendelian patterns. Most males who carry the mutation are retarded and show the typical phenotypic pattern, while about 20% have no obvious symptoms but nonetheless are obligate carriers. Conversely about 33% of heterozygous females show phenotypic effects, but mental retardation only occurs if the mutation is inherited from the mother. Moreover the risk of clinical symptoms and the degree of mental retardation increases in succeeding generations. The explanation lies in the fact that a CGG triplet repeat is found in the first and untranslated exon, and in affected individuals this repeat is expanded to hundreds or even thousands of repeats. Above a certain critical number the gene becomes hypermethylated and is shut off. Further variability is built into the condition by the fact that the expanded repeat is unstable during mitosis, causing extensive somatic mosaicism with respect to the number of repeats in various cell types. The diagnosis of fragile X syndrome should be considered in any child with undiagnosed developmental and/or mental retardation. This can now be done using molecular methodologies that are more efficient and easier to do than the classic cytogenetic analyses.

Clinical features of trisomy 18 (choice **B**) are a prominent occiput and low-set, posteriorly rotated, malformed auricles; clenched hand with overlapping fingers; and rocker-bottom feet. Physical manifestations of trisomy 21 (choice **D**) include epicanthal folds, Brushfield's spots, and simian crease, a wide space between the first and second toes, a short fifth finger, and small ears. In patients with Klinefelter's syndrome (choice **A**), hypogonadism, long extremities, decreased intelligence, and behavioral problems can be seen. The physical features associated with Prader-Willi syndrome (choice **C**) include a narrow face, almond-shaped eyes, a thin upper lip, hypoplastic gonads, small hands and small feet, and truncal obesity after 1 to 4 years of age. These patients also have slow motor development, delayed puberty, mental retardation, and behavioral problems.

24 The answer is A *Medicine*

The patient has a stress fracture of the tibia (choice **A**). It is caused by repetitive overload to the bone, usually from a change in training habits. The junction of the middle and distal thirds of the tibia is a common site.

Chronic exertional compartment syndrome (choice **B**) is caused by elevated pressure within an enclosed leg fascial compartment. There is no localized bony tenderness on examination. In overuse myositis (choice **C**), there is tenderness over the muscle–tendon units instead of along the tibia. Acute compartment syndrome (choice **D**) is caused by a short-term increase in tissue pressure within a fascial compartment. Patients have severe pain, weakness of muscles in the compartment, and elevated compartment pressures. Patients with anterior tibialis tendinitis (choice **E**) have pain over the dorsum of the feet. There is tenderness, and sometimes swelling, over the anterior tibialis tendon.

25 The answer is C *Preventive Medicine and Public Health*

There have been numerous studies concerning risk factors for prostate cancer (PC). The greatest risk as indicated in the vignette is age; however, until death occurs aging is inevitable. Studies also implicate genetics; a study of twins reported 42% of the risk for PC is genetic and 58% is environmental. Contributing to the relatively high genetic component is the role of the *HPC1* gene on chromosome 1 and the *HPC2* gene on chromosome 17; mutation in either of these has been implicated as a cause of PC, but such direct inheritance occurs in fewer than 10% of all cases. The genetic influence is also reflected by the facts that a man has 5-fold greater chance of developing PC if he has a first-degree relative that developed PC before the age of 55 and that male relatives of women with breast cancer also have a greater risk of getting PC. The observation that African Americans have a 30% greater risk of developing PC than white Americans may also be due to genetics, although lifestyle differences may also play a role. However, since we are still unable to change our genetic makeup, many studies have investigated potentially manipulatable ways to influence the risk of getting PC. The sum of these studies indicates that diet provides the single most important controllable risk factor. An appropriate diet (choice **C**) for reducing the risk (which because of its slow growth may translate into delaying the onset) of PC is one rich in fruits and vegetables and low in saturated and *trans*-fatty acids. In contrast, studies of the influence the most suspected sources of carcinogenic potential, primarily smoking and heavy alcohol consumption have shown mixed results at best.

Although testosterone enhances the growth of PC once it is established, there is no good evidence suggesting that it induces the cancer. Therefore even though orchiectomy (choice **A**) is sometimes used to slow the growth of advanced PC, there is no reason to believe it would reduce the risk of developing it in the first place; it also would be a rather radical approach to use to reduce a risk. Although a large double-blind study showed that 5 mg per day of finasteride per day (choice **B**) over a 7-year period reduced the incidence of new cases by 24.8%, 27% of the men who developed cancer had a form of PC that was apparently more aggressive as judged by the Gleason scoring system; thus finasteride seems to trade potential reduction in numbers for greater malignancy, not necessarily a wise or practical choice to reduce risk. Vasectomy (choice **D**) has been demonstrated to have no influence on the rate of PC development, so fear of PC is no reason not to have one done. Although use of zinc supplements has sometimes been claimed to reduce the risk of developing PC, a National Cancer Institute Study involving 47,000 men showed that supplementing a diet with 100 mg or more of zinc daily (choice **E**) actually doubled the risk of developing advanced cancer.

26 The answer is B *Surgery*

The patient has disseminated intravascular coagulation (DIC) (choice **B**) secondary to massive soft-tissue trauma. Release of tissue thromboplastin from the injured tissue activates the extrinsic and intrinsic coagulation systems, leading to the formation of clots in the microvasculature. The consumption of fibrinogen, factors V and VIII, prothrombin, and platelets by the clots renders the patient anticoagulated, so bleeding occurs from all open wounds. Laboratory studies typically reveal the following: decreased plasma fibrinogen and prolonged prothrombin and partial thromboplastin times (PT and PTT, respectively) resulting from the consumption of fibrinogen, factors V and VIII, and prothrombin (hence the term *consumption coagulopathy*); thrombocytopenia; increased fibrinogen degradation products (i.e., fibrin) from activation of the fibrinolytic system; increased d-dimers (cross-linked fibrin degradation products) indicating fibrin-associated clots, because cross-links indicate factor XIII activity in a clot (excludes primary fibrinolysis); and schistocytes in the peripheral blood from damage to the red blood cells (RBCs) by fibrin strands in the microthrombi. The best treatment for DIC is to treat the underlying cause. Fresh frozen plasma replaces all of the coagulation factors. Cryoprecipitate only replaces fibrinogen and factor VIII. Platelet concentrations raise the platelet count. Packed red blood cells (PRBCs) are used if symptomatic anemia is present. Because heparin enhances antithrombin III activity, the neutralization of thrombin produced by the extrinsic and intrinsic pathways prevents clot formation and factor consumption. Therefore, it is used to treat DIC.

Thrombotic thrombocytopenic purpura (TTP) (choice **A**) is not associated with trauma. It is characterized by a pentad of fever, central nervous system (CNS) abnormalities, thrombocytopenia, hemolytic anemia, and renal failure. An unknown circulating plasma factor damages vascular endothelium, resulting in platelet thrombi. There is no consumption of clotting factors, so the PT and PTT are normal. Primary fibrinolysis (choice **D**) is extremely rare. It is associated with primary activation of the fibrinolytic system, most commonly in the setting of open heart surgery and prostate surgery. Fat embolism syndrome (choice **C**) is seen 1 to 3 days after trauma associated with multiple fractures of long bones, most commonly the femur. The embolus can travel to the lungs or to the brain. When it travels to the lungs, dyspnea is an early symptom. When it travels to the brain, confusion and coma prevail. Diffuse bleeding problems like those described in this patient are not usually part of this syndrome. A circulating anticoagulant (e.g., antibody against a clotting factor) (choice **E**) is not associated with thrombocytopenia or d-dimers.

27 **The answer is C** *Medicine*

This patient has epidermolysis bullosa (choice **C**). This is an inherited condition that affects 1 in 50,000 individuals in the United States. The skin breaks down and forms blisters, usually after minor trauma. Even stretching the skin can cause the lesion, and this is done to confirm the diagnosis. Treatment is symptomatic.

Ehlers-Danlos syndrome (choice **A**), of which there are 11 types, is an inherited condition in which there is hyperelasticity of the skin and hypermobility of the joints. The skin does not break down. The incidence is approximately 1 in 5000 births and is higher in African Americans. The symptomatology varies depending on the type of disease and ranges from mild to life threatening. The skin may be very thin, and the subjacent blood vessels may be seen. On the other hand, the skin may look like velvet and have stretch ability that may be extreme (the "rubber man" syndrome). Scars may look like cigarette paper, and hyperpigmentation over the joints is not uncommon. The pattern of inheritance varies with the type of disease, and in most forms, the biochemical defect has to do with collagen synthesis. Osteogenesis imperfecta (choice **D**) also exists in multiple forms, having in common osteopenia (decreased bone mass). The simplest functional classification is: type I, mild; type II, lethal; and type III, moderately severe. Type I commonly is found over several generations in families and is characterized by a triad of blue sclera, brittle bones, and deafness. Joint laxity can also be a problem. Multiple fractures are most common before puberty and in association with premature osteoporosis in the elderly. Fractures are minimally displaced, and soft tissue swelling is minimal. Deafness of the conductance type generally starts in the third or fourth decade. Penetrance of the blue sclera approaches 98%, whereas bone fractures and deafness are expressed less often. Some families with type I (type Ib) osteogenesis imperfecta also have dental abnormalities. Patients with type II osteogenesis imperfecta who do not die in utero or shortly after birth become progressively worse. Some of the subtypes of type III osteogenesis imperfecta do not have blue sclera. The diagnosis is clinical, and x-ray films reveal decreased bone density. This can be confirmed by photon or x-ray absorptiometry. Type I procollagen defects have been noted in most patients. Systemic sclerosis (choice **B**), also known as scleroderma, is a multisystem disorder of unknown etiology in which there is progressive fibrosis of the skin, blood vessels, and visceral organs in the chest and abdomen. The condition may predominantly involve the skin, in which there is rapid symmetric thickening of the skin of the proximal and distal extremities, face, and trunk. The patient may have a grin at all times. In other cases, the patient may have localized sclerosis, the CREST syndrome, which is an acronym for calcinosis, Raynaud's phenomenon, esophageal dysfunction, sclerodactyly, and telangiectasia. Child abuse (choice **E**), while a possibility, is usually associated with fractures in different stages of healing, and retinal hemorrhages seen on ophthalmoscopy. Fractures involving the posterior aspect of the ribs, spiral fractures of the extremities, and bucket-handle fractures of the metaphysis are pathognomonic of child abuse. Skin lesions include bruises; circular burns from cigarettes, especially in the gluteal region; and symmetric scalds involving the lower extremities and gluteal area as a result of immersion in hot water. Distinguishing osteogenesis imperfecta from child abuse is important.

28 **The answer is C** *Preventive Medicine and Public Health*

Summation of *a* + *b* represents the cohort involved in a prospective study group. In cohort designs, the investigator first identifies a study group of individuals who have common characteristics (cohort). Some of these will be exposed to a proposed risk agent for disease, while another group will not. The two are observed forward in time for the development of disease. The investigator then establishes the extent to which the disease develops in the two groups. The group *a* + *b* (choice **C**) represents the cohort (i.e., the study group), while *c* + *d* (choice **D**) represents the control.

The sum *a* + *c* (choice **A**) represents the retrospective study group, which is studied backward in time—from the point of disease to the point of exposure. Note that in a prospective study, one can determine the incidence of the disease, but this is not possible in the case of a retrospective study. The sums *c* + *b* (choice **B**) and (*a* + *c*) + (*c* + *d*) (choice **E**) have no statistical value, because they represent two diverse groups. The cohort who are disease free after exposure are represented by *b*, while *c* represents the control (nonexposed) group who develops disease.

29 **The answer is D** *Surgery*

The patient has central retinal artery occlusion (choice **D**). Retinal artery occlusion could be central or peripheral. The disorder is characterized by a sudden, complete, painless loss of vision in one eye. The patient often notices it when he or she closes one eye. Potential causes include atherosclerotic carotid disease, giant cell arteritis, lipid emboli from trauma, intravenous drug abuse, sickle cell anemia, and hypercoagulable states. Funduscopy reveals pallor of the optic disc, edema of the retina, and a cherry-red spot. The cherry-red spot represents ischemia and edema of the posterior retina, and occurs within hours following the occlusion. The red color is due to perfusion of the choroid through the thinner retinal tissue. Segmentation of retinal vessels giving a boxcar appearance is a feature as well. Initial management is massaging the eyeball. Thereafter, the patient is asked to breathe into a paper bag to increase P_{CO_2}. Doing so will induce vasodilatation of the artery and (one hopes) dislodge the embolus. Definitive treatment involves anterior chamber paracentesis under slit lamp examination. It is the best method to lower intraocular pressure and dislodge the embolus.

Central retinal vein occlusion (choice **A**) is characterized by a sudden, painful, unilateral loss of vision in patients with hypercoagulable states and thrombotic disorders such as deep venous thrombosis. Branch retinal vein occlusion is most commonly seen in systemic hypertension. Funduscopy reveals a "blood and thunder" fundus. That is, dilated tortuous veins, flame-shaped hemorrhages, macular edema, cotton wool spots, and exudates. Neovascularization of the retina or iris can occur and result in secondary glaucoma. Treatment is laser photocoagulation. Acute angle–closure glaucoma (choice **B**) also is usually unilateral, but clinical features include intense ocular pain associated with nausea and vomiting and diminished vision with colored halos around lights. The pupil is mid-dilated and fixed, and perilimbal injection may be present. The anterior chamber is shallow, and this can be confirmed by gonioscopy. Failure to diagnose this condition and treat it in a timely manner will lead to blindness. Treatment involves decreasing intraocular pressure with β-blockers such as timolol, and carbonic anhydrase inhibitors as adjuncts. Miotics such as pilocarpine or cholinesterase inhibitors are also used. Corneal abrasion (choice **C**) is associated with pain and lacrimation, (epiphora) and blepharospasm. Diagnosis is made by fluorescein staining of the cornea and observing it under a slit lamp. Treatment involves removal of the foreign body if present, and topical antibiotics. Optic neuritis (choice **E**) presents with unilateral central visual loss associated with painful eye movements. It is usually seen in patients with demyelinating disease such as multiple sclerosis. Most patients recover spontaneously over time. Funduscopy reveals a normal disc in most patients. Some patient may have edema.

30 **The answer is D** *Obstetrics and Gynecology*

Anemia in pregnancy is a common medical complication. Maternal megaloblastic anemia in pregnancy is most commonly caused by folate deficiency (choice **D**). Vitamin B_{12} deficiency, also a cause of megaloblastic anemia, is associated with infertility and thus is seldom seen with pregnancy. Anticonvulsants are known to decrease folic acid absorption so folate deficiency is associated with their use even when supplemented in the typical multivitamin pill. Fetal congenital malformations due to folic acid deficiency can occur as rare complications of anticonvulsant therapy, specifically treatment with phenytoin. However, phenytoin can diminish absorption of folate, resulting in macrocytosis, as seen in this patient.

All of the other options listed—sickle cell trait (choice **A**), iron deficiency (choice **B**), physiologic anemia (choice **C**), and thalassemia (choice **E**)—are associated with either normal or low mean corpuscular volume (MCV).

31 The answer is C *Obstetrics and Gynecology*

The human ovary can develop a wide variety of tumors. These tumors can be functional, inflammatory, metaplastic, or neoplastic, but most are benign. Benign cystic teratoma (choice **C**), also known as a dermoid cyst, is the most common benign complex ovarian tumor in young women. The scenario describes a probable torsion of this enlarged ovary. Urgent surgical exploration is essential.

A follicular cyst (choice **A**) is probably the most common reason for ovarian enlargement. This is the dominant follicle that is found in all women prior to ovulation. However, these are always simple fluid-filled cysts and never have calcifications. A mucinous cystadenoma (choice **B**) is a benign epithelial ovarian tumor and is frequently multiloculated. They can attain a huge size, often filling the entire pelvis. If they rupture they can cause pseudomyxoma peritonei. However, calcifications are not usually seen. A Brenner tumor (choice **D**) is also a benign epithelial ovarian tumor but it is solid, occurring most often in women over 50 years of age. A serous cystadenoma (choice **E**), another epithelial ovarian tumor, tends to be unilocular but does not show calcifications.

32 The answer is D *Medicine*

Mitral regurgitation (choice **D**) can occur because of a tear of papillary muscle, in which the mitral valve prolapses. This is usually seen in young women between the ages of 14 and 30. Mitral valve prolapse is usually asymptomatic, but in a small number of cases can become symptomatic. This condition may actually encompass a wide spectrum of features ranging from a systolic click, murmur, and mild prolapse of the posterior leaflet of the mitral valve to severe mitral regurgitation due to rupture of the chorda tendineae with massive prolapse of both leaflets of the mitral valve. The condition usually develops slowly over a number of years. Mitral valve prolapse is the most common cause of isolated severe mitral regurgitation. Most often, patients have arrhythmias, dizziness, and syncope. Auscultation most often reveals a middle or late nonejection systolic click. This may or may not be associated with a high-pitched, late, crescendo–decrescendo murmur. Mitral valve prolapse is believed to be autosomal dominant. Causes include heritable connective tissue disorders such as Marfan syndrome, osteogenesis imperfecta, and Ehlers-Danlos syndrome; however, in most cases the cause is unknown. The pathology is believed to be due to decreased production of type III collagen.

Mitral stenosis (choice **A**) is most commonly seen in females. The most common cause is rheumatic fever, and it may rarely be congenital. Cough, paroxysmal nocturnal dyspnea, dyspnea on exertion, and cardiac failure can occur, as the stenosis gets more severe. Atrial fibrillation is commonly seen in patients with mitral stenosis. This could result in recurrent pulmonary emboli. Aortic stenosis (choice **B**) can be congenital, following rheumatic endocarditis, or due to idiopathic calcification, as noted in the elderly. Most cases of aortic stenosis occur in males. Physical examination reveals displacement of the apical pulse because of left ventricular hypertrophy, a thrill, and an ejection systolic murmur conducted to the carotids. The volume of the pulse is decreased, and if the stenosis is severe, there may be evidence of left ventricular failure. Aortic regurgitation (choice **C**) is primarily seen in males, although aortic regurgitation with mitral regurgitation is more common in women. Most of the cases occur after rheumatic fever. Other causes of aortic regurgitation include syphilis, Marfan syndrome, and rheumatoid ankylosing spondylitis. Ventricular septal defects may be associated with aortic regurgitation. The most common and earliest complaint is an awareness of the heartbeat while lying down. Dyspnea, chest pains, and excessive sweating develop later. Physical examination reveals a displaced, forceful apex beat; diastolic thrill; and a high-pitched decrescendo diastolic murmur and an ejection click. The pulse is bounding (Corrigan's pulse). Left ventricular failure could follow. Congestive cardiac failure (choice **E**) usually follows cardiac or pulmonary disease. There is a history of dyspnea, fatigue, and swelling of the ankles. Cyanosis may be present. Auscultation will reveal basal rales. Congestive hepatomegaly, pleural effusion, and ascites may also be features. Pulsus alternans, if present, signifies severe heart failure. This is a condition in which a regular cardiac rhythm results in alternate strong and weak pulses. A third heart sound is usually seen in left ventricular failure or left ventricular overload. A fourth heart sound is often heard in normal individuals. It is also heard in patients with aortic stenosis, hypertension, cardiomyopathy, hyperthyroidism, and anemia. The last two are associated with hyperdynamic circulation.

33 The answer is A *Psychiatry*

The presentation is most suggestive of bipolar disorder (choice **A**), which is characterized by periods of mania with relatively normal function between episodes. A manic episode is suggested by the presence of agitation, pressured speech, grandiose delusions, disorganized behavior, increased psychomotor activity, and decreased judgment. Periods of decreased sleep may be present as well. Brief psychotic disorder (choice **B**) lasts less than 1 month and is usually not preceded by similar episodes. Delusional disorder, erotomanic type (choice **C**), is characterized by delusions about special relationships with relative strangers and minimum thought disorganization. Major depressive disorder with mood congruent psychosis (choice **D**) is characterized by episodes of severe depression with hallucinations or delusions involving worthlessness, sickness, guilt, death, or other depressive themes. Schizophrenia (choice **E**) is characterized by the presence of residual symptoms such as affect blunting, lack of motivation, and social withdrawal between psychotic episodes.

34 The answer is A *Surgery*

The patient has superior vena cava syndrome, which is most commonly secondary to extension of a primary lung cancer (choice **A**) (usually a small cell carcinoma) into the neck, with obstruction of superior vena caval blood flow. Clinical findings consist of puffiness and bluish discoloration of the face, arms, and shoulders, along with distention of the jugular veins. Collateral venous circulation results as evidenced by dilated and tortuous veins over the anterior chest. In addition, there are central nervous system (CNS) signs of dizziness, visual disturbances, and convulsions. Prompt administration of diuretics, fluid restriction, and radiation therapy are useful in restoring blood flow. Surgery is rarely indicated. The mean survival is 6 to 8 months.

Pericardial effusion (choice **B**) distends the neck veins but would not be associated with the degree of venous engorgement noted in this case. Sclerosing mediastinitis (choice **C**) is uncommon and usually results from histoplasmosis. Polycythemia rubra vera (choice **D**) is associated with increased plasma volume and red blood cell (RBC) mass, and a tendency for venous thrombosis. However, thrombosis of the superior vena cava is very unlikely. Right ventricular failure (choice **E**) is not associated with the degree of venous engorgement noted in this patient.

35 The answer is B *Surgery*

Blunt trauma to the upper left abdomen or lower left chest, is frequently complicated by a ruptured spleen, especially in the presence of fractures of the lower ribs (choice **B**). This can be diagnosed by computed tomography (CT) or peritoneal lavage if the diagnosis is equivocal. However, the presence of shock in this patient is an indication for immediate surgical intervention—control of hemorrhage followed by splenorrhaphy. Splenectomy is no longer performed. Loss of the spleen would result in inability to opsonize encapsulated bacteria such as pneumococcus.

Pulmonary contusion with hemorrhage into the pleural cavity (choice **A**) is unlikely in the presence of normal breath sounds. The location of the injury and the presence of hypovolemic shock would argue against rupture of the colon (choice **C**) or transection of the abdominal aorta (choice **D**). Hematuria would be present with a ruptured kidney (choice **E**).

36 The answer is C *Pediatrics*

Subdural hematoma and retinal hemorrhages are common signs of fatal child abuse. In this case, they are signs of "shaken baby syndrome," in which a child is shaken to stop him or her from crying. Initially the patient must be medically stabilized using the ABC's (airway, breathing, circulation) of resuscitation. The next step, if abuse is suspected, is to consult social services and the state agency that deals with this problem (choice **C**).

Ongoing medical care (choice **A**) and notification of the patient's primary care provider (choice **B**) can be obtained after the state agency has been contacted. In cases of suspected child abuse, the physician neither has to inform the parents that child abuse is suspected (choice **E**) nor obtain consent from the parent to admit the child to the hospital (choice **D**).

37 The answer is C *Obstetrics and Gynecology*

The case is strongly suggestive of intrauterine fetal death (IUFD). From a medical standpoint, once the embryo completes formation of all the organs at 10 menstrual weeks, it is referred to as a fetus. However, legally and technically the definition of IUFD is fetal demise on or after 20 weeks' gestation. Prior to 20 weeks it is legally referred to as a *spontaneous abortion*. IUFD complicates approximately 3 per 1000 pregnancies. Real-time ultrasound examination for cardiac motion (choice **C**) is the method of choice for ascertaining fetal death. Failure to visualize cardiac motion is diagnostic. Other signs are overlapping of the skull bones. Maternal assessment of fetal movement (kicking) is not accurate in sensitivity or specificity.

The pregnancy test remains positive for a considerable time because the placenta continues to produce β-human chorionic gonadotropin (HCG), thus, choice **E** is not appropriate. Amniocentesis (choice **B**) is an invasive test that relies on the finding of dark, turbid fluid, which is a late development. It is not appropriate to diagnose IUFD. Exposure of a possibly live fetus to x-rays is not recommended (choice **D**). A nonstress test (choice **A**) is the appropriate next step in management with maternal report of decreased fetal movement but would not be helpful in this case.

38 The answer is E *Psychiatry*

Undoing (choice **E**) refers to the performance of an activity that symbolically reverses some previous behavior or thought. This defense mechanism is commonly present in individuals who feel either conscious or unconscious guilt.

The other choices are defense mechanisms that do not apply as well to this patient. Denial (choice **A**) is a failure to acknowledge a disturbing aspect of external reality. Dissociation (choice **B**) involves sealing off disturbing thoughts or emotions from consciousness. Intellectualization (choice **C**) is the transformation of an emotionally disturbing event into a purely cognitive problem. Sublimation (choice **D**) occurs when unacceptable impulses are channeled into more acceptable activities.

39 The answer is D *Psychiatry*

This patient's symptoms suggest somatization disorder. Numerous studies have demonstrated that morbidity from this illness is significantly decreased with regularly scheduled follow-up medical appointments (choice **D**). The focus of such visits is general, and the physician should avoid arguments about the veracity of symptoms. Such an approach also decreases costs associated with overuse of emergency services without a verbal warning to the patient (choice **B**). Refusal to see the patient again (choice **A**) or simply referring her to another clinician (choice **C**) is unlikely to benefit this patient. Trials of various medications (choice **E**) carry the risk of causing iatrogenic problems and are unlikely to be productive in light of the previous history.

40 The answer is D *Surgery*

The upper outer quadrant of the breast is the most common location for a breast carcinoma (choice **D**); 60% of lesions are located here. In contrast, 6% of breast carcinomas reside in the lower inner quadrant of the breast (choice **A**), 12% of breast carcinomas in the upper inner quadrant (choice **B**), 10% in the lower outer quadrant of the breast (choice **C**), and 12% are located subjacent to the areola (choice **E**). Therefore, it is imperative to examine every quadrant of the breast, including the axillary tail, when ruling out a breast mass, keeping in mind the most common location. The examiner should use the flat of his or her hand to examine the breast. The pectoral muscles must be relaxed, as they are immediately deep to the breast. Failure to do so may result in missing a small lesion. Likewise, it is important to relax the axilla, so as not to miss lymphadenopathy here. Most breast carcinomas manifest themselves as a hard lump, and an indrawn nipple may be an added feature. Carcinoma affects the left breast more often than it does the right. Patients often discover them while they are showering.

41 The answer is F *Medicine*

Children who present with generalized edema (anasarca) associated with a 24-hour urine protein level above 3.5 g have the nephrotic syndrome. Urinary waxy casts consist of a mixture of protein, with or without cells or cellular debris, that is present in the renal tubules, and they form a mold of the renal tubules. Their presence in the urine indicates pathologic processes that are occurring in the kidneys, as in the nephrotic syndrome, rather than in the lower urinary tract. Minimal change disease (nil disease, lipoid nephrosis) is the most common cause of the nephrotic syndrome in children. The syndrome results from the loss of polyanions (negative charge) in the glomerular basement membrane, with massive loss of albumin in the urine. Hypoalbuminemia reduces the plasma oncotic pressure, resulting in generalized pitting edema and ascites (anasarca). In addition, the hypoalbuminemia stimulates liver production of excess cholesterol, resulting in hypercholesterolemia. Some of the cholesterol is lost in the urine where it produces lipiduria, fatty casts (choice **F**), and oval fat bodies (renal tubular cells or macrophages with cholesterol). Fatty casts and oval fat bodies, when polarized, exhibit Maltese crosses due to presence of cholesterol.

42 The answer is B *Medicine*

The white blood cell (WBC) cast (choice **B**) distinguishes acute pyelonephritis from acute cystitis. Acute pyelonephritis is an acute tubulointerstitial disease most commonly secondary to ascending infection (usually by *Escherichia coli*) from the bladder. Acute inflammation results in the presence of neutrophils that form microabscesses in the kidney and in the renal tubules. Lower urinary tract infections like acute cystitis have neutrophils in the urine (pyuria) but do not have casts, which are formed only in the kidney.

43 The answer is E *Medicine*

Waxy casts (choice **E**) are acellular casts that represent the progressive degeneration of a cellular cast. The progression to a waxy cast is as follows: cellular cast (WBCs, red blood cells [RBCs], renal tubular cells) → coarsely granular cast → finely granular cast → waxy cast. They are highly refractile and have sharp borders, unlike a hyaline cast, which has soft features and round borders. Waxy casts are a marker for end-stage chronic renal disease.

44 The answer is A *Medicine*

RBC casts (choice **A**) are a marker for acute glomerulonephritis, which is divided into the nephritic and nephrotic types. The nephritic type is commonly seen in poststreptococcal glomerulonephritis, as in this patient recovering from scarlet fever, and in renal involvement in systemic lupus erythematosus (SLE). RBC casts, hematuria, and mild-to-moderate proteinuria are the hallmarks of the nephritic syndrome. Dysmorphic RBCs (RBCs with irregular projections) are also excellent indicators of a nephritic syndrome. They distinguish hematuria of glomerular origin from all other causes of hematuria (e.g., renal stone, transitional cell carcinoma of the bladder).

41–44 Incorrect Choices

Renal tubular cell casts (choice **D**) are associated with acute tubular necrosis secondary to ischemic or nephrotoxic damage. They are partially responsible for the oliguria associated with acute tubular necrosis. Hyaline casts (choice **C**) are the most common overall cast. When present in small numbers, they have the least clinical significance of all casts. Formed from the protein gel in the renal tubule, these casts are called *Tamm-Horsfall mucoprotein*. One hyaline cast per low-power field is commonly seen in normal urine. However, increased numbers are associated with any condition accompanied by proteinuria (e.g., fever, exercise, renal disease).

45 The answer is K *Psychiatry*

These behaviors are most suggestive of regression (choice **K**), characterized by a return to less mature levels of functioning. This defense mechanism appears when levels of anxiety become high and are not alleviated by more mature defenses such as intellectualization (choice **G**) and humor. In medically ill patients presented with a very poor prognosis, regression is often manifested by the use of denial (choice **C**) or fantasy.

46 The answer is H *Psychiatry*

These behaviors are most suggestive of projection (choice **H**), a defense mechanism that involves attributing to others one's uncomfortable internal feelings, especially anger and guilt. As a result, the person transforms anger at self into anger toward others. Such persons often seem bitter or suspicious.

45–46 Incorrect Choices

Altruism (choice **A**) is the reduction of ones own fears or anxieties by caring for others.
   Blocking (choice **B**) is the sudden repression of anxiety-provoking thoughts in midsentence.
   Denial (choice **C**) is a failure to acknowledge an aspect of external reality.

Displacement (choice **D**) occurs when an unacceptable emotion associated with a given object, person, idea, or activity is transferred to a different object, person, idea, or activity.

Dissociation (choice **E**) involves sealing off disturbing thoughts or emotions from the conscious mind.

Distortion (choice **F**) is the twisting of ones perception of disturbing elements of external reality to make those elements more palatable.

Intellectualization (choice **G**) is transformation of an emotionally disturbing event into a simple cognitive problem.

Rationalization (choice **I**) is a distortion of an unacceptable reality into an act or event that is more acceptable.

Reaction formation (choice **J**) is the transfer of an unacceptable thought or feeling into its opposite.

Repression (choice **L**) is the complete separation of unacceptable aspects of reality from conscious awareness.

Sublimation (choice **M**) is the channeling of unacceptable impulses into more acceptable activities.

Undoing (choice **N**) is performance of an activity that symbolically reverses a previous thought or act.

47 The answer is D *Medicine*

This woman almost certainly has osteoporosis. Her sex (female), age (postmenopausal), ethnicity (Asian), and weight (less than 127 lb) all are risk factors for osteoporosis. Moreover, a common symptom is compression fractures of the spine, which result in shortened stature and a buffalo hump. It seems probable that she is soon headed for a major fracture unless treated. Risedronate is another bisphosphonate clinically available at this time. The bisphosphonates work by inhibiting osteoclastic activity and tip the balance during bone remodeling toward laying down bone from resorption of bone.

48 The answer is A *Medicine*

An analgesic is commonly prescribed as a sequel to a root canal procedure. Two analgesics are listed, ibuprofen and acetaminophen with codeine. Of these, acetaminophen with codeine is a more effective pain modulator and even though it contains the narcotic codeine, it can safely be prescribed for short-term use such as treating pain after a dental procedure. Moreover, the antiinflammatory properties of ibuprofen are rarely relevant with respect to the root canal procedure.

49 The answer is C *Medicine*

Auranofin is an oral gold preparation that is one of the disease-modifying antirheumatic drugs (DMARDS) that can often put rheumatoid arthritis into remission.

50 The answer is F *Medicine*

This man suffers from gout. Most of the symptoms associated with gout are caused by hyperuricemia and the limited solubility of uric acid, which causes it to precipitate in joints and within the kidney. Allopurinol is a completive inhibitor of xanthine oxidase, the enzyme that catalysis the conversion of xanthine to uric acid. Thus as long as the hyperuricemia is caused by overproduction (not by limited excretion) allopurinol increases the concentration of the more-soluble intermediates xanthine and hypoxanthine and decreases the level of poorly soluble uric acid; thereby decreasing the possibility of precipitation. The xanthine and hypoxanthine is then salvaged to form XMP and IMP. These salvage reactions require phosphoribosyl pyrophosphate (PRPP), which is also used for the de novo synthesis of purines. As a consequence, allopurinol also inhibits purine synthesis, further enhancing its effectiveness.

47–50 The Incorrect Choices

Rofecoxib (Vioxx) [choice **B**] is a nonsteroidal antiinflammatory drug (NSAID) that was touted as a wonder drug because it was a specific inhibitor of a cyclooxygenase (COX) isozyme present in connective tissue but not found in high concentration in the stomach. As a consequence, Rofecoxib and other COX-2 inhibitors could be used to treat osteoarthritis and other conditions involving inflammation as well as pain with less concern about developing gastritis. Unfortunately Vioxx was shown to adversely affect the cardiovascular system and was withdrawn from the market and the other COX-2 inhibitors currently are under scrutiny.

Fluoxetine (choice **E**) is a selective serotonin reuptake inhibitor that is most often prescribed as an antidepressant. It, however, is sometimes used for other conditions such as fibromyalgia.

Cyclosporine ophthalmic emulsion (choice **G**) is used to promote tear secretion in patients with Sjögren's syndrome and other cases of severe dry eye (xerophthalmia).

Ibuprofen (choice **H**) is a traditional NSAID that inhibits both the COX-1 and COX-2 enzymes. Thus, despite its analgesic and antiinflammatory action, it must be used with caution to avoid occult blood loss, peptic ulceration, and acute renal failure.

test **4**

Questions

1 A 49-year-old blue-eyed blonde woman was brought to the emergency room with a history of having come down heavily on the right leg while getting off a curb. The paramedics reported that she had vomited once during the trip. The patient stated that she had had a dull ache in the right thigh for the past few weeks and had noticed a "boil" there. She had made an appointment to see her primary care physician for this and for recent onset of hot flushes. The emergency physician noted that she was in moderate distress. Her blood pressure was 90/60 mm Hg, pulse was 98/min regular and thready, her respirations were 22/min, and her temperature was 37.5°C (99.5°F). She had no cyanosis, but had pallor of the mucosa. Cardiovascular examination was unremarkable except for a sinus tachycardia and a capillary circulation longer than 2 seconds. Examination of the respiratory system revealed normal breath sounds bilaterally. Her right thigh was swollen, and she had lateral rotation and shortening of the leg. The right groin was tender to palpation, and movement of the leg induced severe pain. There was a raised papular lesion over anterior midthigh, surrounded by inflammation. The pelvis and the left leg were normal. The most likely reason for her problem is

(A) Chronic osteomyelitis
(B) Osteoporosis
(C) Stress fracture
(D) Osteogenesis imperfecta
(E) Metastatic bone disease

2 A 45-year-old war veteran made an appointment with a clinical psychologist seeking help to deal with recurring nightmares concerning horrific events that he witnessed and participated in during a war almost two decades ago. Lately his reaction to these dreams had intensified; he wakes up screaming and damp from a cold sweat. When prodded by the psychologist he admitted that he has come to feel emotionally distant from other people and uncomfortable in their presence. He states that he considers himself to be rejected by "society" and wants to seek out other veterans with similar experiences in an attempt to "relate." Which of the following is the most appropriate first step in the management of this patient?

(A) Begin psychodynamic psychotherapy to explore his guilt before considering unstructured meetings with other veterans
(B) Cognitively reframe his experiences and focus on the present
(C) Make arrangements for him to join a peer support group
(D) Initiate therapy with a combination of clonazepam and paroxetine
(E) Suggest that he meet with citizens and veterans from the nation he fought against to heal anger and guilt

3 A 30-year-old woman, gravida 3, para 1, aborta 1, is at 30 weeks' gestation by dates. She has been married for 7 years to the same husband. Her first pregnancy ended in a spontaneous first trimester loss. Her second pregnancy was unremarkable until delivery at term when she underwent an emergency low-transverse cesarean section because of double footling breech presentation. She has worked in a child daycare center for the past 5 years. She vacationed in Thailand for 2 weeks last year. On routine prenatal laboratory testing you find that she is hepatitis B surface antigen positive, and anti-HBc IgM negative. She inquires about the significance of this finding concerning herself as well as her baby. Which of the following statements best summarizes what you will say?

(A) Pregnancy accelerates the course of acute hepatitis B in the mother
(B) Mode of delivery has no impact on maternal–neonatal hepatitis B transmission
(C) Breast-feeding does not increase neonatal risk of hepatitis B
(D) Neonates can be protected from hepatitis B by passive immunization at birth
(E) Rapidity of hepatitis B progression is the same in mother and neonate

4 A 4-day-old, 1500-g (3 lb 5 oz), premature infant recovering from a respiratory distress syndrome is noted to have bounding peripheral pulsations and a hyperactive precordium. A continuous machinery murmur is most audible at the left infraclavicular area. Left ventricle hypertrophy (LVH) is present on the electrocardiogram (ECG). The chest x-ray film shows slight enlargement of the heart and increased pulmonary venous markings. Which of the following is the most likely diagnosis?

(A) Patent ductus arteriosus
(B) Atrial septal defect (ASD)
(C) Ventricular septal defect (VSD)
(D) Pulmonic stenosis
(E) Tetralogy of Fallot

5 A 30-year-old female visits her family physician for a routine physical examination. During her interaction with him, she stated that she had unprotected sex with a bisexual male about 6 months previously. She did not suffer from any tiredness, weakness, fever, or untoward health problems during this time. However, she was concerned that she may have contracted acquired immune deficiency syndrome (AIDS) during that encounter. She felt that an AIDS test would be appropriate to assuage her fears. Which of the following parameters described in the standard 2 × 2 table below should be fulfilled by the test that was ordered by the physician?

	Disease Present	Disease Absent	Totals
Exposed to infection	*a*	*b*	*a + b*
Not exposed	*c*	*d*	*c + d*
Totals	*a + c*	*b + d*	

(A) The value of *d* must be much less than that of *c*
(B) The value of *d* must be much greater than that of *b*
(C) The value of *a* must be much greater than that of *c*
(D) The value of *d* must be much less than that of *b*
(E) The value of *a* must be much greater than that of *b*

6 A 75-year-old man was rushed to the emergency room of a local hospital after having collapsed at home. The patient's spouse related that he had complained of sudden severe pain over the left flank. She informed the physician that he had been complaining of backache for a few years, but did not want to see a physician, as he felt that it was "no big deal." Physical examination revealed a conscious male, in acute distress, with definite signs of hypotension, tachycardia, tachypnea, and hypothermia. He had mucosal pallor but no cyanosis. The abdomen was tender to palpation, and a pulsatile supraumbilical mass was present. Bowel sounds were diminished, and peripheral pulses were equal and moderately strong. The patient was given 100% oxy-

gen by mask, at 10 L per minute. The cardiac monitor showed sinus tachycardia with mild ischemia. Which of the following mechanisms is most likely involved in the pathogenesis of this patient's clinical disorder?

(A) Cystic medial degeneration
(B) Defect in collagen
(C) Defect in fibrillin
(D) An immunologic reaction
(E) Atherosclerosis

7 A child is at his pediatrician's office for a well-child check. The patient has been well according to the parents, and there are no complaints. On physical examination no abnormalities are noted. Additionally, the pediatrician performs a developmental screen on the patient. He finds that the child is able to say his first and last name and play interactive games. The patient's mother reports that the patient is toilet trained and is able to pedal a tricycle. He is capable of copying a cross and a circle, but cannot copy a square or triangle. He is also not able to catch a bounced ball or dress without supervision. Which of the following is the most likely age of this child?

(A) 1 year old
(B) 2 years old
(C) 3 years old
(D) 4 years old
(E) 5 years old

8 Denton, USA, has a population of 100,000. During 2005 there were 1600 live births, 85 stillbirths, and 15 neonatal deaths. Among the births that year there were 20 sets of twins and 4 sets of triplets, and four mothers died at the time of delivery. Which of the following represents the perinatal mortality rate in Denton during 2005?

(A) 100/1685
(B) 85/1600
(C) 125/2205
(D) 100/1700
(E) 59/2205

9 A 37-year-old woman, gravida 4, para 4, underwent a routine cervical Pap smear during an annual examination. She has regular menstrual periods and underwent a tubal sterilization surgical procedure after her last delivery 5 years ago. She denies excessive pain with menses or intercourse. She has been watching her diet. She exercises regularly at the local fitness center and has lost 15 lb over the past 6 months. She underwent a divorce 3 years ago but has now remarried. Her husband also was divorced after 10 years of a previous marriage. The cytologic evaluation showed a high-grade squamous intraepithelial lesion (HSIL). She was referred for colposcopy and directed biopsies. Which of the following findings would be an indication for a diagnostic cervical conization?

(A) Intraepithelial neoplasia on biopsy with satisfactory colposcopy
(B) Negative endocervical curettage with satisfactory colposcopy
(C) Cervical biopsy showing mild dysplasia
(D) Cervical biopsy showing carcinoma in situ
(E) Cervical biopsy showing stage IB invasive carcinoma

10 A 24-year-old woman, gravida 4, para 1, aborta 2, is at 28 weeks' gestation by poor dates. She admits to intravenous (IV) drug use and having sex for drugs. She is unsure who the father of this pregnancy is. She has recently undergone treatment for syphilis identified by a positive venereal disease research laboratory (VDRL) test result and confirmed by a positive fluorescent treponemal antibody (FTA) test. On her last prenatal visit she underwent human immunodeficiency virus (HIV) testing by enzyme-linked immunosorbent assay (ELISA), which was found to be positive and was confirmed with a positive Western blot assay. She inquires as to the significance of this finding on herself as well as her baby. Which of the following statements best summarizes what you will say?

(A) Pregnancy accelerates maternal progression from HIV positive to acquired immune deficiency syndrome (AIDS)
(B) Mode of delivery has a significant impact on maternal–neonatal transmission of HIV
(C) Breast-feeding does not increase neonatal risk of becoming HIV positive
(D) Neonates can be protected from HIV by passive immunization at birth
(E) Rapidity of disease progression is the same in mother and neonate

11 A 40-year-old man with a 20-year history of schizophrenia, paranoid type, is brought in by police because local business owners complained that he spends all day outside a particular strip mall where his malodorousness and pacing were driving away customers. He lives in the alley behind the mall in a makeshift shelter. The man adamantly refuses hospitalization or any other help with his living situation. He demands to leave. Which of the following findings would provide the best legal support for hospitalizing the man against his wishes?

(A) He lives in a shelter made from wooden crates and cardboard, and receives money for food from begging.
(B) He believes that members of the central intelligence agency are following him.
(C) He believes that he hears the voice of Elvis Presley.
(D) He is disheveled and shows evidence of poor hygiene.
(E) He has a gun and has threatened to kill himself.

12 A 35-year-old female presents to her family physician with a history of lack of sleep, tremors of her hands, excessive sweating, and a racing heart. She has also noticed that she does not require warm clothing in winter, and her friends have noticed that her eyes seem to be bulging out. The patient has noticed a weight loss, despite a voracious appetite. She also noticed a change in her periods. She has two children, aged 4 and 9, and works as a teller at a local bank. Physical examination reveals a rather nervous woman, whose palms are clammy. She is normotensive, but has a sinus tachycardia and normal respiratory rate. She is afebrile. Fine tremors are noticeable in her fingers. Palpation of the thyroid gland reveals many nodules. In addition, she has mild bilateral exophthalmos. The most likely diagnosis is which one of the following?

(A) Hashimoto's disease
(B) Graves' disease
(C) Papillary adenocarcinoma
(D) Toxic multinodular goiter
(E) Follicular adenoma

13 A 55-year-old male presented to his family physician with fairly rapid progress of failing memory, and impaired cognition. Recently he developed difficulty in walking and jerky movements of his limbs that came on spontaneously, usually in the morning, but also occurred during his sleep. The patient had been diagnosed earlier with coronary artery disease. A few years earlier, he developed visual problems in the right eye as a result of an ocular injury. The problem resolved after a corneal transplant. He had lived all his life in the San Joaquin Valley, where he had been a farmer. The farthest he had traveled was to Nevada. Physical examination revealed a rather disheveled man who demonstrated features of moderate dementia. He had fasciculations of his upper extremities, and during the examination, his limbs jerked uncontrollably in a lightening manner. He also demonstrated cerebellar signs. Magnetic resonance imaging (MRI) shows bilateral areas of increased signal intensity in the caudate and putamen in T2-weighted images. An EEG was reported as showing periodic high-voltage sharp spikes. Which of the following is the most likely diagnosis?

(A) Creutzfeldt-Jakob disease
(B) Bovine spongiform dementia
(C) Parkinson's disease
(D) Alzheimer's disease
(E) Progressive multifocal leukoencephaly

14 A 65-year-old man suffering from dysphagia due to esophageal cancer has been on total parenteral nutrition (TPN) for the past month. At this time he develops alopecia, a maculopapular rash around the mouth and eyes, and taste and smell abnormalities. These symptoms are most likely due to a deficiency of which one of the following nutrients?

(A) Essential fatty acids
(B) Zinc
(C) Selenium
(D) Magnesium
(E) Copper

15 A 40-year-old man is obsessed with dressing in women's undergarments. Although he risks extremely negative reactions from his coworkers, he often wears such apparel beneath his office clothes. He is disturbed by his behavior but says that he cannot resist the sexual arousal associated with it. Which of the following is the best description of this man's behavior?

(A) Exhibitionism
(B) Frotteurism
(C) Gender identity disorder
(D) Transvestic fetishism
(E) Voyeurism

16 A 13-year-old girl comes to the outpatient office complaining of bleeding irregularly for the past 3 months. She denies cramping, pain, nausea, vomiting, or diarrhea with her menstrual periods. She started breast budding 3 years ago, with development of pubic and axillary hair a year later. She underwent menarche 1 year ago and uses tampons regularly. She is a student at the local middle school and is doing well in her studies. Her height is 62 inches (1.57 m) and she weighs 130 lb (59 kg). On general examination she appears well developed, well nourished, and in no distress. General and pelvic examinations are unremarkable. If an endometrial biopsy were performed on this girl, which of the following histologic findings would be most likely seen on microscopic examination?

(A) Serrated endometrial glands with inspissated secretions
(B) Tubular endometrial glands with many mitoses

(C) Back-to-back endometrial glands with prominent nuclei
(D) Decidual reaction forming around endometrial arterioles
(E) Hyperchromatism and loss of cellular polarity

17 A 38-year-old man presents with bouts of severe, right retro-orbital pain lasting one-half hour or more, up to several times a day. The pain often occurs at night and is associated with nasal congestion on the right nostril and right conjunctival injection. Which of the following would be an effective short-term treatment in this patient?

(A) Sublingual nitroglycerin
(B) An alcoholic beverage
(C) Vigorous exercise
(D) Oxygen
(E) A warm pack over the eye

18 A 25-year-old woman comes to the outpatient office complaining of a pruritic, painful vaginal discharge. She is sexually active with two male sexual partners but finds intercourse very uncomfortable because of her vaginal symptoms. For the past 8 months she has been using an estrogen–progestin contraceptive patch. She exercises regularly by walking 2 to 3 miles a day. She is following a low carbohydrate diet and takes a multivitamin preparation. Findings of her general examination are unremarkable. Speculum examination of the vagina shows a foul-smelling greenish, frothy discharge. Vaginal pH, using nitrazine paper, is 6.5. A wet mount of vaginal secretions in a saline suspension reveals a highly motile organism. Which of the following pharmacologic agents would be the most appropriate treatment?

(A) Metronidazole
(B) Clotrimazole
(C) Miconazole
(D) Acyclovir
(E) Spectinomycin

19 While perusing a research article, a student came across a data set composed of the numbers 7, 5, 8, 2, and 8. The set of numbers that gives the correct mean, median, and mode in the appropriate order is

(A) 7, 8, 6
(B) 8, 7, 5
(C) 7, 6, 8
(D) 5, 7, 8
(E) 6, 7, 8

20 A teenage boy was seated in the waiting area of an emergency room when he suddenly became very agitated and had a bizarre look. He then cried out loudly and fell to the floor, and his body began to shake uncontrollably. His arms and legs kept flailing, and there was froth coming out of his mouth. The patient was unconscious and continued to shake. The best initial intervention in this patient would be to:

(A) Insert a tongue blade
(B) Administer intravenous (IV) bolus of 50% dextrose
(C) Secure the airway
(D) Inject 2 mg of IV lorazepam followed by phenytoin infusion
(E) Induce pentobarbital coma

21 An obstetric sonogram is performed on a 22-year-old woman, gravida 2, para 1, who is at 30 weeks' gestation by dates and confirmed by early first-trimester ultrasound crown–rump measurements 9 weeks gestation. Her pregnancy is complicated by gestational diabetes diagnosed at 26 weeks gestation that is being managed by diet alone. Her home blood glucose monitoring shows the following mean values: fasting 85 mg/dL; 1 hour postmeal, <130 mg/dL. The sonogram reveals an anterior-fundal placenta and a normal amniotic fluid volume. There is a single fetus with the head in the right upper quadrant, with his back to the mother's left. Both fetal thighs are flexed and both legs are extended. In this case, which of the following is the correct fetal presentation?

(A) Transverse breech
(B) Complete breech
(C) Double-footling breech
(D) Incomplete breech
(E) Frank breech

22 A 45-year-old woman with polyhydramnios delivers a full-term male infant with a birth weight of 6 lb 12 oz (3.06 kg). The infant's physical examination is pertinent for hypotonia, upward and slanted palpebral fissures and epicanthic folds, a simian crease, and a short fifth finger. A few hours after birth, the infant begins to vomit bile-stained fluid. On physical examination, the abdomen is not distended. Radiographs of the chest and abdomen were obtained, and the results revealed a "double bubble" sign. Which of the following is the most likely diagnosis?

(A) Congenital pyloric stenosis
(B) Duodenal atresia
(C) An intussusception
(D) A diaphragmatic hernia
(E) A perforated viscus

23 A 67-year-old man presents with headache, vomiting, blurred vision, difficulty with speaking and swallowing, and loss of balance. He also complained of numbness in his face. His past history was significant for diabetes mellitus and hypertension. The patient was on metformin for the former and a combination of an ACE inhibitor and diuretic for the latter. The acute problem occurred approximately 2 hours prior to being seen in the emergency room. His blood pressure was 150/100 mm Hg, his pulse was 80/min with a few irregular beats, and his temperature and respiratory rate were normal. The patient was conscious, the left pupil was smaller than the right, and the eyeball appeared to be sunken into the orbit. He also had partial closure of the left upper eyelid. He had no pain sensations over the left side of the face to pinprick. Touch however, was preserved. He had a depressed gag reflex, and the palate was noticeably lowered on the left side with the uvula being pulled to the right when he was asked to say, "aaah." There was a noticeable nystagmus to the left, and he had poor coordination of his left upper and lower extremities. His gait was ataxic. He could not feel pain in the right upper and lower extremities, when tested with a pin. However, the sensation of touch was preserved. A noncontrast computerized tomography (CT) of the brain was normal. Which of the following is the best means of immediate medical management in this patient?

(A) Heparinization and observation
(B) Right carotid endarterectomy
(C) Left carotid endarterectomy
(D) Thrombolytics
(E) Antiplatelet agents

24 A 65-year-old woman went bicycling into the country near Lake Tahoe, California, with a few of her friends. She had not bicycled since her childhood growing up at the foothills of the Ural Mountains in Russia. The front wheel struck a pothole and she fell to the ground. While doing so, her chest struck the handlebar. She was immediately rushed to the local hospital. On arrival, she is conscious and appears to be in moderate distress. Her blood pressure is 140/95 mm Hg, pulse 96/min. Her respirations are shallow and rapid, at 22/min. Bruising over the left anterior hemithorax is observed upon examination of the chest. There is no jugular venous dilatation. The rest of her examination findings are unremarkable. Further examination would most likely yield which of the following?

(A) Increased breath sounds on the left
(B) Egophony on the left
(C) Increased timbre
(D) Increased width of intercostals on the left
(E) Mediastinal structures shifted to the left

25 A 60-year-old man presents to the emergency room with a history of vomiting, increasing confusion, hearing voices, and blurred vision. The patient has a history of congestive cardiac failure and is being treated with a diuretic, enalapril, carvedilol, and digoxin. His blood pressure is 140/95 mm Hg; pulse, 88 irregular; respirations, 22/min; and body temperature is normal. Physical examination confirmed altered mental status, an irregular cardiac rhythm to auscultation, and basilar rales on the left, but there is no cyanosis or pallor. The electrocardiogram shows left axis deviation and paroxysmal atrial tachycardia with block. A chest x-ray film confirms left ventricular hypertrophy with blunting of the left costophrenic angle and diffuse shadowing at the base. Effective management of cardiac dysfunction would include which one of the following?

(A) Raising the serum sodium level
(B) Raising the serum magnesium level
(C) Lowering the serum magnesium level
(D) Raising the serum calcium level
(E) Raising the serum potassium level

26 A 38-year-old female visits her family physician because of her concern about a lump in her left breast, which she noticed after a fall approximately 1 week previously. She does not smoke, drinks wine on social occasions, and takes birth control pills. She is a divorced mother of two and recently returned to the dating scene. There is no family history of breast cancer. Physical examination reveals a rather stocky woman with pendulous breasts. She has a moderate-sized, nontender, irregular lump in the lower outer quadrant of her left breast. The overlying skin appears thickened. No nipple discharge is present, and she has no axillary lymphadenopathy. The right breast and axilla are normal. Mammography reveals increased density in the affected region. Ultrasound-guided fine needle aspiration biopsy (FNAB) was performed. The pathology report was consistent with a diagnosis of fat necrosis. Which of the following is the most appropriate next step in the management of this patient?

(A) Excise the mass
(B) Repeat fine needle aspiration biopsy after 1 month
(C) Repeat mammography in a month
(D) Reassure the patient, and follow up in a few weeks
(E) Mastectomy

27 A 42-year-old man with hyperopia presents with a history of sudden severe pain in the right eye, associated with blurred vision, nausea, and vomiting. Examination of the eye reveals lid and corneal edema, conjunctival injection, and a shallow anterior chamber. Physical examination reveals the pupil to be mid-dilated and fixed. No discharge is present. The examining physician would expect to find which of the following?

(A) Intraocular pressure greater than 22 mm Hg
(B) Blood in the anterior chamber
(C) Corneal abrasion on slit-lamp examination
(D) Papilledema
(E) Bloodless arterioles and a cherry-red fovea

28 A 69-year-old man with a known history of coronary artery disease (CAD), atrial fibrillation, and hypertension presents with sudden onset of right facial weakness and numbness. He also complained of a roaring in the right ear. On examination, he has some difficulty with speech. He does not have a pronator drift, and his grip strength is normal. However, there is weakness of the face on the right side, including the orbicularis oculi. He is unable to appreciate taste on the anterior tongue on the right side. He has normal sensations on the face to touch and pinprick. Which of the following would best explain these findings?

(A) Upper motor neuron lesion
(B) Brainstem glioma
(C) Left middle cerebral artery embolus
(D) Hemorrhage within the left internal capsule
(E) Lower motor neuron lesion

29 A 55-year-old female presents to the emergency room with a history of severe crushing retrosternal chest pain while she was moving some furniture around the house. Electrocardiography shows elevated ST segments in leads II, III and aVF, consistent with an inferior myocardial infarction. This diagnosis is further supported by cardiac enzymes that test positive. The patient is hemodynamically stable. She is moved to the intensive care unit. A few hours later she developed tachyarrhythmia. Treatment with intravenous (IV) boluses of lidocaine controls the arrhythmia only transiently—the arrhythmia disappears within 1 minute only to reappear within 4 minutes of each bolus dose. Plasma levels of lidocaine measured soon after each injection remained within the therapeutic range (1–5mg/L). Which of the following statements is most accurate?

(A) Rapid metabolism of lidocaine is responsible for the short duration of its antiarrhythmic action after the bolus administration.
(B) Laboratory determinations of blood levels of lidocaine after IV administration are frequently in error.
(C) The elimination half-life of lidocaine is approximately 2 minutes.
(D) Lidocaine rapidly redistributes from blood to other tissues.
(E) Cardiac cells rapidly develop tachyphylaxis to lidocaine.

30 A 30-year-old Caucasian male from Scotland met and married a 26-year-old French Caucasian woman. Both of them were healthy and lived a healthy lifestyle. They moved to California after their marriage and worked in the entertainment industry in Hollywood. Three years later, the woman gave birth to a child who had respiratory and gastrointestinal problems. The child was diagnosed with cystic fibrosis. Both parents are convinced that the disease was not inherited and are not concerned that subsequent children will have a substantial chance of acquiring the disease. They support this contention by pointing out that they are not related and there is no history of cystic fibrosis in either of their families. Which of the following statements is most likely true?

(A) The case described is a new mutation.
(B) The degree of penetrance is low; therefore, some of their relatives were genetically affected but did not express the disease.
(C) Both parents are carriers and each subsequent child will have a 25% chance of expressing the disease.
(D) It would be easy to determine if they are carriers using simple physiologic methods.
(E) DNA fingerprinting can be used to determine whether or not each parent carries the unique mutation that causes cystic fibrosis.

31 The paramedics were called to a theme park to attend to a 75-year-old woman who suddenly took ill. She complained of headache and numbness and weakness on the left side of her body. She had a prior history of a mitral valve replacement and was on warfarin. She lapsed into coma on the way to the hospital. The emergency room physician observed a left hemiplegia, with hemi-neglect and conjugate ocular deviation to the left. Which of the following is the most appropriate emergent test to obtain?

(A) Magnetic resonance imaging (MRI) scan of the brain
(B) Computed tomography (CT) of the brain
(C) Electroencephalogram (EEG)
(D) Carotid duplex ultrasonography
(E) Spinal tap

32 An anxious 33-year-old woman, gravida 3, para 1, aborta 1, is seen for her first prenatal visit at 10 weeks' gestation by dates. This was a planned pregnancy, and she discontinued the transdermal contraceptive patch 4 months ago. She is taking prenatal vitamins including iron and folic acid. First-trimester bleeding that progressed to hemorrhage complicated her first pregnancy, necessitating a suction dilatation and curettage at 8 weeks' gestation. Her last pregnancy was uncomplicated prenatally. She went into spontaneous labor at 39 weeks gestation progressing normally in labor with a reassuring electronic fetal heart rate monitor pattern. However, after an uncomplicated spontaneous vaginal delivery with neonatal Apgar scores of 8 and 9 at 1 and 5 minutes, respectively, her female neonate died on the second day of life from overwhelming group B β-hemolytic streptococcal infection. Which of the following statements best expresses what you will tell her about her current pregnancy?

(A) Most women with a positive vaginal culture will have uninfected infants.
(B) A negative vaginal culture means the fetus will not be at risk at delivery.
(C) Appropriate treatment for a positive vaginal culture can eradicate the organism.
(D) The organism is a pathologic bacterium in the female genital tract.
(E) Rapid nonculture assay tests are highly sensitive for the organism.

33 A 4-year-old presents to his pediatrician with left ear pain. His parents state that he had been in his usual state of good health until he started swimming lessons 1 week ago. The patient's vital signs are within normal limits for age. He is afebrile and appears nontoxic. Physical examination of the left ear reveals edema and erythema of the ear canal as well as a greenish otorrhea. Pain is increased by manipulation of the pinna and pressure on the tragus. Which of the following is the most likely pathogen producing this patient's symptoms?

(A) *Haemophilus influenzae*
(B) *Pseudomonas aeruginosa*
(C) *Moraxella catarrhalis*
(D) *Streptococcus agalactiae*
(E) *Escherichia coli*

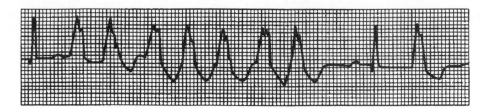

34 The above electrocardiogram (ECG) is from a 65-year-old man with ischemic heart disease. Which of the following is the most likely diagnosis?

(A) Premature atrial contractions
(B) Atrial flutter
(C) Paroxysmal atrial tachycardia
(D) Ventricular tachycardia
(E) Sinus tachycardia

35 A 65-year-old female had a 5-year history of pain in the right hip that had gradually gotten worse. She had reached a point where she hobbled with the help of a cane. Nonsteroidal analgesics did not help her very much. She finally agreed to undergo surgery. An x-ray film of the right hip confirmed severe osteoarthritis. There was no osteoporosis. The orthopedic surgeon recommended hip arthroplasty and she was admitted to the hospital. She was considered a high risk for deep venous thrombosis, and heparin prophylaxis was begun. Which of the following is the best test to monitor heparin therapy?

(A) Thrombin time (TT)
(B) Prothrombin time (PT)
(C) Prothrombin and proconvertin test
(D) Activated partial thromboplastin time (aPTT)
(E) Bleeding time

36 A 34-year-old woman with major depressive disorder, single episode, has responded well to sertraline after 1 month of treatment. There are no significant untoward effects, such as intolerable nausea or other gastrointestinal problems that selective serotonin-reuptake inhibitors (SSRIs) sometimes cause. Which of the following is the most appropriate next step in management?

(A) Continue the sertraline for 6 months
(B) Continue the sertraline indefinitely
(C) Decrease the sertraline gradually until she is medication free, unless depression recurs
(D) Stop the sertraline immediately
(E) Switch to fluoxetine

37 A 58-year old male computer programmer presented to his physician for a routine "check up" after his wife nagged him into it. This was his first visit to a physician in at least a decade. After work he would come home, eat dinner, watch television, and go to bed. He spent his weekends watching sports on television. While doing so, he often ate peanuts, buttered popcorn, or potato chips and downed it with a couple of beers. When asked if this had always been his lifestyle, he replies that prior to turning 40 he played sports and enjoyed dancing with his wife. His subsequent physical examination and laboratory work did not uncover any abnormalities with his heart, lungs, thyroid hormone levels, or kidney function. On the other hand, three different blood pressure readings taken by both the physician and his assistant obtain similar results, namely, an average reading of 178/92 mm Hg. He is 5 feet, 9 inches (1.75 m) tall and weighs 204 pounds (92.5 kg). A fasting blood sugar and lipid profile show a glucose level of 124 mg/dL, total cholesterol (TC) level of 234 mg/dL, and low-density lipoprotein (LDL) level of mg/dL. The most appropriate first line of management in this patient would be which of the following?

(A) Gastroplasty
(B) Prescription of an anorexic drug
(C) Prescription of gemfibrozil
(D) Persuade him to take his wife out dancing at least twice a week.
(E) Prescription of a dietary supplement containing ephedra
(F) Prescription of tolbutamide

38 A young female with phenylketonuria (PKU) who wants to become pregnant asks her physician if any special preparation is required before conception to ensure that her baby is healthy. Her physician tells her that women with PKU who are not on low-phenylalanine diets have a higher risk of spontaneous abortion than the general population and often give birth to infants with mental retardation, microcephaly, and other congenital anomalies; high levels of phenylalanine seem to be the cause of these problems. Therefore, prospective mothers who have PKU should be placed on a low-phenylalanine diet before conception. Which of the following values represents the highest blood phenylalanine concentration that provides a high probability of avoiding untoward complications?

(A) 1 mg/dL
(B) 6 mg/dL
(C) 11 mg/dL
(D) 16 mg/dL
(E) 21 mg/dL

39 A 65-year-old man with a long history of coronary artery disease and recent history of myocardial infarction is seen in the emergency room with a history of sudden onset of pain in the right leg. The patient also complained of numbness in the leg. Physical examination revealed pallor of the right leg, the skin was cool to the touch, and the patient had difficulty in moving his toes. Raising his leg increased the pallor, and the dorsalis pedis pulse could not be felt. These symptoms most likely represent which of the following abnormalities?

(A) Superficial thrombophlebitis
(B) Herniation of a lumbar disk
(C) Arterial occlusion
(D) Deep venous insufficiency
(E) Hypovolemic shock

40 A 3-year-old boy with growth retardation has a long history of recurrent pneumonia and chronic diarrhea. His mother states that he has six to eight foul-smelling stools per day. Physical examination reveals a low-grade fever, scattered rhonchi over both lung fields, crepitant rales at the left lung base and dullness on percussion, mild hepatomegaly, and slight pitting edema of the lower legs. Preliminary laboratory data are as follows:

Analysis	Value
Hemoglobin	7.5 g/dL
WBC count	18,000 cells/mm³, with neutrophilic leukocytosis and 15% bands; occasional hypersegmented neutrophils
Mean corpuscular volume	90 µm³
Red blood cells	Dimorphic population with both microcytic and macrocytic cells
Serum albumin	2.5 g/dL
Serum calcium	7.0 mg/dL
Serum sodium	138 mEq/L
Serum chloride	112 mEq/L
Serum potassium	3.2 mEq/L
Serum bicarbonate	18 mEq/L
Serum alkaline phosphatase	300 U/L
Serum SGOT	115 U/L
Serum SGPT	125 U/L
Total bilirubin	0.9 mg/dL
Urine pH	5
Urine dipstick protein	Negative
Chest x-ray film	Left lower lobe consolidation; generalized osteopenia

The most appropriate next step in arriving at the primary diagnosis would be to order which of the following?

(A) A plasma growth hormone assay
(B) A complete skeletal survey
(C) A sweat chloride test
(D) Endoscope of the upper gastrointestinal (GI) tract
(E) Acute viral serology

Directions for Matching Questions (41 through 50): Each set of matching questions is preceded by a list of 4 to 26 lettered options followed by a brief explanation of the required task and then by a series of numbered statements. For each lettered statement you are to select the ONE lettered option that best fulfills the task as it relates to that statement. Remember each of the listed options might be correctly selected once, more than once, or not at all.

Questions 41–43

(A) Arthropod borne
(B) Coronavirus
(C) Coxsackievirus
(D) Ebola virus
(E) Hantavirus
(F) Lymphocytic choriomeningitis virus
(G) Flavi virus

Select the ONE infectious agent that is most likely responsible for the symptoms described.

41 A 40-year-old Native American, who lives on a Navajo reservation in northern Arizona, develops acute respiratory distress syndrome and renal failure.

42 A 35-year-old missionary in China develops severe pneumonia progressing to multisystem disease shortly after visiting a patient in the hospital.

43 A 38-year-old man in Tulsa, Oklahoma, develops fever and a severe headache. Recently, he picked up and discarded a dead crow that was found in his back yard while he was mowing the lawn.

Questions 44 and 45

Match each disorder with the ONE graph that best describes the course of the disease described.

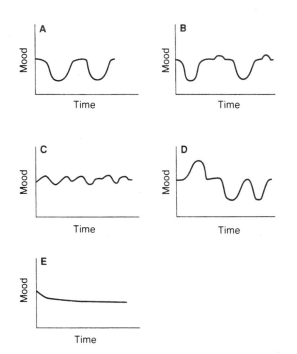

An upward deflection indicates mania; a downward deflection indicates depression. The intensity of the mood is indicated by the degree of deflection.

44 Cyclothymic disorder

45 Bipolar II disorder

Questions 46–48

(A) Iron deficiency

(B) Anemia of chronic disease (ACD)

(C) Thalassemia minor

(D) Lead poisoning

(E) Vitamin B$_{12}$ deficiency

(F) Folate deficiency

(G) Congenital spherocytosis

(H) Autoimmune hemolytic anemia (AIHA)

For each clinical description select the ONE anemia most closely associated.

46 A 3-year-old African-American child presents with abdominal colic and a history of pica. Physical examination shows no localizing signs on abdominal examination. Bone radiographs show densities in the epiphyses. A complete blood count (CBC) shows a hemoglobin (Hgb) of 7.0 g/dL (mean is 11 g/dL), a mean corpuscular volume (MCV) of 70 μm^3 (normal is 80–100 μm^3), and a normal leukocyte and platelet count. An abnormal RBC was observed in the peripheral blood. The corrected reticulocyte count is 4%.

47 A 32-year-old woman with systemic lupus erythematosus (SLE) presents with generalized weakness and malaise. Physical examination shows generalized lymphadenopathy and hepatosplenomegaly. The CBC shows an Hgb of 5.0 g/dL (normal is 12–16 g/dL), an MCV of 103 μm^3 (normal is 80–100 μm^3), and normal platelet and leukocyte counts. Numerous spherocytes are noted in the peripheral blood smear. The uncorrected reticulocyte count is 27%. The direct Coombs' test result is positive.

48 A 42-year-old man with a 20-year history of alcohol abuse presents with hepatosplenomegaly and ascites. The neurologic and mental status examinations yield normal results. A CBC exhibits an Hgb of 7.0 g/dL (normal is 13.5–17.5 g/dL), an MCV of 120 μm^3 (normal is 80–100 μm^3), a leukocyte count of 2500 cells/mm^3 (normal is 4500–11,000 cells/mm^3), and a platelet count of 75,000 cells/mm^3 (normal is 150,000–450,000 cells/mm^3). A peripheral blood smear shows abnormal leukocytes. The corrected reticulocyte count is 1%.

Questions 49 and 50

(A) Acute stress disorder

(B) Agoraphobia

(C) Conduct disorder

(D) Delirium

(E) Generalized anxiety disorder

(F) Obsessive–compulsive disorder

(G) Oppositional defiant disorder

(H) Panic disorder

(I) Posttraumatic stress disorder

(J) Separation anxiety disorder

(K) Social phobia

(L) Specific phobia

(M) Substance-induced anxiety disorder

Match each patient with the ONE correct associated anxiety disorder.

49 The parents of a 4-year-old boy seek marital therapy because they have grown steadily apart since the birth of their only child. They state that they never do things together anymore. It has been years since they left their child and went out to dinner with friends or took a vacation. They have little romantic life. They tried to leave their son with a babysitter several times, but the child became so upset that they canceled the outing. The child sleeps in their bed every night. Occasionally they have tried putting him in his own bed, but he cries or crawls into their bed later.

50 A 35-year-old single male librarian seeks therapy because he is lonely and unhappy. He describes a solitary life spent cataloguing books all day, then remaining alone at night and on weekends. He declines all invitations to dinners or get-togethers because he feels anxious around people. He says that he has tried to meet others but gets so uncomfortable that he goes home quickly.

Answer Key

1	E	**11**	E	**21**	E	**31**	B	**41**	E
2	C	**12**	B	**22**	B	**32**	A	**42**	B
3	D	**13**	A	**23**	D	**33**	B	**43**	G
4	A	**14**	B	**24**	C	**34**	D	**44**	C
5	C	**15**	D	**25**	E	**35**	D	**45**	B
6	E	**16**	B	**26**	D	**36**	A	**46**	D
7	C	**17**	D	**27**	A	**37**	D	**47**	H
8	A	**18**	A	**28**	E	**38**	B	**48**	F
9	C	**19**	E	**29**	D	**39**	C	**49**	J
10	B	**20**	C	**30**	C	**40**	C	**50**	K

Answers and Explanations

1 **The answer is E** *Surgery*

As a result of sustaining a spontaneous fracture of the neck of the femur, this patient is in hemorrhagic shock. Among the choices offered to account for this fracture, metastatic bone disease (choice **E**) is the most probable. Metastases in bone cause lytic lesions, thereby weakening the bone and possibly leading to a spontaneous fracture. The primary cancer may arise in any of several tissues, including breast, small cell carcinoma of the lung, and follicular carcinoma of the thyroid. Lytic lesions are also found in multiple myeloma, which is the most common primary hematologic malignancy of bone and in osteosarcoma, the most common primary cancer of bone. Nonmalignant diseases causing pathologic (spontaneous) fractures include bone cysts, Paget's disease of bone (in which the fractures are usually transverse and usually involve the femur or the tibia), osteogenesis imperfecta, and osteoporosis.

Chronic (not acute) osteomyelitis (choice **A**) results from acute hematogenous infection to the bone that may or may not have been treated adequately. The condition is usually quiescent for several months or even years before it flares up. The patient has fever, prostration, local inflammation, and a draining sinus. This patient had a furuncle on her thigh, not a draining sinus. Fractures are unusual in a setting of chronic osteomyelitis. Treatment is surgical, and cure is difficult. The goal is to remove the sequestrum (dead bone), which is a continual nidus for infection. Osteoporosis (choice **B**) is unlikely. Not withstanding the hot flushes that she has been experiencing recently, the patient is still premenopausal. Declining bone density in women usually commences shortly after menopause, but frank osteoporosis is rare before the age of 65. Colles' fracture, fracture of the proximal humerus, neck of the femur, and collapse of the vertebra are the most common fractures associated with osteoporosis. Only femoral neck fracture and vertebral collapse are not preceded by a history of fall. Stress fractures (choice **C**) are caused by repetitive excessive load on the bones. This can involve the second and third metatarsals (march fracture), which was initially noted in infantrymen during long marches, and femoral neck in the case of young soldiers who have to march for great distances carrying a full, heavily loaded backpack. Stress fractures can also involve the tibiae in runners, especially when they run over uneven surfaces. Physical examination usually reveals localized tenderness without deformity. A radiograph may not show the fracture, especially in the early stages. A bone scan using ^{99m}Tc-labeled bisphosphonate will clinch the diagnosis, by demonstrating increased uptake at the site. Most stress fractures resolve with rest. Osteogenesis imperfecta (choice **D**), also known as brittle bone disease, presents itself in four forms, of varying severity. Type I is the most common form and is associated with a blue sclera 98% of the time (not blue irises, as in this woman); typically fractures are not excessive and primarily occur prior to puberty. Type II manifests in utero or in infancy and is lethal. Type III is relatively rare; fractures abound, causing bone deformities such as scoliosis and deformed limbs and may result in dwarfism. Blue sclera is also a prominent symptom in types II and III. Type IV is similar to type I but much rarer and differs in that blue sclera are not seen. Both types I and IV are associated with childhood fractures after minimal trauma and are easily mistaken for child abuse, particularly type IV in which blue sclera are not present. Although in both type I and IV fractures become less frequent after growth ceases, the bone structure remains less dense than normal, making then susceptible to fractures throughout life and to osteoporosis as the patients age. Types I and IV are autosomal dominant, and commonly, cases can be traced back several generations. In contrast type II and III cases lack a family history and are either autosomal recessive conditions or new mutations.

2 **The answer is C** *Psychiatry*

This patient's symptoms are most suggestive of posttraumatic stress disorder (PTSD), characterized by persistent reexperiencing of traumatic events, coupled with anxiety and emotional numbing. The patient's desire to seek out other veterans with similar experiences is well advised. Peer support groups (choice **C**) permitting collective recall and discussion of traumatic experiences are often effective treatment. Although PTSD is historically associated with war veterans, it can be induced by any traumatic event, and symptoms can persist for a lifetime.

Psychodynamic therapy (choice **A**), cognitive behavioral therapy (choice **B**) as well as hypnotherapy are all acceptable means of nonpharmacologic therapy. However in this case, the patient's expressed preferences for group therapy should take precedence. There is little to suggest that a combination of medications (e.g., clonazepam and paroxetine) (choice **D**) is useful for treating PTSD in the absence of specific symptoms of anxiety or depression, and individuals with PTSD are at higher risk for clonazepam and other benzodiazepine abuse. While meeting with citizens and veterans from the nation he fought against (choice **E**) may be helpful in the future, there is little to suggest that this would be a good initial plan or that it even would be possible to arrange.

3 **The answer is D** *Obstetrics and Gynecology*

Hepatitis B is a serious perinatal viral infection that can be vertically transmitted from mother to neonate, most often at birth. The neonate can be protected from hepatitis B by passive immunization at birth using hepatitis B immune globulin (HBIG) (choice **D**) followed by immunization thereafter. Confirmation of immunization in the infant is carried out approximately a year after birth by testing for HBsAg, anti-HBc, and anti-HBs. The hepatitis B virus is a double-stranded DNA virus that is transmitted via blood, saliva, vaginal secretions, semen, and breast milk, as well as across the placenta. Hepatitis B surface antigen (HbsAg) is the earliest marker of hepatitis B viral infection or carrier state. To clarify further, anti-HBc IgM should also be checked. It is the best marker of acute hepatitis B infection and is seen early. If this had tested positive in the mother, she has acute infection and is not a carrier of the disease. In the vignette presented, she is a carrier of the disease.

Pregnancy does not appear to accelerate acute hepatitis B in the mother (choice **A**). The main route of neonatal infection is by vaginal delivery (choice **B**). The virus can be transmitted through breast milk (choice **C**). Neonatal infection has a higher likelihood of progression to active hepatitis than it does in the mother (choice **E**). Most pregnant women exposed to hepatitis B will become carriers with no active liver disease. However, in the neonate the course of the infection often can be fulminant and lethal.

4 **The answer is A** *Pediatrics*

A patient with patent ductus arteriosus has a continuous machinery murmur (choice **A**). Bounding pulses with hyperactive precordium may be found on physical examination. Although the electrocardiogram (ECG) is usually not helpful, it may show left ventricular hypertrophy (LVH).

Patients with atrial septal defect (ASD) (choice **B**) have a widely split and fixed second heart sound. Patients with ventricular septal defect (VSD) (choice **C**) have a harsh holosystolic murmur heard best over the lower left sternal border. Tetralogy of Fallot (choice **E**) is characterized by the presence of a VSD, right ventricular hypertrophy, pulmonic stenosis, and overriding aorta. The murmur of tetralogy of Fallot is a long, systolic ejection murmur most audible at the midleft sternal border. In patients with pulmonic stenosis (choice **D**), there is a high-pitched systolic ejection murmur, most audible at the upper left sternal border, which transmits fairly well to the back. A systolic thrill may be present at the upper left sternal border and, rarely, in the suprasternal notch.

5 **The answer is C** *Preventive Medicine and Public Health*

In the case presented, the physician would first order the enzyme-linked immunosorbent assay (ELISA) test, which is about 99.5% sensitive (i.e., it usually gives a positive value in the presence of serum samples containing the human immunodeficiency virus [HIV]). High sensitivity is the key feature required of a screening test. Sensitivity is mathematically defined as $a/a + c$. To have a high degree of sensitivity, a must be much greater than c (choice **C**). For example, when $c = 0$ (i.e., when there are no false-negatives [FNs]), $a/a + c = 1$ (i.e., 100% of the patients with the disease will test positive, or the test is 100% sensitive). However, this says nothing about the number of false-positives (FPs) (b). If $b = 0$, there are no FPs. Although the ELISA is highly sensitive, it is not very specific. It provides a large fraction of FPs, or in terms of the 2×2 table, b is a significant, finite number.

In testing for HIV, a positive ELISA result would typically be followed by a Western blot test. The ELISA is used as a sensitive screening test, and the Western blot test as a specific confirmatory test. A highly specific test is one that provides few FP results (i.e., one in which b approaches 0). Specificity is conventionally defined in terms of the ratio $d/d + b$ (choices **B** and **D**). Thus, when $b = 0$, $d/d = 1$ (i.e., 100% of all individuals without the disease will test negative) (choice **B**). There is a limit regarding the lack of specificity that a screening test can tolerate. If $d = 0$, all individuals without the disease will test positive, and the test will have no specificity (i.e., it will be of no value). If $d = b/2$, one half of the normal individuals will test positive; therefore, the test could possibly have value as a screening test (choice **D**).

The practical value of a screening test depends on several factors, including relative cost and the population being tested. Based on these factors, the ELISA is a practical screening test. The ELISA is easier to perform, less time consuming, and significantly less expensive than the Western blot test. Because the ELISA has a very low specificity, it is only used when there is reason to believe that the person was exposed to the virus. In such populations, the total fraction of normals is lower; therefore, the specificity is higher. This principle carries over to all screening procedures.

Other parameters conventionally described by a 2×2 table include the positive predictive value, the negative predictive value, the odds ratio, and the prevalence. The positive predictive value is defined as the probability that a positive test result would actually be associated with a patient who has the disease. In mathematical terms, this is expressed as: $a/a + b$ (choice **E**). In this case, if $b = 0$, the positive predictive value would be 100%. Negative predictive value is defined as the probability that a patient who did not have the disease would test negative, or: $d/c + d$ (choice **A**). In this case, if $c = 0$, the negative predictive value would be 100%. The odds ratio is a measure of the probability that a positive test result would prove that the patient actually has the disease, or $a/a + c \div b/b + d$. Stated in words, the likelihood ratio is the true-positives (TPs) divided by all of the diseased cases, which, in turn, is divided by the FNs divided by the negatives. The likelihood of a positive test result being 100% dependable will then occur when $c = 0$ (no FNs) and when $d = 0$ (no FPs). The prevalence is simply a measure of the proportion of individuals with the disease in the total population. In terms of a 2×2 table, the negative + false-positives divided by the whole sample equals the fraction of positive cases in that particular population at that particular time. Mathematically, this is stated as $a + c/a + b + c + d$.

6 The answer is E *Surgery*

This patient has a ruptured abdominal aortic aneurysm. The abdominal aorta is retroperitoneal. Rupture can be heralded by severe flank or back pain due to bleeding posteriorly into the retroperitoneal space. This is true in 80% of cases, however, in the remaining 20%, the aneurysm ruptures anteriorly into the peritoneal cavity. Hypotension due to blood loss, and a pulsatile mass in the epigastrium are also found. Prior to rupture patients may have a history of backache or a vague discomfort in the epigastric region. Some 95% of cases of abdominal aortic aneurysm are due to atherosclerosis (choice **E**). Other causes include Marfan's syndrome, trauma, mycotic infection, and syphilis. Most aneurysms occur below the renal arteries, as the vasa vasorum are lacking here. Lack of inherent blood supply here leads to tissue hypoxia, atherosclerosis, and weakening of the aortic vessel wall. There may be associated atherosclerosis elsewhere, such as the iliacs, and coronaries.

Cystic medial degeneration (CMD, choice **A**) is involved in the pathogenesis of aortic dissections due to hypertension in elderly men or connective tissue disorders in younger individuals. CMD occurs in the middle and outer part of the aorta and is characterized by elastic tissue fragmentation and the presence of cleft-like spaces containing acid mucopolysaccharides. CMD also occurs in Ehlers-Danlos syndrome, in which there is a defect in collagen (choice **B**) and Marfan's syndrome, in which there is a defect in fibrillin (choice **C**). Aortic dissections are the most common cause of death in these connective tissue disorders. An immunologic reaction (choice **D**) has been implicated in the pathogenesis of some cases of abdominal aortic aneurysms; however, it is rare.

7 The answer is C *Pediatrics*

Most 3-year-old children are toilet trained, play interactive games, give their first and last names, and pedal a tricycle. At age 3 (choice **C**), most children should be able to copy a circle, and some will be able to copy a cross.

A 1-year-old child (choice **A**) would not be able to pedal a tricycle, give his first and last names, or copy a circle or a cross. At age 1, a child should be able to stand momentarily, say "dada" and "mama," and bang two cubes held in his hands. Although some 2-year-old children (choice **B**) may be able to accomplish the tasks noted in the scenario, they would not be able to hop on one foot. Most 4-year-old children (choice **D**) are able to dress without supervision, hop on one foot, and catch a bounced ball. A 5-year-old child (choice **E**) would be able to copy a triangle.

8 The answer is A *Preventive Medicine and Public Health*

$$\text{Perinatal mortality rate} = \frac{\text{Number of fetal deaths} + \text{Number of neonatal deaths}}{\text{Total number of live births} + \text{Total number of stillbirths}}$$

The perinatal mortality rate is calculated by adding the number of fetal deaths, i.e., stillbirths (≥ 20 weeks' gestation), and the number of neonatal deaths (within first 28 days of life), then dividing that sum by the total number of births. In the data presented, the perinatal rate is calculated as follows: 85 (stillbirths) + 15 (neonatal deaths) divided by the sum of 1600 (live births) + 85 (stillbirths). This equals 100/1685 (choice **A**).

Therefore it is apparent that choices **B** (85/1600), **C** (125/2205), **D** (100/1700), and **E** (59/2205) are incorrect because the data sets do not represent the perinatal rate.

9 The answer is C *Obstetrics and Gynecology*

A diagnostic cervical cone biopsy is performed only if the combination of Pap smear, colposcopy, and directed cervical biopsies cannot unequivocally rule out frankly invasive carcinoma. A cone biopsy would be in order if the cervical biopsy showed mild dysplasia (choice **C**), because the high-grade squamous intraepithelial lesion (HSIL) Pap smear suggests a more severe lesion than was identified on colposcopy.

No cone biopsy is indicated for intraepithelial neoplasia on biopsy with satisfactory colposcopy (choice **A**). Satisfactory colposcopy means the entire transformation zone (T-zone) is seen and no lesion or squamous epithelium enters the endocervical canal. A negative endocervical curettage (ECC) result with satisfactory colposcopy (choice **B**) means that the entire T-zone was seen and the ECC pathology report showed normal histologic findings. A cone biopsy is not needed if the cervical biopsy showed carcinoma in situ (choice **D**), because frankly invasive disease is ruled out. When frankly invasive carcinoma is found on cervical biopsy (choice **E**), further confirmation of invasive disease becomes superfluous.

10 The answer is B *Obstetrics and Gynecology*

Infection with the human immunodeficiency virus (HIV) results in the development of the acquired immune deficiency syndrome (AIDS), which has been a recognized disease in the United States since 1981. All pregnant women regardless of HIV RNA viral load and CD4 count should be placed on AZT at 14 weeks and continued on it throughout pregnancy and labor. Mode of delivery is one of the most significant factors that affect maternal–neonatal transmission (choice **B**). Current recommendations are that HIV-positive women should be offered elective cesarean section at 38 weeks to minimize vertical HIV transmission.

Pregnancy does not appear to accelerate progression of HIV to AIDS (choice **A**). Neonates can be infected from HIV-positive breast-feeding mothers (choice **C**). There is no current effective immunization for neonates or for adults for that matter (choice **D**). Disease progression of HIV to AIDS in neonates and infants is more rapid than in adults (choice **E**).

11 The answer is E *Psychiatry*

A person can be involuntarily hospitalized if he is a significant danger to himself or others. Possessing a gun and voicing suicidal intent (choice **E**) suggests such a danger.

Because self-neglect is not sufficient grounds for involuntary hospitalization unless the person is so gravely disabled that he is unable to provide for food clothing or shelter, and as a consequence, has an imminent and significant threat to life, neither living in a makeshift shelter (choice **A**) nor being disheveled and malnourished (choice **D**) can be legal reasons for keeping the man hospitalized against his will. Hallucinations (e.g., hearing voices [choice **C**]) or delusions (e.g., believing he or she is followed by central intelligence agency members [choice **B**]) are seen commonly in patients with schizophrenia but do not necessarily pose a significant danger to self or others or signify grave disability as legally defined.

12 The answer is B *Surgery*

This patient has Graves' disease (choice **B**), also known as diffuse toxic goiter. It usually affects younger women, and eye signs are often noted. The disease affects the entire thyroid gland. Abnormal thyroid-stimulating antibodies lead to hyperplasia and hypertrophy of the thyroid gland. It is the most common cause of hyperthyroidism, the features of which are presented in the vignette. It may be found in patients with other autoimmune disorders such as myasthenia gravis, pernicious anemia, type I diabetes mellitus, rheumatoid arthritis, Addison's disease, chronic hepatitis, idiopathic thrombocytopenic purpura, Sjögren's syndrome and vitiligo.

Hashimoto's thyroiditis (choice **A**) is an autoimmune disease, also known as lymphocytic thyroiditis. It primarily affects women of menopausal age, and usually presents as a multinodular goiter, with evidence of hypothyroidism. Initially, *hyper*thyroidism may be found. Thereafter, hypothyroidism supervenes. Hashimoto's thyroiditis is the most common cause of hypothyroidism. Elevated titers of thyroid antibodies (microsomal and thyroglobulin antibodies) are usually present in the serum. Papillary carcinoma (choice **C**) is the most common primary malignant thyroid tumor (60%). It usually metastasizes to lymph nodes. The tumor is nonfunctional; that is it does not cause hyperthyroidism. Most papillary carcinomas contain a mixture of papillary and colloid-filled follicles. Microscopically, the tumor shows papillary projections with pale empty nuclei. In toxic multinodular goiter (choice **D**); one or more of the nodules become autonomous and secrete excessive amounts of thyroxine. Thus the patient develops symptoms and signs of hyperthyroidism. However, it is far less common than diffuse toxic goiter. Follicular adenomas (choice **E**) are benign, solitary nodules that are usually non-functioning. Follicular adenomas can be distinguished from follicular carcinoma by histology. Lack of capsular invasion or pericapsular blood vessels is noted in follicular adenomas.

13 **The answer is A** *Medicine*

The triad of rapidly progressive dementia, myoclonus and periodic complexes found on EEG are pointers to Creutzfeldt-Jakob disease (CJD), (choice **A**). Magnetic resonance imaging (MRI) shows bilateral areas of increased signal intensity in the caudate and putamen in T2-weighted images. The disease is more common among butchers and farmers. This patient contracted it after a corneal transplant. CJD represents the most common of the prion diseases, or transmissible spongiform encephalopathies, and is rapidly fatal. Prions are highly infectious protein particles that do not contain nucleic acids. They are extremely resistant to heat and formaldehyde. Brain biopsy is the gold standard for diagnosis. It reveals extensive vacuolation (spongiform change) within the neuropil between nerve cell bodies. Most cases of CJD are sporadic in which there is a mutation in the PrP gene, leading to deposition of amyloid. PrP (protease resistant protein) is a membrane bound glycoprotein whose exact function is still unknown. CJD can be inherited as well.

Some cases of spongiform encephalopathies may be transmitted to humans by eating beef obtained from cows suffering from bovine spongiform encephalopathy (choice **B**), also known as "mad cow" disease. This also is a transmissible spongiform encephalopathy caused by prion. The clinical features are similar to CJD, and have been found in young individuals in Britain who consumed contaminated beef. There has been no reported case of "mad cow" disease contracted in the United States to date. Although an infected cow had wandered across the border from Canada, the beef did not make it into the US market. Since this patient never left the United States it makes him a highly unlikely candidate to contract this disease. Parkinson's disease (choice **C**) is due to degeneration of neurons in the substantia nigra that synthesize dopamine, a neurotransmitter involved in voluntary muscle movement. Clinical findings include bradykinesia, cogwheel rigidity, postural instability and resting tremors. Patients have a mask like face, and a monotonous voice. Dementia is a late feature. Alzheimer's disease (choice **D**) is the most common cause of dementia in patients greater than 65 years of age. The disease is due to neuronal destruction by β-amyloid protein, which derives from amyloid precursor protein (APP). Dementia is gradual, involving impairment of memory, cognition, and thought process. Patients show change in behavior and personality, and have difficulty with activities of daily living. Motor function is usually preserved. They often lose their way in their own home. Acetylcholinesterase inhibitors are used in the treatment of mild to moderate Alzheimer's disease, together with adjunctive medications for other associated problems. Progressive multifocal leukoencephalopathy (PML) (choice **D**) is a subacute demyelinating disease, caused by a papovavirus. Destruction of oligodendrocytes leads to demyelination of the white matter. It is usually seen in immune compromised patients, most commonly in those with HIV. Seizures and focal neurologic deficits, such as hemiparesis may be a feature.

14 **The answer is B** *Surgery*

Zinc deficiency is characterized by alopecia, a maculopapular rash around the mouth and eyes, taste (dysgeusia) and smell abnormalities, and problems with healing of wounds.

Essential fatty acid deficiency (choice **A**) is characterized by an eczematous rash and thrombocytopenia. Selenium deficiency (choice **C**) produces muscle pain and a type of cardiomyopathy. Magnesium deficiency (choice **D**) is associated with resistance to activity of parathormone with subsequent hypocalcemia and tetany. Muscle weakness, irritability, delirium, and convulsions are also noted. Alcoholism is the most common cause of hypomagnesemia. Copper deficiency (choice **E**) is associated with iron deficiency anemia, dissecting aortic aneurysm, and kinky-hair syndrome.

15 **The answer is D** *Psychiatry*

This man's behavior is most suggestive of transvestic fetishism (choice **D**), a paraphilia characterized by an obsession with cross-dressing for the purpose of sexual arousal.

Other paraphilias include exhibitionism (choice **A**), in which an individual exposes his genitals to others; frotteurism (choice **B**), in which an individual derives sexual pleasure by rubbing his genitals against an unsuspecting person; and voyeurism (choice **E**), in which a person secretly observes people dressing or engaging in sexual activity. Gender identity disorder (choice **C**) also involves wearing the clothes of the opposite sex, but it is not done for sexual pleasure. Individuals with gender identity disorder feel more comfortable with the opposite gender identity.

16 **The answer is B** *Obstetrics and Gynecology*

The description of this young woman, in the beginning of her reproductive life, is characteristic of anovulation with unopposed estrogen. The expected finding would be a proliferative histologic picture; therefore, tubular endometrial glands with many mitoses, (choice **B**), would be the correct finding in this case.

There will not be evidence of ovulation (serrated endometrial glands with inspissated secretions; (choice **A**), since these findings are characteristic of secretory endometrium seen in the luteal phase of a normal cycle. Secretory changes are dependent on progesterone from a corpus luteum. Since she is not ovulating there is no corpus luteum to produce progesterone. Changes consistent with endometrial carcinoma (back-to-back endometrial glands with prominent nuclei, hyperchromism and loss of cellular polarity [choices **C** and **E**]) essentially are never seen in a pubertal girl. Even though this girl is experiencing the effects of unopposed estrogen, the progression to malignancy takes many years. Endometrial changes of pregnancy (decidual reaction forming around endometrial arterioles [choice **D**]) would not be expected with anovulation.

17 **The answer is D** *Medicine*

This patient is suffering from cluster headaches, often striking young men in the nocturnal hours. Oxygen in a high concentration (choice **D**) is a vasoconstrictor that aborts cluster headaches.

Both nitroglycerin (choice **A**) and alcohol (choice **B**) are vasodilators and may worsen vascular headaches. Exercise (choice **C**) and a warm pack (choice **E**) may distract the sufferer, but do nothing to end the underlying cluster attacks.

18 **The answer is A** *Obstetrics and Gynecology*

The cause of the vaginitis is *Trichomonas vaginalis,* as evidenced by the pruritic discharge and the highly motile protozoan. The elevated vaginal pH and frothy greenish discharge are frequent clinical findings with trichomoniasis. The agent of choice is metronidazole (choice **A**). Due to an antabuse effect of this medication, she should be advised not to drink alcohol while taking it. She also needs to be informed this is a sexually transmitted disease and her sexual partners also need to be treated.

Clotrimazole (choice **B**) and miconazole (choice **C**) are topical intravaginal antifungal agents used to treat vaginal yeast infections. Acyclovir (choice **D**) is an antiviral agent used in genital herpes management. Spectinomycin (choice **E**) is an antibacterial aminocyclitol antibiotic administered intramuscularly for the treatment of gonorrhea.

19 **The answer is E** *Preventive Medicine and Public Health*

$$\text{Mean} = \frac{\text{Sum of all the numbers}}{\text{Total of all the numerals}}$$

Therefore,

$$\text{Mean} = \frac{(7 + 5 + 8 + 2 + 8)}{5} = 6$$

The median is the number equidistant in order from the lowest and highest value in a sequentially ordered set of numbers. The numbers in this question arranged sequentially are 2, 5, 7, 8, 8. The middle number is 7 because there are two numbers of lesser value and two numbers of greater value. Hence, the median is 7. The mode, on the other hand is the most frequently occurring number, which in this set is 8. Therefore, the answer choice that correctly states the mean, median, and mode (numbers 6, 7, and 8) is choice **E**.

Choices **A**, **B**, **C**, and **D** are wrong. They represent the wrong numbers and/or the proper numbers in the wrong order.

20 The answer is C *Medicine*

This boy is in status epilepticus. The initial management always is to secure the airway (choice **C**) by clearing it and inserting an oropharyngeal airway. Ensuring that adequate ventilation (breathing) is occurring follows this, and circulation is checked thereafter—the ABCs of initial airway management.

Insertion of a tongue blade (choice **A**) in a convulsing patient does not contribute to airway management and may lacerate the tongue. A bolus of 50% dextrose (choice **B**) should be preceded by intravenous (IV) thiamine. Lorazepam followed by phenytoin (choice **D**) should be started only after IV thiamine and dextrose have been administered. In case lorazepam is unavailable, diazepam could be substituted. Lorazepam usually stops seizures. However, it should be followed by phenytoin or phosphenytoin infusion, as neither lorazepam nor diazepam alone will prevent their recurrence. If seizures continue, the patient should be intubated. Intravenous *pheno*barbital should be administered and followed by *pento*barbital for maintenance (choice **E**).

21 The answer is E *Obstetrics and Gynecology*

The fetal presentation in this case is a frank breech (choice **E**). In frank breech the thighs are flexed and the legs are extended. This is the only kind of breech in which vaginal delivery may be safely considered. Breech presentation occurs when the fetal buttocks or lower extremities present into the maternal pelvis, a finding in 3–4% of deliveries. Breech presentation is more common in premature fetuses, uterine and fetal anomalies. A major concern with vaginal delivery of fetuses in breech presentation is fetal head entrapment due to inadequate time to mold to the maternal pelvis. Trauma could result to the neck and arms with hasty delivery, and if the fetal head is hyperextended, cervical spine injury could result with tragic consequences. For these reasons many breech fetuses are delivered by cesarean section.

Transverse breech (choice **A**) is not a medical term, but transverse *lie* is. In complete breech (choice **B**) both thighs and knees are flexed. However, if one lower limb is extended at the hip and the knee joints instead, it is called a footling breech. On the other hand, in double-footling breech (choice **C**), both lower extremities are extended at the hip and the knee joints. Incomplete breech (choice **D**) occurs when one or both thighs are extended at the hip joint only and one or both knees are flexed and lie below the buttocks.

22 The answer is B *Pediatrics*

The patient in this question has trisomy 21, or Down syndrome, which is characterized by hypotonia, a simian crease, a short fifth finger, and upward and slanted palpebral fissures and epicanthic folds. These patients will also have differing degrees of mental and growth retardation. Duodenal atresia (choice **B**) is often associated with Down syndrome and appears in the first day of life as bilious vomiting after feedings without abdominal distention. Plain abdominal radiographs typically show the "double bubble" sign, caused by a distended and gas-filled stomach and proximal duodenum. The initial treatment for patients with duodenal atresia is nasogastric or orogastric decompression and intravenous fluid replacement. The definitive treatment is duodenojejunostomy.

Pyloric stenosis (choice **A**) appears at 2 to 3 weeks of age with nonbilious vomiting. Bile-stained emesis may be seen in the later phase of intussusception (choice **C**); however, it is rare under 3 months of age. It is associated with colicky abdominal pain, a sausage-shaped mass, and currant-jelly stool. If a diaphragmatic hernia (choice **D**) presents at birth, the infant usually has a scaphoid abdomen and respiratory distress due to herniation of the abdominal contents into the chest that compresses the lungs. Bowel sounds can be auscultated in the chest, and the presence of abdominal contents in the thorax can be visualized on chest roentgenogram. A perforated viscus, (choice **E**) will cause free air in the abdomen that is evident on plain abdominal radiographs as air under the diaphragm.

23 The answer is D *Medicine*

This patient has had an infarction involving the posterolateral portion of the medulla oblongata as a result of blockage of the posterior inferior cerebellar artery (PICA) on the left side. The condition is also known as the

Wallenberg syndrome. The computerized tomography scan shows no evidence of hemorrhage, and therefore the diagnosis of ischemic infarction is appropriate. Since his condition has been present for less than 3 hours, it is prudent to use a thrombolytic agent (choice **D**) as the initial medication. Recombinant tissue plasminogen activator (rt-PA) must be administered within 3 hours of the onset of the acute event to be efficacious. Up to 90 mg can be administered; 10% is given as an intravenous bolus, the rest in an infusion over an hour. It is contraindicated if the blood pressure is sustained above 185/110. No other antithrombotic treatment should be instituted for 24 hours.

Heparinization (choice **A**) followed by warfarin is appropriate in the management of a patient with a nonhemorrhagic stroke and would have been the choice had it been more than 3 hours after the onset of the acute event. Right or left carotid endarterectomy (choices **B** and **C**) are incorrect, because the problem involves the vertebral circulation. Antiplatelet agents such as aspirin and clopidogrel (choice **E**), are not used in the initial management of infarctions. They have a role to play in the prevention of strokes.

24 The answer is C *Surgery*

This patient has sustained a pneumothorax in the left hemithorax secondary to trauma. A pneumothorax can occur spontaneously or secondary to trauma resulting from a blunt or penetrating injury. A pneumothorax is the presence of air trapped in the pleural space that is unavailable for gaseous exchange. Additional physical findings include hyperresonance to percussion (also known increased timbre) on the side of the problem (choice **C**).

The breath sounds are not increased on the left side (choice **A**) but are absent instead. Egophony (choice **B**) is usually heard in patients with a pleural effusion. It occurs rarely in patients with consolidation of the lung. It is a bronchial sound that is heard when the patient speaks during auscultation. The syllables have an odd nasal or bleating quality. The tonal change is due to compression of the lung and the air passages. The width of the intercostals will not be increased (choice **D**). Widened intercostals spaces are found in patients with chronic obstructive airway disease such as emphysema. Nor will mediastinal shift occur to the left (choice **E**). The shift in fact will occur to the right, especially if the pneumothorax is large or if a tension pneumothorax has occurred.

25 The answer is E *Medicine*

This patient has symptoms of digitalis toxicity in addition to cardiac failure. Digitalis toxicity leads to vomiting, increasing confusion, hallucinations, photophobia, yellow vision, and cardiac arrhythmias that could be potentially dangerous if left untreated, as supraventricular tachycardia (SVT) and atrioventricular (AV) block could supervene, or even worse, ventricular tachycardia and fibrillation. The presence of SVT and AV block signifies cardiotoxicity. Digitalis toxicity may be precipitated by hypokalemia, and therefore, the serum potassium level should be increased (choice **E**), maintaining it between 4.0 and 5.0 mmol/L. There is a strong possibility the patient is on a loop diuretic (such as furosemide), which restricts sodium and chloride reabsorption in the proximal part of the ascending loop of Henle, with resultant excretion of sodium, water, chloride, and potassium. Digitalis administration should be discontinued temporarily. The serum digitalis level does *not* correlate with digitalis toxicity.

Raising the serum sodium level will have no effect on the heart (choice **A**). Sodium has its primary effects on the brain and not the heart. Lowering serum magnesium levels (choice **C**) would aggravate the problem further, as one of the causes of digitalis toxicity is hypomagnesemia. Raising the serum calcium level (choice **D**) would be disastrous, as hypercalcemia promotes digitalis toxicity. Although hypomagnesemia could result from use of loop diuretics, this effect is less common than that of hypokalemia; therefore raising the serum magnesium level (choice **B**) is not indicated. Other causes of digitalis toxicity include hypothyroidism, myocardial ischemia, advancing age, renal insufficiency, volume depletion, and concomitant use of drugs that delay elimination of digitalis, such as amiodarone, verapamil, β-blockers—such as carvedilol (which has been prescribed to this patient) and quinidine, a cinchona alkaloid that is used to treat cardiac arrhythmias. Although with coadministration of ACE inhibitors, such as enalapril, digitalis toxicity can potentially induce hyperkalemia, in the case presented, the electrocardiogram did not show evidence of hyperkalemia (peaked T waves); if it did one would consider lowering the serum potassium level.

26 **The answer is D** *Surgery*

Fat necrosis is usually seen in stocky women with large pendulous breasts. Its importance lies in its ability to mimic breast carcinoma. A history of trauma (such as that from use of a seat belt) may or may not be present. Furthermore, a history of trauma alone is not diagnostic. Trauma on the other hand, may have drawn the attention of the patient to the lump, which is often painless. Fat necrosis usually presents as a nontender, irregular, firm breast lump with thickening of the overlying skin or retraction, giving it the classic *peau d'orange* appearance; and raising doubts about the diagnosis. The lump usually decreases in size with time. However, a residual cyst within the confines of the breast may linger on. The patient should be reassured and followed up in a few weeks (choice **D**). Although mammography may demonstrate nonspecific changes or mimic carcinoma, ultrasound will often prove useful in coming to a diagnosis. The diagnosis can be confirmed by core biopsy under ultrasound guidance as was done in this case. Histologically, the lesion consists of lipid-laden macrophages, scar tissue, and chronic inflammatory cells. Since epithelial tissue is not involved, there is no potential for malignancy.

Excision of the mass (choice **A**) is not indicated, as the mass resolves over time. A repeat fine-needle biopsy (choice **B**) will not contribute to diagnosis in case of doubt. Should the need arise, an open biopsy would be in order. Repeating the mammography after a month (choice **C**) would not be helpful. Mastectomy (choice **E**) is totally uncalled for, and would constitute malpractice.

27 **The answer is A** *Surgery*

The patient has acute glaucoma, which refers to a sudden increase in intraocular pressure in which the tonometer pressures exceed 22 mm Hg (choice **A**); the normal range is between 8 and 21 mm Hg. There are two major types of glaucoma, acute and chronic. Acute, also known as closed-angle glaucoma is characterized clinically by sudden onset, blurry vision; intense pain; and minimal photophobia. The patient may complain of seeing halos around light fixtures and is usually uniocular. Other findings include ciliary injection; a steamy appearing cornea, and lack of discharge from the eye. The pupil is mid-dilated, fixed, and irregular.

A shallow anterior chamber is noted on gonioscopy. Gonioscopy is useful in differentiating between open- and closed-angle glaucoma. The cup to disc ratio is greater than 0.6. The normal cup is one third the size of the disc. Acute-angle closure glaucoma is less common than open-angle glaucoma. It is usually unilateral and occurs as the lens develops cataract, enlarging with age, pushing it forward into the ciliary body narrowing the angle between the iris and the cornea, and eventually closing off the canal of Schlemm. This process is accentuated by inherited anatomic features that also cause farsightedness and by widening of the pupil in dim light, accounting for the transitory attacks noted by this patient. Dilating the pupil can also provoke this latter effect. An attack of closed-angle glaucoma is a medical emergency. Initial treatment is to lower the intraocular pressure with a β-blocker such as timolol, carbonic anhydrase inhibitor such as acetazolamide, and osmotic agents such as oral isosorbide. One of the prostaglandin analogues such as latanoprost, bimatoprost, or travaprost is becoming increasing popular. In most cases, laser iridectomy is necessary. In this procedure a full-thickness opening is created in the peripheral iris to allow the flow of aqueous from the posterior to the anterior chamber. Chronic (open-angle) glaucoma is much more common and is an insidious disease with few clinical symptoms other than elevated intraocular pressure. There is a gradual progressive contraction of peripheral vision that may not be noticed at all. If left untreated, the chronic high pressure damages the optic nerve, resulting in a loss of peripheral vision that occurs so gradually that it may not be noticed until it is too late. Chronic glaucoma is a leading cause of blindness in the United States where about 3% of the population older than 65 years is affected; this amounts to about two million individuals of whom some 60,000 are legally blind. Open-angle glaucoma is eight times more common in African Americans than in other ethnicities. Other risk factors include diabetes mellitus, and prolonged corticosteroid use. Intraocular pressure is lowered with medications already described for angle-closure glaucoma. Surgical intervention is carried out if medical therapy fails and consists of laser trabeculoplasty or filtering surgery.

Blood in the anterior chamber (choice **B**) is called a hyphema and is associated with acute visual loss. The most common cause is ocular trauma. The presence of a hyphema in a small child should always be considered to be secondary to child abuse until proved otherwise. African-American children who present with hyphema should be screened for sickle cell disease or trait. Corneal abrasions (choice **C**) produce blurry vision, pain, moderate photophobia, watery discharge, mild-to-moderate conjunctival injection, a hazy cornea, a positive fluorescein stain, a normal or constricted pupil, a poor-to-normal pupillary light reflex, and normal intraocular pressure.

Papilledema (choice **D**) refers to swelling of the optic disc due to increased intracranial pressure. Patients with papilledema present with venous stasis, prominent disc vessels, a swollen disc with blurred margins, and absence of the physiologic cup. Bloodless arterioles and a cherry-red fovea (choice **E**) characterize a central retinal artery occlusion.

28 The answer is E *Medicine*

This patient has a lower motor neuron lesion (choice **E**) affecting cranial nerve seven—the facial nerve (CN VII) on the right side—and is also known as Bell's palsy. Facial palsy is the most common of the cranial neuropathies. Most cases are due to infection with herpes simplex virus and not idiopathic as was believed earlier. The facial nerve innervates the muscles of the face and the stapedius muscle in the ear and conveys taste fibers to the anterior two thirds of the tongue, via the chorda tympani nerve. The roaring in the ear (hyperacusis) and lack of taste in the anterior portion of the tongue are due to involvement of the aforementioned innervation. The problem with speech is due to dysarthria, resulting from paralysis of the muscles around the mouth. The inability to close his eye can put his cornea, and indeed the eye, in danger. Hence the eyelid should be taped shut or covered with an eye patch. The facial nerve also supplies the lacrimal gland. Absence of tears could result in xerophthalmia (corneal drying) and attendant complications, hence artificial tears are necessary. Corticosteroids are helpful. The disorder usually resolves over time. Other causes of lower motor neuron facial paralysis include lesions in the brainstem, cerebellopontine angle, middle ear infection, multiple sclerosis, HIV infection, Lyme disease, parotid tumor tumors, diabetes mellitus, and trauma to the facial nerve.

An upper motor neuron (choice **A**) lesion of the facial nerve will spare the upper half of the face because of the bilateral innervation to that region. An upper motor neuron VII nerve paralysis is due to involvement of the contralateral motor neurons of the descending corticobulbar pathway or of the pathway used en route to the seventh cranial nerve nucleus in the pons. A brainstem glioma (choice **B**) is unlikely, given the sudden nature of the event, lack of symptoms such as headache, nausea and vomiting, and bulbar signs involving the lower cranial nerves. These patients could have ataxia as well. A left middle cerebral artery embolus (choice **C**) could very well occur given his history of atrial fibrillation. However, embolism involving the middle cerebral artery would be associated with headache, confusion, right hemiparesis or hemiplegia, and an upper motor neuron facial paralysis on the right as well. Hemorrhage into the internal capsule (choice **D**) could occur, given the history of hypertension in this patient. However, the patient would have severe headache, obtundation, and a dense right hemiplegia together with a right upper motor neuron facial nerve paralysis.

29 The answer is D *Medicine*

Rapid (but temporary) control of arrhythmia follows achievement of a therapeutic blood level of lidocaine. This occurs because lidocaine rapidly redistributes from blood to other tissues (choice **D**). In this situation, the reappearance of the arrhythmia reflects the rapid distribution of lidocaine from the blood to highly perfused body tissues, resulting in a decrease in plasma concentration of the drug below therapeutic levels. A similar process, involving redistribution of thiopental from the brain to other highly perfused tissues, is responsible for termination of the anesthetic effects of the intravenous (IV) barbiturate.

Although the liver metabolizes lidocaine extensively, the elimination half-life of the drug is 1 to 2 hours (not 2 minutes [choice **C**]), which cannot account for such a rapid reappearance of the arrhythmia (choice **A**). While the blood levels following IV administration of lidocaine may be variable, this is due to redistribution processes and not to errors in laboratory determination of drug levels (choice **B**). There is no evidence that cardiac cells are capable of rapid (and reversible) changes in sensitivity to any antiarrhythmic drug (choice **E**). Conversely, the lidocaine level may be increased in patients taking cimetidine, and the dosage needs to be reduced in patients with congestive cardiac failure or liver disease.

30 The answer is C *Preventive Medicine and Public Health*

Most recessive diseases (e.g., cystic fibrosis) will present in isolated individuals. When two carriers of a recessive disease have children, those children will have a 25% chance of expressing the disease (choice **C**).

Although new mutations (choice **A**) are a possibility, most often it will turn out that both parents are carriers. It is only in families with many siblings and obvious consanguinity that recessive inheritance can be clearly identified on the basis of genetic evidence alone. As long as outbreeding predominates in a family, the chances of a recessive disease being expressed are remote, largely depending on the incidence in the general population. The recessive gene will be carried from generation to generation, only becoming evident when it shares an allelic site with a second mutated gene. That is, excluding a new mutation, there is zero chance of a recessive disease being expressed if a normal individual mates with a carrier. *Penetrance* is a term primarily used in conjunction with dominant disorders and is a measure of the chance of such a disorder not being expressed clinically (choice **B**). There is often variability in dominant disorders because dominant disease most often involves proteins having a structural function, as opposed to recessive disorders, which most often involve an enzyme. Thus, you can analogize a dominant genetic defect to a house in which every other normal 2×4 stud is replaced by a 1×2 stud. Externally, the two may be indistinguishable until an environmental stress is applied. Currently, it is often easy to identify carriers by simple biochemical techniques. However, there is no simple physiologic method available permitting the identification of carriers of cystic fibrosis (choice **D**). Even analysis involving DNA fingerprinting (choice **E**) is complicated by the fact that more than 400 different mutations in the cystic fibrosis gene have been identified; that is, it is not caused by a unique mutation.

31 The answer is B   *Medicine*

This patient has had a possible hemorrhagic stroke involving the right cerebral hemisphere. This is likely due to the history of treatment with warfarin. The initial investigation is a noncontrast computed tomography (CT) scan of the brain (choice **B**) to establish whether the problem was due to a hemorrhage or an infarct. If it were an infarct, management would include anticoagulants. On the other hand, administering anticoagulants to a patient who has cerebral hemorrhage would be disastrous.

A magnetic resonance imaging (MRI) scan (choice **A**), although helpful, is less sensitive for acute bleeding, takes longer, and is less likely to be available on an emergent basis. The electroencephalogram (EEG) (choice **C**) would be expected to show focal slowing on the right, however it cannot differentiate between an ischemic and a hemorrhagic stroke. Carotid duplex ultrasonography (choice **D**) would be useful to determine if the source of an embolus was a plaque within the carotid artery. However, 80% of emboli are cardiac in origin, and an echocardiogram would be an appropriate initial investigation in such an event. Neither carotid duplex ultrasonography nor echocardiography can distinguish between cerebral ischemic and hemorrhagic stroke. They can only support the diagnosis of ischemic stroke based on CT scan findings in the brain. Finally, a spinal tap (choice **E**) is not helpful in differentiating an ischemic from a hemorrhagic stroke and places an anticoagulated patient at risk for a developing a spinal epidural hematoma with subsequent spinal cord compression. Worse still, if a spinal tap was inadvertently carried out in the presence of raised intracranial pressure, tonsillar herniation and death could ensue.

32 The answer is A   *Obstetrics and Gynecology*

The group B β-hemolytic streptococcus (GBS) neonatal attack rate is only 1–2 cases per thousand women with a positive vaginal culture (choice **A**); most women with a positive vaginal culture will have uninfected infants. However, GBS still has the potential for significant adverse impact on the fetus, neonate, or both, because if neonatal sepsis does occur the mortality rate approaches 50%. This is why screening for GBS is now recommended by the CDC for all women at 36 weeks' gestation with intrapartum penicillin prophylaxis if culture positive.

Even though most infants born to women with a positive GBS culture are not infected, a negative culture does not rule out the presence of the organism at the time of delivery because most GBS carriers harbor the bacterium only intermittently or transiently (choice **B**). Up to 30% of women of reproductive age will have GBS as part of their normal vaginal flora; this is not an infection. Treating carriers is ineffective for eradicating the organism (choice **C**). Up to 30% of women of reproductive age will have colonization with GBS; the organism is part of normal female genital tract flora (choice **D**). Current nonculture assay tests are specific but not very sensitive (choice **E**). The diagnostic modality of choice is a culture.

33 The answer is B   *Pediatrics*

External otitis, or "swimmer's ear," is caused by excessive moisture in the ear canal, which causes the loss of protective cerumen leading to chronic irritation. However, cerumen impaction with trapping of water can also cause infection. The patient presents with ear pain that is worsened by manipulation of the pinna. The ear canal is erythematous and edematous. Otorrhea may be seen. *Pseudomonas aeruginosa* (choice **B**) is the most commonly isolated bacterium in external otitis. Other organisms include *Enterobacter aerogenes*, *Proteus mirabilis*, coagulase-negative staphylococci, *Klebsiella pneumoniae*, streptococci, *Staphylococcus aureus*, diphtheroids, and fungi.

Both *Haemophilus influenzae* (choice **A**) and *Moraxella catarrhalis* (choice **C**) cause otitis media, but not as often as *Streptococcus pneumoniae*. *Streptococcus agalactiae* (choice **D**) has been isolated from middle ear fluid in neonates with otitis media. However, both *S. agalactiae* and *Escherichia coli* (choice **E**) are leading causes of sepsis and meningitis in neonates.

34 The answer is D *Medicine*

Ventricular tachycardia (choice **D**) is defined as three or more beats of ventricular origin that occur in succession at a rate in excess of 100 beats/min, usually between 120 and 220 beats/min. The rhythm may be regular or irregular. P waves may be present, with no fixed relationship to the QRS complexes, or absent, depending on the ventricular rate. The width of the QRS is 0.12 second or above, and the morphology is bizarre, with notching frequently present. This patient's ventricular rate is approximately 150 beats/min, and the rhythm is slightly irregular. A burst of seven consecutive wide complexes follows a normal sinus rhythm and ends with a premature ventricular complex coupled to a sinus complex. The configuration of the premature complex is similar to that of the tachycardia complexes, so this configuration represents a ventricular tachycardia. When prompt therapy is indicated, lidocaine is the treatment of choice.

Premature atrial contractions (choice **A**) originate in the atria outside of the sinus node. The rhythm is irregular because ventricular activation may not occur (nonconduction), resulting in a pause in the cardiac rhythm. Atrial flutter (choice **B**) is a regular atrial rhythm that results from reentry at the atrial level. The atrial rate varies from 220 to 350 beats/min, whereas the ventricular rate varies from 150 to 175 beats/min, indicating atrioventricular (AV) conduction ratios ranging from 2:1 to 4:1. The atrial waves have a "sawtooth" or "picket fence" configuration. Paroxysmal (supraventricular) tachycardia (choice **C**) has a regular atrial rate of 160 to 220 beats/min and a similar ventricular rate if the atrial rate is below 200 beats/min (AV conduction ratio of 1:1). The atrial rhythm is usually regular. P waves are frequently difficult to identify; but when present, they may have different contours than sinus P waves. The P-R and QRS intervals are variable. The QRS complexes are of normal configuration. Carotid sinus massage or the Valsalva maneuver (patients hold their breath) is frequently used to convert paroxysmal tachycardia to normal sinus rhythm. Sinus tachycardia (choice **E**) is caused by an increased rate of discharge from the sinus node. The rate is regular and exceeds 100 beats/min. Each QRS is preceded by an upright P wave in leads I and II, and a Vr.

35 The answer is D *Surgery*

Heparin blocks the intrinsic pathway of the coagulation cascade, and its activity can be measured by determining the activated partial thromboplastin time (aPTT) (choice **D**). The intrinsic system begins with the conversion of factor XII to an active enzyme called XIIa once it has come into contact with negatively charged surfaces. In addition to monitoring adequacy of heparinization, aPTT is used to monitor replacement therapy in hemophilia A and B. The therapeutic range for aPTT is 1.5 to 2.5 times the reference range.

The prothrombin time (PT) (choice **B**) blocks the extrinsic pathway (e.g., after oral anticoagulation). The extrinsic portion of the coagulation cascade is initiated by the interaction between factor VII and tissue factor. The PT is normal in patients who are on heparin alone, because heparin acts on the intrinsic pathway. Thrombin time (TT) (choice **A**) is used to screen for abnormalities of fibrinogen. It measures conversion of fibrinogen to fibrin by thrombin. This is accomplished by polymerization of fibrin polymers to a fibrin gel. TT does not measure fibrinolysis or stabilization of fibrin. The most common cause of prolongation of TT is heparin; however, prolongation can also occur in uremia and defects in fibrin (e.g., dysfibrinogenemia, hypofibrinogenemia). Thus, although heparin prolongs TT, it is not used as a test to monitor heparin therapy. The fact that the TT is not due to heparin can be determined by blocking its action with protamine sulfate or, even better, measuring the reptilase time. Reptilase time is most commonly used to determine the cause of prolonged TT. Reptilase is an enzyme obtained from the venom of a reptile, *Bothrops atrox,* which clots human fibrinogen. Prothrombin and proconvertin test (choice **C**), an assay of prothrombin (factor II) and proconvertin (factor VII), is actually a modified PT in which factor V and fibrinogen are added to it. Thus, the assay is sensitive to defects in factors II, VII, and X. It can be used to monitor oral anticoagulant therapy, not heparin therapy. The test is usually reported in terms of percentage of activity based on a series of normal plasmas diluted with normal saline. This test is no longer used, because it has no advantage over the PT or the international normalized ratio (INR). Furthermore, results from prothrombin and proconvertin tests cannot be converted to INR values. Bleeding time (choice **E**) measures the interaction between platelets and the vessel wall. Defects in platelets or a defect in the vessel wall will result in a prolonged bleeding time. It is the most commonly used test to measure in vivo platelet function. The most common cause for prolonged bleeding time is drug therapy, especially aspirin. Patients with von Willebrand's disease also have prolonged bleeding time due to a deficiency or abnormality in von Willebrand's factor. Von Willebrand's disease is the most common hereditary bleeding disorder.

36 The answer is A *Psychiatry*

Maintenance therapy after response to antidepressants should generally be continued at an effective dose for 6 months after initial response (choice **A**).

Quick relapse is more likely if antidepressants are tapered (choice **C**) or stopped earlier (choice **D**). Some studies suggest much longer treatment after recovery from a depressive episode (choice **B**) if the patient has a history of multiple relapses, but not for a single episode. Therapy should not be switched to fluoxetine (choice **E**) another SSRI, since sertraline has been effective and shows no untoward adverse effects.

37 The answer is D *Medicine*

This patient is in the early stages of developing the insulin resistance syndrome, which when fully developed is characterized by type 2 diabetes, dyslipidemia, hypertension, and obesity. Although only tested once, at this time it is highly probable that he is in a prediabetic state, which is defined as having fasting plasma glucose levels between 100 and 126 mg/dL on two consecutive days. His fasting total cholesterol (TC) and LDL levels are also in the borderline high range. (For TC the normal value is defined as equal to or less than 200 mg/dL [5.2 mmol/L], borderline is between 200 and 240 mg/dL [5.2–6.2 mmol/L], and elevated as equal to or greater than 240 mg/dL [6.2 mmol/L]; whereas for LDL the normal value is defined as equal to or less than 130 mg/dL [3.4 mmol/L], borderline values are between 130 and 160 mg/dL [3.4–4.1 mmol/L], and high as equal to or greater than 159 mg/dL [4.1 mmol/L]). In addition he is definitely hypertensive (systolic/diastolic values reported as mmHg are defined as normal, less than 120/80; prehypertension, 120/80 to 139/89; stage 1 hypertension, 140/90 to 159/99; and stage 2 hypertension, equal to or greater than 160/100). In summary, he is well on his way to becoming a full-blown diabetic, with high total and LDL cholesterol levels, and also is liable soon to be a stage 2 hypertensive and a candidate for severe coronary artery disease (CAD). The primary driving force for these conditions is his obesity created by his lifestyle. His body mass index (BMI) is 30.2 kg/m², calculated using the following formula: BMI = weight in kg divided by height in meters squared, where 1 kg = 2.2046 lb, and 1m = 39.37 inches. A BMI between 25 and 29.9 kg/m² is defined as overweight, and 30 kg/m² or greater as obese. The first step in managing obesity in this patient is to get him off his couch and moving about. Taking his wife out dancing at least twice a week (choice **D**), while not a solution in itself, would be a step in the right direction, and it might be easier to persuade this obviously recalcitrant man to do this to pacify his wife than to initially recommend the more stringent dietary and exercise regimes that will be required. In the interim it also may be possible to persuade him to return to treat his hypertension and incidentally better deal with his lifestyle issues, including the possibility of depression.

Gastroplasty (choice **A**) will cause him to lose weight. However, it requires surgery and has concomitant short- and long-term risks. As a consequence it should be reserved only for the morbidly obese. Although short-term weight loss is enhanced by the prescription of an anorexic drug (choice **B**), patients taking such agents usually end up even heavier than before they started treatment because of a rebound effect. Management in this case clearly entails a lifestyle change, which may require long-term treatment and a great deal of patience. One would prescribe gemfibrozil (choice **C**) as a way to lower triglyceride levels only after they were acutely high and more conservative measures failed. A dietary supplement containing ephedra (choice **E**) would not be a wise move since several studies have shown that it can cause serious reactions including hypertension, which certainly would not be recommended in this case. Ephedra (also known as ma huang) contains the chemical ephedrine, which was used as an asthma medication until the 1980s when it was taken off the market because of its dangerous effects on the heart and blood pressure. Tolbutamide is a first-generation sulfonylurea, oral hypoglycemic agent. Not only are more effective agents available, but also tolbutamide, like all sulfonylureas, runs the risk of inducing hypoglycemia and promotes weight gain. Thus the physician would not likely prescribe tolbutamide (choice **F**). Until recently prediabetes would only be treated by lifestyle changes, diet, and exercise. However, it now is deemed acceptable to be more aggressive and prescribe an oral hypoglycemic agent. Metformin is generally recommended because it neither causes hypoglycemia nor promotes weight gain.

38 **The answer is B** *Pediatrics*

Phenylketonuria (PKU) is caused by a deficiency in phenylalanine hydroxylase, which has a prevalence of 1 case per 11,000 births. The normal pathway is disrupted, so phenylalanine and other metabolites accumulate and cause brain damage. Clinically, affected infants are blond, with fair skin and blue eyes. A mild eczematous rash disappears with age. Vomiting can be confused with pyloric stenosis. Mental retardation is usually severe. The infants have a musty, mousey odor of phenylacetic acid. Screening is recommended after 72 hours of age and after feeding of proteins. Early institution of a diet low in phenylalanine is essential in preventing brain damage. Women who have PKU and want to have children should go on a low-phenylalanine diet before conception and throughout pregnancy to reduce the risk of spontaneous abortion and birth defects. The blood phenylalanine levels should be kept below 6 mg/dL throughout pregnancy (choice **B**).

Pregnant women with PKU and phenylalanine levels above 6 mg/dL (choices **C, D,** and **E**) have a higher risk of spontaneous abortions. Infants born to such mothers may have mental retardation, microcephaly, and/or a congenital heart anomaly. Blood levels of 1 mg/dL (choice **A**) are below the risk level but are not the highest safe level.

39 **The answer is C** *Surgery*

The patient has an acute arterial occlusion (choice **C**), which is associated with the six P's—**P**ain, **P**allor, **P**aresthesias, **P**aralysis, **P**oikilothermia, and **P**ulseless (absence of pulse). The most likely cause is an embolus, but trauma could also be responsible. In an embolic arterial occlusion, there is no antecedent history of claudication pain. Emboli can spring from a recent myocardial infarct, mitral stenosis, artificial heart valve, or an aortic aneurysm. The condition occurs suddenly. The limb is cold to touch, and loss of motor function generally ensues within hours after onset of pain. For this reason, embolic arterial occlusion is an emergency. The first loss of function is the inability to move the toes. (In the case of venous occlusion, on the other hand, motor function is not lost). Heparinization followed by embolectomy and thrombectomy is the preferred treatment. The popliteal artery is the most susceptible vessel for occlusion because it is commonly affected by atherosclerosis and is a small-caliber artery.

Superficial thrombophlebitis (choice **A**) in the saphenous system of the legs presents with pain and tenderness along the course of the vessel. A herniated disk (choice **B**) would not be expected to involve the whole leg nor would it present with the given symptom/sign complex. A history of back pain followed by pain going down the leg would be usual. Findings would include hypesthesia along the lateral or inner aspect of the leg, depending on which intervertebral disk has herniated, and weakness of the plantar or dorsiflexors of the foot. Sciatic stretch sign would be positive, and the deep tendon jerks may or may not be affected, depending on the level of herniation. The pulses will be normal, and skin temperature would be normal. Deep venous insufficiency (choice **D**) is associated with superficial varicose veins and stasis dermatitis around the ankle. Hypovolemic shock (choice **E**) produces hypotension, generalized pallor, and cold, clammy skin.

40 **The answer is C** *Pediatrics*

Cystic fibrosis is a multisystem disease with protean manifestations, and pancreatic exocrine insufficiency is responsible for most of them. Recurrent pulmonary infections, malabsorption, and failure to thrive are hallmarks. It is inherited as an autosomal recessive trait and is the major cause of lung disease in children. Patients with cystic fibrosis exhibit elevated sweat chloride levels. If cystic fibrosis is suspected, a sweat chloride test (choice **C**) is indicated to help establish the diagnosis. More than 60 mEq/L of chloride in sweat is diagnostic of cystic fibrosis when it is associated with a positive family history, typical chronic obstructive pulmonary disease, or documented exocrine pancreatic insufficiency.

Therefore, a plasma growth hormone assay (choice **A**), a complete skeletal survey (choice **B**), endoscopy of the upper gastrointestinal (GI) tract (choice **D**), and acute viral serologies (choice **E**) would not be the most appropriate steps in arriving at the diagnosis.

41 **The answer is E** *Medicine*

The patient has the Hantavirus (choice **E**) pulmonary syndrome. The virus is transmitted by inhalation of urine or feces from deer mice in the southwestern United States. It is particularly prevalent on Indian reservations in New Mexico and Arizona. Patients develop acute respiratory distress syndrome, pulmonary hemorrhage, and renal failure. The diagnosis is obtained by detecting viral RNA in lung tissue. Ribavirin has been used for treatment; however, it is of questionable effectiveness. There is a high mortality rate.

42 **The answer is B** *Medicine*

The patient has severe acute respiratory syndrome (SARS), which is due to a coronavirus (choice **B**) that infects the lower respiratory tract and then spreads systemically. It was first transmitted to humans through contact with masked palm civets in China and then from human-to-human contact through respiratory secretions (e.g., hospitals, families). One third of patients improve and the infection resolves, while others develop severe respiratory infection, and nearly 10% die. The diagnosis is made with viral detection by polymerase chain reaction or by detection of antibodies.

43 **The answer is G** *Medicine*

The patient has encephalitis due to the West Nile virus, which is a flavivirus (choice **G**) that is transmitted by mosquitos. Birds are the reservoir for the virus. Crows and other birds have spread the disease from New York to the west coast. Crows and other birds often die from the disease, as in this case. The encephalitis can be fatal in a minority of cases.

INCORRECT CHOICES

41–43 *Medicine*

Colorado tick fever is an arthropod-borne virus (choice **A**) infection that is transmitted by mosquitos or ticks (the same tick that transmits Rocky Mountain spotted fever [RMSF]). Clinical findings include encephalitis, retro-orbital pain, and severe myalgia. Approximately 10% have a rash that is similar to that of RMSF. A characteristic finding is a biphasic fever pattern with fever for 24 hours → no fever for 2–3 days → fever 2–4 days, which then subsides; this distinguishes the disease from RMSF.

Coxsackievirus (choice **C**) is an RNA virus that is primarily transmitted by the fecal–oral route. It is the most common cause of viral meningitis, myocarditis, and encephalitis. Other diseases include herpangina (vesicles/ulcers on the pharynx and soft palate surrounded by erythema, cervical adenopathy), hand-foot-mouth disease (vesicular rash on hands, feet, and in the mouth), and pleurodynia (fever with pleuritic chest pain).

Ebola virus (choice **D**) infections occur primarily in Africa. It is usually conveyed by secondary transmission in the hospital from patient blood or secretions. It causes a hemorrhagic fever associated with disseminated intravascular coagulation, shock, and hemorrhage from severe thrombocytopenia. Mortality is almost 100%.

Lymphocytic choriomeningitis virus (choice **F**) is endemic in the mouse population. The virus is transmitted to humans by food or water contaminated with mouse urine and/or feces. It produces a severe meningoencephalitis that can produce permanent neurologic damage. Spinal fluid findings include increased protein level, a lymphocyte infiltrate, and normal-to-decreased glucose concentration. The virus can be cultured, and antibody tests are available.

44 **The answer is C** *Psychiatry*

The clinical course of cyclothymic disorder (graph **C**) is characterized by numerous periods of hypomanic symptoms and numerous periods of depressive symptoms. During none of these episodes do patients have full manic or depressive episodes. Cycling is often rapid.

45 **The answer is B** *Psychiatry*

The clinical course of bipolar II disorder (graph **B**) is characterized by depressive episodes and one or more hypomanic episodes.

INCORRECT CHOICES

44–45 *Psychiatry*

Bipolar I disorder (graph **D**) includes both manic and depressive episodes. Graph **A** represents the clinical course of major depressive disorder, recurrent type. Graph **E** represents the clinical course of dysthymic disorder.

46 **The answer is D** *Medicine*

In children, lead poisoning (choice **D**) most commonly occurs by exposure to toys that contain lead in the paint. Other ways to ingest lead may be via a history of pica or contact with contaminated house dust and soil from deterioration of pre-1980 housing and buildings. In adults, inhalation is the most common route of exposure, usually from burning car batteries or painting pottery with lead-based paints. Lead levels of 10 μg/dL or above represent undue exposure to lead and those above 20 μg/dL or higher are considered lead poisoning. Lead inhibits two major enzymes involved in heme synthesis: aminolevulinic acid (ALA) dehydrase and ferrochelatase. This interference with heme production causes a microcytic anemia defined as an anemia in which the RBC mean corpuscular volume (MCV) is less than 80 μm³ as compared to an MCV of 80–100 μm³, or more than 100 μm³ in macrocytic anemias. Lead also inactivates ribonuclease, which breaks down ribosomes in RBCs. Inactivation of this enzyme is responsible for the coarse basophilic stippling in RBCs, which is an extremely good marker of lead poisoning in the setting of a microcytic anemia. Lead also injures the RBC membrane, producing a mild hemolytic component to the anemia, as evidenced by the increase in corrected reticulocyte count in the patient. The anemia is microcytic because whenever hemoglobin (Hgb) synthesis is decreased because of inadequate iron supplies (iron deficiency [choice **A**], in anemia of chronic disease [choice **B**]), or decreased production of heme (lead poisoning), or of globin chains (the thalassemias, choice **C**), extra mitotic divisions in the marrow result in the production of microcytes.

47 **The answer is H** *Medicine*

Patients with autoimmune diseases (e.g., systemic lupus erythematosus [SLE]) are prone to developing other autoimmune diseases. Therefore, in the setting of a patient with known SLE, the presence of anemia with an increased corrected reticulocyte count is most likely an autoimmune hemolytic anemia (AIHA) (choice **H**). The gold standard test for diagnosing AIHA is the Coombs' test, which detects the presence of immunoglobulin G (IgG), C3, or both on the surface of RBCs (direct Coombs' test) or the presence of IgG antibodies against RBC antigens in the serum (indirect Coombs' test). AIHA is subdivided into cold (30%) or warm (70%) types. Patients with SLE account for most cases of warm AIHA (40–50%). Damage to the RBCs inflicted by the macrophages frequently results in the presence of spherocytes in the peripheral blood, which could be confused with congenital spherocytosis (choice **G**) except for the presence of a positive direct Coombs' test result in autoimmune hemolysis. The marked reticulocytosis frequently produces macrocytic indices (folate is used up in producing more RBCs), as exemplified by the increased MCV in this patient. Other causes of warm AIHA include drugs (approximately 20%; e.g., penicillin, methyldopa, quinidine), chronic lymphocytic leukemia, Hodgkin's disease, viral infections, and other collagen vascular diseases. Treatment is extremely difficult and, depending on how the patient responds, progresses in the following manner: corticosteroids to splenectomy to immunosuppressive therapy. Cold AIHA is seen in infections due to *Mycoplasma pneumoniae* and infectious mononucleosis, malignant lymphomas, and chronic lymphocytic leukemia. Alkylating agents are the mainstay of therapy.

48 **The answer is F** *Medicine*

Macrocytic anemias associated with macro-ovalocytes and hypersegmented neutrophils are due to either vitamin B_{12} (choice **E**) or folate deficiency. Folate deficiency (choice **F**) is the more common of the two and is most often associated with excessive intake of alcohol, as in this case. Because vitamin B_{12} and folate are required for DNA synthesis, their absence results in enlarged, immature nuclei in all the nucleated cells in the body. The hematopoietic cells in the bone marrow are enlarged, hence the term *megaloblastic anemia*. These enlarged cells are unable to enter sinusoids to gain access to the peripheral blood and are destroyed by macrophages or undergo apoptosis. Patients present with pancytopenia, in which there is severe macrocytic anemia, neutropenia, and thrombocytopenia.

The incorrect choices are explained in conjunction with the correct ones in the discussions above.

49 **The answer is J** *Psychiatry*

The symptoms are most suggestive of separation anxiety disorder (choice **J**), a condition characterized by fear of separation from caregivers. It can manifest itself as worry about separation, severe protest over separation, or severe anxiety after separation. Often, the presenting complaint involves marital problems caused by these behaviors. Behavioral therapies are often effective for the child. Treatment also involves parent education and therapy to resolve potential ambivalence about allowing the child more independence.

50 The answer is K *Psychiatry*

The symptoms are most suggestive of social phobia (choice **K**), characterized by fear and avoidance of social situations. Individuals with this disorder tend to be solitary and reclusive. Their presenting complaint is often depression and loneliness. Treatment often includes cognitive-behavioral techniques such as assertiveness training in which social interactions are rehearsed.

THE REMAINING INCORRECT CHOICES

Pervasive anxiety in many situations would suggest generalized anxiety disorder (choice **E**). Anxiety after severe emotional trauma, objects (e.g., animals), or situations (other than social situations), would suggest specific phobia (choice **L**). Other disorders associated with childhood behavioral problems are conduct disorder (choice **C**), in which major age-appropriate societal norms are violated, and oppositional defiant disorder (choice **G**), which is characterized by defiance of authority. Delirium (choice **D**), characterized by acute and severe cognitive disturbances, may be associated with anxiety.

There are many disorders associated with anxiety that are not limited to social situations. In panic disorder (choice **H**), attacks of anxiety occur without obvious triggers. Obsessive–compulsive disorder (choice **F**) is often associated with anxiety about the obsessive thoughts or anxiety when the compulsions are resisted.

test **5**

Questions

1 A 21-year-old man presents with auditory hallucinations and the delusion that federal narcotics agents are monitoring his telephone calls. He was dealing cocaine and using large amounts of the substance daily until about 1 week ago when he exhausted his supply and was too frightened to leave his home to get more. Mental status examination reveals an alert and anxious individual who is oriented and coherent. Urine toxicology testing result for cocaine is negative. Which of the following is the most likely fundamental diagnosis?

(A) Cocaine-induced anxiety disorder
(B) Cocaine-induced delirium
(C) Cocaine-induced psychotic disorder
(D) Cocaine intoxication
(E) Schizophrenia, paranoid type

2 A patient with myasthenia gravis that has been well controlled with pyridostigmine for 2 years comes to the emergency department complaining of progressive muscle weakening during the last 24 hours. He has trouble swallowing and suffers from double vision. The patient has had flulike symptoms for the past week. Which of the following is the most appropriate immediate course of action?

(A) Increase the dose of pyridostigmine.
(B) Replace pyridostigmine with physostigmine.
(C) Give a small dose of edrophonium.
(D) Decrease the dose of pyridostigmine.
(E) Administer succinylcholine.

3 A 30-year-old Caucasian female who claims to never have smoked presents with bilateral puffiness and swelling of the fingers and joint pains. Cold exposure and stress cause episodes of blanching or cyanosis of the fingers. She is not on any medications. The mechanism for this patient's disease is most likely the result of which of the following?

(A) Vasospasm and thickening of the digital arteries
(B) Hyperviscosity due to an increase in immunoglobulin M (IgM) antibodies
(C) An immune complex vasculitis
(D) Thrombosis of the digital vessels
(E) An embolism to the digital vessels

4 A 65-year-old woman presents to the emergency department with diffuse abdominal pain and vomiting. She has not had a bowel movement in the past 3 days. Physical examination reveals hyperstasis, tympany to percussion, and no rebound tenderness. Her temperature is 38°C (100.4°F). An abdominal x-ray film reveals distended loops of small bowel with a stepladder pattern of differential air-fluid levels. Which of the following is the mechanism that most likely produced these findings?

(A) Diverticulosis
(B) Adhesions from previous surgery
(C) Torsion of the bowel around the mesenteric root
(D) Intussusception of the terminal ileum into the cecum
(E) Ischemia secondary to thrombosis of the superior mesenteric artery

5 A 62-year-old woman with a history of diabetes and hypertension presents to the emergency department with the right eye deviated outward and an obvious ptosis. She has a slight headache. The pupils are normal size. Which of the following is the most likely diagnosis?

(A) Cavernous sinus thrombosis
(B) Superior oblique palsy
(C) Posterior cerebral artery aneurysm with third nerve impingement
(D) Vasculopathic (noncompressive) third nerve palsy
(E) Internuclear ophthalmoplegia

6 An asymptomatic 3-year-old is brought to the physician because of right cheek swelling. The mother states that the patient had been in his normal state of health until 1 hour ago, when he developed right cheek swelling at a church picnic. The patient is afebrile. Physical examination is unremarkable except for the right cheek, which is erythematous but not warm to touch. On palpation of the right cheek, mildly tender, discrete, indurated masses are appreciated. Which of the following is the most likely cause of this child's problem?

(A) Erysipelas
(B) Cellulitis
(C) Trauma
(D) Panniculitis
(E) Contact dermatitis

7 A worried father brings his 17-year-old daughter to the emergency department in Stockton, California, at 11:15 PM. He informs the triage nurse that his daughter has been experiencing headaches for about 2 days, and today she has been extremely fatigued. He is particularly concerned because she rarely experiences headaches and has always been very active. When seen by the doctor, the daughter tries to make light of her condition. She blames the drowsiness on taking too many acetaminophen/codeine pills prescribed several weeks ago by her dentist. She admits, however, that she took the pills because she has the "mother of all headaches"; she does not recall ever having one of such intensity. She further suggests that her fatigue may also be a consequence of the fact that she has been losing sleep because her headaches wake her up, being particularly intense at night. When asked if her neck is stiff, she gives an ambiguous answer. She is slightly nauseous, but has not vomited. She has never had any major illnesses, has been active in high-school athletics, and does not know of anyone sick with whom she has been in contact.

Physical examination reveals the following results: temperature, 40°C (100°F); blood pressure, 140/70 mm Hg; pulse, 120/min and regular. The cardiovascular, respiratory, gastrointestinal, and genitourinary systems are all normal. The central nervous system (CNS) examination, including funduscopy, seems normal. She is oriented with respect to time and space; however, she is unduly sensitive to bright lights. There is a very slight resistance to the forward flexion of the neck. Neuromuscular tone and reflexes are normal.

The laboratory profile reveals the following: serum white blood cell (WBC) count of 10,500 cells/mm³ (normal 4,800–10,800 cells/mm³), erythrocyte sedimentation rate (ESR) of 20 mm/h (normal female <15 mm/h); electrolyte profile blood sugar level, serum amylase level, and chest x-ray film within normal limits.

On the basis of these data, a lumbar puncture is performed. The following results are obtained: cell count, 28 cells/mm³, 95% lymphocytes (normal is 0–5 cells/mm³ lymphocytes); glucose, 48 mg/dL (normal is 40–70 mg/dL); protein, 85 mg/dL (normal is <40 mg/dL); and chloride, 120 mEq/L (normal is 118–132 mEq/L). Which of the following is the most likely diagnosis?

(A) Bacterial meningitis
(B) Cryptococcal meningitis
(C) *Coccidia immitis* meningitis
(D) Aseptic meningitis
(E) Actinomyces meningitis

8 A 53-year-old man comes to his primary care physician and after some hesitation tells him that recently he has not been able to maintain an erection while trying to make love to his wife of 30 years. His medical history is significant for diabetes mellitus, which was first diagnosed a decade ago. Which of the following is most likely to be true about this patient?

(A) He is maintaining optimum blood sugar levels.
(B) Erection is normal, but orgasm and ejaculatory problems are present.
(C) He has no penile nerve damage.
(D) Ejaculation is normal, but erectile problems are present.
(E) He has no vascular changes in the penis.

9 A 35-year-old man with a long history of dyspepsia experiences sudden onset of severe epigastric distress with associated pain in the right shoulder. Physical examination reveals a patient who appears ill and who has a rigid, quiet abdomen with rebound tenderness. Which of the following is the most appropriate first step in the management of this patient?

(A) Order a barium study of the upper gastrointestinal system
(B) Order upright and supine abdominal films
(C) Perform a peritoneal lavage
(D) Administer antacids
(E) Do an exploratory laparotomy

10 A 2-year-old child attends daycare at a local neighborhood nursery. The parents report that one of his favorite activities at daycare is to play in the sandbox. The parents tell you that the child especially enjoys this activity when the owner's puppies are in the sandbox too. According to the parents, until recently, the patient has been in his usual state of good health, with no significant past medical history, and immunizations up to date. However, at this office visit the patient has wheezing, hepatosplenomegaly, and prominent peripheral blood eosinophilia. Which of the following diagnoses is most likely in this child?

(A) Pinworm infestation
(B) Eosinophilic lung disease
(C) Ascariasis
(D) Visceral larva migrans
(E) Strongyloidiasis

11 A 16-year-old male distance runner presents with complaints of worsening athletic performance and increasing cough and sputum production after running. He is very concerned because the state track meet is only 2 weeks away. Findings of the physical examination are normal. Which of the following is the most appropriate next step in the management of this patient?

(A) Prescribe a β_2-agonist inhaler to be used 5 minutes before activity.
(B) Prescribe theophylline to be taken orally.
(C) Prescribe a cromolyn sodium inhaler to be used 15 minutes before activity.
(D) Prescribe erythromycin to be taken orally for 10 days.
(E) Explain that he has asthma and should refrain from strenuous activities from now on.

12 A 55-year-old Caucasian woman, who has a chronic cough from a 30 pack-year history of smoking, complains of pelvic pressure symptoms. The problem began gradually over the last 2 years. She states that when she increases intraabdominal pressure in having a bowel movement, a mass appears at her vaginal opening. It has been 3 years since her last menstrual period. She is not taking estrogen replacement therapy. She does complain of constipation and has difficulty in stool evacuation, having to press her fingers on her vagina to evacuate her stool. She had three vaginal deliveries, the largest infant weighing 4500 g (9 lb 15 oz). Her postvoiding residual is 60 mL. Which of the following physical findings would be most likely on pelvic examination?

(A) Rectocele
(B) Cystocele
(C) Enterocele
(D) Urethrocele
(E) Vaginocele

13 An obese 18-year-old presents at an emergency clinic in labor and asks for help in delivering her first child. The triage nurse takes a history and determines that the patient has had no prenatal care and cannot recall when her last menstrual cycle was, as she has always had irregular cycles. She further reveals that she first realized that she might be pregnant about 4 months ago; she denies the usage of drugs, alcohol, or tobacco and also denies having any sexually transmitted diseases. The baby was quickly delivered with no untoward incidences. At delivery the infant is noted to be large for gestational age and has cracked, peeling skin. The infant's fingernails are long and its fingers are stained green. There is absence of lanugo. Which of the following is the most likely gestational age of this infant?

(A) 34 weeks
(B) 36 weeks
(C) 38 weeks
(D) 40 weeks
(E) 42 weeks

14 A 40-year-old woman develops an unmanageable fear of snakes while being courted by an avid hiking enthusiast. She has never been married or had any other intimate relationships with men. Prior to being courted by this man, she enjoyed mountain walks and was never concerned with such fears. Although she knows that no poisonous snakes inhabit her area, she can no longer make herself hike anymore. Which of the following is the most commonly postulated psychodynamic defense mechanism in such situations?

(A) Dissociation
(B) Projection
(C) Displacement
(D) Conversion
(E) Resistance

15 A 20-year-old man is stabbed in the left side of his chest, medial to the nipple. His blood pressure is 90/60 mm Hg and his pulse is 130/min. His jugular venous pulse increases on inspiration, whereas his peripheral pulse and blood pressure decrease on inspiration. Breath sounds are normal bilaterally. The patient's chest x-ray film is unremarkable. After receiving 2 L of isotonic saline, his blood pressure remains low, whereas his central venous pressure rises to 32 cm H_2O. Which of the following is the most appropriate next step in the management of this patient?

(A) Insert a chest tube into the left pleural cavity
(B) Increase parenteral fluids until the blood pressure increases
(C) Order an echocardiogram
(D) Decrease venous pressure by administering a venodilator
(E) Decrease venous pressure by administering a loop diuretic

16 A 59-year-old woman has gradual onset of emotional lability, loss of memory (particularly of recent events), forgetfulness (absent mindedness), emotional lability, impulsiveness, and as a consequence difficulty organizing her finances and appointments. Physical examination reveals a bilateral Babinski sign. Which of the following dietary deficiencies most likely causes her symptoms?

(A) Vitamin B_{12}
(B) Vitamin C
(C) Iron
(D) Magnesium
(E) Lecithin

17 A 5-year-old girl with severe mental retardation is brought to the pediatrician for immunizations. According to the history, the patient appeared to be developing normally until 18 months of age, when she acquired dementia and her head circumference plateaued. She wrings her hands, and sighs. She is noted to have ataxia and marked loss of gross motor skills. In addition, she has loss of language milestones. Which of the following is the most likely diagnosis?

(A) Autism
(B) William's syndrome
(C) Rett syndrome
(D) Turner's syndrome
(E) Russell-Silver syndrome

18 A 27-year-old woman, gravida 3, para 0, aborta 2, comes to the outpatient office at 15 weeks' gestation by dates with complaints of exquisite vulvar pain and blisters. The onset of the symptoms was 48 hours ago, and she experienced numbness and tingling in her perineum before any lesions appeared. She states she has had similar episodes prior to the pregnancy for the past 5 years. Her vital signs are as follows: temperature, 37°C (98.6°F); pulse, 95/min; respiration, 20/min; blood pressure, 128/74 mm Hg. On examination you find exquisitely painful vesicles on her left labia minora. Inguinal nodes are negative bilaterally. She has a past history of a right Bartholin's abscess, which was marsupialized. She had a positive cervical chlamydial culture on her first prenatal visit, which was treated with erythromycin tablets. Which of the following statements is true?

(A) She should undergo a cesarean section to protect her infant from infection.
(B) Her fetus has an increased risk of congenital malformations.
(C) Transplacental transmission to her fetus is a significant concern.
(D) Breast-feeding of her infant is probably unsafe and should be avoided.
(E) Decisions regarding route of delivery are best made at the onset of labor.

19 A 19-year-old Caucasian female (illustrated above Right) comes to a walk-in clinic complaining of weakness and general malaise. In presenting her history she informs the physician that over the past month these symptoms have grown progressively worse and that she lost 20 lb (9 kg) during this period but just had no appetite. In addition she states that she has pains in her wrist and finger joints, a stomach ache, and a funny rash on her cheeks that causes her a great deal of embarrassment. Upon examination the physician

notes her vital signs are as follows: temperature, 40°C (100°F); blood pressure, 135/70 mm Hg; pulse, 76/min. Which of the following pairs of antibody tests would be the most specific for diagnosing this patient's disease?

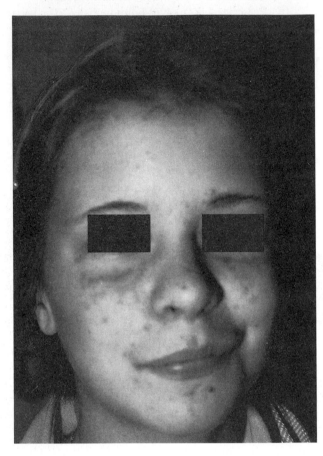

(A) Anti-SSA (Ro) and semi-Sm (Smith)
(B) Antinuclear and anti-ds (double-stranded) DNA
(C) Anti-SSB (La) and anti-ds DNA
(D) Anticentromere and antiribonucleoprotein
(E) Lupus anticoagulant and antihistone

20 A 35-year-old man presents to his physician with a complaint of abdominal discomfort. In providing a history he reveals that both his father and paternal grandmother were hypertensive. Moreover, his father is on renal dialysis, and his paternal grandmother died of a stroke. An ultrasound of the kidney reveals numerous black spaces in both kidneys, but his serum creatinine level is normal. Which of the following is the most likely diagnosis?

(A) Immunoglobulin A (IgA) nephropathy
(B) Goodpasture's syndrome
(C) Staghorn calculus
(D) Alport's syndrome
(E) Polycystic kidney disease

21 The following water deprivation test involves three patients with polyuria and a normal control. Their maximal urine osmolality (Uosm) and plasma osmolality (Posm) after prolonged water deprivation is recorded in addition to the effect of an intramuscular injection of vasopressin (antidiuretic hormone [ADH]) on Uosm.

Patients	Maximal Posm (mmol/kg)	Maximal Uosm (mmol/kg)	Uosm Post Vasopressin (mmol/kg)
Control	290	760	780
Patient A	305	160	400
Patient B	310	125	150
Patient C	290	690	710

Which of the following statements about these results is correct?

(A) Patient A has central diabetes insipidus (CDI).
(B) Patient B has psychogenic polydipsia.
(C) Patient C has nephrogenic diabetes insipidus (NDI).
(D) The Uosm in patient B responds appropriately after administration of vasopressin.
(E) Patients A and B are losing a hypotonic salt solution in their urine.

22 A 52-year-old woman claims that her landlord is pumping poisonous gas into her apartment. Mental status examination reveals anxiety, perseveration, and persecutory ideation. She refuses to cooperate with mental status testing. Which of the following is the most likely diagnosis?

(A) Dementia
(B) Obsessive–compulsive disorder
(C) Panic disorder
(D) Posttraumatic stress disorder
(E) Generalized anxiety disorder

23 A 33-year-old woman, gravida 3, para 2, is at 25 weeks' gestation. Her gestational age was confirmed by a 10-week sonogram performed because of early pregnancy spotting. A 20-week sonogram revealed a normal appearing single male fetus, appropriate size for dates, without any gross congenital anomalies. On examination in the office today her fundal height measures 31 cm. An obstetrical ultrasound examination reveals a single fetus in transverse lie with no part of the fetus touching the uterine wall or placenta. It was determined that there was a 4-quadrant amniotic fluid index (AFI) of 30 cm with the deepest single amniotic fluid pocket

measuring 9 cm. Which of the following maternal conditions does this patient most likely have?

(A) Asthma
(B) Diabetes mellitus
(C) Hyperthyroidism
(D) Seizure disorder
(E) Sickle cell anemia

24 Forty-eight hours after a total hysterectomy for low-staged endometrial carcinoma a 35-year-old woman, with a 20 pack-year history of smoking, presents with the sudden onset of tachypnea, dyspnea, cough, and right-sided pleuritic chest pain. She has a low-grade fever, sinus tachycardia, and a blood pressure of 100/70 mm Hg. Examination of the chest shows scattered, bilateral expiratory wheezes and dullness to percussion at the right lung base. No calf tenderness is present. A chest radiograph shows a small pleural effusion at the right lung base as well as a wedge-shaped area of hypovascularity and atelectasis in the right lower lobe. An electrocardiogram (ECG) shows nonspecific ST and T-wave abnormalities. An arterial blood gas (ABG) sample drawn with the patient breathing room air reveals a pH of 7.50 (normal is 7.35–7.45); a $Paco_2$ of 29 mm Hg (normal is 33–44 mm Hg); a Pao_2 of 70 mm Hg (normal is 75–105 mm Hg); and a bicarbonate level of 21 mEq/L (normal is 22–28 mEq/L). Which of the following is the most appropriate first step in the management of this patient?

(A) Perform a pleural tap
(B) Order a perfusion scan of the lungs
(C) Order a sputum analysis for Gram's stain, culture, and sensitivity
(D) Order pulmonary function tests
(E) Order a consultation for bronchoscopy

25 A 62-year-old man who had a myocardial infarction (MI) is taking 81 mg of aspirin tablet daily and a maintenance dose of warfarin, which is adjusted to give a prothrombin time (PT) of 11–15 seconds. While on vacation, he starts using over-the-counter cimetidine for acid indigestion. A day or two before returning home, he develops a urinary tract infection for which trimethoprim–sulfamethoxazole is prescribed by a local physician. When he returns home, his PT is 27 seconds. Which of the following statements about this situation is most accurate?

(A) The dose of warfarin should be increased to ensure adequate anticoagulation.
(B) The antibiotics have increased the activity of liver enzymes that metabolize warfarin.

(C) The antiplatelet action of aspirin has blocked the effects of warfarin.

(D) Cimetidine has inhibited the hepatic metabolism of warfarin.

(E) Warfarin should not have been prescribed because it is not used prophylactically after an MI.

26 An 80-year-old man with a history of coronary artery disease (CAD) and prostate cancer presents with weakness of both legs that has lasted for a week. Starting yesterday he developed pain in his lower abdomen and had great difficulty emptying his bladder. Examination shows that he has sensory loss from T10 downward and is barely able to move his legs. Which of the following is the proper treatment strategy?

(A) Admit the patient and schedule a magnetic resonance imaging (MRI) study the next day.

(B) Order an emergency MRI study after administering an intravenous (IV) bolus of steroids.

(C) Schedule plasmapheresis for Guillain-Barré syndrome.

(D) Order electromyography (EMG).

(E) Order radiation therapy over lumbar and sacral levels.

27 A 22-year-old woman, gravida 5, para 2, aborta 3, has a history of prenatal substance abuse. Because she had delayed onset of prenatal care (with her first visit in the third trimester), she was too late for maternal serum triple marker screening for fetal anomalies. She is unsure who the father of this pregnancy is. Ultrasound examination of the fetus showed intrauterine growth restriction but normal amniotic fluid volume. At 37 weeks' gestation she underwent a vaginal delivery of a small-for-gestational-age male neonate with short palpebral fissures, epicanthal folds, flat midface, hypoplastic philtrum, and thin vermillion border. These findings are characteristic in offspring born to mothers who prenatally abused which of the following substances?

(A) Tobacco
(B) Alcohol
(C) Marijuana
(D) Amphetamines
(E) Narcotics

28 A 46-year-old man reports for a preemployment physical. He recently moved to California to take up employment as a research scientist at a prestigious university in California. He had had a distinguished career in biochemistry while he lived in Cleveland, Ohio, his place of birth. He did not smoke, drank wine on social occasions, never used recreational

drugs, and had led a healthy lifestyle. He did not have a history of diabetes, hypertension, or coronary artery disease, nor did he have a history of chest pains, shortness of breath, cough, expectoration, or recent weight loss. He was not on any medications. There was no significant history of medical illness on either side of his family. Physical examination revealed a fit man, whose vital signs were normal. He had no pallor, icterus, or cyanosis. No clubbing of the fingers was noted. Cardiovascular examination revealed normal heart sounds, with sinus rhythm and no murmurs or carotid bruits. He did not have distended jugular veins. Examination of the respiratory system revealed a mild right shift of the trachea, good symmetric chest expansion, and absence of adventitious sounds. Examination of the abdomen was unremarkable, and a neurologic examination was normal as well. His Seibert purified protein derivative of tuberculin (PPD) test result was negative and a routine chest radiograph revealed a 0.5 cm concentrically calcified coin lesion in the upper left lobe of the lung. Which of the following is the most likely cause of the lesion?

(A) A primary lung cancer
(B) A bronchial hamartoma
(C) Metastatic cancer
(D) A granuloma
(E) A calcified tuberculosis lesion

29 A 3-year-old child is seen in the emergency department with a lump on his head, which his mother says appeared after he accidentally hit his head. The child did not lose consciousness, and he did not vomit. Examination reveals a tense swelling over the right parietal area and no neurologic deficits. Which of the following is the most likely diagnosis?

(A) Epidural hematoma
(B) Subdural hematoma
(C) Intraventricular hemorrhage
(D) Subgaleal hematoma
(E) Lipoma

30 The data in the following table were obtained from five inhalational anesthetics. Which of the following agents will provide the most rapid rate of recovery?

	Anesthetic	Blood: Gas Partition Coefficient	Minimum Alveolar Concentration (%)
(A)	Nitrous oxide	0.5	>100
(B)	Desflurane	0.4	7
(C)	Sevoflurane	0.7	3
(D)	Isoflurane	1.4	1.4
(E)	Halothane	2.3	0.8

31 A 28-year-old man has rapid onset of insomnia, pressured speech, and hypersexuality. He had a similar episode at age 21 and also had a period of depression and suicide attempts at age 23. Between these episodes, his behavior seems to have been unremarkable. There is no history of substance abuse. Which of the following statements about the pathophysiology of his likely diagnosis is most accurate?

(A) Pathognomonic abnormalities in transportation may occur at the cellular membrane.

(B) Mood-stabilizing medications are used as treatment because they generally block central dopamine receptors.

(C) The etiologic lesion does not appear to be heritable.

(D) Abnormal levels of neurotransmitters have been reported during manic episodes.

(E) Chromosomal abnormalities are often detected.

32 A 22-year-old Asian woman presents for a routine physical examination and a cervical Pap smear. Her menstrual history and physical examination are unremarkable. A stool guaiac test result is negative. A hemogram shows a hemoglobin (Hgb) concentration of 11 g/dL (normal is 12–16 g/dL), a red blood cell (RBC) count of 5.8 million cells/μl (normal is 3.5–5.5 million cells/μl), a mean corpuscular volume (MCV) of 70 μm^3 (normal is 80–100 μm^3), a normal RBC distribution width (RDW; 10 ± 5), and normal leukocyte and platelet counts. The mild anemia in this patient is most likely related to which of the following?

(A) Absent iron stores in the bone marrow

(B) Iron blockade in the macrophages

(C) Hemolysis of RBCs in the spleen

(D) Decreased globin chain synthesis

(E) Decreased heme synthesis

33 A 20-year-old man presents with a history of delayed developmental milestones, problems with impulse control, and an IQ of 65. He was in special education classes during his schooling. There was no history of substance abuse by his mother during the prenatal period and all his first-degree relatives have IQ values above 100. Which of the following is most likely to be revealed by a complete assessment?

(A) Genetic or chromosomal abnormalities

(B) Perinatal insults

(C) Sociocultural deprivation

(D) Maternal substance abuse

(E) Mild mental retardation

34 A mother brings her 12-month-old child to the emergency department because he is having painless rectal bleeding. She tells this physician, new to her, that approximately 2 months ago the patient was evaluated for anemia by his usual pediatrician and was prescribed supplemental iron for presumed iron deficiency anemia. However, the iron deficiency anemia has been refractory to iron therapy. On physical examination the child's stool is repeatedly positive for occult blood. Which of the following is the most likely diagnosis?

(A) Intussusception

(B) Duodenal ulcer

(C) Adhesions

(D) Meckel's diverticulum

(E) Ulcerative colitis

35 A 17-year-old woman has not had a menstrual period for 4 months. She underwent menarche at age 11. She has been sexually active for the past year, but states she has only occasional intercourse. She states that she uses a diaphragm for contraception, but she does not always remember to use it. Her boyfriend occasionally uses a condom. A qualitative serum β-human chorionic gonadotropin (hCG) test is reported back as a negative result. She is given medroxyprogesterone acetate orally for 7 days, and she has a normal withdrawal bleed of 5 days of menstrual flow. Which of the following statements is correct in respect to this diagnostic modality?

(A) It can assess whether the patient is pregnant.

(B) It will indicate whether the endometrium is estrogen primed.

(C) It differentiates primary from secondary amenorrhea.

(D) It can rule out a pituitary adenoma.

(E) It provides no help if the response is only spotting.

36 A 35-year-old man presents with flulike symptoms, malaise, and tender hepatomegaly. Three months ago he had a 10-unit blood transfusion for upper gastrointestinal bleeding due to ulcer disease. Laboratory studies show an atypical lymphocytosis, a serum alanine aminotransferase (ALT) value of 1200 U/L (normal is 8–20 U/L), a serum aspartate aminotransferase (AST) level of 800 U/L (normal is 8–20 U/L), a serum alkaline phosphatase level of 110 U/L (normal is 20–70 U/L), and a normal total bilirubin value. Which of the following is the most likely diagnosis?

(A) Infectious mononucleosis

(B) Hepatitis A

(C) Hepatitis B

(D) Hepatitis C

(E) A cytomegalovirus infection

37 A 72-year-old man with a history of uninterrupted employment as an accountant has insidious onset of difficulty concentrating on tasks and remembering recent events. Physical examination reveals no hypertension, cardiac findings, or focal neurologic signs. Routine laboratory examination is unremarkable. Mental status examination reveals emotional lability, difficulty naming common objects, and recall of only one object of three after 5 minutes. Which of the following is the most likely cause of his symptoms?

(A) Alcoholic dementia
(B) Alzheimer's disease
(C) Cerebrovascular disease
(D) Depression
(E) Normal aging

38 A 34-year-old Hispanic woman, gravida 3, para 2 initiated prenatal care at 14 weeks gestation. Her two previous pregnancies were 5 and 8 years ago. They resulted in spontaneous vaginal deliveries at term of a 9 lb (4082 g) daughter and a 9 lb 8 oz (4309 g) son. Her weight is 180 lb (82 kg). She is 62 inches (157 cm) tall. She underwent a 1-hour 50-g glucose screen at 26 weeks' gestation with a resulting value of 165 mg/dL. After 3 days of carbohydrate loading, she then proceeded to have a 3-hour 100-g oral glucose tolerance test. The resulting values are as follows: fasting, 106; 1 hour, 194; 2 hours, 170; 3 hours, 135. In White's classification of diabetes in pregnancy, she meets the criteria for which of the following categories?

(A) Class A1
(B) Class A2
(C) Class B
(D) Class C
(E) Class D

39 An afebrile 23-year-old woman presents with suprapubic pain, dysuria, and increased frequency of urination. A urinary sediment examination reveals clumps of neutrophils, occasional red blood cells (RBCs), and rod-shaped bacteria. No casts or crystals are present. Assuming that this sediment is representative of the entire specimen, the patient would be expected to have which of the following?

(A) Excessive proteinuria
(B) A positive dipstick for nitrite and leukocyte esterase
(C) A nephritic type of glomerulonephritis
(D) Acute pyelonephritis
(E) A renal stone

40 A 4-month-old infant is brought to the emergency department with sudden onset of lethargy and poor feeding. The mother reports that the infant had been in her usual state of good health until recently when she developed constipation. The mother also states that she has recently stopped breast-feeding and has changed to formula feeding. According to the mother, the infant does not like the formula unless it is sweetened. On physical examination the infant is noted to be afebrile and have generalized hypotonia and weakness, as well as ophthalmoplegia. Which of the following is the most likely diagnosis?

(A) Guillain-Barré syndrome
(B) Hypothyroidism
(C) Werdnig-Hoffmann disease
(D) Infant botulism
(E) Hypomagnesemia

Directions for Matching Questions (41 through 50): Each set of matching questions is preceded by a list of 4 to 26 lettered options followed by a brief explanation of the required task and then by a series of numbered statements. For each lettered statement you are to select ONE lettered option that best fulfills the task as it relates to that statement. Remember each of the listed options might be correctly selected once, more than once, or not at all.

Question 41–50

(A) Cross-over study
(B) Single-blind study
(C) Double-blind study
(D) Meta-analysis
(E) Nonconcurrent prospective study
(F) Cross-sectional study
(G) Case report
(H) Case series report
(I) Case-control study

For each description, select the ONE appropriate investigative method used.

41 A physician reports an unusual clinical presentation in a 50-year-old male with carcinoma of the lung.

42 A physician reports several cases of abdominal pain, neuropathy, and optic neuritis in a coastal population after consumption of fish.

[43] An international multicenter trial was conducted on a new antihypertensive drug to reach a definite conclusion about its efficacy. This involved more than 2000 patients in several hospitals in the United States, Mexico, Canada, Britain, and France.

[44] A researcher interested in establishing the risk factors for a rare collagen disease retraces the illness from its end point to its origin.

[45] An experimental study design was developed to assess differences between two groups of women receiving different treatment for carcinoma of the breast. Neither the investigator nor the participants are aware of the group to which they have been assigned

[46] An investigator conducts a survey to establish the prevalence of bronchial asthma in Los Angeles, California.

[47] An investigator wants to establish the efficacy of a new analgesic. He administers the drug to group A, and a placebo to group B. Thereafter, group B receives the drug, while group A receives the placebo. The results after both studies are recorded.

[48] A clinical trial is conducted for a new drug to treat rheumatoid arthritis. The goal is to observe if the patients improved, became worse, or showed no change with the new medication. Participants and the investigator are oblivious of allocation to the control and treatment group.

[49] An epidemiologist discovers that several workers in a chemical factory became ill after exposure to a chemical. He wants to establish the effect of this exposure and looks back at the health records of workers exposed to the same chemical 30 years earlier.

[50] An investigator wants to establish the effect of a recent radiation leak from a nuclear plant in a group.

Answer Key

1	C	**11**	A	**21**	A	**31**	D	**41**	G
2	C	**12**	A	**22**	A	**32**	D	**42**	H
3	A	**13**	E	**23**	B	**33**	E	**43**	D
4	B	**14**	C	**24**	B	**34**	D	**44**	I
5	D	**15**	C	**25**	D	**35**	B	**45**	C
6	D	**16**	A	**26**	B	**36**	D	**46**	F
7	D	**17**	C	**27**	B	**37**	B	**47**	A
8	D	**18**	E	**28**	D	**38**	A	**48**	C
9	B	**19**	B	**29**	D	**39**	B	**49**	E
10	D	**20**	E	**30**	B	**40**	D	**50**	I

Answers and Explanations

1 **The answer is C** *Psychiatry*

This presentation is most suggestive of cocaine-induced psychotic disorder (choice **C**), characterized by hallucinations and delusions caused by cocaine use. Cocaine-induced psychosis often starts during a binge of cocaine use and persists for 1 or 2 weeks after cessation of cocaine use.

The presence of psychosis explains his anxiety (choice **A**), but the anxiety doesn't cause the psychosis. Delirium (choice **B**) is unlikely because he is alert and oriented. Cocaine intoxication (choice **D**) is unlikely because he last used the substance 1 week ago, and his urine toxicology testing result is negative. Schizophrenia (choice **E**) might present with similar symptoms, but the diagnosis is less likely because of the patient's history of cocaine use.

2 **The answer is C** *Medicine*

The patient may be experiencing a cholinergic crisis from taking an overdose of pyridostigmine or a myasthenic crisis from not taking an adequate dose. Infections in myasthenic patients may alter drug dosage requirements, and because gastrointestinal (GI) upsets are common in "flu," the physician cannot reliably use changes in bowel activity to aid in diagnosis. To determine whether his crisis is due to too much or too little pyridostigmine a small dose of edrophonium (usually 2 mg, 1 hour after the last oral dose of pyridostigmine) should be given (choice **C**). This will inhibit acetylcholine esterase and increase acetylcholine levels. It should be followed by careful observation to see whether muscle strength improves (indicating an inadequate dose of pyridostigmine) or worsens (indicating an excessive dose). In the former case, the dose of pyridostigmine should be increased (choice **A**). In the latter case, the worsening effect is quite brief, lasting only a few minutes. Subsequently, the dose of pyridostigmine should be decreased (choice **D**). Equipment for intubation should be at hand should this be required.

Physostigmine (choice **B**) is a tertiary amine cholinesterase inhibitor that readily enters the central nervous system and the eyes. It is a specific antidote for tricyclic antidepressant and anticholinergic poisoning. It competitively blocks the hydrolysis of acetylcholine by cholinesterase, allowing acetylcholine to accumulate and counter the muscarinic effects of tricyclic overdose. In the case of the eye, it promotes contraction of the ciliary muscle, with resultant miosis and increased outflow of aqueous humor from posterior chamber into the canal of Schlemm. The net effect is lowering intraocular pressure. Hence, it is used in open-angle glaucoma. It has no role in the treatment of myasthenia gravis. Neither is succinylcholine (choice **E**) of any value in the treatment of myasthenia gravis. Succinylcholine is a depolarizing agent that causes neuromuscular blockade, with resultant skeletal muscle paralysis. It is an agonist at the nicotinic end-plate receptor.

3 **The answer is A** *Medicine*

Two forms of scleroderma (sclerosis) exist, limited (in 80% of cases) and diffuse (in 20%). The limited form is usually restricted to the hands and feet and includes the CREST syndrome, and pulmonary hypertension. The limited form of the disease has a better prognosis than the diffuse one. Both systemic sclerosis and localized scleroderma present with Raynaud's phenomenon in almost all patients, often antedating other manifestations of the disease by years. Cold temperatures and stress are stimuli that produce color changes of the fingers (sometimes toes), which first blanch, then become cyanotic, and then red. Vasospasm and thickened digital arteries (choice **A**) are responsible for these changes. CREST syndrome is characterized by **C**alcinosis of the digits, **R**aynaud's phenomenon, **E**sophageal motility dysfunction, **S**clerodactyly of the fingers, and **T**elangiectasia over the digits and under the nails. The anticentromere antibody is positive in about 50% of cases.

Systemic sclerosis is a more generalized disorder of connective tissue, characterized by degenerative and inflammatory changes that result in the subsequent increase of collagen tissue deposition in various tissues. Tightening of the skin of the face and extremities is a universal finding. Esophageal motility problems, with dysphagia for solids and liquids, occur in 80% of patients. Other problems include arthritis (80%), renal involvement–onion skinning of the vessels (60%), pericardial effusions (20–50%), pulmonary fibrosis with restrictive lung disease (35%), and subsequent pulmonary hypertension, and renal crisis (15%). The antinuclear antibody test result is positive in 70–90% of cases. The anti-Scl-70 antibody is specific for systemic sclerosis and is noted in 20–33% of cases. D-Penicillamine may improve long-term survival, as it may improve skin sclerosis. Cryoglobulinemia caused by proteins that precipitate in cold temperatures, cold agglutinins with immunoglobulin M (IgM) antibodies that clump red blood cells (RBCs) in the digital vessels (choice **B**), and immune complexes causing vasculitis (choice **C**) are not present. Other causes of Raynaud's phenomenon are thromboangiitis obliterans (Buerger's disease), which is an inflammatory vasculitis producing thrombosis of the digital vessels (choice **D**) in male smokers, and ergotamine poisoning. Embolism to digital vessels in the hand is uncommon (choice **E**).

4 The answer is B *Surgery*

The patient has a small bowel obstruction, which is most commonly caused by adhesions from a previous surgery (choice **B**). Characteristic physical findings in small bowel obstruction are vomiting, colicky midabdominal pain, abdominal distention, hyperperistalsis, obstipation (i.e., absence of stool and flatus), and a lack of rebound tenderness. Abdominal x-ray films show distended loops of bowel with a "stepladder" pattern of differential air–fluid levels. In some cases, intestinal intubation relieves the entrapped gas and fluids, causing the obstruction to subside. Other cases require surgical intervention.

Diverticulosis (choice **A**) usually causes no symptoms and noninflamed diverticula are generally discovered by chance during an ancillary examination such as a colonoscopy for cancer screening. Torsion of the bowel around the mesenteric root (choice **C**) is a volvulus. It produces obstruction and strangulation of bowel. Intussusception (choice **D**) is uncommon in adults and produces a combination of obstruction and infarction. Generally, a small bowel infarction resulting from thrombosis over an atherosclerotic plaque in the proximal superior mesenteric artery causes bloody diarrhea (choice **A**). "Thumbprinting" from submucosal edema is noted in barium studies.

5 The answer is D *Medicine*

Vasculopathic third nerve palsy due to third nerve deficit (choice **D**) is the correct diagnosis. This causes rotation outward from medial rectus weakness and ptosis from levator palpebrae weakness and is associated with a normal pupillary size.

A compressive lesion, such as an aneurysm (choice **C**) or a tumor, would compress the dorsomedial portion of the third nerve and cause a dilated, unreactive pupil. This distinction is important because a third nerve lesion that spares the pupil is generally nonemergent, whereas lesions that involve the pupil are best considered medical emergencies. Cavernous sinus thrombosis (choice **A**), although possible, is less likely because it would generally involve other cranial nerves as well. A superior oblique palsy (choice **B**) (from fourth cranial nerve damage) can be congenital, but acquired cases are usually caused by trauma. Isolated fourth nerve damage causes upward deviation of the eye and inability of depression on adduction and often first becomes apparent while descending the stairs. Internuclear ophthalmoplegia (choice **E**) is due to interruption of the signal from the sixth nerve nucleus contralateral to the medial rectus nucleus of the third cranial nerve that is conveyed via the medial longitudinal fasciculus. This results in the inability of the medial rectus to contract in a synchronous manner when the lateral rectus does, resulting in diplopia on conjugate gaze. The condition could result from vascular or demyelinating disease.

6 The answer is D *Pediatrics*

Panniculitis is secondary to cold injury to fat and is characterized by the development of indurated lesions that resemble buccal cellulitis. Young children who hold popsicles in their mouths may be prone to panniculitis (choice **D**).

Erysipelas (choice **A**) is a relatively rare acute illness, caused by group A streptococci. In erysipelas there is a well-demarcated infection of the skin with lymphangitis. The patient with erysipelas usually appears ill, with fever, vomiting, and irritability. Cellulitis (choice **B**) usually has distinct margins and is tender, indurated, and warm to touch. There is no history of trauma (choice **C**), nor is there any evidence of bruising or abrasions. Contact dermatitis (choice **E**) has an erythematous or papulovesicular rash in the area that was exposed to the contactant.

7 **The answer is D** *Medicine*

Upon even slight suspicion of meningitis, it is wise to perform a spinal tap, provided of course that there is no evidence of raised intracranial pressure. Features common to most cases of meningitis include headache (often the predominant presenting symptom, and unlike most headaches, it is generally more severe when lying down and resting); photophobia; vomiting; giddiness; fever; and stiffness of the neck, spinal muscles, and hamstrings. This patient presented with sufficient symptoms to suggest that she has meningitis. The analysis of the spinal fluid indicates that she suffers from aseptic meningitis (choice **D**), most typically induced by a viral infection. In viral meningitis, at most there are only few more white blood cells (WBCs) than normal, and as in a normal sample, these primarily are mononuclear lymphocytes. In aseptic meningitis, the spinal fluid glucose level is usually in the low-normal range, and protein levels tend to be elevated as in the case described.

Although the patient presented with sufficient symptoms to diagnose a case of meningitis, many symptoms were marginal, suggesting that it was not a fulminating case, as is often seen in bacterial meningitis (choice **A**). Bacterial meningitis is characterized by a greater number of leukocytes (from 200 to 20,000), which are primarily polymorphonuclear neutrophils. The spinal fluid glucose level is generally significantly lower than normal, and protein levels are elevated to a greater degree than in aseptic meningitis (often above 100 mg/mL). Cryptococcal meningitis (choice **B**) is almost always an opportunistic infection in an immunocompromised host. The patient's history strongly suggests that this is not a relevant factor. Although human immunodeficiency virus (HIV) and herpes simplex virus type 2 infections may cause chronic viral meningitis, her history tends to rule these out as causative agents. Actinomyces meningitis (choice **E**), although uncommon, might be suspected in this case because the patient had recent dental work, a significant risk factor for infection by this anaerobic class of bacteria. However, as discussed above the laboratory results are not characteristic of a bacterial infection. *Coccidia immitis* meningitis (choice **C**), although relatively rare, might also be suspected because the patient comes from the San Joaquin valley in California. However, to make this diagnosis, the glucose level in the spinal fluid should be well below normal. Other pointers to it in the cerebrospinal fluid would be increased cell count, lymphocytosis, the presence of complement-fixing antibodies, and, a positive culture in approximately 30% of cases.

It is critically important to distinguish between bacterial and viral meningitis. If bacterial meningitis is not properly managed, the consequences are severe, often resulting in death, whereas viral meningitis is generally self-limited. Viral meningitis caused by herpes or human immunodeficiency virus (HIV) is a major exception to this rule.

8 **The answer is D** *Medicine*

One fourth to one half of diabetic men suffer from erectile dysfunction; generally ejaculation is normal, but erectile problems are present (choice **D**).

Obviously, if choice **D** is correct, choice **B** (orgasm and ejaculation are less likely to be affected than erection) is incorrect. Microscopic nerve damage (choice **C**) and vascular changes (choice **E**) as well as psychologic factors influence the erectile problems associated with diabetes. Poor metabolic control of diabetes is associated with increased incidence of sexual problems; therefore, this patient is most likely not maintaining optimum blood sugar levels (choice **A**).

9 **The answer is B** *Surgery*

About 5% of ulcer patients develop perforations, most commonly on the anterior wall of the stomach or duodenum and more commonly in males than in females. The incidence of perforations is increasing; it has been hypothesized that this is due to increased use of nonsteroid antiinflammatory drugs (NSAIDs) and/or crack cocaine. Perforation of a peptic ulcer is characterized by the sudden onset of epigastric pain with radiation of the pain into the right shoulder, which results from irritation of the phrenic nerve (C4) by air underneath the diaphragm. Abdominal rigidity, rebound tenderness, and ileus occur as a result of chemical peritonitis. The first step in management is to obtain an upright and supine film (choice **B**) of the abdomen, which shows air beneath the diaphragm in 75–85% of cases; the presence of air establishes a diagnosis. Intravenous cefazolin is given as prophylaxis against infection. Surgical intervention is necessary. Modern minimally invasive laparotomy techniques coupled to postoperative treatment of possible *Helicobacter pylori* infection has reduced the overall mortality to about 5%.

One cannot conclude that there is no perforation if air is not present beneath the diaphragm; as a consequence a follow-up upper gastrointestinal series should be done. However barium studies (choice **A**) should not be performed in patients with suspect perforation. Peritoneal lavage (choice **C**) is usually indicated in the workup of intraabdominal bleeding. Antacids (choice **D**) are not indicated in the treatment of peptic ulcer perforation. Exploratory surgery (choice **E**) is not the initial step in management of abdominal pain.

10 The answer is D   *Pediatrics*

Visceral larva migrans (choice **D**) is caused by infection with *Toxocara* larvae. It is most common in children 1 to 4 years of age, especially if they have pica or have a tendency to place their fingers in their mouth and have close contact with dogs or cats, because *Toxocara* are common parasites of both. Sandboxes are common areas for both pets and children. Symptoms include fever, hepatomegaly, wheezing, pulmonary disease, and eosinophilia.

Eosinophilic lung disease (choice **B**), sometimes called Löffler's syndrome, is a group of disorders, not commonly found in children in the United States, that are linked by the common findings of eosinophilia and pulmonary infiltrates. Anal pruritus and sleeplessness are the presenting complaints in pinworm manifestation (choice **A**). Eosinophilia does not occur in most cases as tissue invasion is absent. Ascariasis (choice **C**) may cause fever, urticaria, allergic symptoms, and granulomatous disease. Vomiting, abdominal distention, and abdominal pain may also be present. Pulmonary infections with *Strongyloides stercoralis* (strongyloidiasis [choice **E**]) are usually mild and may pass unnoticed. However, in immunosuppressed and malnourished children, massive parasite invasion with *S. stercoralis* may cause generalized abdominal pain, fever, and shock due to gram-negative sepsis.

11 The answer is A   *Medicine*

The athlete is suffering from exercise-induced asthma. Common symptoms include postexercise cough, dyspnea out of proportion to the level of exertion, poorer performance than expected, wheezing, chest tightness, and sputum production. The treatment of choice is β2-agonists, usually two puffs to be inhaled 5 minutes prior to exercise (choice **A**).

Cromolyn sodium (choice **C**) is a second-line agent. It is given in the form of two sprays 1 hour prior to exercise. It is used in combination with β2-agonists in the treatment of severe recurrent bronchial asthma. Other uses include the prevention of allergic rhinitis and allergic ocular disorders. A rare but serious complication is angioedema. Theophylline (choice **B**) is usually indicated for rapid relief of symptoms in acute asthma or as a prophylaxis for bronchial asthma and bronchospasm induced by chronic bronchitis and emphysema. It has potentially serious side effects including seizures, hypotension, cardiac arrhythmias, and even respiratory arrest. Erythromycin (choice **D**) should not be part of the treatment plan because there are no signs of an infection. Lifelong abstinence from strenuous activity (choice **E**) would be a gross overreaction.

12 The answer is A   *Obstetrics and Gynecology*

The patient in this scenario has many risk factors for pelvic relaxation: she is white, postmenopausal, without estrogen replacement; is multiparous and has delivered large infants; and she has a long history of smoking. However, her symptom of difficulty in stool evacuation is more referable to lower posterior vaginal relaxation due to a rectocele (choice **A**) that contains the rectum. The diagnosis is made on the basis of inspection at the time of pelvic examination when the patient is asked to cough or perform the Valsalva maneuver (increasing intraabdominal pressure).

Incorrect options include a cystocele (choice **B**) (an upper anterior vaginal relaxation that contains the bladder). This is the most common finding with vaginal wall relaxation and may be associated with urinary stress incontinence. An enterocele (choice **C**) (an upper posterior vaginal relaxation that contains the small bowel), is a more uncommon finding and is associated with rather nonspecific symptoms. A urethrocele (choice **D**) (a lower anterior vaginal relaxation that contains the urethra) may also be associated with urinary incontinence but does not cause defecation symptoms. Vaginocele (choice **E**) is a spurious distracter.

13 The answer is E   *Pediatrics*

Infants born before 37 weeks' gestation (choices **A** and **B**) are preterm. Preterm infants may have lanugo hair; smooth, pink skin with visible veins; faint plantar creases; and ears that are soft with slow recoil. Term infants are defined as those who are born between 37 and 42 weeks' gestation (choices **C** and **D**). Term infants have a small amount of lanugo and some bald areas; smooth, slightly thickened skin; ears that have good recoil; and indentations over more than the anterior third of the plantar area. Postterm babies are born after 42 weeks' gestation (choice **E**). They tend to be large for gestational age and hyperalert. Lanugo is absent, and the skin is cracked and peeling. Fingernails are long. They are at increased risk for meconium aspiration.

14 **The answer is C** *Psychiatry*

The woman's most likely diagnosis is specific phobia, defined as fear of a discrete object or situation. In this case, the object is snakes. The defense mechanism most closely associated with specific phobias is displacement (choice **C**). Displacement occurs when the emotions associated with a psychologically unacceptable object, idea, or activity are transferred to another object or situation, which is often symbolically related to the original one. A psychodynamic explanation for onset of the specific phobia in this case would be the symbolic association between a snake and a penis.

The other choices are defense mechanisms that are not so closely associated with simple phobias. Dissociation (choice **A**) is the fragmentation or separation of aspects of consciousness, including memory, identity, and perception. To some degree such dissociation is normal and may even be a useful defense mechanism; we all have a tendency to forget unpleasant events, and this helps reduce chronic anxiety. However, if a person's consciousness becomes too fragmented, it becomes pathologic. Examples are dissociative: amnesia, fugue, identity disorder, and depersonalization disorder. Projection (choice **B**) is the transfer of uncomfortable inner feelings such as guilt or anger to others; such persons often seem bitter and suspicious. Conversion (choice **D**) is the transfer of emotional conflicts into physical symptoms. Resistance (choice **E**) is the active opposition to bringing unconscious feelings to the conscious level.

15 **The answer is C** *Surgery*

Cardiac tamponade is characterized by decreased cardiac output and increased central venous pressure owing to restriction of blood flow into and out of the heart as fluid in the pericardial sac restricts filling of all the cardiac chambers. An echocardiogram (choice **C**) is the most sensitive and specific noninvasive test to establish the presence of fluid in the pericardial sac. After the diagnosis is established, pericardiocentesis should be performed to immediately reduce intrapericardial sac pressure. Surgery follows to locate the source of the tamponade in those cases that are associated with trauma.

Distention of the neck veins on inspiration is called Kussmaul's sign. Normally, the increase in negative intrathoracic pressure on inspiration sucks blood from the jugular venous system into the right side of the heart. However, if the right side of the heart is restricted by fluid in the pericardial sac, the blood regurgitates into the jugular veins on inspiration.

A drop in the pulse or the blood pressure of more than 10 mm Hg on inspiration is called *pulsus paradoxus*. It reflects the drop in inflow of blood into the right side of the heart, which automatically decreases the outflow of blood from the left ventricle. An increase in central venous pressure without an increase in blood pressure further documents the inability of the heart to receive fluid and pump it out into the systemic circulation; therefore, giving additional fluid (choice **B**) would exacerbate the condition. Inserting a chest tube into the left pleural cavity (choice **A**), decreasing venous pressure by administering a venodilator (choice **D**), and decreasing venous pressure by administering a loop diuretic (choice **E**) would be incorrect steps in management, at least at this time.

16 **The answer is A** *Psychiatry*

This woman's symptoms are suggestive of dementia and neuromotor degeneration secondary to subacute combined degeneration of the cord as a result of vitamin B_{12} deficiency (choice **A**). Causes of vitamin B_{12} deficiency include strict vegetarianism (vegans), alcoholism, and pernicious anemia. It is relatively more common in older adults and should be investigated as part of any workup for dementia, particularly since it is treatable. Although the classic feature of vitamin B_{12} deficiency is a macrocytic, hypochromic anemia, this may be masked by folate supplementation.

The other choices are not commonly associated with dementia. Vitamin C deficiency (choice **B**) presents with hemorrhagic, not mental, symptoms. Clinically significant magnesium deficiency (choice **D**) may present with cognitive changes and weakness but is rare, since magnesium is found in a wide variety of foods. Iron deficiency (choice **C**) presents with lassitude, weakness, and microcytic, hypochromic anemia but not with dementia and neuromotor degeneration. Diet-related deficiencies of lecithin (choice **E**) or its metabolic products are rare. Hereditary absence of the enzyme lecithin–cholesterol acyltransferase prevents the conversion of lecithin to lysolecithin and produces anemia and renal failure.

17 The answer is C *Pediatrics*

Rett syndrome (choice **C**) occurs only in females. Girls with Rett syndrome appear to be developing normally until 6 to 18 months of age, when they manifest dementia, develop microcephaly, and lose purposeful movements of their hands (i.e., hand-wringing). They may also have ataxia, seizures, scoliosis, and loss of gross motor skills. They may have sighing respirations associated with apnea and cyanosis.

Autism (choice **A**) may manifest with great variability in severity and range of symptoms. The usual presenting complaint is regression of language and play without loss of motor skills. Characterizations of William's syndrome (choice **B**) include a depressed nasal bridge, epicanthal folds, prominent thick lips with open mouth, and short stature. Short stature, webbed posterior neck, broad chest with widely spaced nipples, and an increased carrying angle of the arms characterize Turner's syndrome (choice **D**). Key features of Russell-Silver syndrome (choice **E**) are short stature, triangular facies with down-turned corners of the mouth, clinodactyly, and a head that appears disproportionately large.

18 The answer is E *Obstetrics and Gynecology*

The description in this case is that of recurrent genital herpes. The herpes simplex virus has potential for significant adverse impact on the fetus, neonate, or both. Although the herpes simplex virus does not increase the risk of congenital malformations (choice **B**), infectious sequela are possible. The decision about route of delivery cannot be made until the onset of labor (choice **E**). If no lesions are present at the start of labor, this woman can safely undergo labor and vaginal delivery. If lesions are present at the start of labor, cesarean delivery is indicated (choice **A**). Because she has protective antibodies against herpes, she does not experience viremia; therefore, there is no risk of transplacental viral passage (choice **C**). If she has no breast lesions after delivery, she can safely breast-feed (choice **D**).

19 The answer is B *Medicine*

The malar rash, arthralgia, fever, and anorexia are all common symptoms of systemic lupus erythematosus (SLE). The serum antinuclear antibody (ANA) test is the gold-standard screening test used to rule out SLE and other collagen vascular diseases. The major groups of ANAs are antibodies against DNA (both double- and single-stranded), histones and nonhistone proteins, and nucleolar antigens. Some 95–100% of all cases of SLE test positive. However while sensitive, it is far from specific; it also will give a positive test in patients with the following diseases: Sjögren's (95%), diffuse and limited (CREST syndrome) scleroderma (80–95%), polymyositis and dermatomyositis (80–95%), rheumatoid arthritis (30–60%) and Wegner's granulomatosis (0–15%). As a consequence a diagnosis after a positive ANA test result needs to be confirmed using a more specific test. The most specific autoantibody test available for SLE is the anti-native DNA test also known as the anti–double-stranded (ds) DNA test, which has a positive result in some 60% of the patients with SLE and a positive result in fewer than 5% of rheumatoid arthritis cases and in no other of the major autoimmune diseases. Thus positive results obtained with the antinuclear and anti-ds (double-stranded) DNA tests (choice **B**) will almost definitely confirm a case of SLE. Further confirmation can be obtained using an anti-Sm (Smith) test, which is 100% specific for SLE, but its sensitivity is only about 10–25%. Obviously some true cases of SLE will not be confirmed using these tests (false negatives), and as a consequence, the diagnosis will depend upon clinical criteria.

Anti-SSA (Ro) (choice **A**) and anti-SSB (La) (choice **C**) results are both positive in fewer than 20% of SLE patients but are also positive in 60–70% of Sjögren's syndrome patients and in a small minority of patients with rheumatoid arthritis; thus these tests add little to the diagnosis of SLE. Anticentromere antibodies are present in 50% of patients with the CREST syndrome, and antiribonucleoprotein antibodies are seen in most cases of patients with the so-called mixed connective tissue disease (choice **D**), which is also called *overlap connective tissue disease,* since a case will often resolve into one or the other connective tissue autoantibody conditions; however, it is neither as sensitive as the ANA nor very specific for SLE. Despite its name, the lupus anticoagulant test (choice **E**) result is only positive in some 7% of SLE patients. The term is a misnomer in a sense, because the anticoagulant is directed against a phospholipid and not against any specific factor. Hence, the test result is positive in a number of disorders, including rheumatoid arthritis, infections including *Pneumocystis carinii*, lymphoproliferative disorders, drugs, and toxemia of pregnancy. Antihistone antibodies are present in more than 95% of cases of drug-induced lupus but are not in lupus of other causes.

20 The answer is E   *Medicine*

This patient has polycystic kidney disease (choice **E**), which shows up on the ultrasound as black spaces in the kidney parenchyma. Hematuria and hypertension are common presenting complaints. The disease has an autosomal dominant inheritance pattern and affects one newborn in every 800 live births, making it one of the most common hereditary diseases in the United States; half of the affected will have end-stage renal disease by the age of 60 years. Patients with polycystic kidney disease do not have cysts at birth, and renal function is usually retained until the third or fourth decade, at which time many cysts have developed. There is an association with cysts in the liver (30%), berry aneurysms of the circle of Willis (10–15%), and diverticulosis. The grandmother's stroke may have been secondary to a subarachnoid hemorrhage from a ruptured berry aneurysm. Discomfort in the abdomen in this patient could be due to a ruptured cyst, bleeding into a cyst, or an infected cyst. Long-term hemodialysis or renal transplantation is the recommended treatment for these patients.

Immunoglobulin A (IgA) nephropathy (choice **A**) is the most frequent glomerulonephritis in the United States and is even more common in Asia. An episode of hematuria is the usual presenting symptom. It commonly occurs in children and young adults, with males being affected two to three times more often than females. Frequently, microscopic hematuria occurs a few days after an upper respiratory infection, gastrointestinal symptoms, or a flulike illness. Serum IgA levels are increased in 40% of patients. Immunofluorescent stains of glomeruli are strongly positive for IgA, located predominantly in the mesangium. Approximately 50% of patients have a nephritic pattern, with hematuria, red blood cell (RBC) casts, and mild-to-moderate proteinuria; the remainder present with a nephrotic pattern characterized by proteinuria of more than 3.5 g/24 hours. Corticosteroids are not useful in therapy. About half the patients develop renal insufficiency. Goodpasture's syndrome (choice **B**) most often occurs in young men. Antibasement antibodies against pulmonary and glomerular capillaries are present. The disease initially presents with hemoptysis from pulmonary hemorrhage. Renal failure develops shortly thereafter. Glomerular biopsies show crescentic glomerulonephritis and a linear pattern of immunofluorescence. Plasmapheresis is useful in removing the antibodies. Cyclophosphamide is used to suppress antibody synthesis. Kidney transplantation is most successful when the antibasement membrane antibodies are not present. A staghorn calculus (choice **C**) is made up of magnesium ammonium phosphate (struvite). These calculi are commonly associated with urease-splitting organisms, such as *Proteus*, and production of an alkaline pH that favors stone formation. Alport's syndrome (choice **D**) is a genetic disease involving the collagen fibers forming the basement membranes of many organs including the kidney and inner ear, and it causes nerve deafness and glomerulonephritis. It tends to be more common and more severe in boys than in girls. Men usually die of renal failure by 40 years of age, but women frequently have a normal life span.

21 The answer is A   *Medicine*

Differentiation of the polyuria syndromes is best accomplished with the water deprivation test. The polyuria syndromes include central diabetes insipidus (CDI), which involves an absolute deficiency of antidiuretic hormone (ADH); nephrogenic diabetes insipidus (NDI), in which the kidney tubules are not responsive to ADH; and primary polydipsia, in which a person chronically overingests water.

Patients with CDI and NDI present with polydipsia and polyuria owing to the loss of free water (not salt) in the urine (choice **E** is wrong); water loss increases their plasma osmolality (Posm), which stimulates thirst and lowers urine osmolarity (Uosm). However, in primary polydipsia, the patient drinks excessive amounts of water, thus lowering the Posm. The excess water is removed by the kidneys, which produces a low Uosm. Primary polydipsia is usually not difficult to separate from diabetes insipidus because at the outset, the Posm is decreased, as opposed to CDI and NDI, which have an increased Posm secondary to hypernatremia ($\uparrow$ serum Na$^+$ = TBNa$^+$/$\downarrow\downarrow$ TBw; where TBNa$^+$ = total body sodium, and TBw = total body water).

The water deprivation test will cause the Posm in normal controls and in persons with primary polydipsia to reach the upper limit of the normal range, which is 275–295 mmol/kg. Posm is increased in both CDI (patient **A**) and NDI (patient **B**) because the loss of free water concentrates the plasma and increases serum sodium concentration. Uosm is increased in both normal controls and in primary polydipsia (patient **C**), because ADH is available to reabsorb free water and concentrate the urine. However, in CDI and NDI, the Uosm is markedly decreased owing to the loss of free water. Once the maximum Uosm is reached (specimens do not differ by more than 30 mmol/kg), intramuscular vasopressin is administered. Normal controls and patients with primary polydipsia have less than a 9% increase in Uosm. In CDI, the Uosm increases more than 50%, whereas in NDI, it increases less than (not approximate) 45% from the maximum Uosm (choice **D**).

Patient A has CDI, because the maximum Posm is increased, the maximum Uosm is decreased, and the Uosm increase is greater than 50% (160–400 mmol/kg) after administration of vasopressin (choice **A**). CDI is associated with hypothalamic lesions where ADH is synthesized; severance of the pituitary stalk, which interrupts the neuron carrying ADH to the posterior pituitary; or destruction of the posterior pituitary, where ADH is stored.

Patient B has NDI, because the maximum Posm is increased, the maximum Uosm is decreased, and the Uosm does not increase more than 45% (125–150 mmol/kg) after administration of vasopressin consequently (choice **D**) is not correct. NDI can be hereditary or acquired from tubulointerstitial disease (e.g., chronic pyelonephritis) or drugs (e.g., lithium, demeclocycline, alcohol, amphotericin B) (choice **B**).

Patient C has primary polydipsia, because the maximum Posm is normal, the maximum Uosm is increased, the Uosm increases less than 9% (690–710 mmol/kg) after vasopressin administration (choice **C**). The normal control has the same findings.

22 **The answer is A** *Psychiatry*

The patient presents with the psychotic symptom of persecutory delusions. Of the disorders listed, only dementia (choice **A**) commonly presents with psychotic symptoms. Delusions, mood changes (e.g., anxiety, depression), and other thought disturbances (e.g., perseveration) often accompany significant cognitive impairment. Other disorders with similar psychotic symptoms include schizophrenia and delusional disorder. However, in these disorders, obvious cognitive impairment would be absent.

Obsessive–compulsive disorder (choice **B**) may present with anxiety about bizarre ideas, but the individual usually recognizes the irrational nature of the thoughts. Panic disorder (choice **C**), posttraumatic stress disorder (choice **D**), and generalized anxiety disorder (choice **E**) may all present with anxiety but do not explain the presence of psychosis.

23 **The answer is B** *Obstetrics and Gynecology*

The case scenario describes polyhydramnios. Amniotic fluid amount can be quantified using the four-quadrant amniotic fluid index (AFI), which is the sum of the measurements of the deepest amniotic fluid pockets in the four abdominal quadrants, measured by sonography. Polyhydramnios is present when the AFI exceeds 25 cm. or the deepest single amniotic fluid pocket exceeds 8 cm. Excessive amniotic fluid is a result of imbalance of secretion and absorption. The only option listed that is associated with polyhydramnios is diabetes mellitus, (choice **B**), in which polyhydramnios appears to be related to the degree of glucose control.

Asthma (choice **A**), hyperthyroidism (choice **C**), seizure disorder (choice **D**), and sickle cell anemia (choice **E**) are not associated with polyhydramnios.

24 **The answer is B** *Surgery*

This woman has a pulmonary embolus with infarction, a condition most commonly seen in the setting of postoperative recovery associated with stasis of the venous circulation in the proximal (femoral) veins of the leg; the most common location (90%) for thromboembolism. Signs and symptoms depend on the size of the embolus. Large saddle emboli that block four of the five pulmonary artery orifices result in sudden death because of acute strain of the right side of the heart. Small emboli lodge peripherally, where they produce an infarction in fewer than 10% of patients. Infarction is more likely in patients with preexisting lung disease, such as heart failure or chronic obstructive lung disease. Pulmonary angiography is the gold standard test for diagnosing a pulmonary embolus, particularly when other studies give conflicting results. However, most clinicians begin with a perfusion scan of the lungs (choice **B**), which has a high probability of indicating an infarction if a lobar perfusion defect accompanies ventilation mismatch, the latter demonstrated by a ventilation scan. Perfusion defects last 7 to 14 days.

A pleural tap (choice **A**), Gram's stain with culture and sensitivity of sputum (choice **C**), pulmonary function studies (choice **D**), and a bronchoscopy (choice **E**) are noncontributory in the initial workup of a pulmonary embolus.

25 The answer is D *Medicine*

The anticoagulant drug warfarin has been implicated in numerous drug interaction scenarios. Warfarin is documented to exert prophylactic actions after a myocardial infarction (MI) (choice **E**), and the dosage regimen was appropriately adjusted in this patient (choice **A**) to result in an approximate 50% increase in prothrombin time (PT) (normal range is 11–15 seconds). The further increase in PT described is likely to result in a bleeding episode and reflects increased activity of warfarin at the established dose. The histamine (H_2)-blocking drug cimetidine is known to be a potent inhibitor of liver drug-metabolizing enzymes, including those forms of cytochrome P450 that are responsible for the metabolic inactivation of warfarin. Thus, concomitant administration of cimetidine is anticipated to increase PT; by inhibiting the hepatic metabolism of warfarin (choice **D**) it increases its circulating concentration. Other causes that can prolong PT include: inadequate vitamin K in the diet or inadequate absorption, as in Crohn's disease and severe hepatic dysfunction.

Trimethoprim–sulfamethoxazole does not increase the activity of hepatic drug-metabolizing enzymes (rifampin does) and would result in a decreased PT if warfarin metabolism was increased (choice **B**). The antiplatelet action of aspirin does not antagonize the effects of warfarin and may lead to an increased bleeding tendency (choice **C**). Salicylates and sulfonamides may also increase PT by competition with warfarin for plasma protein binding, leading to an increase in the plasma-free fraction of warfarin. Note that many drugs capable of inducing the formation of liver drug-metabolizing enzymes (e.g., barbiturates, carbamazepine, and phenytoin) will decrease PT in patients on warfarin.

26 The answer is B *Medicine*

This patient has neoplastic metastatic epidural cord compression that has arisen from carcinoma of the prostate. The compression has worsened over the past 24 hours but began a week earlier with weakness of his legs. The initial management would be to administer a bolus dose of dexamethasone intravenously (IV) and then perform a magnetic resonance imagining (MRI) study (choice **B**) of the spine with and without gadolinium contrast. The sensitivity of this test is greater than 90%. Thereafter, IV administration of dexamethasone should be continued every 6 hours to combat spinal cord edema. This is a neurosurgical emergency, and immediate decompression should be carried out to salvage neurologic function. The development of urinary bladder problems makes this an even greater reason to act as quickly as possible. Thereafter, the patient should be referred for radiotherapy of the appropriate region.

Waiting for 24 hours before doing an MRI (choice **A**), would only jeopardize neurologic recovery. The patient does not have Guillain-Barré syndrome. This is usually seen in a younger individual, in whom there is a prior history of upper respiratory tract or gastrointestinal infection, following which ascending motor paralysis results. There is no sensory or urinary bladder involvement. Hence, plasmapheresis, (choice **C**) a treatment for Guillain-Barré syndrome is not indicated. Ordering electromyography (choice **D**) would not contribute to diagnosis or management. It would only confirm what is known clinically—that the patient has weakness of his legs due to motor involvement. Even then, abnormalities will be noted approximately 3 weeks after the onset of weakness. Sending him for radiotherapy of the lumbar and sacral spine (choice **E**) is incorrect. Radiotherapy usually follows surgical decompression and has to be done along the extent of the tumor as delineated by the MRI. In some cases however, surgical decompression is not done, and radiotherapy is carried out under steroid cover following a radiologic diagnosis.

27 The answer is B *Obstetrics and Gynecology*

Substance use by an expectant mother can affect reproduction, from fertility through pregnancy and lactation. Research is difficult in this area because of the confounding effects of poor nutrition and exposure to multiple substances. The findings described in the case are consistent with fetal alcohol syndrome (FAS) (choice **B**). In the United States this is the most common preventable cause of mental retardation. Not all children with FAS have the distinctive physical findings, yet they are still at risk for lifelong neurological sequelae such as attention-deficit disorder, hyperactivity, memory difficulties and impulse control.

Prenatal tobacco exposure (choice **A**) is associated with sudden infant death syndrome and childhood behavioral problems but not with any specific syndrome. Prenatal marijuana exposure (choice **C**) is linked to premature births, small birth size, difficult or long labor, and an increase in newborn jitteriness but not to birth defects. Prenatal amphetamine (choice **D**) and narcotics (choice **E**) are associated with neonatal abstinence syndrome (NAS), which refers to the constellation of signs and symptoms exhibited by infants with drug dependencies, but only alcohol has a clearly defined syndrome with intrauterine growth restriction, central nervous system (CNS) effects, and facial anomalies.

28 The answer is D   *Surgery*

About 60% of the solitary coin lesions in the lung are benign. Of the benign causes, granulomas (choice **D**) account for 95%, while the remaining 5% are due to hamartomas or mixed tumors. The patient's midwestern origins strongly suggest histoplasmosis as the cause for the calcified granuloma. Calcification of a coin lesion is more commonly seen in granulomas than in cancer. Absence of growth within 2 years noted on serial radiography of the chest, target or popcorn calcifications, or concentric calcifications strongly favors a benign process. A malignancy would be suggested by indistinct margins, increased growth rate compared with previous films, flecks of calcium in the mass, and sizes greater than 3 cm in diameter. A history of living in an endemic granuloma area and not smoking, in conjunction with no cough, chest pain, weight loss, rhonchi, or hemoptysis all suggest that the lesion is not cancer. Its benign nature also is strongly supported by the fact that it is concentric, calcified, and less than 1 cm in diameter. However, follow-up radiography should be conducted (first yearly, then less regularly) for at least 10 years to make sure the lesion is not growing.

Mixed tumors also known as bronchial hamartomas (choice **B**) are called such because they are pleomorphic and contain epithelial cells, cartilage, and mesenchymal cells. Malignant change is rare in them. Hamartomas are the result of faulty development that results in tissue overgrowth. Indeed, the word *hamartoma* in Greek means fault and was the term used when spear throwers missed their mark. The remaining 40% of the causes of solitary coin lesions in the lung are primary lung cancer (35%) (choice **A**) and metastatic lung cancer (5%) (choice **C**). A negative tuberculosis skin test result proves that it is not a calcified tuberculosis lesion (choice **E**).

29 The answer is D   *Pediatrics*

This patient has a subgaleal hematoma (choice **D**), which is a result of blood collecting subadjacent to the galea. It is seen after minor injury and can be very alarming. It is not associated with loss of consciousness. The best treatment for this condition is to leave it alone. Aspirating the hematoma would only introduce infection, which could be disastrous. The parent should be reassured that no treatment is necessary.

An epidural hematoma (choice **A**) results from blood collecting within the cranial cavity, and is usually seen after a tear of the middle meningeal artery as it courses on the inner aspect of the temporal bone, in which a fracture line is seen. It is associated with a lucid interval and signs of raised intracranial pressure (i.e., headache, vomiting, loss of consciousness, enlarging pupil on the ipsilateral side, and hemiplegia on the contralateral side). A subdural hematoma (choice **B**) results from intracranial hemorrhage within the subdural space. It may be acute or chronic. A fracture may be absent. The patient is comatose from the time of injury and has evidence of cerebral injury. The prognosis is poor. Intraventricular hemorrhage (choice **C**) is associated with coma and may result from trauma. However, it is more commonly seen after hypertensive intracranial hemorrhage, in which the bleeding spreads to the ventricular system. A lipoma (choice **E**) is a benign soft tissue tumor and does not develop suddenly.

30 The answer is B   *Surgery*

With an inhalational anesthetic, both rate of onset and rate of recovery depend on the physiochemical properties of the agent, which are reflected in its blood:gas partition coefficient. Anesthetics with low blood:gas partition coefficients are advantageous because they act rapidly, and the time to recover from their effects is short. As can be seen from the table in the vignette, desflurane (choice **B**) has the lowest blood:gas ratio of all the choices provided. Thus, recovery from the anesthetic effects of desflurane occurs more rapidly than with nitrous oxide (choice **A**), sevoflurane (choice **C**), isoflurane (choice **D**), and halothane (choice **E**). The minimum alveolar concentration is the percentage of anesthetic in the inspired gas that results in immobility in 50% of a patient population exposed to a noxious stimulus. Minimum alveolar concentration is inversely related to the potency of an anesthetic agent and does not influence the kinetics of anesthetic onset or recovery.

31 The answer is D   *Psychiatry*

The case is most suggestive of bipolar disorder; the incident at 23 years of age shows a depressive phase and at 28 years a manic phase. This disorder is characterized by one or more episodes of mania, without known biologic cause and without persisting psychosis between episodes. Evidence of elevated levels of several central nervous system (CNS) neurotransmitters (choice **D**) has been reported during manic episodes in bipolar disorder. The reasons for the antimanic properties of mood-stabilizing medications are unknown.

Family histories of individuals with bipolar disorder suggest that the lesion is heritable (choice **C**), but consistent chromosomal abnormalities have not been detected (choice **E**). Although genetic variations occur in several ion transport mechanisms, no particular abnormality has been clearly identified as a marker for bipolar disorder (choice **A**). Most mood-stabilizing medications, with the exception of antipsychotic drugs, do not block central dopamine receptors (choice **B**).

32 The answer is D   *Medicine*

This patient has α-thalassemia minor, a relatively common cause of microcytic anemia, particularly in the Asian and African-American populations. It is a defect in globin chain synthesis (choice **D**) resulting in decreased production of hemoglobin (Hgb) and is thought to provide protection against falciparum malaria.

The normal globin chains are alpha (α), beta (β), gamma (γ), and delta (δ). Hgb A is the predominant Hgb in adults and accounts for 96 to 98% of the Hgb in red blood cells (RBCs). In adults, Hgb A_2 and F are present in trace amounts (1.5–3% and 0–2%, respectively). All the Hgbs are tetramers; Hgb A is composed of two α and two β chains, Hgb A_2 has two α and two δ chains, and Hgb F consists of two α and two γ chains. The synthesis of α chains is controlled by four genes (two from each parent), and deletions in these genes result in varying severity of disease from mild (1–2 gene deletions) to severe (3–4 gene deletions). A slight decrease in α-chain production (1–2 gene deletions) automatically leads to a proportional decrease in Hgb A, A_2, and F. Because Hgb electrophoresis detects only abnormal Hgb or an increase of a minor Hgb, it is normal in mild α-thalassemia. In severe forms of α-thalassemia (3–4 gene deletions), four β chains combine to form a tetramer called Hgb H (adults) or four γ chains combine to form Bart's Hgb (infants). Because these Hgbs are abnormal, they are detected by Hgb electrophoresis. In β-thalassemia, the decrease in β chains results in a decrease in Hgb A, but there is an increase in Hgb A_2 and Hgb F because α-, γ-, and δ-chain syntheses are unaffected. An unexplained finding in the thalassemias in general is a normal to increased RBC count in the presence of a reduced Hgb concentration and mean corpuscular volume (MCV). This has spawned a number of ratios that are useful in differentiating thalassemia from other microcytic anemias (e.g., iron deficiency and the anemia of inflammation). The Meltzer index is the ratio of MCV to RBC count. A value below 13 is highly predictive for thalassemia, whereas values above 13 usually indicate iron deficiency or anemia of inflammation. In this patient, the ratio is 12 (70/5.8). The RBC distribution width (RDW) is a measure of RBC size variation. When working through the differential diagnosis of a microcytic anemia, iron deficiency, anemia of inflammation, thalassemia, and sideroblastic anemias are the prime suspects. The RDW is most consistently abnormal in iron deficiency, whereas it is usually normal in all the other microcytic anemias.

Mild α-thalassemia, α-thalassemia minor, is a diagnosis of exclusion. If the Hgb electrophoresis result is normal previously and the findings for thalassemia mentioned above are present, the diagnosis is α-thalassemia minor. However, if Hgb electrophoresis indicated an increase in Hgb A_2 and F, the patient has β-thalassemia minor. Results of iron studies are normal in mild α- and β-thalassemia and are not indicated in the initial workup of these patients. Severe forms of either disease (e.g., Bart's Hgb or β-thalassemia major) are uncommon in the United States. There is no specific treatment for thalassemia.

Regarding the other mechanisms listed in the question, absent iron stores (choice **A**) indicate iron deficiency. Iron blockade (choice **B**) is associated with the anemia of inflammation. Hemolysis of RBCs (choice **C**) is present only in very severe forms of thalassemia, such as Hgb H disease with three α-gene deletions. Decreased heme synthesis (choice **E**) characterizes the sideroblastic anemias, which could be due to lead poisoning, pyridoxine deficiency, and, most commonly, the toxic effect of alcohol, to name only a few potential causes.

33 The answer is E   *Psychiatry*

The symptoms suggest a diagnosis of mild mental retardation (choice **E**), defined as mental retardation associated with an IQ of between 50 and 70. Degrees of mental retardation are denoted by IQ: Mild (50–70); moderate (35–50); severe (20–35); and profound (<20). The cause of mild mental retardation is usually idiopathic, with no clear physical or social pathology (e.g., maternal substance abuse [choice **D**], perinatal insults [choice **B**], and sociocultural deprivation [choice **C**]). More severe mental retardation results from known physiologic lesions (e.g., genetic or chromosomal abnormalities [choice **A**]).

34 **The answer is D**   *Pediatrics*

Meckel's diverticulum (choice **D**) usually presents as painless rectal bleeding. The condition is best remembered as the disease of twos; it affects 2% of the population, occurs in the first 2 years of life, and is a sacculation 2 feet proximal to the ileocecal junction. Iron deficiency anemia can result from chronic blood loss. The diverticulum usually consists of ectopic gastric tissue. Diagnosis is made by Meckel radionuclide scan, which is performed after intravenous infusion of technetium-99m pertechnetate. Surgical excision is the treatment of choice.

Intussusception (choice **A**) presents as an acute abdomen with currant-jelly stool. Patients with duodenal ulcers (choice **B**) have pain. Adhesions (choice **C**) are fibrous bands that may cause bowel obstruction after abdominal surgery, causing abdominal pain, nausea, and vomiting. They are not associated with rectal bleeding. Ulcerative colitis (choice **E**) typically presents with bloody diarrhea with mucus.

35 **The answer is B**   *Obstetrics and Gynecology*

This patient meets the criteria for secondary amenorrhea which are absence of menses for 3 months if previous regular menses or absence of menses for 6 months if previously irregular menses. A negative β-hCG test result virtually rules out pregnancy, the most common cause of secondary amenorrhea. The second most common cause of secondary amenorrhea is anovulation. A positive progesterone challenge test result indicates only that the patient has an adequate amount of estrogen to prepare her endometrium for ripening and shedding by progesterone (choice **B**). The patient can be assumed to be anovulatory.

Medroxyprogesterone acetate orally is not helpful as a pregnancy test (choice **A**). The only definitive way to rule out pregnancy is a negative urine or serum β-hCG test result. It also cannot rule out a pituitary adenoma (choice **D**), which requires a screening test with a serum prolactin level followed by a central nervous system (CNS) imaging study of the sella turcica. Even a spotting response is adequate to be a positive result (choice **E**). Primary and secondary amenorrhea can be differentiated from a good history, not from a progesterone challenge test (choice **C**).

36 **The answer is D**   *Medicine*

Hepatitis C virus (HCV) (choice **D**) is the most common cause of posttransfusional hepatitis (90% of cases). There is a 0.3%/unit chance of contracting HCV. HCV has an incubation period ranging from 2 weeks to 6 months. Most cases are anicteric. Approximately 60% of cases progress into chronic hepatitis. There is also a risk for developing cirrhosis and hepatocellular carcinoma. Transaminasemia is the best marker for hepatitis, with serum alanine aminotransferase (ALT) usually higher than serum aspartate aminotransferase (AST). Alkaline phosphatase and γ-glutamyltransferase are better indicators of cholestasis. These enzymes are only mildly elevated in hepatitis unless they are in a transient cholestatic phase. The antibody test for HCV is useful in detecting early disease but is highly specific when the result is positive. It indicates active disease and is not a protecting antibody. Alpha interferon (IFN-α) and virazole are useful in the treatment of chronic HCV infections.

Atypical lymphocytosis is seen in any viral hepatitis and should not always be construed as representing infectious mononucleosis (choice **A**). Hepatitis A (choice **B**) is generally transmitted orally and is rarely contracted by blood transfusion. Hepatitis B (choice **C**) can be transmitted from blood transfusion (1 case/200,000 units), but the screening of blood for hepatitis B surface antigen has markedly decreased the incidence of the disease. Cytomegalovirus (choice **E**) can be transmitted by blood transfusion. It is the most common infectious disease transmitted by blood transfusion, but not the most common cause of hepatitis.

37 **The answer is B**   *Psychiatry*

This man's symptoms are most suggestive of dementia. The most common cause of dementia in this age group is Alzheimer's disease (choice **B**), which is often characterized by a gradual onset of memory impairment and an absence of focal neurologic disease.

Alcoholic dementia (choice **A**) is less likely in the absence of any suggestion of alcohol-related work impairment. Cerebrovascular disease (choice **C**) is less common than Alzheimer's disease and often has a more sudden onset and evidence of focal neurologic impairments or other vascular disease. Depression (choice **D**) may cause difficulty concentrating but is unlikely to interfere with objective testing for agnosia or short-term memory. Aging alone (choice **E**) does not cause significant difficulties with everyday cognitive function.

38 **The answer is A**   *Obstetrics and Gynecology*

Gestational diabetes is a common medical complication of pregnancy with a prevalence of 3–5%. Common risk factors include ethnic background (Hispanic, African American, American Indian, and Pacific Islander), elevated body mass index, and age over 25 years. The patient in this case has many risk factors. The incidence of overt diabetes mellitus in pregnancy is less than 0.5%. If present, it can adversely affect both mother and fetus. The levels in White's classification of diabetes in pregnancy describe increasing perinatal risks as the alphabet letters increase. Class A diabetes is the lowest risk with onset during the pregnancy. The case presentation describes a normal fasting, but abnormal 1- and 2-hour glucose values. This description meets the criteria for class A1 (choice **A**); therefore, the disorder can be treated with diet alone.

Class A2 (choice **B**) is gestational diabetes requiring insulin. Class B (choice **C**) diabetes describes overt diabetes with onset after age 20 and duration less than 10 years. Class C (choice **D**) diabetes describes overt diabetes with onset between ages 10 and 19 years with duration between 10 and 19 years. Class D (choice **E**) diabetes describes overt diabetes with onset before age 10 years and duration over 20 years. All classes beyond Class A1 require additional insulin therapy.

39 **The answer is B**   *Medicine*

The history of suprapubic pain, dysuria, and increased urinary frequency plus the urinary sediment findings of clumps of neutrophils (pyuria), scattered red blood cells (RBCs), and bacteria without the presence of casts or fever is consistent with acute cystitis. The most common cause of pyuria is acute cystitis due to *Escherichia coli.* The absence of white blood cell (WBC) casts, fever, and costovertebral angle pain excludes acute pyelonephritis (choice **D**). In pyuria, the dipstick nitrite test result is positive, because most of the common urinary pathogens (e.g., *E. coli*) are nitrate reducers. The leukocyte esterase test result is positive, because neutrophils contain esterase in their granules. Thus, choice **B** is correct.

Excessive proteinuria (choice **A**) is often associated with hyaline casts or fatty casts, if the patient has the nephrotic syndrome. Proteinuria is the most common urinary finding in renal disease. A nephritic type of glomerulonephritis (e.g., poststreptococcal glomerulonephritis) (choice **C**) is associated with hematuria, RBC casts, and mild-to-moderate proteinuria. Patients with renal stones (choice **E**) have colicky pain emanating from the costovertebral angle and extending anteriorly to the groin. The urinalysis reveals numerous RBCs and occasional WBCs.

40 **The answer is D**   *Pediatrics*

Infant botulism (choice **D**) usually occurs in infants less than 1 year of age, particularly between 2 and 6 months. It occurs after the ingestion of *Clostridium botulinum* spores, which can be found in honey and corn syrup, as well as in soil and house dust. The course of the disease varies but progresses quickly. Typically, the child is afebrile and has been previously healthy. The infant becomes constipated and feeds poorly. A weak cry, hypotonia, and loss of head control are then seen. Descending paralysis progresses over hours to days. Ventilatory support may be necessary.

Guillain-Barré syndrome (choice **A**) consists of weakness that begins in the lower extremities and spreads to the trunk, the upper extremities, and the bulbar muscles. This pattern is known as Landry ascending paralysis, and respiratory failure may result. Although hypothyroidism (choice **B**) and Werdnig-Hoffmann disease (choice **C**) present with hypotonia, it is seen earlier in life, and progression of symptoms occurs more slowly. Hypomagnesemia (choice **E**) usually presents in conjunction with hypocalcemia and manifests as tetany.

41 **The answer is G**   *Preventive Medicine and Public Health*

A case report (choice **G**) is a brief objective report of a clinical feature or outcome from a single patient or event. It is studied retrospectively. Because it pertains to only one case, no statistical analysis or comparison can be made; however, it can form the basis for hypothesis testing. Thus, one can report drug interaction or adverse reaction or even an unusual clinical feature or presentation.

42 **The answer is H**   *Preventive Medicine and Public Health*

A case series report (choice **H**) is an objective report of a number of cases that present with similar features. Its main benefit is in defining the symptoms and signs of a specific disease. A case series report can be a retrospective or a prospective study. The problems in a case series report are the inherent bias built into it and the lack of controls, which prevents generalization of the information.

43 **The answer is D** *Preventive Medicine and Public Health*

One of the problems faced with clinical studies investigating the same phenomenon is the absence of concurrence in terms of conclusion. To obtain a definite conclusion, meta-analysis (choice **D**) is used, wherein the total results of all the studies are pooled so that a single conclusion can be established. To ensure that the meta-analysis is correct, it is analyzed by meta-meta-analysis.

44 **The answer is I** *Preventive Medicine and Public Health*

This is a retrospective study that is also a case-control study (choice **I**). Case-control studies can be retrospective or prospective. A retrospective study follows the group backward in time, from the time of manifestation of disease to the point of initial exposure. Cases with disease and the control group are randomly selected. Interviews are conducted by chart audit; namely, use of questionnaires. A 2 × 2 table is constructed to ascertain whether exposure caused the disease. Thus, a retrospective study compares the frequency of exposure between the two groups—those exposed to the suspected risk factor and those who were not exposed. There are several advantages to conducting a retrospective study: it can be used to establish risk factors for rare diseases, it is relatively inexpensive (does not require long follow-ups), and volunteers are not required.

45 **The answer is C** *Preventive Medicine and Public Health*

This is a clinical trial. These are prospective studies, but are slightly different from observational prospective studies in which the investigator is a passive observer who only records the effect of a factor in a group of individuals exposed to it and in a group who were not exposed (e.g., cigarette smoking). In a clinical trial, the investigator intervenes by withholding intervention in the control group while allowing it in another; thus, the investigator is actively involved. To eliminate bias, which could be introduced by the investigator, the participant, or both, blinding techniques are used. A double-blind study (choice **C**) is used so that neither the investigator nor the participants are aware of whether they have been assigned to the treatment or the control group.

46 **The answer is F** *Preventive Medicine and Public Health*

This is a cross-sectional study (choice **F**), which is used to determine prevalence or to establish etiology. It is most commonly used in surveys designed to establish the distribution pattern of a disease. For example, if one wanted to establish the prevalence of bronchial asthma in a population in Los Angeles, variables such as age, sex, ethnicity, occupation, and place of residence can be incorporated into the study to determine how these influence the disease.

47 **The answer is A** *Preventive Medicine and Public Health*

This is a cross-over study (choice **A**), which is a variation of the double-blind study. In a cross-over study, the two groups have an equal opportunity to receive the intervention and the placebo, so that each group can act as its own control.

48 **The answer is C** *Preventive Medicine and Public Health*

This is another example of a double-blind study (choice **C**). In double blinding, neither the investigator nor the participants are aware of which group they will be assigned (i.e., the control or the treatment group). This is useful if one wants to ascertain the end point of intervention—is there improvement, no change, or does the condition become worse. Double-blinding techniques are used in clinical trials; however, there is no crossover.

49 **The answer is E** *Preventive Medicine and Public Health*

This is a nonconcurrent prospective study (choice **E**), also known as a historical cohort. This study is carried out entirely or partially from existing records. In this type of study, events of interest that include exposure and disease have already occurred. The problem is that bias can enter into the study because one may not be sure in some instances whether the exposure resulted in the disease or whether it occurred de novo.

50 The answer is I *Preventive Medicine and Public Health*

This is a case-control study (choice **I**), which differs from the one presented in question 44 in that it is a prospective study (i.e., it is carried forward in time). A prospective study enables one to ascertain the incidence of a disease. It usually involves a cohort, which is a group that shares a common characteristic or experience within a given time frame (e.g., those who survived a stroke). Sometimes, individuals in a prospective study have to be singled out and studied. Such studies are called *longitudinal studies*. A prospective study involves two groups of individuals: those who have been exposed to the factor and those who have not been exposed (i.e., the control group). The groups are followed until it is possible to establish the number of individuals in the two groups who develop the disease. Bias is low because neither the participants nor the investigator are aware of who will develop the disease and who will not. A prospective study is therefore an observational prospective study, because the investigator is a passive observer and does not manipulate the groups, as he or she would in the case of clinical trials. Disadvantages include attrition (people may not come to follow-up), cost (requires a long period of study), and the need for volunteers (the sample size should be large).

test **6**

Questions

Single Best Choice Directions: This section consists of numbered statements or questions followed by a list of potential answers; you are to select the ONE best answer.

1 A 24-year-old male who had been alcoholic since his early teens underwent rehabilitation therapy during which he suffered severe withdrawal symptoms including a seizure. Subsequently, he had seizures on a regular basis, during which he would turn pale, feel nauseous, become rigid, stop breathing, lose consciousness, and fall to the ground. After a minute, his body would jerk in a violent fashion for an additional 3 or 4 minutes; he would then lapse into a period of flaccid coma, which lasted 30 to 60 minutes more. After recovering consciousness he had a headache, was disoriented and confused, felt nauseated, and had sore muscles but could remember nothing concerning his seizure. Following a detailed diagnostic workup including electroencephalography he was put on medication. Which of the following drugs was most likely used in his initial treatment?

(A) Felbamate
(B) Topiramate
(C) Phenytoin
(D) Ethosuximide
(E) Tiagabine

2 A 14-year-old male comes to the office because his breasts have recently become tender and slightly swollen. He is worried that he is undergoing feminization and will grow up to become a "freak." Upon examination a tender, 2-cm mass is found to be palpable in the subareolar region of both breasts. Which of the following describes the best course of action?

(A) Excise the masses by performing a subcutaneous mastectomy
(B) Incise and drain the masses
(C) Treat the masses with topical steroids
(D) Aspirate the masses for culture and cytology
(E) Leave the masses alone

3 A 20-year-old woman had her ears pierced when she was 16 years old. Since that time she has had only two pairs of earrings, both given to her by her parents; both were 18 karat gold. Last week her 21-year old boyfriend gave her a new pair of earrings for St. Valentine's Day, which she started to wear immediately. Three days latter she developed localized areas of erythema and vesicle formation where she had pierced her ears. The mechanism responsible for this reaction most closely resembles which of the following?

(A) Type I hypersensitivity
(B) An Arthus reaction
(C) A positive purified protein derivative (PPD) skin reaction
(D) Antibody-dependent cell-mediated cytotoxicity
(E) An immune complex disease

4 A 32-year-old woman, gravida 4, para 4, consults a physician because for the past 6 months she has had abnormal vaginal bleeding that occurs intermittently between her predictable menstrual cycles. The bleeding is not associated with cramping, but there are often larger clots of blood. She has to wear panty protection and even a tampon when the bleeding is heavy. She underwent a tubal sterilization after her last delivery 5 years ago. She denies use of any medications other than multivitamins. She also is unaware of a history of bleeding disorders in any family member. A urine β-hCG test result is negative. On physical examination she is well developed and well nourished. Results of a general examination are unremarkable. Pelvic examination reveals normal external genitalia and vagina. No cervical abnormalities are seen. The uterus is slightly enlarged but mobile and nontender. Pelvic imaging studies reveal uterine leiomyomata. Which of the following locations of leiomyomas would be most associated with the kind of bleeding seen in this patient?

(A) Submucosal
(B) Subserosal
(C) Intramural
(D) Intraligamentous
(E) Parasitic

5 A forensic pathologist obtained cerebral spinal fluid (CSF) from three cadavers who died shortly before the samples were taken. One of the individuals died from a heart attack, the second from a self-inflicted gunshot wound, and the third from an intentional overdose of barbiturates. Metabolites derived from which of the following compounds are most likely to be found at a lower concentration in the cadaver who died from the gunshot wound than in the cadavers who died from a heart attack or a barbiturate overdose?

(A) Serotonin
(B) Protein
(C) Norepinephrine
(D) Glucose
(E) Epinephrine

6 A 65-year-old man complains of increasing sadness and inability to find pleasure in anything. He cannot even watch a TV program with his wife without getting so bored he starts fidgeting and then gets up and leaves before the end of the program. He has recently been forced to retire from his job, and he has been diagnosed with hypertension, diabetes mellitus, and glaucoma. Which of the following symptoms is most likely to suggest he may be at risk of committing suicide?

(A) Feelings of hopelessness
(B) Tearfulness
(C) Sleep disturbance
(D) Lassitude
(E) Anorexia

7 Twenty-four hours after an elective cholecystectomy a 5 foot 2 inch (1.57 m) 155 lb (70.3 kg), 45-year-old woman develops a temperature of 101.6°F (38.7°C) and suffers pain and difficulty upon inspiration. Radiologic examination shows elevation of the right diaphragm. Which of the following is the most likely cause of these symptoms?

(A) A wound infection
(B) A urinary tract infection secondary to catheterization
(C) Pulmonary embolus
(D) Intravenous (IV) catheter-related sepsis
(E) A spontaneous pneumothorax
(F) Atelectasis

8 A 23-year-old married woman comes to the office after recent exposure to a person with active hepatitis A. She has a long history of recurrent sinopulmonary infections and bronchial asthma. In addition, after her last pregnancy she received a blood transfusion for severe postpartum hemorrhage. After receiving an intramuscular dose of immune serum globulin as prophylaxis against hepatitis A, she develops an anaphylactic reaction. Which of the following is the most likely cause of this patient's reaction?

(A) Immunoglobulin A (IgA) deficiency with anti-IgA antibodies
(B) A hemolytic transfusion reaction
(C) Contaminated immune serum globulin

(D) A type IV hypersensitivity reaction against a protein in the immune serum globulin
(E) A febrile reaction

9 A 47-year-old man recently consulted a physician about developing weakness, particularly in his right hand. Upon providing a history the man explained that he does house repair and has been working on a neighborhood rehabilitation project for the past several months. In doing this, he sandblasts and sands and scrapes by hand to remove the old paint. These homes were first constructed in the 1920s and since have been covered with several layers of paint. He also revealed that he habitually ate his lunch at the work site, which he described as being dusted with old paint particles. In addition to the weakness in his arm he admitted to sporadic stomachaches, constipation, and said his wife had complained that he is always irritable. He also states until recently he had been in good health. Upon examination he was found to be 6 feet (19.7 m) tall and to weigh 170 lb (77.1 kg). His heart, lungs, and abdomen were normal as were most analytical values, but he did show signs of right wristdrop consistent with radial nerve palsy and his complete blood count (CBC) shows a microcytic anemia; his serum iron levels were found to be normal. Which of the following diagnostic tests would provide the most useful information regarding the appropriate treatment?

(A) Nerve conduction velocity (NCV) study of the right arm
(B) Radiography of the right arm and wrist
(C) Magnetic resonance imaging (MRI) scans of the right arm and wrist
(D) Urine screen for heavy metals (lead, mercury, arsenic)
(E) Screening for diabetes mellitus

10 A 14-year-old female patient, a recent immigrant from Southeast Asia, is diagnosed with uncomplicated pulmonary tuberculosis. She is placed on a three-drug combination regimen with two of the drugs administered daily and one of the agents administered twice weekly. Because of this drug therapy, the patient is also given pyridoxine on a daily basis, and she must undergo periodic tests of ocular function. During her drug treatment, a red–orange coloration of sweat and lacrimal secretions is noticed. Results of her liver function tests are normal. The three drugs that this patient is taking are which of the following?

(A) Bismuth, metronidazole, tetracycline
(B) Ethambutol, isoniazid, rifampin
(C) Clarithromycin, isoniazid, streptomycin
(D) Ethambutol, isoniazid, rifabutin
(E) Isoniazid, pyrazinamide, rifampin

11 A 34-year-old woman has a long history of difficulty forming close interpersonal relationships because she fears rejection. She has an unwarranted low self-esteem and often becomes anxious in the presence of others. According to a psychodynamic theory, which of the following best describes her problem?

(A) It is a response to environmental pressure.
(B) It most likely developed after she left the shelter of her family.
(C) It is caused by childhood problems.
(D) It is unlikely to be responsive to treatment.
(E) It is innate.

12 A 25-year-old female patient of African descent who recently immigrated from Jamaica to the United States presents with intense pain in both hips. A radiograph of her pelvis shows bilateral hip deformities with increased density of the bone, while electrophoresis of a red cell hemolysate reveals predominantly hemoglobin (Hb) S, slightly more than the normal amounts of Hb F and the presence of Hb A_2, but no Hb A. Which of the following is the most likely diagnosis?

(A) Osteomyelitis caused by *Staphylococcus aureus* infection
(B) Aseptic necrosis of the femoral heads
(C) Pathologic bone fracture
(D) Osteoarthritis
(E) Legg-Calvé-Perthes disease

13 A 33-year-old anthropologist from New York had been doing research in a desert region of Arizona for about 6 months. After returning home, he visits his physician complaining of an influenza-like illness with cough, mild chest pain, and occasional fever. He says that the illness started during the last few weeks of his stay in Arizona. Red, tender nodules are present on his shins. Chest x-rays films fail to reveal evidence of pulmonary infiltrates or pleural effusion. Which of the following is the most appropriate next step in the management of this patient?

(A) Delay treatment until culture results are obtained
(B) Begin treatment with fluconazole
(C) Begin treatment with amphotericin B
(D) Aspirate bone marrow and culture
(E) Immediate isolation

14 A 40-year-old man complains of attacks of fear, agitation, a sense of being unable to breathe, and feelings of impending doom. Mental status examination reveals a hyperalert, restless, dysphoric individual. There is no evidence of cognitive impairment, hallucinations, illusions, delusions, or disorganized thinking. Which of the following is the most likely diagnosis?

(A) Delirium
(B) Depersonalization disorder
(C) Dysthymic disorder
(D) Panic disorder
(E) Schizoaffective disorder

15 A 35-year-old Caucasian man presents to the office with a history of abrupt onset of fever, chills, a productive cough, and chest pain on inspiration. Physical examination shows a well-nourished man who is now ill. He demonstrates dullness to percussion; increased tactile fremitus; bronchophony; egophony; and fine, crepitant rales anteriorly over the right lung. A neutrophilic leukocytosis with more than 20% band neutrophils is present. A chest radiograph reveals a lobar consolidation obliterating the outline of the right-heart silhouette. Which of the following is the most likely diagnosis?

(A) Pneumococcal pneumonia involving the right upper lobe
(B) *Klebsiella pneumoniae* of the right lower lobe
(C) Viral pneumonia of the right middle lobe
(D) *Streptococcus pneumoniae* involving the right middle lobe
(E) Primary tuberculosis involving the right upper lobe

16 A 37-year-old male illegal immigrant from Guatemala presents to the emergency room with vomiting and abdominal distension. He reports that he has not had a bowel movement in over a week. Rectal examination reveals the absence of stool in the rectal vault with a dilated colon. He also has a low-grade fever derived from what was diagnosed as Chagas' disease. Further examination would most likely also demonstrate which of the following conditions?

(A) Diverticula
(B) Hirschsprung's disease
(C) Adenomatous polyps
(D) Inflamed colon
(E) Anal fistulas

17 A 48-year-old man complains of a 5-month history of memory impairment; he is afraid of losing his job as a waiter because he has some difficulty in speaking clearly, has difficulty in doing the little but complex maneuvers required, such as folding napkins properly, and he is losing tips because he can no longer recognize favorite customers. Mental status examination reveals an alert and attentive patient with an average vocabulary. He remembers one of three objects after 5 minutes and has marked difficulty with reasoning and abstraction. Which of the following is the most likely diagnosis?

(A) Delirium
(B) Amnestic disorder
(C) Dementia
(D) Major depressive disorder
(E) Mental retardation

18 A 23-year-old African-American male presents to the emergency room with swollen lips, eyelids, and palms and blotchy swellings in his buttocks and genitalia that itch and are painless. He also complains of colicky abdominal pain. He has a history of similar recurrent attacks since his early teens. His family history is strongly positive for a similar problem on his paternal side. Physical examination reveals a young man in apparent respiratory distress due to the swollen lips and tongue. He has large blotchy nontender lesions with indistinct margins in the gluteal areas, and obvious diffuse swelling of his eyelids and hands. Examination of his chest reveals a few scattered rhonchi and rales. His abdomen is soft, but diffusely tender. There is no rigidity, and bowel sounds are present. Which of the following assays would be the best screen for this disease?

(A) C3 complement assay
(B) C4 complement assay
(C) Quantitative immunoglobulins assay
(D) Serum antinuclear antibody assay
(E) Sweat chloride assay

19 A 32-year-old woman, gravida 1, para 0, with a history of infertility, underwent ovulation of induction resulting in a twin pregnancy, now at 31 weeks' gestation. An early obstetric sonogram at 7 weeks' gestation showed dichorionic placentation. She has a positive group B β-hemolytic streptococcus vaginal culture. Because of epigastric pain, vaginal bleeding, and uterine contractions, she is evaluated at the maternity unit. An obstetric sonogram shows twin A to be a female fetus in breech presentation and twin B to be a male fetus in transverse lie with the back down. The sonogram also shows a marginal anterior placenta previa. Her initial vital signs are as follows: temperature, 37.2°C (99.0°F); pulse, 95/min; respiration, 18/min; blood pressure, 165/115 mm Hg. Her urine dipstick test shows 2+ glucose and 3+ albumin. Which of the following is a contraindication to tocolysis in this case?

(A) Multiple gestations
(B) Marginal placenta previa
(C) Pregnancy-induced hypertension (PIH)
(D) Gestational age
(E) Positive group B β-hemolytic streptococcus vaginal culture

20 A 67-year old man who had been successfully medicated for hypertension for the past 15 years develops a diastolic pressure of 110 mm Hg. At that time he was taking hydrochlorothiazide, acebutolol, clonidine, and doxazosin mesylate for his blood pressure and metformin for type 2 diabetes. A serum panel was unremarkable except that his creatinine level was 4 mg/dL (normal, 0.6–1.2 mg/dL), and his blood urea nitrogen (BUN) was 28 mg/dL (normal, 8–20 mg/dL). In an attempt to lower his blood pressure, his physician added enalapril; the patient rapidly developed renal failure. Which of the following choices represents the most likely diagnosis?

(A) Renal arterial stenosis due to fibromuscular dysplasia
(B) Renal arterial stenosis due to occlusive arteriosclerotic disease
(C) Renal vein thrombosis due to a malignant occlusion
(D) Malignant hypertension
(E) Acute renal artery occlusion

21 A 29-year-old nulligravida complains of severe pain with menses for the past 3 years. Her last menstrual period was 10 days ago. She has been married 7 years and has used an intrauterine copper contraceptive system/device until the last couple of years when she and her husband decided to start a family. Intercourse is painful with deep penetration. In spite of 15 months of unprotected twice-weekly intercourse she has been unable to conceive. Her menarche began at age 15, and her menstrual periods have been regular. She is employed as a nurse in a local doctor's office. She has had normal annual Pap smears. Findings of her general examination are unremarkable. On pelvic examination, external genitalia are without lesions. Her vagina is moist and supple. Her cervical os reveals clear, watery mucus. Her uterus is retroverted, tender to palpation and there is nodularity of the uterosacral ligaments on rectovaginal examination. Which of the following will be the most helpful in confirming the diagnosis for this patient?

(A) History
(B) Laparoscopy
(C) Physical examination
(D) Hysterosalpingography
(E) Culdocentesis

22 An 86-year-old woman is taken to the emergency room by her granddaughter because she has become disoriented, confused, and in general is not acting normal. In taking a history, with the aid of the granddaughter, the physician was able to ascertain that the patient complained of ringing in her ears, pain in her stomach, and dizziness. In addition it was ascertained that in the days leading up to this incidence she had been taking two 325-mg aspirin tablets every 4 hours because of arthritic pain. Vital signs were: temperature 101.6°F (38.7°C), respiration 14 breaths per minute, heart rate 150 beats per minute, blood pressure 85/45 mm Hg, and a plasma glucose level of 175 mg/dL. An electrolyte panel shows an anion gap of 18 mEq/L. Salicylate poisoning was suspected, and blood gases were analyzed. Which of the following arterial blood patterns most clearly points to salicylate poisoning?

	pH	$Paco_2$	Bicarbonate
Normal range	7.35–7.45	33–44 mm Hg	22–28 mEq/L
(A)	7.28	53	25
(B)	7.38	22	12
(C)	7.29	58	30
(D)	7.48	70	46
(E)	7.53	30	20

23 A 30-year-old woman seeks treatment for persistent anxiety that has increased since she joined a law firm 4 years ago. She describes worry and rumination that she is inadequate in social situations, concern that she will not be granted partnership next year, and fears that her life will turn out badly. She also complains of difficulty sleeping, trouble concentrating, tenseness, and irritability. She denies any other significant medical problems, any substance abuse, or any history of psychosis. However she admits to worrying a lot since childhood; for example, if her parents left her with a baby sitter she would fear that they would not come home and would be awake until they did. Mental status examination reveals an anxious woman. She is appropriately dressed, and her thought processes are logical. There is no evidence of hallucinations or delusions. She shows no psychomotor retardation. Her

conversation includes no suicidal rumination or feelings of hopelessness. Which of the following is the most appropriate initial pharmacologic treatment for this patient?

(A) Modafinil
(B) Zolpidem
(C) Risperidone
(D) Alprazolam
(E) Venlafaxine

24 A 28-year-old woman, gravida 1, para 0, comes to the outpatient prenatal clinic at 34 weeks' gestation with a twin pregnancy. Her fundal height is 40 cm and the orientation of the fetuses in the uterus is cephalic–breech presentation. She was standing in the kitchen when she experienced a sudden gush of fluid that soaked her panties and created a pool of fluid on the floor. Since then she has had intermittent watery vaginal discharge for the past few days. She has had to wear a perineal pad for comfort. She denies dysuria or urinary burning but admits to urinary frequency. She is having occasional uterine contractions up to three per hour. Which of the following is the most appropriate next step in the management of this patient?

(A) Nitrazine paper on the perineum
(B) Speculum examination for vaginal pooling
(C) Sonogram for amniotic fluid volume
(D) Urinalysis for urinary tract infection
(E) Digital examination for cervical dilation

25 A 56-year-old indigent male had been sent home after undergoing an operation but returns to the hospital's emergency room because of severe abdominal pain that has been getting progressively worse for the past week and has now become totally unbearable. On examination, the emergency physician observes an overweight male who looks much older than his stated years. His blood pressure is 88/68 mm Hg. He has a marked tenderness in the epigastric region along with "bruising" in that area. Laboratory analyses show an elevation of serum amylase. Which of the following is the most likely cause of his symptoms?

(A) A reaction to anesthetic drugs
(B) Hypovolemia
(C) Total parenteral nutrition (TPN)
(D) A common bile duct exploration for gallstones
(E) Postoperative infection

26 A 19-year-old male who fell while playing basketball, fractured the shaft of the right radius and ulna and subsequently underwent closed reduction and application of a cylindrical cast. He now presents with complaints of pain in the right index finger, there is no tingling sensation. Clinical examination reveals no diminution in capillary refill time and no hypesthesia. Cyanosis is absent. Passive movement of the finger elicits pain. The cast appears intact. Which of the following would be the most appropriate next step in the management of this patient?

(A) Reassure the patient
(B) Prescribe analgesics
(C) Prescribe corticosteroids
(D) Cleave the cast
(E) Leave the cast intact and elevate the arm for 24 hours

27 A 65-year-old patient develops aspiration pneumonitis after general anesthesia. Twenty-four hours later, there is a rapid onset of dyspnea, tachypnea, cyanosis, and intercostal refractions. A chest radiograph shows diffuse, bilateral infiltrates with both an interstitial and an alveolar pattern. There is sparing of the costophrenic angles. Air bronchograms are noted. The arterial blood gases (ABGs) on 30% O_2 show a pH of 7.20 (normal, 7.35–7.45), a Pa_{CO_2} of 74 mm Hg (normal, 33–44 mm Hg), and a bicarbonate of 28 mEq/L (normal, 22–28 mEq/L). This patient's clinical and laboratory findings are most likely the result of which of the following mechanisms?

(A) Depression of the respiratory center
(B) Intrapulmonary shunting
(C) Increased compliance of the lungs
(D) Increased elasticity of the lungs
(E) Respiratory alkalosis

28 A 28-year-old man who was in an automobile accident is brought to the emergency department by paramedics. The patient is conscious. Clinical examination reveals no sensations below the level of the umbilicus and absent superficial and deep tendon jerks. Which of the following would be an expected finding in this patient?

(A) Hypertension and tachycardia
(B) Hypotension and bradycardia
(C) Hypertension and bradycardia
(D) Hypotension and tachycardia

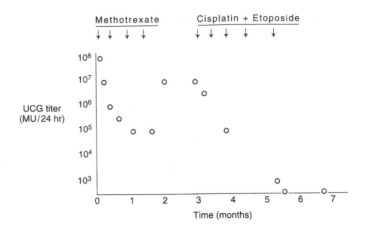

29 The graph above represents two courses of chemotherapy of metastatic choriocarcinoma in a patient monitored by urinary chorionic gonadotropin (UCG) titer (mU/24 h). Both courses represent regimens of drug treatment in a pulsatile mode (indicated by downward arrows). In each course, the drug doses were maximized to the toxicity limit of a 2-log decrease in blood platelets. Which of the following statements about these data is correct?

(A) The effects of chemotherapy on UCG titer bear no relation to cell kill.
(B) The maximal effect of methotrexate is a 2-log decrease in UCG titer.
(C) The drug-induced changes in UCG titer are directly proportional to decreases in platelet count.
(D) The use of UCG titer as a guide to therapy in choriocarcinoma is less valuable than use of chest x-ray films.
(E) The maximal effect of cisplatin plus etoposide is greater than a 4-log decrease in UCG titer.

30 A woman at 7 months' gestation presents for a prenatal examination. She has a history of mild hyperthyroidism, and despite her advanced pregnancy, she is found to have lost 4 lb since her last visit a month ago. She also has developed a fine tremor of her fingers. Her resting heart rate is 120 beats/min, and her thyroid gland is noticeably larger than it was at the time of her last office visit. Management of this patient's condition would be best achieved by treatment with which of the following?

(A) Lugol's solution
(B) Radioactive iodine (^{131}I)
(C) Iodide followed by surgical removal of the gland
(D) Propylthiouracil
(E) Propranolol

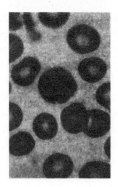

31 The cell depicted in the peripheral smear illustrated above is representative of the majority of cells in an afebrile 75-year-old male with generalized, non-painful lymphadenopathy, hepatosplenomegaly, and petechiae and ecchymoses scattered over his body. His complete blood count (CBC) shows a hemoglobin of 9.0 g/dL (normal for males is 13.5–17.5 g/dL), his red blood cell (RBC) indices are normal, his platelet count is 70,000 cells/μL (normal is 150,000–400,000 cells/μL), and his leukocyte count is 90,000 cells/μL (normal is 4500–11,000 cells/μL). Eighty-five percent of the leucocytes are lymphocytes that are morphologically indistinguishable from small normal lymphocytes. Which of the following scenarios should be expected?

(A) The patient will develop a monocytopenia.

(B) The patient's disease progresses into an acute myelogenous leukemia.

(C) The leukocytes represented in the peripheral smear illustrated above have Auer rods.

(D) Bone marrow infiltration by the cells represented in the peripheral smear illustrated above is manifested by paratrabecular lymphoid aggregates.

(E) Diffuse bone marrow and lymph node infiltration by the cells represented in the peripheral smear illustrated above

32 A 61-year-old male comes to a family physician for the first time after recently moving into town. In providing a history he reveals that he has osteogenesis imperfecta (OGI), a condition that has been in his family for several generations. As a consequence he has had at least a dozen major fractures, all in various long bones. He also disclosed he was diabetic and took metformin, 850 mg, twice daily and that the last time he had a hemoglobin A1c determination, about a year earlier, the value was 5.9%. Additionally, he has been diagnosed as hypertensive and was taking 25 mg hydrochlorothiazide once daily, and 20 mg enalapril as well as 200 mg acebutolol twice daily. At this time his only complaint is various aches and pains, which are particularly bad in his left wrist and ankle, both of which had suffered at least one break. Upon awakening in the morning he feels stiff and has minor pain, but as the day progresses the pain grows worse and, particularly if he had been on his feet for an extended period, the pain in his left ankle becomes excruciating. Examination yielded the following data: temperature 37°C (98.6° F), blood pressure 128/85 mm Hg, respiration 12/min. There was clearly discernible limitation of motion in both the left ankle and wrist, but neither joint was warm to the touch. Examination of his heart and lungs disclosed no abnormalities. At this time which of the following tests is most likely to lead to a treatment protocol that will provide long-term beneficial results?

(A) A bone density determination

(B) Blood test for the rheumatic factor

(C) Radiographic studies

(D) A complete blood count

(E) An erythrocyte sedimentation determination

(F) Blood test for antinuclear antibodies

(G) Arthrographic examination of the affected joints

33 A 75-year-old homeless man develops painful swelling of the right parotid gland 10 days after cholecystectomy. His physician cannot help noticing that he has a bad case of halitosis and that his teeth seem to be poorly cared for. The painful swelling of the right parotid gland is most likely secondary to which of the following?

(A) *Staphylococcus aureus*

(B) Duct obstruction by a stone

(C) A viral infection

(D) Hemorrhage

(E) An immunologic reaction

34 A 29-year-old man is brought to a marriage counselor by his wife, who complains that her husband refuses to attend functions with her; such functions range from PTA meetings to social gatherings that are important to her. Upon interviewing the husband he confesses feelings of extreme anxiety when in social situations. He realizes that as a result, he avoids social gatherings, feels lonely, is not promoted in his job, and is liable to lose his wife, and he feels helpless. Which of the following is the most appropriate initial treatment?

(A) Assertiveness training

(B) Implosion therapy

(C) Psychodynamic psychotherapy

(D) Lorazepam

(E) Systematic desensitization

35 A 52-year-old woman presents to the emergency department because of the recent onset of hallucinations and delirium. Approximately 1 month ago she was diagnosed with type 2 diabetes, and her physician prescribed 250 mg of chlorpropamide daily. At that time the patient told her physician that she was worried about starting a lifetime drug regimen because she had no health insurance and a limited income. Results of physical examination are unremarkable. Her skin turgor is normal. Laboratory studies indicate the following values: serum sodium concentration, 120 mEq/L (normal, 135–147 mEq/L); serum potassium concentration, 3.2 mEq/L (normal, 3.5–5.0 mEq/L); serum chloride concentration, 90 mEq/L (normal, 95–105 mEq/L); serum bicarbonate concentration, 21 mEq/L (normal, 22–28 mEq/L); serum glucose concentration, 140 mg/dL (normal, 70–110 mg/dL); and serum blood urea nitrogen (BUN) concentration, 5 mg/dL (normal, 7–18 mg/dL). Random urine sodium level is 80 mEq/L (normally >20 mEq/L indicates increased loss; <20 mEq/L indicates increased reabsorption). A computed tomography (CT) scan of her head showed small lateral ventricles consistent with cerebral edema. No bleeding was observed. Which of the following would be most appropriate in the management of this patient?

(A) Treat her with a serotonin-reuptake inhibitor (SSRI)

(B) Restrict sodium from her diet

(C) Substitute metformin for the chlorpropamide

(D) Increase her water intake

(E) Add sodium to her diet

(F) Administer demeclocycline, an antidiuretic hormone (ADH) inhibitor

36 A 2-week-old, term infant presents to the pediatrician for a well child check. According to the mother, the patient is a healthy baby; she has been feeding and growing well. Physical examination is pertinent for a slightly jaundiced infant, which after the review of the birth history and laboratory data is attributed to breastfeeding. The total bilirubin is 18 mg/dL (normal is <7 mg/dL), and the direct bilirubin is 0.8 mg/dL (normal is 0–0.4 mg/dL). Which of the following is a true statement about jaundice associated with breast-milk jaundice?

(A) It is seen in the first few days of life.

(B) There is a significant elevation of conjugated bilirubin.

(C) Serum bilirubin falls slowly if breast-feeding is discontinued.

(D) The mother should stop breast-feeding completely.

(E) Mild breast-feeding jaundice requires no intervention.

37 A 26-year-old nulligravid woman comes to the office complaining of increased facial and general body hair. She states that she had no problem until 6 months ago when she began noticing prominent, coarse, dark hair on her upper lip and chin. She says her bra is fitting her much more loosely than it used to. Her menses have always been regular every 30 days, but now she reports her periods are irregular. She is sexually active with her husband of 5 years. She states her libido has increased over the past few months. She denies any family history of excessive body hair. On examination, she presents as a well-nourished, muscular woman with a deep voice. She has copious pubic hair with a male-appearing escutcheon. Examination of her external genitalia reveals clitoromegaly. On bimanual examination a 4 × 5 cm mass is palpated in the left adnexa. Which of the following is the most likely diagnosis?

(A) Granulosa-theca cell tumor

(B) Brenner tumor

(C) Sertoli-Leydig cell tumor

(D) Fibroma

(E) Dysgerminoma

38 A 43-year-old woman becomes listless and apathetic after a series of setbacks in her life. She no longer tries to make her life better, and spends 12 to 14 hours per day in bed. Mental status examination reveals moderate psychomotor retardation, soft speech, and difficulty concentrating. Which of the following is the most accurate behavioral explanation for her symptoms?

(A) Faulty cognitive framework

(B) Object loss

(C) Inadequate exposure to light

(D) Learned helplessness

(E) Double-bind communication

39 A 58-year-old woman presents with vaginal bleeding, which started 1 week ago. Her last menstrual period was 7 years ago, and she has not had any bleeding since that time. She has never been married and has never had any children, nor has she ever used any form of contraception. She is 160 cm (63 in) tall and weighs 86 kg (190 lb). She states she has always been overweight and has a difficult time exercising regularly. Ten years ago she was diagnosed with type 2 diabetes mellitus for which she has been managed with oral hypoglycemic agents. She does not check her blood glucose values regularly. She is taking hydrochlorothiazide for chronic hypertension, which was diagnosed 5 years ago. Which of the following is the diagnostic method of choice in this patient?

(A) Pap smear
(B) Endometrial biopsy
(C) Pelvic examination under anesthesia
(D) Laparoscopy
(E) Colposcopy

40 A 35-year-old woman, gravida 3, para 2, underwent a spontaneous vaginal delivery at 39 weeks' gestation of a 3295-g (7 lb 4 oz) male neonate who has done well. She had a prolonged third stage of labor, resulting in an attempted manual removal of the placenta. The placenta was not completely removed and bleeding progressed to hemorrhage. Ultimately, she underwent an emergency total abdominal hysterectomy due to placenta accreta. She received 5 units of packed red blood cells (PRBCs). Her blood pressure was in the hypotensive range for 30 minutes during the procedure. Which of the following pituitary hormones is most likely to be affected by her clinical course?

(A) Adrenocorticotropic hormone (ACTH)
(B) Prolactin
(C) Thyroid-stimulating hormone (TSH)
(D) Follicle-stimulating hormone (FSH)
(E) Antidiuretic hormone (ADH)

Directions for Matching Questions (41 through 50): *Each set of matching questions is preceded by a list of 4 to 26 lettered options followed by a brief explanation of the required task and then by a series of numbered statements. For each lettered statement you are to select ONE lettered option that best fulfills the task as it relates to that statement. Remember each of the listed options might be correctly selected once, more than once, or not at all.*

Questions 41–45

(A) 47XYY
(B) 47XX + 21
(C) 45X
(D) 47XY + 13
(E) 47XXY

Match the ONE indicated chromosomal aberration listed above with the phenotype described below.

41 Children born alive failed to develop the normal formation of the frontal cortex, a condition called *holoprosencephaly*. They also have a cleft lip and palate, midfacial abnormalities, peculiar punched-out scalp defects, and polydactyly.

42 A male child developed normally into a somewhat taller than expected but otherwise phenotypically normal man. However his parents fear he may become a criminal since males with this chromosomal pattern are found in a higher than expected frequency in mental or penal institutions.

43 A female baby is born with a flattened face and occiput, upward slanting eyes, an extra skin fold at the medial aspect of the eyes, a large tongue and small ears. In addition the newborn is hypotonic.

44 This boy appeared normal at birth and through childhood until puberty, when it became evident that he had small testes and postpubertal gynecomastia that did not resolve.

45 A teenage girl is short for her age, has a webbed neck, and underdeveloped breasts with wide-spread nipples due to a shield-shaped chest. As an infant she had swollen hands and feet.

Questions 46–50

(A) Fractured talus
(B) Tear of the Achilles tendon
(C) Fracture of the calcaneus
(D) Tear involving muscle fibers of the plantar flexors
(E) Torn lateral ligament in the ankle
(F) Fractured metatarsal shafts

Choose the ONE lettered type of injury from the list above that best relates to the symptoms described in the numbered vignettes below.

46 A 27-year old woman running to catch a bus is wearing shoes with 3-inch heels when her heel strikes a pebble and she twist her ankle. As a consequence she can no longer walk without pain.

47 A 46-year-old man has been running for several hours each day in preparation for a local marathon. As a result he has developed some slight pain in the back of the right leg just above the heel. Since it doesn't bother him too much he agrees to play a game of tennis with his girlfriend. She lobs the ball over the net, forcing him to run in close, and then she returns it over his head, making him back up and twist on his right foot. At that moment he hears a pop and feels a sharp pain in his ankle. Subsequently the ankle becomes swollen, and he can only limp along in pain.

48 A 42-year-old ex-minor league pitcher who now makes his living selling insurance was pitching in a pick-up game during a fourth of July picnic. He succeeded in striking out all the opposing batters until there were two out in the 7th inning. By now he was becoming acutely aware that he no longer was in A-1 physical shape. As he pressed on and was throwing a hard fastball he suddenly heard a popping sound in his hind leg (the one he rears on to get force and then extends behind him as he lunges his body and the ball forward). He later says that it felt as if somebody hit him on the calf muscle with a stick followed by rather severe pain that radiated up to his knee and down to his ankle. Within hours the same area was bruised and swollen.

49 A 19-year-old man was washing windows on the second floor of a house when his ladder slipped and he fell to the ground feet first. When he picked himself up he found that he could not bear weight on the right foot, and he is unable to evert that foot.

50 A 73-year-old man decided that walking would be good for his cardiovascular system and started a program of daily walks, increasing the distance regularly. By the second week he developed a pain behind the second toe on his right foot. Figuring he could walk through it he continued walking, but on stepping out of his house during the fourth week, he felt a crackling sensation and the pain intensified. His primary care physician found a tender area on the second metatarsal about an inch below the toe. An x-ray film was negative.

Answer Key

1 C		**11** C		**21** B		**31** E		**41** D
2 E		**12** B		**22** B		**32** A		**42** A
3 C		**13** A		**23** E		**33** A		**43** B
4 A		**14** D		**24** B		**34** A		**44** E
5 A		**15** D		**25** D		**35** C		**45** C
6 A		**16** B		**26** D		**36** E		**46** E
7 F		**17** C		**27** B		**37** C		**47** B
8 A		**18** B		**28** B		**38** D		**48** D
9 D		**19** C		**29** E		**39** B		**49** C
10 B		**20** B		**30** D		**40** B		**50** F

Answers and Explanations

1 The answer is C *Medicine*

Some 0.5% of the population in the United States is afflicted with some form of epilepsy in which seizures generally start between 5 and 20 years of age. Most cases have no known cause, but several types of known triggers also exist; among these, as in the case described, is withdrawal from drugs or alcohol after a period of addiction. Two broad subtypes of epilepsy exist, partial and generalized seizures. The partial seizures are categorized as either simple or complex, while generalized seizures include: absence (petit mal), atypical absence, myoclonic, and tonic-clonic (grand-mal). In the latter case seizures may be isolated, recurrent (with an interval of days, weeks, months or even years between attacks), serial (with a short period of hours or less between attacks), or repeated (with new sets of convulsions without recovering consciousness in between). This latter condition is known as status epilepticus and is a medical emergency. For patients with recurrent forms of epilepsy the goal is to prevent further attacks by administration of an antiepileptic drug. The best drug for initiation of treatment depends upon the type of seizure, and continued use of the same drug depends upon effectiveness and tolerance of side effects by the patient. The symptoms provided in the vignette consist of tonic-clonic seizures clearly suggesting grand mal epilepsy, and phenytoin (choice **C**) is generally used as the drug of first choice. The advantages of this drug include that it is effective in most cases of grand mal usually within 10 days of the initial dose, its side effects can generally be tolerated, and a single daily dose provides the required blood level of 10–20 μg/μL. The latter is important because the less often a drug needs to be taken, the greater the compliance.

Felbamate (choice **A**) can also be used to treat tonic-clonic seizures but is not approved for use as a first-line drug because of the risk of aplastic anemia and hepatic dysfunction. Topiramate (choice **B**) is only approved for adjunctive treatment in cases of partial seizure and secondary generalized seizure; in addition, somnolence is a discouraging side effect and it must be administered twice daily. Use of ethosuximide (choice **D**) is generally reserved for treatment of petit mal, while tiagabine (choice **E**) is an anticonvulsant primarily used as monotherapy for partial seizures.

2 The answer is E *Surgery*

The patient has gynecomastia, the development of breast tissue in males, which is normal in the neonate, pubertal boy, and elderly male. Increased estrogen stimulation (hyperestrinism) of breast tissue is the common factor in all cases of gynecomastia.

Adolescent gynecomastia is usually bilateral, and the tissue averages 2 to 3 cm in diameter. The breast enlargement is transient and most often subsides within 1 year; as a consequence the gynecomastic breast usually should be left alone (choice **E**). The boy should be reassured that he is normal and does not have to worry about developing breasts.

However if the mass is greater than 5 cm or does not regress by 16 to 17 years of age, a subcutaneous mastectomy should be performed (choice **A**). Incision (choice **B**), aspiration (choice **D**), and topical steroids (choice **C**) are not indicated under any circumstances. Gynecomastia in a postpubertal, adult male younger than 70–80 years is not normal and hyperestrinism should be suspected. Hyperestrinism in an adult male is most commonly due to decreased catabolism of estrogen due to liver cirrhosis, most often induced by alcoholism. However, hyperestrinism also can be due to increased synthesis secondary to an adrenal or testicular tumor; increased human chorionic gonadotropin (HCG) from a testicular tumor; the hyperplastic Leydig's cells in Klinefelter's syndrome; decreased androgen activity, which leaves estrogen unopposed (e.g., caused by hypothalamic or pituitary disorders); and by several drugs.

3 The answer is C *Medicine*

It seems highly probable that the earrings given to her by her boy friend were not 18 karat gold, but rather a cheaper alloy containing nickel, and she developed contact dermatitis. Contact dermatitis is a common inflammatory disorder of skin that is associated with exposure to various antigens and irritating substances. Four types have been described—allergic contact dermatitis, irritant contact dermatitis, contact photo-dermatitis, and contact urticaria. Allergic contact dermatitis, of which this case is an example, is a cell-mediated type IV hypersensitivity reaction. Three conditions must be present for this reaction to occur; namely, a genetic predisposition, absorption of sufficient antigen through the skin surface, and a competent immune system. Antigenic substances of low molecular weight penetrate the skin, are phagocytized by Langerhans' cells, and are then transported to regional lymph nodes, where they are presented to T lymphocytes. The T lymphocytes release cytokines that are responsible for the inflammatory response in the tissue. Antigenic substances include rhus (found in poison ivy and poison oak), nickel (earrings, hair dyes), potassium dichromate (household cleaners, leather, cement), formaldehyde (cosmetics, fabrics), ethylenediamine (dyes, medications), mercaptobenzothiazole (rubber products), and paraphenylenediamine (hair dyes, chemicals in photography).

Because allergic contact dermatitis is a type IV hypersensitivity reaction, the positive purified protein derivative (PPD) skin reaction (choice **C**), which involves the interaction of T cells and macrophages, most closely resembles the mechanism of inflammatory response in this patient. Irritant contact dermatitis is not a cell-mediated immune response. It is due to the local toxic effect of the chemical on the skin. Contact photodermatitis is similar to allergic contact dermatitis except that reaction depends on ultraviolet light. Contact urticaria is a wheal-and-flare reaction that may be secondary to a type I hypersensitivity (immunoglobulin E [IgE]-mediated) reaction or a nonimmunologic reaction. The clinical presentation of contact dermatitis, regardless of the mechanism, ranges from localized areas of erythema with vesicle formation to erythematous plaques of thickened skin in chronic disease. The treatment involves removal of the offending agent along with the use of wet compresses with Burow's solution in acute disease, followed by local application of steroid cream to suppress inflammation. Subacute or chronic cases should be treated with local steroid creams without the compresses. Extensive disease may require the use of systemic corticosteroid therapy.

In terms of the other mechanisms listed in the question, type I hypersensitivity (choice **A**) involves the interaction of IgE antibodies developed against specific antigens and mast cells. Reexposure to the antigen causes mast cell degranulation, with the release of histamine and other chemical mediators that produce increased vessel permeability, tissue swelling, and an inflammatory reaction. An Arthus reaction (choice **B**) is a localized immune complex disease (type III hypersensitivity) that activates the complement system to produce anaphylatoxins and chemotactic agents that cause the inflammatory reaction. An example of an Arthus reaction is farmer's lung, in which exposure to thermophilic actinomycetes in the air results in a localized immune complex deposition in the alveoli, with subsequent inflammation and hypersensitivity pneumonitis. Systemic immune complex diseases such as systemic lupus erythematosus (SLE) or serum sickness are also associated with immune complex deposition in various tissues, including the joints, skin, and vessels in the skin and glomerulus. Antibody-dependent cell-mediated cytotoxicity (ADCC) (choice **D**) is a variant of type II hypersensitivity. It involves the presence of antibody against a target tissue, which attracts killer cells, natural killer cells, or macrophages. These cells interact with the antibodies and destroy the target tissue. Warm autoimmune hemolytic anemia (AIHA), with destruction of immunoglobulin G (IgG) antibody-coated red blood cells (RBCs) by macrophages in the spleen, is a classic example of an ADCC reaction. An immune complex disease (choice **E**), such as serum sickness, is a type III hypersensitivity disease.

4 The answer is A *Obstetrics and Gynecology*

The urine β-hCG test rules out pregnancy, the most common cause of abnormal bleeding. Anovulation, another common cause of abnormal vaginal bleeding is associated with unpredictable menstrual cycles rather than predictable ones, as in this case. The history of bleeding between normal predictable menses is classic for a genital tract anatomic lesion. The normal vaginal and cervical examinations rule out lower genital tract lesions. Upper tract lesions include endometrial polyps and submucosal leiomyomas. The latter lesion (choice **A**) causes bleeding by distorting the overlying endometrium, altering its normal response to hormonal changes through the menstrual cycle. This change can lead to abnormal bleeding.

Subserosal myomas (choice **B**) alter the external contour of the uterus, giving the lumpy, bumpy shape but do not cause bleeding. Intramural myomas (choice **C**) located within the myometrial wall are the most common kind of myomas and are generally asymptomatic. Intraligamentous myomas (choice **D**) bulging into the round ligament, and parasitic myomas (choice **E**) attaching to abdominal viscera have no direct impact on uterine bleeding.

5 The answer is A *Psychiatry*

Studies have found lower levels of CSF serotonin metabolites (choice **A**) in postmortem studies of victims of suicide by violent means, but not in victims who die by more passive means, such as heart attack or drug ingestion.

No other biochemical findings (e.g., altered levels of protein [choice **B**], norepinephrine [choice **C**], glucose [choice **D**] or epinephrine [choice **E**] have been consistently found in such studies). Some investigators believe that these findings provide evidence that a low level of central nervous system (CNS) serotonin activity is causally related to depression. However, the relationship to violent suicide is unexplained.

6 The answer is A *Psychiatry*

The presence of hopelessness (choice **A**) as a component of depression greatly increases the chance of suicide. Another high-risk finding would be a suicide plan.

Tearfulness (choice **B**), sleep disturbance (choice **C**), lassitude (choice **D**), and anorexia (choice **E**) are associated with the syndrome of depression, but are not as strongly associated with suicidal behavior.

7 The answer is F *Surgery*

Atelectasis (choice **F**) is the most common cause of fever in the first 24 hours of the postoperative state. Atelectasis refers to collapse of the lung distal to an area of obstruction in the airway. In the postoperative state, the dry secretions imposed by anesthesia and pain-restricted clearance of pulmonary secretions predispose the patient to segmental atelectasis and a nidus of inflammation, resulting in fever. Loss of lung mass leads to elevation of the diaphragm on that side. Deep inspiration on standing is the most effective way of minimizing this complication. Intermittent positive-pressure breathing treatments are too expensive and impose the risk of *Pseudomonas* infection in the lungs.

Wound infections (choice **A**) are more common in the 5- to 10-day postoperative period. Urinary tract infections from indwelling catheters (choice **B**) are common but do not usually cause fever unless pyelonephritis is a complication. Pulmonary embolus (choice **C**) is incorrect. Pulmonary embolus may present with noncharacteristic symptoms such as dyspnea, and palpitations or with characteristic symptoms such as cough, hemoptysis, tachypnea, and tachycardia. There may be evidence of deep venous thrombosis in the lower extremities. The symptoms usually occur within a few days following surgery, rather than soon after. *Candida albicans* is a common cause of intravenous (IV) catheter-related sepsis (choice **D**) and would have a different set of symptoms. A pneumothorax (choice **E**) is usually not associated with fever and is not a common postoperative complication.

8 The answer is A *Medicine*

Immunoglobulin A (IgA) deficiency is the most common immunodeficiency. It occurs in 1 in 500 individuals. There is an intrinsic defect in the differentiation of B cells committed to synthesizing IgA. Although most persons are largely asymptomatic because of a compensatory increase in secreted IgG and IgM, both circulating and secretory IgA are deficient, leaving these patients susceptible to mucosal problems, such as recurrent sinopulmonary infections, allergies, and diarrhea secondary to *Giardia* and other organisms. There is also an increased incidence of autoimmune disease. In some patients, an additional selective deficiency of the IgG subclasses IgG$_2$ and IgG$_4$ predisposes them to bacterial infections. Exposure to blood products containing IgA (through blood transfusion) often sensitizes these patients to IgA, and they develop antibodies against IgA (choice **A**). Reexposure to IgA causes an anaphylactic reaction. Patients should not receive blood products containing IgA. If transfusions are necessary, blood from IgA-deficient patients must be used.

A hemolytic transfusion reaction (choice **B**), contamination of the immune serum globulin (choice **C**), a type IV hypersensitivity reaction (choice **D**) and a febrile reaction (choice **E**) are not associated with the administration of immune serum globulin and would not explain the patient's history of sinopulmonary disease and asthma.

9 The answer is D *Medicine*

His work removing old paint and eating on site very likely exposed him to fine particles of paint that judging by the age of the buildings would have been lead based, so lead toxicity is a likely cause of his weakened state. Moreover, lead is a known inhibitor of heme synthesis, causing a microcytic anemia but not affecting circulating iron levels. Typical early symptoms of lead toxicity include colicky abdominal pain, constipation, headache, irritability, and motor neuropathy, the potential cause of his wrist drop. Thus lead toxicity is suspect, and a urine screen for heavy metals (lead, mercury, arsenic) (choice **D**) will confirm lead poisoning, permitting treatment with either disodium calcium edetate (EDTA) or dimercaptosuccinic acid (DMSA).

A nerve conduction velocity (NCV) study (choice **A**) would only confirm the clinical diagnosis of motor neuropathy, not give the cause. X-rays (choice **B**) and magnetic resonance imaging (MRI) scans (choice **C**) would give uninformative structural information. Diabetes mellitus (choice **E**) is the most common cause of neuropathy and involves the sensory, rather than the motor fibers. Moreover, his age and relatively lean physique makes type 2 diabetes unlikely, and his claim of having been in good health would tend to rule out type 1 diabetes.

10 The answer is B *Medicine*

Ethambutol potentially causes a dose dependent, but optic neuritis which may be reversible while the metabolites of rifampin impart a characteristic red–orange color to body fluids. Thus the need for periodic ocular tests and the presence of a red–orange coloration of sweat and lacrimal secretions indicate that both ethambutol and rifampin were administered. and only choice **B** uses both these compounds. When isoniazid is used in the treatment of tuberculosis, the coadministration of vitamin B_6 prevents the development of neurotoxicity without interfering with the antibacterial action of the drug.

Choices **A** and **D** do not include rifampin, therefore these are incorrect. Moreover, bismuth, metronidazole, and tetracycline (choice **A**) are not used in the treatment of tuberculosis, and the only approved use for rifabutin (choice **D**) is in the treatment of infections due to *Mycobacterium avium-intracellulare*. Pyrazinamide used in choice **E** produces hepatotoxicity, which is not evident in this patient; moreover this combination of drugs does not explain the need for ocular examinations. Clarithromycin (choice **C**) is not used in tuberculosis, but the drug is useful for prophylaxis and treatment of infections caused by *M. avium-intracellulare*.

11 The answer is C *Psychiatry*

Symptoms that include long-term difficulties with interpersonal interaction and distorted self image are suggestive of personality disorder. Psychodynamic theory postulates that the adult personality is, in large part, the product of early childhood experiences (choice **C**). Personality pathology results from various kinds of emotional traumas and conflicts that occur during development. Specific kinds of childhood trauma result in specific kinds of personality disorders.

Psychodynamic theory does not suggest that long histories of difficult interpersonal relationships and low self-esteem are innate (choice **E**), will be unresponsive to treatment (choice **D**), or are a response to environmental pressure (choice **A**). Psychodynamic theory suggests that interpersonal problems often develop during the period a child is raised within the family, not after leaving the shelter of the family (choice **B**).

12 The answer is B *Medicine*

This patient clearly has sickle cell disease. Electrophoresis of red cell lysates from patients with sickle cell disease reveals Hb S as the predominant Hb; in Hb S, valine is substituted for glutamic acid at the sixth position of the β chain. Small quantities of Hb F (fetal Hb), in which a γ chain occurs in place of the β chain, and Hb A_2, in which δ chains replace the β chains, but no Hb A (the predominant normal adult Hb) will be found. Sickle cell disease is a recessive condition that becomes a chronic multisystem disease with eventual death from vital organ failure. With good supportive care death generally occurs in the fourth or fifth decade. Cells in which Hb S is the primary Hb tend to sickle when in a low oxygen environment. Such sickled cells gather in aggregates causing vaso-occlusion that reveals itself as acute pain, low-grade fever and organ necrosis. A common site of sickle cell occlusion is in the marrow of the long bones, resulting in aseptic necrosis in 10 to 25% of patients. The hip joint is most commonly affected, causing bilateral aseptic necrosis of the femoral heads (choice **B**). Heterozygous persons are said to have sickle cell trait, a relatively benign condition in which patients are usually clinically normal, only expressing acute painful episodes under extreme conditions.

In sickle cell disease as with the other hemoglobinopathies, *Salmonella* osteomyelitis is 10 times more common than osteomyelitis caused by other organisms, and ischemic necrosis is 50 times more common than osteomyelitis as a cause of bone pain, consequently choice **A** is not the most likely choice. A pathologic bone fracture commonly results from osteoporosis or metastatic disease to bone and does not commonly occur in sickle cell disease (choice **C**). Osteoarthritis commonly occurs in weight-bearing joints, usually in older individuals, due to chronic wear and tear and is by no means a hallmark of sickle cell disease (choice **D**). Legg-Calvé-Perthes disease is an avascular necrosis of the femoral head that shows a predilection for boys between 4 and 10 years old, not teenaged females suffering from sickle cell disease (choice **E**). Legg-Calvé-Perthes disease is characterized by the insidious development of a limp, with pain in the groin, anterior thigh, or knee initially bringing the patient to a physician. The process is self-limited, and its cause is unknown. Approximately 55% of patients have a full recovery with revascularization of bone; 45% of patients have a permanent hip deformity.

13 The answer is A *Medicine*

This patient most likely has a fungal infection of the lung due to *Coccidioides immitis,* an airborne fungus endemic to dry regions of the southwest United States. Infection of the lungs is often asymptomatic, but after a 10–30 day incubation period, about 40% of infected individuals develop an influenza-like illness. In either case, in an otherwise healthy patient, no drug treatment is indicated unless there are lung lesions or disseminated disease. Thus treatment should be delayed until culture results are obtained (choice **A**) confirming the disease and until an assessment of the patient's clinical status can be made. The painful leg nodules are erythema nodosum, which is a delayed (cell-mediated) hypersensitivity response to fungal (or bacterial) antigens and is a favorable prognostic sign. No organisms are present in the lesions; therefore, erythema nodosum is not a sign of disseminated disease.

If treatment is indicated, intravenous (IV) amphotericin B (choice **C**) is the drug of choice for severe cases. An oral azole such as fluconazole (choice **B**) is used in milder cases and as continuation therapy after an initial positive response to amphotericin B. A bone marrow aspirate with culture (choice **D**) is primarily reserved for ruling out systemic fungi as a cause of fever of unknown origin. Isolation is not required (choice **E**) because the condition is not contagious.

14 The answer is D *Psychiatry*

This patient's symptoms are most suggestive of the anxiety attacks that characterize panic disorder (choice **D**). Other symptoms of panic attacks include hypervigilance, motor tension, and autonomic symptoms such as dyspnea, tachycardia, and diaphoresis. Anxiety can also occur during the course of the other conditions listed; however, additional symptoms are also present.

In delirium (choice **A**), impairment of consciousness is present. In depersonalization disorder (choice **B**), there are illusions involving body distortion. In dysthymic disorder (choice **C**), persistent depression is present. In schizoaffective disorder (choice **E**), both psychotic symptoms and prominent mood symptoms are present.

15 The answer is D *Medicine*

This 35-year-old patient has the classic findings of a typical bacterial pneumonia. They include a history of abrupt onset of fever, chills, a productive cough, and chest pain on inspiration, which correlates with pleuritic inflammation. Physical examination findings of lung consolidation in bacterial pneumonia are dullness to percussion; increased tactile fremitus (increased tactile vibration when a person speaks), bronchophony ("99" becomes clear through the stethoscope), egophony ("eeeeee" sounds like "aaaaaa" through the stethoscope), and fine crepitant rales are present. *Streptococcus pneumoniae* (pneumococcus) is the most common cause of community-acquired bacterial pneumonia. Obliteration of the right-border of the heart (the silhouette sign) indicates involvement of the right middle lobe (choice **D**) rather than the right upper lobe (choice **A**). A neutrophilic leukocytosis with left shift (more than 10% band neutrophils) provides additional evidence of a bacterial pneumonia. A Gram's stain of sputum would likely show gram-positive diplococci. Penicillin G is the drug of choice.

Klebsiella pneumoniae (choice **B**) is more commonly associated with alcoholics and presents with a mucoid-appearing sputum, often tinged with blood. Fat gram-negative rods with a capsule are noted in the Gram's stain of sputum. Viral pneumonias (atypical pneumonias) (choice **C**) are usually associated with a nonproductive cough and have an interstitial pattern on chest x-ray films rather than consolidation. Primary tuberculosis (choice **E**) is rare in a 35-year-old well-nourished Caucasian man in the United States but occurs more frequently in children or immunocompromised patients. It involves the periphery of the lower part of the upper lobe or upper part of the lower lobe in the lungs.

16 The answer is B *Surgery*

Constipation, absence of stool in the vault, and a dilated colon (megacolon) suggest Hirschsprung's disease (choice **B**), which is caused by an absence of ganglion cells in the myenteric plexus of the rectum. In this condition, stool is unable to pass the aganglionic segment, thus producing an obstruction that distally leaves the rectal vault free of stool and causes megacolon due to proximal dilatation of the bowel with concomitant constipation. Classic Hirschsprung's disease is a congenital condition in which babies are born without these ganglionic cells, and such newborns with this disorder are frequently unable to pass their meconium. However, Hirschsprung's disease can also occur in adults, particularly in association with Down syndrome, Chagas' disease, spinal cord injury, Parkinson's disease, and abuse of some narcotics. Chagas' disease is due to *Trypanosoma cruzi* and is endemic in South and Central America and is the probable cause of Hirschsprung's disease in this patient.

The other choices are not accompanied by symptoms similar to those described in the case vignette. Diverticula (choice **A**) produce no symptoms unless inflamed, causing diverticulitis, which is characterized by left flank pain. Adenomatous polyps (choice **C**) also produce no symptoms unless they transform into a carcinoma and the cancer causes problems. An inflamed colon (choice **D**) is more typical of ulcerative colitis. Anal fistulas (choice **E**) may arise from many causes, and although they can be serious, usually they are not.

17 The answer is C *Psychiatry*

The symptoms are most suggestive of dementia (choice **C**), which is characterized by memory disturbance coupled with other cognitive disturbances such as difficulty with abstraction, aphasia (difficulty with articulation), apraxia (loss of ability to execute complex motor behaviors), and agnosia (failure to recognize people or objects). Dementia is often associated with central nervous system damage and is likely to have a protracted course. Clearly this 48-year-old man does not suffer from senile dementia. Although Alzheimer's disease is very unlikely at this age, the dementia could be due to other causes, such as early Parkinson's disease, vitamin B_{12} deficiency, vascular dementia, and hypothyroidism, all of which need to be ruled out.

Delirium (choice **A**) is distinguished from dementia by the additional presence of impaired awareness and attention. It usually has a shorter course than dementia, and symptom severity may fluctuate. Amnestic disorder (choice **B**) is characterized by memory impairment with preservation of awareness and other aspects of cognition. Major depressive disorder (choice **D**) may include complaints of difficulties with memory; however, cognitive testing does not usually reveal marked deficits. Mental retardation (choice **E**) may be characterized by difficulties with reasoning and abstraction. However, vocabulary is usually limited, and a specific complaint of a short history of memory impairment is unlikely.

18 The answer is B *Medicine*

Urticaria is marked by the eruption of wheals or hives on the skin. Angioedema is a urticaria-like condition that involves edema in deeper vessels. The most common cause of angioedema is adverse drug reaction. Hereditary angioedema is rare, occurring in less than 0.4% of all cases of angioedema. It is an autosomal dominant disease characterized by the symptoms and family history described in the vignette; these symptoms generally first start early in the second decade, and as a rule life expectancy is normal, although early death can occur due to asphyxiation caused by uncontrolled laryngeal edema. The abdominal pain is due to edema of the mucosa of the gastrointestinal tract. An angioedema episode usually lasts about 2 to 3 days. The urticarial lesions associated with angioedema have typically indistinct borders. This disease is caused by an inherited C1 complement esterase inhibitor deficiency. The complement system consists of nine proteins, C1 through C9. Activation of C1 starts a cascade that results in the use of some of other members of the complement family. Normally C1 esterase inhibitor acts as a monitor, preventing runaway activation of this system. Absence of this inhibitor results in excessive stimulation of the system, resulting in the release of breakdown products that cause the release of histamine and other vasodilators. These vasodilators increase vessel permeability, resulting in swelling of soft tissue. During the ensuing activation, C4 and C2 are consumed. As a consequence, the best screen is a C4 complement assay (choice **B**). Since C4 complement levels are low in these patients even when they are in a quiescent period, a normal C4 assay value essentially excludes the disease. The diagnosis is confirmed with a C1 esterase inhibitor assay. In acute attacks, maintenance of the upper airways is the most important factor. Recently concentrates of the C1 esterase inhibitor have become available and are used to treat attacks. In its absence, fresh frozen plasma (which supplies the inhibitor) is used. Prophylactic treatment may also be obtained using ε-aminocaproic acid (a nonspecific serum protease and esterase inhibitor) and/or certain synthetic androgens (e.g., danazol or stanozolol) that have immunosuppressive properties and also stimulate the synthesis of C1 esterase inhibitor.

Quantitative immunoglobulin assay (choice **C**), C3 complement assay (choice **A**), serum antinuclear antibody assay (choice **D**), and the sweat chloride assay (choice **E**) for cystic fibrosis are not indicated with this clinical history.

19 The answer is C *Obstetrics and Gynecology*

This twin pregnancy is complicated by preterm contractions and placenta previa as well as preeclampsia. All three of these entities are increased with multiple pregnancies. Although less than 10% of all infants born in the United States are preterm, they account for up to 70% of neonatal morbidity and mortality. Thus, prevention of preterm birth is a high priority unless there are reasons that make tocolysis (i.e., delaying or inhibiting delivery) unsafe for either mother or fetus. Preterm multiple gestation (choice **A**) and preterm placenta previa (choice **B**) are indications for tocolysis. However, if severe PIH (choice **C**) is present, the mother's life and health are jeopardized by prolonging the pregnancy; therefore, tocolysis is inappropriate. Gestational age (choice **D**) and a positive group B β-hemolytic streptococcus culture (choice **E**) are not contraindications for tocolysis.

20 The answer is B *Medicine*

In the general population fewer than 5% of the cases of hypertension result from renal arterial occlusion. However renovascular occlusion accounts for 70% of the cases of hypertension in patients over the age of 60 who have a diastolic blood pressure above 105 mm Hg and a serum creatine value above 2 mg/dL; moreover 80 to 90% of these cases are due to occlusive arteriosclerotic disease (choice **B**). If both kidneys are occluded, provision of an angiotensin-converting enzyme (ACE) inhibitor such as enalapril tends to provoke acute renal failure because the ACE inhibitor decreases angiotensin II production, which is required for effective renal circulation. This is noted on renal function tests by a rising creatinine level.

About 10–15% of the cases of renal arterial stenosis are due to fibromuscular dysplasia (choice **A**). However these cases primarily occur in females who are between the ages of 30 and 50 years. Renal vein thrombosis due to a malignant occlusion (choice **C**) presents with severe back pain and hyperproteinuria; renal stenosis is almost unique among the renal diseases in that it is not accompanied by proteinuria, since the glomerulus is intact and renal arterial pressure is decreased. Symptoms of malignant hypertension (choice **D**) include rapid and extreme increase in blood pressure (systolic pressure over 200 mm Hg), blurred vision, headache, shortness of breath, chest pain, proteinuria, and sometimes seizures. Such an acute attack sometimes occurs for no apparent reason, usually in a person who was being treated for hypertension. It is the extreme increase in systolic pressure that induces the other symptoms, which will get worse the longer the pressure remains elevated. Consequently, this is a medical emergency; the pressure must be reduced immediately, usually by IV administration of antihypertensive agents.

Even though an arthrosclerotic artery is more readily occluded than a healthy one, by definition acute renal artery occlusion (choice **E**) differs from occlusion due to stenosis in that the latter is a chronic event. However, other difference between an acute occlusion and an occlusion due to stenosis are that the acute occlusion generally is unilateral, whereas stenosis is bilateral 70% of the time, and acute occlusion presents with backache and blood in the urine, while stenosis presents with hypertension. An occlusion generally occurs after major surgery or trauma affecting the abdomen or side or in individuals with atrial fibrillation or mitral or valve disease.

21 The answer is B *Obstetrics and Gynecology*

The scenario in this question is characteristic of endometriosis, a benign condition in which endometrial glands and stroma are located outside of the endometrial cavity. The history of secondary dysmenorrhea, dyspareunia, and infertility is classic. This condition affects up to 15% of all women in the United States. Although a history (choice **A**) and pelvic examination (choice **C**) may be suggestive of endometriosis, only a laparoscopy (choice **B**) is definitive. Visualization of the characteristic "powder burns" is typical, along with adhesions, particularly in the cul-de-sac, which cause the fixed, retroverted uterus along with uterosacral ligament nodularity.

A hysterosalpingogram (choice **D**) is not helpful because the findings are extrauterine, and one would not expect an abnormality of the endometrial cavity. A culdocentesis (choice **E**) has been used for identifying non-clotted cul-de-sac blood in cases of ruptured ectopic pregnancy but lacks specificity and sensitivity for diagnosing endometriosis.

22 The answer is B *Medicine*

Salicylate poisoning can result from short-term ingestion of a large dose or by long-term ingestion of more salicylates than can be excreted. In the year 2000 more than 20,000 cases of salicylate intoxication were reported to poison control centers in the United States; these resulted in 55 deaths. Salicylate poisoning most commonly occurs in infants and in the elderly. In infants the sources may seem innocuous such as salicylate-coated teething rings or even breast milk from mothers who use excessive amounts of topical analgesics containing a salicylate. In the elderly, long-term aspirin use coupled to decreased renal function and perhaps forgetfulness can raise plasma levels dangerously. Usually one of the early signs is ototoxicity marked by tinnitus and dizziness. Other symptoms include central nervous effects ranging from mild confusion to coma, emesis, tachycardia, hyperventilation, hypotension, and early hyperglycemia followed by hypoglycemia; death is usually caused by pulmonary edema. Although a tentative diagnosis can be made on the basis of history, symptoms, and the finding of a metabolic acidosis with an increased anion gap, it is confirmed by measurement of serum salicylate levels; the arterial blood gas pattern can also be very revealing, since it is likely to show a mixed pattern, metabolic acidosis plus pulmonary alkalosis (not simply compensation). This is because as the plasma levels increase the central respiratory center is stimulated, causing hyperventilation and inducing respiratory alkalosis, while still further exposure to salicylate causes a cascade of metabolic abnormalities starting with the uncoupling of oxidative phosphorylation and progressing to inhibition of the Krebs cycle dehydrogenases. In turn these events lead to accumulation of acetoacetate, acetate, and lactate and stimulation of gluconeogenesis, resulting in a metabolic acidosis with an increased anion gap as well as initial hyperglycemia. The anion gap is defined as $[Na^+] - ([Cl^-] + [HCO_3^-])$, and any value above 14 is indicative of metabolic acidosis with a positive anion gap. Choice **B** shows a low normal pH and lower than normal Pa_{CO_2} and bicarbonate level. The low bicarbonate level is compatible with both metabolic acidosis and respiratory alkalosis, while the lower than normal Pa_{CO_2} value is compatible with metabolic acidosis and respiratory alkalosis. A double acidosis (respiratory plus metabolic) can be ruled out because the pH would be far below normal, and the anion gap data clearly show metabolic acidosis, a value greater than 14 mEq/L. The decrease in the Pa_{CO_2} is a characteristic of respiratory alkalosis. While respiratory alkalosis is to be expected as compensation for metabolic acidosis, the normal rule is compensation cannot bring the pH back to normal. This "above normal" compensation can best be explained by a mixed acid–base status, namely respiratory alkalosis with metabolic acidosis, a sequel expected in salicylate poisoning. Thus, **B** is the correct choice.

In choice **A** the pH is less than 7.35, the Pa_{CO_2} is elevated, and the bicarbonate value is in the normal range; results consistent with metabolic acidosis with respiratory compensation. Choice **C** also indicates acidemia, but in this case the Pa_{CO_2} and bicarbonate values are greater than normal, indicating respiratory acidosis. In choices **D** and **E** the pH values are above 7.45, indicating alkalemia. In choice **D** the Pa_{CO_2} and bicarbonate values are elevated, suggesting a metabolic basis, while in choice **E** they are decreased, indicating a process driven by the respiratory system.

23 The answer is E *Psychiatry*

The woman most likely suffers from generalized anxiety disorder. The diagnostic feature is poorly controlled anxiety lasting longer than 6 months. Onset is often in childhood and may continue long-term at a low level into adulthood but flare up when exacerbated by stressful conditions. Venlafaxine (choice **E**) is an effective treatment, especially when accompanied by depressive symptoms such as rumination. Buspirone and longer-acting benzodiazepines such as diazepam may also be useful.

Modafinil (choice **A**) is used for disorders associated with excessive sleepiness and may cause anxiety. Zolpidem (choice **B**) is a short-term treatment for insomnia and may cause rebound anxiety. Risperidone (choice **C**) should be reserved for psychosis and manic episodes. Alprazolam (choice **D**) is a shorter-acting benzodiazepine with a higher potential for inducing dependence when used for extended periods.

24 **The answer is B** *Obstetrics and Gynecology*

The clinical scenario strongly suggests premature rupture of membranes (PROM). Accurate assessment of PROM is essential because the outcome of pregnancy can be adversely affected by a positive diagnosis. This question addresses confirmation of PROM by examination, rather than with historic data. A speculum examination (choice **B**) is helpful in determining the extent of vaginal pooling.

Nitrazine paper on the perineum (choice **A**) assesses pH of the fluid. A blue color indicates alkaline pH. While alkaline amniotic fluid will be Nitrazine positive, so can urine, which is often alkaline in pregnancy. Sonographic evidence of oligohydramnios (choice **C**) is often present with PROM; however, it has a low specificity and sensitivity for ruptured membranes. Urinalysis (choice **D**) is not relevant. Digital examination (choice **E**) should never be done until membrane rupture is ruled out, because of the potential increase in infectious morbidity from ascending vaginal flora into the uterus, leading to chorioamnionitis.

25 **The answer is D** *Surgery*

It seems most likely that this man suffers from postoperative pancreatitis, which most commonly is seen after common bile duct exploration for a gallstone (choice **D**) during a cholecystectomy. Both the pancreatic duct and the common bile duct empty into the ampulla of Vater. Emptying is determined by the sphincter tone in the ampulla. Low obstruction in the common bile duct by a stone causes reflux from the bile duct into the pancreatic duct, which can lead to pancreatitis. Endoscopic retrograde cholangiopancreatography is also a cause of pancreatitis.

Anesthetic agents (choice **A**), hypovolemia (choice **B**), total parenteral nutrition (TPN) (choice **C**), and postoperative infection (choice **E**) do not predispose to acute pancreatitis.

26 **The answer is D** *Surgery*

This patient has a compartment syndrome, which occurs as a result of external or internal compression of the neurovascular structures due to soft tissue swelling. Fractures of the leg and forearm region tend to have a high propensity for compartment syndrome; however, it can be found in fractures involving other areas, including those of the calcaneus. After the fracture, tissues begin to swell, but the fascial sheath covering the muscles is unyielding. This leads to pressure on the neurovascular structures, resulting in ischemia to the muscles. Failure to recognize the condition could lead to Volkmann's ischemic contracture, myoglobinuria, and renal failure, hyperkalemia, and even loss of limb due to vascular compromise. Typically, the patient complains of pain in the fingers or toes on movement. Paresthesias may be present. The pulse is normal until late in the process; therefore, viability of the pulse does not exclude impending complications. In cases of compartment syndrome, compartment pressure usually exceeds 35 mm Hg; however, compartment syndrome occasionally may be present with lower pressures. The most important sign to make a diagnosis is the presence of pain on passive movement of the fingers or toes. Treatment involves cleaving (i.e., splitting the cast along its length) (choice **D**) to relieve edema, followed by elevation. Once the swelling has subsided, a full cast can be reapplied.

Reassurance (choice **A**) would be injudicious without concomitant treatment. Administering analgesics (choice **B**) would not address the problem; while it would relieve the pain, it would not in any way stall the relentless march of edema. Although corticosteroids (choice **C**) may initially relieve some of the swelling, they have no role in the management of this condition because the primary problem has to be addressed. Leaving the cast intact and elevating the arm (choice **E**) will help but is insufficient.

27 **The answer is B** *Medicine*

Adult respiratory distress syndrome (ARDS) is marked by the rapid onset of dyspnea within 12 to 24 hours of an initiating event. Initiating events with an increased propensity for ARDS are sepsis (most common), aspiration of gastric contents (this patient), drug overdose, shock, burns, diffuse pneumonias, and oxygen toxicity, to name only a few.

The mechanism of injury is primarily a neutrophil-related event in the lungs, with the release of protease, free radicals, and leukotrienes that produce pulmonary vasoconstriction and increased vessel permeability.

The increased vessel permeability results in leaky capillaries that lose protein-rich fluid into the alveoli to produce hyaline membranes. Lymphocytes and monocytes release cytokines, which also contribute to the inflammatory process. Type II pneumocytes are damaged, thus decreasing the production of surfactant, which results in widespread atelectasis (alveolar collapse). Because atelectasis is a prominent feature of ARDS, the primary defect is intrapulmonary shunting (choice **B**) of blood, accompanied by profound hypoxemia.

Compliance (ability of the lung to expand) is decreased, not increased (choice **C**) by increased inflammation and edema in the interstitium of the lungs. Damage to elastic tissue support would induce a decrease, not an increase (choice **D**) in elasticity (the recoil properties of the lung). In this patient, the $Paco_2$ is 74 mm Hg, a value typical in uncompensated respiratory acidosis; the bicarbonate value of 28 mEq/L, and the pH of 7.20 are also compatible with uncompensated respiratory acidosis, not respiratory alkalosis (choice **E**). The respiratory center is not directly involved (choice **A**).

28 The answer is B *Surgery*

This patient has hypotension and bradycardia (choice **B**) as a result of neurogenic shock. Sympathetic outflow is absent after spinal cord injuries. As a result of sympathetic paralysis, norepinephrine cannot act on blood vessels to induce vasoconstriction; thus, hypotension follows. Failed sympathetic function leads to unopposed parasympathetic action, which causes bradycardia.

A variable degree of hypertension with tachycardia (choice **A**) is seen in patients with acute severe pain; relief of pain lowers blood pressure and heart rate. The combination of hypertension and bradycardia (choice **C**) signifies raised intracranial pressure, as occurs in epidural hemorrhage. Cerebral perfusion pressure, which should be 50 mm Hg at a minimum, depends on the difference between mean arterial pressure and cerebrospinal fluid (CSF) pressure. As intracranial pressure rises, CSF pressure rises; the difference between mean arterial pressure and CSF pressure falls. To maintain the minimum level of cerebral blood flow, the systolic blood pressure has to rise. Bradycardia is a consequence of the resulting hypertension. Hypotension and tachycardia (choice **D**) are seen in hypovolemic shock, in which there is loss of extracellular volume into the third space or elsewhere. In the case of spinal injuries, there is no loss of blood from within the vascular compartment. The blood remains within the system but cannot be distributed due to lack of sympathetic function; hence, there is bradycardia rather than the more typical tachycardia. Furthermore, the treatment of neurogenic shock involves use of vasoconstrictors to drive the blood back into circulation, while hemorrhagic shock requires volume expansion.

29 The answer is E *Medicine*

In questions that ask you to examine the data, do just that. This question includes several statements that may well be true. For example, the effects of chemotherapy may not bear any relationship to cell kill (choice **A**); however, no data concerning cell kill are provided, so the examinee is not in a position to make a judgment concerning the accuracy of the statement. Similarly, it is possible that evaluation of chest x-ray films may be more valuable than monitoring UCG titer as a guide to therapy (choice **D**). Once again, no data are provided to permit such a conclusion. Examining the data, it is clear that the effects of the drug regimens on UCG titer are variable. They cannot possibly be directly proportional to decreases in platelet count (choice **C**) because all drug doses were adjusted to a toxicity limit of a 2-log decrease in platelet count. The methotrexate regimen lowered UCG titer from 10^8 to 10^5, a 3-log decrease (not a 2-log decrease [choice **B**]). Cisplatin plus etoposide lowered UCG titer from 10^7 to less than 10^3, a more than 4-log decrease (choice **E**), the correct answer.

The seemingly small titer changes cause 2- or 4-log changes because the chemotherapeutic agent destroys normal cells as well as malignant ones. Consequently, the platelet count drops considerably. The combination of cisplatin and etoposide has a greater effect than one drug alone.

30 The answer is D *Medicine*

Treatment of hyperthyroidism during pregnancy depends in part on the severity of the disorder. Hyperthyroid females can often tolerate the mild exacerbation of the state that accompanies pregnancy without therapy, and there appears to be no increase in the incidence of fetal loss. If treatment is judged to be required, propylthiouracil (choice **D**) is usually preferred over methimazole, in part because the latter drug enters the fetal circulation more readily and has been reported to cause aplasia cutis. Propylthiouracil also inhibits 5′-deiodinase, decreasing formation of triiodothyronine (T$_3$). The primary objective of drug therapy is to maintain free thyroxin (FT$_4$) and thyroid-stimulating hormone (TSH) at high-to-normal levels using the lowest possible dose of propylthiouracil.

Lugol's solution (iodine and potassium iodide) (choice **A**) exerts only a temporary antithyroid effect. Propranolol (choice **E**) should not ordinarily be given as an adjuvant because it may cause fetal growth retardation and neonatal respiratory depression. Antithyroid agents carry less risk to the patient and the pregnancy than surgery; in any event, surgery is contraindicated during the third (and first) trimester of pregnancy (choice **C**). Radioactive iodine (^{131}I) (choice **B**) should never be given during pregnancy.

31 The answer is E *Medicine*

This patient has chronic lymphocytic leukemia (CLL), a disease primarily affecting the elderly; 90% of patients are over 50, and the median age at presentation is 65 years. The primary clinical characteristic signifying CLL is lymphocytosis with white cell counts usually over 100,000/μL, of which 75 to 98% are lymphocytes. Diagnosis can be confirmed by immunophenotyping in which the B lymphocyte lineage marker CD19 is expressed along with the T lymphocyte marker CD5. The Rai staging system grades CLL as follows: stage 0, lymphocytosis only; stage I, lymphocytosis plus lymphadenopathy; stage II, organomegaly; stage III, anemia; and stage IV, thrombocytopenia. In most cases these lymphocytes are morphologically indistinguishable from normal small lymphocytes; the exception is a CLL variant disease known as prolymphocytic leukemia, in which the lymphocytes are larger and immature and the disease course is more aggressive. More typically CLL follows an indolent pattern, and patients often present with a nonsymptomatic lymphocytosis discovered by chance (i.e., stage 0); other cases commonly first present with fatigue or lymphadenopathy (stage I). Obviously, this man with hepatosplenomegaly, anemia, and thrombocytopenia with petechiae and ecchymoses has already progressed to stage IV. As the disease progresses, the lymph nodes and bone marrow progressively become invaded by small lymphocytes, the latter eventually causing the anemia and thrombocytopenia. Thus, in the case described, diffuse bone marrow and lymph node infiltration by the cells represented in the peripheral smear illustrated (choice **E**) is to be expected. No therapy is required until the disease is well advanced into stage II and of course in stages III and IV. The median survival for patients first diagnosed in stages 0 or I has been 10–15 years. Until recently the mean survival of patients in stages III or IV has been less than 2 years. However, with newer regimens of fludarabine-based therapy, more than 90% of patients live beyond 2 years. Still, treatment of some 5–10% of patients becomes complicated by development of an autoimmune thrombocytopenia or hemolytic anemia or non-Hodgkin's lymphoma.

Nearly all patients with hairy cell leukemia develop a monocytopenia (choice **A**), which is encountered in almost no other disease including CLL. Chronic myelogenous leukemia most commonly terminates as an acute myelogenous leukemia (choice **B**). Auer rods are splinter-to-rod-shaped cytoplasmic inclusions seen in myeloblasts in acute myelogenous leukemia (choice **C**) and are not found in the smear illustrated. Paratrabecular lymphoid aggregates in the bone marrow are a characteristic manifestation of the non-Hodgkin's lymphomas (choice **D**); in CLL lymphocyte invasion is diffuse.

32 The answer is A *Medicine*

OGI is a hereditary osteoporosis due to defective type 1 collagen synthesis. Type I OGI is usually not debilitating, and there are often extensive family histories showing an autosomal dominant mode of inheritance. Fractures most often occur prior to puberty, but like everybody else, as patients age their bone density decreases. Since their bone structure is less than optimal to start out with, this puts them at a greater risk than average of developing age-induced osteoporosis resulting in additional fractures. Among the general population osteoporosis in the elderly is estimated to cause at least 1.5 million fractures annually in the United States. In age-induced osteoporosis the rate of bone formation is usually near normal, but the rate of reabsorption is increased significantly. This results in a greater loss of trabecular bone than compact bone, accounting for the primary clinical features, namely crush fractures of the vertebrae and fractures of the neck of the femur and of the distal end of the radius. These fractures are a leading cause of morbidity among the elderly and indirectly also increase mortality; thus diagnosis and treatment before fractures occur can be of great value. Determination of bone density (choice **A**) in this man, at higher than normal risk for osteoporosis, will have a significant positive effect on his lifestyle and perhaps on his longevity if he is found to have osteopenia or early osteoporosis and this diagnosis triggers the start of treatment. The most probable treatment regimen will be administration of a bisphosphonate that inhibits osteoclastic activity.

Blood test for the rheumatic factor (choice **B**) is not called for because there are no symptoms suggestive of rheumatic arthritis such as symmetric joint involvement, prolonged stiffness, low-grade fever, hot joints, or fatigue. Radiographic studies (choice **C**) could be used to confirm that this patient's joint pain is osteoarthritis, but such studies really are not needed because clinical judgment alone should suffice to reach this conclusion. In any case even if osteoarthritis were confirmed by radiography, it would not lead to a changed treatment modality. A complete blood count (choice **D**) and an erythrocyte sedimentation determination (choice **E**) could be of potential value if this were an inflammatory condition but are essentially irrelevant in this case. A blood test for antinuclear antibodies (choice **F**) has great value in ruling out a number of inflammatory conditions because of its great sensitivity; it is positive in some 30–60% of rheumatic arthritis cases, almost all cases of systemic lupus erythematosus, Sjögren's syndrome, diffuse and limited scleroderma (CREST) syndromes as well as polymyositis/dermatomyositis. However, this patient shows no signs suggesting that he may suffer from any these conditions. Arthrographic examination of the affected joints (choice **G**) is a procedure in which a liquid contrast medium is injected into a joint and its penetration is followed by radiography to see if there are any tears in the cartilage or other tissues. It is rarely used to diagnose a case of nontraumatic osteoarthritis.

33 The answer is A *Surgery*

The patient most likely has acute surgical parotitis (sialadenitis). Surgical parotitis usually occurs 1 week postoperatively in elderly patients who have poor dental hygiene and have been intubated. *Staphylococcus aureus* (choice **A**) is the organism isolated most commonly. Surgical drainage and antibiotics are required.

Acute and chronic sialadenitis can also result from sialolithiasis, which refers to calculi in the major salivary gland ducts, most commonly in Wharton's duct draining the submandibular gland (choice **B**); however the vignette provides no suggestion that this might be the case. Mumps is a common cause of viral parotitis and may be bilateral. However, the advent of vaccination against it has made it very rare indeed. (choice **C**). Hemorrhage (choice **D**) into the parotid gland is rare. Parotid gland enlargement is also associated with Sjögren's syndrome, a collagen vascular disease characterized by immunologic destruction of minor salivary glands with subsequent development of dry eyes and dry mouth (choice **E**); rheumatoid arthritis is frequently present as well.

34 The answer is A *Psychiatry*

This patient's symptoms are most suggestive of social phobia. Assertiveness training (choice **A**) is the treatment of choice for this disorder and involves education, role playing, and desensitization to feared social stimuli. Medications that are useful for social phobia include newer antidepressants such as paroxetine and monoamine oxidase (MAO) inhibitors such as phenelzine. Buspirone is also used occasionally.

Implosion therapy (choice **B**) involves massive exposure to feared stimuli and is not effective for social phobia. Psychodynamic psychotherapy (choice **C**) may bring individuals insight into the reasons for their social phobia, but it has not been demonstrated to reliably decrease the associated symptoms. Lorazepam (choice **D**) and other benzodiazepines are usually ineffective in lessening social avoidance. Systematic desensitization (choice **E**) used alone is less effective than assertiveness training.

35 The answer is C *Medicine*

This woman clearly suffers from hyponatremia, which is defined as a sodium concentration below 130 mEq/L. A urine sodium concentration of 80 mEq/L indicates that the decrease in plasma sodium is due to excess loss into the urine. This typically is caused by hyperfunction of antidiuretic hormone (ADH), also known as vasopressin. Normally, ADH acts to limit water excretion. As a consequence the normal physiologic response is to increase ADH activity only when the body senses increasing osmolarity, as in a hypovolemic state. This woman's skin turgor is normal, and there is a small decrease in concentration of electrolytes other than sodium and chloride, indicating that she is basically euvolemic. Thus this increase in ADH activity is inappropriate, a condition known as the *syndrome of inappropriate ADH* secretion (SIADH). The question then becomes what is causing SIADH in this woman and what can best be done to alleviate this condition. In this case, the obvious solution is to prescribe some drug other than chlorpropamide to treat her diabetes (choice **C**). Although chlorpropamide is an inexpensive and effective long-acting hypoglycemic agent, it rarely is prescribed these days in part because it has a hyponatremic effect due to its propensity to react with kidney ADH receptors and thus enhance ADH activity. This may result in abnormal loss of sodium from the extracellular compartment, which creates an ionic gradient leading to the influx of water into cells throughout the body including the central nervous system, where it causes serious mental distress and accounts for the small vesicles seen on the CT scan.

Choice **A,** administration of a serotonin-reuptake inhibitor, is inappropriate because the cause of her mental problems is the influx of hypoosmotic fluid into the CNS, not a hormonal imbalance. Moreover, several dozen cases of SIADH caused by an SSRI have been reported, albeit mainly in the elderly. Restricting sodium from her diet (choice **B**) or increasing her water intake (choice **D**) makes no sense, since she is already hyponatremic. Adding sodium to her diet (choice **E**) superficially makes sense and might transiently increase circulating sodium levels, but because it does not get at the root cause, any effect provided would not be long lasting. Administering demeclocycline, an ADH antagonist; (choice **F**) is primarily used in patients in whom SIADH is caused by ectopic secretion of ADH by a tumor, such as a small cell carcinoma in which the underling mechanism of SIADH is overproduction of ADH.

36 The answer is E *Pediatrics*

Mild breast-feeding jaundice does not require intervention (choice **E**) from the physician or that the mother stop breast-feeding completely (choice **D**). Breast-milk jaundice may appear in 2% of term, breast-fed infants after the seventh day of life. There is a significant elevation of unconjugated (not conjugated) bilirubin (choice **B**). Bilirubin may be as high as 10–30 mg/dL during the third week. If the mother continues breast-feeding, the hyperbilirubinemia gradually decreases and may persist for 3 to 10 weeks at lower levels. The serum bilirubin level rapidly (not slowly [choice **C**]) declines if nursing is discontinued for 24–48 hours. If nursing is resumed after 24–48 hours the serum bilirubin will not rise to its previously high levels. Breast-feeding jaundice (not breast-milk jaundice) is seen in the first few days of life (choice **A**) and is also associated with increased unconjugated hyperbilirubinemia (>12 mg/dL). Breast-feeding jaundice occurs in 13% of breast-fed infants in the first week of life because of decreased milk intake with concomitant dehydration.

37 The answer is C *Obstetrics and Gynecology*

The scenario described a young woman undergoing virilization, not just hirsutism. Hirsutism is the development of male-pattern hair in a female, whereas virilization is development of male secondary sex characteristics in a female, including deepening voice, increasing muscle mass, and clitoral enlargement. Virilization requires a high level of peripheral androgens, most often from a tumor. The rapid onset, as in this case, is also consistent with a tumor of either the adrenal gland or the ovary. All the choices are ovarian tumors. The ovarian tumor that produces androgens is the Sertoli-Leydig cell tumor (choice **C**).

Another hormone producing non-functional ovarian tumor is the granulosa cell tumor (choice **A**), which produces estrogen and promotes feminizing signs and symptoms. Brenner tumor (choice **B**), fibroma (choice **D**), and dysgerminoma (choice **E**) are not endocrinologically active.

38 The answer is D *Psychiatry*

This woman's symptoms are most suggestive of depression. Learned helplessness (choice **D**) is a behavioral theory of depression in which depression is viewed as a reaction to a perception of one's inability to improve a situation.

Faulty cognitive framework (choice **A**) is a cognitive theory of depression; object loss (choice **B**) is a psychodynamic theory of depression, and inadequate exposure to light (choice **C**) is a biologic theory of depression; none of these is a behavioral explanation. Double-bind communication (choice **E**) refers to incongruity between spoken and unspoken communication in a given exchange. It was a view of family dynamics in schizophrenia that is no longer considered valid.

39 The answer is B *Obstetrics and Gynecology*

With any patient having postmenopausal bleeding, endometrial carcinoma must be ruled out; therefore, endometrial biopsy (choice **B**) is the diagnostic method of choice. Endometrial carcinoma is the most common gynecologic cancer and is most often diagnosed in stage 1 (confined to the uterus) because of vaginal bleeding, the most common symptom.

Cytologic screening by Pap smear (choice **A**) is used for cervical cancer screening, but it misses 60% of endometrial carcinoma cases. Pelvic examination under anesthesia (choice **C**) may be helpful in staging cervical cancer but is not diagnostic for any cancer. Laparoscopy (choice **D**) is useful for diagnosing benign pelvic disease such as endometriosis or pelvic adhesions but not for any kind of cancer. Colposcopy (choice **E**) is used for localization of cervical biopsy sites but is not used for endometrial cancer diagnosis.

40 The answer is B *Obstetrics and Gynecology*

This patient is a candidate for developing Sheehan's syndrome because of hypoperfusion of her anterior pituitary gland. The pituitary hormone most commonly affected is prolactin (choice **B**), resulting in the most common symptom, which is failure of lactation. Although all pituitary trophic hormones are at risk, usually only a few are affected.

If FSH (choice **D**) is involved, the woman will not resume menstrual periods and will experience secondary amenorrhea due to lack of estrogen. Severe involvement of ACTH (choice **A**) may lead to adrenal insufficiency including hypoglycemia, hypotension, and weakness. If TSH (choice **C**) is affected, the patient will experience hypothyroidism. Symptoms of ACTH and TSH deficiency are usually seen in chronic rather than acute Sheehan's syndrome and may take months or years to manifest themselves. Loss of antidiuretic hormone (ADH) (choice **E**), is seldom seen.

41 The answer is D *Pediatrics*

A karyotype is described by first listing the total number of chromosomes followed by the sex chromosomes plus any abnormalities in number or structure. Normal euploid individuals have 46 chromosomes of which two are the sex chromosomes; in other words they are 46XX or 46XY. Thus, 47XY + 13 (choice **D**) describes a male (XY) with 47 chromosomes, the extra one being chromosome 13. Expressed differently, he has three number 13 chromosomes, or trisomy 13. Approximately 1 in 15,000 newborn infants have trisomy 13, and about half of these will die with in the first month of life. Those who survive are severely developmentally and mentally retarded.

42 The answer is A *Pediatrics*

This is a male with one extra Y chromosome (choice **A**). There is no specific name for this condition, but it occurs in about 1 per 1000 male live births, and surveys of mental and penal institutions found that the incidence among inmates was 4–20 per 1000 raising the question whether an extra Y chromosome may be causally related to aberrant behaviors. However, the magnitude of social pathology, if any, has not yet been determined.

43 The answer is B *Pediatrics*

This is a description of a baby girl with Down syndrome due to trisomy 21 (choice **B**). The overall incidence of this disorder is approximately 1 per 900 live births, but it depends on the mother's age. At 20 years the incidence is about 1 per 2300 births, at 30 years about 1 per 1000 births, at 40 years about 1 per 150 births, and at 45 years or older about 1 per 46 births. In about 95% of the cases the cause of Down syndrome is trisomy 21 due to nondisjunction during mitosis. An additional 4% of cases are due to an unbalanced translocation; the remaining individuals with Down syndrome are mosaics having both a 47 + 21 cell line as well as the normal euploid line. In addition to the unusual appearance described, children with Down syndrome will have growth retardation, have some degree of mental retardation, and will show signs of premature aging. They also have a 40% risk of serious heart disease, a 5% risk of serious gastrointestinal problems, and a greater-than-normal risk of leukemia, serious infections, cataracts, and thyroid abnormalities. Individuals who live beyond the age of 35 show signs of Alzheimer's disease.

44 The answer is E *Pediatrics*

The Y chromosome usually carries the genes that code for maleness. As a consequence, this boy has a basic male phenotype despite the fact he is XXY (choice **E**). However, the extra X chromosome does cause some feminization. This condition is known as Klinefelter syndrome and it occurs in about 1 per 1000 male births. In addition to having small testicles and possibly having enlarged breasts, such individuals are usually tall and thin and have arms and legs that are disproportionally long. The testicular tubules are hyalinized, and there is a failure to produce sperm, making them infertile. Despite these signs of feminization, superficially they are phenotypically male with perhaps some small but feminine breasts counterbalanced by a normal sized penis. There is no mental retardation, although the IQ may be somewhat lower than expected. A few men have more than one extra X chromosome, and the greater the number of X chromosomes, the greater the likelihood of frank mental retardation. Their cells have Barr bodies, but at least some cells retain a viable X chromosome.

45 The answer is C *Pediatrics*

This girl has Turner syndrome due to the loss of one X chromosome (choice **C**), a condition that occurs in about 1 in 5000 live births. It is estimated that 99% of concepti with Turner syndrome are spontaneously aborted. In addition to the characteristics noted in the case description, girls with Turner syndrome have an increased carrying angle at the elbow and cardiovascular and renal abnormalities.

46 The answer is E *Surgery*

This patient has a twisting injury to the lateral aspect of the ankle, resulting in a sprained lateral ligament (choice **E**). The lateral ligaments of the ankle consist of the posterior talofibular, the anterior talofibular, and the calcaneofibular ligaments. Although all three ligaments may be involved, usually the anterior talofibular ligament is most severely injured. Sprains are classified as grade I if the ligament involved is simply stretched and not torn, grade II if slightly torn, and grade III if severely torn or ruptured. The ecchymosis (bruising) and swelling in all three grades is due to bleeding from surrounding soft tissue. Injury to these ligaments may occur with or without an associated avulsion fracture of the base of the fifth metatarsal and, rarely, a fracture of the talus. The patient would also be unable to walk on this leg if there were ecchymosis on the dorsolateral aspect of the ankle. She would probably hop, using the good foot.

47 The answer is B *Surgery*

This patient has a tear of the Achilles tendon (choice **B**), just proximal to its insertion in the calcaneus. The prevalence of Achilles tendon tears increases 3- to 5-fold after the age of 40 years, and overall about 2% of Achilles tendon injuries result in a tear that may be partial or complete. Achilles tendon tears often follow tendinitis (patient's slight pain) and can then be caused by even minor additional stress. Patients complain of pain behind the ankle and have difficulty walking on tiptoe. A gap is felt when a finger is run over the skin at the point of tear, and plantar flexion following compression of the bellies of the calf muscles below and behind the knee is weak (Thomson test). There is no pain on compression of the calf muscles. Radiography is irrelevant to the diagnosis, which is clinical. This condition should be differentiated from tears involving the bellies of the calf muscles.

48 The answer is D *Surgery*

This patient has a tear involving some of the muscle fibers of the plantar flexors (i.e., gastrocnemius [most common] and soleus) (choice **D**). Such tears most commonly occur in males in their fourth to sixth decade. Often these men are former athletes who are still well muscled but now no longer work out regularly, so-called weekend warriors. The muscle tears in response to a sudden push-off of the foot, as might occur in hill running, jumping, tennis, or any other activity involving similar movements. Whereas stretching and tears in ligaments are called *sprains,* analogous muscle injuries are called *strains.* Patients who injure the plantar flexors have pain in the calf, and ecchymosis may be present in the overlying skin. Compression of the bellies of the calf muscles causes pain. Plantar flexion is normal with calf compression because most of the muscle fibers are intact, and the insertion to the posterior aspect of the calcaneus is not endangered. Therefore, no gap will be felt in that area. Patients can walk on tiptoe, although with pain. An x-ray film is noncontributory to the diagnosis, which is clinical. This condition should be differentiated from tears of the Achilles tendon.

49 The answer is C *Surgery*

As a result of his fall, this patient has sustained a fracture of the calcaneus (choice **C**), which most commonly occurs from a foot-first fall from a height greater than 6 feet or from an automobile accident in which the patient had the feet firmly braced on the floor. Although the complaint often centers on just one foot, the injury may be unilateral or bilateral, and both legs should be investigated. Also the force is transmitted to the lumbar spine, and often there is an associated compression fracture of the lumbar vertebra. Thus, one must suspect a compression fracture and obtain an x-ray film to exclude it. Failure to do so could have dire consequences, especially if the patient is moved, because an ensuing paraplegia would be irreversible. Due to the presence of fascial compartments restraining the muscles of the foot, which are in four layers in the plantar region, a compartment syndrome and even necrosis of the skin could also ensue. This is due to the edema resulting from trauma impeding blood flow to the tissues.

50 The answer is F   *Surgery*

This patient has a "march" fracture, which usually involves the shafts of the metatarsals (choice **F**), especially the second and third. This condition was initially noted in soldiers who had marched for long distances, hence the name. These patients complain of pain in the foot, which may not become worse with walking. Tenderness over the point of fracture is noted. Although the fracture cannot be seen on x-ray films, a bone scan will reveal the fracture and a second x-ray film taken in about 4 weeks will show the healing fracture.

INCORRECT CHOICES

Choice **A,** fracture of the talus. The talus is a small bone that sits between the calcaneus and the tibia and fibula, forming the subtalar joint. Although the talus may be broken by twisting an ankle, this is relatively rare. It is more commonly broken in falls, automobile accidents, and snowboarding accidents.

test **7**

Questions

Single Best Choice Directions: This section consists of numbered statements or questions followed by a list of potential answers; you are to select the ONE best answer.

1 A 2-year-old boy presents to the pediatrician with a 12-hour history of recurrent and severe paroxysmal colicky pain. The pain is accompanied by straining efforts, loud cries, and vomiting. Abdominal distention and tenderness are present on physical examination. and an oblong mass is palpated in the midepigastrium. Bloody mucus is noted on the examiner's finger as it is withdrawn after rectal examination. Which of the following is the most likely diagnosis?

(A) Meckel's diverticulum
(B) Congenital pyloric stenosis
(C) An intussusception
(D) Meconium ileus
(E) Necrotizing enterocolitis

2 An institute for female felons conducted the following study to confirm that sodium restriction lowered systolic blood pressure in their mix of patients. They divided 300 prisoners into two 150-person groups that are matched with respect to age, ethnicity, and approximate blood pressure values; all were in the prehypertensive range (systolic pressure between 130 and 139 mm Hg, diastolic pressure between 80 and 89 mm Hg), none are diabetic, and none are taking any relevant medication. One group was put on a sodium-restricted diet permitting 2000 mg of sodium daily. The other group was permitted to consume the usual prison fare, which provided an average of 5 g of sodium daily. (The typical daily consumption in the United States is between 4 and 6 g [175–260 mEq] daily). After 2 months on these diets the difference in mean diastolic blood pressure among the 150 subjects in the low-salt diet group and the 150 subjects in the nonrestricted-salt group is 5 mm Hg, a difference significant at a *P* value of .04851. Which of the following statements about the two groups is true?

(A) The blood pressure difference is clinically significant.
(B) The chance that an individual would benefit from a low-salt diet is less than 0.05%.
(C) It is unlikely that random variation accounted for the difference in diastolic blood pressure between the two groups.
(D) Increasing the number of subjects would tend to change the *P* value from significant to nonsignificant.

(E) To show a statistically significant difference, the sodium-restricted group should have been limited to an intake of less than 1000 mg of sodium per day.

3 A 16-year-old boy tells his gym instructor that he just isn't strong enough to do more than one push-up, and he isn't able to run a lap without being left breathless. The instructor suspects malingering but nonetheless sends him to the school physician for evaluation. Physical examination reveals a tall gangly young man who is 5 ft, 10 in (1.8 m) tall and weighs 155 lb (70.3 kg). His has a strikingly narrow face, an arm span of 6 ft 4 in (1.9 m), long legs, long thin fingers, pectus excavatum and is myopic. His heart sounds reveal a pansystolic murmur near the apex of the atrium, with a prominent third heart sound. Which one of the following connective tissue components is most likely abnormal in this young man?

(A) Fibrillin-1
(B) Keratin 5 or 14
(C) Type IV collagen
(D) Type I collagen
(E) Type XI collagen
(F) Fibroblast growth factor receptor

4 A 62-year-old man with Parkinson's disease but no previous psychiatric history is admitted to the hospital with a 1-week history of emotional lability, disinterest in personal appearance, intermittent inattention and confusion, peculiar beliefs about his wife poisoning his food, and intermittent visual hallucinations concerning insects in the house. He is currently taking carbidopa and trihexyphenidyl. He reportedly has a history of alcohol abuse and has been drinking more lately. Mental status examination reveals that the patient is oriented to the year but not the month. Which of the following is the most likely diagnosis?

(A) Alcohol-induced dementia
(B) Alcohol-induced psychotic disorder
(C) Delirium of unknown cause
(D) Dementia due to Parkinson's disease
(E) Mood disorder due to Parkinson's disease

5 A 69-year-old man with a history of coronary artery disease (CAD) and hypertension presents with acute onset of right facial weakness and numbness. On examination, his speech and extremity strength are normal, but he has significant weakness of the right side of the face, including the orbicularis oculi. In addition, he complains of roaring in the right ear, and his taste sensation is absent on the right side of the anterior tongue. Sensation is normal to pinprick. Which of the following would best explain these findings?

(A) Bell's palsy
(B) Brainstem glioma
(C) A stroke due to occlusion of the left middle cerebral artery
(D) Lacunar stroke of the left internal capsule
(E) Parotid tumor

6 A 33-year-old woman complains of being unable to leave her home unless others accompany her. Whenever she is faced with the necessity of traveling beyond her front fence, she calls her friend to help her. She feels discouraged and angry about her condition. Mental examination reveals a normally alert and attentive woman with mild depressive symptoms but no evidence of disorganized thinking or delusions. Which of the following is the most likely disorder associated with this patient's phobia?

(A) Major depressive disorder
(B) Obsessive–compulsive disorder
(C) Panic disorder
(D) Schizophrenia
(E) Somatization disorder

7 An 8-year-old boy is taken to a family physician by his mother who tells the physician that she is worried that her child may have sugar diabetes because he urinates frequently and is almost always thirsty. The mother says she knows that these are signs of diabetes because her 58-year-old husband developed type 2 diabetes earlier this year, and her 76-year-old mother was diagnosed with diabetes only 5 years ago. She asks, "How can my child escape diabetes with such a family history?" During the physical examination the physician notes that the boy is grossly underweight, there is a fruity smell on his breath, and he seems lethargic. His blood pressure is 105/55 mm Hg. The nurse conducts a finger prick blood glucose determination and the resultant value is 325 mg/dL. Which of the fol-

lowing statements concerning this boy and his condition is true?

(A) The boy should be placed on an insulin regime as soon as possible.
(B) It cannot be concluded that the boy has diabetes until a fasting blood glucose value is obtained.
(C) The mother was right to suspect the boy inherited diabetes from either his father or grandmother.
(D) A metabolic syndrome associated with diabetes is liable to make the boy obese as he ages.
(E) The boy can be best treated with oral antihyperglycemic agents.

8 The star quarterback for a university football team presents to the school physician 2 weeks after the onset of symptoms of infectious mononucleosis. He wants to return to playing football and is requesting medical clearance. He states that he feels fine; his muscle aches and fatigue have resolved. Upon examination his heart and lungs are normal, his spleen is not enlarged, he has no temperature, and his liver enzyme values are normal. Which of the following statements is correct regarding when he may return to playing football?

(A) Since he seems fine he may return to football immediately.
(B) He should return next week for another check-up and possible clearance to play.
(C) He should return in 2 weeks for another check-up and possible clearance to play.
(D) He may return to football when the mono-spot test result is negative.
(E) He may return to football when the lymphocyte count returns to normal.
(F) He is out for the remainder of the season (3 months) and may play again next season.

9 A laboratory test has a reference mean value of 20 mg/dL and a standard deviation of 2. Which of the following is the range in which 95% of repeated laboratory determinations would be expected to fall?

(A) 20 to 22
(B) 18 to 22
(C) 16 to 24
(D) 14 to 26
(E) 19 to 21

10 A 26-year-old woman planned to go biking, and as she was dressing she noticed her period had just started, so she inserted a tampon. While biking, a car turned right immediately in front of her; she crashed into it and catapulted over the hood. She was unable to get up, and when she looked at her right leg she found that her knee had traveled more than half way up her thigh. The paramedics approximately realigned the femur, splinted it and transported her to a local hospital where they set the fracture by implanting a metal rod down the shaft of the bone. Because of her blood loss she was administered two units of blood, after which her hemoglobin level was 7 g/dL. After 2 days in the hospital the surgical wound continued to seep blood, but she seemed on the road to recovery and was transferred to a neighboring rehabilitation facility. Because of everything else going on, nobody thought of replacing the tampon. The morning after arriving at the rehabilitation facility she complains of dizziness and a feeling of weakness and seems somewhat disoriented. She has a temperature of 103°F (39.4°C), has a generalized rash that even covers her hands and the soles of her feet. Her skin is warm to the touch, and her blood pressure is 150/90 mm Hg. The duty nurse calls in a physician who arrives 45 minutes later. By the time the physician gets there the patient's skin appears gray and is cold and clammy, she has tachycardia, and the heart sounds are weak, she has a shallow and rapid rate of breathing, her blood pressure is 74/49 mm Hg, her eyes are lusterless, and she is staring without showing signs of recognizing anything. At this time, which of the following choices represents the most probable diagnosis?

(A) Hypovolemic shock
(B) Toxic shock syndrome
(C) Cardiogenic shock
(D) Anaphylactic shock
(E) Shock cause by a gram-negative organism

11 A 20-year-old woman, gravida 2, para 0, aborta 1, is at 25 weeks' gestation with twins. An obstetric ultrasound study notes 30% discordance between the estimated fetal weights of the two fetuses. In addition, the amniotic fluid is significantly increased in the sac of the larger twin, and markedly decreased in the sac of the smaller. Assessment of fetal anatomy is normal in both fetuses, and bladders are seen in both twins.

Which of the following statements is most likely to be true?

(A) The donor twin is more likely to develop hyperbilirubinemia than the recipient twin.
(B) The type of placentation is dichorionic and diamniotic.
(C) The recipient twin often develops signs of volume overload.
(D) The pregnancy was the result of ovulation induction agents.
(E) The fetuses are of opposite gender.

12 A 27-year-old woman who was first diagnosed with schizophrenia at age 18 and has a history of seizures that were reputed to have started at about age 5 is stabilized on divalproex and then clozapine therapy was started. One week later, she complains of sedation and sialorrhea. Which of the following laboratory examinations should be performed immediately?

(A) Clozapine level
(B) Prolactin level
(C) Thyroid function
(D) Divalproex level
(E) White blood cell (WBC) count

13 A patient has Alzheimer's disease, which has advanced to the extent that he can no longer make rational decisions but still enjoys walking in the neighborhood with his caretaker. However he now has difficulty ambulating because of a problem with his knee. His physician believes his knee problem is due to a cartilage injury and wants to conduct a magnetic resonance imaging (MRI) study to determine if surgery is needed and, assuming it is, to follow up with appropriate surgery. Which of the following represents the procedure that takes precedence prior to starting treatment of the knee?

(A) Follow directions the patient expressed in a living will.
(B) Obtain written permission from a person named in a durable power of attorney.
(C) Obtain written permission from the director of the patient's managed care organization.
(D) Invoke the state's involuntary treatment law.
(E) Have the patient sign an informed consent form.

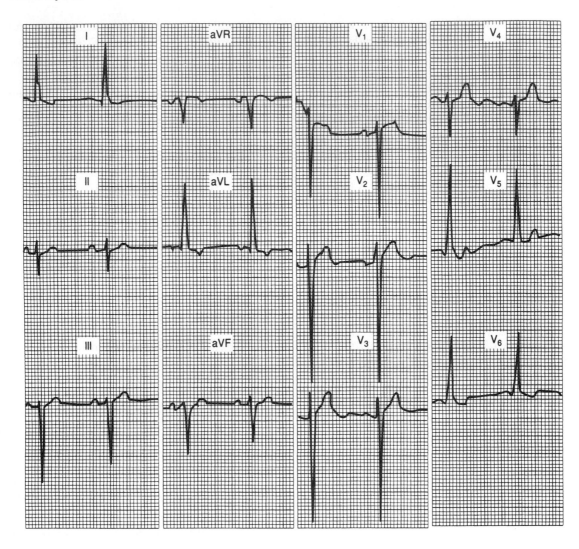

14 A 65-year-old man with multiple myeloma presents with confusion, severe depression, vomiting, constipation, and polyuria. His electrocardiogram (ECG) is shown. Which of the following is the most appropriate first step in the management of this patient?

(A) Give calcium gluconate
(B) Infuse saline
(C) Administer sodium bicarbonate
(D) Infuse furosemide
(E) Initiate mithramycin therapy

15 A 76-year-old female sees her physician with complaints of muscle pain around the neck, a headache particularly intense in the temporal area, a tender scalp, and jaw pain when chewing. She says that these symptoms started some 3 or 4 weeks earlier and seem to be getting progressively worse, and in addition she has felt tired, lost her appetite, and as a result lost 5 lb.

A more recent problem that she finds worrisome is blurred vision in which a single object appears as two. Upon examination she was found to weigh 140 lb (63.5 kg), to be 5 ft 5 in tall (1.65 m), have a temperature of 100.9°F (38.3°C), and a blood pressure of 125/82 mm Hg; her heart rate and rhythms were regular, her lungs clear to auscultation, her abdomen was soft and nontender, liver and spleen were of normal size, her temporal region was tender to touch, and she had small retinal hemorrhages. Which of the following laboratory test or procedures will provide the most significant clue regarding the diagnosis?

(A) A complete blood count (CBC)
(B) A computed tomography (CT) study of her head
(C) An erythrocyte sedimentation rate (ESR) determination
(D) A carotid ultrasound
(E) A lumbar puncture with subsequent culture

16 A 36-year-old woman has a 20-year history of social withdrawal and lack of motivation that began insidiously during high school. She has had several episodes of hallucinations and delusions; however, there have been no clear-cut episodes of depression or mania. There is a history of significant excessive alcohol use from age 20 to age 30. Compared with the general population, which of the following would most likely be found with studies of cerebral morphology and/or functional neuroimaging?

(A) Abnormalities of dopaminergic transmission
(B) Decreased metabolic activity in the prefrontal cortex
(C) Decreased size of the lateral ventricles
(D) Increased cerebral asymmetry
(E) Increased thickness of the corpus callosum

17 A mother presents to the emergency department with her 2-month-old daughter. The child appears lethargic and dehydrated. The mother reports that the patient has not been feeding well for the past few days. The mother says that she changed the infant's feedings from formula to cow's milk because the infant does not care for the taste of formula. Which nutrient normally in high concentration in cow's milk could cause the symptoms seen in this infant?

(A) Linoleic acid
(B) Linolenic acid
(C) Calcium
(D) Protein
(E) B-complex vitamins

18 A 22-year-old woman has had undiagnosed acute intermittent gastrointestinal pains since the age of 17. However, today she presents at an emergency clinic with such severe abdominal pain that the resident on duty seriously considered recommending an emergency laparotomy to find out what is wrong. However, he reconsidered after she complains about pain in both feet, becomes semi-incoherent and starts to act abnormally. Despite her semi-incoherent state he elicited the fact that she recently started having sexual relations with her first serious boyfriend and as a consequence started taking an estrogen-based contraceptive. In addition, to make sure she remained attractive to this, "her one and only love of her life," last week she started a 1200 calorie/day diet. Further questioning disclosed that her father had been bothered by intermittent stomach pains for many years, and although these annoyed him, they never were severe enough to require medical attention. Otherwise both parents, now in their mid-50s, seemed healthy. A physical examination was unremarkable except for borderline hypertension, and

in addition the resident was led to suspect the pain in her feet is due to peripheral neuropathy. A blood panel indicated that she suffered from hyponatremia. On the basis of the foregoing information the resident made a tentative diagnosis, and to confirm his suspicion, he asked the laboratory to run a urine analysis for which of the following elements?

(A) Porphobilinogen
(B) Uroporphyrin
(C) Uroporphyrinogen I
(D) Coproporphyrinogen I
(E) Coproporphyrinogen III
(F) Lead

19 A 59-year-old man made an appointment to see his physician because he had noticed blood in his urine for the past week. Otherwise he felt healthy, and he had no problem voiding his urine. His primary care physician found no other unusual signs or symptoms and referred him to an urologist who conducted a cystoscopic examination of his bladder. A small sample of the bladder wall was removed and examined microscopically. The view obtained is illustrated below.

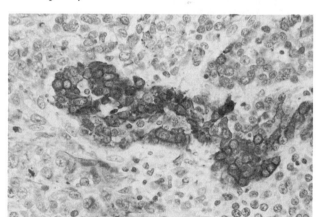

The lesion was evaluated as being a stage T1 papillary carcinoma, which has invaded the lamina propria but has not invaded the superficial layer of the muscularis propria. The lesion was completely excised by transurethral resection. Which of the following is true concerning this condition?

(A) This type of bladder cancer is equally common throughout the world.
(B) The type of carcinogen having the greatest potential of causing this condition is found in smoked foods.
(C) Removal of the growth by transurethral resection usually is not followed by recurrence of the condition.
(D) Usually the condition described is treated by radical cystectomy.

(E) Pelvic pain and difficulty in voiding urine are the earliest signs of bladder cancer.

(F) Women and men have an equal chance of developing bladder cancer.

(G) In the United States, most primary bladder cancers are transitional cell carcinomas.

(H) Bladder cancer is primarily a disease of the middle aged, 40 to 55 years old.

20 After leaving a bar in a five-star hotel a 38-year-old man trips and falls while descending a flight of stairs. Subsequently he feigns severe back pain, seeks medical attention, and then initiates legal action against the hotel in a bid to receive compensation for pain, suffering, and lost wages. Which of the following is the most likely diagnosis?

(A) Conversion disorder
(B) Factitious disorder
(C) Malingering
(D) Pain disorder
(E) Somatization disorder

21 A child is referred to a pediatric endocrinologist for further management of hypophosphatemia. On review of the family history she notes that the patient's mother has fasting hypophosphatemia. Laboratory results show that the patient has a slightly reduced serum calcium level, a moderately reduced serum phosphate level, elevated alkaline phosphatase activity, and no evidence of secondary hyperparathyroidism. On physical examination, the child is noted to have smooth bowing of the lower extremities, coxa vera, genu varum, genu valgum, and short stature. Which of the following is another characteristic seen on physical examination in patients with familial hypophosphatemia also known as vitamin D–resistant rickets?

(A) Tetany
(B) Rachitic rosary
(C) Harrison's groove (pectus deformity)
(D) Myopathy
(E) Waddling gait

22 An 8-year-old boy is brought to his pediatrician by his mother, who disclosed that the patient had been in his usual state of good health until this morning when he awoke covered with bruises and purple dots. The patient has no history of trauma, and there is no history of bleeding disorders in the patient or family. The past medical history is only significant for a mild upper respiratory infection 1 week ago. The pediatrician notes that the boy has petechiae and purpura over his entire body. A complete blood count (CBC) is obtained. The platelet count is 20,000 platelets/μL (normal is 150–450 $\times 10^3$/μL), but the rest of the CBC results are normal. No hepatosplenomegaly is present. A bone marrow aspirate exhibits normal megakaryocytes, but platelet budding is poor. Which of the following is the most appropriate approach to the management of this patient?

(A) Platelet concentrates should be given prophylactically to prevent bleeding.

(B) Whole blood should be administered to prevent bleeding.

(C) Gamma globulin and/or corticosteroid should be administered.

(D) Vitamin C should be administered.

(E) Vitamin K should be administered.

(F) Splenectomy

23 A 16-year-old male died yesterday. His father died from cancer before he was born, and his mother died from cancer a week ago, leaving the boy in a depressed state, and he confessed to his school psychologist that he wasn't sure life was worth living. However even prior to his mother's death he engaged in several antisocial activities. He was a member of a street gang that had recently been conducting a violent turf war with a rival gang; he smoked marijuana, snorted free base cocaine, and loved to drag race while high. Judging by public health statistics among adolescents and young adults between the ages of 15 and 24 years, his death yesterday most probably resulted from which of the following?

(A) Suicide
(B) Homicide
(C) Drug overdose
(D) Automobile accident
(E) Cancer

24 A young mother left her 3-year-old daughter alone in the kitchen while she answered the phone in an adjacent room. In the few minutes she was out of the room the child grabbed a hot frying pan sitting on the stove. The child started to wail and run in a circle waving her hand; the mother panicked, smeared butter on the burned hand and rushed the child to a nearby walk-in clinic. The physician in attendance examined the child and found that the child's thumb, index finger, and the palm of her right hand were red. There was also a 0.5 × 0.25 in (1.27 × 0.64 cm) blister at the base of her thumb and a smaller one on the tip of her index finger. No other injury could be ascertained. Which of the following is the most appropriate first course of action?

(A) Cool the burn site by immediately immersing the hand in ice-cold water

(B) Clean the area and dress it with gauze

(C) Aspirate the fluid underneath the blister

(D) Débride the wound, aspirate the fluid, and apply an antibiotic cream

(E) Provide tetanus prophylaxis

25 A 4-month-old infant is brought to the pediatrician by his mother because he has not been feeding well. The patient has been in his usual state of good health until 1 day earlier. The patient has not had fever and does not attend daycare. There are no ill contacts, pets, or recent travel. Physical examination of the mouth reveals curd-like plaques on the tongue and buccal mucosa that do not scrape off easily. Which of the following is the bodily area most likely to also be affected?

(A) Eyes

(B) Ears

(C) Nose

(D) Scalp

(E) Perineum

26 A 6-year-old female is brought to the pediatrician because of severe dysuria. The history is unremarkable except for the patient having a sore throat. There is no history of hematuria, fever, use of bubble bath, pinworms, tight clothing, nylon underwear, or recent medication. Inspection of the perineum reveals an intense erysipelas-like erythema of the vulva, distal vagina, and perineal area. A serosanguinous vaginal discharge is present. Which of the following is the most likely cause?

(A) *Haemophilus influenzae*

(B) *Neisseria gonorrhea*

(C) *Chlamydia trachomatis*

(D) Group A β-hemolytic streptococcus

(E) *Streptococcus pneumoniae*

27 Prospective parents seek counseling about the risk of having a child with schizophrenia. There is no history of the disease in her family, but an uncle and his son in the potential father's family have been diagnosed with the disease. Which of the following statements should be shared with these prospective parents?

(A) There is no evidence of a familial basis for the disease.

(B) The disease appears to be more prevalent in families that share certain patterns of interpersonal communication.

(C) Climate and season of birth will have no effect on the child's risk of developing the disease.

(D) The child's risk of developing the disease will be less than 10%, but greater than 1%.

(E) The mother should avoid eating wheat gluten during pregnancy.

28 A 27-year-old woman, nulligravida 0, and her 29-year-old husband come to the outpatient office with a 2-year history of infertility. They have been married for 4 years and have been trying for pregnancy for the past 2 years by having regular intercourse twice weekly without using any contraception since she discontinued oral contraceptive pills 48 months ago. They have not undergone any formal medical evaluation but desperately desire children. The family history for both partners is negative for genetic diseases or congenital anomalies. Which of the following causes of infertility would most likely be found in the workup?

(A) Ovulatory factor

(B) Cervical factor

(C) Uterine factor

(D) Tubal factor

(E) Male factor

29 A 32-year-old Mexican-American woman who lives in Phoenix, Arizona, presents with fever, nonproductive cough, flulike symptoms, chest pain, and painful red nodules on both lower extremities. Her hobby is collecting Indian artifacts found in the desert and in caves. A chest x-ray film shows a left lower lobe cavitation and a small pleural effusion. A mild eosinophilia is noted in the peripheral blood. Which of the following is the most likely diagnosis?

(A) Histoplasmosis

(B) *Klebsiella pneumoniae*

(C) Tuberculosis

(D) *Mycoplasma pneumoniae*

(E) Coccidioidomycosis

30 A nonsmoking 42-year-old woman consults her physician after finding a lump in her right breast. Upon examination the physician finds a painless, freely mobile, and well-circumscribed spherical growth with a rubbery consistency. On the basis of this examination he tells her that he is over 99% sure that this lump is due to benign fibrocystic disease, but just to make sure he would recommend a needle biopsy. The woman breathes a sigh of relieve saying she was so worried because her mother died from metastatic breast cancer at the age of 38 years; she thought that was particularly tragic because as a girl and young woman her mother had endured a life of hardship after her Jewish family escaped from eastern Poland when the Nazis

invaded in 1939. She then added: "Doctor I am sure glad that this lump is benign but what do you think my chance of developing a cancer is? Which of the following choices represents the most accurate assessment?

(A) Since she is an otherwise healthy Caucasian woman, she has between a 1 in 8 to 1 in 9 chance of developing a mammary cancer.

(B) She has better than a 44% chance of developing cancer.

(C) Because she is older now than her mother was when she died, she has little risk of developing an inherited form of cancer.

(D) Since she has fibrocystic disease, the probability of ever developing a breast malignancy is reduced.

(E) Since she doesn't smoke, the probability of developing breast cancer is reduced.

31 A 45-year-old woman has a history of many years of reclusiveness and peculiar fantasies about the lives of media celebrities. She does not have a history of hallucinations, delusions, or disorganized behavior. She refuses to interact with other people. There is a history of schizophrenia in two uncles. She has had a trial of antipsychotic medication that decreased her preoccupation with celebrities, but she refused to continue taking it. Which of the following is the most likely diagnosis?

(A) Avoidant personality disorder

(B) Obsessive–compulsive disorder

(C) Schizoid personality disorder

(D) Schizophrenia, residual type

(E) Schizotypal personality disorder

32 A 24-year-old Caucasian female makes an appointment to see an ophthalmologist; she complains that her eyes seep "thick, viscous, yellowish sticky stuff" that tends to mat her eyelashes, making it difficult for her to open her eyes in the morning. In addition, she says her eyes feel gritty when she blinks, and they appear to her to be "bloodshot"; the whites are a "pink-red" color, but they do not hurt, and her vision seems normal, although sometimes she has to wipe "gunk" away from her eyeball. Examination reveals a mild photophobia, a normal pupillary reaction to light, and normal intraocular pressure. This woman most likely has which of the following disorders?

(A) Acute viral conjunctivitis

(B) Optic neuritis

(C) Acute bacterial conjunctivitis

(D) Uveitis

(E) Central retinal artery occlusion

(F) Anterior blepharitis

33 A 30-year-old type 1 diabetic man who has a problem with alcohol is brought to the emergency department suffering from extreme fatigue, nausea, vomiting, abdominal pain and mental stupor. His breathing was rapid and shallow with the fruity odor of acetone. Physical examination reveals yellow papular lesions on the trunk and extremities and retinal vessels that have a milky appearance. Blood collected in a test tube has a milky appearance. A lipoprotein electrophoresis shows an increase in chylomicrons and very-low-density lipoproteins. Which type of hyperlipoproteinemia is present?

(A) Type I

(B) Type II

(C) Type III

(D) Type IV

(E) Type V

34 A 3-year-old child with sickle cell disease presents to the emergency department with a temperature of 40°C (104°F). The mother states that the child had been in his usual state of relatively good health until 4 hours ago. Starting at that time, the mother states that the child became progressively listless. Upon physical examination, the physician notes that the child has nuchal rigidity. The patient has no known ill contacts and takes no medication. Immunizations are up to date. A spinal tap would most likely reveal which of the following pathogens?

(A) *Streptococcus pneumoniae*

(B) Group B streptococcus

(C) *Escherichia coli*

(D) *Listeria monocytogenes*

(E) Group A β-hemolytic streptococcus

35 A 30-year-old woman recently back from a photographic safari trip to Tanzania presents with headache, fever with temperature spikes of 40.6°C (105°F), and scleral icterus. Physical examination reveals tender hepatosplenomegaly. Laboratory data show an increase in the liver transaminases. A complete blood cell count shows a normocytic anemia and an increased corrected reticulocyte count. A direct Coombs' test result is negative. Results of a urine dipstick test for blood are positive. A peripheral blood smear shows many red blood cells with one to three ringlike structures. Which of the following is the most likely diagnosis?

(A) Autoimmune hemolytic anemia

(B) Congenital spherocytosis

(C) Glucose-6-phosphate dehydrogenase (G6PD) deficiency

(D) Hemolytic anemia caused by pyruvate kinase deficiency

(E) *Plasmodium falciparum* malaria

36 A 65-year-old white female slipped and fell on an icy walkway. When seen in the emergency department, she complained of pain in the right hip, and had shortening and external rotation of the right leg. X-ray films confirmed a diagnosis of fractured neck of the femur, for which she underwent arthroplasty. Two days after surgery, she complained of difficulty breathing. On clinical examination, her vital signs were as follows: pulse, 88/min; temperature, 36.9°C (98.4°F); respiration, 18/min; and blood pressure, 130/90 mm Hg. She had distended jugular neck veins. Auscultation of the heart revealed a third heart sound, while that of the chest revealed bibasilar inspiratory crackles. In addition, she had dependent pitting edema. Results of a complete blood cell count including platelet count were normal. Which of the following is the most likely diagnosis?

(A) Endotoxic shock
(B) Cardiogenic shock
(C) Overzealous fluid resuscitation
(D) Fat embolism syndrome
(E) Syndrome of inappropriate antidiuretic hormone (SIADH)

37 A 29-year-old man with a 9-year history of alcoholism recently successfully completes an outpatient drug rehabilitation program. This was the second time he had "dried out." The previous time he vowed he would never touch a drop again but within a month after completing this second program he had "just one night out with the boys" and he starting drinking again. He was arrested for disorderly conduct and ordered to enter an inpatient drug rehabilitation program. He seeks advice about the most effective way to maintain sobriety after discharge. Which of the following is the most accurate advice?

(A) Take disulfiram before participating in a social situation in which he might expect to consume alcohol
(B) Take naltrexone before participating in a social situation, because one drink will make him nauseous
(C) Do not try to totally abstain from alcohol consumption, but rather limit consumption to socially appropriate amounts because this will keep the urge to drink within tolerable limits
(D) Have a definite number of drinks in mind before engaging in a social event involving alcohol
(E) Join a local chapter of Alcoholics Anonymous

Directions for Matching Questions (38 through 50): *Each set of matching questions is preceded by a list of 4 to 26 lettered options followed by a brief explanation of the required task and then by a series of numbered statements. For each lettered statement you are to select ONE lettered option that best fulfills the task as it relates to that statement. Remember each of the listed options might be correctly selected once, more than once, or not at all.*

Questions 38–44

(A) Cervical
(B) Ovarian
(C) Endometrial
(D) Vaginal
(E) Vulvar
(F) Oviduct

For each of the following numbered staging descriptions below, select the ONE most appropriate lettered gynecologic malignancy from the list above.

38 Has no official staging criteria

39 Is clinically staged

40 Has a staging category of IA2

41 Has the highest 5-year survival rate for stage I disease

42 Is epidemiologically considered a sexually transmitted disease

43 Has staging categories of IC, IIC, and IIIC

44 Has the highest overall mortality rate of all gynecologic cancers

Questions 45–50

(A) *Chlamydia trachomatis*
(B) *Chlamydia pneumoniae*
(C) *Rickettsia rickettsii*
(D) *Coxiella burnetii*
(E) *Ehrlichia chaffeensis*
(F) *Mycoplasma pneumoniae*

For each of the following numbered questions below, select the ONE most appropriate lettered organism from the list above.

45 A 13-year-old Boy Scout develops fever, headache, and nausea and vomiting 1 week after a summer camping trip in Oklahoma. Physical examination reveals a petechial rash on the palms. A complete blood cell count reveals absolute neutrophilic leukocytosis with >10% band neutrophils.

46 A 28-year-old man, who is sexually active, presents with tiny papular lesions without ulcerations around the genitals and painful inguinal lymph node adenopathy with draining sinuses.

47 A 64-year-old man with angina pectorales is diagnosed with atypical pneumonia.

48 A 9-year-old boy felt very ill and developed a fever, headache, and muscle pain accompanied by a nonproductive cough approximately 2 weeks after visiting a petting zoo where he was permitted to stroke a goat while she gave birth to six kids.

49 After returning from a hunting trip in eastern Texas, a 56-year-old man found that several "Lone Star" ticks *(Amblyomma americanus)* had dug into his skin. Some 9 days later he developed rigors and nausea, followed by fever, severe headache, and a pleomorphic rash that spared the palm of his hands. He recovered spontaneously.

50 The most common cause of atypical pneumonia

Answer Key

1 C	**11** C	**21** E	**31** E	**41** A
2 C	**12** E	**22** C	**32** C	**42** A
3 A	**13** B	**23** D	**33** E	**43** B
4 C	**14** B	**24** B	**34** A	**44** B
5 A	**15** C	**25** E	**35** E	**45** C
6 C	**16** B	**26** D	**36** C	**46** A
7 A	**17** D	**27** D	**37** E	**47** B
8 C	**18** A	**28** E	**38** F	**48** D
9 C	**19** G	**29** E	**39** A	**49** E
10 B	**20** C	**30** B	**40** A	**50** F

Answers and Explanations

1 The answer is C *Pediatrics*

Intussusception (choice **C**) is the most common cause of intestinal obstruction in children between 3 months and 6 years of age but decreases in frequency after 3 years. The cause is unknown, but it has been associated with gastroenteritis, Meckel's diverticulum, polyps, and sarcoma. Patients have paroxysmal colicky abdominal pain. A sausage-shaped mass can usually be palpated in the right upper abdomen, and bloody, currant-jelly stools are passed. Barium enema reveals a coil-spring sign and may even be therapeutic. However, the use of "air" enemas in the diagnosis and treatment of intussusception has supplanted hydrostatic reduction. If reduction is unsuccessful surgical reduction is necessary.

Pyloric stenosis (choice **B**) is characterized by nonbilious projectile vomiting in a 1- to 3-month-old. Meckel's diverticulum (choice **A**), usually presents as painless rectal bleeding, and symptoms usually arise within the first 2 years of life, but it is not uncommon for initial symptoms to be seen in the first decade. Meconium ileus (choice **D**) and necrotizing enterocolitis (choice **E**) both present in the neonatal period.

2 The answer is C *Preventive Medicine and Public Health*

In biologic systems a *P* value of less than .05 (i.e., the probability that random variation accounted for the difference between the two groups is less than 5 times out of 100) is commonly considered statistically significant; thus, a value of .04851 is statistically significant, meaning that it is unlikely that random variation accounted for the difference in diastolic blood pressure between the two groups (choice **C**).

However as important as this is, without further follow-up studies concerning the health of the participants, it does not prove that this effect is clinically significant (choice **A**). Choice **B** is incorrect for two reasons. First, clinical benefit cannot be determined on the basis of two sets of numbers that do not directly refer to a health-based parameter (e.g., were there significantly fewer myocardial infarcts among the salt-restricted cohort). Second, because as the choice is worded, potential significance would decrease as the *P* value does; that is: to make sense it should say the chance that an individual would benefit from a low-salt diet is more than 0.05%. If the number of subjects were increased (assuming that the means and the standard deviations of the groups remained the same), the *P* value would tend to be lower and would be more, rather than less, statistically significant (choice **D**). Since a 2000-mg diet provided a statistically significant difference, it obviously is not necessary to further reduce sodium intake to prove a statistical difference (choice **E**). In fact, reducing sodium further is liable to be counterproductive because a diet providing 1000 mg or less of sodium per day is difficult for most people to tolerate; thus, even in a prison population, compliance is apt to be low. In contrast, patients on a 2000 mg daily intake for 2 to 3 months often adapt to this diet and actually find excess salt to be unpleasant and often continue to voluntarily restrict salt intake.

3 The answer is A *Medicine*

The features described in the clinical vignette suggest that this boy has Marfan syndrome, a trait that is inherited as an autosomal dominant mutation in the fibrillin-1 gene and results in an aberrant fibrillin-1 protein (choice **A**). Marfan's syndrome is one of the most common connective tissue disorders, with an incidence of about 1 in 5000 births, and about 25% of these cases are due to new mutations. Fibrillin-1 is a major constituent in the elastic fibrillin microfilaments which provide both support and elasticity to connective tissue throughout the body. Persons with Marfan's syndrome may show a wide range of symptoms. Typically they are tall, with abnormally long arms (arm span is greater than height), long legs and fingers (arachnodactyly), and a rather long thin face. (Many believe that Abraham Lincoln expressed the typical phenotype.) In addition to this typical phenotype, affected individuals may show a wide variety of other symptoms, some of which lead to physical weakness and lack of stamina as in the case described. These symptoms may include mitral valve prolapse, aortic root dilation, pectus excavation, scoliosis, joint dislocations, pneumothorax (due to the collapse of a lung), and ectopic lentis. Mitral valve prolapse is the most common symptom (85% of cases); it may eventually contribute to early heart failure and is likely responsible for the unusual heart sounds heard in the patient described. Although heart failure may be responsible for the early demise of Marfan patients; aortic root dilation resulting in eventual dissection is the most common fatal consequence of Marfan syndrome. Prophylactic administration of a β-blocker to slow the heart rate and lower blood pressure is used to help delay expansions of the aorta, and expansion is screened for by annual or even biannual echocardiograms. Once the aortic diameter expands beyond a certain critical diameter, prophylactic surgery can be performed. Similarly, the mitral valve can be surgically replaced if needed. As a consequence, life expectancy of treated Marfan patients is now similar to that of the general population. The major reason for the great variation in symptoms among Marfan patients is that at the molecular level Marfan syndrome is many diseases. The fibril-1 gene is large with 65 exons, and a 1997 study found 85 different mutations among 94 unrelated patients. To add further variety to the mix, even in a given family there can be major differences in the degree that different tissues are affected, presumably because of the nature of other structural connective tissue proteins.

Epidermolysis bullosa (EB) is a constellation of conditions resulting in skin that blisters with minimal trauma. EB is relatively rare; the reported incidence varies from 1 case per 10^6 births in the United States to 54 cases per 10^6 births in Norway. On the physiologic level the common feature of the various forms of EB is a weak connection between the upper and deeper layers of the skin due to aberrant supportive proteins. The worst cases result in death during infancy due to sepsis caused by bacterial invasion. Three major types are recognized: EB simplex (92% of cases), junctional EB (1%) and dystrophic EB (5%); the remaining 2% of cases are unclassified. EB simplex is due to mutations in either keratin 5 or 14 (choice **B**) proteins that form intermediate filaments in basal keratinocytes. A deficiency of, or defects in, these proteins make these cells prone to cytolysis.

Alport syndrome causes inherited kidney disease coupled to extrarenal complications, including sensorial deafness and eye abnormalities and is due to mutations in one of the several genes coding for type IV collagen (choice **C**). Type IV collagen is the major structural component of basement membranes, where it provides a framework for the binding of other basement membrane components and is a substratum for cells. Type IV collagen has the typical collagen triple-stranded structure, and the individual strands are coded for by one or more of six different genes, *COL4A1* through *COL4A6*. About 85% of the cases of Alport syndrome are due to mutations in *COL4A5* located on the X-chromosome. Males with mutations in this gene present with hematuria in infancy, which then progresses to uremic syndrome and end-stage renal disease by the second or third decade. Females are also affected, causing the disease to be classified as X-linked dominant; however, the course of the disease is less severe, and they often die at a normal age without developing end-stage renal disease. *COL4A6* is also located on the X-chromosome, but mutations are less common and are associated with leiomyomatosis in epidermal cells. *COL4A3* and *COL4A4* are located on chromosome 2, and mutations in these genes cause an autosomal recessive form of Alport syndrome. *COL4A1* and *COL4A2* are located on chromosome 13, mutations in these genes cause less than 1% of cases of Alport syndrome, and these are inherited as autosomal dominant traits.

Type I collagen (choice **D**) is composed of 2 α1 and 1 α2 peptides wound in the typical triple-stranded helix. It is the most abundant of the collagens and provides tensile strength to bone and tendons. Any of a number of mutations in either the *COL1A1* or *COL1A2* genes causes osteogenesis imperfecta, a heterogeneous group of conditions generally characterized by easily broken bones, loose and easily torn tendons, and in most cases (about 98%) blue sclera caused by a thin translucent cornea. Although at a molecular level one can describe scores of mutations, clinically they are classified into three or four subtypes. The three major clinical variants are: type I, the most common and least severe form; type II, generally fatal in utero or during the neonatal period; and type III, with severe consequences resulting in deformed limbs and dwarfism. Type I is inherited as an autosomal dominant trait, while types II and III are almost always either new mutations (which if affected individuals were to reproduce would be transmitted in an autosomal dominant manner) or are inherited as recessive traits; the latter likely result from mutations in enzymes that catalyze posttranslational modifications of procollagen. Many investigators also recognize type IV, an uncommon variant similar to type I but in which the sclera are not affected, while others lump these together with the type I cases.

Stickler syndrome is caused by aberrant type XI collagen (choice **E**) or type II collagen due to mutations in the *COL11A1*, *COL11A2*, or *COL2A1* genes that can be inherited as autosomal dominant traits. Affected individuals demonstrate a wide variety of symptoms ranging from subtle to severe. Type XI and type II collagens have a similar tissue distribution and primarily are found in joints, including the temporomandibular, and spinal column, the inner ear, and vitreous fluid of the eye. Persons with Stickler syndrome are generally characterized by a flattened facial appearance caused by underdevelopment of the bones of the middle of the face including the cheekbones and the bridge of the nose. The syndrome may also include cleft palate, myopia, glaucoma, retinal detachment, hearing loss, hypermobile joints, and early-onset osteoarthritis.

Mutations in *FGFR1* or *FGFR2*, the genes that code for the fibroblast growth factor receptor (choice **F**) cause Pfeiffer syndrome, an autosomal dominant condition characterized by premature fusion of skull bones (craniosynostosis), brachydactyly (flat broad thumbs and big toes facing away from the other digits) and syndactyly (webbing between digits). Type I Pfeiffer syndrome may be caused by mutations in either the *FGFR1* or *FGFR2* gene. These mutations cause early maturation of osteoclasts during embryogenesis, resulting in premature fusion of bones in the skull, hands, and feet. Although the craniosynostosis causes an unusual facies with bulging wide-set eyes, an underdeveloped upper jaw, and a peaked nose, most individuals with type I Pfeiffer syndrome have normal intelligence and normal life spans. However, persons with type 2 or 3 Pfeiffer syndrome, always due to mutations in *FGFR2*, suffer more-severe symptoms, often involving the nervous system.

4 The answer is C *Psychiatry*

The symptoms are most suggestive of delirium, which is characterized by disturbances of awareness or attention, cognitive problems, rapid onset, and fluctuations in severity. Associated findings such as hallucinations and persecutory ideation are common. Although possible physiologic causes include L-dopa or anticholinergic toxicity and alcohol withdrawal, no definitive information suggesting a cause is provided. As a consequence, the most specific diagnosis possible is delirium of unknown cause (choice **C**). Patients who are elderly or who have preexisting dementia are much more likely to develop delirium.

Dementias, such as alcohol-induced dementia (choice **A**) or dementia due to Parkinson's disease (choice **D**), would usually present with a history of increasing cognitive problems; however, this patient has no previous history of psychiatric problems. Alcohol-induced psychotic disorder (choice **B**) or mood disorder due to Parkinson's disease (choice **E**) would not be diagnosed in the presence of cognitive problems such as inattention, confusion, and disorientation.

5 The answer is A *Medicine*

Bell's palsy (choice **A**) is idiopathic and nearly always acute. All the patient's deficits are referable to the peripheral nervous system, including the loss of taste (chorda tympani branch of the facial nerve) and hyperacusis (branch of the stapedius muscle of the ear).

The strokes (choices **C** and **D**) are unlikely, because of sparing of the rest of the right side of the body and no other central signs. Although brainstem glioma (choice **B**) and parotid tumor (choice **E**) commonly present with facial nerve weakness, they are unlikely choices considering the sudden onset of the event.

6 The answer is C *Psychiatry*

This patient's symptoms are most suggestive of agoraphobia, which is characterized by a fear of experiencing panic attacks in a place where help would be unavailable. Agoraphobic symptoms are almost always associated with panic disorder (choice **C**), and rarely occur without a history of panic attacks.

Patients with panic disorder often have moderate depressive symptoms (not major depressive symptoms [choice **A**]) as a result of frustration with their condition. Obsessive–compulsive disorder (choice **B**) is characterized by irrational thoughts and urges. Schizophrenia (choice **D**) may present with social withdrawal but also includes psychotic symptoms. Somatization disorder (choice **E**) is characterized by multiple physical complaints.

7 The answer is A *Medicine*

The high blood glucose value, coupled to the boy's age, the fruity breath smell (ketosis), lethargic behavior, and thin physique all point to type 1 diabetes mellitus. That he seems ketotic and lethargic suggests that treatment should be started as soon as possible, and the only treatment for type 1 diabetes is insulin (choice **A**). Naturally a decision should first be made concerning dosage and type of insulin to use, and arrangements must be made to ensure that the possibility of any adverse reaction will be rapidly monitored and addressed.

The American Diabetes Association (ADA) criteria for diagnosing diabetes are any one of the following: (1) one fasting blood value exceeding 125 mg/dL, (2) one random plasma glucose value exceeding 199 mg/dL in the presence of symptoms, or (3) a 2-hour plasma value exceeding 199 mg/dL in an oral glucose tolerance test. Thus choice **B** is incorrect because he meets the ADA diagnostic criterion 2.

Choice **C** the mother was right to suspect the boy inherited diabetes from either his father or grandmother is not correct because the ages of onset indicate that both these relatives have type 2 diabetes. Whereas the risk of contracting type 2 diabetes increases if first-degree family members have the disease, the pathophysiologic mechanisms responsible for type 1 are entirely different, and in terms of inheritance, it is an entirely different disease.

Type 2 diabetes is typically part of the so-called metabolic syndrome characterized by abdominal obesity, hypertension, hyperlipidemia, insulin resistance, and only eventually hyperglycemia. Insulin resistance appears in some way related to the influence of obesity on PPARγ; this is indicated by the facts that some degree of obesity is almost always a precursor event and that the drug thiazolidine lowers blood glucose levels by decreasing insulin resistance via a mechanism involving its interaction with PPARγ. However this boy has type 1 diabetes, which typically is associated with a thin not an obese physique (choice **D**). (PPAR was first discovered as a factor that enhanced peroxisome proliferation and was named the *peroxisome proliferator active receptor* [PPAR]. It was since discovered that there is a super-family of different PPARs all acting as transcription factors when they interact with the proper ligand. PPARγ is the family member implicated as a player in the metabolic syndrome.)

Type I diabetes results from an immunologic reaction that makes the pancreatic β cells incapable of synthesizing insulin; as a consequence endogenous levels fall to zero. The oral antihyperglycemics either increase the ability of the pancreas to secrete insulin more effectively or increase the ability of peripheral cells to use circulating insulin more efficiently. As a consequence, for these oral agents to work, the pancreas must retain the ability to synthesize and secrete some insulin. Since this ability is lost in type I diabetes, oral antihyperglycemic agents cannot be used to treat patients with this disease (choice **E**).

8 The answer is C *Medicine*

Assuming a general state of good health, the present return-to-play recommendation for athletes participating in contact sports who are recovering from infectious mononucleosis is that if the athlete has no splenomegaly or fever, results of liver function tests are normal, and all complications have resolved, he or she may return to contact sports 4 weeks after the onset of symptoms. Since in the case described symptoms started only 2 weeks ago, he needs to wait an additional 2 weeks before he could be given permission, and therefore in 2 weeks he should return for another check-up (choice **C**), and assuming he still is symptom free, he can get clearance to play.

He cannot return to football immediately simply because he feels fine 2 weeks after symptoms began (choice **A**); a possible complication is splenic rupture, which ensues in 0.1–0.2% of cases; the rupture can be spontaneous or trauma related. Rupture only occurs in enlarged spleens, and spleen enlargement may occur between days 4 to 21 after the onset of symptomatic illness; thus a final physical examination is essential no earlier than 4 weeks after the first symptoms. He should return next week for another check-up and possible clearance to play (choice **B**) is incorrect since at this time only 3 weeks will have passed since symptom onset. Had he been participating in a noncontact sport, this would have been a permissible time interval. Approximately 10% of individuals with infectious mononucleosis will not develop a negative mono-spot test result (tests heterophile antibodies); therefore, a negative result should not be grounds for sending him back to play football (choice **D**). In those with a positive test result, it can take anywhere from 1 week to 52 weeks before becoming undetectable. A normal lymphocyte count is not assurance that all complications have resolved or that splenomegaly is not present (choice **E**). There is no reason to keep him from playing football for the remainder of the season (choice **F**), provided he passes the 4-week physical.

9 The answer is C *Preventive Medicine and Public Health*

Assuming a normal distribution, the mean ± 2 standard deviations describes the range in which it can be expected that 95% of repeated observations or determinations would fall. In the scenario described (with a mean of 20 and a standard deviation of 2), the normal range would be 20 ± 4, or 16 to 24 (choice **C**).

Choices **A, B, D,** and **E** are incorrect ranges.

10 The answer is B *Surgery*

Shock is a condition in which peripheral blood flow is compromised, depriving cells of adequate oxygen supply. Several different conditions can cause shock, but there is commonality in the symptoms produced. By the time she is seen by the physician, the patient described is suffering from toxic shock syndrome (TSS) (choice **B**) due to failure to remove the tampon over the course of some 4 days. The early phase, including high temperature, rash, hypertension, and warm skin, reflects the inflammatory effects of toxins caused by bacteria growing in the tampon. In TSS this phase generally lasts some 30 minutes and is then followed by the more typical symptoms of shock due to a toxin-induced shut-down of the vascular system. These typical shock symptoms include: pale or grey skin that is cold and clammy to the touch, tachycardia with weak heart sounds, swallow-rapid breathing, hypotension, lack of focus and confusion, and perhaps delirium. In the 1980s there was a small epidemic of TSS associated with a specific brand of "super-absorbant" tampons that allegedly could be left in place for an extended period. Since that brand was removed from the market, the condition has become much less common and occurs in response to factors other than tampons more often than in menstruating women who use tampons. The hypothesis regarding tampon-induced TSS is that when women leave tampons in place for a long time they may become infected with *Staphylococcus aureus,* which breed in the tampons and produce toxins that induce septic shock. The tampons are a perfect growth medium; the environment is warm and moist, and the blood is a rich source of nutrients. Moreover while in the tampon the bacteria cannot be affected by the normal physiologic defense mechanisms and are even largely immune from the influence of antibiotics.

Hypovolemic shock (choice **A**) can be caused by loss of blood (either externally as by a wound or internally as in gastrointestinal bleeding or a fractured femur) or by dehydration from loss of fluid from extravascular compartments as in vomiting or diarrhea. The symptoms are the same as those described for the patient in shock in the case above, but the onset of shock would not be preceded by the early reaction to toxins. Cardiogenic shock (choice **C**) occurs when the supply of blood to peripheral tissues falls below a critical level because of inadequate pumping ability of the heart. The symptoms again are as those described above, and the condition may be caused by a myocardial infarct, heart failure, cardiac arrhythmias, or cardiac tamponade. Anaphylactic shock (choice **D**) is caused by an allergic reaction to any of a host of potential allergins. As in TSS, shock is preceded by a brief inflammatory period. However, there is no reason to suspect an allergic reaction in the case presented. Shock caused by a gram-negative organism (choice **E**) would represent classic septic shock likely caused by an ingested pathogen or infection from gastrointestinal or urinary tract pathogens. As in TSS and anaphylactic shock, the onset of shock is preceded by a brief inflammatory period. However, gram-negative bacteria are rarely, if ever, associated with tampon-induced shock.

11 The answer is C *Obstetrics and Gynecology*

The scenario describes the clinical findings frequently noted with twin–twin transfusion syndrome (TTTS). TTTS occurs with a shared placenta when an artery from one twin delivers blood to the vein of the other. The recipient twin receives much more blood and because of the increased volume, the recipient twin can develop volume overload (choice **C**). This may result in heart failure and hydropic changes.

Because the recipient twin receives much more blood and becomes polycythemic and plethoric, the recipient twin, not the donor twin (choice **A**), is at higher risk for hyperbilirubinemia. Such placental vascular anastomoses occur with high frequency only in monochorionic (monozygotic) twins, thus are not the result of dizygotic (dichorionic) (choice **B**) pregnancies from ovulation induction (choice **D**). Twins of opposite genders (choice **E**) always are found with dichorionic, diamniotic placentation, consequently TTTS virtually always occurs in twins of the same gender.

12 The answer is E *Psychiatry*

Clozapine monitoring requires weekly white blood cell (WBC) counts (choice **E**) because of an associated 1% risk of agranulocytosis. Sedation and sialorrhea (drooling) are common untoward effects of clozapine treatment.

Clozapine and divalproex levels (choices **A** and **D**) may have clinical significance but are not as immediately required in this patient's treatment. There are no short-term indications in this case for prolactin level determinations (choice **B**) or thyroid function tests (choice **C**).

13 **The answer is B** *Preventive Medicine and Public Health*

Individuals commonly wish to assure they will have a voice in determining what medical treatment they are to receive if they become mentally incapacitated. To do this they create a legal document called an advanced directive. There are two not mutually exclusive types of advanced directives, living wills, and durable powers of attorney for health care. In the latter case, a person while demonstrably of sound mind draws up a legal document in which a person is named to make medical decisions for the patient to be should he/she become mentally incompetent. The person named in such a durable power of attorney (choice **B**) becomes the legal surrogate for a mentally incapacitated patient and the physician must turn to him/her for permission to perform any medical procedure.

A living will (choice **A**), the other type of advanced directive, is a legal document that persons, while still of sound mind, have drawn up to express their wishes for medical treatment should they become mentally incapacitated. Since nobody can predict if they will become mentally incapacitated and what medical problems they will have if they do, such a document needs to be drawn up in general terms (e.g., "I wish to have every conceivable life support measure available used to keep me alive before I am declared dead"). Specifics, such as a knee operation, have to be dealt with as they arise, by a rational being; that being the person named in the durable power of attorney. The director of the patient's managed care organization (choice **C**) may have some practical input in determining the cost–benefit ratio in providing health care but has no legal right to determine whether or not a patient receives any particular treatment. A state's involuntary treatment law (choice **D**) could only be invoked when a patient is a danger to self or others. For a patient's signature on an informed consent form (choice **E**) to have a legal impact, he or she must be of sound mind. If the patient is mentally incapacitated, the person named in a durable power of attorney has the right and obligation to sign, or not sign, the informed consent form. In the absence of a durable power of attorney, a close relative or, in extreme cases, a state representative may sign the informed consent form. However, it is not unheard of for persons to quarrel over who has that right and what should be done, particularly if money is involved in the outcome.

14 **The answer is B** *Medicine*

This patient has clinical and electrocardiographic (ECG) evidence of hypercalcemia. The hypercalcemia is due to the production of osteoclast-activating factor by myeloma cells in the bone marrow. The ECG shows shortening of the QT interval (0.28–0.3), which is the characteristic finding in hypercalcemia. Neuropsychiatric findings in hypercalcemia involve personality changes, confusion, depression, acute psychosis, or coma. Cardiovascular changes include hypertension, potentiation of cardiac glycosides, and shortening of the QT interval. Gastrointestinal signs and symptoms consist of nausea, constipation, peptic ulcer disease (calcium stimulates gastrin release), and acute pancreatitis. Pseudogout can occur in the joints. Metastatic calcification in the kidney produces nephrocalcinosis (calcification in the basement membranes of the tubules), which produces polyuria, natriuresis (leading to volume contraction), and problems with urine concentration. Saline infusion (choice **B**) is the first step in management of hypercalcemia because it corrects volume contraction, which is a stimulus for further calcium reabsorption, and enhances calciuresis.

Once hydration is achieved, a loop diuretic (e.g., furosemide [choice **D**]) is added to potentiate the calciuresis. If saline administration and furosemide are ineffective or if chronic hypercalcemia is anticipated, a number of other options are available. Bisphosphonates are particularly useful in malignancy-induced hypercalcemia because they inhibit bone resorption. Corticosteroids are recommended in hypercalcemia associated with hypervitaminosis D, sarcoidosis, hematologic malignancies, and breast cancer. Mithramycin (choice **E**), an antineoplastic antibiotic, is generally effective but requires close monitoring because of its toxicity. Calcitonin is only effective for 1 or 2 weeks; then, hypercalcemia reappears. Sodium bicarbonate (choice **C**) and calcium gluconate (choice **A**) are useful in the treatment of hyperkalemia, not hypercalcemia.

15 **The answer is C** *Medicine*

The symptoms described suggest giant cell arteritis, also known as temporal arthritis. This is a systemic condition affecting medium-sized and large arteries throughout the body but having the greatest propensity to involve the temporal artery. It is a disease of the aged, with a mean onset in the 70s, and it affects women more often than men. The symptoms are as those described; however, up to 40% of patients have additional symptoms, including cardiac irregularities, thoracic aorta aneurysms and respiratory problems. The nature of these symptoms depends upon which other arteries are involved; in fact classic polymyalgia rheumatica and classic temporal arteritis are believed to be the opposite extremes of a continuum of conditions due to the same underlying cause, with many patients showing symptoms of both entities. In both conditions an exceedingly high ESR (choice **C**) is almost diagnostic. In temporal arteritis ESR values are over 50 mm/h in more than 90% of patients and often exceed 100 mm/h (although the exact value is laboratory specific the normal rates are usually considered to be less than 10 mm/h for males and less than 15 mm/h for females). Although the ESR is increased in most inflammatory conditions, the magnitude of the increase is rarely this great; thus the sensitivity is good but not perfect since about 5% of affected individuals provide false-negative values with ESR values below 40 mm/h. C-reactive protein and interleukine-6, other sensitive markers of inflammation, are also increased, and particularly the latter may prove to be even more sensitive than the ESR; however, the test is more expensive and not widely available and available data are limited. The definitive diagnosis is made by temporal artery biopsy. Treatment with a corticosteroid must be started immediately to prevent blindness even before laboratory of biopsy results are available.

A complete blood count (CBC) (choice **A**) is of limited value. The most significant finding will be a normal white cell count, which will rule out infection and some other inflammatory conditions. A computed tomography (CT) study of her head (choice **B**), a carotid ultrasound study (choice **D**), or a lumbar puncture with subsequent culture (choice **E**) will contribute little to the diagnosis.

16 **The answer is B** *Psychiatry*

The symptoms are most suggestive of schizophrenia. Sophisticated studies of cerebral morphology and functional neuroimaging in schizophrenia have yielded some fairly consistent findings, including decreased metabolic activity in the prefrontal cortex (choice **B**).

Such studies have also found decreased cerebral asymmetry (not increased, choice **D**), decreased size of the corpus callosum (not increased, choice **E**), and increased size of the lateral ventricles (not decreased, choice **C**). Abnormalities of dopaminergic transmission (choice **A**) are not currently measurable with functional neuroimaging. While several abnormalities of dopamine metabolism in schizophrenia have been reported using other experimental techniques, none are found consistently.

17 **The answer is D** *Pediatrics*

Cow's milk is not recommended for children until they are 1 year of age because the high level of protein (choice **D**) causes an increased solute load to the kidneys. It is this overload that led to the lethargic, dehydrated state of the 2-month-old infant.

Linoleic acid (choice **A**), linolenic acid (choice **B**), calcium (choice **C**), and B-complex vitamins (choice **E**) are not present in high concentrations in cow's milk and would not be expected to cause the symptoms noted in this patient.

18 **The answer is A** *Medicine*

A deficiency of uroporphyrinogen I synthetase activity (aka porphobilinogen deaminase) is inherited as an autosomal dominant trait and is responsible for a disease known as acute intermittent proporphyria. This disease is characterized by intermittent bouts of acute gastrointestinal attacks causing extreme pain; sometimes during one of these sessions (which in some patients last for an extended period) there is also constipation, urinary retention, hypertension, and neurologic symptoms that may include neuropathies, seizures, and psychotic episodes. The neural problems are likely caused by hyponatremia, which is in part caused by inappropriate release of antidiuretic hormone and in part due to gastrointestinal loss. After standing, the urine voided during an attack turns dark to a color sometimes described as muddy reddish or purplish. Uroporphyrinogen I synthetase catalyzes the condensation of four molecules of porphobilinogen to form uroporphyrinogen III, the first ring product in heme synthesis. Because uroporphyrinogen I synthetase activity is inadequate during an attack, the substrate, porphobilinogen, accumulates and is excreted in the urine (choice **A**); a finding considered to provide the definitive diagnosis. Although this disease is autosomal dominant, its penetrance is low, and the disease may appear to skip generations. Clinical symptoms are most commonly reported by women beginning in their teens or 20s. Presumably the intermittent nature of the condition reflects the fact that the uroporphyrinogen I synthetase activity inherited from the nonaffected parent is borderline sufficient, and attacks only occur when triggered by some factor that causes a need for greater activity. Such known precipitating factors include a long list of drugs, most, if not all, of which share the property of being metabolized by the P450 heme (cytochrome) system. The implied mechanism is that activation of the P450 enzymes reduces the availability of free heme, a feedback inhibitor of heme synthesis; this releases the heme synthesis sequence of reactions from partial inhibition and produces porphobilinogen at an accelerated rate, producing it faster than the limited activity of the remaining uroporphyrinogen I synthetase activity can use it. Among the drugs that induce an attack are barbiturates, commonly used in test questions as an example, and the estrogens, used as an example in the case presented. However, in addition to being triggered by drugs, attacks are also induced by infections and caloric deprivation (used as an ancillary precipitating factor in the vignette). An acute attack can be life threatening, and emergency treatment by intravenous hematin (an inhibitor of the first step in heme synthesis) and glucose coupled with administration of an analgesic that is not metabolized by the P450 system is often used as the first line of treatment. Long-term treatment is avoidance of known precipitating factors and maintenance on a high-carbohydrate diet, at least 300 g of carbohydrate per day.

Uroporphyrin (choice **B**) accumulates in porphyria cutanea tarda, a condition caused by an inherited deficiency of uroporphyrin decarboxylase; this is the most common of the porphyrias. Uroporphyrinogen I (choice **C**) and coproporphyrinogen I (choice **D**) accumulate in the urine of patients with congenital erythropoietic porphyria, a disease in which uroporphyrinogen III cosynthetase activity is lacking. Coproporphyrinogen III (choice **E**) accumulates in hereditary coproporphyria because of a deficiency of coproporphyrinogen oxidase. Congenital erythropoietic porphyria is inherited as an autosomal recessive trait, the rest of the porphyrias as autosomal dominant conditions. In each of the diseases described with respect to choices **B, C, D,** and **E,** the intermediates that accumulate have the hemelike tetrapyrrole structure, and consequently, patients are photosensitive. This sensitivity is thought to be due to superoxide free radicals produced via the reaction of the tetrapyrrole compound with oxygen in a reaction catalyzed by ultraviolet light. Note that acute intermittent proporphyria is the only porphyria that is not light sensitive, because a tetrapyrrole compound does not accumulate. Lead (choice **F**) is an extremely toxic heavy metal with an affinity for SH groups. As a consequence it inhibits several enzymes, two of which are involved in heme synthesis—δ-aminolevulinic synthase, the first and rate-limiting enzyme in heme synthesis, and ferrochelatase, the last enzyme. Consequently, lead poisoning, among other effects, causes a microcytic anemia.

19 The answer is G *Surgery*

In the United States, primary bladder cancer is the second most common urologic cancer, with some 50,000 new cases per year. Of these, 98% are epithelial malignancies, and 90% of these are transitional cell carcinomas (choice **G**). Adenocarcinomas account for about 2% of cases, and squamous cell cancers constitute about 7%. However, squamous cell carcinoma is the most common type in countries such as Egypt and Sudan, where urinary schistosomiasis due to infestation with *Schistosoma hematobium* is endemic. Consequently, choice **A** is incorrect; the most common type of cancer is not the same worldwide.

About 66% of all transitional cell carcinomas in the United States are believed to be caused by smoking tobacco; in fact, there is little evidence suggesting that carcinogens found in smoked foods (choice **B**) causes bladder cancer. However, workers in the dye, chemical, rubber, and leather industries have a higher prevalence of bladder cancer than the general public because of exposure to aniline-based dyes and organic solvents. One hopes that enforcement of rules laid down by the Environmental Protection Agency (EPA) has caused these to decrease.

Cancers that have not invaded deeply into the bladder wall, such as the one described in this case are removed by cystoscopic resection. However, without further treatment, 50–75% of patients will suffer a recurrence of the condition within 3 years (choice **C** is incorrect). As a consequence, immuno- and/or chemotherapeutic agents are delivered directly into the bladder by catheter after resection. Since the condition described has not invaded deeper layers of the bladder wall, it is unlikely to be treated by radical cystectomy (choice **D**). Such a procedure involves removal of the prostate as well as the bladder in men and the ovaries, uterus, and a portion of the vagina in women. Pelvic pain and difficulty in voiding urine are signs generally associated with more advanced cases of bladder cancer and are usually not the earliest signs (choice **E**). Hematuria, pelvic pain, and voiding difficulties are also common signs of cystitis; therefore both conditions must be carefully considered in making a diagnosis. Bladder cancer is about four times more prevalent in men than in women (choice **F**), and the mean age at the time of diagnosis is 65-years (choice **H**).

20 **The answer is C** *Psychiatry*

In malingering (choice **C**), the patient deliberately produces complaints in the presence of external incentives, such as money. These external incentives are sometimes referred to as secondary gains.

Symptoms in factitious disorder (choice **B**) also are deliberately produced (i.e., made up, self-inflicted, dramatically exaggerated); however, the motivation is not external but internal, so that the patient can assume the sick role, which is sometimes referred to as a primary gain. Symptoms in conversion disorder (choice **A**) are not volitionally produced and involve a loss of sensory or motor function. A person who has pain disorder (choice **D**) experiences actual pain that is largely mediated by psychologic factors. In somatization disorder (choice **E**), there are multiple somatic complaints. Individuals with somatization disorder do not deliberately produce their symptoms for external incentives or to assume the sick role.

21 **The answer is E** *Pediatrics*

Familial, or X-linked, hypophosphatemia (also know as vitamin D–resistant rickets) is the most common non-nutritional form of rickets. It is X-linked dominant, so some mothers as well as fathers may have clinical manifestations of the disease. Hypophosphatemia occurs because of defects in the proximal renal tubular reabsorption of phosphate caused by failure in the conversion of 25-(OH)-vitamin D to 1,25-(OH)$_2$-vitamin D. Bowing of the legs is a common presentation. In addition, these children may have a waddling gait (choice **E**) and short stature. Calcium levels in blood are normal, and thus there is no associated tetany, myopathy, or secondary hyperparathyroidism. Treatment consists of supplementation with phosphate and calcitriol. Two syndromes often confused with X-linked hypophosphatemia are vitamin D-dependent rickets type I and receptor-deficient rickets (formally vitamin D deficient rickets type II). Neither consistently causes hypophosphatemia, and they are autosomal recessive conditions.

Tetany (choice **A**), rachitic rosary (choice **B**), Harrison's groove (pectus deformity) (choice **C**), and myopathy (choice **D**) are present in calcium-deficient rickets. Classic vitamin D–deficiency rickets has become rare in developed countries because of food supplementation and styles that bare much of the body to the sun.

22 **The answer is C** *Pediatrics*

This patient has idiopathic (autoimmune) thrombocytopenic purpura (ITP). ITP is the most common thrombocytopenic purpura of childhood. The disease usually follows a viral infection. The infection seems to trigger an immune mechanism that starts platelet destruction. This destruction is manifested as sudden onset of bruising and petechiae. Other than this condition, the patient looks well. Bleeding into tissues can occur. Platelet counts are depressed, and bleeding time is prolonged, but the white blood cell (WBC) count is normal. Platelet antibodies are commonly seen. Bone marrow examination reveals normal megakaryocytes. The disease is self-limited, with resolution of the petechiae over 1 or 2 weeks, although thrombocytopenia may persist longer. The prognosis for ITP is excellent. Most patients recover within 2 or 3 months. Approximately 90% of children regain normal platelet counts within 9 to 12 months. In cases of mild thrombocytopenic purpura, with no hemorrhages of the retina or mucous membranes, therapy may not be appropriate. However, therapy with intravenous (IV) gamma globulin infusions and/or corticosteroid therapy (choice **C**) can be beneficial. IV gamma globulin infusions induce a sustained rise in platelet counts, while corticosteroid therapy reduces the severity and shortens the duration of the initial phase.

Splenectomy (choice **F**) should be reserved for those patients with chronic thrombocytopenic purpura or severe cases not responding to therapy. Platelet concentrates (choice **A**) are recommended only in life-threatening situations because their short life span is reflected by the temporary nature of the rise in platelet count. Vitamins C (choice **D**) and K (choice **E**) will not ameliorate the disease. The patient's complete blood count (CBC) is normal except for the platelet count. Therefore, it is not necessary to administer whole blood (choice **B**), which should only be used emergently for hypovolemia due to blood loss.

23 **The answer is D** *Preventive Medicine and Public Health*

Accidents are the most common cause of death in youths between the ages of 15 and 24 years, and 75% of these accidents occur in automobiles (choice **D**).

Generally speaking, suicide (choice **A**) and homicide (choice **B**) are the second and third leading causes of death among such youths. Although suicide is a major factor in early death in this age group, and suicidal thoughts are common, actual suicides are uncommon because the overall death rate in this group is so low. In some surveys, homicide is second, and suicide is third. This appears to reflect the group surveyed. In most middle- and upper-class neighborhoods adolescent homicide is almost unheard of. In contrast, homicide is all too common in neighborhoods permeated by gangs. Drug overdose (choice **C**) is a less common cause of death in youths than accidents, suicide, and homicide, although use of drugs, alcohol in particular, is a major contributor to deaths in automobile accidents. In this age group, death from any disease, including cancer (choice **E**), is rare.

24 **The answer is B** *Surgery*

This child suffered first- and second-degree burns on her hand and fingers. The first-degree burns are indicated by the reddened area, second-degree burns by the blisters. The primary treatment should be gently cleaning the burned area with a cool, not cold, antiseptic solution, applying a topical antibiotic, and dressing the injured area with a nonadherent dressing (choice **B**). Following that, a conforming protective material should be applied. The mother suffered from shock at seeing her child suffer and guilt at leaving her unattended and needs to be reassured that luckily the child's burns are minor and should heal without scarring in the course of a couple of weeks. She should also be informed that application of butter or any other greasy substance is not suitable treatment because it traps the heat of the burn, possibly making it worse. She ought to also be advised that a better course of action in the event of any serious accident is to call 911 rather than rush off to a walk-in clinic.

Cooling the burn site by immediately immersing the hand in ice cold water (choice **A**) introduces a risk of compromising circulation to marginally surviving areas of the burn and should not be done for any burn more serious than a first-degree one. For burns covering an extensive area such cooling also creates a risk of hypothermia. On the other hand, washing relatively nonextensive first- or second-degree burns with cool water, about 60–80°F (15–25°C), eases the pain. Most authorities believe the blister should be left intact as long as possible because the skin of a natural blister may act as a natural dressing, protecting the wound against infection and reducing the amount of pain; consequently, choice **C** (aspirate the fluid underneath the blister) and choice **D** (débride the wound, aspirate the fluid, and apply an antibiotic cream) are incorrect. In addition to cooling to reduce pain, an oral analgesia such as acetaminophen (not aspirin) should be provided. Tetanus prophylaxis (choice **E**) is important in all patients with burns in whom the skin is or may be broken. Thus if this child's tetanus immunization is not up to date, it should be brought up to date. The best course of action in this particular case would be to contact and inform the child's regular physician of the accident and treatment, to determine the child's immunization status, and to arrange for a follow-up appointment either at the walk-in clinic or better yet with the child's usual physician. In any case, the child should be seen again within 48 hours to make sure that there is no secondary infection.

25 **The answer is E** *Pediatrics*

Candida species are common causes of oral thrush and diaper dermatitis in infants. Thrush consists of white, curdlike plaques on the tongue, gums, and buccal mucosa that are difficult to remove. The skin manifestations include a beefy-red maculopapular rash that may coalesce and form satellite lesions. Intertriginous areas, especially in the diaper area (perineum), also are usually involved (choice **E**).

Candida infections of the eyes (choice **A**), ears (choice **B**), nose (choice **C**), and scalp (choice **D**) are not usually associated with thrush. Disseminated *Candida* infection is most commonly associated with an immunocompromised host.

26 **The answer is D** *Pediatrics*

Nonvenereal infectious vulvovaginitis is not uncommon in prepubertal patients. Poor perineal hygiene is the most common cause of nonspecific vulvovaginitis and accounts for 70% of all pediatric vulvovaginitis cases. Most of these cases are secondary to fecal contamination. Bacterial vulvovaginitis due to a primary respiratory or skin pathogen may also be found. Group A β-hemolytic streptococcus may be associated with streptococcal nasopharyngitis or scarlet fever or may occur alone. Vulvovaginal symptoms of group A β-hemolytic streptococcal (choice **D**) infection include severe perineal burning, dysuria, and erythema similar in appearance to erysipelas in the perineal area. Most patients will have a serosanguinous or grayish white vaginal discharge.

Streptococcus pneumoniae (choice **E**) and *Haemophilus influenzae* (choice **A**) may cause a purulent vaginal discharge causing vulvovaginitis following, or in conjunction with, an upper respiratory infection. Sexual abuse should be suspected when *Neisseria gonorrhea* (choice **B**) or *Chlamydia trachomatis* (choice **C**) are found in a prepubertal child. In this case, there is no history of bubble bath, pinworms, tight clothing, nylon underwear, or recent medications, all of which have been implicated in vulvovaginitis. Likewise, although there is severe dysuria, there is no history of hematuria or fever, which makes a urinary tract infection less likely.

27 The answer is D *Psychiatry*

Because the potential father's uncle and cousin are second-degree relatives who have been diagnosed with schizophrenia, the risk of the child developing the disease is greater than 1%, the lifetime risk in the general population, but less than 10%, the prevalence rate among first-degree relatives (choice **D**).

Choice **A** is incorrect because there is clear evidence of a familial basis for this disease; namely, there is a 10% chance of a first-degree relative getting the disease and a greater than 50% concordance rate between monozygous twins. However, no particular family communication style appears to cause schizophrenia (choice **B**). For unknown reasons, the risk of developing schizophrenia is higher for individuals born in winter months in temperate regions (choice **C**). Gluten intolerance (coeliac disease) has been associated with higher risks for schizophrenia, but no data suggest that prenatal exposure plays any role (choice **E**).

28 The answer is E *Obstetrics and Gynecology*

Up to 15% of couples experience infertility defined as inability to conceive within 12 months of regular unprotected intercourse. This patient has primary infertility, since she has never successfully conceived. In 40% of couples, multiple causes may be present. The etiology of infertility may involve both partners simultaneously in 20% of cases and in another 30% of the cases, a male factor alone; consequently, of the factors listed, the most common is male factor (choice **E**), which is diagnosed with semen analysis, which may show too small ejaculate volume, too few sperm, no sperm, immobile sperm, or morphologically aberrant sperm.

Other causes of infertility are as follows: ovulatory factor (choice **A**) is seen in 15–20% of couples and is characterized by chronic anovulation, which may be result of hypothyroidism, hyperprolactinemia, or polycystic ovarian syndrome. Cervical factor (choice **B**) is seen in 5–10% of couples and involves unfavorable cervical mucus inhibiting sperm transport into the uterine cavity. Uterine factor (choice **C**) occurs in 5% of couples and involves anatomic defects of the uterine cavity. Tubal factor (choice **D**) is seen in 30% of cases and is diagnosed by hysterosalpingogram revealing anatomic tubal pathology.

29 The answer is E *Medicine*

The conditions described and the symptoms are suggestive of coccidioidomycosis (choice **E**), which is caused by *Coccidioides immitis*, a soil saprophyte predominantly found in the southwestern United States. It is contracted by breathing in arthrospores from the soil, particularly a few days after a rain. Only 40% of infected individuals develop a symptomatic infection. African Americans, Mexicans, and Filipinos are particularly prone to disseminated disease. Clinical presentation consists of fever, cough, chest pain, malaise, and hypersensitivity reactions such as erythema nodosum and eosinophilia. Erythema nodosum presents as raised, erythematous, painful nodules, usually involving the lower extremities. It is not diagnostic of coccidioides infection but is also associated with tuberculosis, sarcoidosis, various drug reactions (sulfonamides, iodides, and birth-control pills), inflammatory bowel disease, and malignancy (Hodgkin's disease). Biopsies of these lesions show an inflammatory panniculitis. *Coccidioides* infection is the most common systemic fungal infection to produce cavitary lesions in the lower lobes. Pleural effusions are commonly present as well. Serologic tests are very useful in screening for coccidioidomycosis. Skin testing is less useful as a screen. Sputum cultures frequently isolate the organism. Primary pulmonary disease usually resolves spontaneously without treatment. More severe cases require fluconazole.

Histoplasmosis (choice **A**) is the most common systemic fungal disease, but it is more common in the central states and is rarely found in the dry climate of the Southwest; rather there is an association with bird and bat droppings in moist soil. It also can be associated with erythema nodosum. Serologic tests and culture confirm the diagnosis. *Klebsiella pneumoniae* (choice **B**) lung infections are usually seen in alcoholics. These infections frequently produce lung abscesses. Tuberculosis (choice **C**), like coccidioidomycosis is a cavitary disease, but reactivation tuberculosis is most commonly located in the upper lobes. *Mycoplasma pneumoniae* (choice **D**) is the most common cause of atypical pneumonia. It does not produce cavitary lesions in the lungs

30 The answer is B *Medicine*

Excluding skin cancers, breast cancer is the most common neoplasm in females; however more females now die from lung cancer. The lifetime chance of developing breast cancer among Caucasian women in the United States is between 1 in 8 and 1 and 9 (choice **A**). However, this woman has additional risk factors. Women whose mothers or sisters have had breast cancer have their risk of developing cancer increased about fourfold; thus this patient's minimal risk is 1 in 9/4 or 44.4% (choice **B**). Since she is an Ashkenazi Jew (her Jewish family comes from eastern Poland) her risk is even greater; this population has a high incidence of the *BRCA1* and *BRCA2* gene mutations, which can increase the lifetime risk to about 85%. In fact, since her mother died relatively young from breast cancer, the chances she had one of these cancer-causing mutations is high, and the physician might well recommend that this patient undergo genetic screening.

Because she is older now than her mother was when she died, choice **C** (she has little risk of developing an inherited form of cancer) is not true. In fact, the risk of cancer increases with age, the incidence increases particularly rapidly between the ages of 40 and 55 years, after which the risk remains constant. Choice **D** (having fibrocystic disease reduces the probability of ever developing a breast malignancy) is not true; in fact it increases the risk slightly. Breast cancer is one of the few cancers that doesn't seem to be increased by smoking, thus the fact she is a nonsmoker doesn't reduce her chance of developing cancer (choice **E**).

31 The answer is E *Psychiatry*

Schizotypal personality disorder (choice **E**) is characterized by social withdrawal, peculiar ideation, and the absence of any history of psychosis. Antipsychotic medication sometimes decreases the peculiar ideation seen in this disorder. Schizotypal personality disorder is associated with a family history of schizophrenia.

Schizophrenia, residual type (choice **D**), would have a very similar presentation, but a history of at least one episode of psychosis is necessary to make this diagnosis. Avoidant personality disorder (choice **A**) is often characterized by reclusiveness, but individuals with this disorder have a desire for human interaction and a fear of rejection. Obsessive–compulsive personality disorder (choice **B**) is characterized by behavioral inflexibility and a preoccupation with meaningless details. Schizoid personality disorder (choice **C**) is characterized by social aloofness without any bizarre ideation.

32 The answer is C *Surgery*

This woman has conjunctivitis. All forms of conjunctivitis share certain features, including a pink or red coloration of the cornea ("pink eye"), a feeling of fine grit in the eye upon blinking, and production of a yellow-tinted exudate. The observation that the exudate is sticky and viscous indicates it caused by a bacterial infection (choice **C**). The three most common infectious agents are *Staphylococcus aureus*, *Streptococcus pneumoniae*, and *Haemophilus* species. The latter two are more common in children; *S. aureus* is most common in adults. Infections are termed *acute* because as a rule they clear up spontaneously within 2 weeks; however, a topical antibiotic can be used to typically cure the infection within a few days.

Acute viral conjunctivitis (choice **A**) can be distinguished from bacterial conjunctivitis by the observation that the discharge is copious and watery with scant exudate; it too resolves spontaneously, but antibiotic treatment does not accelerate recovery. Children most commonly get viral conjunctivitis, the most common infective agent is adenovirus type 3; it is highly infectious, and rapid dissemination to a full classroom is not unknown. Optic neuritis (choice **B**) refers to inflammation of the optic nerve, which may be secondary to multiple sclerosis, glaucoma, or infection as in tuberculosis or syphilis. There is a sudden unilateral loss of vision and pain on eye movements. The optic disc frequently appears swollen and associated with flame-shaped pericapillary hemorrhages. Intravenous (IV) and oral steroid therapies are used for treatment. Uveitis (choice **D**) is an inflammation of the uveal tract, a space formed by the iris, ciliary body, and choroid. Central retinal artery occlusion (choice **E**) is characterized by a sudden, almost complete but painless loss of vision in one eye, most commonly in an elderly patient. Retinal examination reveals pallor of the optic disc; edema of the retina; a cherry-red fovea; bloodless, constricted arterioles. Anterior blepharitis (choice **F**) is a commonly occurring inflammation of the eyelids, skin, eyelashes, and associated glands; it is easily recognized by the red-rimmed eyes with scales hanging onto the lashes. The eyes tend to feel irritated and itchy. There may be small peripheral ulcers caused by staphylococci. Effective home therapy is often achieved by removing the scales from the lid margins on a daily basis with a damp cloth, using baby shampoo as an emulsifier, and by keeping the face and scalp ultraclean. In some cases an antibacterial ointment is also used.

33 **The answer is E** *Medicine*

This man is presenting with ketoacidosis, which likely resulted from poor compliance and/or the effect of excess alcohol consumption on his insulin requirements. In addition this patient has type V hyperlipoproteinemia (choice **E**), which is characterized by an increase in both chylomicrons (containing diet-derived triglyceride) and very-low-density lipoproteins (VLDL, containing liver-synthesized triglyceride). Insulin normally stimulates adipose cells to synthesize and secrete capillary lipoprotein lipase, which is important in removing triglyceride from circulating chylomicrons and VLDL. During a long-term deficiency of insulin (suggested in this patient by the diabetic ketoacidosis), chylomicrons and VLDL accumulate in the blood and produce hypertriglyceridemia. When the concentration of triglyceride exceeds 1500 mg/dL, the blood develops a milky appearance and can produce the hyperchylomicronemia syndrome. The syndrome is characterized by eruptive xanthomas on the skin, lipemia retinalis (milky appearing retinal vessels), abdominal pain, acute pancreatitis, dyspnea (impaired oxygenation in the lungs), and hepatomegaly (fatty liver). Once the insulin levels are restored in the patient, the signs and symptoms disappear.

Type I hyperlipoproteinemia (choice **A**) is a rare disorder that is seen primarily in young children. It is due to a deficiency of apoC-II (activates capillary lipoprotein lipase) or a deficiency in capillary lipoprotein lipase. Chylomicrons are primarily elevated (not VLDL) and can cause the hyperchylomicronemia syndrome. Type II hyperlipoproteinemia (choice **B**) is caused by decreased synthesis of low-density lipoprotein (LDL) receptors, causing an increase in LDL, the vehicle for carrying cholesterol. Chylomicrons and VLDL are not increased. In familial hypercholesterolemia, tendon xanthomas and xanthelasma (yellow patches on the eyelids) are present rather than eruptive xanthomas. Type III hyperlipoproteinemia (choice **C**) is caused by a deficiency of apoE or a mutant form of apoE. ApoE is required to remove chylomicron remnants and intermediate-density lipoprotein (remnant of VLDL hydrolysis). Clinical findings include an increase in both cholesterol and triglycerides and the presence of palmar xanthomas (yellow patches in the creases of the palms) rather than eruptive xanthomas. Type IV hyperlipoproteinemia (choice **D**) is caused by increased synthesis or decreased catabolism of VLDL. Triglyceride levels are markedly increased and may produce eruptive xanthomas and the hyperchylomicronemia syndrome. Chylomicrons, however, are absent.

34 **The answer is A** *Pediatrics*

Patients with sickle cell disease are at increased risk for developing severe pneumococcal disease because of impaired immunologic response to *Streptococcus pneumoniae* (choice **A**). Patients with sickle cell disease should be immunized with the polyvalent pneumococcal vaccine in addition to all other routine immunizations of childhood. The polyvalent pneumococcal vaccine should be administered to asplenic children 2 years of age and older. The pneumococcal vaccine may not be as effective in children under 5 years old as it is in older individuals. Even if patients with sickle cell disease are given prophylactic antibiotics, there is still a chance that they will develop pneumococcal meningitis before 5 years of age.

Escherichia coli (choice **C**), *Listeria monocytogenes* (choice **D**), and group B streptococcus (choice **B**) are more common pathogens in newborns. The most common sites of infection for group A β-hemolytic streptococci (choice **E**) are the upper respiratory tract, skin, soft tissues, and blood.

35 **The answer is E** *Medicine*

There are four *Plasmodium* species that cause malaria: *P. falciparum, P. ovale, P. malariae,* and *P. vivax.* Of these, *P. falciparum* infection is generally the most dangerous. An estimated 30,000 travelers from developed counties to tropical areas are infected with malaria annually, and several hundred die. The patient described in the vignette has *P. falciparum* malaria (option **E**), which is endemic in many east African countries including Tanzania. The peripheral blood findings in the vignette described multiple ring forms, which is a characteristic finding in *P. falciparum* infections. The tertian fever pattern (recurring every other day, with occasional fever spikes) correlates with intravascular hemolysis, which causes hemoglobinuria (positive dipstick test result for blood), and extravascular hemolysis leads to jaundice, as splenic macrophages remove parasitized RBCs and degrade the hemoglobin into unconjugated bilirubin. Hemolytic anemias are all associated with an increase in the corrected reticulocyte count. Hepatosplenomegaly is present after the fourth day in all of the malarias. Malaria is transmitted to humans primarily by the bite of a female *Anopheles* mosquito. *P. falciparum* malaria is the most severe malaria, because it produces a greater degree of parasitism of red blood cells resulting in cytoadherence of parasitized red cells in capillaries and postcapillary venules. Complications include central nervous system hemorrhage, disseminated intravascular coagulation, acute respiratory distress syndrome, and liver cell necrosis with an increase in transaminases. The effectiveness of antimalarial drugs varies depending upon parasite species and stage of the parasite's life cycle. Tissue schizonticides, primarily primaquine, act in the liver to eliminate developing exoerythrocytic schizonts or latent hypnozoites; blood schizonticides such as chloroquine, amodiaquine, proguanil, pyrimethamine, mefloquine, quinine, quinidine, halofantrine, artemisinin, and atovaquone suppress parasite development in the red blood cell; and gametocides, primaquine for *P. falciparum,* kill gametocytes in the blood. There are no true prophylactic drugs, but proguanil, chlorproguanil, atovaquone, and primaquine prevent maturation of early *P. falciparum,* while the blood schizonticides when given weekly for a month after exposure prevent development of *P. falciparum* as well as *P. malariae,* and thereby result in a cure. Resistant *P. falciparum* strains have developed worldwide, particularly to chloroquine in east Africa; otherwise chloroquine is used for prevention of all types of malaria. It is safe during pregnancy, kills blood schizonts, and is gametocidal to all malaria species *except P. falciparum. P. vivax* and *P. ovale* infections are treated with chloroquine plus primaquine. Malarone, mefloquine, or quinine sulfate plus doxycycline or some other drug combination is used for prevention when there are chloroquine-resistant strains of *P. falciparum* present. The treatment of chloroquine-sensitive *P. falciparum* is chloroquine without primaquine.

When autoimmune hemolytic anemia (choice **A**) is suspected, a direct Coombs' test is ordered. It detects IgG and C3b on the surface of the RBCs. The negative Coombs' test result in this patient rules out an autoimmune hemolytic anemia. Congenital spherocytosis (choice **B**) is an autosomal dominant disorder that causes hemolytic anemia with jaundice and splenomegaly. It is not associated with a spiking fever or the intraerythrocytic ring forms that are present in this patient, and erythrocytes have a spherocytic or oval shape. Glucose-6-phosphate dehydrogenase (G6PD) deficiency (choice **C**) is an X-linked recessive disorder (patient is a woman) that causes a predominantly intravascular type of hemolytic anemia that presents with hemoglobinuria. The less predominant extravascular hemolytic component is responsible for producing jaundice. The RBCs do not have intraerythrocytic ring forms. Pyruvate kinase deficiency (choice **D**) is an autosomal recessive disorder associated with a hemolytic anemia. The peripheral blood shows shrunken and spiculated RBCs with no intraerythrocytic inclusions.

36 The answer is C *Surgery*

The patient has volume overload due to overzealous fluid resuscitation (choice **C**) during and after surgery. Volume overload is the most common cause of congestive cardiac failure after surgery. A third heart sound is the first cardiac sign of left- or right-sided congestive heart failure. Bibasilar inspiratory crackles indicate left-sided heart failure, and jugular venous distention and peripheral pitting edema are features of right-sided heart failure. Volume overload can be corrected by administration of a loop diuretic and by restricting fluid volume. It is always important to monitor fluid intake and output carefully in patients to avoid inadvertent fluid overload.

Endotoxic shock and cardiogenic shock (choices **A** and **B**) are incorrect responses because the patient has a normal blood pressure. Fat embolism syndrome (choice **D**) is associated with tachycardia, dyspnea, thrombocytopenia, and petechiae over the chest. The latter two findings are not present in this patient. Syndrome of inappropriate secretion of antidiuretic hormone (choice **E**) is not associated with peripheral pitting edema, because it refers to retention of water without sodium. Serum sodium is usually less than 120 mEq/L; water restriction is the treatment of choice.

37 The answer is E *Psychiatry*

For most adult alcoholics, active participation in alcoholics anonymous (AA) (choice **E**) offers the best chance of preventing relapses. In Alcoholics Anonymous, total abstinence is mandatory.

Naltrexone is an opiate antagonist that may sometimes help prevent relapse by blunting the euphoric effect of alcohol and can be used as an adjunct in the treatment of alcoholism, but would not be recommended in the absence of a supportive program; it would not make him nauseous after one drink (choice **B**). Disulfiram (choice **A**) is a drug known to reduce the chance of relapse by behavioral modification. Normally, alcohol is first oxidized to acetaldehyde by alcohol dehydrogenase (ADH). The acetaldehyde is immediately further oxidized to acetate by low-K_m mitochondrial aldehyde dehydrogenase isoenzymes. Disulfiram acts by being metabolized to diethylthiomethylcarbamate, a suicide inhibitor of the aldehyde dehydrogenase isoenzymes. Inhibition of these enzymes causes the plasma concentration of acetaldehyde to increase, inducing the "acetaldehyde syndrome," largely caused by the vasodilator effects of acetaldehyde. Within 5 to 10 minutes after ingestion of ethanol the aldehyde dehydrogenase isoenzymes become poisoned, and the face feels hot and becomes flushed and scarlet in appearance. This is followed by intense throbbing in the head and neck, a pulsating headache, respiratory difficulties, nausea, copious vomiting, sweating, thirst, chest pain, hypotension, orthostatic syncope, uneasiness, weakness, vertigo, blurred vision, and confusion. Sudden unexplained fatalities have occurred. Clearly, disulfiram should not be used as a therapeutic agent except under careful medical supervision. Some individuals inherit low-activity aldehyde dehydrogenase, which is not able to oxidize acetaldehyde as rapidly as it is formed via the ADH reaction. Consequently, the level of circulating acetaldehyde increases as ethanol continues to be consumed and oxidized by ADH. Although this effect is not as profound as when acetaldehyde dehydrogenase is poisoned by disulfiram, such persons have a genetically based intolerance for alcohol and rarely become alcoholic. Conversely, individuals with a high tolerance to alcohol are at greater risk of consuming large amounts, even if they intend to drink in moderation (choices **C** and **D**). Such individuals have a greater chance of becoming addicted and of relapsing once they have that "first" drink.

38 The answer is F   *Obstetrics and Gynecology*

Fallopian tube, or oviduct, malignancies (choice **F**) are extremely rare and have no official International Federation of Gynecology and Obstetrics (FIGO) staging criteria. However, because they are intraperitoneal organs, intimately related to the ovaries, with a similar mode of metastasis, they are staged with criteria similar to those for ovarian carcinoma (choice **B**).

39 The answer is A   *Obstetrics and Gynecology*

Staging criteria use the best information from a variety of sources to assess the degree of cancer dissemination. All gynecologic cancers use surgical staging methods, with the exception of cervical cancer (choice **A**), which uses only clinical information from noninvasive methods such as pelvic examination, intravenous pyelography, cystoscopy, sigmoidoscopy, and imaging studies.

40 The answer is A   *Obstetrics and Gynecology*

Cervical carcinoma (choice **A**) has three subcategories in stage I (IA1, IA2, and IB). Endometrial (choice **C**) and ovarian (choice **B**) cancer also have three stage I subcategories (IA, IB, and IC). The subcategories were created because the treatment and prognosis is different for each one. Vulvar cancer (choice **E**) has no subdivisions of stage I.

41 The answer is A   *Obstetrics and Gynecology*

Stage I cervical carcinoma has the best 5-year survival rate (90%), largely because it usually is diagnosed in a minimally invasive or microinvasive early stage. The survival rates for the other stage I malignancies are as follows: vaginal (85%) (choice **D**), endometrial (75%) (choice **C**), ovarian (70%) (choice **B**), and oviductal (60%) (choice **F**).

42 The answer is A   *Obstetrics and Gynecology*

Cervical malignancy (choice **A**) of the squamous cell type is associated with human papillomavirus (HPV) subtypes 16 and 18 that are sexually transmitted. Therefore, it is considered epidemiologically to be a sexually transmitted disease.

43 The answer is B   *Obstetrics and Gynecology*

Ovarian carcinoma (choice **B**) is the only gynecologic malignancy that has subcategories A, B, and C for stages I through III. Each of these subdivisions is necessary for directing specific treatment planning.

44 **The answer is B** *Obstetrics and Gynecology*

Cancer of the ovary is the second most common gynecologic malignancy, and the one associated with the highest mortality (choice **B**). There are no early symptoms for ovarian cancer; therefore by the time it is diagnosed it has already spread throughout the peritoneal cavity, making it stage III. Approximately 1% of all women will develop ovarian cancer. It accounts for more deaths than all other primary pelvic cancers combined.

45 **The answer is C** *Medicine*

The patient has Rocky Mountain spotted fever (RMSF) due to *Rickettsia rickettsii* (choice **C**). RMSF is the most common rickettsial disease in the United States, and despite its name, it is more common in the eastern United States than the western United States. It is transmitted by the bite of the wood tick, *Dermacentor andersoni*. Most cases occur in spring and summer. The three classic diagnostic features of RMSF are rash (95% of cases), fever, and a history of tick exposure. All three findings are present in less than 20% of cases. The petechial lesions begin on the palms, unlike other types of rickettsial disease. The organism invades the endothelial cells of small vessels, causing rupture of the vessels. Gastrointestinal findings include nausea and vomiting, diarrhea, abdominal pain, and hepatitis. Central nervous findings include headache, lethargy, delirium, and coma. Laboratory findings include an absolute neutrophilic leukocytosis with a left shift, hyponatremia (50% of cases, possibly due to inappropriate secretion of antidiuretic hormone), and hypoalbuminemia (30% of cases). Spinal fluid studies reveal increased mononuclear cells and neutrophils, a slight increase in protein, and a slight decrease in glucose. The mainstay for diagnosis is serologic testing. The treatment of choice is doxycycline (a shorter course is given to children). Mortality is 20% without treatment.

46 **The answer is A** *Medicine*

The patient has lymphogranuloma venereum (LGV), caused by a subtype of *Chlamydia trachomatis* (choice **A**). It is a sexually transmitted disease characterized by the presence of tiny papules in the genital region without ulceration and inguinal lymphadenitis with granulomatous microabscesses and multiple draining sinuses. After the genital lesions disappear, the infection spreads to lymph nodes in the genital and rectal areas. Inapparent infection and latent disease are not uncommon. In some patients, fibrous stricture formation produces localized lymphedema of the scrotum or vulva and rectal strictures in women. The treatment of choice is doxycycline, but erythromycin is also effective.

47 **The answer is B** *Medicine*

Chlamydia pneumoniae (choice **B**) causes about 10% of cases of community-acquired pneumonia and is second to *Mycoplasma pneumoniae* as a cause of atypical (interstitial) pneumonia. It is transmitted to humans by the respiratory route. There is a strong seroepidemiologic association with coronary artery disease (CAD). The treatment of choice is erythromycin or a tetracycline.

48 **The answer is D** *Medicine*

Q fever is a rickettsial disease caused by *Coxiella burnetii*, (choice **D**) that most often is contracted by individuals involved with the birthing process of sheep, goats, or cattle or who have contact with their excretory products (e.g., abattoir [slaughter house] employees, farmers, veterinarians). It is the only rickettsial disease that is not transmitted by an arthropod vector (e.g., tick). In addition to atypical pneumonia, it can also produce granulomatous hepatitis and endocarditis. The treatment of choice for the acute symptoms is doxycycline, tetracycline, or one of the newer macrolides. If endocarditis results, it is most often treated using a 2-year course of doxycycline plus hydroxychloroquine.

49 **The answer is E** *Medicine*

The tick *Amblyomma americanus* is the major vector of *Ehrlichia chaffeensis* (choice **E**), a rickettsial organism that produces ehrlichiosis. The organism is an obligate intraleukocytic parasite that produces a mulberry-like inclusion called a morula in the cytoplasm. The bite of *Amblyomma americanus* usually results in monocytic ehrlichiosis, which in the United States is primarily seen in the south central, southeastern and mid-Atlantic states. On the other hand, granulocytic ehrlichiosis is primarily transmitted by the bite of ticks belonging to the *Ixodes* species and has a geographic distribution similar to that of Lyme disease, and coinfection does occur.

Both versions have similar clinical manifestations, which can range from mild, as in the case described, to severe. Serous sequela include respiratory failure, adult respiratory disease syndrome (ARDS), encephalopathy, and acute renal failure. Diagnosis is usually made via a fluorescent antibody assay. The treatment of choice is doxycycline.

50 The answer is F *Medicine*

Mycoplasma pneumoniae (choice **F**) is the most common cause of atypical (interstitial) pneumonia. It is transmitted by droplet infection, particularly in crowded conditions (e.g., military personnel, college students, airplanes). It presents as a pneumonia with insidious onset, low-grade fever, nonproductive cough, and no signs of consolidation (e.g., no increased tactile vocal fremitus). Additional associations include cold agglutinins (anti-I IgM antibodies may cause intravascular hemolytic anemia), erythema multiforme, and bullous myringitis. The treatment of choice is doxycycline, erythromycin, or azithromycin.

test **8**

Questions

Single Best Choice: This section consists of numbered statements or questions followed by a list of potential answers; you are to select the ONE best answer.

1 A 4-day-old, 1500-g (3 lb 5 oz) premature infant recovering from respiratory distress syndrome is noted to have bounding peripheral pulsations and a hyperactive precordium. A continuous machinery murmur is most audible at the left infraclavicular area. Left ventricle hypertrophy (LVH) is present on the electrocardiogram (ECG). The chest x-ray film shows slight enlargement of the heart and increased pulmonary venous markings. Which of the following is the most likely diagnosis?

(A) Ventricular septal defect (VSD)
(B) Atrial septal defect (ASD)
(C) Patent ductus arteriosus
(D) Pulmonic stenosis
(E) Tetralogy of Fallot

2 A 48-year-old woman has been married for 8 years and desperately wants to have a child of her own before it is too late. She consults a new obstetrician for help because she has experienced multiple early second-trimester losses due to painless cervical dilation leading to expulsion of immature stillborn fetuses. She reports that she was exposed in utero to diethylstilbestrol (DES), explaining that when her mother was pregnant with her she experienced early pregnancy bleeding and, as a consequence, was treated with DES to prevent the pregnancy from being terminated. At thus time this patient is most likely to demonstrate which of the following conditions on physical examination?

(A) Cervical dysplasia
(B) Breast fibroadenoma
(C) Vaginal adenosis
(D) Müllerian agenesis
(E) Polycystic ovary syndrome

3 A 20-year-old male college student is hospitalized after assaulting a girlfriend whom he accuses of using "radar" to place bizarre thoughts in his mind just after she broke off her relationship with him. He has been increasingly withdrawn and preoccupied over the last year but has no history of substance abuse or other physical problems. Mental status examination reveals an alert, anxious, and oriented male, with dysphoria, suspiciousness, constricted affect, mildly tangential thinking, bizarre ideation, and no memory impairment. Which of the following is the most likely diagnosis?

(A) Delirium
(B) Psychosis
(C) Depression
(D) Anxiety
(E) Mania
(F) Cocaine-induced psychosis
(G) Bipolar disorder
(H) Schizophrenia
(I) Major depressive disorder with psychosis
(J) Shared psychotic disorder

4 A 35-year-old man who is being treated with isoniazid for reactivation tuberculosis develops a microcytic anemia. Laboratory studies show increased serum ferritin, iron, and percentage saturation of transferrin and a decreased total iron-binding capacity (TIBC). A bone marrow examination reveals increased iron stores and numerous ringed sideroblasts. Which of the following vitamin deficiencies is most likely responsible for the anemia?

(A) Folic acid
(B) Vitamin B$_6$
(C) Vitamin B$_{12}$
(D) Vitamin C
(E) Vitamin E

5 A 32-year-old anesthesiologist married with two children and a successful hospital-based practice is discovered by his office assistant to be addicted to fentanyl. He confesses to her that he became addicted after briefly using pentazocine, which was prescribed for pain after minor surgery 2 years ago and that he will voluntarily enter a withdrawal program because he has no intention of losing his good lifestyle for a few hours per day of pleasant relief. Which of the following statements about his case is most accurate?

(A) He is likely to be isolated and lonely as a result of opioid use.
(B) He is likely to develop an opioid-induced psychotic disorder.
(C) His addiction is a fairly common sequel of opioid use for acute pain management.
(D) He will probably recover from his addiction.
(E) Deviant social behavior is unlikely among opioid addicts.

6 A 65-year-old man sees his primary care physician because of pain in his chest that he thinks might indicate heart trouble. He describes the pain as a burning sensation in his chest that radiates into the neck and his left arm. He also reports that he regurgitates a sour-tasting liquid that leaves a feeling of "pins and needles" in his throat and mouth. These symptoms are not aggravated by exercise but are by drinking coffee or chocolate or eating fatty foods. Results of physical examination including his heart sounds and an electrocardiogram (ECG) taken as part of an exercise tolerance test are unremarkable. An upper gastrointestinal barium x-ray study shows the presence of a hiatal hernia. Which of the following is the primary mechanism for this patient's complaints?

(A) Decreased acid production in the stomach
(B) Increased gastric emptying
(C) Decreased esophageal peristalsis
(D) Inappropriate relaxation of the lower esophageal sphincter (LES)
(E) Absence of ganglion cells in the myenteric plexus

7 A 42-year-old woman complains of aching in the shoulder muscles, difficulty with climbing stairs, and difficulty with swallowing solids and liquids from her upper esophagus. Physical examination reveals atrophy of her shoulder and pelvic muscles. There is erythema over the bridge of her nose, with violaceous discoloration and edema of the upper eyelids. Erythematous papules are noted over the proximal interphalangeal joints, metacarpophalangeal joints, elbows, and knees. An electromyogram (EMG) reveals low-amplitude polyphasic potentials, and laboratory testing reveals an increased creatine phosphokinase (CPK). Which of the following is the most likely diagnosis?

(A) Polymyalgia rheumatica
(B) Rheumatoid arthritis
(C) Polymyositis
(D) Dermatomyositis
(E) Systemic lupus erythematosus (SLE)

8 A 31-year-old woman, gravida 4, para 1, aborta 2, presents for prenatal care in the middle of her second trimester. She has a positive history of substance abuse preceding and during this pregnancy. Her first pregnancy ended with an emergency cesarean section delivery at 34 weeks' gestation because of significant painful vaginal bleeding associated with fetal bradycardia. On ultrasound examination, her singleton fetus is noted to have a limb reduction defect of the right lower extremity. Which of the following abused substances is most associated with this fetal anomaly?

(A) Tobacco
(B) Alcohol
(C) Narcotics
(D) Amphetamines
(E) Cocaine

9 A 4-year-old girl fails to develop intelligible speech and simply repeats sentence fragments that she has heard. She spends hours sitting alone, facing a wall, and rocking back and forth. She shows little affection for others and sometimes bangs her head against the floor. Which of the following is the most likely cause for her symptoms?

(A) Childhood exposure to lead
(B) Childhood sexual abuse
(C) Emotionally distant parents
(D) Intrauterine rubella
(E) Maternal cocaine abuse during pregnancy

10 A 48-year-old homeless man, who is an alcoholic, is found supine on a bench in a local park. He is semi-responsive and coughing up foul-smelling sputum. The police call 911, and he is taken to a local emergency department, where he is found to have a low-grade fever, hypotension, tachycardia, and slow shallow respirations. Gram stain of a sputum smear shows a mixture of gram-positive cocci in chains and gram-negative rods. A chest radiograph shows a fluid-filled cavity. This cavity is most likely located in which of the following sites?

(A) Lingula of the left lung
(B) Middle lobe of the right lung
(C) Posterior segment of the right upper lobe
(D) Posterobasal segment of the right lower lobe
(E) Superior segment of the right lower lobe

11 A 30-year-old woman, who is a nonsmoker, presents with bilateral puffiness and swelling of the fingers and joint pains. Cold exposure and stress cause episodes of blanching or cyanosis of the fingers. She is not on any medications, and her liver aminotransferase enzyme activity has always been stable and within the normal range. The mechanism for this patient's disease is most likely the result of which of the following?

(A) Vasospasm and thickening of the digital arteries
(B) Hyperviscosity due to cryoglobulins
(C) An immune complex vasculitis
(D) Thrombosis of the digital vessels
(E) An embolism to the digital vessels

12 A 22-year-old female with cocaine dependence intoxication is brought to the emergency department by the police in a state of extreme agitation. After a brief struggle she is restrained and sedated. A cursory mental evaluation concludes that she probably has persecutory ideation. Physical examination finds hypertension and tachycardia. She is admitted to a medical psychiatric unit for observation and possible treatment. Which of the following statements about this patient is most accurate?

(A) Amphetamines can be used to facilitate her detoxification from cocaine.

(B) Psychologic effects from withdrawal will likely be of short duration.

(C) She is likely to have additional serious psychiatric pathology.

(D) Simultaneous withdrawal from alcohol is unlikely.

(E) Use of antipsychotic medication during her withdrawal is likely to cause a severe toxic interaction with cocaine.

13 A 20-year-old woman in her first pregnancy came to the maternity unit at 39 weeks' gestation after an uncomplicated pregnancy. She had spontaneous onset of labor and progressed normally through the first and second stages of labor. During the second stage of labor the electronic fetal monitor tracing showed frequent prolonged variable decelerations of the fetal heart rate down to 90 beats a minute and lasting 45 seconds. She underwent an outlet forceps vaginal delivery of a 3100-g (6 lb 13 oz) female neonate. One minute after birth, the infant is noted to have acral cyanosis and a weak respiratory effort at a rate of 30 breaths/min. Her heart rate is 105 beats/min, and a systolic murmur is heard. She flexes all four extremities weakly but only after external stimulation. When her nose and mouth are suctioned, she shows no response. She keeps her eyes closed. Which of the following is her assigned Apgar score at 1 minute?

(A) 4

(B) 5

(C) 6

(D) 7

(E) 8

14 An 85-year-old man is found wandering in a confused state in the middle of a busy thoroughfare. He is taken to the nearest emergency department where the physician on duty determines he has a temperature of 102.6°F (39.2°C) as well as chills, a productive cough, and chest pain upon inspiration. His blood pressure is 98/68 mm Hg, his respiratory rate is 28 breaths/min (normal adult rate is 14 to 18 breaths/min), his respiration is labored, and he has pain upon inspiration. Physical examination shows a few bilateral rales and no other abnormality. His white cell count is 10,900/mm³ (normal range, 4.8–10.8 × 10³/μL) with a left shift. A chest x-ray film is ambiguous. His granddaughter is contacted, and she informs the hospital that her grandfather was self-reliant, had no observable memory problems, and still lived alone. However earlier in the week, about 2 days ago, he had been complaining of nausea and loss of appetite. Which of the following is the most likely diagnosis?

(A) Alzheimer's disease

(B) *Klebsiella pneumoniae* pneumonia

(C) Viral pneumonia

(D) *Streptococcus pneumoniae* pneumonia

(E) Primary tuberculosis

(F) Senile dementia due to chronic vascular disease.

15 A 30-year old heroin addict who habitually used shared needles when taking the drug intravenously (IV) tested positive for the human immunodeficiency virus (HIV) by the enzyme-linked immunosorbent assay (ELISA) and then by a Western blot test 4 years ago. He now presents to the physician on duty at a community clinic with fever, dyspnea, tachypnea, and peripheral cyanosis. A chest x-ray film reveals extensive "ground-glass" opacities in the lower zones of both lungs. The physician would expect which of the following?

(A) Organism response to amphotericin B

(B) Organism response to erythromycin

(C) Granulomas in the bone marrow

(D) Organism response to trimethoprim–sulfamethoxazole

(E) Gram's stain of sputum to be diagnostic

16 A 40-year-old man with a 15-year history of intermittent right lower quadrant, colicky pain with diarrhea has a macrocytic anemia with hypersegmented neutrophils. He describes his stools as greasy and foul smelling. Physical examination reveals decreased vibratory sensation in the lower extremities. Which of the following disorders is most likely present?

(A) Chronic pancreatitis

(B) Crohn's disease

(C) Fish tapeworm infestation

(D) Lactase deficiency

(E) Pernicious anemia

17 A 39-year-old woman consults a psychologist because she feels she needs help in dealing with her 62-year old mother. She states that ever since her father died last year her mother constantly nags her about forming a stable relationship by getting married to a professional man. The patient states that she has been living with another woman for the past 10 years in a stable, sexual relationship. The couple purchased a home several years ago, have separate and productive careers, and travel widely. Which of the following statements about this patient is most likely to be true?

(A) She has never had sex with a man.

(B) She would like to have a sex-change operation.

(C) She has never had children.

(D) She has abnormal estrogen levels.

(E) She has a history of satisfying interpersonal relationships.

18 A 50-year-old man is hospitalized after experiencing racing thoughts, insomnia, increasing impulsivity, and grandiosity for 1 month. A 1-month trial of lithium with a blood level of 1.3 mEq/L fails to ameliorate his symptoms. Assuming no contraindications, which of the following is the most appropriate next medication to consider for long-term management of this patient?

(A) A trial of mirtazapine

(B) A trial of divalproex

(C) An increase in the dose of lithium

(D) Addition of olanzapine

(E) A trial of clozapine

19 A 3-year-old child presents to the emergency department via ambulance with seizures followed by coma. The patient is initially stabilized, and diagnostic studies are obtained. The findings of the cerebrospinal fluid (CSF) include a total white blood cell (WBC) count of 250 cells/μL (normal, 0–5 cells/μL) with a predominance of lymphocytes and monocytes. The CSF glucose is 20 mg/dL (normal, 40–70 mg/dL), the total protein concentration is 50 mg/dL (normal, 15–45 mg/dL), and the chloride concentration is 105 mEq/L (normal, 118–132 mEq/L). Results of a Gram stain of spun-down CSF sediment are negative. A computed tomography (CT) scan with contrast shows enhancement at the base of the brain. Which of the following is the most likely diagnosis?

(A) Eastern equine encephalitis

(B) Subacute sclerosing panencephalitis

(C) Tuberculosis meningitis

(D) Cryptococcal meningitis

(E) Meningococcal meningitis

20 One week after having an upper respiratory infection, a 12-year-old boy has several bouts of epistaxis and develops pinpoint areas of hemorrhage over the chest and shoulders. The lesions are nonpalpable and nonpruritic, and they do not blanch under digital pressure. Physical examination reveals no evidence of lymphadenopathy or splenomegaly. Hemoglobin and WBC counts are normal. WBC morphology is normal. The platelet count is 20,000/mm³. Which of the following is the most likely cause of the patient's disorder?

(A) Antibodies directed against a platelet receptor

(B) Deficiency of von Willebrand's factor–cleaving protease

(C) Immunocomplex vasculitis involving small vessels

(D) Infiltrative bone marrow disease with destruction of megakaryocytes

(E) Vessel damage due to a toxin produced by *Escherichia coli*

21 A 55-year-old African-American man with a 5-year history of essential hypertension has a retinal examination revealing an irregular caliber of the arterioles, "copper wiring," and focal areas of arteriovenous nicking. No flame hemorrhages or exudates are present. Which of the following is the most likely diagnosis?

(A) Grade I hypertensive retinopathy

(B) Grade II hypertensive retinopathy

(C) Grade III hypertensive retinopathy

(D) Grade IV hypertensive retinopathy

(E) Grade V hypertensive retinopathy

22 A 32-year-old woman who is 40 weeks pregnant comes to the maternity unit in active labor. She states that she has painful genital blisters and ulcers, which she has experienced intermittently in the past. Pelvic examination reveals exquisitely tender vesicles and ulcers on her labia and vagina consistent with an active genital herpes infection. She is advised by the obstetrician that she should undergo a primary cesarean section delivery because of the increased risk of fetal infection via passage through an infected birth canal. She is mentally competent and tells the obstetrician that she refuses to have a cesarean section because her mother died during a surgical procedure. Although the doctor explains the risks of a vaginal delivery, she still refuses. The obstetrician should do which of the following?

(A) Allow a vaginal delivery

(B) Obtain a court order to perform the cesarean delivery

(C) Perform the cesarean section without her consent

(D) Obtain the consent of the husband to perform the cesarean delivery

(E) Refer her to another physician

23 A 9-month-old child presents for well-child care. The patient's head circumference is noted to be two standard deviations above the norm. In addition, the child also has frontal bossing, translucent skin, and eyes that manifest a "setting sun" sign. A meningomyelocele is also evident on physical examination. A computed tomography (CT) scan of the head would show which of the following?

(A) Type I Chiari malformation

(B) Chronic subdural hematoma

(C) Shaken baby syndrome

(D) Protruding cerebellar tonsils

(E) Leptomeningeal cyst

(F) Epidural hematoma

24 A 17-year-old boy was in his usual state of health until approximately 1 month ago when he developed a painful lump above his right knee. The patient says that he has fatigue and tells you that the leg pain awakens him from sleep. He also states that the leg pain is so bad that he has developed a limp that seems to be worsening. Physical examination reveals a hard, warm, tender mass. A radiograph of the right femur shows an "onion-skin" appearance at the location of the mass. Which of the following is the most likely diagnosis?

(A) Osteomyelitis

(B) Ewing's sarcoma

(C) Osteosarcoma

(D) Chondrosarcoma

(E) Eosinophilic granuloma

25 A 66-year-old woman complains of fatigue, difficulty concentrating, constipation, headaches, and back pain. She says these symptoms have been present for several months. She has been living alone since her husband died 2 years ago, and she has few friends. She has no history of significant medical or psychiatric problems. Physical examination is unremarkable. Mental status examination reveals decreased psychomotor activity, intact memory and cognitive functions, and no evidence of psychosis. She denies feeling depressed or suicidal. Which of the following is the most likely diagnosis?

(A) Delusional disorder, somatic type

(B) Dementia

(C) Factitious disorder

(D) Hypochondriasis

(E) Major depressive disorder

26 A 43-year-old woman, gravida 3, para 2, aborta 1, complains of increasingly worsening pain with menses along with progressively heavier menstrual blood loss. Pelvic examination reveals an asymmetrically enlarged uterus that felt soft and boggy. Results of a quantitative serum β-human chorionic gonadotropin (β-hCG) test were negative. Her symptoms were unresponsive to medical therapy. She underwent a total abdominal hysterectomy with complete resolution of her symptoms. Which of the following statements is correct about her probable diagnosis?

(A) Endometrial glands are found within the myometrium.

(B) Age at diagnosis is usually in the early reproductive years.

(C) Medical therapy is usually successful.

(D) Fertility is unimpaired.

(E) Diagnosis is made by pelvic examination.

27 Three men ranging from 35 to 55 years of age are brought to the emergency department in an ambulance after their friends found them in a hunting lodge that morning. Because of the cold weather the previous evening, they started a fire in a wood-burning stove vented to the outside of the building. Two of the three men are dead on arrival. The third man is unresponsive to verbal commands. Physical examination shows an obese male with alcohol on his breath and a ruddy complexion. Arterial blood gases (ABGs) on room air are reported as normal. Which of the following is the most appropriate first step in the management of this patient?

(A) Administer methylene blue intravenously

(B) Give amyl nitrite, sodium nitrite, and sodium thiosulfate

(C) Intubate the patient and administer 100% oxygen

(D) Administer activated charcoal

(E) Administer ascorbic acid

28 A 3-year-old presents with a history of daily fever with temperature spikes of 39°C for the past 2 weeks. The parents state that the fever is followed by an evanescent rash over the trunk and extremities. In addition, they say that the patient has arthritis-like pains. The patient also has hepatosplenomegaly, lymphadenopathy, and a pericardial effusion. The erythrocyte sedimentation rate (ESR) is elevated, and there is an absolute neutrophilic leukocytosis. Which of the following is the most likely diagnosis?

(A) Acute rheumatic fever

(B) Systemic lupus erythematosus (SLE)

(C) Juvenile rheumatoid arthritis (JRA)

(D) Lyme disease

(E) Ankylosing spondylitis

29. A 3-year-old child with a long history of sinopulmonary disease is noted to have ataxia and dilated vessels in the conjunctiva and skin. In addition, the skin has lost its normal elasticity. Chest radiology reveals an absent thymic shadow. Pertinent laboratory data reveal elevated α-fetoprotein (AFP) levels, decreased serum immunoglobulin G (IgG) levels, and low IgA and IgE levels. Which of the following is the most likely diagnosis?

(A) Wiskott-Aldrich syndrome
(B) Ataxia-telangiectasia
(C) Rendu-Osler-Weber disease
(D) Friedreich's ataxia
(E) Cerebral palsy

30. A 23-year-old college student travels to Mexico on his spring break. Having heard tales about "Montezuma's revenge" from fellow students he was very careful not to eat raw foods or to drink tap water. However he consumed more than his share of drinks cooled with ice cubes provided locally. Two days into the vacation he develops a low-grade fever associated with nausea, vomiting, diarrhea, and abdominal cramps. A stool smear is negative for fecal leukocytes. Which of the following is the mechanism most likely responsible for this patient's diarrhea?

(A) Enterotoxin stimulation of guanylate cyclase
(B) Bacterial invasion of the bowel wall
(C) Enterotoxic damage to the bowel mucosa
(D) Brush border enzyme deficiency
(E) Irritable bowel syndrome

31. A 25-year-old man complains of pain in his buttocks and legs when he walks fast or climbs hills. Physical examination shows +1 dorsalis pedis pulses and +4 radial pulses. Blood pressure measured using his right arm is 160/96 mm Hg. A high-pitched, blowing early diastolic murmur is heard in the right second intercostal space, and it increases in intensity on expiration. An arterial blood gas assay shows a normal PaO_2 and oxygen saturation. What is the most likely diagnosis?

(A) Aortic dissection
(B) Aortic valve stenosis
(C) Patent ductus arteriosus
(D) Postductal coarctation of the aorta
(E) Takayasu's arteritis

32. A 10-year-old child is referred to the pediatrician by the school nurse for a chronic headache. The mother states that the child had been in her usual state of health until 2 weeks ago when she started to complain of a dull continuous headache. The mother states that she has given the patient over-the-counter medication for the headache but nothing seems to make the headache better. In fact, the mother thinks that perhaps the headache seems to be worse. On review of symptoms, the mother states that the patient has had to "pee" with increasing frequency. The physician notes that the child is short and that the patient's height is below the 5th percentile for her age. Bitemporal hemianopia is also present. The physician orders a computed tomography (CT) scan of the head that shows calcifications above the sella turcica. Based on the history and physical examination as well as the result of the CT scan of the head this patient most likely has which of the following?

(A) An astrocytoma of the third ventricle
(B) A pinealoma
(C) A craniopharyngioma
(D) Chromophobic adenoma
(E) Hand-Schüller-Christian disease

33. A 28-year-old woman has a 15-year history of physical complaints, including chronic headaches, backaches, abdominal cramps, genital parenthesis, dizziness, nausea, and lack of energy. She abuses analgesics and benzodiazepines. Several relatives have histories of alcohol abuse and criminal behavior. Which of the following is the most likely diagnosis?

(A) Body dysmorphic disorder
(B) Delusional disorder, somatic type
(C) Factitious disorder
(D) Pain disorder
(E) Somatization disorder

34. A 29 year-old male visits his family physician with a history of pain in his legs. He states that the pain occurs in the evening and even at night, which results in disturbed sleep. He has even tried waking up and walking around to try to get rid of the pain. At times he feels a tingling sensation in the legs, as if something were crawling over them. Recently, he noticed a cramp-like pain while he was driving, and he had to pull over. He had seen a psychiatrist recently and had been prescribed a neuroleptic medication. Based on the presentation, the most likely diagnosis to consider would be which of the following?

(A) Painful legs and moving toes syndrome
(B) Fibromyalgia
(C) Restless leg syndrome
(D) Cauda equina syndrome
(E) Akathisia

35 A 65-year-old woman developed a fever and watery diarrhea while on ampicillin for a urinary tract infection. A colonoscopic examination reveals yellow-white plaques surrounded by hemorrhagic borders on the mucosal surface of the colon. Which of the following is the test of choice for diagnosing the colon disorder?

(A) Gram's stain of the yellowish material
(B) Culture of the yellowish material
(C) Toxin assay of liquid stool
(D) Blood culture
(E) Stool sample examination for ova and parasites

36 A 30-year-old man reports to his physician's office concerned about his well-being because his close friend recently had an acute myocardial infarction (MI). The patient denies a history of chest pain, palpitations, shortness of breath, or swelling of the feet. He does not smoke or consume alcohol, and there is no family history of cardiac disease. His father died of carcinoma of the colon 5 years previously, at the age of 76, and his 74-year-old mother has diabetes, which is controlled with oral medication. Physical examination reveals a 173-cm (68-in) tall white male weighing 81 kg (180 lb), who is not in acute distress. His vital signs are as follows: pulse, 80/min (regular); respirations, 18/min; blood pressure, 128/80 mm Hg. Results of examination of the cardiovascular system and the rest of his physical examination are normal. The patient requests tests to exclude the possibility of him having coronary artery disease (CAD). Which of the following would be the most appropriate next step in the management of this patient?

(A) Order an immediate resting electrocardiogram (ECG) and, if the result is positive, perform an exercise ECG
(B) Immediately order both a resting ECG and an exercise ECG
(C) Schedule the patient for routine ECG screening
(D) Explain to the patient that ECG screening is unnecessary in an asymptomatic patient
(E) Order a total body computed tomography (CT) scan.

37 A 55-year-old woman, gravida 4, para 4, comes to the outpatient office for a routine checkup and Pap smear. She underwent menopause 7 years ago, and initially she experienced hot flushes but they resolved within 2 years of menopause. She is not on any hormone therapy. Her cervical Pap smears since menopause have been read as negative for intraepithelial lesions or malignancy. She is 160 cm (63 in) tall and weighs 64 kg (141 lb). Which of the following endocrinologic profiles (A

through E) (including follicle-stimulating hormone [FSH], gonadotropin-releasing hormone [GnRH], and sex hormone binding globulin [SHBG]) is most likely characteristic of this patient?

	FSH	GnRH	Estrogen	SHBG
(A)	Increased	Decreased	Increased	Increased
(B)	Increased	Increased	Decreased	Decreased
(C)	Increased	Decreased	Decreased	Decreased
(D)	Decreased	Decreased	Decreased	Decreased
(E)	Increased	Increased	Increased	Increased

38 A 27-year-old woman, gravida 1, para 0, presents for a prenatal visit at 32 weeks' gestation. She complains of a severe headache and epigastric pain for 24 hours. The headache is not relieved by acetaminophen. The epigastric pain is unrelieved by antacids. Her blood pressure (BP) today is 165/115 mm Hg. A urine dipstick test shows 3+ proteinuria. Her blood pressure on her first prenatal visit at 12 weeks gestation was 120/70 mm Hg. She experienced severe nausea and vomiting during the first trimester, requiring antiemetic treatment, but her total pregnancy weight gain has been 22 pounds. She has taken thyroid replacement medication after undergoing iodine 131 (^{131}I) treatment for Graves' disease 5 years ago. Which of the following medications would be indicated in the treatment of this patient?

(A) Phenytoin
(B) Magnesium sulfate
(C) Terbutaline
(D) Progesterone
(E) Indomethacin

39 A pediatrician is called to attend a delivery of a 35-year-old primigravida. According to the patient and review of the medical record, the patient has had good prenatal care. And, except for the development of diabetes during the second trimester, the pregnancy has been uneventful. Cultures for sexually transmitted diseases are documented as negative. After many hours of "labor" the patient delivers an infant by spontaneous vaginal delivery with Apgar scores of 8 at 1 minute and 9 at 5 minutes. Birth-weight is 4.5 kg (10 lb). Which of the following injuries is most likely to be found in this newborn?

(A) Cephalhematoma
(B) Facial nerve paralysis
(C) Intraventricular hemorrhage
(D) Brain contusion
(E) Fractured clavicle

40 An afebrile 58-year-old woman with a 30-year history of chronic headaches suddenly develops left colicky flank pain with radiation into the left groin. Urinalysis shows RBCs, WBCs, and mild proteinuria. There are no bacteria, casts, or crystals in the urine sediment. Urine-specific gravity is 1.010 and remains unchanged throughout the day. An intravenous pyelogram shows a ring deformity in the left kidney. Which of the following is the most likely diagnosis?

(A) Acute drug-induced tubulointerstitial nephritis
(B) Chronic glomerulonephritis
(C) Chronic pyelonephritis
(D) Renal papillary necrosis
(E) Ureteral stone

Directions for Matching Questions (41 through 50): *Each set of matching questions is preceded by a list of 4 to 26 lettered options followed by a brief explanation of the required task and then by a series of numbered statements. For each lettered statement you are to select ONE lettered option that best fulfills the task as it relates to that statement. Remember each of the listed options might be correctly selected once, more than once, or not at all.*

Questions 41–47

For the following numbered descriptions of patients with orthopedic injuries, select the ONE lettered condition that is best associated with it from the list below.

(A) Wrist drop may be present
(B) Fractured radius with dislocation of the radioulnar joint at the wrist
(C) Shoulder cannot externally rotate beyond neutral position
(D) Radial pulse should be felt during reduction
(E) Hypesthesia over the lateral aspect of the shoulder may be present
(F) Can be reduced by supination
(G) Fractured ulna with radial head dislocation

41 A 28-year-old football player with anterior dislocation of the right shoulder.

42 A 35-year-old male who presents with suspected posterior dislocation of the left shoulder.

43 A 5-year-old child who was suddenly pulled by his right hand onto the curb by his mother.

44 An 8-year-old boy who fell from a tree and landed on the back of his right elbow.

45 A 30-year-old male who fell off a ladder and fractured the shaft of his right humerus.

46 A 16-year-old male with Monteggia's fracture.

47 An 18-year-old male with Galeazzi's fracture.

Questions 48–50

The lettered values below represent percentage use of various substances by American high school seniors in 2004. Match the closest percentage use with the corresponding substance as described in questions 48–50.

Percentage use

(A) 60.0
(B) 25.0
(C) 20.0
(D) 5.0
(E) 3.5

48 Used anabolic steroids at least once during 2004.

49 Smoked tobacco at least once during the month of the survey

50 Used some form of cocaine at least once during 2004

Answer Key

1	C	**11**	A	**21**	B	**31**	D	**41**	E
2	C	**12**	C	**22**	A	**32**	C	**42**	C
3	H	**13**	B	**23**	D	**33**	E	**43**	F
4	B	**14**	D	**24**	B	**34**	C	**44**	D
5	D	**15**	D	**25**	E	**35**	C	**45**	A
6	D	**16**	B	**26**	A	**36**	D	**46**	G
7	D	**17**	E	**27**	C	**37**	B	**47**	B
8	E	**18**	B	**28**	C	**38**	B	**48**	E
9	D	**19**	C	**29**	B	**39**	E	**49**	B
10	E	**20**	A	**30**	A	**40**	D	**50**	D

Answers and Explanations

1 **The answer is C** *Pediatrics*

A patient with patent ductus arteriosus (choice **C**) has a continuous machinery murmur. Bounding pulses with hyperactive precordium also may be found on physical examination. Although the electrocardiogram (ECG) is usually not helpful, it may show left ventricular hypertrophy (LVH).

Patients with atrial septal defect (ASD) (choice **B**) have a widely split and fixed second heart sound. Patients with ventricular septal defect (VSD) (choice **A**) have a pansystolic murmur. Tetralogy of Fallot (choice **E**) is characterized by the presence of a VSD, right ventricular hypertrophy, pulmonic stenosis, and overriding aorta. The murmur of tetralogy of Fallot is a long, systolic ejection murmur most audible at the midleft sternal border. In patients with pulmonic stenosis (choice **D**), there is a high-pitched systolic ejection murmur, most audible at the upper left sternal border, that transmits fairly well to the back. A systolic thrill may be present at the upper left sternal border and, rarely, in the suprasternal notch.

2 **The answer is C** *Obstetrics and Gynecology*

Diethylstilbestrol (DES) is a nonsteroidal estrogen that was used between 1940 and 1971 for treatment of threatened spontaneous abortion. Vaginal clear cell adenocarcinoma is the most serious consequence of prenatal DES exposure. However numerous nonneoplastic uterine and vaginal anomalies also have been reported in DES-exposed women. Vaginal adenosis (choice **C**), a condition in which columnar epithelium, normally found only around the endocervical canal, extends onto the vaginal fornices, is found in 4% of normal females, but 30% of women exposed to DES in utero have this condition. It is the most common physical finding observed during pelvic examination of DES-exposed women. During colposcopic examination, the immature metaplastic squamous epithelium of the cervix of these women resembles dysplasia with a mosaic and punctate appearance. However, histologic examination demonstrates this epithelium is benign; it is not a true dysplasia, thus choice **A** is not correct.

The following conditions are not associated with prenatal DES exposure: Breast fibroadenoma (choice **B**), which is the most common breast tumor in young women; müllerian agenesis (choice **D**), which is characterized by absence of the oviducts, uterus, cervix, and proximal vagina; and polycystic ovary syndrome (choice **E**), a condition with bilaterally enlarged, smooth ovaries associated with anovulation, infertility, and hirsutism.

3 **The answer is H** *Psychiatry*

The accusations represent bizarre delusions that indicate the presence of psychosis(choice **B**). Schizophrenia (choice **H**) is the most likely diagnosis. Key findings include a history of increasing pathology over the last year, deterioration of function, the presence of constricted affect, mildly tangential thinking, bizarre ideation, and social withdrawal.

The patient's normal awareness and lack of memory impairment make delirium (choice **A**), which also is not a psychosis, unlikely. Although the symptoms of dysphoria and anxiety (choice **D**) are present, they are readily explained by his psychosis, and there is little evidence to suggest that they represent primary mood pathology such as depression (choice **C**) or mania (choice **E**). The lack of significant mood symptomatology makes bipolar disorder (choice **G**) and major depressive disorder (choice **I**) less likely. The patient has no history of cocaine use (thus cocaine-induced psychosis [choice **F**] is not a likely diagnosis), and the girlfriend does not share the content of his delusions (i.e., shared psychotic disorder [choice **J**]).

4 **The answer is B** *Medicine*

The patient has sideroblastic anemia caused by deficiency of vitamin B$_6$ (pyridoxine) (choice **B**). The most common cause of pyridoxine deficiency is isoniazid therapy in patients with tuberculosis. Among many other functions, pyridoxine is a cofactor for δ-aminolevulinic acid synthase, which catalyzes the combination of succinyl-CoA with glycine to form δ-aminolevulinic acid. Since this is the rate-limiting, initial step in heme synthesis, a deficiency of pyridoxine decreases the amount of protoporphyrin that is available to form hemoglobin, and microcytic anemia ensues. Excess iron that normally would be bound to the hemoglobin accumulates in the mitochondria, producing an iron overload condition with an increase in serum ferritin, iron, and percentage saturation of transferrin and a decrease in the total iron-binding capacity (TIBC), as seen in this patient. Since mitochondria are located around the nucleus of red blood cell precursors in the bone marrow, they form a ring around the nucleus, producing ringed sideroblasts.

Deficiency of folic acid (choice **A**) and vitamin B$_{12}$ (choice **C**) produces a macrocytic anemia with hypersegmented neutrophils. The patient has a microcytic anemia. Vitamin C (choice **D**) is involved in both iron and folic acid metabolism. Deficiency of vitamin C may produce a combined microcytic anemia (iron deficiency) and macrocytic anemia (folic acid deficiency). The iron studies in a microcytic anemia show a decrease in serum ferritin, iron, and percentage saturation of transferrin and an increase in TIBC. These findings are not present in this patient. Deficiency of vitamin E (choice **E**) makes red cells prone to undergo a hemolytic anemia caused by damage of the red blood cell membrane by free radicals. The anemia is normocytic (not microcytic) and results of iron studies are normal (patient's results are abnormal).

5 The answer is D *Psychiatry*

Fentanyl is an opioid commonly used to treat cancer-induced and other severe pain. It is available in several forms including a patch, a lollipop to be absorbed sublingually, and an inhalent for use by anesthesiologists. Anesthesiologists are particularly prone to become addicted to fentanyl, which is freely available to them and can satisfy an addictive need when inhaled in such small amounts that it will never be missed during drug inventories or even show up in their urine. However, opioid addiction in a professional of any sort, a physician in particular, is dangerous because impaired judgment accompanies the other effects. Thus it behooves his assistant to make sure he does keep his promise to undergo treatment, which should be successful (choice **D**) because he will be highly motivated. Moreover, there is a high probability he will not relapse. However, his withdrawal will be associated with dysphoric mood, nausea, muscle pains, lacrimation, rhinorrhea, pupillary dilation, piloerection, sweating, diarrhea, yawning, fever, and insomnia and should be supported by proper treatment. Such treatment includes medical support for gastrointestinal and metabolic symptoms, emotional reassurance, and a secure environment. Pharmacologic intervention is not likely to involve tapering the dose of fentanyl, as is done with many other opioids, since presumably he already only inhales a miniscule amount, but methadone might be used for several days to help alleviate neurologic symptoms, and clonidine may be administered to alleviate gastrointestinal symptoms and sweating. If needed, benzodiazepines could be used to decrease severe insomnia.

Opioid addiction is more commonly associated with sociability than with isolation and loneliness (choice **A**), and it rarely is linked to induction of psychosis (choice **B**). Opioid addiction also is not a fairly common sequel of opioid use for acute pain management (choice **C**), because patients are often terminal, and if not, physicians are careful not to continue treatment with opioids for an extended period. Deviant behavior is common in opioid addicts (choice **E**), even if opioids are readily available.

6 The answer is D *Medicine*

Although these symptoms clearly indicate that the patient has gastroesophageal reflux disease (GERD), it is always a wise move to rule out the possibility of cardioarterial disease (CAD) as was done by the exercise tolerance test. GERD is a chronic, recurrent disorder characterized by heartburn, belching, and epigastric pain. The primary mechanism is inappropriate relaxation of the LES (choice **D**). Agents that decrease LES pressure, such as chocolate, coffee, ethanol, fat, peppermint, anticholinergics, theophylline, diazepam, barbiturates, and calcium channel blockers, exacerbate GERD. About 1 in 10 nonpregnant adults complain about heartburn at least once a week, and prevalence of GERD increases with age, is found more commonly in older men than in older women, and is very common during pregnancy; approximately 1 in 4 pregnant women experience heartburn from acid reflux daily during pregnancy. This very high frequency is attributed to impaired LES competence coupled to increased abdominal pressure.

Secondary factors that predispose to GERD include hiatal hernia, acid concentration of the refluxate; delayed acid clearance, which is associated with low-amplitude peristalsis and recumbency; and decreased gastric emptying (not increased [choice **B**]), which aggravates reflux. The acid concentration of the refluxate is the most important factor in determining progression to reflux esophagitis. Complications associated with GERD are reflux esophagitis, stricture formation, and Barrett's esophagus. Barrett's esophagus is a premalignant condition characterized by glandular metaplasia of the distal esophagus. The risk of developing adenocarcinoma is 2 to 10% in the United States, and distal adenocarcinoma of the esophagus has replaced squamous cell carcinoma of the esophagus as the most common esophageal cancer. GERD can also precipitate an asthmatic attack by reflux vagal stimulation or aspiration. Approximately 80% of adults with bronchial asthma have GERD. This percentage appears to be independent of bronchodilator therapy. Chronic aspiration is also linked to pulmonary fibrosis and bronchiectasis. Ambulatory monitoring of esophageal pH for 24 hours, the gold standard, can detect GERD and provide information relative to the potential for chronic aspiration of acid reflux. The treatment of GERD involves reducing gastroesophageal reflux, neutralizing the acid reflux, enhancing esophageal clearance, and protecting the esophageal mucosa from ulceration. Diet modification, weight loss, postural therapy (elevation of the head of the bed), restriction of alcohol, and cessation of smoking, along with pharmacologic treatment are used in a stepwise approach reflecting patient response. A recommended progression of drugs includes antacids and alginic acid → histamine-2 (H_2) receptor antagonists at conventional doses → H_2 receptor antagonists at high doses, omeprazole, or prokinetic agents (metoclopramide) → antireflux surgery.

Absence of ganglion cells in the myenteric plexus (choice **E**) is the key finding in achalasia. Decreased peristalsis (choice **C**) is noted in both achalasia and systemic sclerosis. Decreased acid production in the stomach (choice **A**) is noted in pernicious anemia (destruction of the parietal cells) and *Helicobacter pylori*–induced atrophic gastritis involving the antrum and pylorus.

7 **The answer is D** *Medicine*

The patient has dermatomyositis (DM) (choice **D**), which has some overlapping features with polymyositis (PM). Both disorders are a female-dominant type of myositis, with DM involving skin and muscle in adults and children and PM involving only muscle in adults (choice **C**). Both disorders have muscle pain and atrophy, with the shoulders and pelvic muscles most commonly involved. The pelvic muscle weakness makes it difficult for patients to climb stairs. Dermatologic lesions associated with DM (not PM) include erythema over the bridge of the nose, with violaceous discoloration and edema of the upper eyelids. Erythematous papular lesions are noted over the dorsum of the proximal interphalangeal joints, knuckles, elbows, and knees (present in this patient). Dysphagia for solids and liquids is present, because of weakness of the striated muscle in the upper esophagus. Laboratory findings include a positive serum antinuclear antibody test result in 30% of cases. Anti Jo-1 and anti PM-1 antibodies are present in a small percentage of cases. The serum creatine kinase is increased, and muscle biopsies show a lymphocytic inflammatory reaction with destruction of muscle fibers. The treatment for DM and PM is chronic prednisone therapy. If patients fail to respond to steroid therapy, they may be placed on immunosuppressive agents such as azathioprine, cyclophosphamide, or methotrexate.

Polymyalgia rheumatica (choice **A**) may be associated with proximal muscle aching; however, serum creatine and the electromyogram (EMG) are normal. Likewise, rheumatoid arthritis (choice **B**) does not feature increased in serum creatine kinase or an abnormal EMG. Systemic lupus erythematosus (SLE) (choice **E**) could easily explain the "butterfly rash" but would not explain the myopathic features expressed in the EMG and the increased muscle enzymes.

8 **The answer is E** *Obstetrics and Gynecology*

A frequent adverse effect associated with maternal prenatal use of many substances is intrauterine growth restriction (IUGR) and preterm delivery. However, of all the choices with this case, only cocaine (choice **E**) has clearly defined vascular-disruption anomalies such as intestinal atresia, limb-reduction defects, and brain anomalies. It is also associated with abruptio placenta, which was the most likely cause of the problems that led to the 34-week emergency cesarean described in the scenario. Although the other choices have an adverse impact on pregnancy outcome, they do not cause limb-reduction defects.

Tobacco (choice **A**) is associated with IUGR, alcohol (choice **B**) is associated with fetal alcohol syndrome, and narcotics (choice **C**) and amphetamines (choice **D**) can lead to an addicted newborn.

9 **The answer is D** *Psychiatry*

The symptoms are most suggestive of autistic disorder. Autistic disorder often presents with qualitative disturbances of interpersonal behavior, failure to develop normal communication, and a restricted range of interests. Abnormal behaviors such as rocking and head banging are common. There is a strong association between autistic disorder and intrauterine infections, most commonly rubella (choice **D**). Other prenatal and postnatal factors are also associated with subsequent autistic disorder, including encephalitis and errors of metabolism such as tuberous sclerosis.

Psychosocial factors, such as emotionally distant parents (choice **C**) and childhood sexual abuse (choice **B**), are not causally associated with autistic disorder, although the resultant emotional pathology may mimic some autistic symptoms. Maternal cocaine abuse during pregnancy (choice **E**) and childhood lead exposure (choice **A**) have been associated with behavioral and attention disturbances in children, but not with autistic disorder.

10 The answer is E *Medicine*

The patient has a lung abscess, which is most often caused by aspiration of oropharyngeal material. The microbial pathogens in the aspirated material are a mixture of aerobic (e.g., streptococci) and anaerobic organisms (e.g., *Prevotella melanogenicus*) normally present in oropharyngeal secretions. When the patient is supine, aspirated material localizes in the superior segment of the lower lobe of the right lung (choice **E**). The treatment for anaerobic lung abscesses is intravenous aqueous penicillin G.

Aspiration to the lingula of the left lung (choice **A**) occurs when lying on the left side. Aspiration to the right middle lobe (choice **B**) or the posterior segment of the right upper lobe (choice **C**) occurs when lying on the right side. Aspiration to the posterobasal segment of the right lower lobe (choice **D**) occurs when sitting or standing.

11 The answer is A *Medicine*

The patient has Raynaud's phenomenon. It is the presenting sign of systemic sclerosis (85% of cases) and localized scleroderma, known as the CREST syndrome (95% of cases), often antedating other manifestations of the disease by years. Cold temperatures and stress are stimuli that produce color changes of the fingers (sometimes toes), which first blanch, then become cyanotic, and then red. Vasospasm and thickened digital vessels (choice **A**) are responsible for these changes. Immune complexes are not present in the vessels (choice **C**).

CREST syndrome is characterized by calcinosis of the digits (calcification of subcutaneous tissue), Raynaud's phenomenon, esophageal motility dysfunction, sclerodactyly (tapered fingers), and telangiectasia (small vessel dilation) over the digits and under the nails. The anticentromere antibody is positive in over 50% of cases.

Systemic sclerosis is a more generalized disorder of connective tissue, characterized by degenerative and inflammatory changes that result in the subsequent increase of collagen tissue deposition in various tissues. Tightening of the skin of the face and extremities is a universal finding. Esophageal motility problems, with dysphagia for solids and liquids, occur in 80% of cases. Other problems include arthritis (80%), renal involvement (60% of cases), pericardial effusions (20–50% of cases), and pulmonary fibrosis with restrictive lung disease (35% of cases). The antinuclear antibody test result is positive in 70 to 90% of cases. The anti-Scl-70 antibody (antitopoisomerase) is specific for systemic sclerosis and is noted in 40 to 70% of cases. Penicillamine may improve long-term survival.

Other causes of Raynaud's phenomenon are thromboangiitis obliterans (Buerger's disease), which is an inflammatory vasculitis producing thrombosis of the digital vessels (choice **D**) in male smokers (patient is female and a nonsmoker); and, cryoglobulinemia with proteins that precipitate in cold temperatures (choice **B**). The latter condition is commonly associated with chronic hepatitis C (not present in this patient as demonstrated by her normal, stable liver transaminase levels) and also produces cyanosis of the nose and ears in cold weather that reverses to normal when returning to a warm environment. Embolism to digital vessels in the hand is uncommon (choice **E**) and is most commonly due to infective endocarditis or atrial fibrillation, neither of which are present in this patient.

12 The answer is C *Psychiatry*

Comorbidity for other severe mental disorders is greater than 50% in individuals with severe drug dependence. Mood disorders, anxiety disorders, and psychotic disorders are commonly present, any of which may cause additional serious psychiatric pathology (choice **C**).

Amphetamines play no role in cocaine detoxification (choice **A**). Psychologic effects from cocaine dependence, including mood and sleep disturbances, often continue for several weeks (choice **B**). Alcohol dependence is a common comorbid condition in individuals with cocaine dependence, and alcohol withdrawal may be seen during their hospitalization (choice **D**). Antipsychotic medications are often used to treat psychosis and agitation during cocaine withdrawal without an increased incidence of severe toxic interactions (choice **E**).

13 The answer is B *Obstetrics and Gynecology*

The Apgar score is a five-parameter clinical assessment of the newborn made shortly after birth. The score made at 1 minute indicates the degree of resuscitation that is needed, while the 5-minute score indicates the success of the resuscitation efforts. The five parameters used to assign a score are skin color, respiratory effort, heart rate, muscle tone, and reflex irritability. A score of 7 to 10 is excellent and requires no intervention. A score of 3 or less indicates that immediate life-saving measures are needed. This infant will be assigned 1 point for pink body but blue extremities, 1 point for weak respiratory effort, 2 points for heart rate (because it is over 100 beats/min), 1 point for muscle tone, and 0 for reflex irritability for a total score of 5 (choice **B**).

An Apgar score of 4 (choice **A**), 6 (choice **C**), 7 (choice **D**), or 8 (choice **E**) would be incorrect in this case.

14 The answer is D *Medicine*

The patient most likely has community-acquired bacterial pneumonia as indicated by the abrupt onset of fever, chills, a productive cough, and chest pain upon inspiration. However, pneumonia in the elderly differs in some important ways from the classic findings of community-acquired bacterial pneumonia in younger adults. Commonly the presenting symptoms are acute confusion with rapid breathing. Signs of consolidation such as dullness to percussion are also absent, rales are minimal, and x-ray studies can be difficult to interpret. Although present in the case described, chest pain, productive cough, and chills are not always present. The white cell count is not increased in 50% of cases or, as in this case, increased minimally; however, 95% of cases demonstrate a left shift. As in typical community-acquired bacterial pneumonia. *Streptococcus pneumoniae* (pneumococcus) (choice **D**) remains the most common cause.

Klebsiella pneumoniae pneumonia (choice **B**) is more commonly associated with alcoholics and nursing-home patients. Patients cough up mucoid-appearing sputum that is often tinged with blood. A Gram's stain of sputum shows fat gram-negative rods with a capsule. The treatment of choice is the use of third-generation cephalosporins or fluoroquinolones. Viral pneumonias (atypical pneumonias) (choice **C**) are usually associated with a nonproductive cough and have an interstitial pattern on chest x-ray films rather than a consolidation. Primary tuberculosis (choice **E**) is rare in a 85-year-old otherwise healthy adult and occurs more frequently in children or immunocompromised patients. It involves the periphery of the lower part of the upper lobe or upper part of the lower lobe in the lungs. Alzheimer's disease (choice **A**) and senile dementia due to chronic vascular disease. (choice **F**) can be ruled out because of the sudden onset of symptoms.

15 The answer is D *Medicine*

The patient has a *Pneumocystis carinii* pneumonitis with the characteristic radiographic findings of "ground glass" opacities in the lungs. Methenamine silver stains (not Gram's stain) (choice **E**) of lung tissue or bronchoalveolar lavage specimens frequently demonstrate densely clustered cysts that resemble crushed ping-pong balls. Because the patient is HIV positive and has an opportunistic infection, the patient qualifies as having acquired immune deficiency syndrome (AIDS). *P. carinii* is the most common initial manifestation and cause of death in patients with AIDS. Once considered a protozoan, DNA analysis now shows that the organism is more closely related to a fungus. The organism cannot be cultured. Patients are generally susceptible to infection when their CD4 helper T cell count approaches 200 cells/mm^3. It is contracted in immunosuppressed patients by inhalation and produces an interstitial pneumonitis with extreme hypoxia. *P. carinii* predominantly affects the lungs, but it can also involve other head and neck organs, such as the thyroid or the skin. The treatment for *P. carinii* is trimethoprim–sulfamethoxazole (TMP-SMX), (choice **D**) or pentamidine. Aerosolized pentamidine or low-dose sulfonamides are useful as prophylaxis against the infection. There is a 20% fatality rate with each infection; therefore, lifetime prophylaxis is needed. The infection does not respond to amphotericin B (choice **A**) or erythromycin (choice **B**).

P. carinii is easily confused with *Histoplasma capsulatum,* but *Histoplasma* organisms are located in macrophages. Disseminated histoplasmosis could present with granulomas in the bone marrow (choice **C**). *P. carinii* does not produce granulomatous inflammation. Amphotericin B is the treatment of choice for histoplasmosis.

16 **The answer is B** *Medicine*

The patient has Crohn's disease (choice **B**). The terminal ileum is the primary site for the reabsorption of the intrinsic factor–vitamin B_{12} complex and for bile salts and bile acids. Crohn's disease is an inflammatory condition that involves the terminal ileum in about 80% of cases; therefore, vitamin B_{12} deficiency and bile salt deficiency are potential complications of the disease. Bile salts are required to emulsify the breakdown products of fat digestion and package them into micelles for reabsorption by the villi. Deficiency of bile salts and acids produces malabsorption of fat, which is present in this patient. Vitamin B_{12} deficiency produces a macrocytic anemia with hypersegmented neutrophils and neurologic dysfunction involving the posterior columns of the spinal cord (e.g., decreased vibratory sensation). Bile salts are required to emulsify fatty acids and monoglycerides after hydrolysis of triglyceride by pancreatic lipase in the small intestine. Deficiency of bile salts leads to malabsorption of fat.

Chronic pancreatitis (choice **A**) is incorrect. When vitamin B_{12} is ingested, R factor in the saliva and gastric juice combines with the vitamin to form a complex that cannot be destroyed by acid in the stomach. Pancreatic enzymes are required to cleave R factor from the vitamin B_{12}–R factor complex. This allows intrinsic factor, which is synthesized by the parietal cells in the stomach, to complex with vitamin B_{12} for reabsorption in the terminal ileum. Although chronic pancreatitis is a common cause of vitamin B_{12} deficiency, it does not affect the metabolism of bile salts and acids. Furthermore, chronic pancreatitis produces epigastric pain with radiation into the back rather than right lower quadrant colicky abdominal pain. A fish tapeworm infestation (choice **C**) is incorrect. Fish tapeworms cause vitamin B_{12} deficiency, but they have no adverse effect on bile salt or bile acid metabolism and would not be expected to produce malabsorption of fat. Lactase deficiency (choice **D**) is incorrect. Lactase is a brush border enzyme in the small bowel that cleaves lactose to form glucose and galactose. Deficiency of the enzyme produces an osmotic diarrhea with hydrogen gas formation and an acid stool from colonic bacteria conversion of unmetabolized lactose to lactic acid. Osmotic diarrhea does not produce either vitamin B_{12} deficiency or bile salt deficiency. Pernicious anemia (choice **E**) is incorrect. Pernicious anemia is an autoimmune disease characterized by destruction of the parietal cells in the stomach, causing decreased synthesis of intrinsic factor and gastric acid. Loss of intrinsic factor leads to malabsorption of vitamin B_{12} in the terminal ileum; however, there is no adverse effect on bile salt metabolism. Due to the lack of acid in the stomach, there is maldigestion of protein but not of fat, therefore, fat malabsorption would not likely be present as in this patient.

17 **The answer is E** *Psychiatry*

The ability to maintain a stable relationship and a career over a significant period of time (at least 10 years) suggests that the individual has the general capacity to relate well to others; i.e., she has a history of satisfying interpersonal relationships (choice **E**).

Individuals with gender identity disorder seek sex-change surgery (choice **B**). Homosexual (lesbian) individuals, like this patient, are content with their biologic gender. There is some evidence for a genetic and prenatal hormonal basis for homosexuality; but in adulthood, homosexual individuals have normal sex hormone levels (choice **D**). Homosexual individuals often have experienced heterosexual sex (choice **A**), and many have had children (choice **C**).

18 **The answer is B** *Psychiatry*

This patient's condition is highly suggestive of bipolar disorder, which is not responsive to lithium treatment. This happens in approximately 25% of cases. It would be unwise to increase the lithium dose (choice **C**) in this patient, because his level is already at the top of the therapeutic range. The medication of choice in such circumstances is divalproex (choice **B**), because some patients who do not respond to lithium will respond to it.

Mirtazapine (choice **A**) is a sedating antidepressant that would not be expected to control a manic episode. Olanzapine (choice **D**), clozapine (choice **E**) and other antipsychotic medications may decrease mania, psychotic thinking, and excessive motor activity but have untoward effects that make them less desirable than lithium or divalproex as initial choices for the long-term management of bipolar disorder.

19 **The answer is C** *Pediatrics*

Tuberculosis meningitis (choice **C**) usually presents in recently infected individuals and is usually considered a disease of infants and children. The symptoms develop slowly in three stages. Stage 1 is a prodromal stage with nonspecific symptomatology. Seizures are common in stage 2; coma occurs in stage 3. A high index of suspicion is necessary for rapid diagnosis. A computed tomography (CT) scan of the head may show periventricular lucencies, edema, infarctions, and hydrocephalus. Cerebrospinal fluid (CSF) findings include an elevation in white blood cells (WBCs), usually from 250 to 500 cells/μL, predominantly lymphocytes. The CSF glucose is less than 40 mg/dL, or less than half the serum glucose found simultaneously. Protein concentration is normal or slightly high. Gram's stain is negative because the bacilli are acid-fast. CSF chloride is low.

Cryptococcal meningitis (choice **D**) is associated with elevated protein, hypoglycorrhachia, and mononuclear pleocytosis (rarely >300 cells/mm³). Children with subacute sclerosing panencephalitis (choice **B**) have CSF with normal cell content (may show some plasma cells), normal or slightly elevated protein, and greatly increased γ-globulin. Eastern equine encephalitis (choice **A**) occurs more commonly in young infants, causing serious complications and fatalities. The spectrum and definitive diagnosis of meningococcal meningitis (choice **E**) are made by the isolation of the organism from the CSF.

20 The answer is A *Medicine*

The patient has idiopathic thrombocytopenic purpura, which is caused by IgG antibodies directed against glycoprotein IIb/IIIa fibrinogen receptors on the surface of platelets (choice **A**). Petechiae and epistaxis are common signs of platelet disorders, which are not present in other disorders of hemostasis (e.g., coagulation factor deficiencies). The treatment is to minimize activity to prevent injury or bruising (e.g., contact sports should be avoided) and to avoid medications that increase the risk of bleeding (e.g., aspirin). The platelet count is low enough to warrant the use of prednisone. Platelet infusions should be avoided. Most children recover uneventfully.

A deficiency of von Willebrand's factor–cleaving protease (choice **B**) is found in thrombotic thrombocytopenic purpura (TTP), which usually occurs in women. TTP produces a classic pentad of fever, thrombocytopenia, microangiopathic hemolytic anemia with schistocytes, central nervous system dysfunction, and renal failure. Except for thrombocytopenia, none of these findings are present in this patient. Immunocomplex vasculitis involving small vessels (choice **C**) damages the vessels and causes multifocal areas of subcutaneous hemorrhage (purpura or ecchymoses). The inflammatory reaction causes the affected tissue to swell, and the lesions are palpable. This patient's lesions are not palpable, which excludes an immunocomplex type of vasculitis. Infiltrative bone marrow disease with destruction of megakaryocytes (option **D**) commonly occurs in leukemia, myelofibrosis, and metastatic disease to the bone marrow. In all these conditions, immature abnormal WBCs are present in the peripheral blood. The patient's WBC count is normal. The O157:H7 strain of *E. coli* produces a toxin that damages small vessels (choice **E**), causing a hemolytic uremic syndrome. The patient does not have hemolytic anemia or renal failure.

21 The answer is B *Medicine*

According to the Keith-Wagener-Barker classification of the retinal changes in hypertension, the irregular arterial caliber, "copper wiring," and arteriovenous nicking of this patient's retina would indicate grade II hypertensive retinopathy (choice **B**).

The sequence of events in hypertensive retinopathy is focal spasm of the arterioles, followed by progressive sclerosis and narrowing of the arterioles, leading eventually to flame hemorrhages from rupture of the vessels, formation of exudates, and papilledema. Grayish white exudates that are soft, like cotton wool, are due to microinfarctions, whereas exudates that have clear margins (hard exudates) are due to leakage of protein from increased vessel permeability. Sclerotic changes in the vessels are first described as "copper wiring," because blood is still visible through the vessel wall. When the vessel wall is thickened enough to prevent visualization of the blood, the light reflects back from the vessel wall to produce a "silver wiring" effect. Because the arterioles cross over the venules, the wall of the venule is depressed as arterioles thicken, and arteriovenous nicking defects are produced. Papilledema refers to swelling of the optic disc.

The following table describes normal retinal changes as well as findings in grades I (choice **A**), II, III (choice **C**), and IV (choice **D**) hypertensive retinopathy. Keith-Wagener-Barker classification has no such condition as grade V hypertensive retinopathy (choice **E**).

	Normal	Grade I	Grade II	Grade III	Grade IV
A/V ratio*a*	3/4	1/2	1/3	1/4	Fine cords
Flame hemorrhages	None	None	None	Present	Present
Exudates	None	None	None	Present	Present
Papilledema	None	None	None	None	Present
Copper wiring	None	None	Present	None	None
Silver wiring	None	None	None	Present	None
AV nicking	None	Slight depression	Depression with humping at ends	Right-angle deviation; vein disappears underneath	Same as grade III

*a*A/V ratio refers to the ratio of the diameter of the arteriole to that of the venule.

22 The answer is A *Obstetrics and Gynecology*

The physician should allow the patient to deliver her infant vaginally (choice **A**). Although the infant may contract herpes, the mother can refuse the cesarean section, because competent adults have the right to refuse medical or surgical treatment. In this scenario, the fetus has no rights, the mother is the patient, and a court will not order a surgical procedure against the patient's will (choice **B**). Only the patient can consent to her own surgery. No one, including a husband (choice **D**), can consent to surgery for another person. Performing the cesarean without her consent (choice **C**) is legally considered "assault and battery" and is ethically not a viable option. The physician has the right to refuse treatment and to refer her to another physician; however, this will not solve the problem (choice **E**).

23 The answer is D *Pediatrics*

The symptoms described indicate that this patient has type II Arnold-Chiari malformation. In this condition the hydrocephalus is a noncommunicating one. The fourth ventricle is elongated, there is kinking of the brainstem, and portions of the brainstem and cerebellum are displaced into the cervical spinal canal, causing obstruction of flow of cerebrospinal fluid (CSF). Skull films show a small posterior fossa and widened cervical canal (platybasia). Computed tomography or MRI will show hindbrain abnormalities and cerebellar tonsils protruding downward into the cervical canal (choice **D**). In noncommunicating hydrocephalus, the most frequent cause is aqueductal stenosis or the Arnold-Chiari malformation associated with meningomyelocele.

Type I Chiari malformation (choice **A**) is not associated with hydrocephalus and usually produces symptoms during adolescence or adult life. A leptomeningeal cyst (choice **E**) is a rare and late complication of a linear skull fracture and appears as an expanding pulsatile mass on the surface of the skull. Chronic subdural hematomas (choice **B**) are characterized by headache, personality change, and sudden loss of consciousness. Classically, patients with epidural hematoma (choice **F**) experience a brief period of unconsciousness followed by a variable lucid interval. As the hematoma expands, the patient has progressive loss of consciousness, headache, vomiting, and focal neurologic signs. Retinal hemorrhages would be seen in children who are victims of shaken baby syndrome (choice **C**).

24 The answer is B *Pediatrics*

Ewing's sarcoma (choice **B**) most commonly presents during the teenage years. The radiographic feature of Ewing's sarcoma is a diffuse, mottled, lytic lesion affecting the medullary cavity and cortical bone. An "onion-skin" appearance on radiographic examination is seen when the tumor penetrates the cortex and extends into the periosteum, producing elevations represented by multiple layers of reactive new bone formation.

Osteosarcoma (choice **C**) is the most common malignant bone tumor in children. The diagnosis of osteosarcoma may be suspected from good-quality radiographs. In advanced cases of osteosarcoma, possible findings include cortical destruction; sclerosis; a "sunburst" pattern of new periosteal bone formation; and calcified, soft tissue extensions. Chondrosarcoma (choice **D**) is rare in children. It occurs most commonly in the pelvis. Metastasis is usually by local extension. Eosinophilic granuloma (choice **E**) presents as a painless or mildly painful swelling in the skull, long bones, ribs, pelvis, or vertebra. Radiographs show a lytic lesion with well-defined borders. Osteomyelitis (choice **A**) is an infection of the bone, with the femur and tibia most commonly affected. Radiographs are normal early in the course of osteomyelitis.

25 The answer is E *Psychiatry*

This woman's symptoms are most suggestive of major depressive disorder (choice **E**). Depressive disorders may present as physical complaints, without subjective complaints of mood disturbance by the patient. This sort of clinical presentation is more common in patients who are stoic, are less able to introspect, and come from backgrounds in which emotional pathology is less acceptable. It is sometimes called "masked depression."

Delusional disorder (choice **A**) is characterized by more improbable physical complaints. Dementia (choice **B**) presents with evidence of memory impairment and other cognitive deficits. In factitious disorder (choice **C**), symptoms are deliberately produced by the patient for the purpose of assuming the sick role. In hypochondriasis (choice **D**), a patient misinterprets minor physical complaints as evidence of more serious illness.

26 The answer is A *Obstetrics and Gynecology*

The case scenario is characteristic of adenomyosis, a benign condition, in which endometrial glands are found within the myometrium (choice **A**). Adenomyosis usually develops in the later (not earlier [choice **B**]) reproductive years. Fertility may be impaired (choice **D**) if the site affected is in the region of the tubal ostia, a condition known as salpingitis isthmica nodosa. Although a physical examination finding of an enlarged, soft, boggy, tender, nonpregnant uterus may be suggestive of adenomyosis, the definitive diagnosis is based on histologic findings confirmed at the time of hysterectomy, not based on pelvic examination (choice **E**). The only effective treatment is surgical, not medical (choice **C**). The levonorgestrel-containing intrauterine contraceptive system (Mirena) may hold promise for medical treatment of adenomyosis in some patients.

27 The answer is C *Medicine*

Carbon monoxide (CO) poisoning is a common accidental injury or method of suicide, for example, by inhaling automobile exhaust in a closed space. CO is a colorless, odorless gas produced by incomplete combustion of carbon-containing compounds. Because of its high affinity for hemoglobin (Hb), CO passes straight through the lungs and pulmonary capillaries and attaches to the heme group of the red blood cells (RBCs) without setting up any gradients in the alveoli or arterial blood. Therefore, both the alveolar and arterial P_{O_2} are normal. In the standard blood-gas laboratory, only the pH, Pa_{CO_2}, and Pa_{O_2} are directly measured. The oxygen saturation is calculated from the Pa_{O_2}, which explains why it would be reported as normal in this patient. However, in fact, the oxygen saturation is decreased, because a smaller percentage of heme groups are occupied by oxygen, having been replaced by CO, which has a greater affinity for Hb. This potential error in reported values is usually avoided in modern blood-gas analyzers that have a co-oximeter attachment that directly measures the oxygen saturation, as well as oxygen content, CO level, and methemoglobin level. In CO poisoning, patients may present with symptoms ranging from headache in mild forms of poisoning to coma and death in severe exposure. The blood and skin has a cherry-red color, which is often a good clue for the presence of CO. The first step in the management of CO poisoning is the administration of 100% oxygen (choice **C**) via a nonrebreathing mask or endotracheal tube. The increased oxygen displaces the CO on the RBCs. The half-life of CO on RBCs is less than 1 hour when a patient is on 100% oxygen versus 5 to 6 hours when breathing room air, thus giving a victim oxygen immediately can prevent permanent neurologic damage.

Intravenous (IV) methylene-blue therapy (choice **A**) is the treatment of choice for methemoglobinemia. Methemoglobin refers to the presence of Hb iron in the ferric state, which cannot bind with oxygen. Cyanosis is present. The blood has a chocolate-brown color. As was the case for CO poisoning, the true oxygen saturation is not measured on standard blood-gas instruments. Methylene blue enhances an infrequently used methemoglobin reductase system, which converts iron back into the ferrous state. Ascorbic acid (choice **E**), which is a reducing agent, is also used as an ancillary treatment. Since the three men did not have evidence of cyanosis, methemoglobinemia is excluded. Amyl nitrite, sodium nitrite, and sodium thiosulfate (choice **B**) are used in the treatment of cyanide poisoning. Cyanide is a systemic asphyxiant that blocks cytochrome oxidase in the electron transport chain in the mitochondria. This blockade prevents the synthesis of adenosine triphosphate (ATP). The breath has a bitter almond smell. The ABGs are normal. Nitrites are used in the treatment scheme to oxidize a fraction of the Hb into methemoglobin, which has a high affinity for cyanide and prevents it from binding to cytochrome oxidase. Cyanide poisoning can also be treated with thiocyanate, which combines with cyanide to form a nontoxic thiocyanate, which is excreted. No mention is made of a bitter almond smell emanating from the patients. This is a characteristic finding of cyanide poisoning. A common cause of cyanide poisoning is smoke inhalation in a house fire, where cyanide is released from polyurethane products. Activated charcoal (choice **D**) has great absorptive properties for any orally administered poison with an alkene structural component such as theophylline, phenytoin, salicylates, and phenobarbital. It is not useful in poisonings due to carbon monoxide, alcohols, potassium, lithium, and iron.

28. The answer is C   *Pediatrics*

Juvenile rheumatoid arthritis (JRA) (choice **C**) is an autoimmune inflammatory disease that causes chronic synovitis as well as other extraarticular manifestations. This arthritis is divided into subgroups on the basis of presentation and laboratory findings. Systemic JRA occurs in approximately one fifth of patients and is associated with high fevers, rash, hepatosplenomegaly, pleural and pericardial effusions, and anemia of chronic disease. The erythrocyte sedimentation rate (ESR) is elevated during active disease.

Acute rheumatic fever (choice **A**) can be differentiated from JRA by the evidence of carditis and its transient migratory arthritis. Systemic lupus erythematosus (SLE) (choice **B**) usually has milder joint manifestations and a characteristic malar rash. Lyme disease (choice **D**) should be considered in the differential diagnosis. A careful history and physical examination, searching for tick bites and characteristic rash of erythema chronicum migrans, should be performed. Ankylosing spondylitis (choice **E**) can be mistaken for JRA until spine involvement is seen. Its onset is later in life, and it is much more common in men.

29. The answer is B   *Pediatrics*

Ataxia-telangiectasia (choice **B**) is an autosomal recessive disorder and the most common of the degenerative ataxias. The ataxia usually begins at approximately 2 years of age. It is progressive until full loss of ambulation occurs by adolescence. Telangiectasia (red spots on the skin due to dilated superficial blood vessels) is seen in the eyes, bridge of the nose, ears, and exposed surfaces of the extremities. The skin also loses elasticity. Sinopulmonary infections occur frequently, secondary to abnormal immune function. Low immunoglobulin A (IgA) and IgE levels are seen. The α-fetoprotein (AFP) level is elevated. Children with ataxia-telangiectasia have a much higher risk of developing lymphoreticular and brain tumors.

Wiskott-Aldrich syndrome (choice **A**) is an X-linked recessive syndrome that presents with atopic dermatitis, thrombocytopenic purpura, and an increased susceptibility to infection. Rendu-Osler-Weber disease (also known as hereditary hemorrhagic telangiectasia) (choice **C**) is characterized by angiomas of the skin, mucous membranes, gastrointestinal tract, and liver as well as pulmonary arteriovenous fistulas. Friedreich's ataxia (choice **D**) presents before 10 years of age with progressive ataxia, dysarthric speech, nystagmus, and skeletal abnormalities. Cerebral palsy (choice **E**) is a static encephalopathy that is a nonprogressive disorder of posture and movement. Cerebral palsy may be associated with mental retardation, epilepsy, and behavioral abnormalities.

30. The answer is A   *Medicine*

The patient has traveler's diarrhea, which is most often caused by enterotoxigenic *Escherichia coli,* which is responsible for 50 to 75% of cases. Enterotoxins elaborated by the organism stimulate guanylate cyclase (choice **A**) causing the synthesis of cyclic guanylate monophosphate (cGMP) from GTP. cGMP stimulates ionic pumps in the intestine, causing the loss of an isotonic fluid in the bowel, which is classified as a secretory type of diarrhea. There is no mucosal damage (no enterotoxin damage [choice **C**]) in this type of diarrhea. Most cases of traveler's diarrhea are due to ingestion of contaminated food or water or, as very likely in this case, ice. Drugs that are useful for prophylaxis include doxycycline, trimethoprim–sulfamethoxazole combination, fluoroquinolones, and bismuth subsalicylate. Other causes of traveler's diarrhea include *Shigella* species, *Campylobacter jejuni, Salmonella* species, and rotavirus. Species such as *Shigella* and *Campylobacter* invade the bowel mucosa to produce mucosal injury and an inflammatory diarrhea with production of an exudate.

Invasive diarrheas (e.g., *Campylobacter jejuni,* [choice **B**]) are a low-volume type of diarrhea. Owing to bacterial invasion of the bowel, blood, mucus, and inflammatory cells are present in the stool. A stool smear for fecal leukocytes is an excellent screen that distinguishes an invasive diarrhea from a secretory or osmotic diarrhea. The latter two have a negative fecal smear for leukocytes. The most common brush border enzyme deficiency (choice **D**) is of lactase, which normally converts lactose found in dairy products into glucose and galactose for reabsorption in the small intestine. In the absence of the enzyme, lactose is left unmetabolized. Lactose is osmotically active and draws a hypotonic sodium-containing fluid out of the bowel wall into the lumen. This is classified as a high-volume, osmotic type of diarrhea. Colon anaerobes degrade undigested lactose into lactic acid and hydrogen gas. The gas is responsible for abdominal distention and explosive diarrhea. The fecal smear is negative for leukocytes. Irritable bowel syndrome (choice **E**) is an intrinsic bowel motility disorder that causes abdominal pain in times of stress. There is no fever or systemic signs and symptoms. Constipation and/or diarrhea are present. A colonoscopy examination has normal results.

31 The answer is D *Medicine*

The patient has a postductal coarctation of the aorta (choice **D**). Strong pulses in the upper extremities and diminished pulses in the lower extremities associated with pain in the buttocks and legs with walking fast or climbing hills are signs of claudication due to decreased blood flow to the legs. Proximally there may be dilation of the aorta leading to aortic regurgitation (early diastolic murmur that increases with intensity on expiration). The increased blood pressure is caused by increased blood flow into the upper extremity vessels and reduced renal blood flow leading to activation of the renin-angiotensin-aldosterone system. Aldosterone causes renal retention of sodium, and angiotensin II constricts the peripheral resistance arterioles. There is no shunting of blood between chambers of the heart, and arterial blood gases are normal, as in this patient.

Aortic dissection (choice **A**) occurs in elderly men with hypertension or in young individuals with defects in collagen (e.g., Ehlers-Danlos syndrome) or elastic tissue (Marfan syndrome). Blood enters an intimal tear and dissects proximally and/or distally through the weakened media of the aorta. Aortic dissections produce pain that radiates to the back and are often associated with absent upper extremity pulses, neither of which is present in this patient. Aortic valve stenosis (choice **B**) causes a systolic ejection murmur. The pulse amplitude in the upper extremities is the same as that in the lower extremities, unlike that found in this patient. A patent ductus arteriosus (choice **C**) causes a continuous machinery-like murmur. Once again the pulse amplitude in the upper extremities is the same as that in the lower extremities. Furthermore, this is more likely to be found in newborns rather than adults. Takayasu's arteritis (choice **E**) is an elastic artery vasculitis that occurs in young Asian women. Pulses in the upper extremities are absent, not increased in amplitude as in this patient.

32 The answer is C *Pediatrics*

Craniopharyngioma (choice **C**) is the most common supratentorial tumor of children. About 90% of these tumors show calcifications on plain skull films or on computed tomography (CT) scanning. Many cases are originally discovered during an endocrine workup for short stature secondary to pituitary–hypothalamic involvement. Bitemporal field defects occur because of pressure or injury to the optic chiasm. The tumor can also compress the third ventricle, causing noncommunicating hydrocephalus. With prominent hydrocephalus, papilledema is evident. Polyuria from diabetes insipidus results from interruption of the supraoptic–hypophyseal tract. Treatment consists of surgical removal of the tumor and hormone replacement.

Astrocytoma of the third ventricle (choice **A**) commonly presents with symptoms of increased intracranial pressure (headache, nausea, vomiting, and hydrocephalus) and seizures. A pinealoma (choice **B**) presents with failure of upward gaze (Parinaud's syndrome). Hand-Schüller-Christian disease (choice **E**) is a childhood histiocytosis. Presentation is variable, but skeletal involvement occurs in 80% of patients. Skin lesions, exophthalmos, and hepatosplenomegaly occur in 20% of these patients. Pituitary dysfunction may result in failure to thrive; however, calcifications are not seen on CT. Other central nervous system (CNS) symptoms are uncommon. Chromophobic adenomas (choice **D**) of the pituitary may also cause short stature and diabetes insipidus. Calcifications will not be present.

33 The answer is E *Psychiatry*

The presentation is most suggestive of somatization disorder (choice **E**). Somatization disorder is characterized by a long history of physical complaints from multiple organ systems, commonly including general malaise, gastrointestinal symptoms, neurologic symptoms, and sexual symptoms. It almost always begins before 30 years of age, is often associated with analgesic and sedative-hypnotic abuse, and is more common in women.

In somatization disorder, the individual does not complain of an imagined physical deformity, as would be expected with body dysmorphic disorder (choice **A**). There is no evidence of the somatic delusions present in delusional disorder, somatic type (choice **B**). Also there is no suggestion that the complaints are intentionally produced or feigned, as in factitious disorder (choice **C**). Pain disorder (choice **D**) is diagnosed only when the predominant complaint is pain in the absence of complaints from other organ systems.

34 The answer is C *Medicine*

Restless leg syndrome (choice **C**) is a disorder of unknown etiology that affects both men and women equally. These patients complain of disagreeable sensations in the legs, cramplike pains, sometimes a crawling sensation, or even itching. These patients try to move their limbs to get rid of the pain, even getting up to walk or pace around. While the pain tends to disappear with movement, it returns once again during the resting phase. The pain can disturb sleep. It usually peaks by midnight and thereafter tends to improve by morning. The problem can occur sometimes during the day, either while being sedentary or while driving a car. It may be associated with iron deficiency anemia, diabetes, pregnancy, and chronic renal failure, especially in patients who are on dialysis. Sometimes, the patient may go for months without symptoms. There are no clinical tests, and the diagnosis is based on a history of dysesthesia, motor restlessness, a desire to move the limbs, and worsening of symptoms at night or during periods of rest. Painful legs and moving toes syndrome (choice **A**) does not occur at night and so does not induce insomnia. These patients complain of pain in the legs and feet, and involuntary writhing movements occur during this time. The pain does not get worse at the end of the day or during the night. Fibromyalgia (choice **B**), usually involves a large area of the body, including the axial skeleton. Symptoms generally occur throughout the day, and movement does not improve it. Cauda equina syndrome (choice **D**) is usually associated with low back pain, unilateral motor weakness, and sensory loss, and there may be loss of anal sphincter tone and problems with urination. Akathisia (choice **E**), an inner restlessness condition marked by an irresistible urge to move, is usually induced by medications such as phenothiazines or is a result of diseases such as Parkinson's. These patients have restlessness that tends to affect the entire body, unlike restless leg syndrome, in which the problems are localized to the extremities. Symptoms occur less often at night, so insomnia is not a feature.

35 The answer is C *Medicine*

The patient has antibiotic-associated pseudomembranous colitis, due to an overgrowth of *Clostridium difficile*. Ampicillin and clindamycin are the antibiotics most commonly associated with pseudomembranous colitis. Colonoscopy shows whitish or yellowish plaques surrounded by hemorrhagic borders. The diagnosis is best made with a toxin assay of stool (choice **C**) rather than culture (choice **B**) or Gram's stain (choice **A**) of the yellowish material. Blood cultures (choice **D**) are negative, because the damage to the mucosa and submucosa is toxin-induced and not invasive colitis. The association of this patient's complaints with antibiotic use and the appearance of the lesions argue against a parasitic cause of the diarrhea (choice **E**). Metronidazole is the treatment of choice for pseudomembranous colitis.

36 The answer is D *Preventive Medicine and Public Health*

There is insufficient evidence to recommend for or against screening middle-aged and older men and women for asymptomatic coronary artery disease (CAD) using resting, ambulatory, or exercise electrocardiograms (ECGs). Ischemic heart disease is the leading cause of death in the United States, accounting for approximately 500,000 deaths per year. It is estimated that approximately 1.5 million people have an acute myocardial infarction every year, and one third will not survive the acute event. Nonetheless, routine ECG screening as part of the periodic health visit is not recommended for asymptomatic children, adolescents, or young adults (choice **D**). Therefore, in the case scenario, an ECG would be appropriate for a 30-year-old only if the patient had symptoms (e.g., chest pain) or a positive risk factor. Clinicians should emphasize proved measures for the primary prevention of CAD (e.g., reducing hypertension, lowering the blood cholesterol level) and counsel patients to avoid using tobacco, to consume a healthy diet, and to undertake regular aerobic physical activity.

Accordingly, choices **A, B,** and **C** are incorrect. Although total body CT scans are the rage in some quarters, there is no evidence indicating that they should be recommended for screening for CAD (choice **E**).

37 The answer is B *Obstetrics and Gynecology*

Menopause is characterized by absence of functional ovarian follicles resulting in estrogen levels that are decreased; therefore, choices **A** and **E** are incorrect. With the decline in estrogen levels, as well as loss of inhibin from the ovarian follicles, negative feedback to anterior pituitary gland is lost, resulting in increased follicle-stimulating hormone (FSH) levels; therefore, choice **D** is rejected. Choices **B** and **C** are identical except for the direction of gonadotropin-releasing hormone (GnRH). Because menopause is associated with increased GnRH levels, choice **C** is rejected, and choice **B** is found to be the only correct one. Estrogen levels move in the same direction as sex hormone–binding globulin (SHBG). With the normal fall in estrogen, we can expect SHBG to also be decreased.

[38] The answer is B   *Obstetrics and Gynecology*

Hypertensive disorders of pregnancy are among the main causes of maternal mortality in the United States and require a sustained BP above 140/90 for diagnosis. This patient's findings meet the criteria for severe preeclampsia. She meets the BP criteria of above 160/110 and proteinuria criteria of more than 3+ protein. In addition, the symptoms of persistent headache and epigastric pain support the concern regarding severe preeclampsia. The management priorities in this scenario are stabilization of the mother (by lowering her BP with hydralazine or labetalol to diastolic values between 90 and 100), prevention of seizures (using intravenous magnesium sulfate [choice **B**]), and then prompt delivery.

Phenytoin (choice **A**) is an anticonvulsant used in nonpregnant patients but is not appropriate in pregnant women. Terbutaline (choice **C**) and indomethacin (choice **E**) are tocolytics and would be contraindicated in this patient who needs to be delivered. Progesterone (choice **D**) administration is used for prevention of idiopathic preterm labor but has no demonstrable indication in severe preeclampsia.

[39] The answer is E   *Pediatrics*

The clavicle is the most commonly fractured bone in infants during delivery (choice **E**). This fracture is more common in macrosomic newborns (e.g., infants of diabetic mothers). The newborn generally does not move the arm, giving an absent Moro reflex on the affected side. Crepitus is felt on palpation. Treatment is usually unnecessary, and the prognosis is good.

Cephalhematoma (choice **A**) is a subperiosteal hemorrhage and is confined within the area of the affected cranial bone. Cephalhematomas require no treatment, although phototherapy may be necessary to ameliorate hyperbilirubinemia. Facial nerve palsy (choice **B**) may result from pressure over the facial nerve in utero, from forceps during delivery, or from efforts during callose. A patient with facial nerve palsy will have an eye that cannot be closed, an absent nasolabial fold, a corner of the mouth that droops, and a smooth forehead on the affected side. Prognosis depends on the extent of injury to the nerve. Intraventricular hemorrhage (choice **C**) is caused by rupture of the germinal blood vessels. Predisposing factors are prematurity, hypoxic injury, respiratory distress syndrome, reperfusion injury, and change in volume of cerebral circulation, compromised vascular integrity, hypervolemia (hypertension), and pneumothorax. The incidence of intraventricular hemorrhage increases with decreasing birth weight. Brain contusion (choice **D**) may be associated with a skull fracture.

[40] The answer is D   *Medicine*

The patient has renal papillary necrosis (choice **D**), which is a chronic drug-induced tubulointerstitial nephritis (analgesic nephropathy) caused by ingestion of aspirin and acetaminophen over many years. Aspirin inhibits renal production of prostaglandin E_2, which is a vasodilator of the afferent arteriole, leaving angiotensin II, a vasoconstrictor of the efferent arteriole, in control of the blood flow into the peritubular capillaries extending into the renal medulla. Liver conversion of acetaminophen into acetaminophen free radicals causes further injury to renal tubular cells in the renal papillae. The combination of ischemia and damage from the free radicals causes renal papillary necrosis. The resultant sloughing of the renal papillae into the urine cause the patient's left-sided colicky pain that simulates a renal stone. The ring deformity in the left kidney shown on the intravenous pyelogram indicates absence of the renal papillae. An additional complication of analgesic nephropathy is the loss of renal concentration and dilution in the collecting tubules (specific gravity fixed at 1.010).

Acute drug-induced tubulointerstitial nephritis (choice **A**) is characterized by sudden onset of oliguria (renal failure), fever, and rash shortly after taking a drug (e.g., synthetic penicillin). Other findings include eosinophilia, hematuria, pyuria (WBCs in the urine), eosinophils in the urine, and WBC casts. Withdrawal of the drug reverses these findings. None of these findings is present in this patient. Chronic glomerulonephritis (choice **B**) usually arises from preexisting acute glomerulonephritis. Glomerular sclerosis, tubular atrophy, and renal failure eventually occur. Renal papillary necrosis is not a complication of chronic glomerulonephritis. Chronic pyelonephritis (choice **C**) is a complication of vesicoureteral reflux (reflux of urine from the bladder into the ureter) or postrenal obstruction caused by prostate hyperplasia or a ureteral stone. An intravenous pyelogram shows blunting of the renal calyces underlying cortical scars. Renal papillary necrosis is not a complication of chronic pyelonephritis. A ureteral stone (choice **E**) presents with a sudden onset of colicky pain with radiation to the groin.

41 The answer is E *Surgery*

Anterior dislocation of the shoulder is more common than fracture. Joint stability has been sacrificed for mobility. Therefore, the shoulder joint has a shallow glenoid cavity with a small surface area, while the articular surface of the head of the humerus is disproportionately large. This permits one to move the arm to a great degree in several directions. The capsule of the shoulder joint is weak on its inferior aspect, and forced abduction leads to dislocation of the humeral head to a subglenoid and then a subcoracoid position. The subcoracoid position is the most common location for an anteriorly dislocated shoulder. Pull of the pectoralis major muscle attached to the upper end of the humerus results in displacement of the dislocated head to the subcoracoid position. Very rarely, the head is in the subclavicular position. Due to the proximity of the axillary nerve, it is most important to test for hypesthesia (choice **E**) over the lateral aspect of the shoulder, the presence of which signifies neural compression by the dislocated head. The musculocutaneous nerve is also in the vicinity, and hypesthesia over the lateral aspect of the forearm should also be excluded. Failure to document hypesthesia could result in a lawsuit. Unlike posterior dislocation, an anteriorly dislocated shoulder can be externally rotated. In fact, Kocher's method uses external rotation in reduction of shoulder dislocation.

42 The answer is C *Surgery*

Posterior dislocations of the shoulder are rare and are usually caused by seizures. The posterior group of muscles attached to the humerus induces the dislocation during convulsions. Thus, a woman with eclampsia is more prone to a posterior dislocation of the shoulder than an anterior dislocation. The arm cannot be externally rotated beyond the neutral point (choice **C**). The problem can be missed on a standard x-ray, but a tangential view (transscapular view) will confirm the diagnosis.

43 The answer is F *Surgery*

This patient has had a subluxation of the radial head. The radial head is ensconced within the annular ligament, which is still not fully mature. A sudden pull on the arm of a child (e.g., to prevent him from running onto the street) results in subluxation, in which the head of the radius slips inferiorly. There may be an associated partial tear of the annular ligament. This is not a dislocation of the head of the radius. Normally, no swelling is noted. The condition is reduced by supination of the forearm (choice **F**). The head relocates with a click. No immobilization is required. The child starts using the arm quite quickly. Recurrence is rare; however, after three recurrences, surgical repair is indicated.

44 The answer is D *Surgery*

This child has sustained a supracondylar fracture of the elbow. It usually results from a blow to the back of the lower end of the humerus, just above the medial and lateral condyles. These fractures may be associated with neurovascular trauma, most notably compression of the medial nerve and brachial artery. Normally, there is a great deal of swelling around the elbow. During reduction, the radial pulse should be felt constantly (choice **D**). If the pulse diminishes, the elbow should be extended to the position where the pulse returns to normal. Initially, the patient is kept immobilized in a Dunlop traction, in which the forearm and hand are kept elevated with countertraction while traction is maintained on the arm. Failure to ensure adequate circulation could lead to Volkmann's ischemic contracture, a disastrous complication. In the presence of an occult supracondylar fracture, a positive fat pad sign is noted, wherein the pad of fat normally present posterior to the capsule is pushed back further. Similarly, the pad of fat present anteriorly is pushed forward to form a triangular shape (a positive sail sign).

45 **The answer is A** *Surgery*

Patients who sustain fractures involving the shaft of the humerus can have concomitant injury to the radial nerve, which courses behind the shaft of the radius. In such an event, there may be an associated wrist drop (choice **A**). Sometimes, fractures of the humeral shaft may be associated with dislocation of the shoulder joint.

46 **The answer is G** *Surgery*

This patient has a Monteggia's fracture, in which the shaft of the ulna is fractured and the head of the radius is dislocated (choice **G**). In all cases of fractures, it is important to include the proximal and distal joint in the x-ray film so as not to miss associated joint injuries, as would occur in the case of a Monteggia's fracture.

47 **The answer is B** *Surgery*

This patient has sustained a Galeazzi's fracture, in which the shaft of the radius is fractured and the inferior radioulnar joint is dislocated (choice **B**). Just as in the case of a Monteggia's fracture, it is very important to include the proximal and distal joint while taking an x-ray film so as not to miss associated injuries.

48 **The answer is E** *Preventive Medicine and Public Health*

In a 2004 National Institute of Drug Abuse (NIDA) survey, 3.4% (choice **E**) of high school seniors reported use of anabolic steroids at least once. Although not addictive, use of anabolic steroids is a health hazard. Common side effects include severe acne and trembling; males may also undergo shrinking of the testicles and breast development while females may grow facial hair, stop menstruating, and develop a deeper voice. Both sexes are also liable to irreversibly stunt their growth due to premature closure of their epiphyses. Prolonged use also increases the risk of developing jaundice, liver and/or kidney cancers, and hypertension.

49 **The answer is B** *Preventive Medicine and Public Health*

In 2004, 25% (choice **B**) of senior high school seniors reported that they used tobacco at least once during the previous 30-day period. This is a statistically insignificant increase from 2003, when 24% reported use. However both values show an encouraging decline from 1997 data that reported 36.5% use in a comparable sample. Similar declines in use were also found in the lower grades. Another encouraging observation is that over the same time period, high school students at all grades exhibited increased awareness of the health hazards associated with smoking. Despite these encouraging statistics among high school students, the next older bracket of adults studied in 2003 showed the heaviest use of tobacco products, 44.8%. It will be interesting to see if the apparent decline in use among high school students will carry forward into the future and be reflected by a significant decrease in use among young adults.

50 **The answer is D** *Preventive Medicine and Public Health*

Use of some form of cocaine during 2004 was reported by 5% (choice **D**) of 12th graders. There was a major increase in reported use between 1992 and 1999, from 3.2 to 6.2%, among this group of students. The rate then dropped to 5% in 2000 and has essentially remained steady since. Paradoxically, 12th graders also reported a perceived increase in availability of all forms of cocaine in 2004.

Questions

Single Best Choice Directions: This section consists of numbered statements or questions followed by a list of potential answers; you are to select the ONE best answer.

1 A 25-year-old African-American woman complains of fatigue and exercise intolerance. Physical examination shows conjunctival pallor. A complete blood cell count reveals a moderately severe anemia with a decreased mean corpuscular volume (MCV) and an increased red blood cell (RBC) distribution width (RDW). A stool guaiac test (fecal occult blood test) result is negative. Which of the following laboratory tests is most useful in confirming the cause of her anemia?

(A) Hemoglobin electrophoresis
(B) Serum iron
(C) Serum ferritin
(D) Percentage saturation of transferrin
(E) Serum total iron-binding capacity (TIBC)

2 A 9-year-old boy constantly tests the limits of discipline with parents and teachers by speaking out of turn, flaunting rules about dressing and grooming, and staying out past his curfew. However, he gets along well with his peers, and he completes projects that he likes. He reached all developmental milestones at appropriate ages. He does not have a history of fighting, theft, or destruction of property. Mental status examination reveals an assertive child who tells the examiner that he does not wish to discuss his problems. Which of the following is the most likely diagnosis?

(A) Oppositional defiant disorder
(B) Mental retardation
(C) Conduct disorder
(D) Childhood disintegrative disorder
(E) Attention-deficit/hyperactivity disorder

3 A 53-year-old woman presents with a history of a painless lump in the region of the right parotid gland. The lump has been present for about 6 years and has recently started growing in size. Her husband says that her speech has started to sound "funny." Examination reveals a firm, nontender mass with early evidence of peripheral facial nerve palsy. No lymphadenopathy is noted in the neck. Which of the following is the most likely diagnosis?

(A) Adenoid cystic carcinoma
(B) Adenolymphoma

(C) Pleomorphic adenoma
(D) Mucoepidermoid carcinoma
(E) Acinic cell carcinoma

4 A 48-year-old man with a 20-year history of smoking cigarettes presents with a painless mass in the left scrotal sac that was not present during an annual examination 6 months ago. Physical examination shows an enlarged scrotal sac with distended and tortuous vascular channels. Testicular volume is below normal on the left and normal on the right. Laboratory studies show microscopic hematuria and an absence of serum human chorionic gonadotropin (hCG) and α-fetoprotein (AFP). Which of the following is the most likely cause of the scrotal mass?

(A) Epididymitis
(B) Hydrocele
(C) Renal cell carcinoma
(D) Testicular cancer
(E) Torsion of spermatic cord

5 A 20-year-old woman has had recurrent urinary tract infections since early childhood. She now presents with a temperature of 101.2°F (38.4°C), acute left flank pain, suprapubic discomfort, dysuria, and increased urinary frequency. The urinary sediment examination shows clumps of WBCs, WBC casts, occasional RBCs, and numerous motile bacteria. Which of the following acute conditions is the most likely diagnosis?

(A) Cystitis
(B) Glomerulonephritis
(C) Pyelonephritis
(D) Tubular necrosis
(E) Urethritis

6 A 45-year-old obese woman enters the emergency room complaining of steady, severe, aching pain in the right upper quadrant that radiates to the right scapula. The onset is sudden and occurs 15 minutes after eating. She has nausea and vomiting, but the pain is not relieved by vomiting. Palpation after inspiration reveals right upper quadrant tenderness. Laboratory studies reveal an absolute leukocytosis and a shift to the left. Which of the following is the mechanism most likely responsible for her condition?

(A) An impacted stone in the cystic duct

(B) Chemically induced inflammation of the gall-bladder

(C) An impacted stone in the common bile duct

(D) Biliary dyskinesia

(E) Hydrops of the gallbladder

7 While watching television (TV) a 45-year-old man heard that in the United States prostate cancer is the most common malignancy in men, that in 2003 approximately 220,000 new cases were diagnosed, and that as many as 10% of these were predicted to result in death. He also read on the internet that there is a simple blood test called the prostate specific antigen (PSA) test that will determine if a man does or does not have prostate cancer, and if a man were at risk to develop it, there is a drug called finasteride that can prevent cancer from developing. Consequently he made an appointment to see his primary care physician and berated him, as well as all physicians in general, for not routinely screening all men for prostate cancer and insisting he be tested. He also asked if he should be started on finasteride to prevent prostate cancer if the test results were negative, because he thought he might be at risk since his 68-year-old uncle was diagnosed with the disease last year. Which of the following choices is the most appropriate response?

(A) No health-related organization recommends prostate cancer screening before the age of 60.

(B) The PSA test needs to be used cautiously because false positive results are a potential problem and he is at minimal risk, and finasteride may cause its own problems.

(C) Finasteride is not recommended for use by the general male population because the lifetime risk of getting pancreatic cancer is only about 0.2%.

(D) Transrectal ultrasound is a simpler and better screening method than the PSA test and will soon replace it, so physicians hesitate to recommend the latter.

(E) Despite the endorsement of the PSA on the internet, it is so inaccurate that most physicians would rather use the older, time-tested, digital rectal examination (DRE)

8 A 38-year-old man seeks treatment for a depressive episode. He complains of feelings of hopelessness and despair, with a marked lack of energy. He remarks that on most days he just is too tired to get out of bed in the morning. He denies suicidal plans, stating, "There is really no point in suicide." At which of the following times is the patient most likely to commit suicide?

(A) When the patient admits his feelings of guilt

(B) When the patient completes a course of electro-convulsive therapy

(C) At the start of treatment

(D) When the patient develops untoward effects to antidepressants

(E) When the patient begins to respond to anti-depressant medication

9 A 27-year-old man is arrested after robbing a liquor store. He has multiple tattoos with slogans about racial supremacy. Mental status examination reveals an angry and belligerent individual without evidence of psychosis or cognitive impairment. Which of the following would most suggest a diagnosis of antisocial personality disorder?

(A) A belief that other people are unimportant, coupled with idealization of past tyrants like Hitler

(B) A childhood history of enuresis, fire setting, and cruelty to animals

(C) A history of abuse during childhood and incarceration for substance-related crimes

(D) A long and pervasive pattern of disregard for, and violation of, the basic rights of others

(E) Membership in cults with destructive ideologies and plans for future warfare

10 A 60-year-old man with chronic ischemic heart disease has dyspnea and decreased urine output. Physical examination reveals bibasilar crackles in the lungs. There is no neck vein distention or dependent pitting edema. His serum blood urea nitrogen (BUN) is 60 mg/dL (normal, 7–18 mg/dL), and serum creatinine is 2 mg/dL (normal 0.6–1.2 mg/dL). The patient is not taking diuretics. Which of the following laboratory findings also is most likely present?

(A) Fractional excretion of sodium ($FENa^+$) < 1%

(B) Random urine sodium > 40 mEq/L

(C) Urine osmolality (U_{Osm}) < 350 mOsm/kg

(D) Urine sediment with renal tubular cell casts

11 A 26-year-old woman is admitted to a psychiatric unit with a diagnosis of bipolar disorder. Her medical history, physical examination, and laboratory studies are unremarkable. She is started on lithium 300 mg PO tid. Her manic symptoms remit over 14 days. At discharge from the hospital, she complains of a slight resting tremor but otherwise feels well. Assuming she develops a toxic response to lithium, which of the following findings would most likely be noted when seen in a follow-up clinic 1 month later?

(A) Abnormal liver function
(B) Fever
(C) Hypothyroidism
(D) Leukopenia
(E) Urinary retention

12 A 65-year-old man presents to the emergency department with sudden onset of left retroperitoneal pain. He is 5 ft 9 in tall (1.75 m) and weighs 190 lb (86.2 kg). Physical examination reveals his blood pressure to be 85/45 and a pulsatile mass in the abdomen is palpitated. The pathogenesis of this patient's disease is most closely related to which of the following?

(A) Hypertension
(B) Atherosclerosis
(C) Elastic tissue fragmentation
(D) Immune complex-mediated inflammation
(E) Vasculitis secondary to syphilis

13 A 29-year-old man suffered from hepatitis, splenomegaly, a Coombs-negative hemolytic anemia, and portal hypertension during his adolescent and earlier adult years. Now he is showing signs of behavioral and personality changes with emotional lability. In addition, he has a profound resting tremor, his speech has become slurred and difficult to understand, and he drools and has trouble swallowing. Physical examination shows a rim of brown pigment around the perimeter of the cornea. Which of the following laboratory findings would most likely be reported?

(A) Decreased serum ceruloplasmin
(B) Increased serum ferritin
(C) Increased serum mitochondrial antibodies
(D) Increased total serum copper
(E) Normal serum prothrombin time

14 A 25-year-old woman has type 1 diabetes mellitus, and her grandfather has type 2 diabetes mellitus. Which of the following is a characteristic that is present in both type 1 and type 2 diabetes mellitus?

(A) Antibodies against β islet cells
(B) Association with HLA-Dr3/Dr4
(C) Downregulation of insulin receptor synthesis
(D) Ketoacidosis
(E) Osmotic damage

15 A 19-year-old man born and brought up in Brooklyn, NY, visited his grandfather who lived in western North Carolina. His grandfather, wanting to give him a taste of the life of his ancestors, took him hunting. The fol-

lowing week, after his return to Brooklyn, he presents with fever, lethargy, headache, and abdominal pain. Petechial lesions are noted on the palms of the hand. Which of the following is the arthropod vector most likely responsible for this disease?

(A) Flea
(B) Louse
(C) Mite
(D) Chigger
(E) Tick

16 A 28-year-old woman who habitually fed feral cats is bitten on the hand by one in the neighborhood park. Twenty-four hours later, the hand is swollen, and there is swelling and warmth around the puncture sites of the bite. Which of the following organisms is most likely responsible for these findings?

(A) *Bartonella henselae*
(B) *Pasteurella multocida*
(C) *Staphylococcus aureus*
(D) Group A streptococci
(E) *Pseudomonas aeruginosa*
(F) *Eikenella corrodens*

17 A 15-year-old girl who has had regular menstrual cycles since the age of 12 years makes an appointment to see her primary care physician because of the development of sudden onset of abdominal pain. Physical examination reveals a tender mass in the left adnexa. A pregnancy test has a negative result. Ultrasound examination exhibits a mass lesion of the left ovary, with focal areas of calcification (increased density). Which of the following is the most likely diagnosis?

(A) Follicular cyst
(B) Mucinous cystadenoma
(C) Cystic teratoma
(D) Brenner's tumor
(E) Serous cystadenoma

18 A random sample of 100 female students is selected from the freshmen class of a large university. The women are followed prospectively over 4 years to see if use of oral contraceptive pills is associated with a decrease in ovarian cysts. Which of the following is the proper name of this study design?

(A) Cohort study
(B) Case-control study
(C) Randomized controlled clinical trial
(D) Cross-sectional study
(E) Crossover study

19 A 25-year-old woman without any prior history of psychiatric problems has a 3-week episode of insomnia, increased psychomotor activity, and impulsivity. There is no history of substance abuse or general medical conditions. Prior to this episode, she has worked steadily as a secretary. There have been no recent emotional stressors. She has no history of depressive episodes and has always led an active social life. Physical examination and routine laboratory studies, including thyroid function tests, are unremarkable. Mental status examination reveals a well-oriented female with pressured speech and mood lability, but no psychotic symptoms. Which of the following most closely approximates her lifetime percentage chance of experiencing another similar episode?

(A) 5%

(B) 25%

(C) 50%

(D) 75%

(E) 90%

20 On the day after Thanksgiving a young man brings his 50-year-old mother to the emergency department. The triage nurse notes she has a temperature of 102°F (38.9°C), blood pressure of 90/42 mm Hg, severe right-upper-quadrant (RUQ) pain, and jaundice. She also observes that she seems to have a problem with answering her questions and sometimes babbles incoherently. Her son tells the nurse that after consuming a hearty Thanksgiving meal his mother felt ill, and her pain and symptoms grew worse during the night and early morning, so he thought he ought to bring her in. He also tells her his mother has had two or three earlier episodes of gallbladder trouble but none so severe. Upon examination the patient is also found to have mild hepatomegaly; her heart sounds were normal, but the pulse rate is 125 beats/min. Her white cell count is $13.6 \times 10^3/\mu L$ (normal range, $4.8-10.8 \times 10^3$), her total bilirubin level is 6.6 mg/mL (36.3 μmol/L), (normal range, 0.1–1.2 mg/mL [2.0–21 μmol/L]); her γ-glutamyl transpeptidase (aka γ-glutamyltransferase) activity value is 105 units/mL (normal, 9–85 units/mL), and her alkaline phosphatase value is. 176 units/L (normal range, 41–133 units/mL). Urine analysis was normal. Which of the following is the most likely diagnosis?

(A) Amebic liver abscess

(B) Acute hepatitis

(C) Acute pancreatitis

(D) Ascending cholangitis

(E) Sclerosing pericholangitis

21 A 50-year-old man presents to his physician with dyspnea and cyanosis. He is currently breathing room air. An arterial blood gas reveals the following: pH, 7.20 (7.35–7.45); P_{CO_2}, 72 mm Hg (33–45), HCO_3^-, 28 mEq/L (22–28), and P_{O_2}, 50 mm Hg (80–100). Which of the following conditions is most compatible with the history and laboratory findings?

(A) Acute respiratory distress syndrome

(B) Barbiturate overdose

(C) Chronic bronchitis

(D) Emphysema

(E) Pulmonary infarction

22 A 40-year-old nurse has been complaining for years about long work hours, poor pay, and lack of concern from her supervisors for her well-being. However, despite her constant complaining she reports to work punctually and gets her work done in a yeomanlike fashion. She starts to also complain of recurrent episodes of forgetfulness, associated with bouts of sweating, palpitations, anxiety, tremulousness, and fainting. As a consequence, she asks for a medical leave with pay. Before granting her request she is given a physical examination. Laboratory studies show a serum glucose level of 55 mg/dL (normal, 70–110 mg/dL), elevated serum insulin levels, and a suppressed level of serum C-peptide. Which of the following is the most likely cause of the hypoglycemia?

(A) Benign tumor of β islet cells

(B) Ectopic secretion of an insulin-like factor

(C) Malignant tumor of α islet cells

(D) Pancreatic carcinoma

(E) Injection of human insulin

(F) Factitious disorder

23 A 42-year-old woman with a basal metabolic index (BMI) of 42 kg/m², who does not smoke, presents with diastolic hypertension and menstrual irregularities. Pertinent findings upon physical examination are a full, plethoric appearing face, increased facial hair, predominantly truncal obesity with purple stria around the abdomen, and scattered ecchymoses over the entire body. Laboratory studies indicate a hemoglobin (Hgb) level of 18 g/dL (normal, 12–16 g/dL), a white blood cell (WBC) count of 18,000 cells/mm³ (normal, 4500–11,000 cells/mm³), and a normal platelet count. The leukocyte differential shows an absolute neutrophilic leukocytosis and absolute lymphopenia and eosinopenia. Which of the following screening tests is most useful in the initial workup of this patient?

(A) Captopril-enhanced renal radionuclide test

(B) Plasma cortisol at 8 AM and 4 PM

(C) Clonidine suppression test

(D) Bone marrow aspiration and biopsy

(E) Low-dose dexamethasone suppression test

24. A 35-year-old man is scuba diving in 70 feet of water and suddenly develops stabbing chest pain in the left side with dyspnea while coming to the surface at the appropriate rate of ascent. Physical examination of the left lung shows hyperresonance to percussion, deviation of the trachea to the left, elevation of the left diaphragm, absent vocal tactile fremitus, and absent breath sounds. Which of the following is the most likely diagnosis?

(A) Decompression sickness

(B) Pleural effusion

(C) Pulmonary infarction

(D) Spontaneous pneumothorax

(E) Tension pneumothorax

25. An 18-year-old woman comes to the physician's office stating that she has never had a menstrual period. She has never been sexually active and has never used any contraceptive agents. She started breast development at age 10 years and started her growth spurt at age 11 years. She states she is not on any medications. She graduated from high school a year ago and is a nursing student at the local university. Physical examination reveals normal female breast development, but no uterus can be palpated on pelvic examination. The cause of her amenorrhea can best be discovered by testing for the serum level of which one of the following substances?

(A) Follicle-stimulating hormone (FSH)

(B) Luteinizing hormone (LH)

(C) Prolactin

(D) Testosterone

(E) Progesterone

26. A 19-year-old woman, gravida 2, para 0, aborta 1, comes to the outpatient office for a prenatal visit. She is currently at 30 weeks' gestation confirmed by an 18-week sonogram that showed a single fetus with size appropriate for dates. She states that the fetus is moving well. Pregnancy weight gain to date is 20 lb. Her fundal height today measures 25 cm. Fetal heart tones are heard in the right upper quadrant. An obstetric ultrasound examination reveals a 4-quadrant amniotic fluid index (AFI) of 4 cm. Which of the following fetal conditions is most likely associated with this scenario?

(A) Duodenal atresia

(B) Open spina bifida

(C) Tracheoesophageal fistula

(D) Renal agenesis

(E) Atrial flutter

27. A 7-year-old boy is referred from a school because of poor speaking and reading ability, failure to follow directions, and classroom disruptiveness. He appears to be alert and affectionate with others. He does not appear to be preoccupied with internal stimuli. IQ testing results are in the normal range. Which of the following is the most likely cause of his symptoms?

(A) Autistic disorder

(B) Food allergies

(C) Hearing impairment

(D) Schizophrenia

(E) Seizure disorder

28. A 50-year-old cattle farmer, who recently dug a well for drinking water, presents to his family physician with fatigue, dyspnea, and a headache. Physical examination reveals bluish discoloration of the skin and mucous membranes. Supplemental O_2 does not alleviate his symptoms or alter the skin discoloration. Blood drawn for arterial blood gases has a chocolate brown discoloration. Which of the following laboratory test findings is most likely present?

(A) Decreased arterial O_2 saturation (Sao_2)

(B) Decreased arterial Po_2

(C) Increased alveolar-arterial (A-a) gradient

(D) Increased serum bicarbonate

(E) Normal O_2 content

29. A 23-year-old woman requests reduction mammoplasty because she is convinced that her breasts are grossly large and misshapen. This perception started in her teens but until now she has been inhibited from doing anything about it because she still lived at home and her parents simply pooh-poohed the idea, making fun of her and calling her stupid to even think of such an option. She now dresses in elaborate clothing to hide her shape and avoids situations in which she might be expected to disrobe even partially. Physical examination reveals large well-formed breasts well within the normal range of size and shape. Which of the following is the most likely diagnosis?

(A) Body dysmorphic disorder

(B) Delusional disorder, somatic type

(C) Hypochondriasis

(D) Major depressive disorder, single episode

(E) Somatization disorder

30. A 40-year-old woman complains of episodic "attacks" of headache, palpitations, and profuse perspiration. She has recently experienced substernal chest pain during the attacks. Physical examination reveals multiple pigmented, pedunculated tumors in the axilla and flat,

oval, coffee-colored skin patches over her chest and back. Her pulse is 170 bpm, and the average of three blood pressure readings is 200/120 mm Hg. Which one of the following laboratory studies will most likely identify the underlying cause of the hypertension?

(A) Complete urinalysis
(B) Serum electrolytes
(C) Twenty-four hour urine analysis for free cortisol
(D) Twenty-four hour urine analysis for 17-keto-steroids
(E) Twenty-four hour urine analysis for metanephrine

31. A 62-year-old man is recovering from an acute anterior myocardial infarction (MI). His medications include warfarin and one baby aspirin every other day. He is also taking over-the-counter antioxidants and B-complex vitamins. After 1 month, he develops multiple ecchymoses and black, tarry stools. The international normalized ratio (INR) is well beyond the normal range for appropriate anticoagulation, even though he is taking the prescribed dose of warfarin. Results of liver function tests are normal. Which of the following best explains the cause of his hemorrhagic diathesis?

(A) Aspirin synergism with warfarin
(B) Vitamin A toxicity
(C) Vitamin B_1 (thiamine) toxicity
(D) Vitamin C toxicity
(E) Vitamin E toxicity

32. A 56-year-old known alcoholic with portal hypertension was admitted to the hospital for surgery. He underwent a portacaval shunt procedure. Clinically, the patient was confused and had tremulousness of the hands. The following laboratory data were obtained:

Substance Measured	Observed Value	Normal Range
Serum sodium	148 mEq/L	135–145 mEq/L
Serum potassium	3.8 mEq/L	3.5–5.0 mEq/L
Serum chloride	98 mEq/L	101–112 mEq/L
Serum bicarbonate	26 mEq/L	22–32 mEq/L
Serum cholesterol	230 mg/dL	<200 mg/mL
Serum ammonia	120 µmol/L	11–35 µmol/L
Leukocytes	$12.6 \times 10^3/µL$	$4.8–10.8 \times 10^3/µL$
Arterial pH	7.68	7.35–7.45
$Paco_2$	45 mm Hg	32–48 mm Hg
Pao_2	98 mm Hg	83–108 mm Hg

Which of the following would be the most effective next step for the long-term management of this patient?

(A) Lactulose
(B) Neomycin sterilization of the bowel
(C) Reduced protein intake
(D) Loop diuretic
(E) Infused sodium bicarbonate

33. A 26-year-old woman, gravida 3, para 2, at 14 weeks' gestation by dates complains of severe nausea and vomiting for the past 2 weeks. She has had vaginal bleeding and states that she passed what looked like grapes from her vagina. Her two previous pregnancies were unremarkable prenatally, resulting in term vaginal deliveries of grossly normal neonates who are developing normally. She states that all three of her pregnancies were fathered by her husband. On examination her fundus is palpable at her umbilicus. No fetal heart tones can be heard with a Doppler stethoscope. Cytogenetic studies performed on this tissue would most likely show which of the following karyotypes?

(A) 46 XX
(B) 69 XXX
(C) 46 XY
(D) 45 X
(E) 69 XXY

34. A 35-year-old man complains of rapid onset of a steady unrelenting midepigastric pain with radiation into the back after eating a large meal. He has nausea and vomiting; while vomiting aggravates the pain, leaning forward relieves it. Physical examination reveals a temperature of 99.8°F (37.7°C), epigastric tenderness, and decreased bowel sounds. An abdominal film shows a localized dilation of the upper duodenum and a small collection of fluid in the left pleural cavity. Which of the following tests would be the most useful and cost-effective in the initial workup of this patient?

(A) Upper gastrointestinal barium study
(B) Endoscopy
(C) Serum amylase or lipase analysis
(D) Oral cholecystogram
(E) Hepato-iminodiacetic acid (HIDA) radionuclide scan

35. Which of the following statistical tests would be most appropriate for assessing whether there are significant differences in 1-minute Apgar scores between infants born by emergency cesarean section and those born by spontaneous vaginal delivery?

(A) Student's *t*-test
(B) Analysis of variance
(C) Correlation coefficient
(D) Chi-squared test
(E) Logistic regression

36 A 51-year-old woman, gravida 4, para 4, presents to the outpatient office complaining of painless, continuous leakage of clear fluid through her vagina. She had initially come to the clinic for an annual examination, at which time a Pap smear was obtained for cervical cancer screening. The report came back "consistent with cancer." Colposcopy was performed showing a lesion on the anterior cervix with abnormal vessels. A cervical biopsy was performed with the histology report stating "squamous cell carcinoma with invasion of 6 mm but no vascular or lymphatic involvement." Bimanual pelvic examination did not reveal any vaginal lesions or broad ligament masses. She underwent a radical hysterectomy 3 weeks ago. Which of the following tests would best assess the cause of the complaint?

(A) Cystometric studies
(B) Urine culture
(C) Intravenous (IV) indigo carmine
(D) Pelvic ultrasonography
(E) Urethral pressure measurements

37 A 60-year-old man complains of pain and numbness in the left leg when walking. The pain is relieved by resting. He also complains of impotence. Physical examination reveals atrophy of the left leg muscles, normal reflexes, and a bruit over the femoral artery. Which of the following is the most likely diagnosis?

(A) Leriche's syndrome
(B) A herniated lumbar disc
(C) Osteoarthritis of the hip
(D) Phlegmasia alba dolens
(E) A peripheral neuropathy

38 A 21-year-old nulligravid woman comes to the outpatient office for her first prenatal visit at 12 weeks' gestation by dates. A home urine pregnancy test result was positive 6 weeks ago. A pelvic examination performed today was unremarkable, with uterine size consistent with her dates. Fetal heart tones were heard with a Doppler stethoscope at a rate of 130 beats/min. A prenatal laboratory panel is ordered. Her rubella titer is found to be negative. Which of the following recommendations would be most appropriate in managing this patient?

(A) Provide gamma globulin for prophylaxis after exposure
(B) Administer rubella vaccine in the third trimester
(C) Avoid breast-feeding after postpartum vaccination
(D) Avoid pregnancy for 1 month after vaccination
(E) Offer genetic amniocentesis for amniotic fluid culture
(F) Provide gamma globulin for prophylaxis now

39 A mother was driving her 5-year-old daughter home after the child had a good time at a birthday party when, while making left turn, an SUV ran into the side of the car. The mother emerged with a few scratches, but the daughter was killed instantly. However, when told of her child's death by the paramedics the mother seems oddly calm and says that she feels no emotion. Which of the following mechanisms is this mother using?

(A) Isolation
(B) Depersonalization
(C) Disorientation
(D) Intellectualization
(E) Derealization

Directions for Matching Questions (40 through 50): Each set of matching questions is preceded by a list of 4 to 26 lettered options followed by a brief explanation of the required task and then by a series of numbered statements. For each lettered statement you are to select ONE lettered option that best fulfills the task as it relates to that statement. Remember each of the listed options might be correctly selected once, more than once, or not at all.

Questions 40–47

(A) Deferoxamine mesylate
(B) Atropine sulfate
(C) Oxygen
(D) Fomepizole
(E) Pyridoxine
(F) Methylene blue
(G) Naloxone hydrochloride
(H) *N*-Acetylcysteine
(I) Pralidoxime
(J) Fab antibody fragments

Match the indicated antidote listed above with the description of the ONE appropriate poisoning/toxic sign listed below.

40 A 3-year-old is brought to the emergency center by ambulance. The parents state that the child's adolescent babysitter found him with an empty bottle of prenatal vitamins earlier in the day. The babysitter says that the child thought they were candy, and because they were vitamins, she wasn't concerned. However, 4 hours after the ingestion, the child developed vomiting bloody diarrhea and appears listless.

41 A 5-year-old has an ulnar fracture that needs to be reduced. The orthopedic surgeon decides that this can be done in the emergency center with procedural sedation. Consent is obtained, and the patient is prepped for the procedure. During induction of medication the nurse rapidly injects the medication and the patient develops chest wall rigidity.

42 A 16-year-old is brought to the emergency department via ambulance. The family states that the patient was found with an empty bottle of her father's tuberculosis medicine after getting into a verbal altercation with him about her boyfriend. On arrival the patient complains of nausea. She is tachycardic and seems somewhat somnolent. Paramedics report that she had an unsteady gait at the scene. The patient begins to convulse in the emergency department and a benzodiazepine is administered.

43 A father brings his 30-month-old son to the emergency department for treatment. The father says that he had been in the family garage changing the radiator fluid when his wife called him into the house to answer the telephone. His son had been "helping" him. The father states that he couldn't have been on the phone more than 5 minutes, but when he returned to the garage he found his son playing with a spilled bottle of radiator fluid. He is uncertain if the child ingested any. In the emergency center, the child's urine is examined and tests positive for crystals, and fluoresces when viewed under a Wood's lamp.

44 A 1-month-old infant with severe cyanosis is brought to the emergency department of a local hospital. The mother states that the baby is her firstborn child and was a term infant born by spontaneous vaginal delivery without any complications. The infant had been exclusively breast-fed until 1 week ago, when the mother began supplementing breast feedings with powdered formula feedings. The family lives on a farm and uses well water.

Although 100% oxygen is delivered via non-re-breather, the oxygen saturation remained in the 80s. In addition, the infant is noted to be tachycardic and tachypneic. The lungs were clear to auscultation bilaterally, and no heart murmur was detected. Abdominal examination showed no hepatomegaly, splenomegaly, or tenderness. Neurologic examination did not reveal any deficiency, and the anterior fontanel was normal. The infant's height, weight, and head circumference were at the 25% for age. Radiography and electrocardiography findings were normal. Laboratory tests were ordered, and the nurse tells you that when she drew the blood it looked chocolate brown.

45 A 16-year-old female decided that life was too difficult and too filled with sorrow after her boyfriend told her that he no longer wanted to date her. She "just wanted to die." The patient was found in her bedroom unresponsive, with a note that told her family and ex-boyfriend that she loved them. With the note was an empty bottle of her mother's digoxin tablets. The teenager was taken to the emergency center by ambulance, where it was determined that she had atrioventricular block with extreme bradycardia. An external pacemaker was applied, but the patient developed intractable hyperkalemia (serum potassium of 8.5 mEq/L) with increasing pacing threshold and progressive intraventricular conduction delay.

46 A 10-year-old child comes to the emergency department after a major snowstorm that resulted in power outages. The parents state that for the last few hours they have been using a barbecue grill inside their home for heat and to cook food. Prior to the storm, the patient had been in his usual state of good health but now complains of nausea, vomiting, and headache. Others in the family also have had similar symptoms since the storm. In fact, the patient's 6-year-old cousin is presently in the emergency center being evaluated for a seizure.

47 A 3-year-old ingested acetaminophen that was in his grandmother's medicine cabinet. They were not in a childproof container because the patient's grandmother has arthritis, and she changed containers for ease. The grandmother says that she has used 2 tablets of acetaminophen from this bottle. The bottle originally had 50 tablets. At present, there are 5 tablets left. The patient receives oral charcoal and blood for an acetaminophen level is drawn 4 hours postingestion.

Questions 48–50

(A) *Escherichia coli*

(B) *Salmonella typhi*

(C) *Klebsiella pneumoniae*

(D) *Yersinia enterocolitica*

(E) *Campylobacter jejuni*

(F) *Helicobacter pylori*

(G) *Pseudomonas aeruginosa*

For each numbered disease described below, select the ONE microbial pathogen from the list above that is most likely to be causing the disease.

48 A 25-year-old woman who recently returned from India had a sustained high fever of 40°C (104°F) for

7 days. This was followed in the second week by diarrhea and abdominal pain. Physical examination reveals sinus bradycardia; a faint, erythematous rash on the upper anterior trunk; and painful hepatosplenomegaly. Laboratory studies reveal a leukocyte count of 1500 cells/mm³ (normal range, 4500–11,000 cells/mm³).

49 A 55-year-old postmenopausal woman complains of weight loss, a poor appetite, and epigastric pain. She says that she has had a 10-year history of epigastric pain aggravated by food. Physical examination reveals midepigastric tenderness with no radiation into the back. The pelvic examination reveals bilaterally enlarged, nontender ovaries. Results of a stool guaiac test are positive.

50 A 35-year-old man who recently attended a chicken barbecue develops a fever of 40°C (104°F), severe abdominal pain, and bloody diarrhea. He is also experiencing some low back pain in the sacroiliac area.

Answer Key

1 C		**11** C		**21** B		**31** E		**41** G	
2 A		**12** B		**22** E		**32** C		**42** E	
3 C		**13** A		**23** E		**33** A		**43** D	
4 C		**14** E		**24** D		**34** C		**44** F	
5 C		**15** E		**25** D		**35** A		**45** J	
6 A		**16** B		**26** D		**36** C		**46** C	
7 B		**17** C		**27** C		**37** A		**47** H	
8 E		**18** A		**28** A		**38** F		**48** B	
9 D		**19** E		**29** A		**39** A		**49** F	
10 A		**20** D		**30** E		**40** A		**50** E	

Answers and Explanations

1 The answer is C *Medicine*

The patient has a microcytic anemia (decreased mean corpuscular volume). Since iron deficiency is the most common cause of a microcytic anemia in mensurating women, usually due to menorrhagia (excessive menstrual flow), this is most likely due to iron deficiency anemia. Moreover, iron deficiency anemia is the only microcytic anemia with an increase in the RBC distribution width (RDW). Although not very sensitive, a negative stool guaiac test result tends to rule out a gastrointestinal cause of the anemia. Serum ferritin analysis is the most sensitive screening test for all of the iron-related disorders (choice C). Ferritin is a soluble iron–protein complex that is a storage form for iron in the intestinal mucosa, liver, spleen, and macrophages in bone marrow. A small circulating fraction of ferritin correlates with the amount of storage iron located within these organs. Consequently, in iron deficiency anemia, serum ferritin levels are decreased. Conversely, in conditions in which iron stores are increased, such as anemia of chronic inflammation and hemochromatosis, serum ferritin levels are increased.

Hemoglobin (Hb) electrophoresis (choice A) is only indicated if thalassemia (globin chain deficiency) or an abnormal Hb is suspected (e.g., Hb S) as a cause of anemia. Thalassemia is unlikely, because the RDW is increased. Sickle cell disease is unlikely, because in sickle cell disease the anemia is normocytic not microcytic. Serum iron (choice B) is not as sensitive or as specific a test as serum ferritin in diagnosing iron deficiency. Serum ferritin is the first laboratory test result that is abnormal in the early stages of iron deficiency, before serum iron is decreased or anemia has developed. Furthermore, serum iron levels do not always correlate with the bone marrow iron stores. For example, in anemia of chronic inflammation, which also produces a microcytic anemia, serum iron is decreased and serum ferritin is increased. Transferrin is the circulating binding protein of iron. In the laboratory, the percentage saturation of transferrin (choice D) is reported as the total iron-binding capacity (TIBC) (choice E). Since the normal serum iron is 100 µg/dL and the normal TIBC is 300 µg/dL, the normal percentage saturation of transferrin is 33% (iron/TIBC = percentage saturation). The percentage saturation of transferrin is decreased in iron deficiency anemia; however, it is also decreased in the anemia of chronic disease, so it is not a very good screening test for iron deficiency. Considered from the point of view of the transferrin level, TIBC reflects the amount of transferrin that is present in the blood. Iron stores in the bone marrow have an inverse relationship with transferrin synthesis by the liver. For example, when iron stores are decreased (iron deficiency), transferrin synthesis is increased (increased serum TIBC). When iron stores are increased (e.g., anemia of chronic disease, hemochromatosis), serum transferrin synthesis is decreased (decreased serum TIBC).

2 The answer is A *Psychiatry*

Oppositional defiant disorder (choice A) involves problems in relating to authority figures. Generally, such children get along well with peers and have no other problems of conduct or development.

Mental retardation (choice B) is associated with delayed developmental milestones and other evidence of impaired intellectual abilities. Conduct disorder (choice C) is characterized by violation of age-appropriate social norms, fighting, runaway behavior, theft, and destruction of property and often is a sequel to oppositional defiant disorder. Childhood disintegrative disorder (choice D) involves the development of severe disturbances in social, communicative, and cognitive functions after a period of normal development. Attention-deficit/hyperactivity disorder (choice E) is characterized by inattention, impulsivity, and hyperactivity. Individuals with this disorder would be unlikely to complete projects even if they were interested.

3 The answer is C *Surgery*

This patient has a pleomorphic adenoma (also known as a mixed parotid tumor) (choice C). It is the most common tumor affecting the salivary glands, accounting for approximately 70% of parotid tumors and 50% of all salivary gland tumors. Pleomorphic adenomas are essentially benign and, as in this patient, are often present for more than 6 years. Malignancy can develop and is heralded by a sudden increase in size, pain, and infiltration into the facial nerve, where it traverses the gland.

Adenolymphoma (choice **B**) (also called Warthin's tumor), the second most common benign tumor of the salivary glands, is almost always located in the parotid gland. It most often is cystic and usually affects middle-aged or elderly males. More than one tumor may be found in one or both parotid glands. Mucoepidermoid carcinoma (choice **D**) is the most common malignant tumor of the parotid glands. It has varying degrees of differentiation and growth; the greater the squamous component, the worse the prognosis. When mucoepidermoid carcinoma occurs in the parotid gland, it does not usually cause facial nerve paralysis, because local invasion is limited. Metastasis is also limited to the local lymph nodes. Adenoid cystic carcinoma (choice **A**) is the most common malignant tumor of minor salivary glands and has a tendency to invade perineural tissue. As a result, the patient presents with pain, paralysis of muscles, and areas of anesthesia over involved skin. The tumor may even invade bone, without evidence of it on initial radiography. Thus, like an iceberg, it is far more extensive than encountered on physical examination or perceived on radiography. Acinic cell carcinoma (choice **E**) is a rare malignant tumor that is more common in women than in men. It is most commonly located in the parotid gland. It is slow growing, tends to be soft, is locally invasive, and may metastasize.

4 **The answer is C** *Medicine*

The patient has a varicocele (looks like a "bag of worms") in the left scrotal sac caused by engorgement of the internal spermatic veins above the testis. Varicoceles usually occur on the left side, because the left spermatic vein empties into the left renal vein, imposing increased resistance to blood flow, while the right spermatic vein empties into the vena cava. Sudden development of a left-sided varicocele indicates a lesion blocking blood flow into the left renal vein, such as a renal cell carcinoma associated with invasion of the left renal vein or thrombosis of the renal vein. Of the two choices, a renal cell carcinoma (choice **C**) is the most likely cause, because cigarette smoking is the greatest risk factor and hematuria is the most common presenting sign.

Epididymitis (choice **A**) is associated with scrotal pain with radiation of the pain to the spermatic cord or flank and decreased pain when the scrotal sac is elevated (Prehn's sign). These findings are not present in this patient. A hydrocele (choice **B**) is a collection of fluid between the two layers of the tunica vaginalis. Enlargement of the scrotal sac is caused by distended vascular channels, not fluid. Testicular cancer (choice **D**) presents with a painless mass in the testes. In this patient, testicular volume is reduced, and tumor markers for testicular cancer (hCG and AFP) are absent. An increase in hCG indicates the presence of a choriocarcinoma, while an increase in AFP is associated with an endodermal sinus tumor (yolk sac tumor). Torsion of the spermatic cord (choice **E**) produces a sudden onset of testicular pain. The testicle draws up into the inguinal canal. Stroking the inside thigh on the side of the torsion does not elicit the normal cremasteric reflex (contraction of the scrotal sac). The patient does not have these findings.

5 **The answer is C** *Medicine*

The patient has acute pyelonephritis (choice **C**), which is an acute bacterial infection (usually caused by *Escherichia coli*) that involves the tubules and interstitium. Classic signs include fever, flank pain, and WBC casts accompanied by signs of a lower urinary tract infection (e.g., suprapubic discomfort, dysuria, and urinary frequency). Results of the urine dipstick test for nitrates are positive (most uropathogens are nitrate reducers) and those of the dipstick for leukocyte esterase (a particularly active enzyme in neutrophils) are also positive. Most cases occur in women who have recurrent lower urinary tract infections and vesicoureteral reflux, which involves passage of urine into the ureter during micturition. Infection then ascends into the renal pelvis and into the renal parenchyma, producing microabscesses.

Acute cystitis (choice **A**) is characterized by lower urinary tract infection but not by fever, flank pain, or WBC casts in the urine. Acute glomerulonephritis (choice **B**) is characterized by oliguria (decreased glomerular filtration rate), proteinuria, hematuria, and urine casts (RBC, WBC, or fatty casts), depending on the type of glomerulonephritis. Dysmorphic RBCs (RBCs with projections from the cell membrane) are a characteristic feature of hematuria of glomerular origin. Most cases of acute glomerulonephritis are immune mediated. Flank pain, dysuria, and increased urinary frequency are not present in glomerulonephritis. Acute tubular necrosis (choice **D**) is most commonly caused by ischemia (e.g., decreased cardiac output) or nephrotoxic drugs (e.g., aminoglycosides). Acute tubular necrosis is characterized by oliguria and is associated with renal tubular cell casts rather than WBC casts. Acute urethritis (choice **E**) is a lower urinary tract infection and is not characterized by fever, flank pain, or WBC casts in the urine.

6 The answer is A *Surgery*

The patient has acute cholecystitis, which most commonly (90% of cases) results from a stone impacted in the cystic duct (choice **A**). Ischemic damage to the gallbladder mucosa and secondary invasion by bacteria, usually *Escherichia coli,* result from the impacted stone. Right upper quadrant pain usually occurs within 15 to 30 minutes after eating. Vomiting does not relieve the pain. The pain is steady and aching and often radiates to the right scapula. Right upper quadrant tenderness on palpation after deep inspiration is called Murphy's sign. The gallbladder is palpable in 30 to 40% of patients. The patients are usually febrile. Jaundice occurs in 20% of patients. Absolute neutrophilic leukocytosis with a shift to the left is usually present. A hepato-iminodiacetic acid (HIDA) nuclear scan (i.e., a nuclear scan following an intravenous injection of iminodiacetic acid) is the study of choice to identify the stone in the cystic duct. Assuming that the patient is otherwise in good health, most surgeons recommend surgery within the first 72 hours to reduce overall morbidity. Other surgeons manage the patient expectantly, because most acute attacks (60%) resolve when the stone disengages from the cystic duct.

Chemically induced inflammation of the gallbladder (choice **B**) is more commonly associated with chronic, rather than acute, cholecystitis. A stone in the common bile duct (choice **C**) most often presents with an obstructive jaundice. Biliary dyskinesia (choice **D**) presents with right upper quadrant pain in the absence of stones. It results from abnormal motor function of the gallbladder musculature. Hydrops of the gallbladder (choice **E**) is an accumulation of mucus in the lumen secondary to duct obstruction. It is not an acute disease.

7 The answer is B *Preventive Medicine and Public Health*

Routine screening for prostate cancer is not recommended because it is feared that increased screening will result in unneeded biopsies, which have their own risk of complications, let alone the increased cost, inconvenience, and pain, and although a 2003 study concluded that finasteride reduced the risk of prostate cancer by 25%, it does create its own problems (choice **B**). The cancers that did develop while a patient was on finasteride were more aggressive than usual, and libido was reduced, ejaculate volume was decreased, and reports of erectile dysfunction were increased.

Controversy remains concerning who should or should not be screened and at what age; however, most agencies recommend some screening before the age of 60 (choice **A**). The 2005 Centers for Disease Control and Prevention (CDC) statement on the internet basically summarizes the status. It says that all men have the right to hear the pros and cons concerning routine screening and then to make an informed decision. In addition, they say that for those who believe in routine screening, they recommend that if life expectancy is greater than 10 years, PSA and DRE testing should be conducted annually starting at age 50 or earlier for African Americans and if a brother or father had prostate cancer.

According to 2005 CDC figures, over a lifetime one of every six males (16.6%) will develop prostate cancer, not 0.2% (choice **C**). However, only 1 of every 2500 45-year-old men will have prostate cancer; at age 50, the odds increase to 1 in 476; at age 55, 1 in 200; at age 60, 1 in 43; at 65, 1 in 21; at 70, 1 in 13: and by 75 years of age, 1 in 9. In fact, autopsy data suggest all men would eventually develop prostate cancer, provided they live long enough. Risk development rate is accelerated among African Americans and in men who have an affected brother or father. The good news is that most cases of prostate cancer develop at an indolent rate, and many cancers remain asymptomatic for years, so most men who are first diagnosed in their late 70s or 80s will die of some other disease before their prostatic cancer becomes truly troublesome.

At this time there are basically three methods available to screen for prostate cancer. PSA, DRE, and transrectal ultrasound. Transrectal ultrasound is more expensive than the other two modalities, it has a low specificity (consequently a high biopsy rate), and its sensitivity is no greater. Thus it is not likely to replace DRE and PSA (choice **D**).

PSA is more sensitive than the DRE (not vice versa, choice **E**). Using the standard cutoff of 4 ng/mL the PSA test will find that 2% of men older than 50 have prostate cancer, while the DRE will find that 1.5% do. Although the combined use of DRE and PSA increases the accuracy of prostate cancer diagnosis, problems remain. The DRE is subjective, and even the best diagnosticians cannot detect early cancer. PSA is elevated in benign prostatic hypertrophy (BPH) and other benign conditions, which can increase PSA values into the "gray" risk zone of 4–10 ng/mL or even higher, causing false-positive results triggering biopsy and further studies. Conversely, treatment of BPH with finasteride lowers PSA values and causes false-negative results. Many clinicians believe that testing high-risk subjects (primarily older men) annually and looking for an increase in the PSA value is a more sensitive test than relying on one value. An annual increase of 0.75 ng/mL or more, even if the value remains below 4 ng/mL, denotes a high probability of cancer. Other investigators tout the measurement of free and protein-bound PSA rather than the standard total PSA; cancer patients have a lower percentage of free PSA. A free PSA value of 25% or above means the risk of cancer is low, even if the total PSA value was over 4 ng/mL, while a free value below 10% means the risk is very high. However, once again there is a zone of uncertainty between 10 and 25%, making biopsy inevitable in such cases. Still another approach trying to increase the sensitivity of a PSA test is by establishing age-related cutoff values rather than assuming a value of 4ng/mL fits patients at all ages.

8 The answer is E *Psychiatry*

In major depressive disorder, the greatest risk for suicide occurs after partial response to antidepressants (choice **E**). Usually, energy and motivation return before a subjective improvement in mood. A patient who has been too apathetic to act on suicidal rumination may, at this point, attempt suicide. Also, some antidepressants provide the means for a suicide attempt by overdose. Close assessment of patients during treatment with antidepressant medication is therefore essential.

Admission of feelings of guilt (choice **A**), completion of a course of electroconvulsive therapy (choice **B**), the start of treatment (choice **C**), and development of untoward effects to antidepressants (choice **D**) are all situations that are not closely associated with a risk for suicide.

9 The answer is D *Psychiatry*

A neglect of the basic rights of others (choice **D**) is most characteristic of antisocial personality disorder.

Dismissal of most people and idealization of a few famous or infamous figures (choice **A**) are characteristic of narcissistic personality disorder. A history of earlier abuse during childhood (choice **C**) and other childhood psychopathology (e.g., fire setting, cruelty to animals [choice **B**]) are often found in individuals with several types of adult psychopathology such as borderline personality disorder or dissociative identity disorder. Although a history of incarceration (choice **C**) is common in individuals with antisocial personality disorder, there are many incarcerated individuals without this disorder and many individuals with the disorder that are never incarcerated. The mere belief in violence (choice **E**) does not necessarily indicate antisocial personality disorder.

10 The answer is A *Medicine*

The dyspnea and pulmonary edema with inspiratory crackles indicate the patient has left-sided heart failure. This causes a decrease in cardiac output and leads to a decrease in renal blood flow, glomerular filtration rate (GFR), and oliguria. The serum blood urea nitrogen (BUN):creatinine ratio is 30 (60/2), which is consistent with prerenal azotemia. A decrease in the GFR causes backup of both urea and creatinine in the blood. However, after filtration, some of the urea is reabsorbed back into the blood by the proximal tubule, while creatinine is not reabsorbed. This causes a disproportionate increase in the serum BUN over that of serum creatinine resulting in a BUN:creatinine ratio greater than 15. The $FENa^+$ is a sensitive indicator of tubular function. It represents the amount of sodium excreted in the urine divided by the amount of sodium that is filtered by the kidneys. The calculation is as follows: $FENa^+ = [(UNa^+ \times PCr) \div (PNa^+ \times UCr)] \times 100$, where UNa^+ is a random urine sodium, PNa^+ serum sodium, UCr random urine creatinine, and PCr plasma creatinine. Creatinine is used in the formula, because the amount of sodium filtered depends on the GFR, which closely approximates the creatinine clearance. $FENa^+$ values below 1% indicate intact tubular function, while those above 2% indicate tubular dysfunction. In prerenal azotemia, tubular function is intact, therefore, the $FENa^+$ is less than 1% (choice **A**).

Since tubular function is intact in this patient, reabsorption of sodium in the proximal and distal tubules is normal, and the random urine sodium is less than 20 mEq/L (not >40 mEq/L [choice **B**]). Random urine sodium above 40 mEq/L indicates tubular dysfunction. Furthermore, since tubular function is intact, renal concentration is normal, and the UOsm is greater than 500 mOsm/kg (not <350 mOsm/kg [choice **C**]). A UOsm below 350 mOsm/kg indicates a loss of urine concentration, which is the first sign of tubular dysfunction. In prerenal azotemia, there should be no casts in the urine (no renal tubular cell casts [choice **D**]), which indicate tubular dysfunction in renal failure.

11 The answer is C *Psychiatry*

Lithium-induced hypothyroidism occurs in approximately 5% of individuals on lithium maintenance therapy (choice **C**). Lithium maintenance therapy may also induce weight gain, acneform skin eruptions, tremor, leukocytosis, and polyuria. The latter reflects a low incidence of potential renal toxicity. Consequently, routine monitoring during lithium maintenance therapy includes plasma lithium levels, complete blood count (CBC), blood urea nitrogen (BUN) concentration, creatinine levels, and thyroid function testing.

In contrast to its potential effect on the thyroid, lithium has no reported hepatotoxicity, which would cause abnormal liver function test results (choice **A**). Fever (choice **B**), urinary retention (choice **E**), and leukopenia (choice **D**) are rarely associated with lithium treatment.

12 The answer is B *Surgery*

The patient has a classic triad for a ruptured abdominal aortic aneurysm: an abrupt onset of back pain, hypotension, and a pulsatile mass in the abdomen. An aneurysm is a localized dilatation of a vessel. It is usually caused by structural weakness in the wall of the vessel due to atherosclerosis (choice **B**). Abdominal aortic aneurysms are the most common type of aneurysm in the vascular system, located below the orifices of the renal arteries. Most occur in men over 55 years of age, who are asymptomatic. Each year some 9000 Americans die from a ruptured abdominal aortic aneurysm, and most of these are men over 65 years of age. Ultrasound is the most effective means of making the diagnosis of an aneurysm, and in 2005 the U.S. Preventive Services Task Force (USPSTF) recommended this procedure for routine screening of men between the ages of 65 and 75 who have smoked at least 100 cigarettes during their lifetime. The evidence for nonsmokers is less compelling, but the possibility of screening others is left open. Rupture of the aneurysm is the most common complication. The aorta's normal diameter is less than 3 cm; a value above that is diagnosed as an aneurysm, but the risk of rupture is not great until the diameter exceeds 5 cm. Other risk factors for rupture include hypertension and the presence of chronic obstructive pulmonary disease (COPD). Indications for surgery include any symptomatic aneurysm or any asymptomatic aneurysm larger than 5 cm, because rupture is inevitable with time, and after rupture, mortality rates exceed 90%.

Hypertension (choice **A**) and elastic tissue fragmentation (choice **C**) are associated with dissecting aortic aneurysms. Immune complex–mediated inflammation (immune complex vasculitis) (choice **D**) is the primary pathogenesis of small vessel disease. Vasculitis secondary to syphilis (syphilitic aortitis) (choice **E**) is a late symptom rarely observed since the advent of penicillin.

13 The answer is A *Medicine*

The patient has Wilson's disease, which is an autosomal recessive disease due to genetic aberration in the "Wilson" gene on chromosome 13; the worldwide prevalence is 30 cases per 10^6 persons. More than 200 different mutations have been uncovered leading to some variation in symptoms. However, typically, the disease first presents in adolescence with liver disease plus a variety of hemolytic and other symptoms and then progresses in early adulthood to neurologic problems similar to those described. Once the disease progresses to the neurologic state, a Kayser-Fleischer ring (brown pigment around the perimeter of the cornea) is essentially pathognomic for the condition. The genetic defect affects a copper-transporting ATPase (ATP7B) in the liver and leads to accumulation of copper in the hepatocytes and oxidative damage to hepatic mitochondria. The major physiologic effects are due to a defect in the hepatocyte transport system for copper secretion into bile, leading to increased copper deposition in liver, brain, cornea, and kidneys. In addition, copper cannot be incorporated into an α_2-globulin to produce ceruloplasmin, which is the copper-binding protein. Normally, the total serum copper equals copper that is bound to ceruloplasmin (95% of the total) plus copper that is unbound (free). In Wilson's disease, the total serum copper level is decreased (not increased [choice **D**]) because ceruloplasmin is decreased (choice **A**). However, the free copper level in the serum and urine is increased because of defective excretion in the bile and subsequent accumulation of copper in the serum. Excess copper is deposited in Descemet's membrane of the cornea of the eye (producing Kayser-Fleischer ring) and in the basal ganglia. In the latter location, it may cause parkinsonism, choreiform movements, and dystonia in the bulbar musculature. This latter effect can produce dysarthria (problems with speech and/or drooling) and/or dysphagia.

Increased serum ferritin (choice **B**) in the setting of chronic liver disease is associated with hemochromatosis, an autosomal recessive disease with unrestricted reabsorption of iron from the gastrointestinal tract. Hemochromatosis is not associated with corneal abnormalities or a movement disorder. Increased serum mitochondrial antibodies (choice **C**) is a marker for primary biliary cirrhosis, which is an autoimmune disease characterized by destruction of bile ducts in the portal triads. It is not associated with corneal abnormalities or a movement disorder. Since the patient has chronic liver disease (chronic hepatitis or cirrhosis), the prothrombin time is most likely increased (not normal [choice **E**]) because of decreased synthesis of coagulation factors in the damaged liver.

14 The answer is E *Medicine*

Glucose can be converted to fructose via sorbitol in a two-reaction sequence.

Reaction 1 catalyzed by aldose reductase: Glucose + NADPH + H$^+$ → sorbitol + NADP$^+$

Reaction 2 catalyzed by sorbitol dehydrogenase: Sorbitol + NAD$^+$ → fructose + NADH$^+$ H$^+$

Under hyperglycemic conditions, as in poorly controlled diabetes mellitus whether type 1 or 2, glucose is converted to sorbitol in all tissues containing aldose reductase as long as NADPH is available. Under these conditions sorbitol accumulates in those tissues in which the aldose reductase has a higher intrinsic activity than the sorbitol dehydrogenase. These tissues include Schwann cells, pericytes in retinal vessels, lens, and some kidney cells. This sorbitol cannot cross the membrane and the intracellular amount increases in proportion to the plasma glucose level and draws in water, causing osmotic damage (choice **E**) promoting the development of cataracts, peripheral neuropathy, microaneurysms and nephropathy.

Antibodies against β islet cells (choice **A**) occur in 80 to 90% of patients with type 1 diabetes within the first year of diagnosis. Type 2 diabetic individuals do not have these antibodies. An HLA-Dr3/Dr4 association (choice **B**) is present in patients with type 1 diabetes mellitus. Presence of these HLA types increases the risk for autoimmune destruction of the β islet cells by viruses (e.g., Coxsackie) or other environmental factors. Type 2 diabetes mellitus is more often associated with obesity than is type 1 diabetes mellitus. Increased adipose tissue downregulates insulin receptor synthesis (choice **C**), which contributes to the hyperglycemia that occurs in type 2 diabetes. Ketoacidosis (choice **D**) occurs in type 1 diabetes mellitus where there is absolute insulin deficiency due to autoimmune destruction of β islet cells. In the absence of insulin, there is increased β-oxidation of fatty acids, which provides acetyl-CoA for the liver to synthesize ketone bodies. In type 2 diabetes mellitus, there is enough insulin present to prevent ketone body synthesis but not enough to lower blood glucose. Instead of developing ketoacidosis, if plasma glucose levels increase sufficiently, they could develop hyperosmolar nonketotic coma.

15 The answer is E *Medicine*

All of the insects listed are vectors of rash-producing diseases caused by microorganisms in the Rickettsiae family. The man in the case described has Rocky Mountain spotted fever, which is due to the bite of a hard tick (*Dermacentor andersoni,* choice **E**) a vector for *Rickettsia rickettsii*. A diagnostic triad for the disease is rash, fever, and history of exposure to a tick. The incubation period is approximately 2 to 12 days after exposure. Unlike the other rickettsial organisms, which cause a rash extending from the trunk to the extremities in centrifugal fashion, the rash of Rocky Mountain spotted fever begins on the palms and soles and spreads to the trunk. The rash is due to a vasculitis caused by the rickettsial organisms invading the endothelial cells of small vessels and producing petechial lesions. Oklahoma and North Carolina share the lead for the highest incidence of Rocky Mountain spotted fever. The diagnosis is best made serologically using indirect immunofluorescent techniques rather than the outdated Weil-Felix reaction, which has a positive *Proteus vulgaris* OX-2 and OX-19 reaction. Doxycycline is the treatment of choice. The mortality rate is 20% without treatment and 5% with treatment.

The vector for murine typhus and the plague is the flea (choice **A**) and the disease-causing agent is *R. typhi*. The typical hosts are mice and rats, but the disease has also been transmitted by cats and opossums. In the United States, approximately 100 cases are recorded each year, primarily in southern California and Texas. The disease-causing agent for the plague is *Yersinia pestis*. The typical host is the rat, but it is also carried by other rodents, including the ground squirrel. Historically, plague epidemics killed millions, but since 1950, outbreaks have been sporadic and isolated due to modern sanitation, rodent control, and use of antibiotics. The typical vector for epidemic typhus is the human body louse (choice **B**). The disease-causing organism is *R. prowazekii*. Epidemic typhus is typically transmitted from human to human via the louse, under unsanitary conditions, and epidemics are often associated with wars. Mites (choice **C**) carry rickettsial pox. The primary host is the mouse, and the causative agent is *R. akari*. Mites also cause severe pruritic conditions, but directly by their bite rather than serving as vectors. Scrub typhus is transmitted by mites (choice **D**). The disease-causing organism is *R. tsutsugamushi*, a distinct genus and species, which is in the Rickettsiae family. Cases of scrub typhus primarily occur in Oceania and the Far East.

16 **The answer is B** *Medicine*

Pasteurella multocida (choice **B**) is the organism that most commonly infects the deep puncture wounds characteristic of cat bites. Signs of infection arise within 24 hours. There is also a potential for developing tendinitis and osteomyelitis. *P. multocida* responds to amoxicillin, penicillin G, or ampicillin.

 Staphylococcus aureus (choice **C**), *Pseudomonas aeruginosa* (choice **E**), and group A streptococci (choice **D**) are not common pathogens in cat bites with symptoms in the first 24 hours. *Bartonella henselae* (choice **A**) is the cause of cat-scratch fever. In this disease, there are granulomatous microabscesses in lymph nodes draining the infection site.

 In all bites (animal and human), the mainstay of therapy is proper cleansing of the wound with soap and water. All bites on the extremities should be treated aggressively because of the potential for septic arthritis and tenosynovitis. Antimicrobial amoxicillin prophylaxis is recommended for all human bites (due to *Eikenella corrodens*) (choice **F**) and most cat bites. High-risk dog bites requiring antibiotic prophylaxis (e.g., amoxicillin) are those on the hand, those associated with puncture wounds, and wounds that are more than 6 to 12 hours old.

 The risk of tetanus is always greater in contaminated wounds, puncture wounds, and wounds that come late to medical attention. In general, tetanus toxoid protects a person for 10 years. Tetanus immunoglobulin is reserved for dirty wounds in persons who have never been immunized (never received the primary series of three doses of tetanus toxoid) or whose status is unknown. For a dirty wound (bite), a tetanus booster should be administered if more than 5 years have elapsed since the last booster shot.

 The decision for rabies prophylaxis in animal bites depends on the circumstance of the bite and the local prevalence of rabies. In this country, rabies is most commonly contracted from the bites of bats, skunks (most common), raccoons, and squirrels rather than dogs. In dogs or cats, a period of 10 days is sufficient to determine whether the animal is rabid. Strays or wild animals should be sacrificed and examined for rabies. If postexposure prophylaxis is required, washing the wound with soap and water is the first step in management. Half the dose of rabies immune globulin should be administered in the wound site and the other half in the gluteal region. Rabies vaccine is administered the same day and given at varying time intervals. Without treatment, there is a 100% fatality rate.

17 **The answer is C** *Obstetrics and Gynecology*

Ovarian tumors are more likely to be benign than malignant in women less than 45 years old. They are classified in the following categories: surface-derived (65–75% of tumors), germ cell (15–20% of tumors), sex-cord stromal (3–5% of tumors), and metastatic (5% of cases). Surface-derived cancers arise from coelomic epithelium and induce the greatest number of malignant ovarian tumors. Germ cell tumors derive from primitive cells that differentiate along gonadal cell lines (e.g., dysgerminoma, most common malignant germ cell tumor), somatic cell lines (e.g., teratoma), and extraembryonic lines (e.g., yolk sac tumor, most common malignant germ cell tumor in children). Sex-cord stromal tumors derive from stromal cells and may be hormone producing (e.g., estrogens, androgens). Breast cancer and stomach cancer are the most common cancers that metastasize to the ovaries. Risk factors for malignant tumors include the following: nulliparity (increased number of ovulatory cycles increases the risk for surface-derived cancers), genetic factors (e.g., mutations of *BRCA1* and *BRCA2* suppressor genes), chromosomal aberrations (e.g., Turner's syndrome), and smoking cigarettes. Oral contraceptives decrease the risk for surface-derived cancers by decreasing the number of ovulations.

 Clinical presentations for ovarian tumors vary. Malignant surface-derived tumors often spread by seeding and produce malignant ascites and increased abdominal girth. Recall, that the ovaries of a postmenopausal woman are not usually palpable, because they undergo atrophy. Therefore, a palpable ovary in a postmenopausal woman is likely to be a primary ovarian cancer or an ovary with foci of metastatic cancer.

 Malignant pleural effusions are a common presentation of ovarian tumors. A number of ovarian tumors produce calcifications that are visible on x-ray films; these include cystic teratomas (this case), gonadoblastomas, and fibromas. Finally, ovarian tumors may present with signs of feminization (estrogen-secreting tumors, e.g., granulosa cell tumor) or masculinization (androgen-secreting tumors, e.g., Sertoli cell tumor). CA 125 is a tumor marker for surface-derived tumors.

The patient in this question has a cystic teratoma (choice **C**), which has undergone torsion, causing abdominal pain. Teratomas are the most common benign germ cell tumor. Common ectodermal derivatives include hair, sebaceous glands, teeth, and neuroepithelium. Examples of endodermal derivatives include gastrointestinal tissue and thyroid tissue. Common mesodermal derivatives include muscle, cartilage, and bone. Most of these derivatives are found in a nipplelike structure in the cyst wall called a Rokitansky tubercle. In rare cases, squamous epithelium in a teratoma may undergo malignant transformation and produce a squamous cell carcinoma. A struma ovarii type of teratoma has functioning thyroid tissue and is a rare cause of hyperthyroidism. The treatment for a cystic teratoma is surgical removal of the tumor.

A follicular cyst (choice **A**) is the most common ovarian mass in young women. It is due to an accumulation of fluid in a follicle or previously ruptured follicle. They may rupture and produce a sterile peritonitis with abdominal pain. Ultrasonography is useful in identifying the cyst. There are no calcifications. A mucinous cystadenoma (choice **B**) is a benign surface-derived tumor that is lined by mucus-secreting cells (recapitulates endocervical epithelium). An ultrasound scan shows a large, multiloculated tumor without calcifications. A Brenner's tumor (choice **D**) is a benign surface-derived tumor that contains Walthard rests (transitional-like epithelium). It is commonly associated with benign mucinous cystadenomas. Ultrasonography shows a solid ovarian mass without calcifications. A serous cystadenoma (choice **E**) is the most common benign tumor of the ovaries. It is a surface-derived tumor that is commonly bilateral. It is lined by ciliated cells (recapitulates fallopian tube epithelium). Ultrasonography shows a cystic mass without calcifications.

18 **The answer is A** *Preventive Medicine and Public Health*

This is a cohort study (choice **A**) because all subjects are free of illness at the start of the study.

In a case-control study (choice **B**), ill subjects (cases) and well subjects (controls) are compared with respect to a risk factor. In a randomized controlled clinical trial (choice **C**), some members of a cohort with a specific disorder are given one treatment and other members of the cohort are given a different treatment or a placebo. In a cross-sectional study (choice **D**), subjects are studied at a specific point in time. In a crossover study (choice **E**), some subjects receive the drug first while others receive the placebo first; later in the study the groups switch treatments.

19 **The answer is E** *Psychiatry*

This patient's presenting symptoms are most suggestive of a manic episode, which is characterized by an irritable, elevated, or euphoric mood, coupled with increased psychomotor activity, decreased need for sleep, grandiosity, and deterioration of judgment. Her most likely diagnosis is bipolar disorder, manic phase, single episode. Bipolar disorder is characterized by one or more episodes of mania that are not substance induced or due to a general medical condition. It is usually first evident in the third decade, but many exceptions exist. Its incidence is between 0.5 and 2%, and it is equally common in both sexes. There is no relationship to socioeconomic status. In bipolar disorder, the lifetime chance of another episode is greater than 90% (choice **E**).

Therefore, choices **A** (5%), **B** (25%), **C** (50%), and **D** (75%) are incorrect. The chance of developing further episodes of other mental disorders varies. For example, the lifetime chance of another episode of depression following major depressive disorder, single episode, is approximately 50%. The chance of schizophrenia following the onset of schizophreniform disorder is between 33 and 50%.

20 **The answer is D** *Surgery*

The patient has ascending cholangitis (choice **D**), which results from concurrent biliary tract infection and obstruction (e.g., by a stone, stricture, or neoplasm). Attacks are often precipitated by heavy fatty meals. The classic Charcot triad is colicky, right upper quadrant pain; fever; and jaundice to which in cholangitis can be added mental statis change and sepsis. Laboratory studies reveal an absolute neutrophilic leukocytosis, direct hyperbilirubinemia, and elevation of alkaline phosphatase and γ-glutamyltransferase, which are increased in obstructive jaundice. Infection and subsequent sepsis may result from infection by *Escherichia coli*, *Klebsiella* species, enterobacteria, enterococci and/or group D streptococci. Although 95% of the patients who present this way have common duct stone obstruction, only a small minority of patients with acute cholecystis present in this manner. This presentation is associated with infection, which often results from repeated attacks, as in the case described in the vignette. Septicemia frequently occurs as infected bile regurgitates into the liver and the liver sinusoids, and the tachycardia and hypotension are signs of septic shock. Ascending cholangitis is the most common cause of liver abscesses, because the infection extends into the portal triads. The initial treatment is with intravenous antibiotics. If the inflammation does not subside, then surgery is indicated to decompress the common bile duct and remove the source of obstruction. The mortality rate approaches 90% in untreated patients.

Acute hepatitis (choice **B**) is not associated with colicky pain and has a mixed indirect and direct hyper-bilirubinemia. Acute pancreatitis (choice **C**) presents with a steady, boring, midepigastric pain, with radiation into the back or periumbilical area. Jaundice is unusual. An amebic liver abscess (choice **A**) does not present with colicky pain or jaundice. The organisms drain into the liver via the portal vein from a primary site of infection in the cecum. Sclerosing pericholangitis (choice **E**) is most commonly associated with ulcerative colitis.

21 The answer is B *Medicine*

The arterial blood gas determination reveals an acute, uncompensated respiratory acidosis with hypoxemia: pH, 7.20 (acidemia); $PaCO_2$, 72 mm Hg (respiratory acidosis); HCO_3^-, 28 mEq/L (normal); PO_2, 50 mm Hg (hypoxemia). To determine whether the hypoxemia is pulmonary or extrapulmonary in origin, a calculation of the alveolar-arterial (A-a) gradient is required. The alveolar PO_2 is calculated as follows: 0.21 (room air) $\times$ 713 mm Hg (atmospheric pressure – water vapor pressure) 72 mm Hg (arterial $PaCO_2$)/0.8 (respiratory quotient) = 60 mm Hg. Since the PaO_2 is 50 mm Hg, the A-a gradient is $60 - 50 = 10$ mm Hg. An A-a gradient greater than 30 mm Hg is medically significant. Hypoxemia in the presence of a normal A-a gradient indicates an extrapulmonary cause of hypoxemia that involves hypoventilation (respiratory acidosis) due to depression of the respiratory center in the brain (e.g., barbiturates, [choice **B**]) or chest wall dysfunction (e.g., neuromuscular disease, kyphoscoliosis, obesity, paralysis of the diaphragms). Hypoxemia in the presence of an increased A-a gradient indicates a primary disease in the lungs (e.g., atelectasis, ventilation-perfusion defect, pulmonary vascular disease) or congenital heart disease with a right to left shunt (e.g., tetralogy of Fallot; reversal of a ventricular or atrial septal defect).

The acute respiratory distress syndrome (choice **A**) is associated with acute respiratory acidosis leading to severe hypoxemia. It is characterized by neutrophil damage to the alveoli (ventilation–perfusion defect), atelectasis (decreased surfactant from destruction of type II pneumocytes causing intrapulmonary shunting of blood), and noncardiogenic pulmonary edema with hyaline membranes (diffusion defect). All of these lung findings cause an increase in the A-a gradient. Chronic bronchitis (choice **C**) is an obstructive lung disease associated with chronic respiratory acidosis leading to severe hypoxemia. Inflammation and mucus plugs blocking the terminal bronchioles interfere with clearance of CO_2, causing an increase in alveolar PCO_2 and a corresponding decrease in alveolar PO_2 and PaO_2. The proximal small airway obstruction produces a major ventilation–perfusion mismatch, causing an increase in the A-a gradient.

Emphysema (choice **D**) is an obstructive lung disease that produces destruction of the respiratory unit (respiratory bronchioles, alveolar ducts, alveoli) and the pulmonary vascular bed leading to a ventilation–mismatch causing hypoxemia and an increased A-a gradient. Arterial blood gases either show a normal $PaCO_2$ or slightly decreased $PaCO_2$, the latter due to respiratory alkalosis from hyperventilation. Pulmonary infarction (choice **E**) is associated with an acute respiratory alkalosis (alkaline pH, decreased PCO_2) and mild hypoxemia. Thromboembolism originating from the femoral vein is the most common cause of a pulmonary infarction. Obstruction of pulmonary vessels produces a perfusion defect leading to an increase in dead space in the lungs, causing a mild hypoxemia and an increase in the A-a gradient.

22 The answer is E *Medicine*

When preproinsulin in the β islet cell is delivered to the Golgi apparatus, proteolytic reactions generate insulin and a cleavage peptide called C-peptide. Therefore, C-peptide is a marker for endogenous synthesis of insulin. Injection of human insulin (choice **E**) increases serum insulin and produces hypoglycemia. Hypoglycemia suppresses β islet cells, causing a decrease in endogenous synthesis of insulin and a corresponding decrease in serum C-peptide. In this case, the nurse was titering her glucose level so that she would show clear symptoms of hypoglycemia without invoking serious central nervous consequences (serum levels below 50 mg/dL). Her motivation is to get time off with pay; an external motivation. Consequently, she is malingering. It is not a factitious disorder (choice **F**) because to be so the motivation must be internal, driven by a psychologic need.

Benign tumors of the β islet cells (choice **A**), or insulinomas, synthesize excess insulin, causing a severe fasting hypoglycemia. Both serum insulin and serum C-peptide levels are increased. Serum C-peptide is decreased in this patient. Ectopic secretion of an insulin-like factor (choice **B**) that causes hypoglycemia is most often produced by a hepatocellular carcinoma. Since the insulin-like factor is not measured in the serum as insulin, hypoglycemia suppresses β islet cells, resulting in a decrease in serum insulin and C-peptide. The patient has an increase in serum insulin and a decrease in C-peptide. Malignant tumors of α islet cells (choice **C**) secrete glucagon, which produces hyperglycemia by stimulating gluconeogenesis. The patient has hypoglycemia. Pancreatic carcinomas (choice **D**) usually develop in the head of the pancreas, causing obstruction of the common bile duct and an obstructive type of jaundice. The patient does not have jaundice. Furthermore, pancreatic carcinomas do not secrete insulin or insulin-like factors to produce hypoglycemia.

23 **The answer is E** *Medicine*

The patient has Cushing syndrome, which is a state of hypercortisolism. There are several causes. Iatrogenic Cushing syndrome, which occurs most commonly in a patient taking corticosteroids, is the major nonpathologic cause. Pituitary Cushing syndrome is the most common pathologic cause of Cushing syndrome (~60% of cases). It is most often due to a benign pituitary adenoma secreting adrenocorticotropic hormone (ACTH). Adrenal Cushing syndrome and ectopic Cushing syndrome account for the remainder of causes of the syndrome. Adrenal Cushing syndrome is most often due to a benign adenoma secreting cortisol. The excess cortisol suppresses plasma ACTH. Ectopic Cushing syndrome is most often caused by a small cell carcinoma of the lung with ectopic production of ACTH.

Clinical findings in Cushing syndrome are protean and parallel the excessive production of cortisol, weak mineralocorticoids (e.g., deoxycorticosterone), and 17-ketosteroids, which are weak androgens (e.g., dehydroepiandrosterone sulfate). Truncal obesity is a characteristic finding. Excess fat is distributed in the face ("moon face"), cervical area ("buffalo hump"), and abdomen, with sparing of the extremities. This peculiar distribution is due to the lipogenic effect of insulin, which is released in response to hyperglycemia caused by hypercortisolism (cortisol is a gluconeogenic hormone). Since most of the substrates for gluconeogenesis derive from amino acids and amino acids are in abundance in muscle tissue, muscle catabolism is prominent in the arm and leg muscles. Wide purple striae are secondary to weak subcutaneous tissue and vessel instability, leading to ecchymoses and bleeding into the stretch marks. This tissue instability is the result of the inhibitory effect of cortisol on collagen synthesis. Hypertension in Cushing syndrome is associated with increased release of weak mineralocorticoids and subsequent retention of sodium. Hirsutism is due to an increased concentration of 17-ketosteroids, which are weak androgens. The plethoric face is due to vessel engorgement from secondary polycythemia induced by cortisol-enhanced erythropoiesis. Severe osteoporosis can result from cortisol's potentiation of the effects of parathyroid hormone and vitamin D on bone. Menstrual irregularities (usually amenorrhea) and mental aberrations round out the clinical picture. Hypercortisolism has an effect on the leukocyte count. Cortisol decreases neutrophil adhesion to endothelial cells, resulting in a neutrophilic leukocytosis; increases adhesion of lymphocytes in efferent lymphatics, which produces lymphopenia; and is cytotoxic to eosinophils, causing eosinopenia.

Laboratory testing for pathologic causes of Cushing's syndrome involves the use of screening tests to establish the diagnosis and other tests to determine the type of Cushing syndrome. After documenting an increased level of serum cortisol, most clinicians screen for Cushing syndrome with a low-dose (1-mg) dexamethasone (an analogue of cortisol) suppression test (choice **E**) to see if the high-baseline cortisol can be suppressed to less than 5 µg/dL. Patients with pituitary, adrenal, and ectopic Cushing syndrome do not suppress cortisol below 5 µg/dL. False-positive results can occur in stressed patients and in obese patients. There is an increased false-positive loss of the normal diurnal rhythm of serum cortisol (high at 8 AM and low at 4 PM) in stressed or obese individuals; therefore, loss of a diurnal rhythm is not a useful screening test (choice **B**). Another excellent screening test is a 24-hour urine collection for free cortisol. This test, along with a low-dose dexamethasone suppression test clearly confirms the presence of Cushing syndrome; however, they do not provide information as to the cause of the syndrome.

To determine the type of Cushing syndrome, the high-dose dexamethasone test (8 mg/day) has the highest specificity. Hypercortisolism in pituitary Cushing syndrome can be suppressed, whereas that associated with adrenal and ectopic Cushing syndrome cannot be suppressed. Plasma ACTH is also a useful study. Patients with adrenal Cushing syndrome have decreased levels; those with pituitary Cushing syndrome have normal to slightly increased levels; and patients with ectopic Cushing syndrome have extremely high concentrations.

A captopril-enhanced renal radionuclide test (choice **A**) is used to document renovascular hypertension, which is most commonly due to atherosclerosis of the renal artery in elderly men or fibromuscular hyperplasia of the renal artery in young to middle-aged women. Other than hypertension, renovascular hypertension has no other parallel signs and symptoms with Cushing syndrome. The clonidine suppression test (choice **C**) is used to confirm pheochromocytoma caused by a tumor secreting excess catecholamines. Clonidine is a centrally acting adrenergic drug that cannot suppress the excessive catecholamines associated with a pheochromocytoma. A pheochromocytoma presents with paroxysmal hypertension, drenching sweats, and excessive anxiety, findings that are not present in this patient. A bone marrow examination (choice **D**), ostensibly as a workup of polycythemia in this patient, is not indicated.

24 The answer is D   *Medicine*

The patient has developed a spontaneous pneumothorax (choice **D**). This is a pulmonary complication of scuba diving that is due to rupture of a preexisting intrapleural bleb or a subpleural bleb, causing a perferation of the pleural which causes loss of negative pressure in the pleural cavity, leading to collapse of the lung. Physical findings include hyperresonance to percussion, tracheal deviation to the side of the collapse, elevation of the diaphragm, and absent breath sounds, all of which are present in this patient. The treatment of a spontaneous pneumothorax is supplemental oxygen, which increases the rate of pneumothorax absorption. A symptomatic pneumothorax, as in this patient, also requires chest tube placement under water seal drainage with suction to restore the negative intrathoracic pressure permiting reexpansion of the lungs.

Decompression sickness (gas embolism; choice **A**) is a complication of scuba diving. As a diver descends, nitrogen gas under increased pressure moves from the alveoli and dissolves in tissue and blood. Rapid ascent forces nitrogen to come out of the tissue and blood in the form of bubbles, causing ischemic damage. The treatment is to recompress them and push the nitrogen gas back into the tissue and then to slowly decrease the atmospheric pressure. The patient did not ascend rapidly. Furthermore, the type of pain that developed in this patient is localized to the lung, while the pain in decompression sickness is often generalized and commonly occurs around joints. Although a pulmonary thromboembolism leading to a pulmonary infarction (choice **C**) with a pleural effusion (choice **B**) is a complication of scuba diving, it usually occurs when the diver is stationary and in deep water. Physical findings of a pleural effusion include dullness to percussion, deviation of the trachea to the contralateral side, and absent breath sounds. A tension pneumothorax (choice **E**) is not a common cause of dyspnea in scuba diving. Unlike a spontaneous pneumothorax, a tension pneumothorax is associated with a flaplike pleural tear. Inspiration causes the flap to open and allow air to enter the pleural cavity. However, the flap closes on expiration and prevents the air from leaving the cavity. Increased intrapleural pressure to a value greater than the atmospheric pressure causes compression of the lung (atelectasis) and deviation of the trachea to the contralateral side. The diaphragm is depressed. The treatment of a tension pneumothorax is needle decompression, in which a large-bore needle is inserted into the second intercostal space in the midclavicular line. This relieves the excess positive pressure. This is followed by insertion of a chest tube.

25 The answer is D   *Obstetrics and Gynecology*

Primary amenorrhea is defined as absence of menses by age 14 without breast development or age 16 with breast development. It can be classified into four groups based on the presence or absence of normal breast development and a palpable uterus. This woman, with normal breast development but without a uterus, has either testicular feminization syndrome or congenital uterine absence. In the former syndrome, a genetic male has a congenital lack of androgen receptors, and so the normal male levels of testosterone are unrecognized. Normal female hormonal status is associated with congenital uterine absence, including low levels of testosterone. Thus, measurement of serum testosterone (choice **D**) would be the most useful test for this patient.

Follicle-stimulating hormone (FSH) determination (choice **A**) is helpful for differentiating the cause of primary amenorrhea with absent breasts but uterus present. An elevated FSH level indicates absence of functional follicles, whereas a low FSH level indicates a hypothalamic–pituitary problem. Luteinizing hormone (LH) assay (choice **B**) is not helpful because it normally fluctuates significantly during a normal menstrual cycle. Prolactin (choice **C**) and progesterone (choice **E**) levels do not contribute to the workup of primary amenorrhea.

26 **The answer is D** *Obstetrics and Gynecology*

The case describes oligohydramnios, or decreased amniotic fluid. Sonographic criteria include AFI less than 5 cm or a maximum vertical single amniotic fluid pocket of less than 2 cm. Marked deficiency in amniotic fluid volume may occur with decreased production or excessive removal of fluid. A serious consequence of oligohydramnios, regardless of cause, is umbilical cord compression leading to fetal hypoxia. The only option of the five provided that leads to oligohydramnios is renal agenesis (choice **D**).

Polyhydramnios, with increased amniotic fluid, is found with each of the other options: duodenal atresia (choice **A**) (more common with Down syndrome), open spina bifida (choice **B**) (often diagnosed by an elevated maternal serum α-fetoprotein test), tracheoesophageal fistula (choice **C**) (especially when the esophagus is a blind pouch), and atrial flutter (choice **E**) (resulting in nonimmune hydrops).

27 **The answer is C** *Psychiatry*

Hearing impairment (choice **C**) is the most likely cause for this boy's poor communication ability and classroom problems. Sensory impairment is an important differential diagnosis for symptoms that suggest mental retardation, learning disorders, or communication disorders. Such children may appear to learn more slowly because they miss many cues. They may become frustrated and develop other behavioral disturbances.

Autistic disorder (choice **A**) is unlikely because the boy is affectionate and engaged with his environment. Food allergies (choice **B**) have not been clearly linked to behavioral problems. Schizophrenia (choice **D**) is very rare in children of this age and would often be manifested by a preoccupation with internal stimuli. Seizure disorder (choice **E**) might cause cognitive disturbances, but these should be detectable with IQ testing.

28 **The answer is A** *Medicine*

The patient has methemoglobinemia. Methemoglobinemia results from exposure to chemicals that oxidize heme iron in hemoglobin (Hb) from its ferrous (Fe^{2+}) state to a ferric (Fe^{3+}) state. Oxidizing agents include nitrate and nitrite salts and sulfur-containing drugs or chemicals (e.g., dapsone, trimethoprim–sulfamethoxazole). The patient was most likely exposed to nitrate and nitrite salts in the well water. Since O_2 only binds to heme iron in the ferrous condition, the SaO_2 (percentage of heme groups on Hb occupied by O_2) is decreased (choice **A**). The increase in deoxyhemoglobin (Hb lacking O_2) gives blood a chocolate-colored appearance and causes cyanosis (bluish discoloration of the skin and mucous membranes) that does not respond to supplemental O_2. The treatment of choice is methylene blue, which directly reduces iron back to the ferrous state and also enhances NADPH methemoglobin reductase. Ascorbic acid, a reducing agent, is used as adjunctive therapy.

The arterial PO_2 is normal in methemoglobinemia (not decreased [choice **B**]), because gas diffusion from the lungs into the pulmonary capillaries is normal. The alveolar–arterial (A-a) gradient is obtained by subtracting the measured arterial PO_2 from the calculated alveolar PO_2. Because of a disparity between ventilation and perfusion in different portions of the lung, the arterial PO_2 is always less than the alveolar PO_2, which causes the A-a gradient. The gradient is increased when there is a further disparity between alveolar and arterial PO_2. This occurs most often with ventilation–perfusion defects due to primary lung disease (e.g., emphysema) or in congenital heart disease with right to left shunts. In methemoglobinemia, the A-a gradient is normal (not increased [choice **C**]), because there is no alteration in either the alveolar or the arterial PO_2. Increased serum bicarbonate indicates the presence of metabolic alkalosis, either as compensation for respiratory acidosis or as a primary disorder. In methemoglobinemia, a decrease in SaO_2 causes tissue hypoxia (lack of O_2 in tissue), which results in anaerobic glycolysis. Lactic acid is the end product of anaerobic glycolysis and produces metabolic acidosis with a decrease in serum bicarbonate (not increased [choice **D**]). The O_2 content represents the total amount of O_2 that is being carried in the blood. It is calculated with the following formula: $1.34 \times Hb \times SaO_2 + 0.003 \times PaO_2$. Since the SaO_2 is decreased in methemoglobinemia, the O_2 content is decreased (not normal [choice **E**]), and the total amount of O_2 that is available to tissue is decreased.

29 **The answer is A** *Psychiatry*

The symptoms are most suggestive of body dysmorphic disorder (choice **A**), a pathologic preoccupation with an imagined (or very minor) defect in appearance. The body parts most often involved are the nose, breasts, and thighs. The increased availability and effectiveness of reconstructive surgery have made diagnosis of this disorder more important. Surgical intervention is often ineffective in resolving it.

Delusional disorder, somatic type (choice **B**), is distinguished from body dysmorphic disorder by the presence of patently false beliefs about one's body. Delusional disorder may be associated with body dimorphic disorder. However, the onset of delusional disorder is generally in middle age or later, whereas body dysmorphic disorder generally starts in adolescence. Hypochondriasis (choice **C**) is characterized by misinterpretation of physical signs or symptoms. This patient shows no clear symptoms of depression (choice **D**). Somatization disorder (choice **E**) is characterized by the presence of many physical symptoms, especially pain.

30 **The answer is E**   *Medicine*

The patient has neurofibromatosis complicated by hypertension due to a pheochromocytoma. Neurofibromatosis is an autosomal dominantly inherited disease. The skin lesions in neurofibromatosis include pigmented, pedunculated tumors (neurofibromas) and flat, oval-shaped, coffee-colored patches (café au lait patches). There is an increased incidence of pheochromocytoma among patients having neurofibromatosis; this relationship is not surprising considering the neural origin of adrenal tissue. The classic triad of headache, palpitations, and excessive perspiration strongly predicts a pheochromocytoma. Catecholamine excess causes vasoconstriction of the coronary arteries, which produces subendocardial ischemia resulting in angina (as occurred in this patient). Hypertension is characterized as sustained, sustained with paroxysms (most common), or paroxysmal only. Twenty-four-hour urine tests for metanephrine, the most sensitive test (choice **E**), and vanillylmandelic acid, the degradation product of norepinephrine and epinephrine, are the most useful screening tests. Other associations with neurofibromatosis include acoustic neuromas (sensorineural hearing loss), meningiomas (seizure activity), and optic nerve gliomas (visual loss).

Although a urinalysis (choice **A**) is useful in the workup of hypertension related to renal disease (e.g., red blood cell casts, proteinuria), it provides no information that is specific for a pheochromocytoma. Serum electrolytes (choice **B**) are most useful in diagnosing primary aldosteronism as a cause of hypertension. Excess aldosterone causes hypernatremia, hypokalemia, and metabolic alkalosis. There is no characteristic electrolyte pattern in a pheochromocytoma. An increase in urine free cortisol (choice **C**) and urine 17-ketosteroids (choice **D**) is present in Cushing syndrome. Cushing syndrome is associated with hypertension; however, the patient lacks the truncal obesity, abdominal stria, and thin extremities characteristic of hypercortisolism. An increase in urine 17-ketosteroids (dehydroepiandrosterone and androstenedione) in a woman produces hirsutism and possible virilization (hirsutism plus male secondary sex characteristics). These findings are not present in this patient.

31 **The answer is E**   *Medicine*

The patient has vitamin E toxicity (choice **E**). Warfarin acts as an anticoagulant by inhibiting epoxide reductase, which converts vitamin K into active vitamin K_1 in the liver. Loss of vitamin K activity leaves the patient anticoagulated, because the vitamin K-dependent coagulation factors II (prothrombin), VII, IX, and X are not γ-carboxylated, which is necessary for calcium binding of the factors in forming a fibrin clot. The international normalized ratio (INR) is a standardized way of reporting the prothrombin time when a patient is taking warfarin. Since the patient is taking the prescribed dose of warfarin, the most likely cause for prolongation of the INR is vitamin E toxicity resulting from the antioxidants he is taking. Most over-the-counter antioxidant preparations contain β-carotene (converted to vitamin A), vitamin C, and vitamin E. Toxic doses of vitamin E (over 1100 units) decrease the synthesis of the vitamin K-dependent factors in the liver, causing anticoagulation of the patient. This has a synergistic effect with warfarin and is most likely responsible for prolonging the INR ratio.

Aspirin (choice **A**) irreversibly inhibits platelet cyclooxygenase, causing decreased synthesis of thromboxane A_2, which prevents platelets from aggregating to form a platelet thrombus. This reduces the risk for developing a coronary artery thrombosis. Since platelet function is not evaluated with the INR or any other coagulation factor test, aspirin is not a cause of prolongation of the INR. β-Carotenes are precursors for retinol, which is converted in the cytosol of target cells into retinoic acid (vitamin A). Vitamin A excess (choice **B**) is associated with liver cell necrosis, which can prolong the prothrombin time. However, results of the liver function tests are normal, so vitamin A toxicity is unlikely. Water-soluble vitamin toxicity is uncommon, since the excess vitamin is easily excreted in the urine. Furthermore, thiamine (choice **C**) is not involved in reactions that influence coagulation factor synthesis or function. Vitamin C toxicity (choice **D**) is associated with diarrhea and the formation of renal stones. It does not interfere with coagulation factor function or synthesis.

32 **The answer is C** *Surgery*

Hepatocellular failure is most commonly caused by alcoholic cirrhosis and chronic active hepatitis. Hepatic encephalopathy, one of many complications associated with hepatocellular failure, is a potentially reversible metabolic disorder characterized by diffuse slowing of brain waves on an electroencephalogram (EEG), altered levels of consciousness, asterixis (a peculiar characteristic, also called flapping tremor, elicited when a patient holds the arms outstretched, leading to dorsiflexion of the wrists), and reversal of the day–night sleep rhythm. Possible causes include increased levels of abnormal neurotransmitters (octopamine, γ-aminobutyric acid [GABA]), reduced levels of branched-chain amino acids, increased levels of aromatic amino acids, and increased levels of serum ammonia. The laboratory data show metabolic alkalosis and abnormally high serum ammonia levels, indicating ammonium toxicity. The safest and most effective way of reducing serum ammonia levels is to reduce protein intake (choice C). This decreases the amount of protein available for bacteria to break down into absorbable ammonia (NH_3).

Lactulose (choice A) given orally is broken down by colonic bacteria, producing hydrogen ions (H^+). These bind with NH_3 to form ammonium (NH_4), which cannot be reabsorbed in the bowel mucosa and thus is of value for the short-term management of ammonia toxicity. Neomycin (choice B) eliminates the bacteria that produce the ammonia and thus also reduces ammonia levels. It again may be used for short-term treatment but is not safe or effective when used long term. A loop diuretic (choice D) could potentially precipitate hepatic encephalopathy, because metabolic alkalosis and hypokalemia are common complications. Sodium bicarbonate (choice E) is sometimes used to treat metabolic acidosis and will make the metabolic alkalosis worse.

33 **The answer is A** *Obstetrics and Gynecology*

The case scenario describes vaginal passage of grapelike vesicles, which are the markedly hydropic avascular villi found with a complete mole. Most hydatidiform moles are "complete," and have a 46,XX karyotype (choice A). All molar chromosomes have paternal origin. Most complete moles arise from an anuclear ovum that is fertilized by a haploid sperm, which then duplicates its own chromosomes.

About 10% of complete moles have a 46 XY chromosomal pattern (choice C). This karyotype arises from fertilization of an anuclear ovum by two spermatozoa. While the chromosomes in the complete mole are entirely of paternal origin, the mitochondrial deoxyribonucleic acid (DNA) is of maternal origin. A 45 X karyotype (choice D) is characteristic of gonadal dysgenesis, with the X chromosome maternally derived; the opposite of molar pregnancy. "Incomplete," or partial, moles often present with a coexistent fetus and have triploid karyotypes, most commonly 69 XXY (choice E) and less commonly 69 XXX (choice B).

34 **The answer is C** *Surgery*

The patient has acute pancreatitis. Approximately 70% of cases are related to alcohol abuse or biliary tract disease. Other causes include metabolic conditions (hypertriglyceridemia, uremia, and hypercalcemia), drugs (azathioprine, sulfasalazine, corticosteroids, thiazides, l-asparaginase, sulfonamides, and estrogen preparations), a penetrating posterior duodenal ulcer, and infection (usually viral—e.g., coxsackie, mumps). Patients present with an acute onset of midepigastric pain that is described as steady and boring. The pain radiates into the back or periumbilical area. Leaning forward often relieves the pain, whereas vomiting aggravates it. Physical examination reveals abdominal tenderness without guarding or rebound. Diminished bowel sounds result from a localized ileus, which corresponds to a dilated sentinel loop on an x-ray film. Low-grade fever is present in 70 to 85% of patients. Shock resulting from loss of isotonic fluid from the peripancreatic third space is present in 20 to 40% of patients. Turner's sign (purplish discoloration of the flank) and Cullen's sign (purplish discoloration around the umbilicus) indicate a hemorrhagic pancreatitis. A left-sided pleural effusion rich in amylase is noted in 10% of patients. The serum amylase (choice C) is elevated in 95% of acute attacks during the first 12 to 24 hours. It increases within 2 to 6 hours after the onset of pain, peaks within 12 to 30 hours, and declines after 2 to 4 days as the glomerular filtration rate (GFR) increases and clears the enzyme. A urine amylase test is most useful when the serum amylase is normal after 2 to 4 days, because it remains elevated for 7 to 10 days after the onset of pain. A serum lipase test (also choice C) is slightly more sensitive and specific than an amylase assay. Ultrasonography is also an excellent screen for pancreatitis. Stippled calcification in the pancreas results from enzymatic fat necrosis. Abdominal radiography reveals a localized ileus (sentinel loop) in the small bowel next to the pancreas.

An upper gastrointestinal series (choice **A**), HIDA nuclear scans (choice **E**), oral cholecystogram (choice **D**), and endoscopy (choice **B**) are not usually part of the workup of acute pancreatitis.

35 The answer is A   *Preventive Medicine and Public Health*

The question relates to assessing the statistic validity of differences in a continuous variable, which in this question are Apgar scores between two groups, babies born vaginally and those born by cesarean delivery. Statistically, comparison of continuous variable data between two groups can best be assessed by the student's *t*-test (choice **A**), which, by the way, is named after a Dr. Student.

If the comparison were between two groups with a categorical variable, a chi-squared test (choice **D**) would be correct. If the comparison were among three groups with a continuous variable, analysis of variance (choice **B**) would be correct. A correlation coefficient (choice **C**) assesses the strength of association, not differences between groups. Logistic regression (choice **E**) is used to assess a categorical outcome for a continuous predictor.

36 The answer is C   *Obstetrics and Gynecology*

The clear fluid leaking through the patient's vagina is probably urine. The history of painless, continuous vaginal leakage of urine with a recent pelvic surgery suggests the diagnosis of a fistula between the vagina and the urinary tract. Fistulas between the urinary tract and reproductive tract occur more frequently after radical pelvic surgery or pelvic radiation therapy. Intravenous (IV) indigo carmine (choice **C**), which is excreted in the urine and discolors a vaginal pack, is the diagnostic modality of choice.

The other choices contribute nothing toward ruling out a fistula. Cystometry (choice **A**) assesses bladder pressure–volume relationships. Urine culture (choice **B**) identifies a urinary tract infection. Pelvic sonography (choice **D**) looks for pelvic masses. Urethral pressure measurements (choice **E**) are helpful in working up genuine stress incontinence.

37 The answer is A   *Surgery*

The patient has Leriche's syndrome (choice **A**). This is due to aortoiliac atherosclerotic disease and is characterized by claudication on walking, atrophy of the calf muscles, diminished or absent femoral pulses, and impotence from involvement of the hypogastric arteries.

A herniated lumbar disk (choice **B**) would not have a claudication history or problems with femoral pulses. Motor and sensory deficits would be present as well. Osteoarthritis in the hip (choice **C**) produces pain that is relieved by the use of a cane. It is not associated with vascular findings including impotence. Phlegmasia alba dolens (choice **D**) is a variant of femoral vein thrombosis in which there is femoral artery spasm, which produces a pale, cool leg with increased pulses. A peripheral neuropathy (choice **E**) has both sensory and motor abnormalities. It does not disappear with rest.

38 The answer is F   *Obstetrics and Gynecology*

Rubella is a highly contagious viral syndrome with potentially disastrous pregnancy impact. With the presence of rubella antibodies, there is lifelong immunity, and a fetus in a subsequent pregnancy is protected. Without antibodies present, as in this scenario, the fetus is susceptible. First trimester infections are particularly hazardous for the fetus. At this time the best course of action is (choice **F**) to provide gamma globulin for prophylaxis now and recommend that she avoid exposure to rubella if possible. However, the best course of action would have been checking her rubella titer before she got pregnant and then avoiding pregnancy for 1 month after vaccination with the attenuated but live virus (choice **D**). However this obviously is impossible at this time since she has been pregnant for some 12 weeks.

Gamma globulin (choice **A**) is not helpful to prevent infection after exposure. Because the vaccine is a live virus, it is inappropriate to administer it to a pregnant woman (choice **B**). Breast-feeding is not contraindicated after maternal vaccination (choice **C**). Amniocentesis offers no benefit to offset the risk in a noninfected gravida (choice **E**).

39 The answer is A   *Psychiatry*

Isolation (choice **A**) describes the separation of a thought from its attached emotional tone, thereby making it tolerable. This defense mechanism is often used during highly stressful events. Depersonalization (choice **B**) and derealization (choice **E**) are other defenses that involve dissociation of mental functions, but both are more often accompanied by anxiety. Disorientation (choice **C**) and intellectualization (choice **D**) are not accompanied by odd calmness.

40 The answer is A   *Pediatrics*

This patient ingested prenatal vitamins (i.e., iron), which is one of the most common causes of childhood poisoning, often causing death. The antidote for iron poisoning is deferoxamine mesylate (answer **A**) and should be administered regardless of the serum iron level if the patient has moderate-to-severe symptoms (e.g., bloody diarrhea, hypotension, drowsiness) or if the patient's serum iron level exceeds 500 μg/dL, whether symptoms are present or not.

41 The answer is G   *Pediatrics*

This patient most likely received fentanyl, a synthetic opioid. Rapid IV administration can lead to a rigid chest wall and difficulty breathing. This effect may be reversed with naloxone hydrochloride (answer **G**) or may require a depolarizing muscle relaxant and intubation.

42 The answer is E   *Pediatrics*

This patient took isoniazid (INH). Initial manifestations may include nausea and vomiting, ataxia, tachycardia, mydriasis, and CNS depression, which may mimic an anticholinergic toxidrome. Acute INH overdose is associated with a triad consisting of: seizures that are refractory to conventional therapy, severe metabolic acidosis, and coma.

When the diagnosis of INH overdose is established, or at the time it is strongly suspected, pyridoxine (vitamin B_6) (answer **E**) should be administered. INH is metabolized to hydrazines that in overdose cause a functional pyridoxine (vitamin B_6) deficiency. This occurs by inhibition of pyridoxine phosphokinase, the enzyme that converts pyridoxine to active B_6. Activated B_6 is required by glutamic acid decarboxylase to convert glutamic acid to γ-amino butyric acid (GABA), an inhibitory neurotransmitter. Decreased levels of GABA are thought to lead to seizures. Administration of pyridine alleviates seizures and may reverse coma and lactic acidosis.

43 The answer is D   *Pediatrics*

The fluorescence of the urine with a Wood's lamp confirms that the patient did ingest the radiator fluid, or ethylene glycol. Many commercial antifreeze products have sodium fluorescein as an additive. Sodium fluorescein is renally excreted up to 6 hours after ingestion and may be detected when illuminated with a Wood lamp. Fomepizole (answer **D**) is an effective competitive antagonist of alcohol dehydrogenase inhibiting metabolism of ethylene glycol to toxic products. Its ease of dosing and lack of side effects are the major advantages of using fomepizole rather than ethanol. However, if not available ethanol can still be used as an antidote. Both fomepizole and ethanol can also be used as an antidote for methanol poisoning.

44 The answer is F   *Pediatrics*

This patient has methemoglobinemia, a blood disorder caused when nitrite interacts with the hemoglobin of the red blood cells. The nitrite can come from nitrate in drinking water, or from food (e.g., bacon, hot dogs), from some drugs, or from other sources. Blood samples appear chocolate brown and do not turn pink when exposed to air. A methemoglobin level can confirm the diagnosis. Methemoglobin can accumulate in red cells for three reasons: (1) a dominantly inherited abnormality in hemoglobin that prevents the reduction of methemoglobin to hemoglobin; (2) a recessively inherited deficiency in the enzyme methemoglobin reductase; or (3) exposure to hemoglobin-oxidizing chemicals or drugs, such as nitrates or nitrites contained in water and in some vegetables (such as carrots, spinach, zucchini, cauliflower, red beets), Xylocaine, or benzene derivatives. Infant methemoglobinemia, or blue baby syndrome, can be found in infants less than 6 months of age who are susceptible to methemoglobinemia because they have smaller amounts of the enzyme, NADH-cytochrome b_5 reductase, which converts methemoglobin back to hemoglobin. Nitrates in drinking water have been reported to be a primary cause of infantile methemoglobinemia. However, there have been reports of infantile methemoglobinemia in infants who became ill after being fed formula that was reconstituted with vegetable soup and nitrate-free water. The antidote for methemoglobinemia is methylene blue (answer **F**).

45 **The answer is J** *Pediatrics*

This patient has advanced digoxin toxicity and should receive purified digoxin-specific Fab antibody fragments (answer **J**) for rapid reversal. This antidote should be used for life-threatening digoxin toxicity and is indicated for life-threatening tachyarrhythmias, sinus bradyarrhythmias, severe AV blocks unresponsive to conventional therapy, and patients with serum potassium levels above 5 mEq/mL.

46 **The answer is C** *Pediatrics*

The patient has carbon monoxide poisoning as a result of indoor burning of charcoal briquettes. There are many reported cases of carbon monoxide poisoning secondary to indoor burning of charcoal briquettes for the purpose of either home heating or cooking. Most of these cases occur in the months of October through January, commonly during power outages or when electricity was intentionally disconnected.

Carbon monoxide toxicity occurs by (1) displacing oxygen (it has an affinity for hemoglobin 250 times that of oxygen), (2) impairing the ability of hemoglobin to release oxygen, and (3) impeding oxygen use by binding cytochrome oxidase in tissues. These mechanisms cause tissue hypoxia. The antidote for carbon monoxide poisoning is 100% oxygen (answer **C**) via non-re-breather or hyperbaric oxygen in severely poisoned patients. Early symptoms are nonspecific and can be confused with the flu, while higher concentrations can cause seizures, coma, respiratory instability, and death. Delayed therapy may cause permanent neurologic sequelae.

47 **The answer is H** *Pediatrics*

Acetaminophen overdose causes hepatic toxicity. Acetaminophen is rapidly absorbed from the gastrointestinal tract, with peak plasma levels usually occurring by 4 hours. Once absorbed, acetaminophen is metabolized by the liver by glucuronidation (60%) or sulfation (30%), and a small amount (4–7%) is excreted unchanged in the urine. Approximately 4% of the ingested dose is metabolized by a hepatic cytochrome P450 mixed-function oxidase to an active toxic intermediate metabolite (NAPQI), which is normally detoxified by conjugation with glutathione. In cases of overdose, glutathione is rapidly depleted, and free unconjugated NAPQI can produce a centrilobular hepatic necrosis, which may progress to fulminant hepatic failure. There are four clinical stages of acetaminophen poisoning:

Stage 1 occurs between 12 and 24 hours and is manifested by nausea, anorexia, vomiting, and diaphoresis.
Stage 2 occurs between 24 and 48 hours and is characterized by resolution of above, right upper quadrant pain, and elevation of transaminases and the prothrombin time (PT). There may also be oliguria.
Stage 3 occurs at 72 to 96 hours, and it is during this time that peak liver function abnormalities are seen, and nausea and vomiting may return.
Stage 4 occurs at 4 days to 2 weeks and there is either resolution of hepatic dysfunction or complete liver failure.

Although charcoal reduces the level of acetaminophen it will still be in the toxic range and *N*-acetylcysteine (answer **H**) is the antidote for acetaminophen toxicity, and indications for *N*-acetylcysteine include (1) toxic level on the Rumack-Matthew nomogram (a plot of the log of acetaminophen concentration versus hours after ingestion [a toxic level is one greater than the reference line]); (2) an ingested dose greater than 140 mg/kg with no level available within 8 hours; (3) elevated liver function test results with a history of acetaminophen poisoning; and (4) acetaminophen-induced hepatic injury.

INCORRECT CHOICES

Atropine (answer **B**) and pralidoxime (answer **I**) are antidotes used for organophosphate poisoning. Atropine is given for the muscarinic effects (SLUDGE) salivation, lacrimation, urination, defecation, gastrointestinal problems (abdominal pain and diarrhea), and emesis. Pralidoxime is administered for the nicotinic effects such as muscle weakness and fasciculations.

48 **The answer is B** *Medicine*

The patient has typhoid fever due to *Salmonella typhi* (choice **B**). In general, *Salmonella* species have animal reservoirs that carry the organisms in nature (e.g., poultry [common], turtles, iguanas, and domestic livestock).

Transmission to humans is by the fecal–oral route. *S. paratyphi* is associated with septicemia (e.g., osteomyelitis in sickle cell disease). *S. choleraesuis* produces septicemia and metastatic abscesses. *S. enteritidis* causes enterocolitis and food poisoning; it does not have a septicemic phase.

S. typhi is transmitted to humans by the fecal–oral route or contact with an asymptomatic chronic carrier. Humans are the reservoir for the disease. In the initial infection, bacteria enter macrophages in Peyer's patches in the first 24 hours. The first week is characterized by a bacteremic phase with sustained high fever, as in this patient. The blood culture is positive. The second week is associated with a faint, erythematous rash on the upper anterior trunk called a "rose spot" (10% of cases). Diarrhea or constipation is usually present in 30–50% of cases. There is a positive stool culture. There is a classic triad of hepatosplenomegaly, sinus bradycardia, and absolute neutropenia, which is evident in this patient. The third week is noteworthy for a potential for bowel perforation. The fourth week is characterized by resolution of the disease or development of the chronic carrier state, which usually involves proliferation of organisms in the gallbladder. The treatment of choice is a fluoroquinolone or ceftriaxone. Preventive measures include vaccination and food precautions. A cholecystectomy may be necessary in the chronic carrier state.

49 The answer is F   *Medicine*

The patient has weight loss and anorexia due to a gastric adenocarcinoma with metastasis to both ovaries (Krukenberg tumors). She has a long history of epigastric pain that is aggravated by food. This is compatible with peptic ulcer disease, the most common cause of which is *Helicobacter pylori* (choice F). The organism is a gram-negative curved rod that colonizes the pylorus and antrum of the stomach. It is present in the mucous layer and does not invade into the gastric mucosa. The organism produces urease (converts urea into ammonia), mucolytic proteases, and cytotoxins, all of which destroy the bicarbonate-rich mucous layer causing chronic atrophic gastritis and peptic ulcer disease (duodenal ulcers > gastric ulcers). Intestinal metaplasia (i.e., goblet cells, Paneth cells) develops as a reaction to injury. This is a precursor lesion for gastric adenocarcinoma (*H. pylori* is the most common risk factor). The inflammatory infiltrate in the stomach primarily consists of lymphocytes with prominent germinal follicles. This may be a precursor lesion for a low-grade B cell malignant lymphoma (*H. pylori* is the most common risk factor). Transmission of *H. pylori* to humans is by ingestion and from person to person. It is common in areas of poor sanitation. Many tests are available to identify *H. pylori*. The CLO-test is performed on tissue removed by endoscopy. It detects urease produced by *H. pylori*. Serologic tests are highly sensitive and specific; however, results remain positive over an extended period, which limits their usefulness for detection of recurrences. In the radiolabeled urea breath test, ^{14}C-urea is swallowed, and urease releases radioactive ammonia, which is detected in the breath. It is an excellent test, but it is expensive. Many treatment regimens are available for *H. pylori*. One treatment modality uses omeprazole (proton blocker) plus amoxicillin plus clarithromycin (efficacy, 80–95%). Another regimen is bismuth plus omeprazole plus tetracycline plus metronidazole (efficacy, 90–99%). Since *H. pylori* is the most common cause of gastric adenocarcinoma and B cell lymphomas in the stomach, treatment of *H. pylori* infections reduces the risk for developing these cancers.

50 The answer is E   *Medicine*

The patient has enterocolitis due to *Campylobacter jejuni* (choice E), which is a gram-negative curved or S-shaped rod. It is the most common cause of invasive enterocolitis in the United States. Animal reservoirs for the bacteria include cattle, chicken, and puppies (common source for children). Transmission to humans is via contaminated water, poultry, and unpasteurized milk. The organism invades the jejunum, ileum, and colon and produces a secretory and invasive diarrhea. Crypt abscesses and ulcers resemble ulcerative colitis. There is bloody diarrhea with leukocytes (fecal smear of stool is positive for leukocytes), and organisms are readily identified in stool with Gram's stain. Complications include Guillain-Barré syndrome (ascending paralysis), hemolytic uremic syndrome, and HLA-B27–positive seronegative spondyloarthropathy. The treatment of choice is erythromycin.

INCORRECT CHOICES

Escherichia coli (choice A) is the most common cause of upper and lower urinary tract infections, nosocomial septicemia (usually from an indwelling urinary catheter), spontaneous peritonitis in cirrhotics with ascites, traveler's diarrhea (enterotoxigenic strain that stimulates guanylate cyclase), hemolytic uremic syndrome (cytotoxic serotoxin produced by O157:H7 serotype *E. coli*), acute cholecystitis, and acute appendicitis. It is a common cause of nosocomial pneumonia, neonatal meningitis, and otitis media in infants less than 2 months old. It can be treated with amoxicillin clavulanate.

Klebsiella pneumoniae (choice **C**) is a fat gram-negative rod surrounded by capsule. It is the most common cause of pneumonia in nursing homes and is a common cause of lobar pneumonia in alcoholics and of upper and lower urinary tract infections. The treatment of choice is fluoroquinolones.

Yersinia enterocolitica (choice **D**) is a gram-negative coccobacillus that produces mesenteric lymphadenitis in children that simulates acute appendicitis, septicemia in iron-overload disorders (e.g., hemochromatosis), and septicemia in contaminated blood transfusions. It is one of the pathogens associated with HLA-B27–positive seronegative spondyloarthropathy.

Pseudomonas aeruginosa (choice **G**) is a green-pigment-producing gram-negative rod. It is a water-loving bacterium that is the most common contaminant in respirators that are used in hospitals. It is the most common cause of nosocomial pneumonia in intensive care patients (respirators), hot tube folliculitis, malignant external otitis in diabetics, ecthyma gangrenosum (often seen in ulcerative colitis patients), and osteomyelitis due to puncture wounds through rubber footwear. It is the most common cause of death in patients with third-degree burns and in cystic fibrosis patients. It is a common cause of purulent conjunctivitis in lens wearers, septicemia in immunocompromised hosts, and urinary tract infections. Infections are treated with antipseudomonal aminoglycosides.

Questions

Single Best Choice Directions: This section consists of numbered statements or questions followed by a list of potential answers; you are to select the ONE best answer.

1 A 68-year-old man presents at the emergency department because of such severe abdominal pain that he "just could not stand it any longer." He tells the triage nurse that he hadn't been feeling well for the past couple of months, primarily because he had been having abdominal pain about 30 minutes after eating and as a consequence lost almost 10 lb, but last night he suddenly developed "a stomachache from hell." He also has been vomiting and has had several episodes of bloody diarrhea. Upon physical examination the physician confirms the abdominal pain and notices abdominal distention. However, bowel sounds are absent, and there is no rebound tenderness present or other relevant findings upon abdominal examination. Laboratory data reveal an absolute neutrophilic leukocytosis and left shift plus lactic acidosis, hypotension, and elevation of the serum amylase level. Which of the following is the most likely diagnosis?

(A) Acute ulcerative colitis
(B) Hemorrhagic pancreatitis
(C) Aortoenteric fistula
(D) Acute small bowel infarction
(E) Toxic megacolon

2 Soon after birth, a term newborn is noted to be cyanotic with feeding. The infant was born to a 24-year-old primigravida who had excellent prenatal care. There is no history of tobacco, alcohol, or use of illicit drugs. Review of the mother's medical record shows that results of all diagnostic studies for sexually transmitted diseases have been negative. The delivery was uncomplicated. The infant weighed 6 lb 13 oz, and Apgar scores at 1 and 5 minutes were 8 and 9, respectively. Examination of the newborn reveals that crying relieves the cyanosis. Which of the following is the most likely diagnosis?

(A) A tracheoesophageal fistula
(B) Bronchopulmonary dysplasia
(C) Respiratory distress syndrome
(D) Choanal atresia
(E) A patent ductus arteriosus

3 A 54-year-old man presents to his physician for a physical examination. He is 5 ft 11 in tall and weighs 229 lb (body mass index [BMI] 33 kg/m²). His blood pressure is 165/80, pulse is 75 beats/min and regular. Otherwise, results of his physical examination are unremarkable. He was asked to have a fasting blood sample taken for a lipid profile. The next week the following data are reported: total cholesterol, 225 mg/dL; triglyceride level, 200 mg/dL; low-density lipoprotein, 145 mg/dL; and high-density lipoprotein, 40 mg/dL. Because his BMI defines him as being class I obese and because his total cholesterol is borderline high, the physician puts him on a diet and prescribes a cholesterol-lowering medication. Since starting the medication the patient experienced problems with constipation and a bloating sensation that is relieved by increasing dietary fiber. Which of the following metabolic alterations is expected from the drug he is taking?

(A) Decreased activity of hydroxymethylglutaryl (HMG)-CoA reductase
(B) Decreased synthesis of triglyceride in hepatocytes
(C) Increased activity of capillary lipoprotein lipase
(D) Increased excretion of free cholesterol in feces
(E) Increased synthesis of hepatocyte low-density-lipoprotein receptors

4 A 62-year-old woman suffers a myocardial infarct (MI) while being examined in her physician's office. He attempts cardiopulmonary resuscitation, administers oxygen, and a bolus of epinephrine, all to no avail. The woman dies. Her family files a malpractice suit. For this claim to have merit, which of the following must the family prove about the doctor?

(A) He was improperly educated.
(B) He intended to cause the patient harm.
(C) He committed a crime.
(D) He overcharged the patient for the care given.
(E) He deviated from the established standard of care.

5 A 48-year-old obese woman was admitted to the hospital with upper-right-quadrant pain and vomiting. She had no diarrhea or constipation. Clinical examination revealed tenderness in the right upper quadrant, and appropriate investigations demonstrated the presence of a stone in the common bile duct. Attempts to dislodge the stone endoscopically proved futile, so she underwent common bile duct exploration. Six days after surgery she developed a temperature of 38°C (101°F). Which of the following is the most likely cause of her fever?

(A) Resorption of blood from the peritoneum
(B) Endotoxic shock
(C) Atelectasis
(D) A wound infection
(E) Renal failure

6 A 6-month-old African-American girl presents with low-grade fever and acute onset of painful swelling of the hands and feet. Radiographs taken at the onset of symptoms reveal soft tissue swelling. A peripheral blood smear was made and is illustrated below. The findings described for this infant most likely correlate with which of the following events?

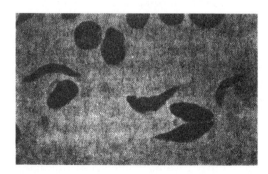

(A) A hemolytic crisis induced by an aberrant glucose-6-phosphate dehydrogenase (G6PD)
(B) Infection of the digital bones by salmonella
(C) Replacement of fetal hemoglobin (Hb F) with Hb A
(D) A coxsackievirus infection
(E) Lymphedema of the hands and feet caused by the deletion of a chromosome

7 A 3-year-old girl with autistic disorder has a buccal smear for chromosomal analysis. Her 14-year-old brother is retarded, with an unusually narrow face, a prominent forehead, large protruding ears, a prominent jaw, unusually large testes, and a high-pitched voice. The 55-year-old maternal grandfather of these children has had an inattention tremor for at least the past 5 years. With which of the following chromosomal abnormalities is the girl most likely afflicted?

(A) Cri du chat syndrome (deletion of short arm of chromosome 5)
(B) Fragile X syndrome
(C) Klinefelter syndrome (XXY)
(D) Down syndrome (trisomy 21)
(E) Turner syndrome (XO)

8 A 42-year-old man complains of headaches when he wakes up in the morning. He reveals that has had these headaches for maybe as long as a year, but they have been occurring more often and are getting progressively worse. He also feels as though he is losing his strength and that he sometimes has trouble placing his feet where he wants to without looking down at the ground. The physician observes him to have an unusually prominent jaw with spaces between the teeth, and large hands and feet. By asking him to press against his arm the physician confirms muscle weakness. Upon physical examination his blood pressure was found to be 135/95 mm Hg and his nonfasting blood glucose value was 195 mg/dL. Which of the following would be expected in this patient?

(A) Chest radiograph with normal-sized heart
(B) Normal-sized sella turcica
(C) Lack of suppression of glucose with an oral glucose challenge
(D) Decreased concentration of insulin-like growth factor-1
(E) Decreased serum growth hormone

9 During a routine examination, a 65-year-old woman complains to her gynecologist that she has not been sleeping well for the past 5 or 6 months because of a sensation of pressure and burning in the middle of her chest. Further questioning reveals that she also feels the pressure and burning intermittently during the day; however, it is not induced by exercise and is relieved by antacids. The patient's blood pressure is 135/82 mm Hg, her pulse is 96/min and regular, and her temperature is 37.0°C (98.6°F). Her heart sounds are normal, and her lungs are clear. Palpation of her abdomen reveals no abnormalities. Which of the following is the most appropriate first step in the management of this patient?

(A) Refer her to a psychologist

(B) Prescribe cisapride

(C) Prescribe ranitidine, cimetidine, nizatidine, or famotidine

(D) Order an electrocardiogram (EKG)

(E) Prescribe antibiotics to control gastric *Helicobacter pylori*

(F) Prescribe omeprazole, lansoprazole, rabeprazole, esomeprozole, or pantoprazole

10 A 25-year-old man was thrown to the ground in a motorcycle accident. The paramedics transported him to the nearest emergency department. The physician on duty notes bruising about the orbit and blood in the external auditory meatus. Clear fluid exudes from his ear. The physician suspects that it is cerebrospinal fluid (CSF). Chemical analysis of the fluid compared with that of serum would be expected to show which of the following?

(A) A higher protein concentration than serum

(B) A higher chloride concentration than serum

(C) A higher glucose concentration than serum

(D) More white blood cells (WBCs) in the CSF than in the serum

(E) Absence of prealbumin on CSF electrophoresis

11 A 4-year-old spent a week on vacation with his parents at a Lake Michigan beach. During this time he learned to swim and spent many hours swimming and playing in the water. He spent most of the night after returning home fussing and crying because of left ear pain. The following day his mother takes him to his pediatrician who finds his left ear canal to be edematous and erythematous, and it contains a greenish otorrhea. Pain is increased by manipulation of the pinna and pressure on the tragus. The tympanic membrane is normal in appearance and mobility. Which of the following is the most likely pathogen producing this patient's symptoms?

(A) *Haemophilus influenzae*

(B) *Pseudomonas aeruginosa*

(C) *Moraxella catarrhalis*

(D) *Streptococcus agalactiae*

(E) *Escherichia coli*

12 A grossly underweight 52-year-old woman with chronic malnutrition is due to undergo major surgery. It is decided to start total parenteral nutrition (TPN) as part of the initial therapy. While introducing a central venous catheter into the right subclavian vein, the patient develops sudden dyspnea. Which of the following is the most likely diagnosis?

(A) Air embolism

(B) Pulmonary embolism

(C) Fat embolism

(D) Acute anxiety

(E) Pneumothorax

13 A 56-year-old woman is taken to the emergency department with severe sunburn and dehydration. Her husband is in a similar condition. They explain that they have been living in their car in the desert for several weeks to elude a band of alien creatures disguised as humans. The husband has a history of one past psychiatric hospitalization 10 years ago with a diagnosis of delusional disorder. The wife has never been hospitalized. For the past 7 years, the couple has led an isolated existence, living in cheap motels for several months at a time before moving on. Mental status examination reveals a middle-aged woman who states that aliens have been pursuing her husband. Further questioning reveals that she has not actually seen the aliens herself, but that her husband frequently spots them. The woman's thought processes are otherwise logical, and there is no evidence of cognitive deficits. Which of the following is the most appropriate initial step in treatment for this woman?

(A) Behavioral psychotherapy

(B) Cognitive psychotherapy

(C) Conjoint psychotherapy

(D) Ziprasidone

(E) Separation from her husband

14 A mother brings her 7-year-old son to an emergency clinic because he has been vomiting and has had diarrhea for the past 3 days. Upon taking a history the attending physician determines that the emesis was nonbilious and nonbloody, and the diarrhea was nonbloody, loose, and watery. The patient states that he vomited more than 10 times, and the number of times for his diarrhea are too numerous to count. He is in the second grade and has had no ill contacts and no recent travel. There is no exposure to pets. On clinical examination the physician determines that the patient is dehydrated with a loss of less than 5% of his total body water (TBW). Which of the following choices represents the next best step in management of this patient?

(A) Give the patient a bolus of 20 mL/kg of isotonic crystalloid over 20 minutes.

(B) Give the patient no less than 60 mL/kg of isotonic crystalloid to restore perfusion.

(C) Give the patient maintenance fluids of 5% dextrose and 0.45 N saline to replace the fluid deficit and to accommodate on-going losses.

(D) Give the patient an antiemetic.

(E) Give the patient an antibiotic to treat the infectious process.

15. A 42-year-old man with a 4-month history of increasing occupational and marital stress fails to return home from work at his usual hour of 6:00 PM, causing his spouse to file a missing persons report the next day. Based on a license plate and physical description, police find him in a bar in a neighboring metropolitan area during the following evening, alert, and sitting without a drink. He says that he lost his wallet, is unsure of who he is, and can't remember how he got there. Which of the following is the most likely diagnosis?

(A) Psychosis due to a general medical condition

(B) Conversion disorder

(C) Dissociative fugue

(D) Major depressive disorder

(E) Delirium

16. A 23-year-old woman presents with crampy left-lower-quadrant pain, bloody diarrhea with mucus, and a history of tenesmus. Fecal culture reveals no contaminating organisms. The table below summarizes clinical findings.

Symptom/Sign	Patient	Normal
Bowel movements	5 to 6 per day	3 per week to 2 per day
Pulse beats per minute	<85	95
Hematocrit (percent)	31	35–45 (young adult female)
Weight loss in last 3 months	5%	0%
Temperature (°F)	100.0	98.6
Erythrocyte sedimentation rate	25 mm/h	<15 mm/h (female)
Albumin (g/dL)	3.2	3.4 to 4.7

Which of the following is the most likely diagnosis?

(A) Ulcerative colitis

(B) Crohn's disease

(C) An anal fissure

(D) Ischemic bowel disease

(E) Solitary ulcer syndrome

17. A 65-year-old man has moderately severe, drug-resistant diastolic hypertension that has been present for the past 5 years. Physical examination reveals hypertensive retinopathy, diminished pulses in both lower extremities, and a bruit in the epigastric area. A renal arteriogram shows narrowing of the left renal artery orifice. Radioisotope renography, after a dose of captopril, shows a small left kidney with decreased uptake and excretion of the isotope. Which of the following findings would be expected in this patient?

(A) Hypokalemia and metabolic acidosis

(B) A decrease in plasma renin activity over the baseline after taking captopril

(C) Decreased plasma aldosterone

(D) Decreased plasma renin activity from the right renal vein

(E) Fibromuscular hyperplasia of the left renal artery

18. A 72-year-old female is seen in the emergency department with a history of sudden, severe, colicky midabdominal pain and nausea and vomiting over the past 3 hours. During the examination, she vomits a bile-stained vomitus. Physical examination reveals generalized abdominal tenderness with diminished bowel sounds. Radiography of the abdomen shows a radiopaque mass in the distal small bowel on the right side, with dilated loops proximally. No free air is noted under the diaphragm, but air is present in the biliary tree. Which of the following is the most likely diagnosis?

(A) Lymphoma of the small bowel

(B) Acute pancreatitis

(C) Acute appendicitis with radiopaque fecalith

(D) Gallstone ileus

(E) Intussusception

19. For the past 6 months, a 55-year-old man with a 35-year history of smoking cigarettes has complained of persistent frontal headaches. For several days, he has had projectile vomiting and bilateral blurry vision. Physical examination shows bilateral papilledema. A magnetic resonance imaging (MRI) study shows a mass lesion involving the corpus callosum that has spread to both cerebral hemispheres. The patient dies a few days later of a transtentorial herniation. Which of the

following underlying conditions is the most likely cause of the lesion?

(A) Cerebral infarction
(B) Glioblastoma multiforme
(C) Intracerebral hemorrhage
(D) Medulloblastoma
(E) Metastatic lung carcinoma

20 An article concerning the relative ability of a new drug to lower systolic blood pressure describes a study in which age- and ethnicity-matched male patients are divided into three groups. One group receives a well-recognized drug at a standard dose. The other two groups receive the new drug, but at different doses. At the end of 30 days, the systolic blood pressure of each group was determined, and the significance of the differences in the mean values was tested statistically. Which of the following statistical tests would provide the greatest confidence in the results?

(A) Student's *t*-test
(B) Analysis of variance
(C) Correlation coefficient
(D) Chi-squared test
(E) Logistic regression

21 Psychiatric consultation is requested for a 51-year-old woman on a surgical ward undergoing postoperative treatment for a mesenteric infarction. The consultation request notes "altered mental status; rule out delirium versus schizophrenia." Which one of the following combinations is more typical of schizophrenia than of delirium?

(A) Social withdrawal and a family history of psychopathology
(B) Memory impairment and waxing and waning of symptoms within a period of hours
(C) Visual and auditory hallucinations
(D) A family history of psychopathology and waxing and waning of symptoms within a period of hours
(E) Social withdrawal and waxing and waning of symptoms within a period of hours

22 A 35-year-old man with sarcoidosis complains of excessive thirst and increased frequency of urination. He always carries a gallon jug of water around to quench his thirst. A magnetic resonance imaging (MRI) study of his brain reveals lesions in the medial hypothalamic area. Which of the following laboratory test results is expected if the patient is deprived of water?

(A) Decrease in plasma osmolality
(B) Increase in serum sodium

(C) Increase in urine osmolality (U_{Osm})
(D) No significant increase in U_{Osm} after injection of vasopressin

23 A 19-year-old quarterback for a community college football team was hit hard just above his left knee. Although bruised, there did not seem to be a serious injury. However, pain persisted during the following months, and the area began to swell. Physical examination disclosed that the swollen area was hard to the touch. An x-ray film revealed a lesion with the appearance of a sun ray. A biopsy specimen of the lesion examined histologically is illustrated below.

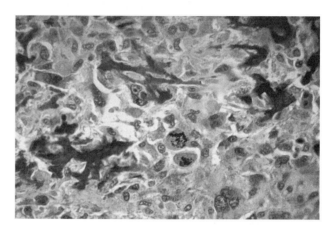

Which of the following is the most likely diagnosis?

(A) Ewing's sarcoma
(B) Legg-Calvé-Perthes disease
(C) Acute osteomyelitis
(D) A slipped capital femoral epiphysis
(E) Neurogenic arthropy
(F) Osteogenic sarcoma
(G) Osteitis deformans

24 A young lactating mother is found to have a red, hot, painful, inflamed right breast consistent with mastitis. In addition, she has a temperature of 38.4°C (101.1°F), headache, and nausea. Her physician prescribes rest, antibiotics, plenty of fluids, and cold packs for the affected breast. The patient is concerned about breast-feeding. Which of the following is the best advice that the physician can give to the patient?

(A) Stop breast-feeding immediately because the baby may become infected
(B) Stop breast-feeding immediately because she will be taking an antibiotic
(C) Continue breast-feeding using the left breast only
(D) Continue breast-feeding using both breasts
(E) Change the infant to a commercially prepared formula

25 A 28-year-old woman who works as a computer analyst in a large company and does not exercise at all is concerned about the possibility of developing a myocardial infarction. This stems from the fact that her oldest brother, who is 42 years old, has already undergone coronary bypass surgery, and her mother died at 50 years of age after an acute myocardial infarction. She denies a history of chest pains, palpitations, or shortness of breath. The patient does not smoke, does not consume alcohol, and does not take any regular medication. Physical examination reveals an obese woman who is 163 cm (64 in) tall and weighs 112 kg (247 lb). Her vital signs reveal the following: heart rate, 92 beats/min; respirations, 18/min; blood pressure, 125/90 mm Hg. A serum lipid panel yields the following values: total cholesterol, 250 mg/dL (normal, <200 mg/dL); high-density lipoprotein (HDL), 32 mg/dL (normal >60mg/dL); low-density lipoprotein (LDL) (normal, <130 mg/dL), triglyceride (TG), 185 mg/dL (normal, <150 mg/dL); and very-low-density lipoprotein (VLDL), 260 mg/dL (normal <125 mg/dL). Based on this information, which of the following is the best step in the management of this patient?

(A) Start her immediately on 3-hydroxy-3-methyl-glutaryl-coenzyme A (HMG-CoA) reductase inhibitors

(B) Start her on bile acid sequestrants and exercise

(C) Commence a diet for 6 months and exercise

(D) Start her on the American Heart Association step 2 diet and exercise

(E) Commence a combination of niacin, exercise, and diet

26 A 14-year-old girl complains bitterly that her mother intrudes into every aspect of her life and tries to control her. The mother admits that she closely monitors her daughter and sets many rules. The father has largely withdrawn from trying to control her behavior and is deeply involved in his work. The child has recently withdrawn from family interaction, refusing to speak to her parents or spend mealtimes with them. The mother has redoubled her efforts to maintain control. The cause of which one of the following disorders is most often ascribed to family dynamics similar to that described?

(A) Anorexia nervosa

(B) Dissociative identity disorder

(C) Narcissistic personality disorder

(D) Schizophrenia

(E) Separation anxiety disorder

27 A 65-year-old woman develops compression fractures of the vertebrae in the spinal column. Radiography of the spine shows generalized osteopenia and narrowing of the disk spaces. The serum calcium and phosphorus levels are normal. Which of the following most accurately describes the underlying pathogenesis responsible for this patient's radiographic findings?

(A) Vitamin D deficiency

(B) Increased secretion of parathyroid hormone-related peptide

(C) Imbalance between osteoclastic and osteoblastic activity

(D) Secretion of osteoclast activating factor by macrophages

(E) Increased secretion of parathyroid hormone

28 A 23-year-old woman has tearing and moderate pain in her left eye. Her pupillary light reflex is normal. She recently was placed on topical corticosteroids for suspected allergic conjunctivitis. A Gram's stain and Giemsa stain are negative for organisms. A fluorescein stain of the eye exhibits a shallow ulcer with a dendritic appearance and irregular borders. Which of the following topical treatments would be most appropriate?

(A) Ketoconazole

(B) Trifluridine

(C) Phenylephrine

(D) Erythromycin

(E) Sulfacetamide

29 A 30-year-old woman with a history of intravenous drug abuse died of complications related to septicemia. She had a history of fever and erythematous, painful lesions on the pads of several fingers; splinter hemorrhages under several fingernails; and a pansystolic murmur and third and fourth heart sounds that increased in intensity on inspiration. The liver was enlarged and pulsatile. Which of the following valvular disorders and pathogens most likely caused this patient's death?

(A) Aortic regurgitation and *Staphylococcus aureus*

(B) Mitral regurgitation and viridans streptococci

(C) Mitral stenosis and viridans streptococci

(D) Tricuspid regurgitation and *Staphylococcus aureus*

(E) Tricuspid regurgitation and *Staphylococcus epidermidis*

30 A 64-year-old widow with substantial savings develops Alzheimer's disease. She has a 36-year-old son who still lives at home and is looking forward to a substantial inheritance. His mother is beginning to require around-the-clock supervision; consequently, the son started to look into residential care options. He was appalled by the cost, but a friend told him not to worry because at her age Medicaid will pick up the tab. Which of the following statements about her potential use of the federal Medicare or Medicaid program to finance her care is most accurate?

(A) Medicaid will not cover the cost of her medications.

(B) Medicaid will not pay for her residential care.

(C) She will become eligible for Medicaid only if she has contributed to the program through federal withholding of her wages.

(D) She will become eligible for Medicaid only upon turning 65.

(E) She will become eligible for Medicaid only if impoverished.

(F) In another year Medicare will pay the cost of residential care.

31 A 32-year-old man with a long history of substance abuse blames his parents for his inability to live without drugs. He insists that he obviously inherited his addictions from them. On this basis, he rejects any discussion about how changing the way he relates to others might decrease his drug cravings. While the man's conclusions about treatment may be wrong, for which of the following drugs is his surmise of heritability dependency best supported by clinical evidence?

(A) Opiate

(B) Cocaine

(C) Heroin

(D) Tobacco

(E) Benzodiazepine

(F) Alcohol

(G) Psychostimulant

32 A girl is repeatedly sexually molested from age 7 through age 14 by her father, who warns her never to tell anyone or she will be killed. Although it seems hard to understand why she was not at least suspicious, the mother claims she never had an inkling that this type of deviant behavior was going on in her household. Which of the following has been most commonly suggested as a sequel to this situation?

(A) Dependent personality disorder

(B) Autistic disorder

(C) Dissociative identity disorder

(D) Hypochondriasis

(E) Major depressive disorder

33 A 35-year-old fireman was badly burned when the roof of a house collapsed on him. He had second-degree burns involving 15% of his body surface and third-degree burns involving 20% of his body surface.

He was rushed to the nearest emergency department and then transferred to a burn unit. A week later he develops fever, and black patches are noted in the burn wounds. Biopsy and culture of one of the wound sites would most likely reveal which of the following organisms?

(A) *Staphylococcus aureus*

(B) *Pseudomonas aeruginosa*

(C) *Candida albicans*

(D) Group A streptococcus

(E) *Streptococcus pneumoniae*

34 A 47-year-old man is described by coworkers as being intensely competitive, driven, hostile, distrustful, excitable, and anxious. The man complains of being tense, easily bored, and unhappy. Mental status examination reveals increased psychomotor activity with many quick shifts of posture, pressured speech, and irritability. According to psychosomatic theory, which of the following disorders is most likely to occur in such a person?

(A) Cancer

(B) Coronary artery disease (CAD)

(C) Emphysema

(D) Migraine

(E) Peptic ulcer disease

35 A 50-year-old man with a 20-year history of alcohol abuse presents to his family doctor with a complaint of diminished taste and smell. Physical examination reveals an acneiform rash across his face, head, and neck. In addition, there is poor healing of a skin incision site on the back of his right hand, where a squamous cell carcinoma was excised 2 weeks ago. Which of the trace metals is most likely deficient?

(A) Chromium

(B) Copper

(C) Fluoride

(D) Selenium

(E) Zinc

36 A 30-year-old woman complains of colicky abdominal pain and vomiting. She has had multiple laparoscopic surgeries for endometriosis. A plain abdominal radiograph is taken of the patient in an erect position and shows multiple air–fluid levels with a stepladder configuration. Which of the following is the most likely cause of the abdominal pain?

(A) Direct inguinal hernia

(B) Intussusception

(C) Large bowel infarction

(D) Small bowel adhesions

(E) Volvulus

37 A 70-year-old man with chronic back pain develops urinary retention as a result of prostate hyperplasia. A transurethral resection is performed to relieve the obstruction. Shortly after the procedure, there is profuse bleeding from the penis. Coagulation studies show a partial thromboplastin time (activated, APTT) of 30 seconds (25–40 seconds is normal), a prothrombin time (PT) of 14 seconds (11–15 seconds is normal), a bleeding time >15 minutes (normal is 3–7 min), and a platelet count of 350,000/mm³ (normal range is 150,000–400,000/mm³). The d-dimer assay is negative. Which of the following is most likely responsible for the bleeding disorder?

(A) Antiphospholipid antibodies
(B) Circulating anticoagulant
(C) Coagulation factor deficiency
(D) Platelet function disorder
(E) Primary fibrinolytic disorder

38 A 45-year-old man states that when he defecates, a painless mass protrudes from the anus that reduces spontaneously. Occasionally, there is bright red blood on the toilet paper or in the toilet bowl and a mucoid perianal discharge that often soils his underwear. Which of the following is the most likely diagnosis?

(A) Internal hemorrhoids
(B) Angiodysplasia
(C) Colorectal cancer
(D) Anal fissure
(E) Ischemic colitis

39 A 55-year-old woman had a modified radical mastectomy 10 years ago. She now has pain in the pelvic girdle and point tenderness over the lower lumbar vertebra. A complete blood cell count shows a normocytic anemia, an increased total WBC count, and a normal platelet count. The peripheral blood shows nucleated red blood cells and immature WBCs, including metamyelocytes and myelocytes. No myeloblasts are present. Which of the following is the most likely diagnosis?

(A) Acute myelogenous leukemia
(B) Chronic myeloproliferative disorder
(C) Leukemoid reaction
(D) Malignant plasma cell disorder
(E) Metastatic disease to the bone marrow

40 A 23-year-old woman with an 18-year history of insulin-dependent diabetes is brought to the emergency department by her date who became alarmed by her acute mental confusion and sudden-onset bizarre behavior. He explains that they spent the day at the beach where she had been very active playing volley ball and swimming and that they missed lunch but were on their way to eat dinner when this sudden change in behavior occurred. He states over and over again that they had not been using drugs or drinking alcohol. The triage nurse notes perspiration, increased salivation, restlessness, and tachycardia. Which of the following is the most appropriate next step in the management of this patient?

(A) Order a complete blood count (CBC)
(B) Order an immediate blood glucose analysis
(C) Order serum electrolytes analysis
(D) Order an immediate drug screen
(E) Order arterial blood gases (ABGs) analysis

Directions for Matching Questions (41 through 50): Each set of matching questions is preceded by a list of 4 to 26 lettered options followed by a brief explanation of the required task and then by a series of numbered statements. For each lettered statement you are to select ONE lettered option that best fulfills the task as it relates to that statement. Remember each of the listed options might be correctly selected once, more than once, or not at all.

Questions 41–50 (Obstetrics and Gynecology)

(A) Ectopic pregnancy
(B) Vaginal foreign body
(C) Endometrial carcinoma
(D) Submucous leiomyoma
(E) Molar pregnancy
(F) Cervical carcinoma
(G) Simple hyperplasia without atypia
(H) Sarcoma botryoides
(I) Uterine adenomyosis
(J) Ovarian carcinoma

For each of the numbered questions below (41 to 50) select the ONE lettered condition above to which it relates best.

41 A 3-year-old girl who has been experiencing vaginal bleeding is brought for evaluation by her worried mother. The girl's medical history is unremarkable with normal physical growth and appropriate developmental landmarks. She has had all the recommended immunizations. On visual examination of the perineum bleeding, multiple cystic masses resembling grapes are seen at the introitus.

42 A 32-year-old multiparous woman complains of intermittent vaginal bleeding between normal menstrual periods over the past 6 months. The bleeding is painless and is not associated with cramping. She denies postcoital bleeding. Her last Pap smear, 6 months ago, was negative for dysplasia or malignancy. She underwent a tubal sterilization after her last pregnancy 3 years ago. Pelvic examination reveals normal external genitalia and vulva. Her vagina and cervix are without lesions. Her uterus is asymmetrically enlarged, about 8-week size, and nontender. Results of a urine quantitative β-hCG are negative.

43 A 39-year-old woman multiparous woman complains of heavy vaginal bleeding with her menstrual periods increasing over the past 9 months. She states that her cramping with menses is also getting worse. Two years ago, after workup for American Society of Cytology Pap smear, she underwent cryotherapy for biopsy which confirmed cervical intraepithelial neoplasia grade I (CIN 1). Subsequent follow-up Pap smears have been negative. Her pelvic examination is unremarkable except for a diffusely enlarged, globular, soft, tender uterus. Results of a urine quantitative β-hCG are negative.

44 A 14-year-old girl complains of irregular, unpredictable heavy menstrual bleeding. She denies pain or cramping. Her first menstrual period was at age 13, and they have always been irregular, but the bleeding seems to be getting heavier. She has no chronic health problems and states she has never been sexually active. She appears well developed and well nourished, with normal female secondary sexual characteristics. Inspection shows normal female external genitalia. Results of a urine quantitative β-hCG are negative.

45 A 39-year-old multiparous woman complains of intermittent vaginal bleeding between normal menstrual periods that has been going on for the past 4 months. The bleeding is painless and occurs after sexual intercourse. She has had three cesarean sections along with a tubal sterilization with her last delivery. She has a 30 pack-year history of cigarette smoking. She is currently in a monogamous sexual relationship but has had multiple sexual partners in the past. She has not been regular in her annual examinations. Her last Pap smear was 5 years ago.

46 A 6-year-old girl states that she has had vaginal bleeding for the past 3 days. She is brought to the office by her worried mother. The mother states that the child has no medical problems and is not on any medications. She denies headache or visual changes. General physical examination is consistent with a normal 6-year-old female without breast budding. External genitalia are unremarkable with no pubic hair.

47 A 63-year-old woman nulligravid woman comes to the outpatient office complaining about intermittent painless vaginal bleeding. Her last menstrual period was 10 years ago. She is not on hormone therapy. She has never used oral contraceptives. She has struggled with overweight all her life. Her last Pap smear a year ago was negative for dysplasia or malignancy. Her pelvic examination is unremarkable without vulvar, vaginal, or cervical lesions. Her uterus is small, mobile, and nontender. No adnexal masses are palpable.

48 A 21-year-old nulligravid woman complains that she has nonmenstrual vaginal bleeding and left-sided lower-abdominal pain. Her last menstrual period was 7 weeks ago. She is sexually active with multiple sexual partners. She uses barrier contraception irregularly and was treated with antibiotics 6 months ago for bilateral lower-abdominal pelvic pain. Her vital signs are stable. On pelvic examination she has dark blood in the vagina with no active bleeding. Her uterus is slightly enlarged but nontender. She has left adnexal tenderness to palpation without an obvious mass.

49 A pregnant 15-year-old refugee girl from the Darfur region of Sudan presents with irregular uterine bleeding and vaginal passage of grapelike clusters of enlarged edematous villi. Ultrasonography of the uterus shows a "snow storm" image with no fetus or placenta.

50 A 38-year-old woman presents with abdominal pain, blotting and ascites.

Answer Key

1	D	**11**	B	**21**	A	**31**	F	**41**	H
2	D	**12**	E	**22**	B	**32**	C	**42**	D
3	E	**13**	E	**23**	F	**33**	B	**43**	I
4	E	**14**	A	**24**	D	**34**	B	**44**	G
5	D	**15**	C	**25**	C	**35**	E	**45**	F
6	C	**16**	A	**26**	A	**36**	D	**46**	B
7	B	**17**	D	**27**	C	**37**	D	**47**	C
8	C	**18**	D	**28**	B	**38**	A	**48**	A
9	D	**19**	B	**29**	D	**39**	E	**49**	E
10	B	**20**	B	**30**	E	**40**	B	**50**	J

Answers and Explanations

[1] The answer is D *Surgery*

Acute small bowel infarction (choice **D**) is indicated by the sudden onset of severe abdominal pain with vomiting and abdominal distention out of proportion with the physical findings, absent bowel sounds, a striking neutrophilic leukocytosis with left shift, lactic acidosis, hypotension, and increased serum amylase concentration of bowel origin. The increased serum amylase concentration is sometimes misinterpreted as representing acute hemorrhagic pancreatitis. Barium studies reveal "thumbprinting" of the mucosa due to submucosal hemorrhages and edema. Peritoneal signs (e.g., rebound tenderness) are generally late findings. These signs of acute infarction are often preceded by abdominal angina (mesenteric angina) 30 minutes after eating. Because of the pain, patients tend to have a fear of eating, and they lose weight. In 50% of cases acute small bowel infarction occurs in elderly patients with atherosclerotic disease; usually the pathogenesis relates to sudden occlusion of the superior mesenteric artery by thrombosis over an atherosclerotic plaque, less often to an embolism from the left heart (mitral valve disease, atrial fibrillation or left ventricular mural thrombosis), and rarely from vasculitis. In about 25% of cases, nonocclusive infarction can occur from a low rate of blood flow as in vasospasm or shock. Causes of vasospasm include ergot or cocaine poisoning and sympathomimetic drugs, such as digitalis. Shock can be induced by hypovolemia and hypotension as may be caused by cardiac failure, or loss of blood as would occur with aortic aneurysm repair, or dissections of the aorta (uncommon). The remaining 25% of cases of small bowel infarction may result from superior mesenteric vein occlusion related to hypercoagulable states, which could be associated with polycythemia rubra vera, oral contraceptives in females, malignancy, or one of the hereditary hypercoagulable states (e.g., antithrombin III deficiency, protein C and S deficiencies). Whatever the underlying mechanism, transmural, hemorrhagic infarctions damage the integrity of the mucosa, thus predisposing the bowel to secondary bacterial penetration and generalized peritonitis. The reestablishment of blood flow frequently results in further damage due to reavailability of oxygen to help form free radicals. Treatment of the ischemic bowel must occur within 12 hours; otherwise, a 100% mortality rate can be expected. Surgery is always indicated if a grossly obvious hemorrhagic infarction has already occurred. Visible peristalsis is the best way to determine if the bowel is viable or dead. Embolectomy and intraarterial vasodilators are also used, depending on the cause of the ischemia.

The situation in this case is an unlikely clinical presentation for acute ulcerative colitis (choice **A**); moreover, ulcerative colitis is most often seen in young adults. Although hemorrhagic pancreatitis (choice **B**) involves an elevated serum amylase concentration, it is not associated with diffuse abdominal pain and bloody diarrhea. An aortoenteric fistula (choice **C**) is usually a late complication of repair of an abdominal aortic aneurysm. Toxic megacolons (choice **E**) are associated with ulcerative colitis.

[2] The answer is D *Pediatrics*

Choanal atresia (choice **D**) should be suspected in any infant who develops cyanosis that occurs with feedings or at rest but is relieved by crying. The cyanosis occurs because newborns are obligate nose breathers, and this congenital anomaly consists of a unilateral or bilateral bony or membranous septum between the nose and the pharynx. Diagnosis is made by failure to pass a catheter through the nasal passages.

Tracheoesophageal fistula (choice **A**) is characterized by choking with feeding. An orogastric tube curls up and does not pass to the stomach. Bronchopulmonary dysplasia (choice **B**) is a complication of respiratory distress syndrome (choice **C**) and appears later in the infant's life. Cyanosis is not relieved by crying in either entity. A patent ductus arteriosus (choice **E**) is a left-to-right shunt and is not associated with cyanosis.

[3] The answer is E *Medicine*

The patient is most likely taking a bile acid-binding resin (e.g., cholestyramine) to lower his cholesterol level. These resins work by binding bile acids in the intestine to form an insoluble, nonabsorbable complex that is excreted in the feces along with the resin. This action reduces circulating cholesterol levels and causes a compensatory increase in the synthesis of hepatocyte low-density lipoprotein receptors (choice **E**) to more efficiently recover reduced levels of cholesterol from the blood. Recovered cholesterol is then converted to bile acids to replenish the bile acids that are lost in the stool. The most common complaints are constipation and bloating that are relieved by increasing fiber or mixing psyllium seed with the resin. Heartburn and diarrhea are occasionally reported. Problems may also arise from the resin forming complexes and promoting the excretion of other substances such as digitalis, folic acid, thiazides, and warfarin.

Normally, cholesterol is effectively reabsorbed from the intestine as part of the bile acids and is not excreted as the free compound. A bile acid-binding resin does not change this condition; however, now rather than being reabsorbed as an integral part of the bile acid, it is excreted as a component in a bile acid–bile acid-binding resin complex, not as free cholesterol; increased excretion of free cholesterol in feces (choice **D**) does not happen. The "statin" drugs (e.g., lovastatin) inhibit HMG-CoA reductase (choice **A**), the rate-limiting enzyme of cholesterol synthesis. This decreases the synthesis of cholesterol. Rare side effects of statin drugs include hepatic toxicity with an increase in transaminases, and a myopathy with an increase in creatine kinase; however, evidence suggests that the statins are also antiosteoporotic, an unexpected boon. Fibric acid derivatives (e.g., gemfibrozil) and nicotinic acid lower serum triglyceride (TG) levels. Fibric acid derivatives decrease hepatic TG synthesis (choice **B**) and also interfere with the formation of very-low-density lipoproteins (VLDLs) in the liver. Complications that might be associated with fibric acid derivatives include rash and myopathy, the latter sometimes causing rhabdomyolysis with marked elevation of creatine kinase and myoglobinuria. Nicotinic acid is also used in the treatment of hypertriglyceridemia (also hypercholesterolemia). The drug interferes with the formation of VLDL in the liver. Flushing is the major side effect of nicotinic acid and is diminished by taking a nonsteroidal 30 minutes before taking the drug. Flushing is not present in this patient. Fibric acid derivatives and nicotinic acid both activate capillary lipoprotein lipase (choice **C**), promoting increased delivery of fatty acids to the adipose.

4 **The answer is E** *Preventive Medicine and Public Health*

Malpractice is generally defined as deviation from the established standards of professional care (i.e., professional negligence). For a claim of malpractice, the patient must prove that the doctor was negligent by deviating from the established standard of care (choice **E**) and that this deviation caused injury (not necessarily deliberately). Additionally, the physician has to have a duty to the patient because of their professional relationship.

Neither the doctor's education (choice **A**) nor how much he charges the patient (choice **D**) is related to malpractice claims. Malpractice is a civil wrong (a tort), not a crime (choice **C**), and intent to cause harm does not have to be shown (choice **B**).

5 **The answer is D** *Surgery*

The patient most likely has a postoperative wound infection (choice **D**), which occurs in 2 to 5% of patients who have had biliary tract surgery. The infections are usually the result of contamination of the wound either during or after surgery; there rarely is an infection prior to surgery. Although infections can become evident within 1 day in a grossly contaminated wound, they generally first emerge 5 to 10 days postoperatively. Operative wounds are classified as clean (no gross contamination), clean-contaminated (e.g., in gastric or biliary tract surgery), contaminated (e.g., in unprepared colon surgery), or dirty and infected (infection encountered during the surgery). The risk for wound infection increases if the wound is located in the abdomen, the surgery lasts longer than 2 hours, or contamination of the wound is encountered during surgery. One of the key factors that predisposes to infection is decreased oxygen tension in the tissues. Attention to careful surgical techniques (reduced trauma to tissue, less suture material, removal of foreign bodies) and prophylactic use of antibiotics in certain types of surgeries reduce the chance of infection. Cefazolin is the drug of choice for prophylaxis during surgery when both aerobes and anaerobes are a concern. Antibiotic prophylaxis is only given in selected clean or clean-contaminated procedures, because antibiotic use in contaminated and dirty wounds is considered therapeutic. A single preoperative dose should be administered intravenously at the time of induction of anesthesia. Additional doses may be given after surgery but are usually discontinued within 24 hours. Treatment of wound infection involves opening the wound and allowing drainage. Antibiotics are reserved for invasive infections.

Atelectasis (choice **C**) is the most common cause of fever within 24 hours of surgery. Endotoxic shock (choice **B**) would be accompanied by warm shock, due to vasodilation of peripheral vessels, and would be an unlikely cause of this woman's fever. Resorption of blood (choice **A**) is not associated with fever. Renal failure (choice **E**) is associated with oliguria, not fever.

6 **The answer is C** *Pediatrics*

With an incidence of 1 case per 400 births, sickle cell disease is the most common hemoglobinopathy in the African-American population. The blood smear illustrated as part of the case history confirms a diagnosis of sickle cell disease in this girl, since it shows numerous boat-shaped sickle cells. Dactylitis is the most frequent initial manifestation of sickle cell disease, with a typical onset of symptoms at an age of 4 to 12 months; this time range approximately coincides with the replacement of hemoglobin (Hb) F with Hb A (choice **C**). Dactylitis is characterized by soft tissue swelling of the hands, feet, or both, with associated heat and tenderness over the metacarpals, tarsals, and proximal phalanges. Radiographs made at the onset of disease only show soft tissue swelling. After 1 to 2 weeks, infarction and necrosis of the underlying bones are noted secondary to sickling of red blood cells (RBCs) in the sinusoids. This is followed by subperiosteal new bone formation. Absorption of the infarcted bone results in radiolucent areas. These areas of infarction are restored to normal within a few months, but recurrent disease is common.

A hemolytic crisis induced by an aberrant G6PD (choice **A**) may be caused by infection (most common) or by oxidizing drugs. The mutation resulting in this aberrant enzyme occurs on the X chromosome and is inherited as a recessive trait; consequently, it is very unlikely to occur in a female infant. The G6PD gene is very susceptible to mutation; over 400 hundred different genetic variants of G6PD have been described. Nonetheless, most black Africans express the "normal" A variant while most Caucasians carry the "normal" B variant. However, about 11% of African Americans express the A⁻ variant, which affords protection against falciparum malaria. Individuals carrying the A⁻ form are essentially normal except when their red cells are exposed to oxidative stress. This is because the primary function of the hexose monophosphate shunt in red cells is to produce NADPH via the G6PD reaction to keep glutathione (GSH) in the reduced state; this GSH protects the red cell membrane and the hemoglobin (Hb) from oxidative denaturation. The residual activity of the A⁻ variant suffices to maintain healthy red cell function for almost their full normal life span. However as red cells age the activity of their enzymes decline, and G6PD activity falls below a critical limit at which NADPH production can no longer maintain GSH levels in stressed cells. Consequently, some of the Hb is denatured, forming Heinz bodies that react with the cell membrane, causing a distortion that is recognized by and destroyed in the spleen; this causes a hemolytic crisis. This crisis is self-limiting, even in the continued presence of the agent causing the stress, because only a variable population of older cells is affected. The B⁻ variant, also known as the Mediterranean form, is commonly expressed by people originating from the malaria zones abutting the northern, southwestern, and western Mediterranean Sea. It too protects against malaria, but the residual activity is lower, and a hemolytic crisis can be life threatening; the mutation sometimes also makes itself evident in the newborn via excessive jaundice. Individuals carrying the B⁻ variant also suffer severe crises when exposed to fava beans, the common Mediterranean flat bean. As noted above, there are more than 400 known variants of this enzyme. Expression of many of these produce symptoms, some incompatible with life; others cause a chronic hemolytic anemia or chronic granulomatous disease. However, since most of these impart severe symptoms and have no benefit they are very rare conditions.

Salmonella paratyphi is the most common cause of osteomyelitis (choice **B**) in sickle cell disease, and infection tends to occur when functional hyposplenism is present from autoinfarction of the spleen. However, hyposplenism is unlikely to occur in a 6-month-old infant. The highest risk of infection is after age 1 year to 10 years of age. Coxsackieviruses (choice **D**), an enterovirus, are associated with hand, foot, and mouth disease, a highly contagious condition that primarily affects children in preelementary school groups. It is called hand, foot, and mouth disease because of the typical ulcers on the tongue and oral mucosa and vesicles that do not ulcerate on the palms and soles. It is also accompanied by a temperature of 101 to 104°F (38.3–40°C), and although most often self-limiting, in rare cases, usually in neonates, it causes life-threatening myocarditis or encephalitis. Turner syndrome, a sex chromosome abnormality with an XO pattern (choice **E**), is associated with nuchal lymphedema and painless lymphedema of the hands and feet in newborns; there is no fever, and no sickle cells are seen in a peripheral smear.

7 **The answer is B** *Psychiatry*

The phenotype described for the boy is typical of fragile X syndrome, the most prevalent inherited cause of mental retardation in males. It is caused by the expansion of a CGG repeat near a gene located on the X chromosome. Once the number of repeats goes beyond 52, chance of further expansion during oogeneses or spermatogenesis is great. Because it is X-linked, males are generally more severely affected than females, but females sometimes do show psychologic symptoms such as autism and mild mental retardation (choice **B**). In this family, the grandfather was a so-called premutation carrier, with minimal expansion, the only obvious symptom being tremor. The number of repeats probably increased in the mother and then again in her children. The mother was completely protected by her second X chromosome, and the daughter was partly protected.

Cri du chat syndrome (choice **A**) is associated with severe mental retardation. Klinefelter syndrome (choice **C**) is associated with cognitive and emotional difficulties. Down syndrome (trisomy 21) (choice **D**) is associated with mental retardation and Alzheimer's disease. Turner syndrome (choice **E**) is associated with various cognitive, social, and behavioral problems.

8 The answer is C *Medicine*

The patient has acromegaly secondary to a benign pituitary adenoma with excess secretion of growth hormone (not decreased [choice **E**]) by the anterior pituitary and of insulin-like growth factor-1 (not decreased [choice **D**]) from the liver. If the condition occurs before fusion of the epiphysis, gigantism occurs.

Clinical findings associated with acromegaly include:

- Generalized enlargement of bone, cartilage, and soft tissue, resulting in large hands and feet, frontal bossing, a prominent jaw, an increase in hat size, spaces between the teeth, and hypertrophy of the left ventricle observed by chest radiography (not a normal-sized heart [choice **A**]). This hypertrophy may lead to cardiomegaly and cardiomyopathy with congestive heart failure (the most common cause of death)
- Diastolic hypertension (observed blood pressure is 135/95 mm Hg)
- Muscle weakness (his perception confirmed by the physician)
- Peripheral neuropathies (he can't be sure where his feet are, loss of proprioception)
- Diabetes mellitus from the gluconeogenic properties of growth hormone
- Headaches and visual field defects from encroachment on the optic chiasm

The laboratory findings include:

- Hyperglycemia (40%) (his serum glucose level is 195 mg/dL.)
- Inability to suppress glucose with an oral glucose tolerance test (choice **C**)
- A paradoxical increase of serum growth hormone concentration with injection of thyrotropin-releasing hormone (TRH)
- No stimulation of growth hormone release with L-dopa (normal persons have an increase in GH)
- Before fusion of the epiphysis occurs, increased serum phosphate associated with growth spurts
- Enlargement of the sella turcica in more than 90% of patients (not a normal-sized sella turcica [choice **B**])

Treatment consists of transsphenoidal surgery or the use of a somatostatin analogue called octreotide, which produces clinical improvement in 70% of cases.

9 The answer is D *Medicine*

The differential diagnosis of this patient resides among gastroesophageal reflux disorder (GERD), peptic ulcer with associated reflux disease, an esophageal motility disorder, panic disorder, and some type of myocardial disease. GERD is suggested by pain that is not induced by exercise and is relieved by antacids. However, a myocardial disorder (e.g., atypical angina) is still a possibility and could be life threatening. Therefore, an electrocardiogram (EKG) should be performed immediately (choice **D**).

Referral to a psychologist (choice **A**) would be a proper course of action for panic disorder, which is often associated with chest discomfort. However, the absence of other symptoms makes this an unlikely diagnosis. Cisapride (choice **B**) decreases reflux activity by acting as a prokinetic motility agent that increases the strength of esophageal peristalsis, raises the lower esophageal sphincter pressure, and increases the rate of gastric emptying; however, not only should potential cardiac problems be ruled out first, but cisapride was voluntarily withdrawn from the market in 2000 because of potential side effects. The histamine blockers mentioned in choice **C** or the proton pump inhibitor listed in choice **F** lower acid secretion. However, after heart problems are ruled out, the first line of treatment recommended by the American College of Gastroenterology is a series of lifestyle changes. Controlling gastric *Helicobacter pylori* infection (choice **E**) is part of the standard treatment used to cure peptic ulcers, not GERD.

10 **The answer is B** *Surgery*

Bruising about the orbit (raccoon sign) and blood in the external auditory meatus indicate that the patient has a basilar skull fracture. Cerebrospinal fluid (CSF) is an ultrafiltrate of plasma primarily derived from the choroid plexus in the lateral ventricles and is resorbed by the arachnoid granulations. The patient has otorrhea with suspected loss of CSF. When compared with serum concentrations, CSF has a higher chloride (118–132 vs. 94–106 mEq/L) (choice **B**), a lower protein (<4 vs. 6.0–7.8 g/dL) (choice **A**), a lower glucose concentration (about 60% of the plasma; 40–70 vs. 70–110 mg/dL) (choice **C**), and fewer white blood cells (0–5 vs. 4,500–11,000 leukocytes/μL) (choice **D**). Prealbumin is present in CSF electrophoresis (choice **E**) but cannot be distinguished on routine serum protein electrophoresis.

11 **The answer is B** *Pediatrics*

External otitis, or "swimmer's ear," is caused by excessive moisture in the ear canal, which causes chronic irritation, inducing the loss of protective cerumen and making the canal susceptible to infection. The patient presents with ear pain that is worsened by manipulation of the pinna; the ear canal is erythematous and edematous, and otorrhea is seen. These are signs of external otitis, which is most commonly caused by *Pseudomonas aeruginosa* (choice **B**). Other organisms sometimes found include *Enterobacter aerogenes*, *Proteus mirabilis*, *Klebsiella pneumoniae*, streptococci species, *Staphylococcus epidermidis*, and fungi.

Both *Haemophilus influenzae* (choice **A**) and *Moraxella catarrhalis* (choice **C**) cause otitis media. *Streptococcus agalactiae* (choice **D**) has been isolated from middle ear fluid in neonates with otitis media. However, both *S. agalactiae* and *Escherichia coli* (choice **E**) are leading causes of sepsis and meningitis in neonates.

12 **The answer is E** *Surgery*

Pneumothorax (choice **E**) can inadvertently occur while introducing a subclavian venous catheter. The patient will complain of sudden dyspnea. A chest x-ray film should always be taken after subclavian catheter placement, to determine the position of the tip of the catheter and to exclude the possibility of pneumothorax.

Air embolism (choice **A**) is not usually seen during introduction of a subclavian venous catheter, because the patient is placed in a Trendelenburg position (head end down, foot end up) so that venous pressure is increased, and air cannot be sucked into the right atrium. However, should this be attempted with the patient lying flat, or if the line is disconnected when the patient is upright, a fatal air embolism could result. The patient will have tachypnea, hypotension, and a continuous murmur. Pulmonary embolism (choice **B**) is unlikely, as no particulate matter has been introduced through the catheter at this point in time. Fat embolism (choice **C**) most often results from fractures of the long bone. If acute anxiety were to cause the dyspnea (choice **D**) an attack would be expected to precede the introduction of the catheter.

13 **The answer is E** *Psychiatry*

This woman's symptoms are most suggestive of shared psychotic disorder, characterized by the acceptance of delusional beliefs from a psychotic individual with whom one has a close relationship, often called the inducer. Shared psychotic disorder most often occurs in individuals who are in close company of a dominant person with delusional beliefs and who are isolated from others. She is less likely to suffer from delusional disorder in so much as there is little evidence of delusions not connected with those of the husband.

Shared psychotic disorder is most successfully treated by separation from the inducer (choice **E**). When this is accomplished, symptoms usually fade quickly. Separation may be difficult or impossible because of the wishes of the patient.

There is little evidence to suggest that behavioral psychotherapy (choice **A**), cognitive psychotherapy (choice **B**), conjoint psychotherapy (choice **C**), or ziprasidone (choice **D**) are useful treatments for this disorder.

14 **The answer is A** *Pediatrics*

As the patient is dehydrated, fluid replacement is warranted. However since total body water loss is minimal, aggressive therapy is not called for, and a bolus of 20 mL/kg of isotonic crystalloid (choice **A**) is the most appropriate choice.

Accordingly, more aggressive fluid management (answer **B**) is not warranted. Likewise, administering maintenance fluids (answer **C**) would be inappropriate for this patient and for the emergency medicine setting. Most likely an initial bolus will be adequate therapy; therefore giving an antiemetic (choice **D**) would not be the next best step. Additionally antiemetics are not widely used in the pediatric population. Antibiotic therapy (answer **E**) is also incorrect because the first step in management is to administer fluids and because antibiotics should not be administered until it is determined that there is a bacterial infection.

15 The answer is C *Psychiatry*

Dissociative fugue (choice **C**) is characterized by sudden travel away from home, inability to recall one's past, and a disturbance of identity. It often occurs during the course of severe stress.

Memory impairment may or may not be present with psychosis due to a general medical condition (choice **A**), but no psychotic symptoms are present in the case description. Conversion disorder (choice **B**) is characterized by loss of sensory or motor function—not simply memory loss. Subjective memory problems sometimes occur during major depressive disorder (choice **D**), but identity disturbance would be very unusual in this condition. Delirium (choice **E**) may present with memory impairment but also involves a disturbed level of awareness.

16 The answer is A *Surgery*

The clinical presentation of a young adult female with fever, left-sided abdominal pain, multiple daily bowel movements, bloody diarrhea with mucus, and rectal bleeding is strongly suggestive of ulcerative colitis (choice **A**). This diagnosis will be confirmed by sigmoidoscopy (colonoscopy is not recommended for fear of perforation). Sigmoidoscopy will reveal a granular, hyperemic, and friable mucosa that bleeds easily on minimal contact. The disease is confined to the rectum in up to 50% of cases. However, in about 30% of patients inflammation extends up the left colon in a continuous fashion (no skip lesions) to the splenic flexure, and 20% will have even more extensive colitis. The disease is slightly more common in females than males, and surprisingly, smoking seems to impart some protection against this disease. Its etiology is unknown, and the clinical profile is highly variable. Mild cases are defined as having fewer than four bloody bowel movements per day, moderate case have four to six, and severe cases more than six. The severity of the anemia, the elevation of the sedimentation rate, and the decrease in serum albumin level also reflect the severity of the disease. Typically, ulcerative colitis is a recurring disease with attacks precipitated by stress.

There are several goals in the treatment of ulcerative colitis. First is to stop an attack in progress. In the typical case limited to the distal part of the tract this is done using mesalamine and hydrocortisone suppositories or enemas. In more extensive cases, mesalamine tablets are used along with sulfasalazine and balsalazide. Very severe cases are treated with IV methylprednisolone. The second aim of treatment is to return the patient to a more healthy state by evaluating and treating the anemia, hypovolemia, and malnourishment that is likely to have developed. A final goal is to try to prevent further sudden attacks. This is done by a high-fiber diet, which also limits the intake of caffeine and gas-producing vegetables. Prophylactic use of antidiarrheal agents is sometimes recommended, and a maintenance daily dose of sulfasalazine with mesalamine has been shown to reduce relapse rate to about 33%, compared with a rate of 75% for patients not on maintenance therapy. Although medical management permits most patients to live an almost normal life, some 25% will need surgery to remove the affected segment of rectum and colon or to remove observed dysplasia or carcinoma. (The disease makes patients more prone to develop colon cancer).

Crohn's disease (choice **B**) is an ulcer causing inflammatory bowel disease. About half the cases involve the small bowel, usually the terminal ileum and the adjacent colon (ileocolitis). Crohn's disease usually presents with right lower quadrant pain, fever, and diarrhea. However, in other cases more distal areas are affected, and in about 30% of cases there is perianal involvement. In contrast to ulcerative colitis, the diarrhea is nonbloody and cigarette smoking is a definite risk factor. Anal fissures (choice **C**) produce severe rectal pain on defecation, bleeding, and anal tenderness. Ischemic bowel disease (choice **D**) presents with diffuse abdominal pain and bloody diarrhea. The solitary ulcer syndrome (choice **E**) is characterized by mucosal prolapse with ischemic ulceration.

17 The answer is D *Medicine*

The patient has renovascular hypertension secondary to atherosclerotic narrowing of the left renal artery orifice. The diagnosis of renal artery stenosis should always be considered when the following are present:

- Hypertension develops after 50 years of age
- Vascular bruits are heard in the abdomen

- Hypertension is resistant to therapy
- Advanced retinopathy is present
- The serum creatinine concentration is increased
- Abrupt deterioration of renal function occurs after an angiotensin-converting enzyme (ACE) inhibitor is given
- Peripheral vascular disease

Renovascular hypertension is the most common secondary cause of hypertension. In young to middle-aged women, it is most commonly caused by fibromuscular hyperplasia of one or both renal arteries. In elderly men, it is most commonly caused by atherosclerosis (not fibromuscular hyperplasia [choice **E**]) causing decreased blood flow through the renal artery orifice. In fibromuscular hyperplasia, the renal arteriogram shows a characteristic beading effect along the course of the artery. In patients with atherosclerosis, there is narrowing of the renal artery orifice, as in this patient. In either condition, reduced blood flow to the kidneys causes activation of the renin–angiotensin–aldosterone system. Hypertension is due to the release of angiotensin II, which vasoconstricts peripheral resistance arterioles, and to an increase in aldosterone (not a decrease [choice **C**]), which increases the reabsorption of sodium and water. The increase in aldosterone is also responsible for hypokalemic metabolic alkalosis (not metabolic acidosis [choice **A**]), because of enhanced exchange of potassium and hydrogen ions for sodium in the distal tubule. Loss of hydrogen ions in the urine causes an increase in the reabsorption of bicarbonate in the plasma, leading to metabolic alkalosis. In renovascular hypertension, captopril blocks the production of angiotensin II, which has a negative feedback on renin; therefore, plasma renin activity increases significantly over the baseline high values (not a decrease in plasma renin activity [PRA] [choice **B**]). However, if the patient has bilateral renal artery stenosis, captopril causes abrupt deterioration in renal function. This change is caused by the block in angiotensin II, which is important in maintaining renal blood flow in both kidneys.

The captopril stimulation test with radionuclide scan is a good first step in the workup of renovascular hypertension. The test result is positive if a small kidney shows delayed uptake and excretion of a radioisotope after captopril administration. Angiography is the definitive test, and is usually accompanied by a split renal vein sampling of PRA from the right and left renal veins. In this patient, the left renal vein renin levels would be increased, whereas those on the right should be suppressed (choice **D**), because the excess angiotensin II and volume overload from aldosterone will shut off renin production from the right kidney. If the ratio of PRA from the arteriographically abnormal kidney is 1.5 times higher than that of the PRA obtained on the normal (uninvolved) side, patients are likely to benefit from surgery or angioplasty. However, if both sides have increased PRA levels, the "normal" kidney also has vascular disease, most commonly nephrosclerosis with small vessel disease due to hypertension (hyaline arteriolosclerosis). These changes occur because the "normal" kidney experiences a significant increase in blood flow and systemic blood pressure owing to reduced flow to the stenotic kidney by the stenotic segment in the artery. In these difficult cases, the "normal" kidney is often removed, and the renal artery is repaired in the involved kidney.

18 **The answer is D** *Surgery*

This patient has a mechanical obstruction of the bowel caused by a large gallstone (>2.5 cm) lodged within its lumen of the ileus, i.e., gallstone ileus (choice **D**). These stones are usually radiopaque. Gallstone ileus is most commonly seen in elderly women who have a chronically inflamed gallbladder that adheres to the bowel. This results in a cholecystenteric fistula, which connects the gallbladder with either the duodenum or hepatic flexure of the colon, both of which are in the vicinity of the gallbladder. In 40% of cases, air is seen in the biliary tree because bowel air is transported to that location via the fistula. Emergency laparotomy and enterotomy to remove the stone should be undertaken. A second stone may be present proximally and should be removed to avoid recurrence. The fistula should be left alone, because it is not the cause of this patient's symptoms, and it closes off by itself. Cholecystectomy might be undertaken at a later date, if the patient has symptoms.

Tumors of the small bowel (e.g., lymphoma of the small bowel [choice **A**]) are rare. The most common location is the terminal ileum, and they are not radiopaque. Lymphoma is the most common primary malignant tumor of the small intestine. It may present with rectal bleeding or intussusception. Acute pancreatitis (choice **B**) presents as an acute abdomen, but it is not associated with a radiopaque mass in the small bowel. It is more common in males and in a younger age group. A plain abdominal x-ray film shows a sentinel loop, which represents a dilated proximal loop of jejunum adjoining the pancreas. Intussusception (choice **E**) is a telescoping of a segment of the bowel into the adjacent segment. This usually involves the terminal ileum telescoping into the proximal large bowel. It is the most common cause of intestinal obstruction in children. It is associated with a sausage-shaped mass in the midabdomen and red, currant-jelly stool. If it cannot be reduced by barium enema, surgery is required. Acute appendicitis with radiopaque fecalith (choice **C**) has a different clinical presentation. The patient would complain of nausea, vomiting, constipation, and periumbilical pain that radiates and settles in the right lower quadrant. Physical examination would elicit tenderness and guarding in the right lower quadrant. Finally, fecaliths are not radiopaque.

19 The answer is B *Medicine*

The patient has a glioblastoma multiforme (choice **B**). This is the most common primary cancer of the brain in adults (peaks in the 40- to 70-year-old age bracket) and either arises de novo or from a preexisting low-grade astrocytoma. The tumors are located predominantly in the cerebral hemispheres and are classified as grade IV astrocytomas. There is no causal relationship with cigarette smoking. The distribution of this lesion and the history of headache, projectile vomiting, and bilateral papilledema are classic signs and symptoms of glioblastoma multiforme. The MRI shows a mass lesion extending across the splenium of the corpus callosum and into the adjacent cerebral hemisphere bilaterally. These tumors rarely metastasize out of the neuraxis. Radiation and chemotherapy are used for treatment. There is a 25 to 40% 5-year survival rate.

Cerebral infarctions (choice **A**) are most commonly caused by a thrombus overlying an atheromatous plaque, which causes a pale infarction that extends to the periphery of the cerebral cortex. The lesion in this patient does not adhere to this distribution. Intracerebral hemorrhages (choice **C**) usually are due to hypertension (not recorded in this patient), which produces small-vessel aneurysms that result in rupture of the vessel and hemorrhage into the brain. The basal ganglia area is the most common site for the hemorrhage. Medulloblastomas (choice **D**) usually are located in the midline of the cerebellum in children. Metastases to the brain (choice **E**) usually are multifocal and occur primarily at the junction of the gray and white matter near the periphery of the brain.

20 The answer is B *Preventive Medicine and Public Health*

The question relates to assessing differences among three groups of a continuous variable, which in this question is systolic blood pressure. To assess the significance of differences in data derived from three or more groups it is necessary to use analysis of variance (choice **B**).

If the comparison were between only two groups, a Student's *t*-test (choice **A**) would be correct. A correlation coefficient (choice **C**) assesses the strength of association, not the differences between groups. The chi-squared test (choice **D**) assesses differences among groups of categorical variables. Logistic regression (choice **E**) is used to assess a categorical outcome for a continuous predictor.

21 The answer is A *Psychiatry*

Social withdrawal and a family history of psychopathology (choice **A**) are both more commonly associated with schizophrenia than with delirium.

Memory impairment and waxing and waning of symptoms within a period of hours (choice **B**) are both more suggestive of delirium. Hallucinations (choice **C**) are common in both delirium and schizophrenia. Visual hallucinations are more commonly associated with delirium, while auditory hallucinations are more often described in schizophrenia, but there is much overlap. A family history of psychopathology is more common in schizophrenia, but waxing and rapid waning of symptoms is a characteristic of delirium; hence choice **D** is incorrect. Similarly, choice **E** is wrong because social withdrawal suggests schizophrenia, while rapid fluctuation of symptoms suggests delirium.

22 The answer is B *Medicine*

Two important polyuria syndromes are central diabetes insipidus (CDI) in which there is an absolute deficiency of antidiuretic hormone (ADH) and nephrogenic diabetes insipidus (NDI) in which the kidney tubules are not responsive to ADH. In either case, the patient cannot concentrate urine (cannot reabsorb water out of the urine), and consequently, the urine's osmolality (U_{Osm}) is decreased and the loss of water in the urine causes a corresponding increase in both plasma osmolality (P_{Osm}) and serum sodium, because P_{Osm} correlates closely with the serum sodium concentration.

The patient has sarcoidosis, which is a multisystem granulomatous disease of unknown etiology. Although the primary target organ is the lung, the central nervous system can also be involved. In this case, there is granulomatous inflammation in the medial hypothalamus, where the paraventricular nucleus and supraoptic nucleus contain cells that synthesize ADH. The resultant inability to synthesize ADH results in CDI. Differentiation of CDI from NDI is best accomplished with a water deprivation test. In CDI, water deprivation results in an increase in P_{Osm} (not a decrease [choice **A**]), an increase in serum sodium (choice **B**), and a decrease (not increase [choice **C**]) in U_{Osm}. Injection of vasopressin (ADH) produces an increase in U_{Osm} (not no response to vasopressin [choice **D**]) that is usually greater than 50% of the baseline U_{Osm} after deprivation. In NDI, water deprivation results in an increase in P_{Osm}, an increase in serum sodium, and a decrease in U_{Osm}. Injection of vasopressin does not significantly increase the U_{Osm}, because the collecting tubules are resistant to ADH. The following table summarizes changes in the P_{Osm} and U_{Osm} in CDI and NDI after a water deprivation test.

	Maximal P_{Osm}	Maximal U_{Osm}	U_{Osm} Postvasopressin
Normal	↑	↑↑	No significant change
CDI	↑↑	↓↓	↑↑
NDI	↑↑	↓↓	No significant change

23 The answer is F   *Surgery*

Osteogenic sarcoma (choice **F**) (aka osteosarcoma) is the most common primary cancer of bone. Typically it affects adolescents who present with persistent pain and swelling. Development of an osteosarcoma has no known hereditary component except in patients who have hereditary retinoblastoma, who are a high risk of also developing an osteogenic carcinoma. The most common site is the distal end of the femur and proximal end of the tibia close to the metaphysis, sometimes affecting the knee joint. Although a relationship has not been proved, symptoms often are first noted after an injury to the affected area, often causing diagnosis and treatment to be delayed. Radiographic study frequently reveals a "sun ray" pattern, which while suggestive is not pathognomonic. The final diagnosis is made by histologic examination of a biopsy sample. Three or four decades ago the survival rate was 15%, and at that time, the only "cure" was amputation. Today the survival rate is over 75%, and most limbs are saved by resection, followed by chemotherapy and radiation and then by surgical repair including provision of an endoprosthetic device or a bone graft.

Ewing's sarcoma (choice **A**) also is primarily a disease of adolescence but is far less common than osteosarcoma and is as likely to originate in almost any bone on the body. X-ray films are likely to show an "onion-peel" pattern rather than a sun-burst pattern, but again this is not pathognomonic; the definitive diagnosis once again depends upon histologic examination, which will show small round cells. Primitive neuroectodermal tumors (pPNETs) show a histologic pattern similar to that of Ewing's sarcoma, respond similarly to chemotherapy, and both are characterized by a 11,12 chromosomal translocation. In spite of resection, chemotherapy, and irradiation, Ewing's carcinoma still has a 50% mortality rate.

Legg-Calvé-Perthes disease (choice **B**) primarily affects children between the ages of 3 and 12 years and is more common in boys than in girls. It presents as a slowly evolving, painless limp. Pain is most frequently referred to the groin area. The leg is shorter on the affected side. Radiographs reveal increased density in the femoral head, but magnetic resonance imaging (MRI) is preferred for making the diagnosis. Treatment varies from observation to surgery, in which the joint is braced so proper remodeling of bone can occur.

Acute osteomyelitis (choice **C**) is an infection accompanied by fever and an extremely high erythrocyte sedimentation rate (ESR). Aspiration of bone and culture of lesion tissue is essential for diagnosis. The infection is usually difficult to treat; most patients are treated by débridement of necrotic tissue and prolonged and massive antibiotic treatment.

A slipped capital femoral epiphysis (choice **D**) is most commonly seen in obese adolescent boys from 9 to 15 years of age. Pain is classically located on the medial aspect of the knee. The secondary erosion of a joint caused by diminution of proprioception and perception of pain due to peripheral neuropathy is called *neurogenic arthropathy* (choice **E**) and can be responsible for "Charcot's joint," in which, as muscle tone and protective reflexes are lost, a joint undergoes secondary degeneration; cartilage is lost, the joint becomes boggy, osteophytes develop, and accumulated debris impairs function. Osteitis deformans (choice **G**), aka Paget's disease of bone, is a disease with a higher prevalence among the elderly, and it is characterized by one or more bony lesions created by areas of high turnover resulting in disorganized osteoid creating a dense expanded appearance upon radiography. Although often asymptomatic, it can cause a variety of unpleasant effects depending upon its location and the number of lesions.

24 The answer is D *Pediatrics*

Mastitis is not a contraindication to breast-feeding (choice **D**). The infant will not become ill if nursed on the affected breast (choice **A**). The most important fact to remember about mastitis is that early antibiotic treatment and continued breast feeding or pumping are essential to its cure. However, the mother should be treated with antibiotic therapy and analgesics that do not put the infant at risk (choice **B**). Frequent nursing on the affected breast will keep the breast from becoming engorged (choice **C**). In many cases, this will keep mastitis from progressing to a breast abscess. Changing to a commercially prepared formula (choice **E**) is not necessary because mastitis is not a contraindication to breast-feeding. Other supportive therapy for mastitis may include rest, plenty of fluids, and cold packs on the painful breast.

25 The answer is C *Preventive Medicine and Public Health*

Despite the fact that this woman is young and has no signs or symptoms of coronary artery disease (CAD), her obesity, lipid profile, and family history put her at risk for early disease; therefore, she is a prime subject for preventive measures. Regardless of the serum cholesterol level, high-density lipoprotein (HDL) level, or any other relevant laboratory value, the first step in management for primary prevention is 6 months of diet and aerobic exercise (choice **C**).

The patient should always begin with the American Heart Association step 1 diet, not the step 2 diet (choice **D**). If after 3 months there is no change in lipid profile, the patient should be changed to the step 2 diet. Pharmacologic intervention (choices **A, B,** and **E**) should be considered only after 6 months of aerobic exercise and diet.

26 The answer is A *Psychiatry*

Family dynamics are strongly implicated in the development of anorexia nervosa (choice **A**). Patients' mothers are often seen as overly controlling and fathers are seen as inhibited and compulsive. Food restriction and weight loss are postulated to be attempts to regain some control and perhaps avoid sexual issues. Psychotherapeutic intervention often involves family therapy.

Dissociative identity disorder (choice **B**) is associated with childhood sexual abuse. Narcissistic personality disorder (choice **C**) and schizophrenia (choice **D**) are not associated with a particular set of family dynamics. The onset of separation anxiety disorder (choice **E**) in childhood is sometimes associated with the death or other loss of a primary family member.

27 The answer is C *Medicine*

Osteoporosis is the most common metabolic abnormality of bone in the United States. There is a reduction in normal mineralized bone, resulting in decreased bone mass and bone density. Decreased bone mass and density is reflected as osteopenia in bone radiography. Estrogen deficiency after menopause is the most common cause of primary osteoporosis in women. Most of the bone is lost in the first 3 to 6 years after menopause. A partial list of secondary causes of osteoporosis includes estrogen deficiency associated with exercise-induced amenorrhea or anorexia nervosa, primary hyperparathyroidism, Cushing syndrome, chronic metabolic acidosis, heparin therapy, osteogenesis imperfecta, and the lack of gravity in space. In primary osteoporosis in women, an imbalance occurs between the resorption of bone (osteoclastic activity) and the formation of bone (osteoblastic activity) (choice **C**). Normally, estrogen inhibits osteoclast development in the bone marrow as well as osteoclast activity and increases osteoblastic activity in bone. Therefore, a deficiency of estrogen increases osteoclastic resorption of both cortical and trabecular bone and decreases osteoblastic bone formation. Osteoporosis increases the risk of compression fractures of the vertebral bodies, Colles' fractures, other pathologic fractures, a decrease in overall height, and "dowager's hump" of the cervical spine.

Serum phosphate and calcium levels are normal in osteoporosis. The latter finding excludes vitamin D deficiency (choice **A**), which produces hypocalcemia, secretion of PTH-related peptide (choice **B**) and PTH (choice **E**), which produce hypercalcemia; and, also rules out increased secretion of osteoclast-activating factor by macrophages (choice **D**), since that produces lytic bone lesions and hypercalcemia.

28 **The answer is B** *Medicine*

The patient has herpes simplex keratoconjunctivitis. A fluorescein stain exhibits the classic dendritic type of shallow ulcer with an irregular edge. Herpes labialis may or may not be present. Corneal involvement is frequently precipitated by topical corticosteroids or systemic corticosteroid therapy. Steroid therapy frequently results in deeper penetration of the ulcer. Topical trifluridine (choice **B**) is used for treatment. Ophthalmologists frequently denude the infected corneal epithelium to enhance recovery.

Topical phenylephrine (choice **C**) is a decongestant. Topical ketoconazole (choice **A**) is used in fungal corneal ulcers, which are rare. Topical erythromycin (choice **D**) and sulfacetamide (choice **E**) are both useful for bacterial conjunctivitis.

29 **The answer is D** *Medicine*

The fever and painful lesions on the pads of the fingers (Osler's nodes) are clinical characteristics of acute bacterial (infective) endocarditis. In patients with a history of intravenous drug abuse, bacterial endocarditis usually involves the tricuspid valve and is caused by *Staphylococcus aureus* (choice **D**) (not *Staphylococcus epidermidis* [choice **E**]). The pansystolic murmur and the S3 and S4 heart sounds that increases on inspiration indicate tricuspid regurgitation, a result of damage caused by the large, friable vegetations that infect the valve. Recall that all right-sided murmurs and abnormal heart sounds increase in intensity on inspiration, while left-sided murmurs and abnormal heart sounds increase in intensity on expiration. The patient also has jugular neck vein distention and a pulsatile liver, which are also signs of tricuspid regurgitation. The treatment of *S. aureus* infection involving the tricuspid valve is nafcillin plus gentamicin if the organism is methicillin sensitive or vancomycin if the organism is methicillin resistant.

Aortic regurgitation (choice **A**) is associated with a high-pitched diastolic blowing murmur that occurs immediately after the second heart sound. It increases in intensity on expiration. The aortic valve is the second most common valve involved in acute bacterial endocarditis in intravenous drug abusers. *S. aureus* is again the most common pathogen. Mitral regurgitation (choice **B**) is associated with a pansystolic murmur that increases on expiration. Although viridans streptococci are the most common pathogens causing infective endocarditis, *S. aureus* is the most common pathogen in intravenous drug abusers. The heart sounds associated with mitral stenosis (choice **C**) begin with an opening snap followed by a middiastolic rumbling murmur (unlike the murmur in this case). The bacterial endocarditis is marked by tricuspid involvement (indicated by the pansystolic murmur increasing on inspiration). However, the causal agent is not likely to be *S. epidermidis,* because *S. epidermidis* is most common in bacterial endocarditis associated with prosthetic heart valves, not intravenous drug abuse.

30 **The answer is E** *Preventive Medicine and Public Health*

Medicaid eligibility is a means-tested program, and eligibility is generally determined by the presence of financial hardship. In most states this means that to be eligible, a person's net worth must be less than $2000 (choice **E**). This often requires an individual to expend personal resources for health care before Medicaid can be used. A potential loophole is that a sum of money, usually $10,000 or less, can be transferred to a family member not sooner than 3 years before residence is established. The 3-year requirement can sometimes be at least partially averted if it can be shown that a person, usually a family member, has been providing nursing care and can document valid expenses.

In contrast to Medicaid, Medicare is a Social Security–linked program, and all persons who or whose spouses paid into Social Security are eligible for benefits at an age of 65 years. There is no financial requirement, but Medicare will only pay for doctor care, hospital stays, and usually 10 to 20 days of posthospitalization rehabilitation care. Since 2006, it contributes to payment of prescription drugs. It will not contribute toward the cost of residential care (choice **F**). In contrast, Medicaid almost always covers the cost of medications (choice **A**) and the cost of long-term residential care (choice **B**). It also differs from Medicare in that eligibility does not depend on prior payment into the system (choice **C**) or on reaching a particular age (choice **D**). Specific regulations for Medicaid vary by state, but the federal aspects of both programs are run by the Centers for Medicare and Medicaid Services (CMS) a division of the U.S. Department of Health and Human Services.

31 **The answer is F** *Psychiatry*

About 20% of adult sons of alcoholics are also alcoholic. That this is due to a component of heritability is supported by twin studies and studies of adopted children in which the biologic parent does not raise the child (choice **F**).

Although there is speculation about heritability of other substance dependencies, including cocaine (choice **B**), heroin (choice **C**), and benzodiazepines (choice **E**), the data are much less compelling. Social factors, rather than genetics, appear to be of great significance in causing opiate (choice **A**), psychostimulant (choice **G**), and tobacco (choice **D**) dependency.

32 **The answer is C** *Psychiatry*

Patients with dissociative identity disorder (choice **C**) (formerly called multiple personality disorder) report a much higher incidence of childhood sexual abuse. Such a history is also associated with borderline personality disorder and antisocial traits.

Dependent personality disorder (choice **A**), hypochondriasis (choice **D**), and major depressive disorder (choice **E**) are not so clearly associated with a history of childhood sexual abuse. Children with existing emotional disturbances are more likely to be abused than other children; however, autistic disorder (choice **B**) is not known to be a sequela of abuse.

33 **The answer is B** *Surgery*

Infection is the most common complication of burns. *Pseudomonas aeruginosa* (choice **B**) is the organism most frequently involved and the most common cause of death in burn patients. This organism will cause black patches; however, charred fat can also result in black patches. Burn patients who develop fever do not always have an infection. Thermal injury releases interleukin-1 (IL-1), which can produce fever by stimulating the hypothalamus to synthesize prostaglandins, which in turn stimulate the thermoregulatory center in the brain. This underscores the need for biopsy of suspicious burn wounds for culture to ascertain whether infection is the cause of fever. Antibiotics are not recommended for prophylaxis in burn patients.

Staphylococcus aureus (choice **A**), *Candida albicans* (choice **C**) (usually involved in catheter-related sepsis), and group A streptococcus (choice **D**) are less common offenders. *Staphylococcus pneumoniae* (choice **E**) is rarely involved.

34 **The answer is B** *Psychiatry*

The signs and symptoms are most suggestive of "type A" behavior, described as a constellation of personality traits that include anger, ambition, competitiveness, hostility, and impatience. Such behavior has been associated with an increased risk for coronary artery disease (CAD), at least in middle-aged U.S. citizens (choice **B**).

Cancer (choice **A**), emphysema (choice **C**), migraine (choice **D**), and peptic ulcer disease (choice **E**) have not been as convincingly associated with these traits.

35 **The answer is E** *Medicine*

The patient has zinc deficiency (choice **E**). Zinc is a coenzyme for reactions associated with maintenance of skin and mucosal integrity, wound healing, spermatogenesis, and growth in children. Zinc deficiency commonly occurs in alcohol abuse, rheumatoid arthritis, and acute and chronic diseases. Clinical findings include problems with taste (dysgeusia) and smell (anosmia) and development of an acneiform rash on the face. In addition, there are problems with wound healing, since zinc is a coenzyme for collagenase, which is important in remodeling a wound involving the replacement of type III collagen with type I collagen.

Chromium (choice **A**) is a component of glucose tolerance factor, which helps maintain a normal glucose level. It also facilitates the binding of insulin with its receptors located in adipose tissue and muscle. Deficiency of chromium is associated with impaired glucose tolerance and peripheral neuropathies, neither of which is present in this patient. Copper (choice **B**) is important in scavenging oxygen free radicals, wound healing (provides cross-bridges in collagen and elastic tissue), and iron metabolism (binds iron to transferrin). Copper deficiency most often results from total parenteral nutrition. Clinical findings include iron deficiency, aortic dissection, and poor wound healing. Fluoride deficiency (choice **C**) is associated with dental caries, which are not present in this patient. Selenium (choice **D**) is a cofactor for glutathione peroxidase, which neutralizes hydrogen peroxide and peroxide free radicals in cells (e.g., red blood cell). Deficiency is associated with muscle pain and weakness as well as a cardiomyopathy with biventricular heart failure, none of which are present in this patient.

36 The answer is D *Medicine*

The patient's history of colicky pain (pain followed by a pain-free interval) is characteristic of a small bowel obstruction. It is likely that the patient has developed small bowel adhesions (choice **D**), the most common cause of small bowel obstruction, from previous laparoscopic surgeries for endometriosis. A radiograph in small bowel obstruction shows multiple air–fluid levels with a stepladder configuration.

Direct inguinal hernias (choice **A**) produce a bulge in the middle of the triangle of Hesselbach, which is located above the inguinal ligament. The bulge appears when the patient is standing and disappears when the patient is lying down. This type of hernia is not associated with entrapment of bowel leading to small bowel obstruction. An intussusception (choice **B**), or telescoping of a portion of bowel into another portion of bowel, is uncommon in adults. The nidus for intussusception in adults usually is a polyp or cancer. Obstruction and ischemic damage with bloody diarrhea usually are present. The patient does not have bloody diarrhea. Large bowel infarctions (choice **C**) cause bloody diarrhea (not present in this patient) and localized, noncolicky abdominal pain. Atherosclerosis of a mesenteric artery is the most common cause of large bowel infarction. Volvulus (choice **E**) occurs when bowel (sigmoid colon or cecum) twists around the mesenteric root, resulting in obstruction and strangulation. The affected bowel is distended and visible on a plain abdominal radiograph. In a sigmoid volvulus, the concave portion of dilated bowel points to the left lower quadrant and a barium enema reveals a "bird's beak" due to tapering of the bowel toward the origin of the volvulus. In a cecal volvulus, the distended cecum looks like a coffee bean, and the concavity points to the right lower quadrant.

37 The answer is D *Medicine*

The patient has a qualitative platelet disorder (choice **D**), most likely associated with the use of nonsteroidal antiinflammatory drugs (NSAIDs) for chronic back pain. NSAIDs inhibit platelet cyclooxygenase, which prevents the synthesis of thromboxane A_2 (TXA_2), a platelet aggregator and vasoconstrictor of small vessels. TXA_2 is mainly responsible for producing a temporary platelet plug that stops bleeding in small vessel injury. The temporary plug consists of aggregated platelets held together by fibrinogen. Therefore, blocking the synthesis of TXA_2 causes severe bleeding from small vessel damage incurred by the prostate surgery, because the vessels do not have temporary platelet plugs. The bleeding time, which evaluates platelet function up to the formation of the temporary platelet plug, is prolonged in this patient. The platelet count is a quantitative measurement of platelets and does not evaluate platelet function. The platelet count is normal in patients taking NSAIDs. The APTT evaluates the intrinsic coagulation system (factors XII, XI, IX, and VIII), and the PT evaluates the extrinsic coagulation system (factor VII). NSAIDs do not interfere with the coagulation system, which explains why results of both studies are normal in the patient.

Antiphospholipid antibodies (choice **A**), such as anticardiolipin antibodies and lupus anticoagulant, are directed against phospholipids bound to plasma proteins. These antibodies are more often associated with thrombosis syndromes (e.g., strokes, recurrent spontaneous abortions) than with bleeding disorders, as in this patient. Circulating anticoagulants (choice **B**) are antibodies that inhibit specific coagulation factors (e.g., antibodies against factor VIII), causing prolongation of the APTT and/or PT. However, the patient has a normal APTT and PT, which excludes a circulating anticoagulant from the differential diagnosis. In a coagulation factor deficiency (choice **C**), the APTT and/or the PT are prolonged. The patient has a normal APTT and PT, which exclude a coagulation factor deficiency from the differential diagnosis. The prostate gland is rich in fibrinolytic agents (e.g., urokinase) that activate plasminogen, causing the release of plasmin. Plasmin destroys some of the coagulation factors (e.g., fibrinogen, factor V, factor VIII), which prolongs the APTT and PT. However, since the patient has a normal APTT and PT, primary fibrinolysis is excluded as a cause of bleeding (choice **E**).

38 The answer is A *Medicine*

The patient has prolapsing internal hemorrhoids (choice **A**). Internal hemorrhoids are a plexus of superior hemorrhoidal veins located above the dentate line, which are covered by mucosa. The most common cause is straining at stool, often causing the hemorrhoids to protrude from the anal opening. The protrusion reduces spontaneously. Passage of bright red blood per rectum and a mucoid perianal discharge that often soils the underwear are common problems. Unless there is thrombosis of the prolapsed hemorrhoids, there usually is no pain.

Anal fissures (choice **D**) cause acute anal pain in adults. A tearing or cutting type of pain is associated with defecation. However, anal fissures are often associated with bright red blood. Angiodysplasia (dilated vascular channels in the submucosa) (choice **B**) typically develops in the cecum of older individuals. Angiodysplasia is associated with intermittent hemorrhage (hematochezia) with the passage of bright red blood. Colorectal cancer (choice **C**) is associated with blood coating and mixing with stools. There is no prolapse of the cancer through the anal opening or soiling of the underwear by a mucoid discharge. Ischemic colitis (choice **E**) occurs in older individuals. Ischemic colitis is associated with pain in the splenic flexure after eating and with bloody stools.

39 The answer is E   *Medicine*

The patient most likely has breast cancer that has metastasized to the bone marrow (choice **E**) causing displacement of immature erythrocytes and leukocytes from the bone marrow into the peripheral blood; this will result in a "leukoerythroblastic smear." In women, breast cancer is the most common cancer that metastasizes to bone. The vertebral column is the most common site due to the Batson venous plexus. This plexus extends along the entire length of the vertebral column and has branches that connect to the vena cava and branches that extend into the vertebral bodies. Therefore, a tumor embolus in the venous system has easy access to the vertebral column. The treatment of choice for pain due to bone metastasis is radiation.

Although acute myelogenous leukemia (choice **A**) occurs in this patient's age bracket, it usually causes thrombocytopenia, generalized lymphadenopathy, and hepatosplenomegaly and is characterized by the presence of myeloblasts in the peripheral blood. None of these findings are present in this patient. Chronic myeloproliferative disorders (choice **B**) include polycythemia vera, chronic myelogenous leukemia, myelofibrosis and myeloid metaplasia, and essential thrombocythemia. They are all associated with splenomegaly, which is not present in this patient. A leukemoid reaction (choice **C**) is a benign increase in leukocytes, often exceeding 50,000/mm^3. It usually occurs in response to infection (e.g., tuberculosis) and is not associated with anemia, which is present in this patient. The most common malignant plasma cell disorder is multiple myeloma (choice **D**). It produces lytic lesions in the bone and prominent rouleaux (RBCs with a stack of coins appearance), the latter are not present in this patient.

40 The answer is B   *Medicine*

The clinical findings in this patient are due to hypoglycemia. The most common overall cause of hypoglycemia is excessive insulin in a person with insulin-dependent diabetes. Hypoglycemia is precipitated by administration of an excessive dose of insulin, increased physical activity, delay in eating a meal, fluctuations in absorption in various administration sites, and autonomic neuropathy impairing counterregulatory mechanisms. The adrenergic symptoms of hypoglycemia include perspiration, tachycardia, increased salivation, and restlessness. These symptoms can be blunted if the patient is taking a β-blocker (e.g., propranolol), thus making the diagnosis more difficult. Lack of Kussmaul's respiration (deep respiration) and no smell of ketones on the breath are clues that ketoacidosis is not present in this patient. Immediate measurement of blood glucose (choice **B**) with glucose oxidase-impregnated paper strips or a glucometer is easily accomplished in the emergency department, so therapy can be initiated. Patients who are conscious should be given oral feedings of fruit juice. Comatose patients are usually given an intravenous (IV) infusion of 50% dextrose in water. If IV glucose is not available, 1 mg of glucagon is given intramuscularly.

A complete blood count (CBC) (choice **A**), serum electrolytes (choice **C**), a drug screen (choice **D**), and arterial blood gas (ABG) determination (choice **E**) are not appropriate initial steps in the management of patients with insulin-dependent diabetes and the classic adrenergic symptoms of hypoglycemia.

41 The answer is H   *Obstetrics and Gynecology*

The most common cause of vaginal bleeding in a prepubertal girl is a vaginal foreign body. However, a cystic grapelike mass at the introitus suggests a more worrisome cause. Sarcoma botryoides (choice **H**), also known as rhabdomyosarcoma of the vagina, is a malignancy in infants and young children that arises from embryonal rhabdomyoblasts (ancestral muscle cells). The tumor resembles a bunch of grapes. It has a generally good prognosis with conservative surgery followed by chemotherapy. It is a rare malignant tumor of the female reproductive tract, most commonly seen in girls under 8 years of age. The most common symptom is abnormal vaginal bleeding.

42 The answer is D *Obstetrics and Gynecology*

Intermittent vaginal bleeding between normal menses is suggestive of an anatomic lesion. The absence of postcoital bleeding makes it unlikely that the bleeding is caused by invasive cervical carcinoma. The normal pelvic examination rules out a lower genital tract lesion such as vulvar neoplasms, vaginal varicosities, or cervical polyps. Upper tract causes of vaginal bleeding include endometrial polyps or submucosal leiomyomas. The presence of an asymmetrically enlarged, firm, nontender uterus is suggestive of subserosal or intramural uterine myomas. The presence of bleeding suggests the likelihood of a submucosal leiomyoma (choice **D**) as the cause.

43 The answer is I *Obstetrics and Gynecology*

The key in identifying the most likely cause of the increasing vaginal bleeding in this case is its linkage to increasing pain with her menses. Pain with menses is known as dysmenorrhea, and this scenario describes secondary dysmenorrhea. Secondary dysmenorrhea is caused by anatomic abnormalities such as endometriosis, chronic pelvic inflammatory disease, leiomyomas, or adenomyosis. The finding of a diffusely enlarged, globular, soft, tender uterus is classic for adenomyosis (choice **I**). Ordering a β-hCG test is critical to rule out pregnancy, the most common cause of an enlarged uterus in the reproductive years. The history of treatment for cervical dysplasia is only an incidental historical finding.

44 The answer is G *Obstetrics and Gynecology*

The history of irregular, unpredictable menstrual bleeding is strongly suggestive of an anovulatory cause. The absence of cramping and pain is consistent with anovulation. (Ovulatory cycles typically are associated with cramping from the release of prostaglandins triggered by the necrosis from endometrial spiral arteriolar spasm caused by the decrease in progesterone production from the corpus luteum.) With anovulation, the unopposed estrogen results in simple endometrial hyperplasia without atypia (choice **G**). Management is by administering cyclic progestins or combination oral contraceptives.

45 The answer is F *Obstetrics and Gynecology*

A history of intermittent vaginal bleeding between normal menses is suggestive of an anatomic lesion. The additional finding of painless postcoital bleeding makes one highly suspicious for a cervical lesion such cervical polyps or invasive cervical carcinoma (choice **F**). She has many risk factors for cervical neoplasia including multiple sexual partners and a long history of cigarette smoking. The long gap to the present from her last Pap smear is troublesome. She will need colposcopy and a cervical biopsy for diagnosis.

46 The answer is B *Obstetrics and Gynecology*

The most common cause of vaginal bleeding in a prepubertal girl is a vaginal foreign body (choice **B**). To confirm that this is the case requires visual inspection of the vagina by a speculum or a fiberoptic scope, usually under sedation. In this case, the lack of pubertal changes on examination (e.g., breast budding, pubic hair) makes precocious puberty unlikely, and the absence of a growth as in case 41 tends to rule out other possible causes of bleeding. Although an unlikely possibility in a 6-year-old, the ingestion of steroid contraceptives could stimulate the endometrium resulting in bleeding; this possibility could be checked by obtaining a medical history.

47 The answer is C *Obstetrics and Gynecology*

Vaginal bleeding in a postmenopausal woman must be assumed to be endometrial carcinoma (choice **C**) until proved otherwise. A complete workup will require endometrial biopsy and hysteroscopy. The presence of a normal-sized uterus on pelvic examination cannot rule out endometrial cancer. The most likely cause of endometrial carcinoma is long periods of unopposed estrogen. This patient has many risk factors that include never being pregnant (with 9 months of high progesterone levels), absence of oral contraceptive use (which provides regular progestin effects that stabilize the endometrium) along with obesity (with peripheral adipose cell conversion of adrenal androgens to estrogens).

48 **The answer is A**   *Obstetrics and Gynecology*

This scenario displays the classic triad of ectopic pregnancy (choice **A**): vaginal bleeding, unilateral lower abdominal pelvic pain, and amenorrhea. If this triad is accompanied by hypotension and tachycardia, the diagnosis would be ruptured ectopic pregnancy with hemoperitoneum, and the management would be emergency laparotomy to stop the bleeding. With stable vital signs, this case is suggestive of unruptured ectopic pregnancy. The diagnosis is confirmed by failure to see an intrauterine gestational sac with transvaginal sonography plus the presence of a quantitative serum β-hCG titer above 1500 mIU. (A gestational sac from a normal intrauterine pregnancy would be visible when the serum β-hCG titer is above 1500 mIU.) The most likely site of the ectopic pregnancy is in the distal oviduct. Management is by parenteral methotrexate if the pregnancy is early (serum β-hCG titer below 6000 mIU) and by laparoscopy surgery if the pregnancy is an advanced pregnancy (serum β-hCG titer above 1500 mIU).

49 **The answer is E**   *Obstetrics and Gynecology*

This girl shows the classic symptoms of gestational trophoblastic disease and is probably carrying a hydatiform mole (choice **E**). In the United States the frequency of trophoblastic disease is 1 per 1500 pregnancies. However in some developing countries the rate is 1 per 125 pregnancies. The risk is increased with lower economic status and age below 18 or above 40 years.

50 **The answer is J**   *Obstetrics and Gynecology*

This woman has an advanced case of an ovarian carcinoma (choice **J**). The overall lifetime risk of a woman developing ovarian cancer is 1.6%, if one first-degree relative has had it, the risk is 5%, with two affected first-degree relatives the risk is 7%; if a woman carries a *BRCA2* gene her lifetime risk is 25%, but a *BRCA1* gene raises the risk to 45%. Unfortunately, most early ovarian neoplasms, whether benign or malignant, are essentially asymptomatic. Some are discovered during routine physicals, and many benign ones resolve without treatment; transvaginal sonography and CA 125 testing are used to screen very high risk women but are too insensitive to use on the general population. As a consequence of all these factors, some 75% of women are first diagnosed with ovarian cancer at an advanced stage. The overall 5-year survival is 17% with advanced disease with distal spread, 36% with local metastases, and 89% if discovered early.

test 11

Questions

Single Best Choice Directions: This section consists of numbered statements or questions followed by a list of potential answers; you are to select the ONE best answer.

1 A 21-year-old nulligravid woman who has been married and sexually active for 2 years comes to the outpatient office complaining of pain with intercourse. She explains that the pain is worse with deep penetration. Although they have frequent sex and neither she nor her husband used any type of contraceptive since her marriage, she has not been able to get pregnant. The onset of her menarche was at age 11. Her menses were originally irregular but were regular and predictable for the past 8 years. She has had pain with her menses as well as pain with bowel movements for the past 4 years. Laparoscopic examination shows diffuse involvement of her peritoneal surfaces with thickened, scarred, "powder-burn" implants of various sizes. Which of the following statements is correct about her probable diagnosis?

(A) The most common site is the uterosacral ligaments.
(B) Medical treatment is seldom curative.
(C) The average age of onset is older than 35 years.
(D) The chance of malignant transformation is high.
(E) It is associated with uterine leiomyomata.

2 At a routine well child visit a mother reports that her infant is able to babble, coo, and form a social smile. When supine, the infant is able to follow an object 90° from the midline through an arc of 180°. When prone, the infant is able to lift its head 45°. The infant is also able to roll from the prone to the supine position. Which of the following is the most likely age of this infant?

(A) Newborn
(B) 1 month
(C) 2 months
(D) 3 months
(E) 4 months

3 A 3-year-old Caucasian boy of Scandinavian descent, who had been developing normally, contracted otitis media. Because he had not felt well he missed two meals. Suddenly he became lethargic, started vomiting, had a violent seizure, and became comatose. His parents called 911, and he was put on a saline IV drip and taken to the emergency department, where they immediately ordered a complete blood count, a liver panel, a chemistry panel and a urinalysis. A finger prick test showed that the child was hypoglycemic but not ketonic. In taking a history from the mother, the attending physician finds out that what would have been an older sibling died mysteriously in her sleep as an infant. He immediately orders the saline IV drip to be changed to a 10% glucose solution, and shortly thereafter, the patient starts to recover. Several hours latter when the laboratory results become available; it was determined that his serum glucose value had been 35 mg/dL and that he had slightly elevated serum BUN, ammonia, and uric acid levels; an anion gap metabolic acidosis; and his liver enzyme values were also elevated; however, both his serum and urine ketone levels were zero. The child most likely has which of the following?

(A) Glucose 6-phosphatase deficiency
(B) Medium chain acyl-CoA deficiency
(C) Carnitine acyltransferase deficiency
(D) Primary hyperinsulinemia
(E) Acute intermittent porphyria

4 A 32-month-old male child had been unresponsive to normal stimuli since birth. He didn't smile or babble and was indifferent to his mother's attempts to kiss, hug, or socialize with him. He also had bizarre behavior patterns including repeating meaningless motions and banging on the floor or walls, and although able to talk, his choice of words and protosentence structure was peculiar. However, he did like to play with his toy piano and could produce simple melodies. Physically he seemed healthy. In which of the following ways does this developmental pattern trend typically describe diagnostic features of autistic disorder?

(A) It is a qualitative disturbance of normal development.
(B) It shows progressive deterioration of function over the developmental period.
(C) There is an absence of metabolic diseases.
(D) He showed evidence of a potential musical talent, presence of areas of brilliant accomplishment.
(E) Although noncommunicative, he seems of normal intelligence.

5 In 1955, a now 54-year-old woman contracted a mild case of poliomyelitis from which she completely recovered. In high school and during college she participated in sports, and after college, she participated in an annual local marathon until 1986 when she had to pull out of the race because of fatigue, which she attributed to a normal consequence of aging and not being in top physical shape. Since then there has been a slow progressive weakening of her leg muscles that was not noticeable on a day-by-day basis. However, she now consults a physician because her calf muscles have begun to atrophy, and she has trouble straightening her back. The most probable diagnosis is which of the following?

(A) Postpolio syndrome
(B) Amyotrophic lateral sclerosis
(C) Osteoarthritis
(D) Tendinitis
(E) Guillain-Barré disease

6 The peripheral smear shown below is from a 65-year-old man who complains of tiredness and generalized weakness. A complete blood count (CBC) reveals a hemoglobin level of 7.0 g/dL (normal, 13.5–17.5 g/dL), a mean corpuscular volume (MCV) of 62 mm³ (normal, 80–100 mm³), a red cell distribution width (RDW) of 20 (normal, 10 ± 5), a leukocyte count of 8500 cells/mL (normal, 1500–11,000 cells/mL), and a platelet count of 650,000 cells/mL (normal, 150,000–450,000 cells/mL). The leukocyte differential is unremarkable except for the presence of absolute monocytosis. The serum alkaline phosphatase concentration is 225 U/L (normal, 20–70 U/L), the γ-glutamyltransferase is 175 U/L (normal, 6–35 U/L), and the lactate dehydrogenase concentration is 250 U/L (normal, 45–90 U/L). The total bilirubin and transaminase levels are normal. In the course of the patient's workup, a barium enema reveals a polypoid mass in the ascending colon. Additional studies on this patient should reveal which of the following?

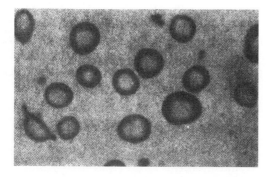

(A) Normal percentage iron saturation
(B) Increased serum ferritin level
(C) Metastatic lesions to the liver
(D) Decreased total iron-binding capacity (TIBC)
(E) Normal red blood cell distribution width (RDW)

7 A newborn infant is noted to be cyanotic at 24 hours of age. A loud, harsh, systolic ejection murmur is transmitted widely but is heard best at the head at the upper sternal border. A workup for heart disease is initiated. A coeur en sabot image of the heart is seen on chest roentgenogram. The electrocardiogram demonstrates right axis deviation and evidence of right ventricular hypertrophy. A two-dimensional echocardiogram establishes the definitive diagnosis to be consistent with tetralogy of Fallot. Which of the following characteristics primarily determines the prognosis in this patient?

(A) Degree of pulmonic stenosis
(B) Overriding aorta
(C) Level of hypoxemia at birth
(D) Size of the ventricular septal defect
(E) Degree of right ventricular hypertrophy

8 A pediatrician is examining a 2-week-old infant who is brought by his mother for a well child check. Review of the medical record shows that the mother is a 28-year-old who had prenatal care. She did not smoke, take drugs, or use alcohol during her pregnancy. Results of all diagnostic studies for sexually transmitted diseases are negative. The infant was born by spontaneous vaginal delivery and weighed 7 lb 6 oz (3.3 kg). At this visit the baby weighs 7 lb 12 oz (3.5 kg). The mother states that she is breast-feeding the infant without difficulty. During the physical examination the physician noted that the infant symmetrically abducts and extends his extremities after a loud noise and then begins to cry. This reflex is known as which of the following?

(A) Asymmetric tonic neck reflex (ATNR)
(B) Parachute reflex
(C) Moro reflex
(D) Hand-grasp reflex (grasping reflex)
(E) Protective equilibrium reflex

9 An 18-year-old male left the Amish community in Lancaster County, Pennsylvania, in a rebellious mood and joined the army. He passed the preinduction physical with no problems but subsequent postinduction studies raised questions. The following data were obtained: red blood cell count, 3.4 × 10⁶/μL (normal range, 4.7–6.1 × 10⁶/μL); hematocrit, 26% (normal range, 39–49%); hemoglobin concentration, 9 g/dL (normal range, 13.6–17.5 g/dL); reticulocyte count, 8% (normal range, 1–2%); white cell count,

$5.0 \times 10^3/\mu L$ (normal range, $4.8\text{--}10.8 \times 10^3/\mu L$), indirect bilirubin value, 2 mg/dL (normal range, 0.1–0.7 mg/dL). Additionally, the basic red cell morphology is normal with no Heinz bodies but a few crenated forms. Electrophoresis shows no abnormal hemoglobin (Hb) with a normal ratio of Hb A, Hb A_2, and Hb F. Results of the Coombs, Ham, and Donath-Landsteiner antibody tests were all negative, and no cold agglutinins were found. This young man most likely had which of the following conditions?

(A) Paroxysmal nocturnal hemoglobinuria
(B) Pyruvate kinase deficiency
(C) Hereditary spherocytosis
(D) Glucose 6-phosphate dehydrogenase deficiency
(E) Hemoglobin C disease
(F) Paroxysmal cold hemoglobinuria
(G) Autoimmune hemolytic anemia

10 A 35-year-old man has repeated sinus infections, chronic cough, and dyspnea. He does not smoke cigarettes. A chest radiograph shows multiple nodular masses in the lungs, some of which have central cavitation. Urinalysis shows numerous red blood cells (RBCs) and RBC casts. The serum blood urea nitrogen (BUN) and serum creatinine levels are both increased. Which of the following laboratory findings is also most likely present?

(A) Anti-streptolysin O (ASO) antibodies
(B) c-Antineutrophil cytoplasmic antibodies
(C) Hepatitis B surface antigen (HBsAg)
(D) p-Antineutrophil cytoplasmic antibodies
(E) Serum antinuclear antibodies (ANA)

11 A 65-year-old woman comes to the office with a 2-day history of fever, chills, and a cough productive of purulent sputum. She has a history of smoking two packs of cigarettes a day for the last 45 years. A chest x-ray shows a right lower lobe consolidation. Which of the following organisms is the most likely cause of her infection?

(A) *Mycoplasma pneumoniae*
(B) *Haemophilus influenzae*
(C) *Streptococcus pneumoniae*
(D) *Legionella pneumophila*
(E) *Coccidioides immitis*

12 A 36-year-old man complains of stomach pain. When the physician tries to ask him questions, he answers, "You're the doctor; you figure it out." He also states that he does not like the physician's attitude and will sue if he is not treated appropriately. "If you make me leave the hospital," he adds, "I'll slit my wrists in the parking lot and it will be your fault." Which of the following is the best first response to this patient?

(A) "Without better cooperation, I'll be forced to order a stat barium enema and then probably have to do exploratory surgery."
(B) "You make me feel unable to help you, and that hurts me personally."
(C) "You seem angry with me, and I'd like to know why."
(D) "You're an irritating person, and that makes me angry."
(E) "I'm sure that you'd like my colleague better—I'll page her right away."

13 A mother becomes concerned as her daughter approaches puberty, because her husband has always played a prominent role in raising her and she always looks to him for signs of affection. The mother fears that their obvious intimacy will lead to sexual abuse, particularly as the girl develops more prominent womanly attributes. As a consequence of her fears, she attends a seminar concerning childhood sexual abuse with her husband during which they learned about many facets concerning the subject. Which of the following statements did they learn is the most accurate?

(A) Increased involvement of fathers in raising children decreases the risk of sexual abuse.
(B) More men than women have a history of being abused.
(C) More traditional, less democratic families are associated with a decreased risk of childhood sexual abuse.
(D) Mothers who sexually abuse children are often gregarious and socially active.
(E) Most abused children were abused by fathers or stepfathers.

14 A 28-year-old female who is an Olympic cyclist is seen in the orthopedic clinic with complaints of numbness in her fingertips and pain in her left hand that occasionally radiates up her arm. She is often awakened by the symptoms. On physical examination, there is decreased sensation over the radial 3½ digits of the hand and results of the Phalen's test are positive. Which of the following is the most likely diagnosis?

(A) Carpal tunnel syndrome
(B) Pronator syndrome
(C) Cubital tunnel syndrome
(D) Ulnar nerve entrapment at the wrist
(E) De Quervain's disease

15 A 62-year-old man was a passenger in a car driven by his son when they crashed into a car making an illegal left turn. He was not wearing a seat belt and he hit his head on the dashboard. Within minutes the paramedics arrived on the scene of the accident. When they examined him they determine that his heart rate is 120 beats/min, and his blood pressure is 80/60 mm Hg. In addition his skin is cold and clammy. Which of the following hemodynamic changes is most likely present?

(A) Decreased hemoglobin concentration
(B) Decreased red blood cell (RBC) count
(C) Increased left ventricular end-diastolic pressure
(D) Increased pulmonary capillary hydrostatic pressure
(E) Increased total peripheral arteriolar resistance

16 A married couple has been trying to have children of their own for the past 22 years and thinking that impossible are seriously considering adoption at this time. They think they may be getting a little old to get a newborn infant and consider an older child, but they worry about the psychologic stability of a child who may have been or at least feel he or she was abandoned by the biologic parent or who may have been overlooked in the past by other couples looking to adopt. Which of the following statements about adoptees is most accurate?

(A) About 50% of adoptions are considered "successful".
(B) Improved family environments rarely raise IQ scores in such individuals.
(C) Narcissistic injury is a significant psychologic issue in such individuals.
(D) Rates of psychopathology among adopted individuals are comparable to the rates among individuals reared by their biologic parents.
(E) The relationships of adoptees with their adoptive parents are generally no more troubled than the relationships of individuals with their biologic parents.

17 A 2-year-old child has gait abnormalities, appears awkward, and frequently falls. Physical examination is pertinent for hypotonic extremities and absent deep tendon reflexes bilaterally. A lumbar puncture is performed and shows increased cerebrospinal fluid (CSF) protein with a normal glucose and cell count. The patient's urinary sediment stains positively with toluidine blue. The physician tells the parents that the prognosis is poor and that they should expect deterioration in the child's intellectual function and developmental milestones, as well as swallowing and feeding difficulties. Death usually occurs in these patients by age

5–6 years. Which of the following is the most likely diagnosis?

(A) Phenylketonuria
(B) Metachromatic leukodystrophy
(C) Krabbe's disease
(D) Fabry's disease
(E) Adrenoleukodystrophy

18 A 40-year-old African-American woman complains of difficulty with breathing and blurry vision in the right eye. Physical examination reveals a miotic right pupil and circumcorneal ciliary body congestion, a violaceous rash on the nose and cheeks, and dry, late inspiratory crackles at both lung bases. A chest radiograph shows bilateral hilar adenopathy and reticulonodular densities throughout both lung fields. Which of the following results of pulmonary function tests would most likely be reported?

(A) Decreased arterial pH
(B) Increased forced expiratory volume in 1 sec to forced vital capacity ratio (FEV_1/FVC)
(C) Increased functional residual capacity (FRC)
(D) Increased residual volume (RV)
(E) Increased total lung capacity (TLC)

19 A 67-year old man bought an old home near Shreveport, Louisiana, and decided to clean out an adjacent shed that was dark and dank and obviously had not been disturbed for a long time. While working he feels a slight stinglike burning sensation on his arm, but thinks nothing of it. Later that day while washing up after his days work he notices a reddish spot with a clear center, like a bull's eye, on the underside of his forearm. The following morning the spot has formed a pustule that filled with blood, which breaks 3 days later, forming a necrotic craterlike lesion. He then develops generalized symptoms including malaise, an itchy rash, headache, nausea with vomiting, and low-grade fever, inducing him to consult a physician who makes a diagnosis and prescribes dapsone and rest. The doctor further tells him the systemic symptoms should clear up shortly, but if they don't, to make another appointment. He also recommends icing the arm to reduce pain and tells him the sore on his arm will continue to fester for a while but should heal spontaneously in 6 to 8 weeks; in the meantime it is best to simply keep it clean and leave it alone. Which of the following is the most probable diagnosis?

(A) A red fire ant bite
(B) A black widow spider bite
(C) A bite by the deer tick, *Ixodes scapularis*
(D) A brown recluse spider bite
(E) A scorpion sting

20 A 52-year-old man who is a cattle rancher complains that he has become terrified of flying in private planes since an acquaintance of his was killed in one. However, flying is a necessary part of running his enterprise. He knows his fear is irrational, but no matter how important to him, he fears that he will not be able to make himself fly. An amateur psychologist friend tells him his problem reflects a fear of being abandoned because his father ran out of the family when he was a child. Which of the following would indicate a specific phobia in this patient?

(A) Patient believes his fear is irrational.

(B) Patient has a history of separation anxiety from childhood.

(C) Patient has no detectable unconscious symbolism behind his fear.

(D) Patient is not able to fly even when absolutely necessary.

(E) Patient's fears are well grounded in reality.

21 A 50-year-old woman complains of generalized pruritus. Physical examination shows nontender hepatomegaly and excoriation marks in areas where she has been scratching. Initial laboratory studies show increased serum alkaline phosphatase and γ-glutamyl transferase (GGT) levels, and a normal total bilirubin value. Results of a serum antinuclear antibody (ANA) test is negative. Ultrasonography of the gallbladder is negative for gallstones. Which of the following additional laboratory findings is most likely to be reported?

(A) Antimitochondrial antibodies

(B) Anti–smooth muscle antibodies

(C) Increased serum α-fetoprotein

(D) Increased serum IgG

(E) Increased triglycerides

22 Findings of a routine physical examination of an asymptomatic 20-year-old African-American woman are normal. Urinalysis shows RBCs; however, casts are not present. Phase contrast microscopy of the RBCs in the urine shows uniformly normal-appearing RBCs. Results of a urine culture are negative and those of a peripheral smear and renal ultrasonography are normal. Laboratory studies show normal serum blood urea nitrogen, serum creatinine, and hemoglobin levels. Which of the following tests should be ordered?

(A) Bone marrow examination

(B) Cystoscopy

(C) Renal biopsy

(D) Serum ferritin

(E) Sickle cell screen

23 A 17-year-old woman, gravida 1, para 0, has come to the outpatient office for a routine prenatal visit. She is currently at 25 weeks' gestation with a singleton pregnancy. She has a 10-year history of asthma but is not requiring any pharmacologic bronchodilator therapy. She is not currently having respiratory complaints or symptoms. An obstetric sonogram performed 3 weeks ago showed a female fetus with grossly normal anatomic findings and appropriate size for gestational age. The patient is scheduled to undergo pulmonary evaluation and spirometry testing today. Which of the following statements regarding her current spirometry findings are most likely to be true compared with her last pulmonary assessment prior to pregnancy?

(A) Respiratory rate is increased

(B) Vital capacity is decreased

(C) Minute ventilation is increased

(D) Function residual capacity remains unchanged

(E) Tidal volume is decreased

24 A 7-year-old boy presents to the emergency department with his father, complaining of pain and decreased ability of the boy to bear weight on his right foot. There is no evidence of cellulites. The father states that 5 days ago the patient stepped on a rusty nail that not only pierced through his tennis shoe but also punctured his right foot. At that time, the patient's foot was cleaned with soap and water. The patient's immunizations are up to date. The physician suspects that the child has osteomyelitis. Which of the following is the most likely pathogen in this patient?

(A) *Staphylococcus saprophyticus*

(B) *Clostridium tetani*

(C) *Staphylococcus epidermidis*

(D) *Pseudomonas aeruginosa*

(E) *Streptococcus pyogenes*

25 A 13-year-old boy presents to his physician with a sore throat. The patient had been in his usual state of good health until 2 days ago, when he started to developed this sore throat. He has been taking acetaminophen for the pain without relief. In fact, according to the patient's mother he appears to be getting worse. On physical examination, he is noted to have a temperature of 103°F (39.4°C). He appears quiet and uncomfortable. Additional pertinent findings are torticollis, trismus, and drooling. You are unable to visualize the patient's throat adequately. However, when answering questions the patient's speech is muffled. Which of the following is the most likely diagnosis?

(A) Epiglottitis

(B) Croup

(C) Peritonsillar abscess

(D) Tonsillar lymphoma

(E) Uvulitis

26 A 16-year-old boy has the onset over several weeks of disorganized thinking. His utterances are clearly enunciated but impossible to understand, and he seems perplexed by events around him. He seems agitated, unable to sit or stand still, and suspicious of the actions and thoughts of others. Which of the following would suggest that the boy's symptoms include a flight of ideas?

(A) The sudden disappearance of thoughts from consciousness

(B) Catatonic excitement

(C) Illogical thought processes

(D) Rapid shifting from one thought to another

(E) An irrational belief that one has special powers

27 A 33-year-old man with a history of bipolar disorder is brought into the hospital with a self-inflicted stab wound. He admits to suicidal intent. He had been on lithium therapy for the past 4 years. However, because he had been doing well since starting therapy, he decided he was cured and stopped taking the drug 2 months ago. For purposes of determining treatment for this acute mood episode, which of the following will best distinguish mania from depression?

(A) An altered level of activity

(B) The presence of psychosis

(C) The quality of mood

(D) The presence of insomnia

(E) The presence of known pathophysiology

28 A 24-year-old woman, gravida 1, para 0, is 20 weeks' pregnant. She recently had a mononucleosis-like syndrome with right upper quadrant tenderness. Laboratory testing showed elevation of liver enzymes. While working as a nurse in a neonatal intensive care unit, she had been taking care of a newborn that was small for gestational age and had hepatosplenomegaly. Workup of the neonate showed chorioretinitis, microcephaly, and intracranial calcifications. Which of the following statements is true regarding the probable infection this woman acquired from the neonate?

(A) No specific treatment exists.

(B) Cesarean delivery of her baby is recommended.

(C) Risk of fetal infection is highest during the first trimester.

(D) Gamma globulin is useful for prophylaxis after exposure.

(E) Most infected infants are asymptomatic.

29 A 52-year-old woman, gravida 4, para 4, comes to the outpatient office complaining of hot flashes, which occur without warning. At night the episodes result in profuse diaphoresis, leaving her nightgown and bed sheets wet. She is experiencing less lubrication and vaginal secretions with intercourse, leading to pain and discomfort. She also is having mood swings and difficulty concentrating. Her last menstrual period was 3 months ago. She is 168 cm (66 in) tall and weighs 61 kg (135 lb). She smokes one pack of cigarettes a day and is a social user of alcohol. Which of the following is most likely to be found on laboratory blood testing?

(A) Elevated cortisol

(B) Decreased luteinizing hormone (LH)

(C) Elevated follicle-stimulating hormone (FSH)

(D) Decreased free thyroxin

(E) Elevated androstenedione

30 A 24-year-old woman complains of chronic and diffuse body pain since a bicycle accident 6 months ago in which she sustained abrasions and a wrist sprain. Despite lack of objective findings, she refuses to engage in even minimal exercise and says that she can't drive. Which of the following features would be most important in making a diagnosis of pain disorder?

(A) The pain is largely mediated by psychologic factors.

(B) A physical lesion will be determined by imaging studies.

(C) No personality pathology is present.

(D) There is not a good response to biofeedback therapy.

(E) Worker's compensation and legal issues are not involved.

31 A 26-year-old woman seeks medical attention because of amenorrhea and back pain. She weighs 88 pounds (40 kg) and she has fine downy hair on her face and back. When asked how she feels about her appearance, the woman says that she feels fat. Results of a urine test for pregnancy are negative. Which of the following laboratory findings would most likely be reported?

(A) Decreased concentration of serum adrenocorticotropic hormone

(B) Decreased concentration of serum cortisol

(C) Decreased concentration of serum gonadotropins

(D) Decreased concentration of serum growth hormone

(E) Increased concentration of serum gonadotropin-releasing hormone

32 A 53-year-old man of Scotch-Irish ancestry consults a physician because in the past few months he has developed joint and abdominal pains. Moreover he lacks energy, feels so tired that even getting up in the morning is difficult, has lost interest in sex, and has had chronic diarrhea with greasy stools. Physical examination reveals a pale grayish bronze skin color, hepatosplenomegaly, and an irregular heart rhythm. A finger stick glucose analysis shows a serum glucose value of 452 mg/dL. Which of the following laboratory findings will also most likely be present?

(A) Decreased serum ceruloplasmin
(B) Decreased serum iron
(C) Decreased small bowel reabsorption of D-xylose
(D) Increased serum ferritin
(E) Increased total iron-binding capacity

33 A 60-year-old man, who is an alcoholic and a cigarette smoker for the past 40 years, complains of difficulty swallowing solids but not liquids. In addition, he has progressive weight loss and weakness. A barium swallow reveals an obstructive lesion in the midesophagus. Which of the following is the most likely diagnosis?

(A) Diffuse esophageal spasm
(B) Zenker's diverticulum
(C) Achalasia
(D) Squamous cell esophageal carcinoma
(E) Plummer-Vinson syndrome
(F) An esophageal adenocarcinoma

34 Sigmund Freud is often described as the father of modern psychiatry, and throughout most of the 20th century his theories were refined by others such as Jung and Klein, all of whom used the process of psychoanalysis to root out and cure the subconscious factors underlying the problem. During the last quarter of the 20th century, psychoanalytic therapy started to be replaced by various schools of psychotherapy including somatic, psychodynamic, behavorial, cognitive, and humanistic. Which of the following is the most common component shared by the various schools of psychotherapy and psychoanalysis?

(A) An explanation of pathologic behavior
(B) A firm concept of the unconscious
(C) A long duration of treatment
(D) A dependency on drugs to alter behavior
(E) A belief that the privacy of the interpersonal experience must take precedence over other considerations

35 A centrally located lung mass is removed from a 60-year-old man who has smoked two packs of cigarettes a day for 30 years. A hematoxylin and eosin–stained section of a bronchoscopy biopsy specimen shows eosinophilic staining cells with keratin pearls. Which of the following findings is frequently associated with this type of tumor?

(A) Hypercalcemia
(B) Hypocalcemia
(C) Hypercortisolism
(D) Hyponatremia
(E) Polycythemia

36 Ever since she was a toddler a girl was nagged by her mother to stand up straight. As she became older she had little interest in sports because of shortness of breath. She also constantly complained that the shorts and slacks her mother purchased for her were shorter in one leg than the other. In the sixth grade at the age of 12 years, a school nurse asked her to strip to the waist and bend forward at a 90° angle while she looked at her back. On the basis of this examination the nurse called in her parents to recommend that the girl see an orthopedic surgeon. Which of the following is the most likely diagnosis suspected by the nurse?

(A) Ankylosing spondylitis
(B) Pott's disease of the spine
(C) Idiopathic scoliosis
(D) Osteomyelitis
(E) Neurofibromatosis

37 A 52-year-old man with chronic bronchitis due to cigarette smoking is being treated with theophylline. He also has peptic ulcer disease and is taking cimetidine to control gastric acidity. It is determined that in this man the normal therapeutic drug level for theophylline is in the toxic range. Assuming that the patient is taking the appropriate dose of theophylline, what is the most likely cause for the toxic levels of the drug?

(A) Decreased liver metabolism of the drug
(B) Decreased liver uptake of the drug
(C) Increased gastrointestinal reabsorption of the drug
(D) Increased renal excretion of the drug

38 A 29-year-old woman has retro-orbital pain and blurry vision in the left eye. Physical examination shows flame hemorrhages around the disc vessels and a swollen optic disc. After treatment with systemic corticosteroids, the patient's vision is restored to normal. A few months later, the patient has slurred speech, an ataxic gait, and weakness and paresthesias in the arms and legs that eventually remit without sequelae. Which of the following findings is most likely present in the cerebrospinal fluid (CSF)?

(A) Decreased glucose
(B) Increased neutrophils
(C) Normal protein
(D) Oligoclonal bands
(E) Positive Gram's stain

39 A young mother brings her 4-year-old son to the pediatrician because he had daily nosebleeds for the past few days. The mother states that during these episodes the nose bleeds slowly but freely, usually from the left nostril. She is able to stop the bleeding by applying pressure for a few minutes to the nares of the child. She denies that the patient had any traumatic injury or exposure to dry heat. She states that there are no bleeding disorders in the patient's family. The patient was in his usual state of health until 3 days ago when the epistaxis started. Growth parameters for both height and weight are in the 25 percentile. The patient's immunizations are up to date. Which of the following is the most common cause of epistaxis in the pediatric population?

(A) Allergic rhinitis
(B) Nose picking
(C) Von Willebrand's disease
(D) Idiopathic thrombocytopenic purpura (ITP)
(E) Nasal angiofibroma

40 A 19-year-old woman sees her physician because of a severe sore throat. Three weeks later, she complains of fever, pains in the knees, and a rash on the arms that consists of a circular ring of erythema around normal skin. Other findings on physical examination include bibasilar inspiratory crackles, an S_3 heart sound, and a pansystolic murmur at the apex that radiated into the axilla. The heart murmur and S_3 heart sound increase in intensity on expiration. Which of the following is the most likely diagnosis?

(A) Acute bacterial endocarditis
(B) Acute rheumatic fever
(C) Libman-Sacks endocarditis
(D) Nonbacterial thrombotic endocarditis
(E) Subacute bacterial endocarditis

Directions for Matching Questions (41 through 50): Each set of matching questions is preceded by a list of 4 to 26 lettered options followed by a brief explanation of the required task and then by a series of numbered statements. For each lettered statement you are to select ONE lettered option that best fulfills the task as it relates to that statement. Remember each of the listed options might be correctly selected once, more than once, or not at all.

Questions 41–50

(A) Acetaminophen
(B) Diazepam
(C) Scopolamine
(D) Ethanol
(E) Amitriptyline
(F) Barbiturates
(G) Nicotine
(H) Sertraline
(I) Amphetamines
(J) Cocaine

Match each numbered description below with the ONE lettered drug or agent above.

41 In acute oral overdose, signs and symptoms may include dilated pupils; nystagmus; hot, dry skin; decreased bowel sounds; confusion; hallucinations; and seizures. Characteristic cardiotoxic effects include tachycardia, QRS prolongation, hypotension, and cardiac arrhythmias.

42 Symptoms of acute oral overdose include diarrhea, myoclonus, diaphoresis, elevated temperature, facial flushing, and tremor. Depending on the dose ingested, the patient may become agitated, confused, and hypertensive. Hyperreflexia can occur and progress to seizures. These symptoms may occur at conventional doses if the patient is also using monoamine oxidase inhibitors.

43 An over-the-counter drug that is the most common cause of hepatic failure in the United States.

44 A fat-soluble substance that crosses the blood–brain barrier, where it acts on the limbic system to potentiate dopamine transmission in the basal nuclei. The rush obtained from this substance lasts for less than 30 minutes when it is smoked.

45 An anticholinergic substance commonly used to combat motion sickness.

46 The drug that indirectly results in the greatest drug-related medical expenditure in the United States.

47 The number one drug problem in the Unites States in terms of direct observable effects.

48 A potentially habit-forming drug that is the prototype of a family of drugs presently having widespread medical use including treatment of anxiety, panic, posttraumatic stress, and sleep disorders as well as substance withdrawal symptoms.

49 The first member of this class of so-called sedative, hypnotic drugs was synthesized in 1903, and until the 1970s, members of this class were the primary drugs used as sedatives to treat anxiety and epilepsy. Taking an overdose was a favored means of committing suicide, particularly for women. They still have medical use but have in large part been replaced by newer, safer drugs.

50 Their medical use includes appetite suppression in weight loss programs, treatment of narcolepsy and depression, and in children treatment of attention deficit and hyperactivity (ADH) syndrome. Despite profound health hazards, they also are gaining popularity as recreational drugs because they are easily synthesized from readily available materials.

Answer Key

1 B	**11** C	**21** A	**31** C	**41** E
2 E	**12** C	**22** E	**32** D	**42** H
3 B	**13** A	**23** C	**33** D	**43** A
4 A	**14** A	**24** D	**34** A	**44** J
5 A	**15** E	**25** C	**35** A	**45** C
6 C	**16** C	**26** D	**36** C	**46** G
7 A	**17** B	**27** C	**37** A	**47** D
8 C	**18** B	**28** E	**38** D	**48** B
9 B	**19** D	**29** C	**39** B	**49** F
10 B	**20** A	**30** A	**40** B	**50** I

Answers and Explanations

1 The answer is B *Obstetrics and Gynecology*

This woman has the classic symptoms of endometriosis, namely, dysmenorrhea (painful menses), dyspareunia (painful intercourse), dyschezia (painful defecation), and infertility. Endometriosis is a benign condition in which the endometrial glands and stroma are present outside the uterus and uterine cavity. Currently, surgery is the only definitive treatment; medical treatment is seldom curative (choice **B**).

The condition typically occurs in the early reproductive years, not after 35 years of age (choice **C**). The most common sites of occurrence, in order of frequency, are ovaries, cul-de-sac, uterosacral ligaments (choice **A**), broad ligaments, and oviducts. Endometriosis is not associated with endometrioid carcinoma of the ovary or a high chance of malignant transformation (choice **D**). Endometriosis is not associated with uterine leiomyomata (choice **E**), but in 15% of cases is associated with adenomyosis, a benign condition in which islands of endometrial glands and stroma are found within the myometrium without a direct connection to the endometrial cavity.

2 The answer is E *Pediatrics*

Rolling over from the prone to supine position usually does not occur until 4 to 6 months of age (choice **E**). From the age of newborn (choice **A**) to 1 month, an infant (choice **B**) may be able to regard a face, respond to a bell, and have equal movements. In addition, a 1-month-old may follow to midline. Babbling and cooing occur by 2 months of age (choice **C**). The social smile also is present by this time. Lifting the head and chest occurs by 3 months of age (choice **D**). A 2-month-old infant can use the eyes well enough to follow an object through 180°.

3 The answer is B *Medicine*

The first step in the β-oxidation of fatty acids is catalyzed by an acyl-CoA dehydrogenase. There are at least four classes of acyl-CoA dehydrogenases: those that act on very long chain fatty acids (e.g., the 20-carbon arachidonic acid); those that act on long-chain fatty acids, C12 to C18; those that act on medium-chain fatty acids, C6 to C12; and, those acting on shorter-chain fatty acids, less than C6. Inborn errors inhibiting the activity of each of these dehydrogenases have been reported; these all are inherited as autosomal recessive traits, and all but medium-chain acyl-CoA dehydrogenase (MCAD) deficiency (choice **B**) are extremely rare. MCAD deficiency has a reported incidence of 1 per 6,500 births among North European Caucasians and from 1 per 9,000 to 1 per 17,000 births in the general U.S. population. Among certain ethnic groups the presence of a mutant gene has been reported to be as high as 1 per 40 individuals. The prevalence of the disease is as at least as high as that of phenylketonuria, yet newborn screening is only required in a few states. The *MCAD* gene is located on chromosome 1p31, and 26 different mutant forms have been characterized. However, the K304E *MCAD* mutation accounts for 90% of cases; 81% of these cases are homozygous for this gene, and 18% are compound heterozygotes.

Typically, the deficiency is characterized by sudden attacks after infection and/or fasting for some 8 to 16 hours. The pathophysiology results from an inability to accomplish the first step in β-oxidation of midchain fatty acids, either those ingested (minor contribution) or longer-chain fatty acids that have been partially metabolized to some 10 to 12 carbons and thus become the normal substrates for MCAD. Attacks are provoked by any situation that normally requires increased fatty acid oxidation, such as fasting or an illness. Since increased fat metabolism is not possible, continued existence in MCAD patients depends entirely upon glucose metabolism, and hypoglycemia results. To make matters worse, gluconeogenesis is inhibited because acetyl-CoA cannot be formed but is required for the activity of pyruvate carboxylase to produce oxaloacetate from pyruvate, thus amino acids cannot be used as a fuel. Furthermore, since acetyl-CoA cannot be formed, ketone bodies also cannot be synthesized, and the brain is also deprived of this alternate fuel. The final insult is provided by the cell's attempt to metabolize the accumulated fatty acids by an endoplasmic reticular detoxifying P450 cytochrome mixed oxidase system that converts them into shorter-chain dicarboxylic acids by sequentially oxidizing and then removing the ω-carbon by ω-oxidation. This results in the accumulation of several unusual and abnormal mono- and dicarboxylic acids, which causes an anion-gap metabolic acidosis that will increase as more of these acids accumulate. Octanoic acid is one of these abnormal acids, and it is a mitochondrial toxin suspected of inhibiting the urea cycle, causing an elevated BUN and hyperammonemia; the latter may induce an encephalopathy.

About 25% of babies succumb to respiratory or cardiac arrest during the first attack, which usually occurs between the ages of 6 to 24 months. Subsequent attacks are seldom fatal but are characterized by vomiting, seizures, lethargy, and sometimes coma and encephalopathy. In the long term, individuals may have developmental and behavorial problems, chronic muscle weakness, attention deficit disorder, or cerebral palsy or may seem normal. The penetrance is unknown, and it is believed that an unknown number of homozygous individuals never developed symptoms. Because infants who die during the first attack generate few physical clues relating to the cause of death, it was postulated that such cases are a common cause of the sudden infant death syndrome (SIDS). However, subsequent studies have shown that only 0.01% of SIDS cases are due to MCAD. Screening for MCAD is typically done by determining the presence of abnormal fatty acids and other metabolites, using tandem mass spectrophotometry, and more recently in some laboratories by genetic analysis using the polymerase chain reaction, which however will only recognize the presence of the more prevalent *K304E* gene.

Glucose 6-phosphatase deficiency (choice **A**), also known as type I glycogen storage disease or Von Gierke's disease, also causes a severe fasting hypoglycemia and hepatomegaly, but the latter is due to accumulated glycogen, whereas in MCAT all carbohydrate stores are depleted. Carnitine acyltransferases I and II are required to shuttle fatty acids in and out of the mitochondria. As a consequence, carnitine acyltransferase deficiency (choice **C**) results in an inability to use long-chain fatty acids as fuel, causing myoglobinemia and weakness following exercise. Although hypoglycemia occurs in hyperinsulinemia (choice **D**), a metabolic sequence similar to that described is not caused by fasting or illness. Acute intermittent porphyria (choice **E**) is characterized by unexplained abdominal crises, acute peripheral or central nervous system dysfunctions, recurrent psychiatric illness, hyponatremia, and porphobilinogen in the urine during an attack.

4 The answer is A *Psychiatry*

The distinguishing feature of autistic disorder is a qualitative disturbance in development (choice **A**), as opposed to retardation of development. Qualitative disturbances include lack of attachment to others; restrictive, repetitive, and stereotyped behavior patterns; and peculiar use of speech. The onset of such deficits occurs before the age of 3 years, and it occurs at a 5:1 male-to-female ratio.

Although autistic individuals may have normal intelligence (choice **E**) or may even be gifted in certain areas (choice **D**), some 75% have concurrent mental retardation. The prognosis for autistic disorder is most severe when associated with mental retardation or failure to speak by age 5. Depending on the cause of the disorder, there may, but need not, be progressive deterioration of function (choice **B**). Autistic disorder has multiple causes, including intrauterine infection, errors of metabolism (choice **C**), and encephalitis. A genetic component in at least some cases is suggested by the observation of an increased incidence of autism among family members.

5 The answer is A *Medicine*

Poliomyelitis, also known as infantile paralysis, was the scourge of the first half of the 20th century. Ironically its prevalence increased as sanitation improved, because prior to that, persons were first exposed to the virus as infants while still protected by antibodies in their mother's milk; consequently, the most severe aspects of infection were mitigated, and they developed long-term immunity. By the 1920s through the 1950s, polio epidemics occurred annually until Salk developed an injectable killed vaccine first widely used in 1954 and 1955; this was followed by Sabin's attenuated virus oral vaccine in 1963. Consequently, there has not been a case of polio in an American resident since 1979 (on occasion it has been observed in an immigrant), and routine vaccination in the U.S. is no longer required. However, the effects of poliomyelitis are still with us. Some 10 to 40 years after having had paralytic polio, individuals tend to develop a condition known as postpolio syndrome (choice **A**), characterized by slowly developing but progressively worsening symptoms that include fatigue and muscle weakness; commonly, joint pains and scoliosis also occur. Although the condition can be debilitating, it is only life threatening if it affects the muscles of respiration. It is thought that postpolio syndrome is caused by fatigue of motor neurons, which serve more muscle fibers than normal after what were their partner neurons were killed by the virus; one line of thought is that the condition can be aggravated by excess use. No known treatment modality exists, and most experts recommend limited nonfatiguing exercise.

Amyotrophic lateral sclerosis (choice **B**), sometimes called Lou Gehrig's disease, is also a disease of motor neurons, but usually of unknown cause. It starts somewhat innocuously with weakness in a hand, foot, or leg, but then progresses; causing degeneration throughout the brain and spinal cord; usually within 2 to 10 years after diagnosis, death ensues. The drug riluzole tends to slow, but does not stop, progression of the disease. Although most cases have no known cause, a mutated *SOD1* gene has been implicated in 2% of the cases, and about 20% of the cases have a familial connection. Osteoarthritis (choice **C**) and tendinitis (choice **D**) are both conditions that can develop because of overuse but usually at an older age, rarely is there a history of polio and neither is characterized by fatigue or muscle weakness of the kind associated with postpolio syndrome. Guillain-Barré disease (choice **E**), also known as acute idiopathic polyneuropathy, is characterized by weakness that usually begins in the legs and spreads upward, frequently to the arms and face. Typically, it is symmetric, and the extent of weakness varies from case to case. It primarily affects motor neurons, but distal paresthesias and dysstasias commonly occur. Onset of the disease frequently follows immunizations, surgical procedures, or infections; an association with *Campylobacter jejuni* enteritis has been particularly well documented. Most patients recover spontaneously over a period of months, but some 10–20% retain some degree of disability.

6 The answer is C   *Medicine*

The patient has iron deficiency anemia secondary to blood loss from a polypoid mass in the ascending colon, which on biopsy would most likely reveal an adenocarcinoma. The photograph of the peripheral smear shows red blood cells (RBCs) with increased central pallor, indicating a decrease in hemoglobin synthesis. In addition, there is laboratory evidence for metastasis to the liver. Iron deficiency in an adult more than 50 years of age is most likely due to colon cancer, which is the second most common cancer in adults. The iron studies would likely reveal a decreased serum iron level, increased total iron-binding capacity (TIBC) (not decreased [choice **D**]), decreased percentage iron saturation (not normal [choice **A**]), and a decreased serum ferritin level (not increased [choice **B**]). The RDW (measure of size variation of RBCs) is increased in iron deficiency (not normal [choice **E**]), because some RBCs are normocytic, while others are microcytic. Carcinomas located in the ascending colon tend to bleed and produce iron deficiency, while those in the descending tend to obstruct. A positive stool guaiac test result secondary to blood loss should be expected in this patient. As the age of the patient increases, there is a higher predictive value for occult blood indicating cancer (18% at 40–49 years vs. 83% at 70+ years). Recent studies indicate a 33% reduction in the mortality rate from colorectal cancer in those patients who have a yearly stool guaiac test. Based on these studies, it is recommended that asymptomatic patients over 50 years of age should have an annual stool guaiac test and a flexible sigmoidoscopy examination or colonoscopy every 3 to 5 years, depending on the risk factors in the patient. Colonoscopy is considered the gold standard for the workup of positive stool guaiac test results. Barium studies are not as sensitive in detecting colon cancer as is endoscopy performed by a skilled physician.

Serum enzyme studies in this patient reveal an increase in serum alkaline phosphatase, γ-glutamyltransferase, and lactate dehydrogenase, whereas the total bilirubin and transaminase concentrations are normal. This pattern is highly predictive for liver metastasis (choice **C**). Both serum alkaline phosphatase and γ-glutamyltransferase are excellent indicators of cholestasis in the presence of diffuse liver disease or focal disease in the liver due to granulomas or metastatic cancer. When tumor nodules in the liver compress the bile ducts, there is increased synthesis of alkaline phosphatase and γ-glutamyltransferase. Lactate dehydrogenase is a nonspecific enzyme marker of malignancy, because it is so widespread in tissue. The total bilirubin and transaminase levels are normal because there must be diffuse liver disease before they are increased. The increase in γ-glutamyltransferase is highly predictive of the alkaline phosphatase being of liver rather than bone origin, because γ-glutamyltransferase is not present in bone. This is a much easier way of distinguishing alkaline phosphatase of bone origin versus liver origin than using isoenzyme analysis of alkaline phosphatase or heat stability tests.

Absolute monocytosis in this patient is due to malignancy. Monocytes are part of the immune surveillance system against tumors. Monocytosis is also a feature of chronic infections (e.g., tuberculosis) and chronic inflammation (e.g., autoimmune diseases). Thrombocytosis (increased platelet count) is commonly present in chronic iron deficiency and in disseminated cancer.

7 The answer is A   *Pediatrics*

Classic tetralogy of Fallot consists of pulmonic stenosis, overriding aorta, right ventricular hypertrophy, and ventricular septal defect. Fallot's tetralogy is the most common congenital heart disease presenting with cyanosis, although cyanosis may not be present at birth. Typical chest x-ray films show a boot-shaped heart (coeur en sabot) with diminished pulmonary vascular markings. The electrocardiogram findings include right axis deviation and right ventricular hypertrophy. A dominant R wave appears in the right precordial chest leads. The P wave is tall and peaked and may be bifid. Patients are at higher risk for cerebral thromboses and brain abscess. Treatment is surgical. Prognosis depends on the degree of pulmonic stenosis (choice **A**), which determines the degrees of hypoxemia (choice **C**) and right ventricular hypertrophy (choice **E**). Overriding aorta (choice **B**) and size of the ventricular septal defect (choice **D**) do not relate significantly to the prognosis.

8 The answer is C   *Pediatrics*

The Moro reflex (choice **C**) is initiated by loud noise or sudden motion. It involves abduction of the extremities and extension of the elbows and knees, followed by flexion. The Moro reflex appears at birth and disappears at approximately 4 months of age. If the reflex is asymmetric, this suggests extremity fracture or peripheral nerve injury.

The asymmetric tonic neck reflex (ATNR) (choice **A**) appears at approximately 2 weeks of age and disappears at approximately 6 months of age. There is flexion of the arm and leg on the occipital side and extension on the chin side, creating a "fencer position." The parachute reflex (choice **B**) appears at about 8 to 9 months of age and persists voluntarily. The child is placed in the examiner's hands and is permitted to free fall in ventral suspension. The child extends his extremities symmetrically to distribute his weight for landing. The grasping reflex (choice **D**) appears at birth and disappears at about 3 months of age. This is when the infant reflexively grasps at an object placed in his palm. The protective equilibrium reflex (choice **E**) appears at 4 to 6 months of age and persists voluntarily. The child is pushed laterally by the examiner and flexes his trunk toward the force to regain equilibrium while he extends one arm to protect against falling.

9 The answer is B   *Medicine*

In the red blood cell (RBC), pyruvate kinase (PK) catalyzes the net ATP-producing reaction, and the major function of this ATP is to maintain activity of the sodium-dependent ATPase that sustains the ionic equilibrium of the cell. As a consequence, when ATP levels fall, cells tend to become hypoosmotic, crenate, and be hemolyzed in the spleen. Thus, the primary symptom of pyruvate kinase deficiency (PKD) is a chronic hemolytic anemia. Surprisingly, most individuals with PKD do well despite being very anemic, similar to the man described in the vignette. This is because a limitation in the rate of flux of intermediates at the level of PK causes the concentration of intermediates proximal to this block to increase. The resultant increase in 2,3-diphosphoglycerate concentration shifts the O_2:Hb saturation curve to the right, increasing the efficiency of O_2 transfer to tissues; thus even though less Hb is present, what is there is more efficient. In addition, some compensation is also provided by the increased circulating reticulocyte count. Consequently, most affected individuals are nearly symptom free for much of their lives.

However, more than 100 different mutant PK variants have been described, and symptomology varies with the type of mutation. Some mutations affect the V_{max}, some the K_m, some the affinity for activators, some sensitivity to product inhibition, and some stability. Moreover, PKD is inherited as an autosomal recessive trait, and most nonconsanguineous cases are in compound heterozygotes. In addition, symptoms generally are more severe during the neonatal period and early childhood. Consequently, neonates often present with anemia, an abnormally severe and prolonged jaundice, and a delayed growth pattern. Cholecystolithiasis may develop after the first decade, but relatively few adults suffer the fatigue and other symptoms that usually are associated with profound anemia.

PKD (choice **B**) has a relative high prevalence among the Amish in Lancaster County, a factoid pointing toward PKD in the case described; however, selecting this choice depends more logically upon eliminating the other choices by using the data provided in the vignette. Paroxysmal nocturnal hemoglobinuria (choice **A**) is a disorder that results in abnormal sensitivity of the RBC membrane to lysis by complement. The underlying disorder is a defect in the phosphatidylinositol class A gene, which results in an aberrant glycosyl-phosphatidylinositol anchor for cellular membrane proteins, particularly the CD55 and CD59 complement-binding ones. The negative Ham test result rules out this possibility.

Hereditary spherocytosis (choice **C**) is a dominant trait resulting in a hemolytic anemia in which hemolysis is caused by destruction of the less supple spherocytic erythrocyte in the sinuses of the spleen. Clearly the man described in the vignette did not suffer from hereditary spherocytosis because the red cell morphology is normal.

Glucose 6-phosphate dehydrogenase (G6PD) deficiency (choice **D**) is the most common disease producing RBC enzymopathy in the world; both the African (A⁻) and the Mediterranean (B⁻) varieties are inherited as X-linked recessive traits that impart partial resistance to falciparum malaria. Except for perinatal jaundice, males carrying the mutated gene are asymptomatic until subjected to an oxidative stress that will induce an acute hemolytic crisis, which is more severe in the Mediterranean form. Clearly the man described in the vignette is not suffering from an acute episode of hemolysis.

Hemoglobin C disease (choice **E**) is a hemoglobinopathy analogous to sickle cell disease in which a lysine rather than a valine substitutes for the normal glutamate in position 6 of the β-globin chain. Although this causes a chronic mild hemolytic anemia and a low level of chronic jaundice, this disease is ruled out by the finding of a normal electrophoretic pattern; Hb C runs more slowly toward the anode than either Hb A or Hb S.

Paroxysmal cold hemoglobinuria (PCH) (choice **F**) is a rare condition that primarily affects children after a viral disease, although it sometimes occurs in adults with certain neoplastic conditions. At one time it was more common, as it is also associated with congenital syphilis in neonates and in adults having stage 2 or 3 syphilis. The pathophysiology relates to the binding of biphasic IgG to the "P" antigen, a glycosphingolipid that normally binds early complement components. In PCH, the P antigen is defective, and a change in temperature such as might occur in the hands or feet causes release and activation of the complement sequence, causing hemolysis. In the case described in the vignette, there is no clue suggesting such a system could be active, and results of the Donath-Landsteiner antibody test, which can be used to confirm PCH, are negative.

Autoimmune hemolytic anemia (choice **G**) is due to the formation and binding of an IgG autoantibody to RBC membranes. The Fc portion of the antibody is "bitten off" by macrophages along with a piece of the membrane. The damaged RBC takes on a spheroid shape and is hemolyzed in the spleen. In addition, when large amounts of IgG are attached to the membrane, complement components become "fixed" to the cell and the C3b factor is recognized by C3b receptors on hepatic Kupffer cells, which also participate in the hemolytic process. Half the cases are idiopathic; the remaining cases are associated with systemic lupus erythematosus, chronic lymphocytic leucemia, or lymphomas. The negative Coombs test result rules out autoimmune hemolytic anemia as a possibility.

10 The answer is B *Medicine*

Wegener's granulomatosis is defined by a triad consisting of upper respiratory disease, lower respiratory disease, and glomerulonephritis. It follows that this patient most likely has Wegener's granulomatosis, since he demonstrates this triad of symptoms: the upper airways (sinus infections), the lower respiratory system (nodular masses with cavitation in the lungs), and kidneys (hematuria and RBC casts). Wegener's granulomatosis causes a necrotizing vasculitis of muscular arteries, arterioles, venules, and capillaries in the lungs and upper airways and necrotizing granulomas in the upper respiratory tract and lungs. Cytoplasmic c-antineutrophil antibodies (choice **B**) are specific for Wegener's granulomatosis. The antibodies are directed against neutrophilic granules in the cytosol, and destruction of neutrophils by antineutrophil cytoplasmic antibodies (ANCAs) releases enzymes that contribute to the inflammatory lesions. The renal disease in Wegener's has a nephritic presentation with hematuria and RBC casts. Biopsy specimens reveal crescentic glomerulonephritis, which rapidly progresses to renal failure (increases blood urea nitrogen and creatinine). Cyclophosphamide and corticosteroids are the treatment of choice.

Anti-streptolysin O antibodies (choice **A**) develop in infections associated with group A streptococci (e.g., rheumatic fever). Rheumatic fever is an immunologic disease that primarily targets the heart, joints, skin, and basal ganglia, none of which are targeted in this patient. Hepatitis B surface antigenemia (choice **C**) is associated with classic polyarteritis nodosa in approximately 30% of cases. Polyarteritis nodosa causes vasculitis of muscular arteries (e.g., renal and coronary arteries), leading to vessel thrombosis and infarctions or aneurysm formation caused by weakening of the vessels. It does not affect the pulmonary arteries. It produces renal infarctions, not glomerulonephritis, as in this patient. p-Antineutrophil cytoplasmic antibodies (choice **D**) are directed against myeloperoxidase in neutrophils and are associated with microscopic polyangiitis. Microscopic polyangiitis causes vasculitis of small vessels (capillaries, venules, arterioles) in multiple target organs, including the lungs and kidneys (glomerulonephritis). It is not associated with necrotizing granulomas in the upper airways and lungs, as this patient exhibits. Serum antinuclear antibodies (choice **E**) are directed against nuclear antigens. These antibodies are increased in autoimmune disorders (e.g., systemic lupus erythematosus) and are not present in Wegener's granulomatosis.

11 The answer is C   *Medicine*

Typical community-acquired pneumonia is most commonly caused by *Streptococcus pneumoniae,* which is a gram-positive diplococcus. Azithromycin is the treatment of choice. Other organisms, such as *Haemophilus influenzae* (choice **B**) or *Moraxella catarrhalis,* are commonly found in smokers with chronic bronchitis or those with underlying lung disease, but *S. pneumoniae* remains the most common. There is now concern about the rising percentage of *S. pneumoniae* strains that are resistant to penicillin. The best way to protect elderly patients and those with underlying lung disease from pneumonia is by use of the pneumococcal vaccine, which is recommended for all persons over age 65 and those younger who have underlying lung disease or who are asplenic. Infections caused by *Mycoplasma pneumoniae* (choice **A**), *Legionella pneumophila* (choice **D**), and *Coccidioides immitis* (choice **E**) are not associated with cough or signs of lung congestion.

12 The answer is C   *Psychiatry*

This man is demonstrating passive-aggressiveness, which is described as covert aggression expressed through passivity, masochism, and self-defeating behavior. Such an individual often is angry—and often angers others. The usual result is further deterioration of the interaction, with even greater anger and passive-aggressiveness. The most effective way to deal with covert communication is to bring it into the open and discuss it (choice **C**). This technique is called "identifying the process."

Threats (choice **A**) and expressions of anger (choice **D**) or hurt (choice **B**) are generally not useful. Because personality traits are generally stable in various environments, it is unlikely that a different clinician (choice **E**) would be spared this patient's passive-aggressiveness.

13 The answer is A   *Psychiatry*

Increased involvement of fathers in raising children decreases the risk of sexual abuse. More women than men have a history of being abused (choice **B**). More traditional, less democratic families are associated with an increased, not decreased (choice **C**), risk of abuse. Mothers who sexually abuse children are often lonely and emotionally deprived, not gregarious and socially active (choice **D**). Contrary to popular wisdom, only a minority of childhood sexual abuse is perpetrated by fathers and stepfathers (choice **E**). However, the abuser is often another relative or family member.

14 The answer is A   *Surgery*

Carpal tunnel syndrome (choice **A**) is caused by compression of the median nerve at the level of the wrist. The median nerve supplies sensation to the radial 3½ digits of the hand as well as innervation of the thenar musculature. Symptoms include numbness and tingling in the fingertips and pain that can awaken the patient at night and that can travel proximally up the arm. Hyperextension of the hand or tapping over the nerve reproduces the findings. There can be sensory loss in the median nerve distribution and muscle weakness in the thumb.

Pronator syndrome (choice **B**) is a median nerve entrapment in the proximal forearm. It is a pure sensory syndrome. The cubital tunnel is a groove in the posteromedial aspect of the elbow that contains the ulnar nerve. Cubital tunnel syndrome (choice **C**) is an ulnar nerve neuropathy. Ulnar nerve entrapment (choice **D**) can occur at the wrist in Guyon's canal. In both of these conditions, patients may complain of numbness in the ulnar 1½ digits and have weakness of the intrinsic muscles. De Quervain's disease (choice **E**) is usually caused by repetitive use of the thumb for some activity. Patients have pain and tenderness at the region of the radial styloid.

15 The answer is E   *Medicine*

The patient has hypovolemic shock caused by blood loss (tachycardia with weak pulse; cold, clammy skin; decreased blood pressure). In the initial phase of acute blood loss, the hemoglobin and RBC count are normal (not decreased [choices **A** and **B**, respectively]), because whole blood containing both RBCs and plasma is lost;

the amount decreases, but the concentration is not yet affected. Within a few hours, plasma begins to be replaced, and the RBC count and hemoglobin level drop. A decrease in cardiac output causes underfilling of the aortic arch, which activates the sympathetic nervous system, subsequently releasing catecholamines. Catecholamines cause venoconstriction, increased myocardial contraction, increased heart rate, and vasoconstriction of the smooth muscle cells of the peripheral-resistance arterioles (choice **E**). Decreased renal blood flow activates the renin–angiotensin–aldosterone system, causing the release of angiotensin II and peripheral arteriolar vasoconstriction. Vasoconstriction of arterioles in the skin shunts blood to more important areas of the body, causing cold, clammy skin. Left ventricular end-diastolic pressure and pulmonary capillary hydrostatic pressure are decreased in hypovolemic shock (not increased [choices **C** and **D,** respectively]).

16 The answer is C *Psychiatry*

Narcissistic injury (choice **C**), the emotional pain from having been rejected as a child, often plays a significant role in the emotional life of adoptees. It sometimes manifests itself as insecurity about acceptance by others and requires sensitive care and patience on the part of new adoptee parents. Over 80% (not 50%, choice **A**) of adoptions are considered successful, and IQ scores have been demonstrated to rise in adoptive environments that provide enriched intellectual and social stimulation (choice **B**). However, the rate of psychopathology is higher among adoptees (choice **D**), as is the rate of parent–child problems (choice **E**).

17 The answer is B *Pediatrics*

Metachromatic leukodystrophy (choice **B**) is a disorder of myelin metabolism in which arylsulfatase A activity is deficient. Six disorders are included in the metachromatic leukodystrophic group of diseases. These are classified by age of onset and specific enzyme deficiency. All are characterized by gait disturbances that progress to complete inability to walk. The extremities become hypotonic, and deep tendon reflexes are lost. Speech becomes slurred, and nystagmus is present. Feeding and swallowing are impaired, and death from bronchopneumonia occurs by 5 to 6 years of age. Cerebrospinal fluid (CSF) shows elevated protein. Metachromatic granules in urine are suggestive of metachromatic leukodystrophy and not of the other choices presented.

Infants with Krabbe's disease (choice **C**) tend to be hypertonic. Globoid histiocytes are seen in the white matter. Fabry's disease (choice **D**) is X-linked recessive, and manifestations occur at adolescence. Skin eruptions around the navel and buttocks are characteristic. Patients with phenylketonuria (choice **A**) usually have fair skin and blue eyes. Some may have an eczematoid or seborrheic rash. These children also have a musty odor. Adrenoleukodystrophy (choice **E**) is an X-linked genetic disorder that causes accumulation of long-chain saturated fatty acids in the skin, adrenals, and white matter of the central nervous system (CNS), resulting in dysfunction. There are seven phenotypes of adrenoleukodystrophy; three of which are expressed in children, in whom they induce hyperactivity, impaired auditory discrimination, visual disturbances, and seizures.

18 The answer is B *Medicine*

The patient has sarcoidosis, which is a multisystem granulomatous disease of unknown etiology that accounts for ~25% of chronic interstitial lung diseases. It has an increased incidence in women, African-American blacks, and nonsmokers. Sarcoidosis is a disorder of immune regulation in genetically predisposed individuals. CD4 Th cells interact with an unknown antigen leading to the formation of noncaseating granulomas, which are a characteristic finding in the disease. Although other organs including the central nervous system can be affected, the lungs are the primary target organs. Noncaseating granulomas develop in the lung interstitium and incite a fibrous tissue reaction primarily along the lymphatics and around the bronchi and blood vessels. Granulomas also develop in the mediastinal and hilar lymph nodes. Dyspnea is the most common symptom, but eye lesions are common, particularly inflammation of the uveal tract (uveitis), which causes blurry vision, glaucoma, and corneal opacities with the potential for blindness. Findings include a miotic pupil with a poor light reflex and circumcorneal ciliary body vascular congestion, as described for this patient. Skin lesions are also a common finding. Nodular lesions containing granulomas develop on the skin, and a violaceous rash called *lupus pernio* occurs on the nose and cheeks, again described in this patient. Other findings include granulomatous hepatitis, hypercalcemia (5%), enlarged salivary and lacrimal glands, cranial nerve palsies, and diabetes insipidus. Sarcoidosis is a progressive or intermittent disease with periods of activity and remissions. Most patients respond well to corticosteroid therapy, and approximately 70% of patients recover with minimal or no residual changes; 10–15% develop severe interstitial fibrosis, leading to cor pulmonale and death.

Regarding laboratory tests, increased angiotensin-converting enzyme (ACE) levels are a good marker of disease activity and response to corticosteroid therapy; however, this is *not* used as a screening or confirmatory test. There is cutaneous anergy to common skin antigens (e.g., *Candida*). Arterial blood gases usually show a respiratory alkalosis (not a decreased arterial pH [choice A]) with hypoxemia. Pulmonary function tests show a restrictive pattern due to the interstitial fibrosis, which decreases compliance (filling of the lung with air) and increases elasticity (rapidly expels air). The FEV1/FVC ratio is increased (choice B) in restrictive lung disease. The FEV_1, or the amount of air expelled from the lungs in 1 second after a maximal inspiration, is decreased (e.g., 3 L vs. the normal 4 L) because of decreased compliance. However, the FVC, or total amount of air expelled after a maximal inspiration, is also decreased (e.g., 3 L vs. the normal 5 L), and the ratio of FEV_1 to FVC is increased (e.g., 3:3 = 100% vs. 4:5 = 80%). Due to the increase in lung elasticity, the FEV_1 and FVC are often the same. The FRC is the total amount of air in the lungs at the end of a normal expiration. It is the sum of the expiratory reserve volume (amount of air forcibly expelled at the end of a normal expiration) and the residual volume. It is decreased (not increased [choice C]) in restrictive lung disease, because all volumes and capacities are due to the decrease in lung compliance. Therefore, the RV and the TLC are also decreased (not increased [choices D and E, respectively]).

19 The answer is D *Medicine*

The brown recluse spider (choice D), *Loxosceles reclusea* is also known as the violin or fiddleback spider because of a dark violin-shaped design on its back. It has a habitat limited to the southcentral part of the United States centered near Shreveport, Louisiana. It is a shy creature that prefers dark undisturbed areas but will bite if disturbed, and its bite is venomous with symptoms varying from only an erythematous spot that clears up almost unnoticed to symptoms similar to those described, which may also include generalized pruritus, arthralgias, and as it heals severe pain; a death has never been reported. At one time surgical débridement was recommended, but that was found to delay recovery. There is no antivenom or other recommended treatment other than oral administration of the antibiotic dapsone. Whereas the range of the true recluse spider *L. reclusea* is limited to an area roughly extending into eastern Texas to Alabama on the south and up north paralleling the Mississippi into Missouri, there are another 12 species of *Loxosceles* belonging to the recluse family. The habitat of most of these spiders extends across the Southwest from Louisiana to the Pacific, mostly in desert areas, while another species the "Hobo spider" inhabits the Northwest, primarily in Washington and Oregon. These spiders have habits similar to *L. reclusea*, but their bite usually is not as toxic, and the violin on their backs may be difficult, or even impossible, to see.

Red fire ants (*Solenopsis invecta*) (choice A) were introduced into Mobile Bay in the ballast of ships coming from South America in the late 1920s or early 1930s and since have spread across the southern tier of states from the Atlantic to the Pacific. They are a very aggressive species, an expensive nuisance, and their bite is painful. It creates a red swollen area that will become a sterile pustule. Other than a remote chance of anaphylactic shock (<5%), the bite is not a health hazard. Six *Latrodectus* species of black widow spiders (choice B) live in the United States. In all species the females have yellow-to-red markings on their abdomen, which clearly looks like an hourglass among the southern species but less so among the northern ones. All are shy, nocturnal, web-weaving animals in which the females inject a neurotoxic venom that is 15 times more toxic than prairie rattlesnake venom. However, they inject so little that it is only mortally dangerous to the very young, old, and debilitated. Nonetheless, even healthy adults will develop severe abdominal pain, muscle pain, pain under the soles of their feet, alternating periods of dry mouth and excess salvation, perfuse sweat, swollen eyelids, and partial paralysis of the diaphragm. Typically, symptoms decrease in a day or so and clear up within several days. There is antivenom available. A deer tick, *Ixodes scapularis*, bite (choice D) in and of itself does little harm but may transmit *Borrelia burgdorferi*, the organism that transmits Lyme disease. The habitat of this tick is in the northeast and north central states. In the far west, *Ixodes pacificus* serves as the vector spreading Lyme disease. There are some 90 scorpion species in the United States, but only one, *Centruroides exilicauda*, has a venomous sting (choice E). *C. exilicauda*'s habitat is in the deserts of Arizona and eastern California, and its venom causes severe but rarely fatal symptoms. Antivenom is available.

20 The answer is A *Psychiatry*

Adults with specific phobia believe that their fear is irrational (choice A). Other features of specific phobia include fear of an object or situation that is excessive or unreasonable, efforts to avoid the feared object or situation, and extreme anxiety if the object or situation cannot be avoided. The objective or actual degree of danger is not relevant to a diagnosis of phobia.

It is difficult to determine that a particular fear has no associated unconscious symbolism (choice **C**). A history of separation anxiety in childhood (choice **B**) is not associated with specific phobia; however, it is associated with the later development of panic disorder. Individuals may be able to force themselves to confront the feared situation (choice **D**) but will experience severe anxiety in such instances. While some phobias make logical sense, many have no basis in reality (choice **E**).

21 The answer is A   *Medicine*

The patient has primary biliary cirrhosis (PBC), which is an autoimmune disease associated with granulomatous destruction of bile ducts in the portal triads. Deposition of bile salts in the skin, causing generalized pruritus, is a common early finding of this disease. Jaundice is a late finding, because not all the bile ducts are simultaneously destroyed. The presence of antimitochondrial antibodies (choice **A**) and an increase in serum IgM (not IgG [choice **D**]) are characteristic markers for PBC. Serum alkaline phosphatase and γ-glutamyltransferase are enzymatic markers of bile duct obstruction (cholestasis) and are markedly increased in PBC. Diseases associated with PBC include rheumatoid arthritis, Sjögren's syndrome, Hashimoto's thyroiditis, and renal tubular acidosis. Treatment includes the use of ursodeoxycholic acid and cholestyramine. Other drugs that have been used include cyclosporine, colchicine, and methotrexate.

Anti–smooth muscle antibodies (choice **B**) are present in autoimmune hepatitis, which is commonly associated with other autoimmune diseases (e.g., rheumatoid arthritis, Sjögren syndrome). In these autoimmune diseases, results of the serum antinuclear antibody test are usually positive (not negative as in this patient), and the concentration of serum IgG is increased. The resulting hepatic cell necrosis releases aminotransferases (e.g., alanine transferase) rather than alkaline phosphatase and γ-glutamyltransferase, as in this patient. Increased serum α-fetoprotein (choice **C**) occurs in hepatocellular carcinoma, which may occur in PBC. However, the patient does not show signs of ascites and weight loss, which commonly occur in hepatocellular carcinoma. Obstruction of bile flow causes reflux of bile into the blood. Cholesterol is the primary lipid excreted in bile (not triglyceride [choice **E**]) and frequently produces cholesterol deposits in the eyelids (xanthelasma).

22 The answer is E   *Medicine*

The patient most likely has sickle cell trait, which causes recurrent microscopic hematuria. In sickle cell trait, the percentage of sickle hemoglobin is 40–45%, and the remainder of the hemoglobin is hemoglobin A. There are no sickle cells in the peripheral smear in sickle cell trait; therefore, a sickle cell screen is required to induce sickling of RBCs containing sickle hemoglobin. The oxygen tension in the renal medulla is low enough to induce sickling of RBCs in the peritubular capillaries. This creates microinfarctions in the renal medulla, causing microscopic hematuria. Repeated infarctions in the renal medulla may cause renal papillary necrosis. A sickle cell screen (choice **E**) in African Americans is always indicated whenever there is unexplained hematuria.

A bone marrow examination (choice **A**) is not warranted, because the patient does not have anemia or evidence of intrinsic bone marrow disease. If results of the sickle cell screen are negative, cystoscopy (choice **B**) may be necessary to determine the cause of the hematuria. Similarly, if results of the sickle cell screen are negative, a renal biopsy (choice **C**) may be necessary to rule out primary renal disease, particularly IgA glomerulonephritis, which is commonly associated with episodic hematuria. However, since the phase contrast microscopy of urine does not demonstrate dysmorphic RBCs (RBCs with protrusions from the membrane), a glomerular origin for the hematuria is unlikely. Although the serum ferritin level (choice **D**) is decreased in the early stages of iron deficiency when anemia is not present, hematuria is rarely a cause of iron deficiency.

23 The answer is C   *Obstetrics and Gynecology*

This patient does not currently have any respiratory complaints or symptoms; therefore, she will undergo the normal changes in respiratory physiology that occur during pregnancy. Respiratory rate is unchanged (not increased [choice **A**]). Tidal volume is increased (not decreased [choice **E**]). Minute ventilation is the product of respiratory rate and tidal volume, thus it increases. This is the correct answer (choice **C**). Vital capacity (the sum of inspiratory reserve volume, tidal volume, and expiratory reserve volume) remains unchanged (not decreased [choice **B**]). The enlarging uterus elevates the resting position of the diaphragm, resulting in the functional residual capacity decreasing (not remaining unchanged [choice **D**]).

24 **The answer is D** *Pediatrics*

The most likely pathogen to cause osteomyelitis of the foot after a puncture wound is *Pseudomonas aeruginosa* (choice **D**). The pathogen is frequently colonized in tennis shoes and can be inoculated into a puncture wound. However, *Staphylococcus aureus* is another pathogen that must also be considered for this type of injury. Appropriate antibiotic treatment should be given to cover for both organisms.

The hallmarks of tetanus, caused by *Clostridium tetani* (choice **B**), are trismus and opisthotonus. *Streptococcus pyogenes* (choice **E**) is not as common in osteomyelitis as *P. aeruginosa*. *Staphylococcus saprophyticus* (choice **A**) is a cause of urinary tract infections. *Staphylococcus epidermidis* (choice **C**) is associated with abscesses, wound infections, and subacute bacterial endocarditis.

25 **The answer is C** *Pediatrics*

A peritonsillar abscess (choice **C**) surrounds the tonsil and extends onto the soft palate. Clinical signs associated with a peritonsillar abscess are torticollis; limitation of mouth opening, i.e. trismus; drooling; and thick, muffled speech, or "hot potato" voice. Physical examination reveals an asymmetric tonsillar bulge with displacement of the uvula away from the affected tonsil. In some cases, physical examination may be limited because of trismus, and computed tomography of the neck is helpful to reveal the abscess. Treatment includes surgical drainage and antibiotic therapy against the most common pathogens, group A streptococci and oropharyngeal anaerobes.

Tonsillar lymphoma (choice **D**) presents with painless dysphagia. Inflammation and edema of the uvula characterize uvulitis (choice **E**). Patients with uvulitis have throat pain, difficulty swallowing, and a gagging sensation. Stridor, hoarseness, and a loud "barking" or "seallike" cough characterize croup (choice **B**). Clinical signs of epiglottitis (choice **A**) include high fever, sore throat, dysphasia, and extended neck.

26 **The answer is D** *Psychiatry*

Flight of ideas refers to a rapid flow of thoughts (choice **D**), often unconnected or tenuously related to one another. This condition is commonly associated with pathologically accelerated psychomotor activity, such as is seen in the manic phase of bipolar disorder.

Catatonic excitement (choice **B**) and illogical thought processes (choice **C**), examples of disorganized thinking and behavior, are seen in many psychotic disorders. The sudden disappearance of thoughts from consciousness (choice **A**) is called thought blocking and may represent unconscious psychologic conflict. An irrational belief about possessing irrational powers (choice **E**) is an example of a grandiose delusion, often associated with psychotic episodes in schizophrenia or bipolar disorder, manic phase.

27 **The answer is C** *Psychiatry*

The quality of mood distinguishes mania from depression (choice **C**). Mood pathology during a manic episode includes elation, expansiveness, and irritability. Mood pathology during a depressive episode includes dysphoria and loss of the ability to experience pleasure.

Sleep disturbances (e.g., insomnia [choice **D**]), psychotic symptoms (choice **B**), and altered levels of activity (choice **A**) may be present during both manic and depressive episodes. Both mania and depression may be caused by known pathophysiology (choice **E**), such as endocrinopathies and steroid use.

28 **The answer is E** *Obstetrics and Gynecology*

Cytomegalovirus (CMV) is the most common congenital viral syndrome in the United States. The triad of chorioretinitis, microcephaly, and intracranial calcifications is characteristic for neonatal CMV infection. Specific treatment does exist (choice **A**) in the form of ganciclovir. Cesarean delivery is not effective in the prevention of transmission of CMV to the fetus (choice **B**). The risk of fetal infection from a maternal primary infection is the same in all trimesters (choice **C**), approximately 40 to 50%. Gamma globulin prophylaxis is ineffective (choice **D**). However, 85% of infected infants are asymptomatic, with only 5% of them later developing symptoms (choice **E**).

29 **The answer is C** *Obstetrics and Gynecology*

The case scenario is characteristic of perimenopause. This is caused by increasing depletion of ovarian follicles and decreasing estrogen levels. With the lack of estrogen feedback to the anterior pituitary, there is an increase in follicle-stimulating hormone (FSH) levels (choice **C**), the correct answer. In addition, the other gonadotropin hormone, luteinizing hormone (LH), will also elevate (not decrease, as in choice **B**). Cortisol (choice **A**), thyroxin (choice **D**), and androstenedione (choice **E**) do not change in normal reference values after menopause.

30 The answer is A   *Psychiatry*

By definition, pain disorder is characterized by pain that is largely mediated by psychologic factors (choice **A**). There is often an underlying physical lesion, but the resultant pain is disproportional to the nature of the lesion.

In individuals with chronic, physiologically mediated physical pain, as in individuals with pain disorder, physical lesions may be difficult to find (choice **B**), personality pathology may emerge (choice **C**), there is often a good response to biofeedback therapy (choice **D**), and economic and legal issues are involved (choice **E**). Consequently, not any of these factors clearly discriminate between pain disorder and physiologically mediated pain conditions. Worker's compensation issues may raise additional concerns about malingering.

31 The answer is C   *Medicine*

The patient has anorexia nervosa (self-starvation). Features include loss of muscle mass and subcutaneous tissue, fine downy hair (lanugo hair), distorted body image (feeling fat), and secondary amenorrhea. Excessive loss of body weight (>25% of ideal weight) leads to decreased secretion of gonadotropin-releasing hormone (not increased [choice **E**]) from the hypothalamus and a corresponding decrease in the concentration of serum gonadotropins (follicle-stimulating hormone and luteinizing hormones) (choice **C**). The stress hormones adrenocorticotropic hormone, growth hormone, and cortisol are increased (not decreased [choices **A, B, D**]). Amenorrhea is caused by decreased ovarian synthesis of estradiol, which may lead to osteoporotic changes resulting in compression fractures in the vertebral column, which may cause back pain, as in this patient.

32 The answer is D   *Medicine*

The patient has hemochromatosis, an autosomal recessive disease that is relatively common among individuals of northern European ancestry. Most cases are due to a mutation in the *HFE* gene on chromosome 6. About 7% of northern Europeans carry the defective gene, with a 0.5% prevalence of the homozygous condition; it is diagnosed 5 times more often in men than in women, and is rarely found in Asian or African Americans. The homozygous condition causes unrestricted reabsorption of iron from the small intestine, leading to iron overload in the liver (where it causes cirrhosis), pancreas (where it causes type 1 diabetes and malabsorption leading to diarrhea), and skin (where it increases the production of melanin, causing increased skin pigmentation). The term "bronze diabetes" is often applied to this condition because affected patients often present with type 1 diabetes and have a bronze skin color. The disease has a slow onset and is not generally diagnosed in men until the fifth decade and later in women because menstrual blood loss protects them. It is postulated that in former times it had survival value when it helped protect against iron deficiency anemia and the diseases of late middle-age were of less consequence because of the shorter life expectancy. Once diagnosed, it is treated by phlebotomy and as long as the secondary organ damage described has not yet reached an irreversible stage, prognosis is good. An excellent screening test is the serum ferritin level; ferritin is a soluble iron–protein complex that reflects the iron stores in the bone marrow macrophages, and serum ferritin levels are increased (choice **D**) in iron overload diseases.

A decreased synthesis of ceruloplasmin (choice **A**) is found in Wilson's disease, an autosomal recessive disorder characterized by defective secretion of copper into bile and reduced synthesis of ceruloplasmin in the liver. The accumulation of excess copper in the tissues causes chronic liver disease and a movement disorder. Although excess copper deposition in tissues does not cause skin discoloration or pancreatic insufficiency, it does cause cirrhosis, a finding that is also present in hemochromatosis. Patients with iron overload diseases such as hemochromatosis have an increase in serum iron (not decreased [choice **B**]), ferritin, and percentage saturation of transferrin (>50% transferrin saturation after an overnight fast). Transferrin is the iron-binding protein. D-Xylose absorption is an excellent screening test for malabsorption caused by small bowel disease. Decreased absorption of orally administered D-xylose into the blood occurs in small bowel disease (e.g., celiac disease) because of flattening of the villi. The reabsorption of D-xylose (choice **C**) is normal in pancreatic disease associated with hemochromatosis, because pancreatic enzymes are not required to degrade xylose for reabsorption by the small bowel. Patients with iron overload diseases have a decrease in total iron-binding capacity (not increased [choice **E**]). The total iron binding capacity (TIBC) is decreased, because increased iron stores in the bone marrow cause decreased synthesis of transferrin (binding protein of iron) in the liver.

An increase in serum TIBC is only present in iron deficiency, because decreased iron stores in the bone marrow cause increased synthesis of transferrin by the liver.

33 The answer is D *Surgery*

The patient has an esophageal carcinoma. Squamous cell carcinoma (choice **D**) accounts for most midesophageal cancers. The major predisposing factors are smoking and alcohol. However, other factors such as lye strictures, Plummer-Vinson syndrome, diverticular diseases, nitrosamines, and achalasia are also risk factors. Dysphagia for solids but not liquids, weakness, and weight loss are the usual presenting complaints. These cancers initially spread locally by lymphatics and drain into surrounding lymph nodes. Distant metastasis is to the liver (70%), lungs (60%), and adrenal glands (35%). Approximately 50% of esophageal carcinomas are resectable at the time of presentation. An esophagectomy is usually performed followed by radiation and chemotherapy. Because early symptoms are easy to overlook, many patients have a stage IV disease at the time of diagnosis, with a 5-year survival rate of only 5% despite such extensive treatment.

Currently in the United States, most esophageal cancers are distal (not midesophageal) adenocarcinomas (choice **F**) arising from gastric metaplasia (Barrett's esophagus) in a patient with gastroesophageal reflux disease (GERD); the survival rate is similar to that of patients with squamous cell carcinoma. Diffuse esophageal spasm (choice **A**), or "nutcracker esophagus," produces dysphagia and chest pain that is often relieved with nitroglycerin. A barium study reveals a "corkscrew" esophagus. A Zenker's diverticulum (choice **B**) is the most common acquired diverticulum of the esophagus and is treated by surgery. Because of stagnant food collected in the pouch, the patient has halitosis. Achalasia (choice **C**), a motor disorder of the distal esophagus due to failure of relaxation of the lower esophageal sphincter, is associated with dysphagia for solids and liquids. The proximal esophagus is dilated and aperistaltic. It is treated with pneumatic dilatation, drugs that decrease lower esophageal sphincter tone (e.g., nifedipine), or surgery (esophagocardiomyotomy) in 20 to 25% of patients. Plummer-Vinson syndrome (choice **E**) is more common in elderly women with iron deficiency. Findings include an esophageal web, spoon nails, and achlorhydria.

34 The answer is A *Psychiatry*

Most effective psychotherapies and psychoanalysis have specific explanations for the genesis of pathologic behavior (choice **A**). However psychoanalysis tends to focus on subconscious factors initiated during early childhood while the modern psychotherapies focus on specific factors directly affecting behavior in the here and now.

Since psychoanalysis needs to probe the subconscious, it is often a lengthy process (choice **C**), but since the brief psychotherapies focus on the immediate, they are not. Moreover, the explanations and treatment techniques differ between psychoanalysis and psychotherapy as well as among schools of psychotherapy. For instance, interpersonal psychotherapies may emphasize interpersonal experiences over unconscious conflicts or biologic factors (choice **E**); psychodynamic psychotherapy like psychoanalysis may center on a concept of unconscious processes (choice **B**); and cognitive psychotherapy focuses on ways to change a person's way of looking at problems. In general, use of drugs in therapy is limited to certain conditions such as the psychoses, bipolar disorder, anxiety states, and depression, and therapies for substance abuse that are based on the recovery model often include a warning to avoid drug treatment (choice **D**).

35 The answer is A *Surgery*

The patient has a primary squamous cell carcinoma of the lung (eosinophilic staining cells with keratin pearls) that ectopically secretes parathyroid hormone-like peptide causing hypercalcemia (choice **A**) and a decrease in serum parathyroid hormone (suppression by hypercalcemia). These tumors are centrally located within the lung and are strongly associated with smoking.

Hypocalcemia (choice **B**) may occur in medullary carcinomas of the thyroid that secrete calcitonin. Calcitonin inhibits osteoclasts, which prevents lysis of bone. Hypercortisolism (choice **C**) may be caused by small cell carcinoma of the lung and medullary carcinoma of the thyroid, both of which ectopically secrete adrenocorticotropic hormone (ACTH). Small cell carcinomas of the lung have round- to spindle-shaped basophilic staining cells. They are neuroendocrine tumors that derive from Kulchitsky cells and more often secrete antidiuretic hormone (ADH) producing hyponatremia (choice **D**) rather than ACTH. Like primary squamous cancer of the lung, they are centrally located tumors that have a strong association with smoking; however, the histologic appearance of the tumor in the patient is that of a squamous cancer.

Renal cell carcinoma and hepatocellular carcinoma are tumors that ectopically secrete erythropoietin-producing polycythemia (choice **E**). No primary lung cancer ectopically secretes erythropoietin.

36 The answer is C *Surgery*

The nurse suspects that the patient has idiopathic scoliosis (choice **C**). The school screening test for this disorder is called the Adam's forward-bending test. By assuming this near 90° bent position, abnormal lateral curvature (S or C shape) of the spine is easy to observe. Confirmation is generally made by an imaging study in which the degree of curvature is determined by a geometrical process called the Cobb method. A curvature greater than 25° is considered significant, greater than 45–50° is considered severe. In the United States, the prevalence of scoliosis greater than 25° is 1.5 cases per 1000; most states have mandatory screening by a school nurse by the 5th or 6th grade. Scoliosis is most commonly idiopathic and often is first diagnosed in adolescent girls from 10 to 16 years of age. Scoliosis refers to lateral displacement of the spine, while kyphosis refers to forward displacement (e.g., hunchback) of the spine. A third type of unusual spinal shape is called lordosis (aka sway back); this is not considered pathologic as long as the back remains flexible.

Pott's disease of the spine (choice **B**) refers to tuberculosis involving the vertebral column. Ankylosing spondylitis (choice **A**) is a human leukocyte antigen (HLA)-B27–positive arthropathy that is more common in men. Sacroiliitis and fusion of the spine (bamboo spine) are prominent features of this disease. Forward bending of the spinal column becomes increasingly more pronounced as the disease progresses. Osteomyelitis (choice **D**) does not typically produce spinal abnormalities. Neurofibromatosis (choice **E**) is associated with kyphoscoliosis; however, café au lait spots are likely to be present as well.

37 The answer is A *Medicine*

Cimetidine, an imidazole compound that blocks histamine receptors, also inhibits cytochrome enzymes in the liver microsomal P450 mixed-function oxidase system. This system is located in the smooth endoplasmic reticulum (SER) and is responsible for the catabolic detoxification of many drugs and other products. Competitive inhibition of the system may lead to drug toxicity (choice **A**), particularly if the therapeutic window is small, as is the case of theophylline.

Cimetidine inhibits the metabolism of this drug in the liver by the microsomal mixed-function oxidase system and does not affect the uptake of the drug into hepatocytes (choice **B**). Although increased drug reabsorption in the gastrointestinal tract is a potential cause of drug toxicity (choice **C**), the most likely cause in this patient is decreased metabolism of the drug in the liver. Increased excretion in the kidneys (choice **D**) is more likely to cause decreased levels of the drug in the serum rather than increased levels.

38 The answer is D *Medicine*

The patient has multiple sclerosis, an autoimmune disease characterized by destruction of the myelin sheaths caused by the production of antibodies that are directed against myelin basic protein. The episodic course of acute relapses with optic neuritis (blurry vision), scanning speech, cerebellar ataxia, and sensory and motor dysfunction, followed by remissions, are often characteristic of this disease. The demyelinating plaques in multiple sclerosis occur in the white matter of the cerebral cortex. The plaques usually have a perivenular distribution and are accompanied by a perivascular lymphoid and plasma cell infiltrate with microglial cells containing phagocytosed myelin. CSF shows an increase in CSF protein (not normal [choice **C**]). High-resolution electrophoresis of CSF shows discrete bands of immunoglobulins in the gamma-globulin region called oligoclonal bands (choice **D**). They indicate a demyelinating process.

The CSF glucose level (choice **A**) is normal in multiple sclerosis. T lymphocytes are increased in the CSF in multiple sclerosis (not neutrophils [choice **B**]). A Gram's stain (choice **E**) is negative in the CSF, because multiple sclerosis is an autoimmune disease, not an infectious one.

39 The answer is B *Pediatrics*

Nose picking (choice **B**) is the most common cause of epistaxis in the pediatric population. The significance of knowing this is that the practitioner can avoid doing unnecessary laboratory work in patients with the habit of nose picking. In the case of nose picking no further diagnostic studies are necessary when the patient does not have a family history of bleeding or any pertinent findings on physical examination. Pertinent physical findings to exclude in a patient with epistaxis would include abnormal finding of the nasal cavity, hypertension, pallor, enlarged nodes, organomegaly, and petechiae.

Trauma and irritation (e.g., colds, allergic rhinitis [choice **A**]) are less common causes of epistaxis in this population. Bleeding disorders (e.g., von Willebrand's disease [choice **C**], idiopathic thrombocytopenic purpura [choice **D**]) are rarely causes of epistaxis and usually have other manifestations. Nasal masses associated with epistaxis may rarely signal a nasal angiofibroma (choice **E**).

40 The answer is B   *Medicine*

The patient has acute rheumatic fever (ARF, choice **B**). It is an acute, immune-mediated multisystem disease that follows a group A streptococcal pharyngitis after an interval of a few weeks. Antibodies develop against group A streptococcal M proteins that cross-react with similar proteins in human tissue, producing a type II hypersensitivity reaction with destruction of tissue. Blood cultures are negative (not positive as in acute bacterial endocarditis [choice **A**] or subacute bacterial endocarditis [choice **E**]). Clinical findings include carditis, polyarthritis, subcutaneous nodules, erythema marginatum, and Sydenham's chorea. Carditis refers to inflammation of all layers of the heart (pericardium, myocardium, and endocardium). The mitral valve is the valve most commonly involved in ARF, followed by the aortic valve. The patient has a pansystolic murmur at the apex that is caused by mitral regurgitation due to endocarditis and bibasilar inspiratory crackles and an S_3 heart sound caused by left-sided heart failure due to myocarditis. Note that the murmur and abnormal heart sound increase in intensity on expiration, a sign of a left-sided valvular abnormality. Recurrent infections of the mitral valve and aortic valve lead to mitral stenosis (most common) and aortic stenosis, respectively. Migratory polyarthritis, the most common presenting symptom of ARF, occurs in large joints (knees) and small joints (e.g., wrists). There is no permanent joint damage associated with the arthritis. Subcutaneous nodules occur on extensor surfaces and are similar to rheumatoid nodules. The patient exhibits erythema marginatum, which is characterized by an evanescent circular ring of erythema that develops around normal skin. Sydenham's chorea is a reversible late manifestation of ARF and is characterized by rapid, involuntary movements affecting all muscles.

The diagnosis of ARF is best made with the revised Jones criteria. Major criteria include an increased antistreptolysin O titer, positive throat culture, or a recent history of scarlet fever. Minor criteria include a previous history of rheumatic fever or rheumatic heart disease, fever, arthralgia, an increase in acute phase reactants (e.g., fibrinogen causing an increase in the erythrocyte sedimentation rate, C-reactive protein, leukocytosis), and a prolonged PR interval. One major and two minor criteria if supported by evidence of an antecedent group A streptococcal infection confirm the diagnosis. Short-term therapy involves a course of penicillin to eradicate throat carriage of group A streptococcus. Long-term therapy involves secondary prevention of recurrences and includes monthly intramuscular injections of benzathine penicillin (erythromycin is used if allergic). Myocarditis is the most common cause of death in ARF, while complications related to mitral stenosis are the most common cause of death in chronic rheumatic fever.

Libman-Sacks endocarditis (choice **C**) occurs in a minority of patients who have systemic lupus erythematosus (SLE). Sterile vegetations develop on the mitral valve. This patient has none of the classic findings of SLE (e.g., malar rash, morning stiffness in the hands). Nonbacterial thrombotic endocarditis (NBTE, choice **D**) is characterized by the presence of sterile lesions on the mitral valve that are very similar to those seen in ARF. However, NBTE is usually associated with a mucin-secreting adenocarcinoma of the pancreas, which is not present in this patient.

41 The answer is E   *Preventive Medicine and Public Health*

The "3 Cs"—cardiotoxicity, convulsions, and coma—are the most common causes of death after overdose of tricyclic antidepressants, such as amitriptyline (choice **E**). Many of the signs and symptoms of poisoning caused by a tricyclic antidepressant are similar to those seen with drugs that have atropine-like actions, including scopolamine (choice **C**) and the phenothiazines. However, widening of the QRS complex to more than 1 second on the electrocardiogram (ECG) is an important diagnostic feature of tricyclic overdose. Multiple dosing with activated charcoal may prevent absorption of tricyclics. Key interventions include correction of the acidosis with bicarbonate, control of cardiotoxicity with phenytoin, and use of intravenous diazepam or lorazepam for control of seizures.

42 **The answer is H**   *Preventive Medicine and Public Health*

Given the widespread use of selective serotonin-reuptake inhibitors (SSRIs) in the management of major depressive disorders, it is hardly surprising that their toxicity in overdose has been designated a "serotonin syndrome." Diaphoresis, diarrhea, myoclonus, tremor, and confusion are characteristics of overdoses of fluoxetine, sertraline (choice **H**), and most other SSRIs. In extreme situations, the toxic syndrome may be life threatening, with seizures, marked hyperthermia, and possible ventricular arrhythmias. The syndrome may occur at conventional doses of the SSRIs with concomitant administration of monoamine oxidase inhibitors, levodopa, meperidine, lithium, or dextromethorphan (in over-the-counter cough medications). Management is supportive, with the possible use of phenytoin or lidocaine for cardiac arrhythmias and benzodiazepines for seizures.

43 **The answer is A**   *Preventive Medicine and Public Health*

Acetaminophen is the most widely used analgesic in the United States. In addition to being sold as an individual product under several trade names, the most common being Tylenol, it is found as an ingredient in at least 100 compounded products. Its widespread use makes it one of the most common causes of accidental poisoning. When ingested at a toxic level, either as a single dose or because of accumulation associated with long-term consumption, acetaminophen (choice **A**) is a hepatotoxin and is the most common cause of liver failure requiring transplantation in the United States and Great Britain. Normally acetaminophen is conjugated in the liver and excreted in the urine. However, if the amount of acetaminophen exceeds the liver's ability to conjugate it, the excess is oxidized by a P450 mixed oxidase to N-acetyl-p-benzoquinone-imine (NAPQI), a toxic byproduct that binds with SH groups on glutathione, vital enzymes, and membrane proteins; the result being centrilobular liver necrosis. N-Acetylcysteine is used as an antidote. Most vulnerable to being overdosed are children given adult doses, individuals with renal problems, alcoholics with already compromised livers, and arthritic elders with concomitant memory problems.

44 **The answer is J**   *Preventive Medicine and Public Health*

Cocaine (choice **J**) is a drug that is available in many forms, can be ingested in many ways, and has many physiologic effects. A strong psychologic addiction is primarily caused by its effect on the limbic system, which results in irresistible feelings of euphoria and pleasure. These effects last for a limited time—when snorted or swallowed with ethanol, usually for less than 4 hours and when smoked or taken intravenously, for less than 30 minutes (the latter modes of consumption are popular because they induce an almost immediate high). The profound feelings of well-being that are induced and its limited duration leads to a desire to repeat the experience as soon as possible, causing "bingeing." In addition to these pleasant central nervous system (CNS) effects, cocaine has several other physiologic effects. A primary one is blockade of norepinephrine reuptake, resulting in release of norepinephrine and α-adrenergic hyperactivity causing hypertension. β-Receptor stimulation via epinephrine causes tachycardia and vasoconstriction. The net result is an increase in myocardial infarcts, aortic dissections, and other medical emergencies, making cocaine abuse the most frequent drug-related visit to emergency departments. Use of cocaine among pregnant mothers, particularly during the first trimester, when many don't even realize they are pregnant, can have disastrous results on the fetus. The vasoconstrictor properties of cocaine still find medical use as a way to stop nose bleeds, and it also still finds limited use as a local anesthetic. The latter effect is due to the drug's blockade of voltage-gated fast sodium channels, which reduces permeability to sodium and results in increasing the threshold of excitability and decreasing the rise rate of the action potential. Cocaine, when used recreationally, is commonly taken in conjunction with other drugs, including alcohol, diazepam, or heroin. The latter combination is called speed balling; the heroin is used to increase the length of a pleasant experience.

45 **The answer is C**   *Preventive Medicine and Public Health*

Scopolamine (choice **C**) is an anticholinergic drug commonly used to combat motion sickness and is provided as a dime-sized patch, usually worn behind the ear. It causes dry mouth in most users and may also induce temporary blurred vision and dilation of the pupils. Other medical uses include treatment of ataxia in Parkinson's disease, muscle spasms of the stomach and intestines, and irritable bowel syndrome.

46 **The answer is G** *Preventive Medicine and Public Health*

Nicotine, primarily in the form of cigarettes, has been estimated to cost more than 150 billion dollars per year in medical costs as well as an even greater amount in indirect cost, making its use the greatest drug-related medical expenditure in the United States (choice **G**). Diseases to which tobacco consumption has been linked include: carcinoma of the lung, larynx, mouth, pharynx, stomach, liver, pancreas, bladder, uterine cervix, and brain; emphysema; chronic bronchitis; asthma; bacterial pneumonia; tubercular pneumonia; asbestosis; coronary artery disease; hypertension; aortic aneurysm; arterial thrombosis; stroke; carotid artery atherosclerosis; intrauterine growth retardation; spontaneous abortion; fetal and neonatal death; abruptio placenta; bleeding in pregnancy not yet discovered; placenta previa; premature rupture of the membranes; prolonged rupture of the membranes; preterm labor; preeclampsia; sudden infant death syndrome; congenital malformations; low birth weight; frequent respiratory and ear infections in children; higher incidence of mental retardation; peptic ulcer disease; osteoporosis; Alzheimer's disease; wrinkling of the skin ("crow's feet" appearance on the face); and impotence.

47 **The answer is D** *Preventive Medicine and Public Health*

Ethanol abuse (choice **D**) is considered by many to be the greatest drug problem in the United States. It may be argued that tobacco is a greater problem in terms of diseases induced and cost for medical care, but alcohol is certainly the greatest in terms of direct observable effects. In any given year, 5 to 7% of the population has an alcohol-related problem, and some 13% have had a problem during their lifetime. Two levels of problems are recognized. The initial level is alcohol abuse in which alcohol consumption continues even though use has already caused failure to meet obligations, accidents (automobile being paramount), legal problems, and/or relationship problems. The next level is alcohol dependency. At this stage, withdrawal causes severe physiologic symptoms (said to be more severe than those in heroin withdrawal). Ethanol-dependent individuals also take extreme actions to avoid withdrawal symptoms such as drinking early in the morning or in desperation drinking anything they think may contain ethanol as an ingredient. Another symptom of alcohol dependence is a change in tolerance, either increased or decreased. Environmental issues and genetic imprinting play a role in determining if a person will have alcohol-related problems. Concordance studies show that the rate of alcoholism between fathers and sons, brothers, and identical twins is very high.

48 **The answer is B** *Preventive Medicine and Public Health*

Diazepam (choice **B**), the generic name for Valium, was put on the market in the 1960s as the prototype member of the benzodiazepine family of anxiolytics. Presently, there are about 15 commonly prescribed drugs in this family, the choice of which is often determined by the length of action. All potentiate the action of γ-aminobutyric acid (GABA) as a neurotransmitter by binding to its receptor. The major resultant effect is sedation, anxiolysis, and striated muscular relaxation; the latter effect makes them useful as anticonvulsants. In psychiatry, they are used to treat anxiety, panic, posttraumatic stress, and sleep disorders, as well as substance-withdrawal symptoms. All have adverse effects including impairment of concentration and memory and possible induction of confusion, ataxia, hypotension, bradycardia, and vertigo. Although rarely fatal alone, they may cause cardiac arrest, particularly in the elderly. All are also potentially addictive, and withdrawal symptoms include anxiety, insomnia, and tremors; after withdrawal from prolonged use, delirium and seizures may also occur. In 2003 there were 60,014 emergency department visits related to benzodiazepine use, and 0.04% of these resulted in death, most of which involved use of a benzodiazepine in conjunction with another drug, often ethanol.

49 **The answer is F** *Preventive Medicine and Public Health*

Veronal, the first barbiturate, was synthesized in 1903, and during most of the 20th century the barbiturates (choice **F**) were widely prescribed as sedatives, anxiolytics, and antiseizure drugs. Although largely replaced by the benzodiazepines, phenytoin, or other drugs, they still have medical uses today. Commonly used barbiturates include phenobarbital (Nembutal), seconal, and mephobarbital. Like the benzodiazepines, they act by binding to the GABA receptors to cause CNS inhibition. They also are highly addictive, with profound withdrawal symptoms including irritability, fainting, nervousness, nausea, and convulsions and are commonly abused, either because they provide a feeling of euphoria or because withdrawal is uncomfortable. Long-term use causes impaired thinking, poor reflexes, depression, reduced sex drive, and deterioration of the liver, pancreas, and brain. They have been implicated in many suicides. On the street they are often used in combination with caffeine, heroin, or methamphetamine to enhance the euphoric effects.

50 **The answer is I** *Preventive Medicine and Public Health*

The amphetamines (amphetamine, dextroamphetamine, and especially methamphetamine) are CNS stimulants that act by releasing dopamine. Their medical use includes control of excessive appetite in weight loss programs, treatment of narcolepsy and depression. Paradoxically, their widest use is to calm children who have the attention deficit and hyperactivity (ADH) syndrome. They were first introduced to the general public during World War II, when the army used them to keep tired and hungry soldiers going. They then became popular as drugs to permit late night cramming. Some continue to use them because they produce a feeling of euphoria and can be purchased relatively cheaply because they can be synthesized in "kitchen" laboratories, and during the past decades there has been a virtual explosion in use. In 2003, 6.2% of high school seniors, 5.2% of 10th graders, and 3.9% of 8th graders used an amphetamine regularly. Unfortunately, once hooked they become addicted, and a tolerance builds, causing persons to consume more and more. Progressively, they cause appetite loss, aggressiveness, delusions, paranoid personality disorder, hallucinations, and eventual true paranoid psychotic events. In addition to these negative psychologic manifestations, they also have profound physical effects: they wreak havoc with the circulatory system, damaging blood vessels, causing irregular heartbeat, and high blood pressure, all of which may induce a stroke or cardiac collapse. To get "better highs," an amphetamine is often "speed-balled" by mixing with other drugs, usually a barbiturate, cocaine, or heroin, and sometimes lysergic acid (LSD) or phencyclidine (aka PCP, angel dust, peace pill or hog).

Questions

Single Best Choice Directions: This section consists of numbered statements or questions followed by a list of potential answers; you are to select the ONE best answer.

1 A 35-year-old man arrives in the emergency department bleeding profusely from a knife wound in the right side of the chest. The wound was inflicted about 30 minutes ago. The patient has hypotension; cold, clammy skin; and tachycardia. Which of the following laboratory parameters is most likely to be outside the normal range?

(A) Arterial pH, arterial PO_2 (PaO_2), arterial PCO_2 ($PaCO_2$)
(B) Hemoglobin (Hb) and hematocrit (Hct)
(C) Central venous pressure
(D) Arterial O_2 saturation (SaO_2)
(E) Red blood cell (RBC) count

2 A 25-year-old man has fever, fatigue, and a sore throat. Findings on physical examination include exudative pharyngitis, hepatosplenomegaly, and tender generalized lymphadenopathy. Laboratory findings include an increased WBC count with atypical lymphocytes as illustrated below, normal hemoglobin concentration, and normal platelet count. Which of the following additional laboratory studies would be most useful in the diagnosis?

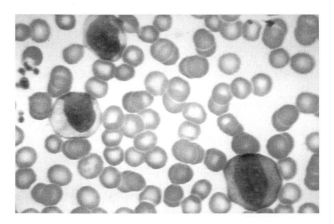

(A) Bone marrow aspiration biopsy
(B) Heterophil antibody test
(C) Lymph node biopsy
(D) Serum antibody screening
(E) Serum transaminase tests

3 A 10-year-old child had an upper respiratory infection 5 days ago and was given symptomatic treatment and an antipyretic (i.e., aspirin for fever). She had seemingly recovered but now presents with fever, protracted vomiting, and lethargy. Physical examination reveals mild hepatomegaly. Total bilirubin, serum transaminases, and serum ammonia are increased. Cerebrospinal fluid (CSF) is obtained and is normal except for elevated pressure. Which of the following is the most likely diagnosis?

(A) Hepatitis A virus (HAV)
(B) Drug-induced hepatitis
(C) Reye syndrome
(D) Infectious mononucleosis
(E) Gilbert syndrome

4 During a routine visit to his physician, a 71-year-old man complains about a persistent pain in his back and abdomen that started some weeks ago and has been getting progressively worse. He adds that "sometimes feels a heart beat around his belly button." In reviewing his history the physician notes that he has smoked since his teens, he has hypertension, and although he finally brought his total cholesterol level down below 200 by taking a statin he did have hypercholesterolemia for many years. After determining that his vital signs were stable, the physician has his patient lie on his back on the examination table with his knees slightly flexed and palpates his abdomen; a pulsating mass near the midline between the xiphoid process umbilicus is felt. Which of the following tests is best to conduct next?

(A) A computed tomographic (CT) scan
(B) Abdominal radiography
(C) A magnetic resonance imaging (MRI) study
(D) Abdominal ultrasonography
(E) An upper gastrointestinal series

5 A 26-day-old infant is brought to the emergency department with a temperature of 39.0°C (102.2°F). The mother is a 25-year-old gravida 2, para 2 who had good prenatal care. Culture of the cerebrospinal fluid (CSF), blood, and urine are sent for analysis. Prophylactic antibiotics are started. It is of paramount importance that the antibiotic treatment provides protection against which of the following pathogens?

(A) *Escherichia coli, Streptococcus pneumoniae,* and *Listeria monocytogenes*

(B) *Streptococcus pneumoniae, Neisseria meningitides,* and *Listeria monocytogenes*

(C) *Streptococcus agalactiae, Escherichia coli,* and *Listeria monocytogenes*

(D) *Streptococcus agalactiae, Escherichia coli,* and *Neisseria meningitides*

(E) *Neisseria meningitides, Streptococcus pneumoniae,* and *Streptococcus agalactiae*

6 A 5 ft 2 in (1.57 m), 31-year-old woman who weighs 186 pounds (84.4 kg) (basal metabolic index = 34 kg/m²) complains to her physician that she has been trying to get pregnant for the past 5 years, and while she has stopped having periods and has gained a lot of weight, it is all fat, no baby. Examination shows no major physical disorder other than hirsutism. Ultrasonography of the ovaries reveals bilaterally enlarged ovaries with subcortical cysts. Which of the following laboratory findings will most likely also be found?

(A) Decreased serum estrone

(B) Increased dehydroepiandrosterone (DHEA) sulfate

(C) Increased follicle-stimulating hormone (FSH)

(D) Increased luteinizing hormone (LH)

(E) Increased serum prolactin

7 A 45-year-old male presents to the emergency department with a history of difficulty breathing and palpitations. On inquiry, he states that he cannot walk more than a couple of blocks, because he becomes short of breath. He has also noticed some swelling of his feet. Physical examination reveals no pallor or cyanosis. His pulse is 88/min, his respiratory rate is 20/min, and his blood pressure is 110/80 mm Hg. A third heart sound is present on auscultation of the heart. A large pulsatile mass is present below the groin. The mass is compressible, and a continuous machinery murmur is heard on auscultation. Which of the following is the most likely cause of this lesion?

(A) A penetrating injury

(B) Blunt trauma

(C) A previous femoral artery bypass

(D) A mycotic aneurysm

(E) A congenital malformation

8 A 40-year-old woman, who enjoys walking barefoot on the beach and in the area around her home, also enjoys taking hiking trips into the Florida Everglades. However, she presents to her physician complaining about such severe fatigue that she has had to curtail her hiking. Physical examination reveals pale conjunctiva. Results of a stool guaiac test are positive for blood. Laboratory studies show a microcytic anemia, eosinophilia, and decreased serum ferritin. An ova and parasite study of stool is positive. Which of the following pathogens is most likely present in the stool sample?

(A) *Ascaris lumbricoides*

(B) *Entameba histolytica*

(C) *Enterobius vermicularis*

(D) *Necator americanus*

(E) *Trichuris trichiura*

9 A 40-year-old man presents to a physician complaining of erectile disfunction. In taking a history it is determined that he started drinking alcohol at the age of 14 years and has continued since. Presently he starts his day by having a beer or two with his breakfast and carries a flask with him to help him get thorough the day. In the evening he often polishes off a pint of whiskey before going to bed. However, he also states he has a "hollow leg" and the alcohol doesn't affect his functioning in any way. Physical examination reveals a distended abdomen and dependent pitting edema. He also has numerous radially oriented vessels around a central core on his face, neck, and upper trunk. Which additional physical finding in this patient has the same pathogenesis as the skin lesion?

(A) Ascites

(B) Asterixis

(C) Caput medusae

(D) Esophageal varices

(E) Gynecomastia

10 A 34-year-old female presents to the outpatient clinic with swelling in the lower anterior aspect of her neck. She does not complain of insomnia, weight loss, or increased appetite, and she does not express decreased tolerance to heat or increased tolerance to cold. Clinical examination reveals a solitary nodule in the right lobe of the thyroid gland. The nodule is nontender and firm. No additional signs (e.g., lid lag, proptosis, tremulousness of the hands) are present. Which of the following would be the most likely indication that this nodule is malignant?

(A) Evidence of a cold nodule on an iodine-131 (¹³¹I) scan

(B) Cystic on fine-needle aspiration

(C) History of previous irradiation of the neck

(D) History of hyperthyroidism

(E) History of Hashimoto's thyroiditis

11 An afebrile 50-year-old woman complains of watery diarrhea and facial flushing. Physical examination reveals an enlarged, nodular liver. A computed tomography (CT) scan of the liver shows multiple nodular masses in the liver parenchyma consistent with metastasis. A small bowel barium study shows a mass lesion in the terminal ileum. A fecal smear for leukocytes is negative. Which of the following laboratory studies is most useful for confirming the diagnosis?

(A) Liver function tests
(B) Serum α-fetoprotein
(C) Serum electrolytes
(D) Stool culture
(E) Urine test for 5-hydroxyindoleacetic acid

12 A 56-year-old alcoholic male with chronic pancreatitis has recurrent attacks of abdominal pain that radiates into his back. The pain is controlled with medical therapy. He has lost 30 lb (13.6 kg) in the past 3 months because of chronic diarrhea. Examination of the abdomen reveals no masses. Computerized tomography (CT) of the pancreas reveals multiple calcifications but no mass lesions. The serum glucose determination is normal. A qualitative stool test for fat has positive results. Antigliadin antibodies are not present. Which of the following would be the most appropriate treatment?

(A) Total pancreatectomy
(B) Broad-spectrum antibiotic therapy
(C) Gluten-free diet
(D) Oral pancreatic enzymes before, during, and after meals
(E) Administration of lactulose

13 A 30-year-old man with AIDS develops focal epileptic seizures. A magnetic resonance imaging (MRI) study shows multiple ring-enhancing lesions in the gray matter of the cerebral cortex. The CD4 helper T-cell count is 50 cells/mm^3. Treatment with an antibiotic causes some resolution of the lesions. Which of the following is the most likely pathogen?

(A) *Cryptococcus neoformans*
(B) Cytomegalovirus (CMV)
(C) Epstein-Barr virus (EBV)
(D) Herpes simplex type 1
(E) *Toxoplasma gondii*

14 A 36-year-old woman complains of severe episodes of headache, tremulousness, palpitations, and anxiety. The patient has noted a change in her voice, and she has difficulty swallowing solids. On physical examination there is a palpable, nontender swelling in front of her neck that moves with deglutition. No cervical

lymphadenopathy is noted. Laboratory studies show serum hypercalcemia. An x-ray film of the cervical region reveals irregular calcification in the mass, while magnetic resonance imaging (MRI) of the abdomen confirms the presence of bilateral adrenal lesions. Which of the following would be the best screening test for the thyroid mass in this patient?

(A) An iodine-123 (^{123}I) scan
(B) Measurement of the serum thyroid-stimulating hormone (TSH) level
(C) Measurement of the serum thyroxine (T$_4$) level
(D) Measurement of the serum calcitonin level
(E) Measurement of the serum parathormone level

15 A 52-year-old woman is seen with a history of a mass in the right breast. She states that it resulted from trauma. Physical examination reveals a firm, nontender mass with no evidence of involvement of the overlying skin. The ipsilateral axilla does not contain enlarged lymph nodes. The contralateral breast and axilla are normal. A biopsy confirms the diagnosis of traumatic fat necrosis; however, it also reveals evidence of an in situ lobular carcinoma. Which of the following best characterizes this breast cancer?

(A) Increased incidence of negative estrogen- and progesterone-receptor assays
(B) Aggressive natural history with early invasion of the breast stroma
(C) Increased likelihood of cancer developing in the other breast
(D) Increased incidence of chest wall involvement by this tumor
(E) Increased incidence of breast cancer in first- and second-degree relatives

16 A 40-year-old man has had a problem with alcohol since his early 20s. He has been arrested twice for driving under the influence, and just a few months ago his wife left him and filed for divorce. About a month ago he started feeling poorly and found that his tolerance for alcohol had decreased. As a consequence, he made an appointment to see a physician to whom he presents with fever, painful hepatomegaly, and jaundice. A liver biopsy shows fatty change, a neutrophilic infiltrate, and eosinophilic staining material within hepatocytes. Which of the following laboratory findings also would most likely be reported?

(A) Conjugated bilirubin percentage <20%
(B) Increase in serum aspartate aminotransferase
(C) Normal serum γ-glutamyltransferase
(D) Positive anti–hepatitis A virus IgM
(E) Positive serum antimitochondrial antibody

17 A 30-year-old man with a history of chronic diarrhea describes his stools as greasy and foul smelling. He recently developed pruritic vesicular lesions involving the elbows. A quantitative stool test for fat shows an increased amount of fat. An oral D-xylose absorption test reveals decreased reabsorption of xylose into the blood. Which of the following tests would be most useful in identifying the cause of the diarrhea?

(A) Antigliadin antibodies

(B) Antinuclear antibodies

(C) Fecal smear for leukocytes

(D) Stool for ova and parasites

(E) Stool osmotic gap

18 A 16-year-old adolescent with normal secondary female sex characteristics has primary amenorrhea. Physical examination shows discrete masses in both inguinal canals. Speculum examination of the vagina shows it ending in a blind pouch. Which of the following laboratory findings is most likely present?

(A) Buccal smear with one Barr body

(B) Chromosome study with XO genotype

(C) Chromosome study with XY genotype

(D) Decreased serum testosterone

(E) Increased serum gonadotropins

19 A 71-inch tall (1.8 m), 57-year old man weighs 208 pounds (94.3 kg) feels healthy and wants to take out life insurance. Consequently, he is subjected to a physical examination with subsequent laboratory analyses. The following data are obtained: blood pressure, 155/84; fasting blood glucose, 115 mg%; total cholesterol, 265 mg/dL; triglycerides, 157 mg/dL; HDL, 39 mg/dL; LDL, 125 mg/dL. Which of the following is also most likely true regarding this man?

(A) His plasminogen activator inhibitor-1 (PAI-1) is lower than normal

(B) His insulin levels are higher than normal

(C) Glucose uptake into his muscles is inhibited

(D) Glucose uptake into his adipose tissue is inhibited

(E) His uric acid level is lower than normal

20 The son of a 65-year-old woman whose husband died more than 2 years ago consults a physician about his mother's current behavior. She had her husband's body cremated and keeps the urn in the bedroom, spending an inordinate time there talking to his ashes. She also has ceased socializing with her friends and in fact doesn't get dressed or sometimes even get up out of bed. Which of the following behaviors would the physician most likely consider normal under these circumstances?

(A) Brief periods of longing for her husband

(B) Feelings of worthlessness

(C) A suicide attempt

(D) Inability to work

(E) Despair

21 A 21-year-old soldier returns from a 15-month overseas tour of duty during which time he participated in close-quarter and bloody combat. Since returning home 3 months ago, his parents note that he stays in his room all day and does not return calls from friends. They find him awake in the kitchen at night, looking anxious and sweaty. He says he can't sleep because he keeps thinking about his war experiences. Which of the following might be the medication with which to treat him?

(A) Olanzapine

(B) Sertraline

(C) Eszopiclone

(D) Topiramate

(E) Atomoxetine

22 A bereaved family just returned from a funeral for their 20-year old son. In her grief, the mother began to reminisce to her mother. "He was such a healthy baby until he reached his third birthday. Then he stopped running and started walking like a duck. Next he couldn't stand without climbing up on somebody or something, and by his eleventh birthday we had to get him a motorized wheelchair. Even then he was doing well, finished high school, enrolled in City College, was a member of the chess team, and took an interest in politics. Then he caught what seemed just to be a cold and died." The grandmother replied, "Yes it is so tragic. I can't understand what happened. Nobody else in the family ever had anything like his disease. Not his sisters, your sisters, or my sisters." Which of the following diseases did this young man have?

(A) Becker muscular dystrophy

(B) Myotonic muscular dystrophy

(C) Facioscapulohumeral muscular dystrophy

(D) Limb girdle muscular dystrophy

(E) Digital muscular dystrophy

(F) Duchenne muscular dystrophy

23 A pediatrician performs a physical examination on a newborn he is asked to evaluate. The pertinent findings he notes include severe hypotonia, generalized weakness, and absent tendon stretch reflexes. The baby lies flaccid with little movement, but there appears to be preservation of the extraocular muscles. The patient is also observed to have fasciculations of the tongue, and the nurse informs the pediatrician that the infant has had trouble feeding. Which of the following is the most likely diagnosis?

(A) Myotonic dystrophy
(B) Werdnig-Hoffmann disease
(C) Infant botulism
(D) Infantile myasthenia gravis
(E) Duchenne's muscular dystrophy

24 The pediatric intern is called to the nursery to examine a small-for-gestational-age newborn. The mother had one prenatal visit during her entire pregnancy. Physical examination is pertinent for hepatosplenomegaly, jaundice, cataracts, and widespread maculopapular lesions of a reddish-blue color. Diagnostic studies are indicative of hepatitis and thrombocytopenia. Which of the following is the most likely cause of these findings?

(A) Toxoplasmosis
(B) Rubeola
(C) Rubella
(D) Varicella
(E) Syphilis

25 A 52-year-old woman with type 2 diabetes mellitus presents with altered mental status to the emergency department. She is taking 250 mg of chlorpropamide daily. Physical examination is unremarkable. Her skin turgor is normal. Laboratory studies indicate the following values: serum sodium concentration of 110 mEq/L (normal, 135–147 mEq/L), serum potassium concentration of 3.2 mEq/L (normal, 3.5–5.0 mEq/L), serum chloride concentration of 90 mEq/L (normal, 95–105 mEq/L), serum bicarbonate concentration of 21 mEq/L (normal, 22–28 mEq/L), serum glucose concentration of 140 mg/dL (normal, 70–110 mg/dL), and serum blood urea nitrogen (BUN) concentration of 5 mg/dL (normal, 7–18 mg/dL). Random urine sodium level is 80 mEq/L (normally, >20 mEq/L indicates increased loss, <20 mEq/L indicates increased reabsorption). Which of the following would be most appropriate in the management of this patient?

(A) Restrict both water and sodium from the diet
(B) Restrict only sodium from the diet
(C) Restrict only water from the diet
(D) Add sodium to the diet
(E) Increase water intake

26 A 55-year-old man presents to the emergency department with massive hematemesis. Physical examina-

tion reveals abdominal distention, shifting dullness on percussion of the abdomen, and spider angiomata over the face and upper chest. An emergency endoscopic examination reveals blood rapidly filling the distal esophagus. The hematemesis is most likely due to which of the following?

(A) Pyloric obstruction
(B) Ruptured esophageal varices
(C) Gastric ulcer
(D) Esophageal carcinoma
(E) Duodenal ulcer

27 A dental hygienist notes white patches on the lateral borders of both sides of the tongue of 66-year-old man and suggests that he consult his physician. Upon taking a history, the physician determines that the patient has no problems with mastication or swallowing, and that the lesions are painless. Further examination reveals that the discrete white patches are raised and they do not scrape off. Which of the following is the greatest risk factor for developing these types of lesions?

(A) Excessive consumption of alcohol
(B) Glossitis due to *Candida albicans*
(C) Glossitis due to Epstein-Barr virus
(D) Glossitis due to vitamin B_{12} deficiency
(E) Smoking cigarettes

28 A 60-year-old man has a 30-year history of productive cough and occasional bouts of hemoptysis. A chest x-ray film shows crowded bronchial markings extending to the lung periphery. A high-resolution computerized tomography (CT) scan shows dilation of the bronchi and bronchioles. Which of the following is the most likely cause of the lung disease?

(A) Chronic infection
(B) Emphysema
(C) Immotile cilia syndrome
(D) Inhalation of mineral dust
(E) Primary lung cancer

29 A 42-year-old male executive complains of upper abdominal pain, diarrhea, and a 30-lb (13.6 kg) weight loss in 3 months. He states that he is under considerable stress at work, consumes a large amount of caffeine, and smokes a pack of cigarettes every day. He has no history of shortness of breath, swelling of the feet, chest pain, or allergies. He has not been on any long-term medications. Further inquiry reveals that the pain is very intense at night, waking him from sleep. It also occurs between meals and is relieved by drinking milk or consuming a bland diet. Spicy foods aggravate the condition. On one occasion he vomited

blood. Standard laboratory parameters are within normal limits. However, a gastric analysis reveals a basal acid output (BAO) of 60 mEq/h (normal, <5 mEq/h), a maximal acid output (MAO) of 100 mEq/h (normal, 5–20 mEq/h), and a serum gastrin level of 1000 pg/mL (normal, <300 pg/mL). Which of the following is the most likely diagnosis?

(A) Ménétrier's disease (giant hypertrophic gastritis)
(B) Gastric adenocarcinoma
(C) Glucagonoma
(D) Zollinger-Ellison syndrome
(E) Pernicious anemia

30. A 77-year-old man who prides himself as having been in prime physical health all his life despite seldom seeing a doctor and who claims the only medication he ever takes is aspirin, has a sudden severe headache, vertigo, and a loss of balance that makes standing and walking difficult. Consequently, he has a fall and bumps his head. His worried daughter takes him to the nearest emergency department where he is examined. He is found to be a thin man who is relatively muscular for his age. Although still unable to stand or walk, there is no evidence of muscle weakness. He remains fully conscious, is fully cognizant of his surroundings, and can answer questions quickly and lucidly. His heart and lungs are normal as is an electrocardiogram (ECG). A finger stick blood glucose determination reads 152 mg/dL of glucose. His blood pressure remains between 165 and 185 mm Hg systolic over 75–85 mm Hg diastolic. Which of the following is the most likely underlying cause of his problem?

(A) An epidural hemorrhage
(B) Ménière's syndrome
(C) Isolated systolic hypertension
(D) A cerebral infarct
(E) A pulmonary thromboembolism

31. A low-birth-weight infant presents to his pediatrician at 2 months of age. The mother states that the infant has not been eating well. Upon physical examination the infant is noted to be pale and tachycardic. The lungs are clear to auscultation, and there is no hepatosplenomegaly. A complete blood count (CBC) shows a hemoglobin (Hb) level of 6 g/dL. Which of the following is the most likely cause of anemia in this infant?

(A) Megaloblastic anemia
(B) Sickle cell anemia
(C) Anemia of prematurity
(D) α-Thalassemia
(E) Homozygous β-thalassemia

32. A 51-year-old woman presents with an episode of dysphoria, sleep difficulty, psychomotor agitation, and rumination about mistakes she has made in her life. She has delusions of guilt about indirectly causing the deaths of many people. She has a history of two previous episodes with similar symptoms, but no history of manic episodes. Between episodes, she is asymptomatic. Which of the following is the most likely diagnosis?

(A) Bipolar disorder, depressed phase
(B) Dysthymic disorder
(C) Major depressive disorder, recurrent
(D) Schizoaffective disorder, depressive type
(E) Schizophrenia

33. A child was in her usual state of good health when she developed a focal seizure while playing with her sister. The mother, a registered nurse, states that the seizure lasted approximately 5 minutes. The 911 Emergency Services were called and the child arrived postictal to the emergency department approximately 1 hour after the seizure first occurred. On physical examination the vital signs are stable, but the patient is noted to have weakness and hemiparesis. Remarkably, within 24 hours the weakness and neurologic deficits disappear. Which of the following is the most likely diagnosis?

(A) Hemiplegia complicating a migraine headache
(B) Spastic hemiplegia
(C) Postviral encephalitis
(D) Todd's paralysis
(E) Infratentorial tumor

34. A 38-year-old woman, gravida 1, para 0, delivers an appropriate-for-gestational-age infant by spontaneous vaginal delivery in the vertex position. The mother had excellent prenatal care and denies any history of tobacco, alcohol, or drugs. The infant weighs 8 lb 6 oz (3.8 kg). The Apgar score is 8 at 1 minute and 9 at 5 minutes. On physical examination the infant is noted to have edematous swelling of the soft tissue of the scalp that crosses the midline. Which of the following is the most likely diagnosis?

(A) Cephalohematoma
(B) Subcutaneous fat necrosis
(C) Fracture of the skull
(D) Caput succedaneum
(E) Overriding of the parietal bones

35. A blue-eyed Caucasian 75-year-old man has had gradual loss of vision for the past 5 years. He initially had trouble reading fine print and road signs, and

similar distant objects appeared blurred. The vision loss has progressed to the point that if he looks directly at a book or an object he cannot make out what it is. However, he found that he can compensate to a large extent by looking at things using side vision. As a consequence, he can still walk around and even cross a street safely unaided. Which of the following is the most likely cause of his visual loss?

(A) Macular degeneration
(B) Trauma
(C) Cataract surgery
(D) Optic neuritis
(E) Diabetic retinopathy

36 A 17-year-old male football player reports to the school clinic complaining that he feels poorly. In fact, he has not felt well for the past 2 days. He is nauseous and vomited twice before coming to the clinic. He describes a pain in the middle of his belly that recently moved to the right lower quadrant and became more severe. Because of a poor appetite, he ate very little for supper last night and nothing for breakfast. Upon physical examination, the patient looks ill. His temperature is 38.1°C (102.2°F). Although both the left and right quadrants have significant tenderness, the pain is much greater on the right side. Rebound tenderness is present. Which of the following is the most likely diagnosis?

(A) Ulcerative colitis
(B) Crohn's disease
(C) Acute appendicitis
(D) Irritable bowel syndrome
(E) Psychogenic pain

37 A 57-year-old man has a prosthetic aortic valve. He develops a normocytic anemia with an increased reticulocyte count. A peripheral blood smear shows an increased reticulocyte count and numerous irregularly shaped red blood cells (RBCs). Measurement of the changes in the concentration of which of the following

serum proteins would be most useful for following the severity of this patient's anemia?

(A) Ceruloplasmin
(B) Albumin
(C) C-reactive protein
(D) Transferrin
(E) Haptoglobin

38 A 49-year-old man comes to the emergency department complaining that a worm is eating the bone marrow in his "leg bone." He indicates a small scab over his right femur and insists this is where the worm entered while he was asleep several days ago. There is no previous history of psychiatric hospitalization or substance abuse. Mental status examination reveals an alert, oriented individual whose thought processes are coherent. Which of the following is the most likely diagnosis?

(A) Body dysmorphic disorder
(B) Delusional disorder, somatic type
(C) Hypochondriasis
(D) Schizophrenia
(E) Somatization disorder

39 A 14-year-old previously well patient is diagnosed with clinical sinusitis by his physician. A prescription for antibiotics was made out for the patient and given to his parents to treat this condition. The patient's parents had the prescription filled at the pharmacy. Unfortunately, the teenager, who does not like to take medication, was not always compliant and missed many doses of the antibiotic. Presently he is being evaluated in the emergency department for fever, confusion, extraocular palsies, and proptosis of the eye. Which of the following is the most likely diagnosis?

(A) Hand-Schüller-Christian disease
(B) Graves' disease
(C) Cavernous sinus thrombosis
(D) Acute bacterial conjunctivitis
(E) Temporal lobe abscess

Directions for Matching Questions (40 through 50): Each set of matching questions is preceded by a list of 4 to 26 lettered options followed by a brief explanation of the required task and then by a series of numbered statements. For each lettered statement you are to select ONE lettered option that best fulfills the task as it relates to that statement. Remember each of the listed options might be correctly selected once, more than once, or not at all.

Question 40–46

(A) Granulosa cell tumor
(B) Brenner tumor
(C) Serous adenocarcinoma
(D) Endodermal sinus tumor of the ovary
(E) Gynandroblastoma
(F) Nongestational choriocarcinomas of the ovary
(G) Dysgerminoma

For each of the following numbered description, select the ONE type of ovarian cancer listed above to which it relates best.

40 Cancer antigen 125 (CA-125)

41 Testosterone secretion

42 Increased serum lactate dehydrogenase (LDH) activity

43 α-Fetoprotein (AFP)

44 β-Human chorionic gonadotropin (β-HCG)

45 Estrogen secretion

46 Has no tumor marker

Questions 47–50

Match each drug with the related graph from those below, which illustrate sleep patterns. Graph A represents normal sleep architecture.

47 Often associated with major depressive disorders

48 Diazepam

49 Benzodiazepine rebound

50 Barbiturates

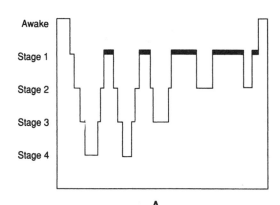

A

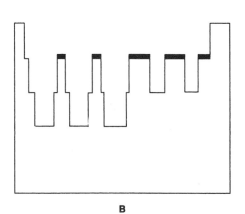

B

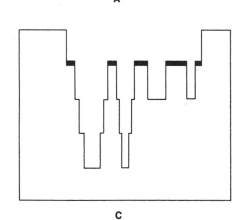

C

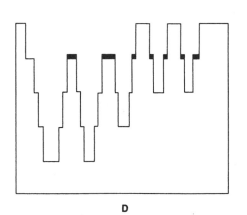

D

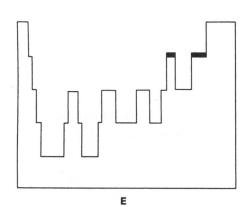

E

Answer Key

1 C	**11** E	**21** B	**31** C	**41** E
2 B	**12** D	**22** F	**32** C	**42** G
3 C	**13** E	**23** B	**33** D	**43** D
4 D	**14** D	**24** C	**34** D	**44** F
5 C	**15** C	**25** C	**35** A	**45** A
6 D	**16** B	**26** B	**36** C	**46** B
7 A	**17** A	**27** E	**37** E	**47** D
8 D	**18** C	**28** A	**38** B	**48** B
9 E	**19** B	**29** D	**39** C	**49** C
10 C	**20** A	**30** C	**40** C	**50** E

Answers and Explanations

1 The answer is C *Surgery*

Volume loss from hemorrhage is first detected by a drop in the central venous pressure (choice **C**) or capillary wedge pressure in the lungs. The hemoglobin (Hb) and hematocrit (Hct) (choice **B**) and RBC count (choice **E**) often remain normal in the initial stages of blood loss, because an equal amount of plasma and red blood cells (RBCs) are lost, and the vascular tree contracts around the reduced volume of blood. Plasma is the first to be restored as fluid moves from the interstitial space into the blood vessels. This uncovers the deficit in RBCs, resulting in a drop in the Hb, Hct, and RBC count. Intravenous (IV) administration of isotonic (normal) saline dilutes the blood faster and uncovers this deficit faster. An increased reticulocyte count reflects effective erythropoiesis in the bone marrow, which will, in 5 to 7 days, replace the deficit in RBCs in the peripheral blood.

Blood loss leading to a normocytic anemia does not alter the arterial pH, PaO_2, or $PaCO_2$ of blood (choice **A**). However, it does reduce the total amount of oxygen available to tissue, thus producing tissue hypoxia. The SaO_2 (choice **D**), which represents the total number of binding sites on Hb that are occupied by oxygen, is normal in anemia, because there is normal oxygenation of Hb in the pulmonary capillaries. The problem in anemia is a decrease in Hb, which automatically lowers the total oxygen content of blood.

2 The answer is B *Medicine*

The patient has infectious mononucleosis, which is caused by the Epstein-Barr virus (EBV). Infectious mononucleosis is usually transmitted by saliva; although called the "kissing" disease, transmission requires a deep kiss in which saliva is exchanged and is probably more often transmitted by shared eating utensils or food. Symptomatic infectious mononucleosis is usually observed in the late teens or twenties, and the symptomatic individuals represent the relatively few who did not get a nonsymptomatic infection during early childhood. By the age of 30 years, over 95% of individuals in the United States would test positive for EBV virus. EBV is a herpesvirus and will remain latent after an infection only to reactivate later; in the reactivated state, individuals have no symptoms but are infective and it is believed that most infections are spread by seemingly healthy individuals.

As illustrated in the figure, larger than normal lymphocytes with prominent nucleoli and dark-staining coarse chromatin are present; these represents an antigenically stimulated T cell that is responding to B cells infected by the virus. Hepatosplenomegaly and painful generalized lymphadenopathy are invariably present in mononucleosis. In about 95% of cases recovery is spontaneous, fever disappears in 10 days, and lymphadenopathy and splenomegaly clear up in 4 weeks, although debility sometimes lingers for 2–3 months. The most dangerous complication is spleen rupture, which can occur if infected persons engage in active sports or other rough activities.

The heterophil antibody test (choice **B**) is useful in the diagnosis of infectious mononucleosis, because it confirms the presence of IgM heterophil antibodies (e.g., anti-horse or sheep red blood cell antibodies) that are specific for the disease. Typically in the clinical setting, the mono spot test is used in which a drop of blood is added to reagent on a microscopic slide. This will give a positive result from 2 to at least 9 weeks after infection. If deemed necessary, more-quantitative immunologic studies using more-specific antigen can also be run in a laboratory. There are three EBV antigens: early antigen, viral capsid antigen, and nuclear antigen. Depending upon the antigen used and the antibody formed, IgM or IgG, it can be determined with reasonable certainty whether an individual has never been infected with EBV, has a primary infection, has an old latent infection, or has an old infection that has reactivated.

Bone marrow aspiration biopsies (choice **A**) are performed to rule out leukemias. A lymphocytic leukemia is not likely in this case, because the patient's hemoglobin concentration and platelet count are normal, and the peripheral blood smear shows an atypical lymphocyte that is not neoplastic. A lymph node biopsy (choice **C**) is usually performed when a neoplastic process (e.g., malignant lymphoma, or metastatic disease) is suspected. A neoplastic process produces painless enlargement of lymph nodes, which is not present in this case; rather this patient's painful lymphadenopathy indicates a benign, reactive process. Standard serum antibody screening (choice **D**) detects antibodies directed against Rh and other antigens that occur normally on the surface of human RBCs, but it does not detect the antibodies present in infectious mononucleosis. Tests for serum transaminases (e.g., alanine aminotransferase; choice **E**) are useful in the diagnosis of hepatitis, which is invariably present in patients with infectious mononucleosis. Thus, markedly elevated levels of serum transaminases would be expected in this patient, but they would not help diagnose the specific cause of the hepatitis.

3 The answer is C *Pediatrics*

Reye syndrome (choice **C**) shows a very high association with the ingestion of aspirin-containing medicines during influenza-like illnesses or varicella. Reye syndrome has a biphasic course. It usually presents in a previously healthy child who had an upper respiratory infection (90%) or varicella (5–7%). After the child seems to have recovered, the symptoms of vomiting, lethargy, and confusion can appear and progress quickly. The patient may also be combative. Liver enzymes and ammonia level are elevated. Treatment requires early recognition and control of increased intracranial pressure. Prognosis depends on duration of disordered cerebral function.

Hepatitis A virus (HAV) (choice **A**) is an RNA-containing virus. It is a member of the Picornaviridae family and is spread predominantly by the fecal–oral route. In the United States, there is increased risk of infection with HAV in daycare centers, in contacts of children who attend daycare centers, and in the homosexual population. The diagnosis of HAV infection should be considered when a history of jaundice exists in the patient's contacts, or if the patient or his or her family has traveled to an endemic area. The acute infection is diagnosed by the presence of immunoglobulin M (IgM) anti-HAV. Although elevation may be found in the bilirubin and serum transaminase levels, they do not help to differentiate the cause. Drug-induced hepatitis (choice **B**) is not the correct answer, because the patient in this scenario has a history of aspirin usage, and aspirin is excreted by the kidney. Infectious mononucleosis (choice **D**) is a clinical syndrome caused by the Epstein-Barr virus (EBV). Clinical symptoms in children are often mild, but patients may have fatigue, fever, sore throat, and generalized lymphadenopathy. Splenomegaly may be prominent, causing left upper quadrant abdominal tenderness. Hepatomegaly may be present in a small number of patients. Symptomatic hepatitis or jaundice is uncommon. A mononuclear lymphocytosis with atypical-appearing lymphocytes is associated with infectious mononucleosis. Gilbert syndrome (choice **E**) is an inherited, benign, unconjugated hyperbilirubinemia that is transmitted as an autosomal dominant disease. The hyperbilirubinemia is mild, and the bilirubin level may fluctuate. Jaundice is intermittent and may be noted on routine physical examination. Results of liver biopsy and other liver function tests are normal.

4 The answer is D *Medicine*

The described symptoms suggest an expanding abdominal aortic aneurysm, and the patient has the primary risk factors—age, a long history of smoking, hypertension and probable arthrosclerosis (high cholesterol for years)—and the finding of a palpable pulsatile mass in the abdomen is almost diagnostic. The most appropriate next test is abdominal ultrasonography (choice **D**), which indeed has been recommended by the U.S. Preventative Task Force (USPSTF) as a screening test for all men over 65 years old who have smoked for years, particularly if the risk has been compounded by hypertension or arthrosclerosis or if a first-degree relative has had an aneurysm. Ultrasonography is available at most hospitals, is relatively inexpensive, does not require exposure to radiation, reveals details of the aortic wall, and permits accurate measurement of shape and size of the aneurysm. An aneurism larger than 5.5 cm (2¼ inch) is in danger of rupture and is usually surgically repaired as soon as possible, either by open surgery or more recently by less invasive endosurgery procedures. One less than 3 cm (1½ inch) is generally committed to watchful waiting. Whether surgery should be done on aneurysms of intermediate size depends upon the assessment of risk of rupture, including size, evidence of recent expansion, family history, and the patient's general health. The goal is to avoid rupture because once ruptured, there is a 90% fatality rate. Some 9,000 to 15,000 Americans are estimated to die from an abdominal aortic aneurysm annually.

A CT scan (choice **A**), abdominal radiography (choice **B**), or a MRI study (choice **C**) all can be used to diagnose an aneurism but are either more expensive, are less convenient, or provide less information and are therefore no longer recommended as first-choice diagnostic modalities. An upper gastrointestinal series (choice **E**) would be inappropriate.

5 The answer is C *Pediatrics*

The infectious disease that the physician would be most concerned about is meningitis. The treatment must be designed to prevent or, if already fulminating, cure this disease. *Streptococcus agalactiae* (group B streptococcus) is a common inhabitant of the maternal genitourinary tract. It is acquired by newborns via vertical transmission, and it is the most common cause of neonatal meningitis, followed by *Escherichia coli* and *Listeria monocytogenes*. Early-onset disease is associated with sepsis; late onset is associated with meningitis. Consequently, *S. agalactiae, E. coli,* and *L. monocytogenes* (choice **C**) is the correct answer.

Streptococcus pneumoniae (part of choice **A, B,** and **E**) and *Neisseria meningitidis* (part of choice **B, D,** and **E**) are seen in older age groups.

6 The answer is D *Medicine*

The patient has polycystic ovary syndrome (PCOS), which affects 4–6% of reproductive-age women. In this disorder, patients have a steady production of estrogen rather than the normal fluctuating rate that occurs during the menstrual cycle. Commonly this excess estrogen is due to conversion of ovarian and adrenal androgens to estrogen in the body fat, although there also may be an underlying endocrine disorder. The excess synthesis of estrogen causes a steady rate of luteinizing hormone (LH) production, leading to a relative increase (choice **D**); this causes excessive stimulation of the ovaries with increased synthesis of 17-ketosteroids (dehydroepiandrosterone [DHEA] and androstenedione) and testosterone. An increase in these androgen compounds causes hirsutism (excess hair in normal hair-bearing areas). Thus in obese patients, a vicious circle is established; this androgen excess is converted to still more estrogen by the aromatase in the excess number of adipose cells (e.g., androstenedione is converted to estrone and testosterone is converted to estradiol). An increase in estrogen has a negative feedback on the release of FSH and a positive feedback on the release of LH; therefore, LH is still further increased and FSH is decreased (not increased [choice **C**]). Decreased FSH causes degeneration of the ovarian follicles, which results in the formation of subcortical cysts. In PCOS, the LH-to-FSH ratio usually exceeds 2:1, and 80% of cases present with amenorrhea or abnormal menstruation, 50% with hirsutism, 40% with obesity, and 20% with virilization. In addition, patients are generally infertile (although they may ovulate on occasion), show insulin resistance putting them at risk for type 2 diabetes, and are at risk for endometrial and breast cancer because of the unopposed action of estrogen. In obese patients, weight loss will often break the vicious circle and restore normal ovulatory function.

Serum estrone is increased in PCOS (not decreased [choice **A**]) because of increased conversion of androstenedione to estrone by aromatase in the adipose cells. DHEA sulfate (choice **B**) is a 17-ketosteroid that is primarily synthesized in the adrenal cortex (95%) and is not increased in PCOS. However, there is an increase in DHEA in PCOS, because the nonsulfated form is synthesized in the ovaries. This explains why an increase in DHEA sulfate is used as a marker for hirsutism caused by adrenal cortical hyperfunction (e.g., Cushing syndrome). Prolactin levels (choice **E**) are not altered in PCOS.

7 The answer is A *Surgery*

The patient has an arteriovenous (AV) fistula, which is most commonly results from a penetrating injury (e.g., knife wound) (choice **A**). Other causes of AV fistulas include congenital causes, which can result in hemihypertrophy of an extremity; erosion of an arterial graft or aneurysm into a subjacent vein; and bone disease such as Paget's disease of the bone, in which the remodeling of bone creates intramarrow AV communications. A continuous machinery murmur is usually heard on auscultation of an AV fistula. Proximally, the arteries and veins are dilated. The distal pulse is usually diminished in amplitude. Compression of the mass results in slowing of the pulse rate. This is called Branham's sign. Because an AV fistula bypasses the microcirculation, there is an increase in venous return to the right heart, which results in a high-output failure, which is present in this patient (third heart sound). Magnetic resonance imaging (MRI) and angiography are very useful in delineating these lesions. Heart failure in this patient is an indication for surgical removal or embolization of the lesion under radiographic control.

Blunt trauma (choice **B**), previous femoral artery bypass (choice **C**), a mycotic aneurysm (aneurysm caused by a microbial pathogen; choice **D**), and a congenital malformation (choice **E**) are all possible causes of an AV fistula; however, they are not as common as a penetrating injury.

8 The answer is D *Medicine*

The patient has a hookworm infection due to *Necator americanus* (choice **D**), which is the most common parasite causing iron deficiency. Filariform larvae in soil penetrate skin when persons walk barefoot. There is a larval phase in lungs, and organisms are swallowed and develop into adult worms. The cutting plates of adult worms attach to villi, and the worms feed on blood. Since the worms are invasive, eosinophilia is present. The treatment is albendazole or mebendazole.

The adult worms of *Ascaris lumbricoides* (choice **A**) cause intestinal obstruction and do not cause bloody diarrhea. Since the adult worms are noninvasive, there is no eosinophilia. The treatment is albendazole or mebendazole. *Entameba histolytica* (choice **B**) is a protozoan that produces bloody diarrhea, however, blood loss is not chronic, and therefore, iron deficiency does not occur. There is not eosinophilia. The treatment is metronidazole. *Enterobius vermicularis* (choice **C**) is the most common helminth in the United States. It primarily causes anal pruritus when the adult worms lay eggs in the anal region. Additional complications include urethritis in girls and appendicitis. There is no eosinophilia, because the adult worms are noninvasive. The Scotch tape test of perianal skin identifies embryonated eggs (flat on one side). The treatment is albendazole or mebendazole. *Trichuris trichiura* (choice **E**), or whipworm, is the parasite most commonly causing rectal prolapse in children. Eosinophilia is present; however, it does not cause iron deficiency. The treatment is albendazole.

9 The answer is E *Medicine*

The patient has cirrhosis of the liver (history of alcohol abuse, ascites, and dependent pitting edema). The skin lesions are spider angiomas, which have a central spiral arteriole with a group of small vessels radiating from the arteriole. Spider angiomas are associated with hyperestrinism, which is a complication of cirrhosis. In cirrhosis, the dysfunctional liver is unable to metabolize estrogen, which produces hyperestrinism. Hyperestrinism in men causes gynecomastia (development of breast tissue in males; choice **E**) and female secondary sex characteristics (palmar erythema, soft skin and female hair distribution).

Factors that contribute to the development of ascites (choice **A**) include portal hypertension (increase in hydrostatic pressure), hypoalbuminemia (decrease in oncotic pressure), secondary aldosteronism (salt retention), and increased lymphatic drainage into the peritoneal cavity. Asterixis (choice **B**), or flapping tremor, refers to the inability to sustain posture. It is a sign of hepatic encephalopathy, which is caused by an increase in ammonia and false neurotransmitters (e.g., γ-aminobenzoic acid). Caput medusae (choice **C**) are dilated periumbilical veins that are associated with increased venous pressure caused by portal hypertension. Esophageal varices (choice **D**) are dilated left gastric coronary veins, which normally drain the distal esophagus and proximal stomach and empty into the portal vein. An increase in portal vein pressure leads to dilation of the gastric veins (varices), which commonly rupture.

10 The answer is C *Surgery*

In adult women, most (60%) solitary nodules in the thyroid gland are not neoplastic and represent cysts or goiter. Approximately 25% are follicular adenomas, and the remaining 15% are malignant. Factors that suggest malignancy in a solitary nodule are as follows: a history of previous irradiation of the neck (choice **C**); a hard, irregular nodule with cervical lymphadenopathy, or one that is greater than 3 to 4 cm; a serum thyroglobulin level above 100 ng/dL; and a family history of a medullary carcinoma of the thyroid suggesting multiple endocrine neoplasia (MEN) IIa or IIb syndrome. Any solitary nodule in a man or a child also is suspicious. Fine-needle aspiration (FNA) is the first step in the workup of a thyroid nodule. If the FNA is positive for cancer, surgery is performed. If it is inconclusive, a thyroid scan is ordered.

A cold nodule (nonfunctioning nodule; choice **A**) is treated by surgery. A hot nodule (functioning nodule) is surgically removed as a cure for hyperthyroidism; such hot nodules are rarely malignant and may be associated with a history of hyperthyroidism (choice **D**). Solitary nodules are not commonly present in Hashimoto's thyroiditis (choice **E**). Cysts (choice **B**) are usually part of a multinodular goiter and are generally benign. Multinodular goiters are first treated with thyroxine to reduce the size of the gland and to achieve a euthyroid state. Surgery is required if compressive symptoms persist.

11 The answer is E *Medicine*

The patient has the signs and symptoms of a carcinoid syndrome (facial flushing, diarrhea). In most cases of carcinoid syndrome, a carcinoid tumor that secretes serotonin must metastasize to the liver (the *exception* is a bronchial carcinoid tumor). The most common primary site of a carcinoid tumor that has the capacity to metastasize to the liver is the terminal ileum. In this patient, the small bowel barium study shows a mass lesion in the terminal ileum, and the CT scan of liver shows metastatic disease. Tumor nodules in the liver release serotonin directly into the hepatic vein tributaries; these empty into the vena cava and thus into the systemic circulation. In the systemic circulation, serotonin produces vasodilation (facial flushing) and increases bowel motility, causing a watery type of diarrhea. 5-Hydroxyindoleacetic acid (choice **E**), a metabolic end-product of serotonin metabolism in the liver, is increased in patients with the carcinoid syndrome and confirms the diagnosis.

Liver function test results (choice **A**) are usually normal in the presence of liver metastasis. Furthermore, liver function tests do not confirm the diagnosis of carcinoid syndrome. α-Fetoprotein (choice **B**) is a tumor marker for hepatocellular carcinoma. This primary liver cancer usually develops in a background of cirrhosis, which is not present in this patient. Furthermore, hepatocellular carcinoma does not secrete compounds that produce facial flushing and watery diarrhea. Although serum electrolytes (choice **C**) would likely show hypokalemia and metabolic acidosis due to the loss of potassium and bicarbonate in the diarrheal fluid, these findings do not confirm the diagnosis of carcinoid syndrome. A stool culture (choice **D**) is ordered to rule out a bacterial cause of diarrhea. Since most bacterial causes of diarrhea produce an inflammatory response in the bowel mucosa, the fecal smear is usually positive for leukocytes. The fecal smear is negative in this patient, because the diarrhea is not caused by a bacterial pathogen but by increased peristalsis initiated by serotonin.

12 The answer is D *Surgery*

Chronic pancreatitis produces steatorrhea (increased fat in the stool), because the intestine is lipase deficient. Consequently, undigested lipid and fat-soluble vitamins are lost in the stool. Oral pancreatic enzyme preparations (choice **D**) high in lipase, before, during, and after the meal, with concurrent administration of a histamine (H_2) antagonist to block inactivation of the enzyme by acid, facilitate absorption of fats. In addition, the patient should be on a low-fat diet.

Total pancreatectomy (choice **A**) is a treatment option in chronic pancreatitis if intractable pain is present and is not amenable to medical therapy. The patient's pain is controlled with medical therapy. A broad-spectrum antibiotic (choice **B**) does not enhance lipid absorption, because bacterial overgrowth is not part of the pathophysiology of chronic pancreatitis. Bacterial overgrowth produces bile salt deficiency, which leads to steatorrhea. A gluten-free diet (choice **C**) is the therapy of choice for celiac disease, which is an autoimmune disease that has antibodies directed against the gliadin fraction in gluten. These antibodies are not present in the patient. Lactulose (choice **E**) is used to lower blood ammonia levels and has no role in the treatment of steatorrhea.

13 The answer is E *Medicine*

The patient has toxoplasmosis due to the protozoan *Toxoplasma gondii* (choice **E**). *T. gondii* is the most common cause of space-occupying lesions in the brain in AIDS patients, especially when the CD4 helper T-cell count is 50 cells/mm³ or below. Histologic sections of brain show a mononuclear cell infiltrate in multifocal areas of the cerebral cortex gray matter. Pseudocysts or individual tachyzoites of *T. gondii* are located at the periphery of the lesions. Treatment includes pyrimethamine plus sulfadiazine plus folinic acid (prevents folate deficiency). Primary prevention of toxoplasmosis is obtained with trimethoprim–sulfamethoxazole.

Cryptococcus neoformans (choice **A**) is the most common systemic fungus causing chronic meningitis in patients with AIDS. It does not cause space-occupying lesions in the brain. Treatment for cryptococcal meningitis in AIDS includes amphotericin B plus flucytosine followed by fluconazole. CMV (choice **B**) causes encephalitis in immunocompromised patients. It does not cause space-occupying lesions in the brain. Ganciclovir is the treatment for CMV. The Epstein-Barr virus (choice **C**) is responsible for the genesis of most AIDS-related primary B-cell lymphomas of the brain. The MRI shows multifocal, ring-enhancing lesions located in the same areas as in *T. gondii* encephalitis. Malignant lymphoma is excluded, because the lesions responded to antibiotic therapy. Herpes simplex type 1 (choice **D**) produces an encephalitis characterized by hemorrhagic necrosis of the temporal lobes and orbital frontal areas. This pattern of inflammation is not present in this patient. The treatment is acyclovir.

14 The answer is D *Surgery*

This woman has bilateral pheochromocytoma (bilateral adrenal lesions), a parathyroid adenoma (hypercalcemia and ectopic calcium deposits), and an oversized thyroid (a palpable, nontender swelling in front of her neck). This by definition is an example of multiple endocrine neoplasia (MEN). There are three such multigland syndromes, called MEN 1 (aka Wermer's syndrome), MEN 2a (aka Sipple's syndrome), and MEN

2b. All are inherited as autosomal dominant traits. MEN 1 is due to a mutation in a tumor suppressor gene on chromosome 11; in this germline mutation, tumors form in cells in which the normal allele is suppressed. Both MEN 2a and 2b are due to mutations in a gene that codes for a protooncogene called *RET*, which is only expressed in cells with a neurocrest origin, such as medullary thyroid C-cells and chromaffin cells. (C-cells are sometimes also found in parathyroid tissue.) The *RET* gene is located on chromosome 10, and a given kindred will have a mutation in a specific codon that will correlate with a variation in clinical expression such as age first expressed. This probably also accounts for the unique characteristics of MEN 2b, which include gastrointestinal and mucosal neuromas, a Marfan-like phenotype with skeletal abnormalities, as well as medullary carcinoma and pheochromocytoma. Genetic testing can identify 95% of persons with a mutated gene and is of value for genetic counseling and for identification of affected family members before symptoms arise; the latter permits a prophylactic thyroidectomy. Among adults worldwide the prevalence of all three types of MEN is estimated to be between 0.2 and 2 cases per 10^5 individuals; about 90% of cases are MEN 1, and MEN 2a makes up almost all of the remainder (MEN 2b is extremely rare). There is a 2:1 male-to-female ratio.

The approximate degree to which the various organs are affected is as follows. MEN 1: parathyroid >80%, pancreas 75%, pituitary, 60%; MEN 2a: medullary thyroid carcinoma >90%, parathyroid 20–50%, pheochromocytoma 20–35%; MEN 2b: mucosal and gastrointestinal gangliomas >90%; medullary thyroid carcinoma 80%, pheochromocytoma, 60%, and parathyroid, rarely. Accordingly, the woman described in the vignette has MEN 2a. Medullary carcinomas of the thyroid derive from C cells, which synthesize calcitonin. For MEN 2a, serum calcitonin is the best screen (choice **D**). A provocative stimulation test using omeprazole, pentagastrin or calcium can be used on family members to identify those who are at risk for developing medullary carcinoma. Although medullary carcinomas of the thyroid arising from MEN 2a are usually not highly aggressive, eventually death will ensue unless the thyroid is removed; thus early identification by genetic screening of children in affected families is important.

Serum thyroid-stimulating hormone (TSH) (choice **B**) and serum thyroxine (T_4) (choice **C**) levels are normal in patients with medullary carcinoma. An iodine-123 (^{123}I) scan (choice **A**) and measurement of the serum parathyroid hormone level (choice **E**) are of no additional value in determining a diagnosis in this patient and would only identify half the cases.

15 **The answer is C**   *Surgery*

Lobular carcinoma is the most common malignancy of the terminal lobule. It accounts for 5 to 10% of all breast cancers and is usually nonpalpable on self-examination. It is not a complication of traumatic fat necrosis. Left untreated, lobular carcinoma in situ tends to become invasive in 20 to 30% of patients over a prolonged period (10–15 years) (not early invasion [choice **B**]). It is most commonly associated with a high degree of bilaterality in the same quadrant of the contralateral breast (choice **C**), which underscores the need for mammography of the contralateral breast at regular intervals. The contralateral tumor can be another lobular cancer or a ductal cancer. Simultaneous bilateral breast cancer occurs in less than 1% of cases.

Most in situ lobular carcinomas are estrogen and progesterone receptor positive (not negative [choice **A**]). Chest wall involvement is uncommon in cases of lobular carcinoma (not increased incidence of involvement [choice **D**]). There is an increased incidence of breast cancer in first-degree relatives but not in second-degree relatives (not both first- and second-degree relatives [choice **E**]).

16 **The answer is B**   *Medicine*

The patient has alcoholic hepatitis. It is characterized by fatty change, loss of the normal liver architecture, scattered neutrophils, and eosinophilic staining material within hepatocytes consistent with Mallory's bodies. These findings, plus the clinical findings of fever, painful hepatomegaly, and jaundice, are compatible with alcoholic hepatitis. Alcohol is toxic to mitochondria, and aspartate aminotransferase (AST) (choice **B**) is located in mitochondria. This transaminase is released in greater amounts than is alanine aminotransferase (ALT), which is located in the cytosol.

Alcoholic hepatitis causes a mixed hyperbilirubinemia with a conjugated bilirubin percentage of 20–50% (not <20% [choice **A**]). Unconjugated bilirubin is increased because of decreased uptake and conjugation; conjugated bilirubin is increased because of destruction of intrahepatic bile ducts with release of conjugated bilirubin into the sinusoidal blood. Alcohol induces the cytochrome P450 system within the smooth endoplasmic reticulum in the liver, leading to increased synthesis of γ-glutamyltransferase (not normal [choice **C**]).

An increase in this enzyme and an aspartate aminotransferase level that exceeds that of alanine aminotransferase are characteristic of alcoholic hepatitis. Fatty change, neutrophils, and Mallory's bodies are not present in viral hepatitis (choice **D**). Antimitochondrial antibodies (choice **E**) are present in primary biliary cirrhosis, which is an autoimmune disease associated with granulomatous destruction of bile ducts in the portal triads. Fatty change, neutrophils, and Mallory's bodies are not present in primary biliary cirrhosis.

17 The answer is A   *Medicine*

The patient has celiac disease, an autoimmune disease with antibodies directed against the gliadin fraction in gluten (choice **A**), which is present in wheat products. The antibodies cause an inflammatory reaction in the villi, resulting in villous atrophy (flat mucosa) leading to malabsorption of fat (greasy stools), carbohydrates, and protein. In addition, this patient has an increased quantitative stool test result for fat and abnormal results in the D-xylose reabsorption test, which is an excellent screening test for documenting small bowel disease as a cause of malabsorption. The vesicular lesion on the patient's elbow is dermatitis herpetiformis, which is an autoimmune skin disease that has an almost 100% correlation with underlying celiac disease. Other antibodies present in celiac disease include antiendomysial and antireticulin antibodies. The treatment of choice is to eliminate gluten from the diet.

Antinuclear antibodies (choice **B**) directed against nuclear proteins are not present in celiac disease. A fecal smear for leukocytes (choice **C**) is used for evaluating diarrhea that may be caused by invasive microbial pathogens (e.g., *Campylobacter jejuni*, *Shigella sonnei*). The presence of leukocytes presumes an invasive enterocolitis and would not be expected in celiac disease. Testing the stool for ova and parasites (choice **D**) is always recommended in the workup of a patient with chronic diarrhea. Giardiasis is the most common cause of chronic diarrhea associated with malabsorption; however, the presence of dermatitis herpetiformis, excludes a parasitic cause of the chronic diarrhea. A stool sample to calculate the osmotic gap (choice **E**) is used for high-volume diarrheal states when a secretory or osmotic type of diarrhea is suspected rather than malabsorption. The stool osmotic gap is obtained by measuring potassium and sodium in the diarrheal fluid, adding them together, and multiplying the number by 2 (i.e., 2 × [potassium + sodium]). This value is then subtracted from 300 mOsm/kg, which represents the osmolality of plasma. Secretory diarrheas are characterized by isotonic diarrheal fluid, therefore, the osmotic gap in stool will be less than 50 mOsm/kg. Causes of a secretory type of diarrhea include certain types of laxatives and enterotoxigenic bacteria such as enterotoxigenic *E. coli* and *Vibrio cholerae*. Osmotic diarrhea is characterized by a hypotonic stool due to the presence of osmotically active solutes drawing more water than electrolytes out of the enterocytes. The classic example of an osmotic diarrhea is lactase deficiency, leading to an increase in lactose, which is osmotically active. The osmotic gap in osmotic diarrheas exceeds 100 mOsm/kg.

18 The answer is C   *Medicine*

The patient has testicular feminization syndrome, which is an X-linked recessive disorder (choice **C**) with absence of the androgen receptors. The testes are present and either remain in the abdominal cavity or present as masses in the inguinal canal. Concentrations of testosterone and dihydrotestosterone (DHT) are normal (not decreased [choice **D**]), but the lack of androgen receptors prevents the development of male secondary sex characteristics and external genitalia. Testosterone effects normal development of the epididymis, seminal vesicles, and vas deferens. DHT converts female-appearing external genitalia into a penis and scrotal sac. Hence, the external genitalia are female. There are no müllerian structures (fallopian tubes, uterus, cervix, upper one third of vagina), because müllerian inhibitory factor produced by the fetal Sertoli cells in the testes activates apoptosis. The vagina ends as a blind pouch, because the lower two thirds of the vagina develops from the urogenital sinus. Breast development and female secondary sex characteristics are normal, because estrogen receptors are present.

One Barr body (inactivated X chromosome; choice **B**) is present in a normal female (patient is a male). An XO genotype occurs in Turner's syndrome. Gonadotropins are normal (not increased [choice **E**]), because the testosterone level is normal.

19 The answer is B   *Medicine*

Syndrome X (sometimes called the metabolic syndrome, insulin resistance syndrome, or the deadly quartet) is a prediabetic condition in which there is: hyperglycemia (but not to the level that diabetes can be diagnosed), hypertension, dyslipidemia, and hyperinsulinemia. The man as described in the vignette has HYPER-GLYCEMIA (fasting serum glucose, 115 mg/dL [normal, <110 mg/dL; impaired glucose tolerance, 110–125 mg/dL, and diabetic, >125 mg/dL]); HYPERTENSION (BP, 155/84 mm Hg [normal, <120/<80, prehypertensive, 120–139/80–89, stage 1 hypertensive, 140–159/90–99; stage 2 hypertensive, >160/>100]); and DYS-LIPIDEMIA (total cholesterol, 265 mg/dL [desirable, <200 mg/dL, high risk, >240 mg/dL]; triglycerides, 157 mg/dL [desirable, <150 mg/dL, high risk, >200 mg/dL]; HDL, 39 mg/dL [desirable, >60 mg/dL, high risk, <40 mg/dL]; LDL, 125 mg/dL [optional, <100 mg/dL, desirable, <130 mg/dL, high risk, >160 mg/dL]). Consequently, it is highly probable that he has HYPERINSULINEMIA (choice **B**); the final principal component in the syndrome. In addition, this man's height and weight correspond to a body mass index (BMI) of 29 kg/m², which is classified as overweight, borderline obese; obese is anything above 30 kg/m². Overweight is an important factor in the development of the syndrome but is of itself not a causative factor as shown by the fact that many obese individuals do not develop it; the syndrome is caused by an interaction between a genetic predisposition and a lifestyle leading to overweight. The complex of abnormalities making up the syndrome often precedes type 2 diabetes, sometimes as much as by 9 to 10 years, and during this time some of the vascular complications such as retinopathy and nephropathy may begin. Thus the condition should be treated before frank diabetes manifests. The first line of treatment is usually diet and exercise. As little as a 15-lb weight loss can make remarkable changes and even prevent the development of diabetes.

Although the four factors described are the ones usually associated with the syndrome, there are others. One is an increase in plasminogen activator inhibitor-1 (PAI-1) (it is not lower than normal, choice **A**). This inhibits fibrinolysis and along with hypertension and dyslipidemia further promotes development of coronary and other artery disease. Although muscle and adipose tissues become resistant to insulin, glucose uptake into muscle (choice **C**) or adipose cells (choice **D**) is not inhibited, because the resistance to insulin is compensated for by an increase in its concentration as well as by a minimal hyperglycemia. That uptake of glucose into adipose cells is not inhibited is clearly demonstrated by the fact that pre-type 2 diabetics gain weight. Not all cells become insulin resistant, thus the hyperinsulinemia causes a metabolic imbalance that causes the symptoms associated with the syndrome. This state of affairs continues until the ability of the pancreas to compensate becomes limited; when it does, the circulating glucose levels increase until frank diabetes occurs. An increase in serum uric acid levels, not a decrease (choice **E**), also occurs in syndrome X.

20 The answer is A   *Psychiatry*

Brief periods of longing for the lost person are seen in normal bereavement (choice **A**), even many years after the event, especially on holidays or on the anniversary of the death. Feelings of worthlessness (choice **B**), suicide attempts (choice **C**), inability to work or as in this case to socialize and get out of bed (choice **D**), or feelings of despair (choice **E**) 2 years after an event indicate depression rather than a normal grief reaction.

21 The answer is B   *Psychiatry*

The patient's symptoms are most suggestive of posttraumatic stress disorder, characterized by traumatic recollections, emotional numbing, and increased arousal that follow a traumatic event and persist for at least 1 month. While treatment involves psychotherapy and emotional support, sertraline (choice **B**) and other selective serotonin reuptake inhibitors have been shown to be effective pharmacologic interventions. Other antidepressants may also be useful.

Olanzapine (choice **A**) is an antipsychotic medication that has not been demonstrated to be useful for PTSD. Eszopiclone (choice **C**) is a nonbenzodiazepine hypnotic that can be used for chronic insomnia but has not been studied as a treatment for PTSD. Topiramate (choice **D**) is an anticonvulsant that may be useful for treating bipolar disorder but not PTSD. Atomoxetine (choice **E**) is a treatment for attention-deficit/hyperactivity disorder (ADHD) and may exacerbate insomnia.

22 The answer is F   *Medicine*

There are nine major variant types of muscular dystrophy with several subtypes. The common feature is a progressive form of muscular weakness. The most common of these is Duchenne (choice **F**), the disease that killed the boy described in the vignette. It has an estimated incidence of 1 case per every 3500 live boys born in the United States. It is due to a major deletion on the short arm of the X-chromosome (Xp21), is inherited as a sex-linked recessive trait, and results in the nonproduction of dystrophin, a very large protein (427 kDa) that is part of the contractile apparatus of muscle cells. In addition to making the muscles weak, the absence of a dystrophin molecule makes the muscle cell leaky; which leads to a marked increase in the serum creatine kinase activity and contributes to the ultimate death of muscle cells. Affected boys seem normal until the age of 2 to 5, when they develop a peculiar ducklike waddling gait, due to weakness of the pelvic girdle muscles. The weakness then progresses first down the legs, forcing them into a wheelchair by their teens, and then to the upper body. During the early period their lower legs often increase in diameter, but it is not muscle, only fat and connective tissue. By their late teens their respiratory muscles and/or heart also weaken, and they succumb to a respiratory disease or cardiac failure not too long afterward. There is no treatment. The literature often reports that they are mildly retarded with an average IQ of 85, but there are many exceptions to this, as in the case described.

Becker muscular dystrophy (choice **A**) also results from a mutation in the dystrophin gene, but the mutation permits production of dystrophin protein, which however is defective. The result is a muscular dystrophy similar to Duchenne but not as severe. First symptoms usually occur during the late teens or early 20s, and affected persons are able to walk into their 30s. However, they too will eventual die from either respiratory or cardiac failure. Naturally, it too is also inherited as an X-linked recessive disorder. The incidence in the United States is about 1 case per 30,000 live male births.

Myotonic muscular dystrophy (choice **B**) is an autosomal dominantly transmitted disease in which symptoms usually first become evident in the 20s or 30s. It is sometimes also called Steiner's disease. It is due to a mutation of a gene on chromosome 19 and results in a defective myotonin protein kinase. Symptoms start with prolonged spasms in the finger and facial muscles and a slowly progressing weakness that eventually result in droopy eyelids and facial muscles, a floppy-footed, high stepping gait, cataracts, and cardiac and endocrine problems; affected members are said to be slightly mentally retarded and to have an indifferent psyche. However, even in the same family, symptoms may vary greatly from individual to individual, and severe symptoms usually do not manifest themselves until 15 or 20 years after the onset. Mothers with the mutation who seem normal at that time or are only slightly affected may give birth to a baby with a congenital variation of the disease, which is more severe. The tonic aspect of the disease is treated with phenytoin, quinine sulfate, or procainamide.

Facioscapulohumeral muscular dystrophy (choice **C**) is an autosomal dominant condition that usually starts in the teens or early adulthood. It first affects the face and shoulder girdle and then the pelvic girdle, legs, and abdomen. Clinically its effects vary from very mild to severe; about 50% of patients can walk until they die at a normal age.

Limb girdle muscular dystrophy (choice **D**), considered from the molecular viewpoint, is in fact several different diseases with similar clinical symptoms. It can be inherited in either an autosomal dominant or an autosomal recessive fashion. First symptoms usually start in teens or early adulthood as weakness in the hips. It then slowly progresses, first to the shoulders, then to the arms and legs. Some 20 years after the first onset of symptoms, it becomes hard to walk.

Digital muscular dystrophy (choice **E**) is very rare autosomal dominant condition that is more common in Sweden and among persons of Swedish ancestry in the United States. It starts in the hands during adulthood, and individuals in the same family can be affected to markedly different degrees. One member may live a long, essentially normal life with little more than what appears to be arthritis of the hands, while another will be bedridden by the age of 40.

23 **The answer is B** *Pediatrics*

Werdnig-Hoffmann disease (choice **B**) is a spinal muscular atrophy caused by a pathologic continuation of a process of programmed cell death that occurs normally in embryonic life, but not postnatally. It is inherited in an autosomal recessive fashion. Infants can be symptomatic at birth. Sparing of the extraocular muscles and sphincters is characteristic. Fasciculations are a sign of denervation of muscle and are best seen in the tongue. Infants assume a flaccid "frog-leg" posture. Most die by 2 years of age.

A neonatal form of myotonic dystrophy (choice **A**) appears in infants born to mothers with myotonic dystrophy. Clubfoot and contractures are common. Fasciculations are not seen. Infant botulism (choice **C**) has a peak onset at 2 to 6 months of age. Sources for spores include honey, corn syrup, soil, and dust. Infantile myasthenia gravis (choice **D**) can be transient—as in those infants born of mothers with myasthenia gravis—or, very rarely, a congenital manifestation of the disease itself. Fasciculations are not seen, and the extraocular muscles are not spared. Duchenne's muscular dystrophy (choice **E**) is rarely symptomatic at birth.

24 **The answer is C** *Pediatrics*

Congenital rubella syndrome (choice **C**) occurs after German measles infection during pregnancy and causes a variety of congenital malformations. These manifestations may include hepatosplenomegaly, thrombocytopenia, hepatitis, jaundice, cataracts, widespread maculopapular lesions of reddish blue color (i.e., "blueberry muffin" rash), and neurologic depression.

Rubeola (choice **B**), measles, during pregnancy is not associated with congenital abnormalities. Congenital varicella (choice **D**) can be acquired early or late in pregnancy. If acquired in the first half of pregnancy, it may cause limb hypoplasia, microcephaly, seizures, and cataracts in the newborn. If transmitted in the last 3 weeks of pregnancy, varicella can be mild or can involve fever and pneumonia. Clinical manifestations of congenital toxoplasmosis (choice **A**) are chorioretinitis, hepatosplenomegaly, jaundice, convulsions, and cerebral calcifications. Hepatosplenomegaly and generalized lymphadenopathy may be seen in a newborn with congenital syphilis (choice **E**). In addition, the mucocutaneous lesions of syphilis produce snuffles (a purulent and blood-tinged nasal discharge).

25 **The answer is C** *Medicine*

The patient has the syndrome of inappropriate secretion of antidiuretic hormone (SIADH), which is secondary to factors that stimulate antidiuretic hormone (ADH) release from the hypothalamus (e.g., chlorpropamide, trauma, tumor), infections in the lungs (e.g., tuberculosis), or neoplastic conditions that ectopically secrete excess amounts of ADH (e.g., small cell carcinoma of the lung). In SIADH, there is increased reabsorption of water from the late distal and collecting ducts of the kidneys, leading to concentration of the urine and the addition of water to the extracellular fluid (ECF) compartment, causing dilutional hyponatremia. Because the serum sodium approximates the ratio of total body sodium (TBNa) to total body water (TBW), an increase in TBW produces a dilutional hyponatremia. According to the law of osmosis, water moves from the point of low solute concentration, in this case the ECF compartment, to high solute concentration, which is the intracellular fluid (ICF) compartment. This influx of water into the brain produces cerebral edema, which is responsible for the altered mental status in this patient. A rough estimation of the TBNa can be determined by physical examination because TBNa is primarily located in the ECF compartment (vascular compartment plus the interstitial place). A normal TBNa is reflected by the presence of normal skin turgor, as evident in this patient. A decrease in TBNa is clinically reflected by signs of volume depletion (i.e., dehydration), such as dry mucous membranes, tenting of the skin (poor skin turgor), and hypotension. An increase in TBNa is manifested as dependent pitting edema and effusions into body cavities (e.g., ascites). Because the patient's TBNa is normal, restriction of sodium (choices **A** and **B**) or addition of sodium (choice **D**) is not warranted.

In SIADH, there is an increase in arterial blood volume, which increases peritubular capillary hydrostatic pressure in the kidneys. This decreases the reabsorption of all solutes that are normally removed by the proximal tubule, such as sodium (60–80%), urea, uric acid, potassium, and glucose. Furthermore, the increase in arterial blood volume decreases the release of renin and, ultimately, aldosterone; therefore, additional sodium is lost in the distal tubules (10–20%) as well. This loss in sodium is reflected by an increased level of random urine sodium, as evident in this patient.

Finally, the dilutional effect of excess plasma water affects not only the sodium concentration but also other electrolytes, such as potassium, chloride, and bicarbonate. Serum urea and uric acid concentrations are decreased, because they are lost in the urine by the mechanism discussed above. Therefore, the classic triad for diagnosing SIADH is severe hyponatremia (invariably ≤120 mEq/L), decreased serum blood urea nitrogen (BUN), and decreased serum uric acid. All of these findings are present in this patient.

The best treatment for SIADH is water restriction (choice **C**), because the patient is water overloaded. This patient also should be taken off chlorpropamide and given another oral hypoglycemic agent that does not produce SIADH. Giving the patient water would only further exacerbate her condition (choice **E**). Use of hypertonic saline infusions to raise serum sodium is only a temporary measure, because the sodium is eventually excreted in the urine by the mechanism discussed above.

26 **The answer is B** *Surgery*

The patient has cirrhosis of the liver complicated by ascites (shifting dullness in the abdomen) and portal hypertension, the latter causing esophageal varices that have ruptured (choice **B**), producing hematemesis. The most common cause of portal hypertension is alcoholic cirrhosis. Approximately 50% of the deaths in cirrhosis are due to ruptured varices.

The left gastric coronary vein, a branch of the portal vein, normally drains blood from the distal esophagus and proximal stomach to the portal vein for drainage into the liver. However, in portal hypertension, blood flow backs up into the vein causing distention (varices) and the potential for rupture. Bleeding varices cannot be diagnosed on the clinical presentation alone and require an emergency endoscopy to localize the source of bleeding. Endoscopy also is useful in therapy with variceal ligation, banding, or sclerotherapy. Ancillary management may include the use of intravenous octreotide, which decreases splanchnic blood flow and portal vein pressure, or intravenous vasopressin plus nitroglycerin, the latter reducing cardiac afterload and coronary artery resistance induced by vasopressin. In recalcitrant cases, a transjugular intrahepatic portosystemic shunt (TIPS) may be required to stop the bleeding. A metal stent is inserted that connects the hepatic vein with the portal vein. This reduces portal pressure; however, it increases the risk for developing hepatic encephalopathy by increasing blood ammonia levels. Other options include caval shunting, in which the portal vein is anastomosed to the inferior vena cava (side-to-side or end-to-side), or a distal splenorenal shunt.

Pyloric obstruction (choice **A**) is associated with vomiting due to retention of food in the stomach. Hematemesis is not a feature of the disease. Although hematemesis is most frequently associated with peptic ulcer disease (most commonly duodenal ulcers [choice **E**] followed by gastric ulcers [choice **C**]), the endoscopic findings are most compatible with bleeding varices. Esophageal carcinoma (choice **D**) does not usually present with massive hematemesis. Dysphagia for solids, weakness, and weight loss are the usual presenting signs and symptoms.

27 **The answer is E** *Medicine*

The term for the raised white patches on both sides of the patient's tongue that do not scrape off is *leukoplakia*. They should be biopsied to rule out squamous dysplasia and/or squamous cancer. Cigarette smoking (choice **E**) is the greatest risk factor for these patches, and their possible transformation into a squamous cell cancer in the mouth. Pipe smoking and smokeless tobacco are also risk factors. Smoking and alcohol have a synergistic effect and predispose a patient to squamous cell cancer in the oral cavity, upper and midesophagus, and larynx.

Alcohol excess alone (choice **A**) is a risk factor for squamous cell cancer in the mouth, but it is not as strong a risk factor as smoking. Glossitis due to *Candida albicans* (choice **B**) is characterized by the presence of a white pseudomembrane overlying the surface of the tongue. The pseudomembrane does scrape off (leukoplakia does not) and leaves a bloody base. Glossitis due to Epstein-Barr virus (choice **C**) is called hairy leukoplakia, and it is commonly seen as white patches located on the lateral border of the tongue in the setting of HIV infection. Hairy leukoplakia frequently occurs when the CD4 helper T-cell count is 200–500 cells/mm^3. It is not a precancerous lesion. Glossitis due to vitamin B_{12} deficiency (choice **D**) is incorrect. The glossitis in vitamin B_{12} deficiency is characterized by atrophy of the papillae, resulting in a smooth-surfaced tongue without leukoplakic lesions. It too is not a precancerous lesion.

28 **The answer is A** *Medicine*

The patient has bronchiectasis, which is an obstructive lung disease that involves mainly the bronchi and terminal bronchioles. It is caused by a combination of obstruction of airways (i.e., mucus plugs, proximally located cancer) and chronic infection (choice **A**), leading to weakening of the bronchial wall that results in dilation and trapping of purulent material. Cystic fibrosis complicated by pneumonia due to *Pseudomonas aeruginosa* and *Staphylococcus aureus* is the most common cause of bronchiectasis in the United States. Other pathogens unrelated to cystic fibrosis include those for tuberculosis (most common cause in developing countries), for histoplasmosis, and adenoviruses. The cough is productive of copious sputum. Hemoptysis is common and may be massive. Fever, empyema, lung abscesses, digital clubbing, and metastatic abscesses to the brain are common findings. A chest x-ray film shows crowded bronchial markings extending to the lung periphery. High-resolution CT is excellent in defining bronchiectasis. The treatment is postural drainage, antibiotics, and surgery for disease localized to segments or lobes.

Emphysema (choice **B**) is an obstructive lung disease characterized by destruction of elastic tissue in all or part of the respiratory unit (respiratory bronchiole, alveolar duct, alveoli), leading to permanent distention of the distal airway, not the bronchioles or bronchi as in bronchiectasis. The immotile cilia syndrome (choice **C**) is associated with bronchiectasis, but it is extremely rare. The cilia lack the dynein arm, which contains ATPase for cilia motility. Lack of cilia in the airways causes stasis of mucus and eventual infection. Other findings include sinusitis, infertility, and situs inversus, none of which are present in this patient. Inhalation of mineral dust (choice **D**) causes pneumoconiosis. Mineral dusts include coal dust, silica, asbestos, and beryllium. Mineral dusts cause restrictive disease of the lung with increased interstitial fibrosis; however, they are not associated with destruction of elastic tissue and cartilage leading to bronchiectasis. A proximally located primary lung cancer (e.g., squamous cell carcinoma or small cell carcinoma; choice **E**) that completely obstructs the bronchus usually leads to bronchiectasis distal to the obstruction. The patient has had a productive cough for a lengthy period; therefore, cancer is an unlikely cause of the bronchiectasis.

29 The answer is D   *Surgery*

The patient has Zollinger-Ellison (ZE) syndrome (choice **D**), which is caused by a malignant tumor that secretes excessive amounts of gastrin. Approximately 85% are located in the pancreas, and the remainder are in the duodenum. A characteristic clinical pentad is epigastric pain, weight loss, peptic ulceration (most are solitary duodenal ulcers rather than multiple ulcers), acid hypersecretion, and diarrhea (acid inactivates pancreatic enzymes). In 20–30% of cases it is associated with multiple endocrine neoplasia type 1 (MEN 1) syndrome. In ZE a gastric analysis shows basal acid output (BAO) above 20 mEq/h (normal, <5 mEq/h), maximal acid output (MAO) above 60 mEq/h (normal, 5–20 mEq/h), and a BAO:MAO ratio above 0.60 (normal, 0.20:1). Serum gastrin levels are above 300 pg/mL (normal, <300 pg/mL). The patient has an increase in all of these parameters. An intravenous secretin test shows a paradoxical increase (>200 pg/mL) despite an already high serum gastrin level. Treatment options include surgical removal (about 20–25% can be completely removed), parietal cell vagotomy, high doses of H_2-blockers or proton pump inhibitors (most effective medical treatment), and chemotherapy for metastatic disease (streptozocin, 5-fluorouracil).

Ménétrier's disease (giant hypertrophic gastritis) (choice **A**) is characterized by giant rugal hypertrophy secondary to the collection of protein-rich fluid in cysts in the submucosa and glandular epithelium. The mucosa is atrophic (decreases BAO and MAO), and achlorhydria is the rule. Loss of protein-rich fluid from the mucosa is often associated with hypoalbuminemia (protein-losing enteropathy). A gastric adenocarcinoma (choice **B**) is associated with achlorhydria and would not be expected to be associated with an increase in BAO and MAO. A glucagonoma (choice **C**) is a malignant islet cell tumor that presents with diabetes mellitus and migratory necrolytic erythema. It is not associated with increased gastrin release or peptic ulcer disease. Pernicious anemia (choice **E**) involves autoimmune destruction of parietal cells; hence, the BAO and MAO are decreased. Decreased acid increases serum gastrin.

30 The answer is C   *Medicine*

Isolated systolic hypertension (choice **C**) is a condition that often affects the elderly; in fact it is so common that it was once believed that normal systolic pressure is equal to 100 plus a person's age. However, trial studies have conclusively demonstrated that elevated systolic blood pressure is a more significant underling cause of cardiac disease and stroke than is elevated diastolic pressure; 30% of women and 20% of men older than 65 years have this condition. The underlying reason is a loss of arterial elasticity that occurs with aging. The man described most likely is suffering from a cerebellar stroke, which typically is associated with headache and ataxia.

An epidural hemorrhage (choice **A**) is a consequence of trauma and could conceivably have resulted from his fall. However, his fall occurred after the symptoms first appeared, and typically an epidural hematoma is characterized by coma after a lucid interval, and there is no mention of loss of consciousness. Ménière's syndrome (choice **B**) is a cause of vertigo induced by distention of the endolymphatic compartment of the inner ear. Although usually idiopathic, it can be caused by head trauma or syphilis. It is not age associated, and there is no evidence presented in the vignette that this patient might have Ménière's syndrome. A cerebral infarct (choice **D**) would not have only primary symptoms relating to ataxia but would rather have loss of muscular strength or cognitive function. A pulmonary thromboembolism (choice **E**) is usually accompanied with signs of dyspnea, chest pain, hemoptysis, and/or syncope. Except for syncope, the man had no other of these symptoms. Moreover, there is no indication of a predisposition for venous thrombosis, and the one drug this man uses is aspirin.

31 The answer is C   *Pediatrics*

Anemia of prematurity (choice **C**) occurs in low-birthweight infants approximately 1 to 3 months after birth. It is caused by the physiologic effects of the transition from fetal to neonatal life, as well as factors such as shortened red blood cell (RBC) survival, rapid growth, and frequent phlebotomy for blood tests. Hemoglobin (Hb) levels in anemia of prematurity are below 7 to 10 g/dL. Clinical manifestations may include feeding problems, tachypnea, tachycardia, and pallor.

Megaloblastic anemia of infancy (choice **A**) usually is caused by a deficiency of folic acid and has its peak incidence between 4 and 7 months of age. Infants with folate deficiency are irritable, have poor weight gain, and have chronic diarrhea. Newborns with sickle cell anemia (choice **B**) rarely exhibit clinical manifestations until 5 to 6 months of age, when the γ-globin of fetal Hb is replaced by the β-globin of adult Hb. Acute sickle dactylitis (i.e., painful swelling of the hands and feet) is usually the first evidence that sickle cell disease is present in an infant. The thalassemias are a group of heritable, hypochromic anemias. α-Thalassemia (choice **D**) is caused by abnormalities in the synthesis of the α chains of Hb and is manifested as microcytosis of the newborn (mean corpuscular volume [MCV] <95 pg). Homozygous β-thalassemia (choice **E**) usually manifests as a severe, progressive hemolytic anemia in the second 6 months of life, (once again after Hb A replaces Hb F) requiring regular blood transfusion.

32 The answer is C *Psychiatry*

The history and findings are most suggestive of major depressive disorder, recurrent (choice **C**), with mood-congruent psychosis. The absence of a history of manic episodes makes bipolar disorder (choice **A**) unlikely. Dysthymic disorder (choice **B**) is less likely because it is usually characterized by long periods of depressed mood, but without the full features of a depressive episode or psychosis present in this case. Schizoaffective disorder (choice **D**) is diagnosed only when psychosis persists for at least 2 weeks in the absence of mood episodes. In schizophrenia (choice **E**), psychotic symptoms and emotional blunting persist in the absence of mood symptoms and are usually more prominent than any associated mood pathology.

33 The answer is D *Pediatrics*

Todd's paralysis (choice **D**) commonly occurs after a seizure. The hemiparesis lasts minutes to hours but resolves within 24 hours. It can easily be confused with a stroke except for its duration.

Hemiplegia complicating migraine headaches (choice **A**) also shows recovery within a few hours without seizures, but residual neurologic effects are associated with transient hemiparesis/plegia. The disorder usually involves a strong maternal history of classic migraine. Neurologic deficits would not disappear after 24 hours in patients with infratentorial tumor (choice **E**). In postviral encephalitis (choice **C**), focal neurologic signs may be stationary, fluctuating, or progressive. Spastic hemiplegia (choice **B**) occurs in patients with cerebral palsy who have decreased spontaneous movements on one side of their body. These patients may also demonstrate hand preference at a very early age. This problem is not transient.

34 The answer is D *Pediatrics*

Caput succedaneum (choice **D**) is a diffuse swelling of the soft tissues of the scalp. It extends across suture lines, and the edema starts to resolve over the first few days.

Underlying skull fractures (choice **C**), not seen in caput succedaneum, are occasionally associated with cephalohematomas (choice **A**). The hemorrhages caused by cephalohematomas are subperiosteal; therefore, they are limited to one bone and do not cross suture lines. Cephalohematomas tend to increase in size over the first few days and resorb in approximately 3 months. Subcutaneous fat necrosis (choice **B**) of facial or scalp tissue may be associated with a forceps delivery. Overriding of the parietal bones (choice **E**) occurs when the bones of the scalp overlap at the suture line. The examiner would feel the overlap of bone, not a soft tissue swelling.

35 The answer is A *Surgery*

Macular degeneration (choice **A**) is the most common cause of permanent loss of visual acuity in the elderly. It is a strongly age-related phenomenon (prevalence of 25–30% by 75 years of age). Predisposing conditions include sex (slightly more common in females than in males), Caucasian ethnicity, a genetic propensity as demonstrated by family history, occupational exposure to chemicals, blue eyes, cardiovascular disease, smoking, diastolic hypertension, and left ventricular hypertrophy. There are two basic types: atrophic (or dry) and exudative (or wet). The dry form progresses slowly and is usually bilateral. The wet form progresses more rapidly, and affects the eyes sequentially. The wet form is usually more severe and is accompanied by accumulation of serous fluid or blood that separates the retina. The wet form is responsible for 90% of the blindness associated with macular degeneration but if caught earlier can be treated by laser therapy.

Diabetic retinopathy (choice **E**) is the most common cause of blindness in the United States, but its development is associated with uncontrolled diabetes, either type 1 or 2, and it does not have a primary predilection only for the elderly population. Neovascularization of the retinal vessels portends a poor prognosis. Optic neuritis (choice **D**) is a cause of sudden, unilateral loss of vision. The vignette provides no reason to suspect trauma (choice **B**) or cataract surgery (choice **C**), and neither of these are associated with a high rate of permanent loss of visual acuity.

36 The answer is C   *Surgery*

The patient has acute appendicitis (choice **C**). Low-grade fever with absolute neutrophilic leukocytosis and left shift, and pain beginning in the umbilicus and finally moving to McBurney's point between the umbilicus and the anterior iliac spine, strongly suggest acute appendicitis. Other signs and symptoms include rebound tenderness at McBurney's point (Blumberg's sign); pain in the right lower quadrant on palpation of the left lower quadrant (Rovsing's sign); abdominal pain on extension of the right thigh with the patient on the left side (Psoas sign); abdominal pain on internal rotation of the flexed right thigh with the patient supine; and pain preceding nausea and vomiting. Facial flushing may occur in children due to the release of serotonin. Diarrhea is absent in all but retrocecal appendicitis. Complications include perforation with peritonitis, periappendiceal abscess, pylephlebitis (inflammation of the portal vein), subphrenic abscess, and septicemia. Treatment is surgery.

Ulcerative colitis (choice **A**) presents with left lower quadrant pain and bloody diarrhea. Crohn's disease (choice **B**) presents with colicky, right lower quadrant pain with diarrhea. Irritable bowel syndrome (choice **D**) is associated with stress-induced diarrhea, constipation, or both, with mucus in the stools. Psychogenic pain (choice **E**) is usually periumbilical.

37 The answer is E   *Medicine*

Prosthetic heart valves often damage red blood cells (RBCs) and produce a normocytic anemia secondary to intravascular hemolysis. As expected in a hemolytic anemia, the reticulocyte count is increased in response to the loss of peripheral RBCs. The blood smear shows numerous irregularly shaped RBCs called schistocytes, which are the result of intravascular damage incurred by hitting the prosthetic valve. Haptoglobin (choice **E**) is synthesized in the liver in response to increased free hemoglobin in the circulation. Its main function is to bind free hemoglobin to form a haptoglobin–hemoglobin complex. This complex is removed by macrophages in the liver, which results in a decreased concentration of serum haptoglobin, making measurement of haptoglobin level (choice **E**) a useful marker of intravascular hemolysis. Hemoglobinuria is also present in intravascular hemolysis. Chronic loss of hemoglobin in the urine may produce a microcytic anemia due to iron deficiency. The patient has a normocytic anemia; however, it is likely that serum ferritin levels are decreased.

Ceruloplasmin (choice **A**), a binding protein for copper; albumin (choice **B**), a binding protein for calcium and free fatty acids; and, transferrin (choice **D**), a binding protein for iron are not useful markers for intravascular hemolysis. C-reactive protein (choice **C**) is an acute phase reactant in the liver and a marker of necrosis. It has no usefulness in gauging the severity of intravascular hemolytic anemia.

38 The answer is B   *Psychiatry*

This patient's symptoms are most suggestive of delusional disorder, somatic type (choice **B**), which is characterized by clearly false beliefs about bodily symptoms, sensations, or functions.

Unlike individuals with schizophrenia (choice **D**), individuals with delusional disorder are often coherent and show no other signs of thought disturbance. Body dysmorphic disorder (choice **A**) is characterized by an exaggerated perception of a slight physical anomaly. Hypochondriasis (choice **C**) is characterized by a misinterpretation of physical symptoms. Somatization disorder (choice **E**) is characterized by multiple physical complaints.

39 The answer is C   *Pediatrics*

Cavernous sinus thrombosis (choice **C**) is a complication of sinusitis. Symptoms of cavernous sinus thrombosis include ophthalmoplegia and loss of accommodation. Sinusitis also can be complicated by meningitis, epidural or subdural abscesses, optic neuritis, periorbital and orbital cellulitis and abscess, and osteomyelitis of surrounding bones. Complications develop secondary to local extension of the infection.

Hand-Schüller-Christian disease (choice **A**) has a variable presentation. It may involve skeletal abnormalities, skin lesions, exophthalmos, hepatosplenomegaly, or pituitary dysfunction. Proptosis is not a feature.

Graves' disease (choice **B**) is a hyperthyroid state characterized by irritability, excitability, crying easily, restlessness, and tremors of the fingers. Acute bacterial conjunctivitis (choice **D**) presents with generalized conjunctival hyperemia, edema, mucopurulent exudate, and various degrees of ocular discomfort. Temporal lobe abscess (choice **E**) does not present with proptosis.

40 **The answer is C** *Obstetrics and Gynecology*

The epithelial tumors of the ovary (serous, mucinous, and endometrioid adenocarcinoma) (choice **C**) are associated with cancer antigen 125 (CA-125). CA-125 is the only epithelial tumor marker that has adequate sensitivity and specificity to be clinically useful in identifying regression as well as recurrence of the tumor.

41 **The answer is E** *Obstetrics and Gynecology*

The gonadal–stromal tumors of the ovary produce sex steroids. Sertoli-Leydig cell tumors, lipid cell tumors, and gynandroblastomas (choice **E**) produce testosterone. These endocrinologically active, rare tumors may lead to virilization due to the elevated peripheral androgen production. They are most commonly diagnosed early (stage I) before distant spread has occurred.

42 **The answer is G** *Obstetrics and Gynecology*

Dysgerminomas (choice **G**) are the only gonadal–stromal tumors of the ovary that are associated with increased lactate dehydrogenase (LDH) activity. They occur predominantly in younger women and are the most common ovarian tumors found in women younger than 20 years of age.

43 **The answer is D** *Obstetrics and Gynecology*

Endodermal sinus tumors of the ovary (choice **D**) produce α-fetoprotein (AFP). These tumors are most common in young women and girls and are highly responsive to chemotherapy.

44 **The answer is F** *Obstetrics and Gynecology*

β-Human chorionic gonadotropin (β-HCG) is produced by nongestational choriocarcinomas of the ovary (choice **F**).

45 **The answer is A** *Obstetrics and Gynecology*

Granulosa cell tumors (choice **A**) and thecomas of the ovary produce estrogen. These endocrinologically active tumors are seen in all ages and often lead to clinical symptoms of abnormal bleeding during prepubertal, reproductive, and postmenopausal years.

46 **The answer is B** *Obstetrics and Gynecology*

Brenner tumor (choice **B**) is the only tumor listed that is not associated with a measurable tumor marker.

47 **The answer is D** *Psychiatry*

Graph **D** represents early morning awakenings, which are often associated with major depressive disorder.

48 **The answer is B** *Psychiatry*

Diazepam decreases stage 4 sleep (graph **B**), which makes this medication useful in treating sleep disorders characterized by pathology during this stage. Sleep terror and sleepwalking are examples of such pathologies.

49 **The answer is C** *Psychiatry*

Benzodiazepine rebound causes increased sleep latency (time to fall asleep) (Graph **C**), which is one mechanism that leads to addiction.

50 **The answer is E** *Psychiatry*

Graph **E** represents suppression of rapid eye movement (REM) sleep, which is caused by barbiturates and some antidepressants.

Questions

Single Best Choice: This section consists of numbered statements or questions followed by a list of potential answers; you are to select the ONE best answer.

1 A well-dressed, middle-aged male enters a doctor's office asking to see the doctor. When the receptionist inquires as to why he is there, the man replies in a slightly puzzled manner, "Didn't you know that the posted name and address in the foyer was a message specifically telling me that the doctor wished to see me?" This man most likely suffers from which of the following?

(A) Reference delusion
(B) Grandiose delusion
(C) Bizarre delusion
(D) Somatic hallucination
(E) Auditory hallucination

2 A 28-year-old has been having night sweats, is running a low but chronic fever and has lost 45 lb over the last 3 months. A disproportional amount of the weight loss was due to muscle loss. However, the symptom that brings him to see a physician are painless, erythematous, raised nonpruritic purplish red lesions on the right side of the neck, his hard palate, and his left leg. Which of the following is the most likely causal organism?

(A) *Bartonella henselae*
(B) Cytomegalovirus
(C) Epstein-Barr virus
(D) Human herpesvirus 8
(E) Human immunodeficiency virus

3 An 8-year-old patient presents to the pediatrician complaining of profuse, watery rhinorrhea; difficulty breathing; and itching of the nose and palate. There is a family history of atopy. During the physical examination, the child has paroxysmal sneezing. The physician suspects that the patient has allergic rhinitis. To substantiate the diagnosis, the physician should perform which of the following tests?

(A) A radioallergosorbent test (RAST)
(B) A Coombs' test
(C) A nasal smear for eosinophils
(D) A scratch test
(E) Immunoglobulin E (IgE) levels

4 A concerned daughter brings her 73-year-old father to a physician because recently he started showing profound symptoms of short-term memory loss and has started wandering around the neighborhood having a difficult time finding home. The incident that troubled her most was last week when he took the car to get groceries and got so lost that he drove around until after midnight and was finally brought home by the police. The physician examined the man and found him to be socially charming, but he failed recall testing and was unable to copy a geometric design on paper. The patient's vascular system showed no signs of deterioration nor were there any other observable physical problems. The physician prescribed donepezil. Which of the following will be the most likely effect?

(A) It will be remarkably effective in reversing his rate of cognitive decline.
(B) It will be somewhat effective in reducing his symptomatology.
(C) It will become increasingly effective over several years of treatment.
(D) It will decrease his renal function.
(E) It will increase levels of dopamine in his hippocampal region.

5 A child who has a diagnosis of neurofibromatosis presents to the ophthalmologist with the chief complaint of decreased visual acuity. The mother states that the patient has been in his usual state of health until 1 month ago. At that time she received a call from the patient's teacher who noticed that the child appeared to be having difficulty with his vision. On physical examination of the eyes the patient is noted to have a unilateral decrease in visual acuity, pallor of the disc, and exophthalmos. Which of the following is the most likely diagnosis?

(A) Craniopharyngioma
(B) Optic nerve glioma
(C) Medulloblastoma
(D) Cavernous sinus thrombosis
(E) Cerebellar astrocytoma

6 A 32-year-old man with eunuchoid proportions and arachnodactyly comes to the emergency department complaining of sudden onset of severe substernal chest pain with searing pain radiating into his back. He lacks a pulse in both arms. A chest radiograph reveals widening of the aortic diameter. The pathogenesis of this man's disease is most closely related to which of the following?

(A) Atherosclerosis
(B) Cystic medial degeneration
(C) Vasculitis secondary to syphilis
(D) Granulomatous inflammation
(E) Coronary artery thrombosis

7 A 58-year-old woman presents with a rapidly enlarging, painful breast mass. The overlying skin exhibits edema, warmth, and erythema. There is nonpainful adenopathy in the ipsilateral axilla. Which of the following is the most likely diagnosis?

(A) Breast cancer with plugging of the dermal lymphatics by tumor
(B) Paget's disease of the breast
(C) Phyllodes tumor
(D) Erysipelas due to group A streptococci
(E) Breast abscess

8 In response to a community-wide influenza A epidemic, residents of a nursing home were vaccinated with inactivated (killed virus) influenza vaccine containing antigens identical or similar to the currently circulating influenza A and B viruses. Six days later, an ambulatory and sociable 74-year-old resident developed a temperature of 38.8°C (102°F), severe headache, myalgia, nausea, and weakness over a 24-hour period. Which of the following would be the most appropriate response on the part of the nursing home administration?

(A) Take no further prophylactic measures, because the residents have already been vaccinated
(B) Prophylactically treat all residents with ampicillin
(C) Prophylactically treat all residents with amantadine or rimantadine
(D) Attempt to isolate all residents with whom the patient had been in contact during the past week
(E) Give all residents a booster influenza vaccination to ensure that their antibody titer is high

9 A 21-year-old woman, gravida 1, para 0, at 39 weeks' gestation comes to the maternity suite complaining of uterine contractions. Five hours ago her contractions were mild and irregular, but they are now intense and regular (every 3 minutes). She has had some bloody vaginal discharge. Her prenatal course was complicated at 30 weeks' gestation with gestational diabetes managed successfully by diet therapy. In addition, she has had recurrent urinary tract infections requiring prophylactic antibiotics. She has a total of 10 prenatal visits. Which of the following is most helpful in deciding whether she should be admitted to the maternity unit?

(A) Character of pain
(B) Progressive descent of fetus to birth canal
(C) Regular uterine contractions
(D) Bloody show
(E) Progressive effacement and cervical dilation

10 A homeless 30-year-old man dressed in tattered clothes is brought into the emergency department by police after he was found haranguing passersby in a residential neighborhood. Which of the following additional findings is most suggestive of psychosis?

(A) Hyperreligiosity and ascetic living habits
(B) Rumination about the meaninglessness of material things
(C) A belief that his thoughts are controlled via secret television messages
(D) Disorientation to time and place
(E) An unfounded suspicion that others are plotting against the government

11 A 25-year-old woman who has not menstruated for the past 9 months complains of a milky nipple discharge that has been present for the past 5 months. She is not taking any prescribed or over-the-counter medications. Physical examination is otherwise unremarkable. A pregnancy test result is negative. Serum thyroid-stimulating hormone (TSH) level is normal. Which of the following is the most likely diagnosis?

(A) Cushing syndrome
(B) Graves' disease
(C) Hypopituitarism
(D) Primary hypothyroidism
(E) Prolactinoma

12 A 35-year-old male has flulike symptoms for a few days and noticed the appearance of painless lump on his neck and is now concerned about his health. As a consequence, he made an appointment to see his physician. Upon presentation he admits to having had unprotected intercourse with multiple same-sex partners during the past year, the last encounter being last week. The physician orders an enzyme-linked immunosorbent assay (ELISA) test for human immunodeficiency virus (HIV) and the results come back negative. Which of the following is the most appropriate next step in the management of this patient?

(A) Inform him that there is nothing to worry about because the sensitivity of the ELISA test is 100%; thus, if negative, it rules out the diagnosis of acquired immune deficiency syndrome (AIDS)

(B) Advise him to have the ELISA test repeated immediately

(C) Explain that the median interval between infection and seropositivity is 2 weeks, so the test should be repeated at that time

(D) Explain that the median interval between infection and seropositivity is 3 months, with 95% seroconversion within 6 months

(E) Advise him to have a Western blot test

13 A 10-year-old girl worries every day that she will be abducted after classes and never see her family again. This worrying interferes with her ability to work or play in school. She voices no other worries. Which of the following is the most likely diagnosis?

(A) Generalized anxiety disorder

(B) Pervasive developmental disorder

(C) Separation anxiety disorder

(D) Specific phobia

(E) Social phobia

14 A 61-year-old man with a 40-year history of smoking cigarettes develops weight loss, jaundice, and light-colored stools. Physical examination reveals a palpable gallbladder. The total bilirubin is 10 mg/dL (normal, 0.1–1.0 mg/dL) and conjugated bilirubin is 8 mg/dL (normal, 0.0–0.3 mg/dL). Computerized tomography shows a mass in the head of the pancreas and dilation of the common bile duct. Which of the following sets of laboratory data is most likely present?

	Urine Bilirubin	Urine Urobilinogen
(A)	0	+1
(B)	0	+2
(C)	+2	0
(D)	+2	+2
(E)	0	0

15 A 26-year-old woman, gravida 0, para 0, comes to the outpatient office requesting an infertility evaluation. She has been married for 3 years and has regular intercourse with her husband one or two times per week. She has never used any contraception. She states that her menses have always been irregular and unpredictable. She seldom has any cramping with her periods. On pelvic examination, her uterus is midline, anteverted, freely mobile, and nontender. Her ovaries are easily palpable, slightly enlarged, and smooth. Pelvic ultrasonography confirms the pelvic examination findings. Both her ovaries are noted to have a "necklace" of multiple peripheral cysts. Which of the following statements is most likely to be true regarding this patient's condition?

(A) She has a low body mass index (BMI).

(B) She has evidence of virilization.

(C) Androgen production is primarily from adrenals.

(D) Gonadotropins are tonically elevated.

(E) Age of menarche is delayed.

16 A 36-year-old African American presents to a physician because of an itchy, darkly pigmented lesion in his axilla, which is illustrated below. He knows of no family history of a similar lesion, has no other symptoms of disease, and appears to be in good health. Physical examination found no abnormalities. The physician was particularly concerned about possible malignancy or diabetes but found no evidence of either. However, his serum insulin level was elevated. Which of the following is the most probable diagnosis?

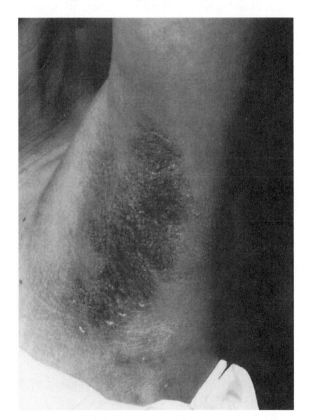

(A) Pityriasis rosea

(B) Erythema multiforme

(C) Erythema nodosum

(D) Acanthosis nigricans

(E) Keratoacanthoma

(F) Urticaria

17 A 46-year-old man underwent an emergency operation to repair a left lung laceration from a knife wound received during a brawl while intoxicated in a bar. A few days later, while still hospitalized, he develops anxiety, tremor, hallucinations, overactivity, and seizure activity. Which of the following is the most likely diagnosis?

(A) Reaction to the anesthetic drugs
(B) Delirium tremens (DT)
(C) Postoperative psychosis
(D) Intensive care unit (ICU) syndrome
(E) Hypoglycemia

18 An 89-year-old patient lives with her son and has mild Alzheimer's disease. Her son brings her to see a physician because she constantly complains about pain in her right arm. Her son suggests she is hallucinating but thought she should be examined anyway. A brief physical examination reveals bruises on both arms, and a fractured right humerus. She appears disheveled and smells of urine. Which of the following is the most appropriate first step in the management of this patient?

(A) Administer a pain reliever
(B) Call for an orthopedic consult
(C) Contact the state agency that deals with elder abuse
(D) Obtain consent from her son to admit her to the hospital
(E) Call for psychiatric consult

19 A measles outbreak at a daycare center has been confirmed in your community. Hearing this news, a mother brings her 7-month-old child to the pediatrician's office for measles vaccine. The mother is extremely worried, as she and her cousin had measles as children and her cousin developed panencephalitis from measles and died. The child's immunization record shows that the child's immunizations are up to date for age. The child appears to be very healthy. All growth parameters are at the 75th percentile, and the physical examination is unremarkable. Which of the following is the most appropriate next step in the management of this patient?

(A) Tell the mother not to worry because the child appears to be in good health and his immunizations are already up to date
(B) Tell the mother not to worry because her child does not attend the daycare center where the outbreak occurred
(C) Tell the mother that exposure to measles is a contraindication to receiving the vaccine

(D) Give the child monovalent measles vaccine, but do not use the measles, mumps, rubella (MMR) vaccine because it is contraindicated
(E) Reassure the mother that her child is considered protected by maternal antibody.

20 Although a 74-year-old patient goes to bed each night at 11 PM and wakes up at 7 AM, he feels sleepy all day, tends to drift off to sleep while watching television or writing on the computer, and often feels a need for an afternoon nap. His wife reports that he snores loudly and sleeps fitfully. Which of the following is the most likely diagnosis?

(A) Narcolepsy
(B) Sleep–wake schedule disorder
(C) Insomnia
(D) Kleine-Levin syndrome
(E) Sleep apnea

21 Children are more responsive to environmental influences than are adults. Consequently, it is more difficult to distinguish between behaviors that represent childhood psychopathology and those that represent response to environmental influences. Which of the following concepts refers to the requisite environment for the development of emotionally healthy children?

(A) "As if personality"
(B) "Lock and key"
(C) "Goodness of fit"
(D) "Good-enough mothering"
(E) "Emerging competencies"

22 A now 76-year-old man, who worked as a roofer with his father starting in his late teens until he retired at the age of 62, consults a physician because of a chronic cough. In taking a history the physician determines that he never smoked cigarettes or used any other form of tobacco. As part of his physical workup he was given chest radiography, which shows no mass lesion in the hilum or the periphery of the lung but does show calcifications in the diaphragm, parietal, and visceral pleural. What is the most likely diagnosis?

(A) Benign pleural plaques
(B) Diffuse interstitial fibrosis
(C) Pleural mesothelioma
(D) Primary bronchogenic carcinoma

23 An obstetrician requests a consult with a pediatric resident on a case involving a pregnant woman at 32 weeks' gestation by a date, who is scheduled for an elective cesarean section. The woman has not received prenatal care. The gestational age of the fetus as shown by ultrasound examination is 34 weeks. The obstetrician reports that an examination of the amniotic fluid was performed. The lecithin-to-sphingomyelin (L:S) ratio measures more than 2, and phosphatidylglycerol (PG) is present in the amniotic fluid. Which of the following courses of action should the pediatric resident recommend?

(A) The cesarean section should be canceled

(B) The cesarean section should be performed as scheduled.

(C) The mother should be given beclomethasone for 24 hours.

(D) The mother should be given beclomethasone for 48 hours.

(E) The infant should be placed on mechanical ventilation immediately after delivery.

24 A 12-year-old boy with cystic fibrosis presents to the emergency center with temperature 102°F (38.9°C), wet cough, and tachypnea. A radiograph is obtained and *Staphylococcus aureus* is suspected. Administration of appropriate intravenous antibiotics is initiated, and the patient is admitted to the hospital ward. The patient complains of shortness of breath and chest and shoulder pain. He then suddenly develops increased respiratory distress, decreased breath sounds in the left chest, and tracheal deviation to the right. Which of the following is the most likely diagnosis?

(A) Emphysema

(B) A pleural effusion

(C) A ruptured tension pneumatocyst

(D) Adult respiratory distress syndrome (ARDS)

(E) A pulmonary infarction

25 A 59-year-old man apparently fully recovers from a myocardial infarct and is sent home. Two weeks later he returns to the emergency room because of chest pains. He informs the physician on duty that the pain radiates to his neck and shoulder but tends to come and go. Moreover, it makes his chest feel tight, leaves a crushing sensation, and makes breathing difficult. He also says he simply feels "poorly," is extremely tired, and every joint in his body seems to ache. He thought it might be a bad case of indigestion and took several antiacids to no avail. His temperature is 38°C (100.4°F), his blood pressure is elevated, as might be expected because of his hyperanxious state. On physical examination it is noted that deep breathing increases the pain, while standing upright relieves it. Examination of the heart reveals tachycardia, distant heart sounds, and a rubbing sound (not a murmur).

Radiography shows evidence of some pleural infusion. His erythrocyte sedimentation rate (ESR) is elevated, his cardiac enzymes are not elevated, and he has a leukocytosis. Which of the following choices represents the most probable diagnosis?

(A) Dressler's syndrome

(B) Postmyocardial infarction pericarditis

(C) A reinfarction

(D) Prinzmetal's angina

(E) Gastroesophageal reflux disease (GERD)

26 A 19-year-old woman, gravida 2, para 0, aborta 1, is found upon routine maternal serum α-fetoprotein (MSAFP) screening to have a positive-high result. The blood sample was drawn at 17 weeks' gestation by dates. She has not undergone any obstetric sonography up to this point. Her pregnancy was documented by a home pregnancy test. Fetal heart tones were heard by Doppler stethoscope on her first prenatal visit at 13 weeks' gestation. She presents now at the prenatal diagnostic center for genetic counseling for ultrasound assessment of fetal age as well as assessment of fetal anatomic normality. Which of the following combinations of standard fetal measurements will be used in assessment of gestational age: abdominal circumference (AC), biparietal diameter (BPD), crown–rump length (CRL), femur length (FL), head circumference (HC), humerus length (HL), transcerebellar diameter (TCD)?

(A) AC, BPD, CRL, FL

(B) HC, BPD, AC, FL

(C) BPD, HC, AC, CRL

(D) BPD, HC, AC, TCD

(E) BPD, CRL, FL, TCD

27 A 73-year man awoke with an intense pain on the left side of his temple, which was diagnosed as a possible migraine by his Christian Science practitioner. Two days later a series of grouped, tense, deep-seated vesicles appear on that side of his face and further down; this painful eruption follows along the tract of the trigeminal nerve. It approaches, but does not enter, his eye. This condition is caused by which of the following organisms?

(A) Herpes simplex 1

(B) Herpes simplex 2

(C) Herpes varicella

(D) Human herpesvirus 6 (HHV-6)

(E) Epstein-Barr virus

(F) Cytomegalovirus

(G) Human herpesvirus 7 (HHV-7)

(H) Human herpesvirus 8 (HHV-8)

28 A 36-year-old woman with a long history of problematic interpersonal relationships is undergoing psychotherapy for this problem. She becomes increasingly frustrated with what she perceives as her slow rate of therapeutic progress and expresses this to her therapist. He replies, "I wonder if you are attempting to devalue my skills because you have always resented people that come across as 'experts.'" Which of the following does this intervention represent?

(A) Behavioral psychotherapy
(B) Cognitive psychotherapy
(C) Humanistic psychotherapy
(D) Psychodynamic psychotherapy
(E) Supportive psychotherapy

29 An 18-year-old male vacationed at a resort with some of his buddies to celebrate his graduation from high school. While there he had his first sexual encounter, unprotected intercourse with a young woman also on vacation. Three weeks after coming home he began to feel ill. Initially he developed conjunctivitis, and then stiffness and pain in his knees, ankles, and feet. Feeling concerned, he consulted his primary care physician who took a careful history and discovered that the patient also had pain in his lower back and had an increased need to urinate; urination created a burning sensation, and recently there has been a small discharge from his penis. He also had a low-grade fever but otherwise tested normal. The physician took a sample of synovial fluid and blood for further analysis and made appointments for the patient to see a rheumatologist and a radiologist for x-ray examination. By the time the boy saw the rheumatologist the laboratory and radiology data were available. He tested positive for infection with *Chlamydia trachomatis*, negative for rheumatoid factor and antinuclear antibodies (ANAs), and positive for human lymphocyte antigen-B27 (HLA-B27). The synovial fluid sample tested negative for bacteria. He also had an elevated erythrocyte sedimentation rate (ESR) and a neutrophilic leukocytosis. The radiologic report indicated possible early arthritic changes in the sacroiliac region, along his spine, and in his knees. Which of the following is the most probable diagnosis?

(A) Ankylosing spondylitis
(B) Crohn's disease associated arthritis
(C) Psoriatic arthritis
(D) Nongonococcal acute bacterial (septic) arthritis
(E) Reactive arthritis (Reiter's syndrome)

30 Obstetric sonography is performed on a 22-year-old woman, gravida 2, para 1, who is at 30 weeks' gestation by dates and confirmed by early first-trimester ultrasound crown–rump measurements at 9 weeks' gestation. Her pregnancy is complicated by gestational diabetes diagnosed at 26 weeks' gestation that is being managed by diet alone. Her home blood glucose monitoring shows the following mean values: fasting, 85 mg/dL; 1 hour postmeal, <130 mg/dL. The sonogram reveals an anterior-fundal placenta and a normal amniotic fluid volume. There is a single fetus with the head in the right upper quadrant; back is to the mother's left. Both fetal thighs are flexed and both legs are extended. Which of the following is the correct name for the fetal presentation?

(A) Frank breech
(B) Complete breech
(C) Incomplete breech
(D) Double-footling breech
(E) Transverse breech

31 A pediatrician is called to the nursery to examine a newborn infant with excessive drooling. The nurse reports that in addition, the infant has coughing and choking with feeding. Cyanosis is present and is unrelieved by crying. Bilateral pulmonary rales are present. There is abdominal distention with tympany on percussion. The birth history is unremarkable, and the baby was born term via vaginal delivery. The Apgar scores were 9 at 1 minute and 9 at 5 minutes. The birth weight was 7 lb 12 oz. Which of the following is the most likely diagnosis?

(A) Choanal atresia
(B) Respiratory distress syndrome
(C) Zenker's diverticulum
(D) A tracheoesophageal fistula
(E) Duodenal atresia

32 A 40-year-old woman comes to the outpatient office complaining of a pruritic, cheesy vaginal discharge. She states that her vagina is tender and sexual intercourse is painful. Six years ago she was diagnosed with type 2 diabetes mellitus for which she is being treated with oral hypoglycemic agents. Pelvic examination reveals an erythematous, edematous labia minora and vagina. A whitish vaginal discharge is present. Which of the following diagnostic tests is most useful for identifying the cause of this condition?

(A) Wet saline prep
(B) Gram's stain
(C) Vaginal pH
(D) Vaginal culture
(E) A potassium hydroxide (KOH) preparation

33 The pediatrician visits a mother in the hospital after delivery of an infant with a cleft lip. The patient was full term and born by repeat cesarean section. The patient weighed 6 lb 13 oz (3.1 kg) and had Apgar scores of 7 at 1 minute and 8 at 5 minutes. At birth the patient was noted to have a cleft lip, otherwise the physical examination is unremarkable. The mother states that the patient has been feeding slowly, and she is worried that the infant may not be taking adequate nourishment, as it is difficult for the infant to latch onto the nipple. She asks when the infant will be ready to have the cleft repaired. The physician then tells the mother that the cleft lip can be repaired when the child reaches which of the following milestones?

(A) 1½ months, weighs 8 lb (0.36 kg), and has a hemoglobin level of 10 g/dL

(B) 2½ months, weighs 10 lb (4.5 kg), and has a hemoglobin level of 10 g/dL

(C) 3½ months, weighs 12 lb (5.4 kg), and has a hemoglobin level of 10 g/dL

(D) 4½ months, weighs 12 lb (5.4 kg), and has a hemoglobin level of 10 g/dL

(E) 5½ months, weighs 13 lb (5.9 kg), and has a hemoglobin level of 10 g/dL

34 At a routine prenatal visit, a 28-year-old woman, gravida 5, para 4, at 28 weeks' gestation reports that she has not felt the baby move for 2 days. She first felt fetal movement at 17 weeks' gestation. She denies any vaginal bleeding or fluid leakage. Her pregnancy has been complicated by chronic hypertension, for which she is being treated with twice-daily tablets of α-methyldopa. She is afebrile, and her vital signs are stable. On physical examination the fundal height measures at an appropriate 30 cm. Four weeks ago the fundus measured 26 cm. Leopold's maneuvers reveal the fetus to be in transverse lie. Her blood pressure is 145/85 mm Hg. A urine dipstick test is negative for albumin. You are unable to obtain fetal heart tones with a Doppler fetoscope. Which of the following is the most accurate way to assess the condition of the fetus?

(A) Nonstress test

(B) Amniocentesis

(C) Maternal assessment

(D) Maternal abdominal radiologic assessment of the fetus

(E) Quantitative β-human chorionic gonadotropin (HCG) determination

(F) Ultrasound assessment for cardiac motion

35 A 43-year-old African-American male presents with a history of increased tiredness, lack of appetite, nausea, and pruritus. He is unable to sleep at night because of a constant need to void. He has no history of increased bruising or prolonged bleeding since the onset of his illness. Clinical examination reveals pallor of the mucous membranes, tachycardia, and a few bibasilar rales. In addition, he has bilateral peripheral pitting edema and a pericardial friction rub. Laboratory data support the evidence for chronic renal failure. Despite prolonged therapy, the patient fails to respond to medical measures, including dialysis, and a renal transplant is considered. Which of the following pretransplant tests is most relevant to prevent hyperacute rejection of a donor kidney?

(A) Proper matching of the ABO groups of the recipient with the donor

(B) Proper matching of the human leukocyte antigen (HLA)-A loci of the recipient with the donor

(C) Proper matching of the HLA-B loci of the recipient with the donor

(D) Proper matching of the HLA-C loci of the recipient with the donor

(E) Proper matching of the HLA-D loci of the recipient with the donor

(F) Proper matching of CD4 T helper cells of the recipient with the donor

36 A 32-year-old Japanese-American woman with two children comes to the office for a routine physical examination. She is in good health, does not smoke, drinks only at social occasions, and leads a healthy lifestyle. She is concerned about developing breast cancer and wishes to know about significant risk factors. Which of the following is a significant risk factor for breast cancer in Japanese-American women?

(A) History of smoking cigarettes

(B) Typical Japanese diet

(C) Late menarche

(D) Early menopause

(E) History of endometrial carcinoma

37 A 67-year-old woman presents to the outpatient office with intense pruritus of the vulva for the past 9 months. The itching is so severe it interferes with sleep as well as daily activities. Sexual intercourse is extremely painful and even urination causes burning and pain. On examination, the vaginal introitus is stenotic, with the skin appearing thin, wrinkled, and parchmentlike. A biopsy shows both epidermal and dermal atrophy with loss of rete pegs. Which of the following treatments is most appropriate?

(A) 5-Fluorouracil
(B) Clobetasol cream
(C) Fluorinated corticosteroids
(D) Miconazole
(E) Estrogen cream

38 Items included in this volume provide many examples of the health hazards associated with cigarette smoking, and answer 46 in Test 11 provides a long list of diseases in which tobacco smoking is a major contributor. Recent data (2003) from the Centers for Disease Control and Prevention show that there are more than 430,000 annual deaths from tobacco use, making it a factor in about two thirds of death from preventable causes in the United States. If tobacco use is the leading preventable cause of mortality, which of the following is second?

(A) Illicit drug use
(B) Fire arms
(C) Unsafe sexual behavior
(D) Alcohol
(E) Motor vehicle accidents
(F) Poor diet and physical inactivity

39 A 3-year-old boy with puffy eyes presents to the pediatric emergency department. His physician had treated the patient for allergies, but symptoms have not improved. Upon physical examination, the patient is noted to have edema. The physician suspects nephrotic syndrome. Which of the following characteristics would support the diagnosis of nephrotic syndrome?

(A) Hyperproteinemia
(B) Heavy proteinuria
(C) Hypolipidemia
(D) Hyperalbuminemia
(E) Hypertension

40 A 27-year-old man is brought to the emergency room with such severe agitation that he was put into restraints. He has slurred speech, ataxia, circumoral numbness, and horizontal nystagmus. Friends report that he was recently using crack cocaine and possibly other drugs as well. Which of the following substances most likely caused the findings noted on examination?

(A) Cannabis
(B) 3,4-Methylenedioxymethamphetamine (MDMA)
(C) Methamphetamine
(D) Phencyclidine
(E) Volatile inhalants

Directions for Matching Questions (41 through 50): Each set of matching questions is preceded by a list of 4 to 26 lettered options followed by a brief explanation of the required task and then by a series of numbered statements. For each lettered statement you are to select ONE lettered option that best fulfills the task as it relates to that statement. Remember each of the listed options might be correctly selected once, more than once, or not at all.

Questions 41–50

(A) Alemtuzumab
(B) Vincristine, doxorubicin, and dexamethasone
(C) Daunorubicin and cytarabine
(D) Imatinib mesylate
(E) Cladribine hydrochloride
(F) Mitotane
(G) Melphalan and prednisone
(H) Bortezomib
(I) Etoposide and cisplatin
(J) Bacillus Calmette-Guérin (BCG)
(K) Hydroxyurea
(L) Fludarabine phosphate
(M) Paclitaxel
(N) Rituximab
(O) Thalidomide

Select the ONE drug from the lettered list above that would be used to treat the clinical condition describe in questions 41 through 50 below.

41 A 67-year-old female presents with pain in the back, chest, and head. She recently fell and sustained a fracture of the neck of the left femur. Paraprotein is noted on serum protein electrophoresis, and rouleaux formation in the red blood cells.

42 A 39-year-old male presents with a history of fatigue, mild fever, and night sweats. Physical examination reveals splenomegaly and sternal tenderness. The white cell count is markedly elevated. Myeloid series and a positive Philadelphia chromosome are identified.

43 A 62-year-old female sees her family physician for fatigue and bleeding from the gums and nose. Clinical examination reveals pallor, evidence of bleeding from the gingiva, and tenderness in the sternum and tibia. Blast cells containing eosinophilic needlelike inclusions in the cytoplasm are found in the peripheral smear.

44 A 49-year old male goes to his primary care physician with a history of passing blood in his urine. He states that a few months ago the same thing happened. He ignored it, thinking it had something to do with the beet root he had eaten. He denies pain. Cystoscopy confirms carcinoma in situ.

45 A 60-year old male goes to his family physician for recurrent chest infection. During the examination, a painless mobile lump is found in his neck. Initial chemotherapy did not provide any benefit.

46 A 30-year-old male has confirmed inoperable carcinoma of the adrenal gland.

47 A 53-year-old man has a history of progressive fatigue, recurrent upper respiratory infection and massive splenomegaly. The lymph nodes are not palpable. A peripheral blood smear reveals numerous cells with cytoplasmic projections.

48 A 39-year old female goes to her primary care physician with a history of gradual increase in abdominal girth. She has also started to feel pelvic pressure and pain. An ovarian mass felt on pelvic examination is confirmed by ultrasonography. Serum CA 125 is markedly elevated. The patient undergoes a staging laparotomy followed by hysterectomy, bilateral salpingo-oophorectomy, omentectomy, and selective lymphadenectomy.

49 A 28-year-old male sees his primary care physician with a history of an enlarging testis. Physical examination reveals an enlarged right testis that does not cause pain when compressed. Computerized tomography confirms retroperitoneal disease, with lymph node involvement more than 3 cm in size. An orchidectomy is performed.

50 A 74-year-old male sees his family physician for increasing fatigue, loss of weight, and bruising easily. Physical examination reveals pallor of the mucosa, and hepatosplenomegaly. A complete blood count confirms anemia, and the erythrocyte sedimentation rate is raised. Serum protein electrophoresis reveals a monoclonal spike, due to IgM. The urine contains kappa chains. Initial chemotherapy is ineffective.

Answer Key

1	A	**11**	E	**21**	D	**31**	D	**41**	G
2	D	**12**	D	**22**	A	**32**	E	**42**	D
3	C	**13**	C	**23**	B	**33**	B	**43**	C
4	B	**14**	C	**24**	C	**34**	F	**44**	J
5	B	**15**	D	**25**	A	**35**	A	**45**	A
6	B	**16**	D	**26**	B	**36**	E	**46**	F
7	A	**17**	B	**27**	C	**37**	B	**47**	E
8	C	**18**	C	**28**	D	**38**	F	**48**	M
9	E	**19**	E	**29**	E	**39**	B	**49**	I
10	C	**20**	E	**30**	A	**40**	D	**50**	L

Answers and Explanations

1 **The answer is A** *Psychiatry*

A delusion of reference (choice **A**) involves the assignment of personal significance to neutral events. Such a delusion, along with delusions of persecution and jealousy, are often a component of paranoia. They are common in paranoid schizophrenia and delusional disorders.

An irrational belief that one has a special mission is a grandiose delusion (choice **B**). A belief that others are reading one's thoughts is a bizarre delusion (choice **C**). Formication, the belief that ants are crawling on one's body, is a somatic hallucination (choice **D**) that is classically described during alcohol withdrawal. Hearing strange sounds in the wind might represent auditory hallucinations (choice **E**) or might simply be the product of an active imagination.

2 **The answer is D** *Medicine*

The patient has the acquired immune deficiency syndrome (AIDS), and the lesions are Kaposi sarcoma, a vascular malignancy closely associated with AIDS and caused by human herpesvirus 8 (HHV-8) (choice **D**). Kaposi sarcoma is the most common malignancy in patients with AIDS. Lesions appear most often on the skin but may also occur in the intestinal tract, particularly on the hard palate. They often clear up if AIDS treatment results in a significant increase in CD4 helper T cells.

Bartonella henselae (choice **A**) is a gram-negative bacterium that causes bacillary angiomatosis, a disease that occurs almost exclusively in patients with AIDS. It produces highly vascular skin lesions that can mimic the lesions of Kaposi's sarcoma. Silver stains of a biopsy specimen demonstrate the organisms. Systemic signs of the infection include fever, lymphadenopathy, and hepatomegaly. These findings are not present in this patient. (*Bartonella henselae* also causes cat-scratch disease.) Drugs that are used in treatment include erythromycin or doxycycline. Cytomegalovirus (CMV) (choice **B**) is not an oncogenic virus and does not produce vascular lesions on the skin or in the gastrointestinal tract. In patients with AIDS, CMV is the most common cause of blindness, biliary tract disease, and pancreatitis. The Epstein-Barr virus (choice **C**) does not cause vascular skin lesions, although it does cause hairy leukoplakia (glossitis), primary central nervous system lymphoma, and Burkitt's lymphoma. The human immunodeficiency virus (choice **E**) is not oncogenic and does not produce vascular skin lesions. In patients with AIDS, it is associated with generalized lymphadenopathy, destruction of CD4 helper T cells, and central nervous system findings (e.g., AIDS dementia).

3 **The answer is C** *Pediatrics*

Finding a predominance of eosinophils on nasal smear (choice **C**) substantiates the diagnosis of allergic rhinitis. The Coombs' test (choice **B**) is used to detect hemolytic anemia due to blood group incompatibility. The radioallergosorbent test (RAST) (choice **A**) helps determine antigen-specific immunoglobulin E (IgE) concentrations in serum. The RAST is less sensitive than direct skin testing but brings no risk of allergic reactions. IgE levels (choice **E**) are increased in allergic disease. A scratch test (choice **D**) is used to determine sensitivity to certain allergens (e.g., foods, drugs). The side of a beveled, sterile needle is used to break the skin with a scratch that is 1 cm long. A drop of test material is then placed on the scratch. A positive reaction is a wheal-and-flare response, usually obvious 15 to 20 minutes after application.

4 **The answer is B** *Psychiatry*

Dementia is the fourth leading cause of death in the Unites States and has a prevalence that doubles every 5 years after the age of 55 and affects an estimated 35 to 50% of the population at an age of 85 years. Alzheimer's disease accounts for over two thirds of these cases, with vascular problems accounting for essentially all the rest; this patient had no signs of vascular aberrations and undoubtedly has early Alzheimer's disease. Donepezil has been moderately effective in improving cognitive performance in patients with mild Alzheimer's dementia (choice **B**). Its therapeutic effectiveness is due to its inhibition of acetylcholinesterase and resultant higher levels of acetylcholine in the central nervous system (CNS).

Donepezil is rarely remarkably effective in reducing the rate of cognitive decline (choice **A**) and is less effective in individuals with more severe symptoms. It does not become more effective over time (choice **C**). It has no known effect on levels of dopamine in the hippocampus (choice **E**), and it is not associated with renal toxicity (choice **D**).

5 The answer is B   *Pediatrics*

Optic gliomas are present in approximately 15% of patients with neurofibromatosis-1 (von Recklinghausen's disease), and they are one of the criteria used in diagnosing the disease. Most patients with optic gliomas are asymptomatic, but approximately 20% show signs of visual disturbances. Optic nerve gliomas (choice **B**) present with decreased visual acuity and pale discs.

Children with craniopharyngioma (choice **A**) may have short stature and bitemporal visual field defects. Medulloblastoma (choice **C**) is the most prevalent brain tumor in children under 7 years of age, but it is not associated with neurofibromatosis. Cavernous sinus thrombosis (choice **D**) may occur as a complication of an orbital infection. Symptoms may include venous engorgement of the lids and orbital tissues, ptosis, ophthalmoplegia, and loss of accommodation. Symptoms of increased intracranial pressure and hydrocephalus are seen with cerebellar astrocytoma (choice **E**).

6 The answer is B   *Surgery*

The patient has Marfan syndrome complicated by an aortic dissection that has extended into the proximal aorta and reduced blood flow to the upper extremities. Marfan syndrome is an autosomal dominant disease with a defect in fibrillin in the connective tissue, which weakens collagen. Eunuchoid proportions (i.e., span greater than height), arachnodactyly, lens dislocation, and a predisposition for aortic dissections (the most common cause of death in these patients) commonly round out the clinical picture. In aortic dissections, weakening of the middle and outer layers of the aorta is due to cystic medial degeneration (CMD) (choice **B**), which is characterized by elastic tissue fragmentation and mucoid degeneration. CMD occurs in elderly patients with hypertension or in younger individuals with connective tissue disorders such as Marfan syndrome or Ehlers-Danlos syndrome involving elastic tissue and collagen, respectively. An intimal tear occurs, causing blood to dissect through the areas of weakness in the aorta. It may extend proximally, distally, or in both directions. Eventual sites of egress of the blood include the pericardial sac (the most common cause of death), mediastinum, peritoneum, or reentry through another tear to create a "double-barreled" aorta. Patients present with an acute onset of severe retrosternal chest pain that is often described as "tearing." Pain radiates into the back rather than down the arm or into the jaw, which occurs in a myocardial infarction due to a coronary thrombosis (choice **E**). In addition, a proximal aortic dissection often occludes the orifices of the arch vessels, causing loss of the arterial pulses or stroke. Some 80% of the time, the diagnosis is established by noting an increased aortic diameter on a chest x-ray film. Retrograde arteriography is considered the gold standard for confirming the diagnosis. Treatment consists of using immediate antihypertensive measures (e.g., nitroprusside) to decrease the head of pressure causing the dissection. This is followed by surgery and insertion of a graft. The overall long-term survival rate is 60%.

Atherosclerosis (choice **A**) is the most common cause of abdominal aortic aneurysms. It does not predispose to dissections. Syphilitic aortitis involves the arch of the aorta. It produces vasculitis (choice **C**) of the vasa vasorum with ischemic damage to the aortic wall, resulting in aneurysmal dilation leading to aortic regurgitation. It does not predispose to aortic dissection. Granulomatous inflammation (choice **D**) involving the aorta (Takayasu's arteritis) can predispose to a dissection; however, it is an uncommon vasculitis that occurs primarily in young Asian women.

7 The answer is A   *Surgery*

The patient has inflammatory carcinoma of the breast. This cancer is characterized by a painful breast, with the overlying skin exhibiting lymphedema, warmth, and erythema due to plugging of the dermal lymphatics by tumor (choice **A**). Although it accounts for less than 3% of all cases, it is the most malignant type of breast cancer; metastases occur early, and the prognosis is extremely poor. Approximately 75% of patients already have axillary node involvement at presentation. Modified radical mastectomy is rarely performed. Radiation, hormone therapy, and chemotherapy are the mainstays of treatment.

Paget's disease of the breast (1% of breast cancers) (choice **B**), most commonly occurs in elderly women and presents as a scaly, eczematous rash usually involving the nipple. Unlike extramammary Paget's disease involving the vulva, the breast variant is always associated with an underlying ductal carcinoma in situ, which extends up into and invades the epidermis. A phyllodes tumor (choice **C**) is a stromal tumor of the breast that produces massive breast enlargement. The stroma is hypercellular, but the epithelial elements are benign. Whether low- or high-grade in histologic appearance, it rarely metastasizes to the axillary nodes and is treated with simple mastectomy. Erysipelas is a brawny cellulitis associated with group A streptococci (choice **D**). Although it can simulate inflammatory carcinoma, it responds rapidly to antibiotics. A breast abscess (choice **E**) is most commonly associated with breast-feeding.

8 The answer is C *Preventive Medicine and Public Health*

The index case is most likely suffering from influenza A. Because the infected patient is ambulatory and sociable and living in a closed community, the risk of spreading the disease among the other residents is very high. In addition, the mortality rate and the incidence of serious complications are increased in the elderly. Therefore, the nursing home medical staff should take advantage of every preventive measure available. Assuming a vaccine is prepared from viruses similar to the ones responsible for the epidemic (which it was in this case), prophylactic vaccination has been demonstrated to reduce the number of infected individuals by 50–80%. Moreover, the severity of complications among those who still get infected is, in general, reduced. However, it takes approximately 2 to 4 weeks after vaccination for antibody levels to build up to an effective level, so the vaccination received 6 days ago will be ineffective. Therefore, other prophylactic measures should be considered (choice **A** is wrong). Administration of either amantadine or rimantadine has been shown to be an effective prophylactic measure in the prevention of influenza A, which has little or no effect on the immune response to the virus or vaccine. Therefore, all residents should be treated with one of these drugs (choice **C**).

Treatment with ampicillin or any other antibiotic would be ineffective against a viral infection (choice **B**). Isolation of contacts would be a difficult and likely futile exercise (choice **D**). The residents were just immunized, so administration of a booster shot would not be appropriate (choice **E**).

9 The answer is E *Obstetrics and Gynecology*

Labor is a process in which, over time, in the presence of uterine contractions, progressive cervical dilation and effacement take place (choice **E**). Distinguishing between true and false labor is a difficult task prospectively because many features are found in both. Character of pain (choice **A**) is not a differentiating criterion since both may have significant pain. Descent of the fetus (choice **B**) will occur with true labor, but engagement of the fetus often occurs in primigravidas prior to labor. Regular contractions (choice **C**), and bloody show (choice **D**) occur in false labor. The combination of progressive effacement and cervical dilation is the key distinguishing feature of true labor.

10 The answer is C *Psychiatry*

Psychosis is identified by the presence of hallucinations, delusions, or disorganized speech or behavior. A delusion is a patently false belief and would include the belief that one's thoughts are controlled by secret television messages (choice **C**).

Suspiciousness (choice **E**), hyperreligiosity (choice **A**), and philosophical rumination (choice **B**) are not necessarily delusions. Depending on the context, these characteristics may be present in both disturbed and emotionally healthy individuals. Disorientation to time and place (choice **D**) suggests a cognitive disorder that affects short-term memory.

11 The answer is E *Medicine*

The patient has a prolactinoma (choice **E**), which is the most common functioning tumor of the anterior pituitary gland. Hyperprolactinemia suppresses the release of gonadotropin-releasing hormone from the hypothalamus. This, in turn, causes secondary amenorrhea (absent menses) as a result of decreased synthesis of follicle-stimulating hormone (FSH) and luteinizing hormone (LH) by the anterior pituitary gland. Prolactin also stimulates milk production in the breasts, causing galactorrhea. Other causes of increased prolactin secretion include primary hypothyroidism (15–30% of cases), drugs (e.g., estrogen, cimetidine, plus many more; the patient in question is not taking any drugs), pregnancy (pregnancy test is negative), chronic stimulation of the nipple (e.g., suckling, nipple piercing), and pituitary stalk transection or injury (loss of inhibitory effect of dopamine on prolactin). Laboratory findings in a prolactinoma include serum levels of prolactin over 200 ng/mL (height of prolactin correlates with tumor mass), decreased gonadotropins, decreased estradiol, and decreased testosterone. Most patients respond to treatment with a dopamine analogue (e.g., cabergoline bromocriptine), which restores gonadal function in 70–80% of cases and shrinks the tumor mass in less than 50% of cases. Surgery is used if the sella turcica is enlarged or if the condition doesn't respond to the dopamine analogue. Although hyperprolactinemia is less common in men, they do get prolactinomas, in which case symptoms include erectile dysfunction, loss of libido, and in some cases gynecomastia but not galactorrhea.

Cushing syndrome (choice **A**) is characterized by signs of hypercortisolism (e.g., truncal obesity with purple striae, hypertension), which are not present in this patient. Furthermore, hypercortisolism does not produce galactorrhea or amenorrhea. Graves' disease (choice **B**) is characterized by exophthalmos and thyromegaly, which are not present in this patient. Excess thyroid hormone causes menstrual irregularities, but it does not cause galactorrhea. Hypopituitarism (choice **C**) is associated with amenorrhea as a result of decreased synthesis of FSH and LH. However, other expected findings of anterior pituitary hypofunction (e.g., decreased serum TSH in secondary hypothyroidism) are not present in this patient. Serum prolactin levels are decreased in hypopituitarism.

Primary hypothyroidism (choice **D**) may cause amenorrhea and galactorrhea, because a decrease in serum thyroxine increases both serum TSH and thyrotropin-releasing hormone. Thyrotropin-releasing hormone is a potent stimulator of prolactin release. Since the serum TSH level is normal in this patient, primary hypothyroidism is excluded.

12 The answer is D *Preventive Medicine and Public Health*

The initial test to detect antibodies to human immunodeficiency virus (HIV) is the enzyme-linked immunosorbent assay (ELISA). In patients with clinical acquired immune deficiency syndrome (AIDS), the sensitivity of ELISA is close to 100%, but individuals with recent infections will not develop detectable antibodies for periods of weeks to months after infection. The median interval between infection and seropositivity has been estimated at 3 months, with 95% seroconverting at 6 months. Therefore, a negative ELISA does not rule out the diagnosis of AIDS at this time and will not until there is a 6-month interlude between his last unprotected sexual encounter and taking the test (choice **D**).

Since he had sex as recently as 2 weeks ago, AIDS cannot be ruled out (choice **A**) at this time. Whereas ELISA is nearly 100% sensitive, it is not highly specific. Therefore, the Western blot test is used to determine if a patient who tested positive using ELISA is truly infected with HIV. Although the Western blot test is almost 100% sensitive and specific, it is not used as a screening test because it is too difficult and expensive to perform on a routine basis. In the case presented, it would be senseless to perform a Western blot test (choice **E**) because it has already been determined that the results would be negative (i.e., ELISA, which is essentially 100% sensitive, was negative). Because it takes 3 months for 50% of individuals to raise antibody titers to detectable levels, repeating the test before this time would not be recommended (choices **B** and **C**).

13 The answer is C *Psychiatry*

Separation anxiety disorder is characterized by worry about being separated from caregivers, severe protest on impending separation, or severe anxiety after separation. Such worry often takes the form of fantasies about how the separation will occur (choice **C**). Homesickness is another form of this disorder.

Generalized anxiety disorder (choice **A**) involves multiple worries that are difficult to control. Pervasive developmental disorder (choice **B**) involves qualitative disturbances of development. Specific phobias (choice **D**) involve fears of objects or situations other than social situations or the fear of being helpless during a panic attack. Social phobia (choice **E**) is characterized by fear of social situations.

14 The answer is C *Surgery*

The patient has carcinoma of the head of the pancreas, which is most commonly due to carcinogens that are present in cigarette smoke. Since the common bile duct (CBD) passes through the head of the pancreas, there is complete obstruction of the CBD, leading to distention of the CBD and gallbladder. The bile containing conjugated bilirubin refluxes back into the hepatocytes and out into the sinusoids. Since conjugated bilirubin (CB) is water soluble, bilirubin is filtered and excreted in the urine. Urobilinogen (UBG) in the stool derives from degradation of CB by colonic bacteria. Urobilin, its oxidation product, is responsible for the color of stool. A small fraction of UBG is recycled back into the blood where it is taken up by the liver (90%) and filtered in the kidneys (10%). The normal yellow color of urine is due to urobilin. Therefore, normal findings in the urine include no CB and a small amount (+1) of UBG (choice **A**). Laboratory findings associated with obstruction to bile flow include light-colored stools, owing to the absence of UBG in stool, absence of UBG in the urine, and an increase in CB (choice **C**).

Absence of bilirubin in the urine and an increase in UBG (choice **B**) occurs whenever there is an increase in unconjugated bilirubin presented to the liver for conjugation. This occurs in extravascular hemolytic anemias in which there is macrophage destruction of RBCs leading to an increase in unconjugated bilirubin. Examples include congenital spherocytosis, sickle cell anemia, ABO and Rh hemolytic disease of the newborn, and warm autoimmune hemolytic anemia. More unconjugated bilirubin is converted to CB, more CB is converted to UBG in the colon, and proportionately more UBG is recycled to the kidneys. Unconjugated bilirubin is lipid soluble; therefore, the kidneys do not filter it. The presence of bilirubin in the urine and an increase in UBG (choice **D**) occurs in hepatitis. In hepatitis, there is disruption of bile ductules in the liver, which allows CB to enter the sinusoids of the liver and gain access to the systemic circulation. Furthermore, the UBG that is normally recycled to the liver is redirected to the kidneys, causing an increase in urine UBG. As long as the urine is concentrated enough to have a slight yellowish color it will contain some urobilinogen, thus, choice **E** is not logical.

Summary Table

Urine Bilirubin	Urine Urobilinogen	
0	+1	Normal
0	+2	Extravascular hemolytic anemia
+2	0	Obstructive jaundice
+2	+2	Hepatitis

15 **The answer is D** *Obstetrics and Gynecology*

The scenario describes a patient with polycystic ovarian syndrome (PCOS). The underlying mechanism in PCOS is tonically elevated gonadotropins (choice **D**). The elevated follicle stimulating hormone (FSH) leads to a stable estrogen level that prevents the luteinizing hormone (LH) surge. Anovulation results from the elevated luteinizing hormone (LH) level that never peaks or surges.

Excessive stimulation of androgen production from the follicular theca cells leads to hirsutism but not virilization (increased muscularity, voice deepening, clitoral enlargement) (choice **B**). In patients having PCOS the body mass index is usually high, not low (choice **A**). The androgen production is largely from the ovary, rather than the adrenals (choice **C**). Age at menarche is unaffected (choice **E**).

16 **The answer is D** *Medicine*

Acanthosis nigricans (choice **D**) is a verrucoid, pigmented, sometimes pruritic skin lesion that most commonly occurs in the axilla, groin, or the folds at the back of the neck that commonly accompany an overweight state and occasionally elsewhere, including oral mucosal membranes and on or around the eyelids or cornea. In susceptible individuals, it is caused by a factor that stimulates proliferation of epidermal keratinocytes and dermal fibroblasts. Most commonly, the underlying growth-inducing factor is higher than normal insulin levels; however, other growth factors may also be responsible including insulin-like growth factor, other endocrine factors, and factors generated by malignancies; in the latter case acanthosis nigricans lesions often appear before any of the more sinister signs of cancer become evident. Why acanthosis nigricans only develops in a select number of individuals is unknown. The reported prevalence is less than 1% among Caucasians, 5.5% among Hispanics, and 13.3% among African Americans, and it is also observed among Native Americans. As mentioned above, the most common underlying factor is elevated insulin levels, and as in the case presented, it may occur in susceptible insulin-resistant individuals before there is any other sign of impending diabetes, as well as in overt type 2 diabetics. As might be expected considering the relationship between obesity and the insulin-resistance syndrome, obesity is also a risk factor. Upon presentation, affected individuals should be screened for the underlying cause; although not a common cause, it is critical to look for signs of an underlying malignancy, since those that do stimulate acanthosis nigricans are usually very aggressive. The treatment of acanthosis nigricans involves treatment of the underlying cause.

Pityriasis rosea (choice **A**) is a common eruptive dermatitis that mainly affects young adults. The cause is unknown but is speculated to be viral, because many patients have a history of an upper respiratory infection preceding the skin lesion. The lesion initially presents as a single, pruritic erythematous, oval-shaped plaque on the trunk, called a "herald patch," Days or weeks later, an erythematous papular eruption develops on the trunk that follows the lines of cleavage in a "Christmas tree" distribution. Topical antipruritic agents, oral antihistamines, calamine lotion, ultraviolet treatments, and topical corticosteroids (e.g., triamcinolone cream) are used for treatment. Most cases resolve in 6 to 8 weeks, but in severe cases, systemic steroids may be necessary. Erythema multiforme (choice **B**) is a hypersensitivity reaction that may accompany infections (e.g., Herpes simplex, *Mycoplasma pneumoniae*), pregnancy, malignancy, or any of a host of drugs including sulfonamides, penicillins, and barbiturates. Vesicles and bullae have a "bulls-eye" appearance. Clinically it is divided into two types, erythema multiforme minor and major. Common locations of erythema multiforme minor are the palms, soles, and extensor surfaces. Erythema multiforme major also is called Stevens-Johnson syndrome and involves two or more mucous membranes, either oral or conjunctiva, and is often triggered by *Mycoplasma pneumoniae*. Severe cases of erythema multiforme major should be treated in a burn unit; however, identification and withdrawal of the triggering substance before blistering will reduce symptom severity. Potent topical corticosteroids (e.g., betamethasone dipropionate) or systemic steroids are used for treatment. Erythema nodosum (choice **C**) is the most common inflammatory lesion of subcutaneous fat. Women between the ages of 20 and 30 years are most likely to be affected. It results from a cell-mediated immune reaction to a variety of stimuli. It is characterized by the presence of raised, erythematous, painful nodules, usually located on the extensor surfaces of the lower extremities. Many factors may activate development of erythema nodosum lesions, including oral contraceptives, pregnancy, coccidioidomycosis, histoplasmosis, tuberculosis, leprosy, streptococcal infection, and sarcoidosis. The nodules usually darken during the resolution phase and resolve within 8 weeks. Keratoacanthoma (choice **E**) is a rapidly growing, crateriform benign tumor with a central keratin plug. It develops in sun-exposed areas of the body and is more common in men than women. Locations include the cheeks, nose, ears, and dorsa of the hands. Histologically, they are difficult to distinguish from a well-differentiated squamous cell cancer. However, keratoacanthomas regress spontaneously in a few months with scarring, while squamous cancers persist. Urticaria (choice **F**) is a common condition characterized by pruritic transient wheals (hives) as a result of vasodilation and subsequent fluid leakage into the dermis. It may be caused by IgE-mediated reactions (i.e., mast cell release of histamine) associated with intake of certain foods (e.g., peanuts), insect bites, or drugs (e.g., penicillin, morphine) or it may be caused by an immunocomplex-mediated reaction (e.g., serum sickness prodrome in hepatitis B). Other clinical findings include dermatographism (i.e., urticaria develops in areas of mechanical pressure on skin and angioedema) (i.e., diffuse subcutaneous swelling), which can cause obstruction of the airway and death. Treatment is to avoid agents that precipitate urticaria and the use of both H_1 and H_2 blockers.

17 The answer is B *Surgery*

The patient is most likely an alcoholic who has delirium tremens (DT) (choice **B**) as a result of abrupt withdrawal of alcohol. A full-blown attack is often precipitated by a respiratory alkalosis caused by hyperventilation during surgery. The chance of inducing an attack is enhanced by a chronic nutritional deficit. The attack is characterized by anxiety, tremor, hallucinations, hyperactivity, and seizures. The end effect may result in dehiscence of the wound. Management of DT is geared toward reducing agitation and anxiety. This is accomplished by the administration of diazepam or chlordiazepoxide. In addition, attention must be given to correcting underlying nutritional deficiencies. Hypomagnesemia is particularly common in alcoholics and is associated with tetany secondary to hypocalcemia (magnesium normally enhances parathyroid activity). Thiamine deficiency is also common in alcoholics. Infusion of an intravenous (IV) solution containing glucose can precipitate acute Wernicke's encephalopathy, characterized by confusion, agitation, and nystagmus. The glucose is converted into pyruvate. The pyruvate is converted into acetyl coenzyme A (CoA) via pyruvate dehydrogenase, which uses thiamine pyrophosphate as a cofactor. Hence, the already low thiamine levels become further depleted, potentially causing Wernicke's encephalopathy.

Intensive care unit (ICU) syndrome (choice **D**) is associated with the typical ICU environment of bright lights, noise, and sleep deprivation, which can produce confusion and subsequent development of delirium in patients. Postoperative psychosis (choice **C**) is an uncommon stress-induced psychosis that is seen particularly in elderly patients with chronic disease. Many of these patients have preexisting mood disturbances. Stress, drugs, and high β-endorphin levels are also contributing factors. Delirium occurs in approximately 20% of cases. Although uncommon, it is most commonly associated with thoracic or abdominal surgery. Hypoglycemia (choice **E**) produces adrenergic signs and symptoms without hallucinations. Reactions to anesthetic drugs (choice **A**) would have occurred immediately after surgery rather than a few days later.

18 The answer is C   *Preventive Medicine and Public Health*

This patient is showing signs of elder abuse. The most likely person to have abused this patient is her son with whom she lives. Therefore, the first thing that the physician should do is to contact the state agency that deals with such issues (choice **C**).

A physician does not have to obtain consent from her son to admit her to the hospital (choice **D**). Medical care (choices **A** and **B**) and a psychiatric consult (choice **E**) can be obtained after the state agency has been contacted.

19 The answer is E   *Pediatrics*

Although the child is in good health and immunizations are up to date, the child has not been immunized against measles, which would normally be administered at 1 year of age (choice **A**). In children less than 1 year of age, the risk of complication resulting from measles is high. Infants 6 months or younger born to immune mothers are considered protected by maternal antibody. Infants 6 months or younger born to nonimmune mothers should receive immune globulin. During an outbreak, monovalent measles vaccine or measles–mumps–rubella (MMR) vaccine (if monovalent measles vaccine is not available) may be given to infants as young as 6 months of age (choice **D**). Exposure to measles is not a contraindication to immunization. (choice **C**). Live virus measles vaccine, if given within 72 hours of measles exposure, will provide protection in some cases. Infants should be vaccinated regardless of their proximity to the location where the outbreak occurred (choice **B**). However, the child will need to be revaccinated at 12 to 15 months of age and again at 11 to 12 years of age. Seroconversion rates for measles, mumps, and rubella antigen are lower in children vaccinated with MMR before 12 months of age.

20 The answer is E   *Psychiatry*

Poor sleep efficiency (time actually sleeping/time in sleep period) and resultant daytime drowsiness is a characteristic of sleep apnea (choice **E**). The stimulus of anoxia following each apneic episode repeatedly awakens such individuals. Obese individuals and older adults are at higher risk for sleep apnea.

In narcolepsy (choice **A**), a patient falls asleep suddenly during the daytime. In insomnia (choice **C**), the person has difficulty initiating or maintaining sleep. In sleep–wake schedule disorder (choice **B**), patients sleep at the wrong time. Kleine-Levin syndrome (choice **D**) includes periods of hypersomnia and hyperphagia.

21 The answer is D   *Psychiatry*

"Good-enough mothering" (choice **D**) refers to Winnicott's widely accepted description of the minimum threshold for acceptable mothering, which is sensitive and responsive enough to allow the child to develop a healthy relationship with the outside world.

"Lock and key" (choice **B**) and "goodness of fit" (choice **C**) describe properties of the caregiver–child relationship. "Emerging competencies" (choice **E**) refers to innate abilities that become evident at given ages. "As if personality" (choice **A**) refers to a particular type of pathologic relationship to the environment.

22 The answer is A   *Medicine*

The patient has been exposed to asbestos as a roofer. There are two geometric forms of asbestos—serpentine (i.e., curly and flexible fibers, e.g., chrysotile) and amphibole (i.e., straight and rigid, e.g., crocidolite). In both fiber types fibrogenesis is initiated by macrophages that attempt to phagocytose fibers and in this process release cytokines. Both types of fiber are associated with asbestos-related disease. Crocidolite fibers are more likely to produce disease than serpentine fibers, because they enter the distal respiratory unit where they penetrate epithelial cells and reach the interstitium, and they are the most likely cause of malignant mesotheliomas. The two life-threatening diseases associated with exposure to asbestos fibers are such mesotheliomas and lung carcinoma. Lung involvement begins around respiratory bronchioles and alveolar ducts and extends into the alveoli. Asbestosis is a nodular interstitial fibrosis characterized by dyspnea, inspiratory crackles, and in severe cases clubbing and cyanosis. The most common lesions are benign (nonmalignant) pleural plaques. These plaques are often calcified (visible on x-ray films) and involve the parietal and visceral pleura as well as the dome of the diaphragm, as in this patient (choice **A**). Starting during World War II, asbestos was regarded as the wonder mineral; it doesn't burn and is tough, and consequently, it was used wherever feasible. However, in the late 1970s the health hazards associated with asbestos became appreciated, and its use has been sharply curtailed since the 1980s. Sources of asbestos exposure include insulation around pipes in ships and elsewhere, roofing material used over 20 years ago (this patient), demolition of old buildings (serious problem in the 9/11 bombing), automobile brake shoes, and asbestos mining.

Diffuse interstitial fibrosis (choice **B**) is a manifestation of asbestos exposure. It involves the respiratory bronchioles, alveolar ducts, and alveoli. The pleura are not involved. A malignant mesothelioma of pleura (choice **C**) is the second most common primary cancer. It has no etiologic relationship with smoking, but 80% of patients with malignant mesothelioma report a history of asbestos exposure, and 8% of individuals in asbestos-related industries develop malignant mesothelioma. The tumor arises from the serosal cells lining the pleura (80%) or peritoneum (20%) and encases and locally invades the subpleural lung tissue. A benign pleural plaque is *not* a precursor lesion for a mesothelioma, which requires 25–40 years to develop. Primary bronchogenic carcinoma (choice **D**) is the most common cancer, regardless of whether the patient is a smoker or nonsmoker; however, the risk of lung carcinoma is increased 65 to 100% in individuals exposed to asbestos fibers who also smoke. Primary bronchogenic carcinoma is liable to develop within 20 years after asbestos fiber exposure. The patient has no mass lesion in the hilum or the periphery of lung, ruling out bronchogenic carcinoma.

23 **The answer is B** *Pediatrics*

The fetal lung secretes surfactant into the amniotic fluid. Analyzing amniotic fluid for surfactant-associated phospholipids can assess fetal lung maturity and can usually be done by measuring the lecithin-to-sphingomyelin (L:S) ratio. When the ratio is greater than 2, the fetal lungs are most likely mature. A ratio of 1.5:2 is indeterminate, and a value below 1.5:2 predicts immaturity. Phosphatidylglycerol (PG) also predicts lung maturity. An L:S ratio greater than 2 and the presence of PG further confirm fetal lung maturity.

If there is no PG and the L:S ratio is below 1.5:2, the obstetrician considering elective cesarean section should probably delay it until the lungs are mature (choice **A**). If surfactant is immature (which it isn't), fetal lung maturity and the production of pulmonary surfactant may be hastened by giving the mother a steroid such as beclomethasone over a 24-hour period (choice **C**), not 48 hours (choice **D**). Administration of corticosteroid 48 to 72 hours before delivery, to fetuses 32 weeks of age or less, has reduced the incidence and mortality from hyaline membrane disease. The infant should be delivered (choice **B**) and will not need mechanical ventilation (choice **E**), because the L:S ratio is greater than 2 and PG is present in the amniotic fluid, which indicates mature lungs.

24 **The answer is C** *Pediatrics*

Sudden deterioration of respiratory status should lead one to suspect pneumothorax. Clinically, decreased breath sounds are heard on the affected side. Radiography shows extrapulmonary air, with deviation of the trachea away from the affected side. *Staphylococcus aureus* frequently causes pneumatocyst, which can rupture and cause a pneumothorax (choice **C**).

Emphysema (choice **A**) and pleural effusions (choice **B**) are also caused by *S. aureus*, but these effusions have a different radiologic appearance. Adult respiratory distress syndrome (ARDS) (choice **D**) is an acute respiratory failure associated with impaired oxygenation, increased permeability, pulmonary edema, and normal cardiac function (noncardiogenic pulmonary edema). Although it is known as adult respiratory failure, this is a misnomer, because it has been identified in patients as young as 1–2 weeks of age. The more common causes of ARDS in the pediatric patient include sepsis, shock, and near-drowning. Widespread infiltrates on chest radiographs can be seen in ARDS patients. Patients with sickle cell disease may have a pulmonary infarction (choice **E**) associated with pneumonitis or microscopic fat emboli from bone marrow infarction. In addition to the difference in symptomology, this choice is made very unlikely by the fact that cystic fibrosis affects Caucasian's, while sickle cell disease affects African Americans.

25 The answer is A *Medicine*

Dressler's syndrome (choice **A**) is a relatively rare postcardiotomy pericarditis that manifests itself some 5 days up to months after a myocardial infarct. The signs and symptoms are as described in the vignette (except rather than the ischemic crushing pain described in this case sometimes the pain is described as a pleuritic one, i.e., sharp and stabbing). The syndrome may cause large pericardial effusions and accompanying pleural effusions. It is thought to be caused by an immune reaction to dead tissue. Treatment is nonsteroidal antiinflammatory drugs (NSAIDs) or in severe cases steroids or colchicine. As a rule, resolution occurs without any complications, but symptoms may recur. Dressler's syndrome may also follow any surgical procedure in which heart tissue is injured. Cardiac tamponade is sometimes an additional feature in such cases but rarely occurs in post-myocardial pericarditis.

Postmyocardial infarction pericarditis (choice **B**) is a more immediate pericardial inflammatory reaction to necrotic tissue. Symptoms are similar, albeit less severe, than those described for the Dressler syndrome. This is a more common syndrome (17–25% of postinfarct patients) and can be distinguished from Dressler' syndrome by the fact that symptoms occur earlier, between 2 to 5 days after an infarction. Spontaneous resolution occurs within a few days. The condition described in the vignette can be distinguished from a reinfarction (choice **C**) by the nonelevation of cardiac enzymes. Prinzmetal's angina (choice **D**) is an angina variant in which chest pain occurs in the absence of the factors that usually precipitate an attack of angina pectoris, such as exercise, and it is associated with an ST elevation rather than the usual depression. An attack tends to occur early in the morning, awakening a person from sleep, and it commonly affects women under the age of 50 years. Gastroesophageal reflux disease (GERD) (choice **E**) can produce chest pain that simulates a myocardial infarct or aspects of pericarditis but is not accompanied by the ancillary symptoms described. Moreover, pain can usually be quickly relieved by an antiacid.

26 The answer is B *Obstetrics and Gynecology*

One of the most effective tools in evaluating gestational age by dates is sonographic evaluation of the fetal parameters. Assessment of gestational age by head circumference (HC), biparietal diameter (BPD), abdominal circumference (AC), and femur length (FL) (option **B**) correctly includes the four standard measurements combined to assess gestational age and fetal weight. These measurements are used mainly in the second and third trimesters. The accuracy of dating using these measurements is plus or minus 7 days up to 18–20 weeks.

Crown–rump length (CRL) (included in choices **A, C,** and **E**) is a first-trimester parameter, thus would not be used at 17 weeks. The CRL is accurate to plus or minus 5 days. Humerus length (HL) is similar to femur length (FL) but is not a standard measurement. Transcerebellar diameter (TCD) (choices **D** and **E**) may be used for estimating gestational age but is not a standard measurement for gestational dating.

27 The answer is C *Medicine*

This man has a case of the shingles, also known as herpes zoster, which is caused by herpes varicella (choice **C**), the same organism that causes chicken pox. After an initial exposure to the varicella virus, which may or may not cause a full-blown case of chicken pox, the virus retreats into the dorsal ganglia of an infected nerve and lies dormant only to be reactivated by some unknown factor and to then reemerge many years later, mainly in older individuals. An outbreak is preceded by a painful prodrome that follows the track of the affected nerve, as in the case described in the vignette; this prodrome is sometimes misdiagnosed as a migraine, acute abdomen, myocardial infarction, etc. depending upon the nerve affected. In 24–48 hours the lesions erupt; they remain extremely painful. The eruptions persist for some 2–3 weeks and rarely reoccur. Rarely a motor nerve is affected, causing temporary palsy. Rare complications that may occur include loss of vision if the infection gets into the eye (an ophthalmologic emergency), bladder and bowel dysfunction from sacral shingles, scaring, encephalitis, and paralysis of specific affected muscles. However, the most common lingering problem is neuralgia, which most typically occurs in patients over 55 years old with trigeminal nerve involvement. Treatment is with an antiviral such as acyclovir, famciclovir, or valacyclovir. The earlier treatment is started, ideally before eruptions appear, the less likely is postinfection neuralgia or other complications. Pain is sometimes controlled with nerve block and/or oral corticoids.

Herpes simplex 1 (choice **A**) causes cold sores. Over 85% of the population in the United States has serologic evidence of a herpes simplex 1 infection, which usually is acquired in early childhood. After an initial often asymptomatic infection, the virus retreats into a nerve ending where it may be reactivated by sun exposure, orofacial surgery, or an infection. Herpes simplex 2 (choice **B**) is a similar organism that has a proclivity for genital mucosa. About 25% of the population has serologic evidence of infection, which is acquired by sexual contact and can be transmitted during periods of asymptomatic shedding. Because of changing sexual customs, about 25% of genital herpes infections are now due to herpes simplex 1. Herpes simplex 1 or herpes simplex 2 may also cause herpes gladiatorum by direct skin-to-skin contact as occurs in certain sports such as wrestling and rugby. Human herpesvirus 6 (HHV-6) (choice **D**) is the causative agent of exanthema subitum, also known as roseola infantum or sixth disease. It is the most common cause of infantile febrile seizures, particularly in babies under 2 years of age. Epstein-Barr virus (choice **E**) is also known as human herpesvirus 4 and is associated with mononucleosis. Cytomegalovirus (CMV) (choice **F**) is also a member of the herpes family and evidence of CMV infection can be found in most persons, but almost all are asymptomatic. Exceptions are immunocompromised individuals and those with CMV inclusion disease, which is a neonatal condition sometimes (about 10%) acquired in utero from infected mothers during pregnancy. It causes jaundice, hepatosplenomegaly, thrombocytopenia, periventricular central nervous system calcifications, mental retardation, motor disability, and purpura. Human herpesvirus 7 (HHV-7) (choice **G**) is a T cell lymphotropic virus serologically associated with roseola. Human herpesvirus 8 (HHV-8) (choice **H**) is associated with Kaposi's sarcoma.

28 **The answer is D** *Psychiatry*

The therapeutic intervention used by this therapist is an interpretation of transference, defined in psychodynamic theory (choice **D**) as the feelings about a therapist that a patient has transferred from those associated with earlier relationships. In psychodynamic psychotherapy, transference interpretations are believed to provide therapeutic insight to the patient regarding unconscious thoughts and feelings.

This intervention does not represent behavioral (choice **A**), cognitive (choice **B**), humanistic (choice **C**), or supportive (choice **E**) psychotherapy.

29 **The answer is E** *Medicine*

The seronegative spondyloarthropathies are psoriatic arthritis, ankylosing spondylitis, arthritis associated with inflammatory intestinal diseases, and Reiter's syndrome, recently renamed *reactive arthritis*. These are immune syndromes that have in common presentation typically before the age of 40 years, absence of serum autoantibodies, high degree of association with HLA-B27, absence of the rheumatoid factor, inflammatory arthritis of the spine and/or large joints, and usually an elevated erythrocyte sedimentation rate (ESR). Reactive arthritis (Reiter's syndrome) (choice **E**) is an arthritic syndrome also frequently involving the eyes and urogenital system. It is called reactive because it is a reaction to a sexually transmitted infection with *Chlamydia trachomatis* or an enteric infection with any of several bacteria. It most commonly is acquired between the ages of 20 and 40 years, and 75–80% of affected individuals test positive for HLA-B27. The prevalence is 3.5 per 100,000 Caucasians (it is rare among African Americans who also are less often HLA-B27 positive [about 4 vs. 8% in the general population]) and the male-to-female ratio is 5–10 to 1 if associated with a chlamydial infection and 1 to 1 if associated with an enteric infection. The syndrome itself is not contagious, but of course the underlying infection is. There is no specific test for Reiter's disease other than a high degree of suspicion based on signs and symptoms and elimination of other possibilities.

In addition to the symptoms outlined in the vignette, others may appear. Some of these include balanitis in men (small shallow sores on the end of the penis); inflammations in the fallopian tubes, uterus, vagina, or cervix in women; mouth ulcers and keratoderma blennorrhagia (a rash on the palms or the soles of the feet) in either sex, and among 10% with prolonged disease cardiac problems, commonly aortic regurgitation or pericarditides. As the disease progresses the arthritic changes, typically in the vertebrae, the sacroiliac joint, the knees, ankles, and feet become more evident. As a rule, affected joints show inflammation where the tendon joins the bone (enthesopathy), which may cause osteoporotic changes. Generally the acute phase of the disease lasts 2 to 6 months. Afterward some 30–50% of HLA-B27–positive patients are left with some signs of ankylosing spondylitis, 15–50% will have chronic arthritis, and 15–50% will get recurrent attacks. Treatment consists of antibiotics to clear out the underlying infection (if done early this can lessen symptoms of the syndrome). The inflammatory aspects are treated with nonsteroidal antiinflammatory drugs (NSAIDs) or aspirin and, in refractory cases, with corticosteroids or DMARDS ("disease modifying antirheumatic drugs") such as sulfasalazine. Corticosteroids are also commonly injected into badly inflamed joints. During the early acute phase, bed rest is typically prescribed, followed by a measured exercise program.

Although not a specific test, 90% of patients with ankylosing spondylitis (choice **A**) are HLA-B27 positive. The disease is more common and progresses more frequently in males than in females, and generally first symptoms appear in the late teens or early 20s, with low back pain or stiffness that radiates to the thighs. Sacroiliitis is usually an early manifestation, and about 20% of patients will develop anterior uveitis, which actually may be the presenting symptom. Arthritic symptoms slowly progress upward from the sacroiliac joint, affecting the length of the spine, and may eventually limit motion of the chest wall. Ossification of the anterior aspect of the spine causes stiffening and bends it forward; in extreme cases the body will assume a nearly 90° immobile forward bend. However, the course of the disease is variable, ranging from creating only an inconvenience to creating severe disability. Imaging studies of more advanced cases will show a characteristic "bamboo spine" pattern.

Approximately 20% of patients with inflammatory intestinal disease also develop arthritis, which happens more commonly in Crohn's disease (choice **B**) than in ulcerative colitis. Two forms of arthritis occur. The first is a peripheral one affecting large joints in a manner that parallels the activity of the bowel disease. The second is a spondylitis, which is independent of the bowel symptoms and is indistinguishable from ankylosing spondylitis; about 50% of patients with this form are HLA-B27 positive.

About 80% of the time, psoriatic arthritis (choice **C**) follows the onset of the skin disease, and 20% of the time the two aspects present at about the same time. The presence of skin disease makes diagnosis relatively easy. However, on occasion skin lesions are small and are on a part of the body not readily viewed and must be sought, and in other cases, the skin lesions may be in remission, making a careful history essential. Nail pitting may remain as evidence of psoriasis. The arthritis primarily affects the distal interphalangeal joints and may be accompanied by severe osteolysis, which gives the appearance of a sharpened pencil. HLA-B27–positive individuals often have a spondylotic form in which there is sacroiliitis and spinal involvement. Unlike ankylosing spondylitis, in such cases there is no ossification in the anterior aspects of the spine; hence the bamboo spine pattern, and the forward bend is also absent. Uric acid levels are often elevated because of the high turnover of skin lesions. Treatment is symptomatic. Arthritic conditions tend to improve if the skin lesions are in remission.

Nongonococcal acute bacterial (septic) arthritis (choice **D**) is ruled out in the case presented by the negative test result for bacterial infection in the synovial fluid sample.

30 **The answer is A** *Obstetrics and Gynecology*

Breech presentation occurs when the fetal buttocks or lower extremities present into the maternal pelvis, a finding in 3–4% of deliveries. Breech presentation is more common in premature fetuses, uterine anomalies, and fetal anomalies. Major concerns with vaginal delivery of fetuses in breech presentation are fetal head entrapment due to inadequate time to mold to the maternal pelvis, trauma to nuchal arms with too rapid delivery, and cervical spine injury if the fetal head is hyperextended. For these reasons many breech fetuses are delivered by cesarean section. In frank breech (choice **A**), as in this case, the thighs are flexed and the legs are extended. This is the only kind of breech in which vaginal delivery may be safely considered.

In complete breech (choice **B**) both thighs and knees are flexed. A complete breech becomes a footling breech if the thighs and knees are extended. Incomplete breech (choice **C**) occurs when one or both thighs are extended and one or both knees lie below the buttocks. In double-footling breech (choice **D**), the knees and thighs are both extended. Transverse breech (choice **E**) is not a medical term.

31 **The answer is D** *Pediatrics*

Choking and cyanosis with feedings are the hallmarks of tracheoesophageal fistula (choice **D**). Rales can be heard and are caused by aspiration; abdominal distention results from swallowing air. In the presence of a tracheoesophageal fistula a feeding tube will fail to pass into the stomach.

Choanal atresia (choice **A**) presents as cyanosis relieved by crying. Cyanosis, grunting, and rales are seen in respiratory distress syndrome (choice **B**), but they are unrelated to feedings. Zenker's diverticulum (choice **C**) does not appear in the newborn period. Duodenal atresia (choice **E**) is characterized by bilious vomiting without abdominal distention.

32 **The answer is E** *Obstetrics and Gynecology*

The symptom history in this diabetic patient, combined with the gross description, is most consistent with *Candida* vaginitis. Although a wet saline preparation (choice **A**) can show up the mycelia if they are profuse enough, the potassium hydroxide (KOH) preparation (choice **E**) that removes the epithelial debris would give the promptest diagnosis in the simplest way.

Gram's stain (choice **B**) and culture (choice **D**) are more expensive and time-consuming. A low pH (choice **C**), while characteristic of *Candida* vaginitis, is not adequate for diagnosis.

33 The answer is B   *Pediatrics*

Cleft lip results when the medial nasal and maxillary processes fail to join. The treatment for a cleft lip is surgical closure. This usually occurs by 3 months of age, when the infant has shown satisfactory weight gain and is free of any infection. A good rule to follow for cleft lip repair is the "rule of tens." The patient should be at least 10 weeks of age, weigh at least 10 lb, and have a hemoglobin level of 10 (choice **B**). Choices **A, C, D,** and **E** do not fit all of these criteria.

34 The answer is F   *Obstetrics and Gynecology*

The case is strongly suggestive of intrauterine fetal death (IUFD). From a medical standpoint, once the embryo completes formation of all the organs at 10 menstrual weeks, it is referred to as a fetus. However, legally and technically the definition of IUFD is fetal demise on or after 20 weeks' gestation. Prior to 20 weeks it is legally referred to as a spontaneous abortion. IUFD complicates approximately 3 per 1000 pregnancies. Real-time ultrasound examination for cardiac motion (choice **F**) is the method of choice for assessing fetal death. Failure to visualize cardiac motion is diagnostic. Maternal assessment of fetal movement is not accurate with respect to sensitivity or specificity (choice **C**).

The pregnancy test remains positive for a considerable time because the placenta continues to produce β-human chorionic gonadotropin (HCG); thus, choice **E** is not appropriate. Amniocentesis (choice **B**) is an invasive test that relies on finding dark, turbid fluid, which is a late development; it is not appropriate to diagnose IUFD. Exposure of a possibly live fetus to x-rays is not recommended (choice **D**). A nonstress test (choice **A**) is the appropriate next step in management with maternal report of decreased fetal movement but would not be helpful in this case.

35 The answer is A   *Surgery*

Hyperacute rejections of transplants are either due to a mismatch in ABO groups between a recipient and a donor or the presence of anti-human leukocyte antigen (HLA) antibodies in the recipient against HLA antigens in the donor graft. These reactions occur instantaneously once the circulation is established through the graft. Using an ABO mismatch as an example, if a type A person receives a B donor graft, the anti-B immunoglobulin M (IgM) antibodies normally present in the A recipient will attack the B antigen in the endothelial cells of the graft. This activates complement, which damages the endothelium, resulting in thrombosis and immediate rejection of the graft. This is an example of a type II hypersensitivity reaction. A proper ABO match between the donor and recipient is the single most important factor for graft survival (choice **A**). A lymphocyte crossmatch between the recipient's serum and donor lymphocytes is used to detect the presence of anti-HLA antibodies in the recipient.

The lymphocyte microcytotoxicity test is a serologic test that identifies HLA-A, B, C, and some D loci on the recipient and donor lymphocytes. Mixed lymphocyte reaction testing further identifies compatibility of the D loci of the donor and recipient. A modification of the test is used to evaluate the potential for a graft-versus-host reaction, which is particularly common in bone marrow and liver transplantation. Tests that determine the compatibility of the HLA loci are useful in preventing cellular rejection (type IV hypersensitivity) of the graft. However, HLA compatibility (choices **B, C, D,** and **E**) is not as critical for graft survival as ABO compatibility and the absence of anti-HLA antibodies in the recipient. This is mainly true because an immunosuppressant, such as cyclosporine, can block the release of interleukin-2 (IL-2) by CD4 T helper cells, which play a pivotal role in graft rejection. Matching of CD4 T helper cells also is not most relevant for preventing hyperacute rejection of a donor kidney (choice **F**).

36 The answer is E   *Surgery*

Breast cancer is the most common cancer in adult women and the second most common cause of death due to cancer. It occurs in approximately one in nine women in the United States. Predisposing factors for breast cancer in all women, including Japanese-American women, include: a family history of a first-degree relative with breast cancer or mother with breast cancer; previous history of contralateral breast cancer; early menarche and late menopause (not late menarche or early menopause [choices **C** and **D**]), both of which expose women longer to estrogen; a low-fiber, high-fat diet (the Japanese diet [choice **B**] is high in fiber and low in saturated fat); nulliparity, which leaves women exposed to more estrogen without the benefit of the 9 months of progesterone; a history of endometrial carcinoma (choice **E**), which is also an estrogen-induced cancer; increasing age (the most important risk factor for breast cancer in the absence of a positive family history or a previous breast cancer); a history of smoking cigarettes (choice **A**), while a risk factor, is not as significant for breast cancer as a history of endometrial cancer.

37 The answer is B *Obstetrics and Gynecology*

The lesion described is that of lichen sclerosis. The key finding is the atrophic skin description. The treatment of choice is clobetasol cream (choice **B**). 5-Fluorouracil (choice **A**) is used for neoplasias. Fluorinated corticosteroids (choice **C**) are indicated for hyperplastic dystrophies of the vulva. Miconazole (choice **D**) is an antifungal agent. Estrogen cream (choice **E**) is not effective for lichen sclerosis.

38 The answer is F *Preventive Medicine and Public Health*

Centers for Disease Control and Prevention (CDC) data (reported in *JAMA,* 2004) show that the annual deaths (to the closest round number) attributable to preventable causes at the time of the survey are as follows: (the percentage of death relative to total preventable deaths is shown in parenthesis): tobacco, 400,000 (38%); poor diet and physical inactivity (measured as overweight and obesity) 250,000 (28%); alcohol 100,000 (10%); microbial agents 90,000 (8%); toxic agents, 60,000 (6%); firearms, 35,000 (4%); (unsafe) sexual behavior 30,000 (2%), motor vehicle accidents, 25,000 (2%), and illicit drug use 20,000 (<2%).

These data confirm tobacco's dishonorable rank as the number one killer in the United States. However, this is the first survey to show that poor diet and physical inactivity (obesity) (choice **F**) ranks second. In doing this it displaces alcohol use as the reported second most preventable cause of death in the United States; although this may be due to the fact the CDC had not reported obesity as a cause in the past. It also is true that during the past two decades there has been a dramatic increase in overweight and obesity. Between a 1976–1980 survey and a 1999–2000 survey, the percentage of overweight persons (BMI >25 kg/m^2) in the Unites States has increased from 46 to 64.5%, the percentage obese (BMI, 30–40 kg/m^2) from 14.4 to 30.5%, and although not reported in the 1976–1980 survey, in 1999–2000 there were an additional 4.7% of individuals who are severely obese (BMI, >40 kg/m^2).

Relative to nonobese individuals, obesity increases the risk of noninsulin-dependent diabetes 12.9-fold among woman and 5.2-fold among men; the risk of hypertension 4.2-fold among women and 2.6-fold among men; the risk of myocardial infarction 3.2-fold among women and 1.5-fold among men; and the risk of colon cancer 2.7-fold among women and 3.0-fold among men. Dealing with obesity is difficult because it involves genetic, metabolic/physiologic, cultural, environmental, and psychologic factors. Consequently, some $13 billion is spent annually by Americans in their effort to remain slim, with obvious poor results.

Among the other categories listed, illicit drug use (choice **A**) ranks 9th; firearms (choice **B**) ranks 6th; sexual behavior (choice **C**) ranks 7th; alcohol (choice **D**) ranks 3rd; and motor vehicle accidents (choice **E**) ranks 8th.

39 The answer is B *Pediatrics*

Nephrotic syndrome is characterized by hypoproteinemia (serum albumin <2.5 g/dL) (not hyperproteinemia [choice **A**]), heavy proteinuria (choice **B**) (>40 mg/m^2/h in a 24-hour urine sample), edema, and hyperlipidemia (predominantly triglycerides and cholesterol) (not hypolipidemia [choice **C**]). *Primary nephrotic syndrome* is the term applied to diseases limited to the kidney. *Secondary nephrotic syndrome* is the term applied to a multisystem disease in which the kidney is involved. Hypertension (choice **E**) is rarely seen in nephrotic syndrome. Diarrhea is commonly seen. Patients with nephrotic syndrome have hypoalbuminemia, not hyperalbuminemia (choice **D**).

40 The answer is D *Psychiatry*

The man's symptoms suggest phencyclidine (PCP) intoxication (choice **D**), which is characterized by agitation, aggression, impulsiveness, nystagmus, hypertension, and/or tachycardia, numbness, ataxia, dysarthria, hyperacusis, and perceptual distortions. Cannabis (marijuana) (choice **A**) may cause ataxia and slow speech, but does not cause nystagmus. 3,4-Methylenedioxymethamphetamine (MDMA) (choice **B**) more commonly known as Ecstasy, can cause dry mouth, but does not present with the symptoms described. Methamphetamine (choice **C**) may cause autonomic arousal and excitement, but not the other findings in this case. Volatile inhalants (choice **E**) can cause slurred speech, ataxia, and nystagmus, but not circumoral numbness.

41 **The answer is G**   *Medicine*

This patient has multiple myeloma. It is a malignancy of the plasma cells. As a consequence, these cells produce an inordinate amount of intact monoclonal immunoglobulin, most often IgG, or free monoclonal κ (kappa) or λ (lambda) chains. The latter spill into the urine and are known as Bence Jones proteins. Multiple myeloma usually occurs during the sixth and seventh decades of life, and the most common presentation is bone pain. Rouleaux formation on peripheral smear and pathologic fractures due to osteolytic activity can result. Initial treatment is with melphalan and prednisone (choice **G**). Melphalan is phenylalanine mustard. It is an alkylating agent that induces cytotoxicity by forming cross-links of strands of DNA and RNA. As a result, protein synthesis is disrupted.

42 **The answer is D**   *Medicine*

This patient has chronic myelogenous leukemia. Fatigue, night sweats, and low-grade fever are presenting complaints. Marked enlargement of the spleen and sternal tenderness are prominent features. In addition to presence of the Philadelphia chromosome, in some cases an aberrant *bcr-abl* gene is responsible. Imatinib mesylate (choice **D**) is the treatment of choice. The Philadelphia chromosome creates an abnormal tyrosine kinase, *Bcr-abl* tyrosine kinase. This in turn triggers the abnormal growth of myeloid cells. Imatinib mesylate targets *Bcr-abl* tryosine kinase, thereby preventing abnormal growth of myeloid cells.

43 **The answer is C**   *Medicine*

This patient has acute lymphoblastic leukemia (ALL). ALL is the most common leukemia in childhood. In adults, it occurs around the sixth decade of life. The incidence increases thereafter. The presence of eosinophilic needlelike inclusion bodies in the cytoplasm (Auer rods) is pathognomonic of acute lymphoblastic leukemia. The initial goal is to achieve complete remission. For this, daunorubicin (or idarubicin) together with cytarabine (choice **C**) is used. Following remission, treatment is continued with combination chemotherapy, involving daunorubicin, vincristine, prednisone, and asparaginase. Thereafter, autologous or allogeneic bone marrow transplantation is done. The choice will depend on age, clinical status, and type of leukemia. Daunorubicin is an anthracycline antibiotic. It accomplishes its antineoplastic action by interposing itself between the DNA base pairs and unwinding the DNA helix. It also inhibits RNA polymerase activity. It also is the first-line cytotoxic agent for advanced AIDS-related Kaposi's sarcoma. Cytarabine is an antimetabolite that enters the cell, where it gets converted to its active form. Thereafter, it competes with DNA polymerase and upsets normal production of DNA.

44 **The answer is J**   *Medicine*

Bacillus Calmette-Guérin (BCG) (choice **J**) is both an antituberculous and antineoplastic agent. It is used as intravesical immunotherapy in the treatment of carcinoma of the urinary bladder. It is the treatment of choice in patients with carcinoma in situ. It is believed that BCG induces a local inflammatory response in the cancerous region. As a result, histiocytes and leukocytes enter the area. However, the exact mechanism has not been established. Thiotepa is an alternative agent that is used similarly. Its low molecular weight precludes enhanced absorption and the danger of blood dyscrasias. Other chemotherapeutic agents are used in combination, for example, methotrexate, vinblastine, doxorubicin and cisplatin (M-VAC, in which A stands for Adriamycin, which is another name for doxorubicin) or the three-drug regimen cisplatin, methotrexate, and vinblastine (CMV).

45 **The answer is A**   *Medicine*

This patient has chronic lymphocyte leukemia (CLL), which is often diagnosed by accident. He has not responded to treatment. Alemtuzumab (choice **A**) is the medication that is used to treat cases refractory to other drugs. Alemtuzumab is a monoclonal antibody that causes lysis of leukemic cells after binding to the cell surface.

46 The answer is F   *Medicine*

Mitotane (choice **F**) is used in the treatment of inoperable carcinoma of the adrenal cortex. It is derived from the insecticide DDT and causes direct necrosis and atrophy of the adrenal cortex. It also modifies the peripheral metabolism of steroids. Thus, its main action is to suppress adrenocortical function. Therefore, patients should be prescribed steroids.

47 The answer is E   *Medicine*

This patient has hairy cell leukemia. The disease is very slow growing. Patients have recurrent infections and gradually develop pancytopenia. Its name comes from the numerous cytoplasmic projections that are seen on peripheral smear. Cladribine hydrochloride (2-CdAMP) (choice **E**) is the drug of choice. Cladribine crosses the cell membrane passively, where it is converted into its active metabolite 2CdATP. Malignant lymphocytes and monocytes have low levels of activity of deoxycytidine kinase and deoxynucleotidase. Cladribine kills the cells by promoting the accumulation of toxic deoxynucleotides within them. One of the dreaded complications of cladribine hydrochloride is permanent paraparesis.

48 The answer is M   *Medicine*

Paclitaxel (choice **M**) has largely replaced cyclophosphamide in the treatment of ovarian carcinoma. It is extracted from the Pacific Yew tree. Paclitaxel prevents depolymerization of the microtubules, thereby preventing them from arranging themselves during mitosis. It is the first-line drug in the treatment of ovarian carcinoma and is combined with cisplatin or carboplatin. Paclitaxel is generally administered prior to cisplatin or carboplatin, to decrease the chance of myelosuppression. The response rate is about 70%. Other uses for it include treatment of AIDS-induced Kaposi's sarcoma, advanced carcinoma of the breast in which combination chemotherapy for metastatic disease has failed, and the first treatment for advanced non–small-cell carcinoma of the lung.

49 The answer is I   *Medicine*

The presence of an enlarging testis that is painless points to the diagnosis of testicular cancer. The presence of retroperitoneal nodes requires combination chemotherapy following orchidectomy. Etoposide and cisplatin (choice **I**) are used. Failure to respond requires a combination known as CIBE, namely, cisplatin, ifosfamide, bleomycin, and etoposide. Etoposide arrests dividing cells during metaphase and inhibits DNA and RNA synthesis during the G_2 portion of the cell cycle. Other uses for it include treatment of small cell carcinoma of the lung, and Kaposi's sarcoma associated with AIDS. Cisplatin causes its effects primarily by binding with the DNA and inhibiting its synthesis. It also has a minor effect on RNA and protein synthesis. It is an adjunct in the treatment of metastatic testicular and metastatic ovarian cancers.

50 The answer is L   *Medicine*

This patient has Waldenström's macroglobinemia. The disorder results from plasma cells producing excessive amounts of IgM (unlike multiple myeloma in which IgG is usually produced). This is confirmed by serum protein electrophoresis. The urine contains κ (kappa) light chains (unlike multiple myeloma that contains either κ or λ light chains). Those who are asymptomatic do not require treatment. This patient had fatigue, bleeding diathesis, and hepatosplenomegaly. Unlike patients with multiple myeloma whose predominant symptom is bone pain, those with Waldenström's macroglobinemia do not have bone pain. Initial treatment involves a combination of chlorambucil and prednisone. Thereafter, a combination of melphalan, cyclophosphamide, and prednisone is used. Fludarabine phosphate (choice **L**), a purine analogue, is reserved for refractory cases.

CHOICES NOT USED

Vincristine, doxorubicin, and dexamethasone (choice **B**) are used in the treatment of multiple myeloma if there is no response to melphalan and prednisone, which are the initial drugs of choice.

Bortezomib (choice **H**) is used for patients with multiple myeloma who have relapsed or are refractory to treatment. It has also been used in patients with refractory low-grade lymphomas. Bortezomib is a reversible proteosome inhibitor. It inhibits proteosome 26S. The function of proteosome 26S is to degrade ubiquitinated proteins by its chymotrypsin-like activity. The ubiquitin–proteosome pathway is essential for the regulation of intracellular concentration of specific proteins. By inhibiting proteosome 26S, degradation of proteins and cell death is prevented.

Hydroxyurea (choice **K**) is the drug of choice in the treatment of polycythemia vera. It is also used in the treatment of essential thrombocytosis and sickle cell disease, where it is used for relief of pain. For patients who are unable to tolerate the first-line drug imatinib mesylate in chronic myelogenous leukemia (CML), hydroxyurea is the alternative. Hydroxyurea is an antimetabolite that inhibits the incorporation of thymidine into DNA, thereby inhibiting its synthesis. Unlike cisplatin, hydroxyurea does not affect RNA or protein synthesis.

Rituximab (choice **N**) is a monoclonal antibody (hence the suffix "mab"). It is a chimeric antibody against the B lymphocyte antigen CD20. Its role is in the treatment of resistant low-grade lymphomas and those that have relapsed. It has been used in combination with cyclophosphamide, doxorubicin (hydroxydaunomycin or Adriamycin), vincristine (Oncovin), and prednisone (also known by the acronym CHOP) in initial treatment of patients with diffuse large B cell lymphomas. The response rates are better than with CHOP alone.

Thalidomide (choice **O**) is used for the treatment of refractory cases of multiple myeloma. At the time of writing, the drug is still experimental. Thalidomide is an immunomodulator that has been very effective in the treatment of leprosy. It gained notoriety in the late 50s when pregnant women consumed it to prevent morning sickness. The teratogenicity that resulted from its use led to unfortunate consequences such as absence of limbs.

test **14**

Questions

Single Best Choice: This section consists of numbered statements or questions followed by a list of potential answers; you are to select the ONE best answer.

1 A 23-year-old man became aware of a feeling of heaviness in his testicles. As a consequence he probed them while in the shower and felt a pea-sized lump in the left one. He did not immediately make an appointment to see a physician because there was no pain. However, he did ask a nurse that he was dating who convinced him to get it checked out. In taking a history the physician determined that his left testis did not descend at birth and he had an orchiopexy as a child. Physical examination showed him to be in good physical shape and confirmed the presence of the pea-sized mass. The physician arranged for him to have a scrotal ultrasound study. Which of the following is the most probable diagnosis?

(A) Testicular cancer
(B) Epididymitis
(C) Spermatocele
(D) Varicocele
(E) Hydrocele
(F) Orchitis

2 A 4-year-old child is evaluated by his physician at the community clinic for the chief complaint of an upper respiratory illness. The mother states that for the past 2 days the patient has had a low-grade temperature of 100°F (37.8°C) and clear rhinorrhea. The mother also tells the physician that the child attends preschool, and other children in the classroom have similar symptoms. Physical examination supports the diagnosis of an upper respiratory infection. However, other pertinent physical examination findings in this child are mental retardation, eczema, hypopigmentation, and blue eyes. These additional physical findings most likely support the diagnosis of which of the following?

(A) Down syndrome
(B) Tuberous sclerosis
(C) Phenylketonuria
(D) Cretinism
(E) Galactosemia

3 A 22-year-old man was hiking in the mountains when he suddenly had to step back from the road because of an oncoming car. Unknown to him his left foot was wedged between two rocks and as he turned he twisted his knee with his foot held immobile. He immediately felt a popping sensation in his knee followed by intense pain. The following day the knee was very swollen; he consulted an orthopedic surgeon who obtained a positive result to a McMurray's test but was unable to observe any evidence of a fracture by radiography. Which of the following is the most likely diagnosis?

(A) Tear of the medial collateral ligament
(B) Tear of the anterior cruciate ligament
(C) Osteoarthritis of the knee
(D) Tear of the medial meniscus
(E) Osteochondritis dissecans

4 A 42-year-old woman finds a palpable mass in her breast while taking a shower. She makes an appointment with her primary care physician saying she wants a mammogram because that will be able to confirm whether or not the lump is cancer. The physician explains that the primary usefulness of mammography is which of the following?

(A) Detects nonpalpable breast masses
(B) Assigns a clinical stage for breast cancer
(C) Reliably distinguishes benign from malignant breast cancer
(D) Reduces the role of excisional biopsy in diagnosing breast cancer
(E) Replaces fine-needle aspiration of breast masses

5 A 71-year-old man presents to a physician with a complaint about his ability to urinate. His urinary stream is weak and becomes interrupted. He strains to start urinating, often feels as if his bladder has not completely emptied, and often has to urinate a second time within an hour. As part of the workup, the physician has his serum blood urea nitrogen (BUN) and creatinine levels determined; the values respectively are 40 mg/dL (normal range, 7–18 mg/dL) and 2 mg/dL (normal range, 0.6–1.2 mg/dL). Which of the following additional laboratory test findings also is most likely present?

(A) Fractional excretion of sodium (FENa+) is less than 1%
(B) Random urine sodium is more than 40 mEq/L
(C) Urine osmolarity (U_{Osm}), <350 mOsm/kg
(D) Urine sediment with renal tubular cell casts

6. A 39-year-old woman is being seen for prenatal care with a pregnancy complicated by type 2 diabetes mellitus and chronic hypertension. Her diabetes is being managed with twice-daily subcutaneous injections of mixed insulin, and her home blood glucose values are within the target ranges. She is not on any antihypertensive agents, with home blood pressure readings averaging 140/80. Her sister gave birth to a neonate with trisomy 18, and she is interested in screening to see whether this fetus has the same anomaly. She defers amniocentesis and requests triple-marker screening. Which one of the following panel combinations would be most consistent with this anomaly?

(A) Maternal serum (MS) α-fetoprotein (AFP) ↓, estriol↓, human chorionic gonadotropin (hCG) ↓
(B) MS-AFP↑, estriol↓, hCG↓
(C) MS-AFP↓, estriol↓, hCG↑
(D) MS-AFP↓, estriol↑, hCG↓
(E) MS-AFP↑, estriol↑, hCG↓

7. A 46-year-old woman has hypertension and also has problems with her weight. This is not only a cosmetic and health problem, but she feels it is important for her continued employment and advancement as a flight attendant. She has tried just about all the popular diets but always gains back more than she lost. In desperation, she consults a surgeon asking for bariatric surgery. He gauges her height and weight and calculates her body mass index (BMI) to be 27 kg/m² and consequently refuses, pointing out that while somewhat overweight, she is a long way from being morbidly obese. Moreover, he adds, such surgery has a significant inherent risk, with a 0.5% mortality rate and a 15% surgical complication rate plus nutritional and other postsurgical complications. Instead he recommends a dietary and exercise regime plus an appetite suppressor that has minimal metabolic side effects. Which of the following drugs does he most likely recommend?

(A) Ephedra
(B) Orlistat
(C) Fexofenadine
(D) Dexfenfluramine
(E) Fenfluramine

8. A 5-year-old child with severe asthma is being treated with continuous short-acting β_2 agonist in the emergency department. Review of previous medical records shows that this child has had multiple hospital admissions but has never been admitted to the intensive care unit or intubated. The child is slowly becoming sleepy and less responsive. Examination of the chest reveals less wheezing than on admission. At this time which of the following actions is most appropriate in the care of this patient?

(A) Send the child home with the mother
(B) Order a chest x-ray film
(C) Order a bolus of normal saline solution
(D) Order arterial blood gas (ABG) studies immediately
(E) Order a complete blood count (CBC)

9. A 63-year-old house painter who is looking forward to retiring at 65 and collecting full Social Security benefits presents to his physician with a complaint of extreme fatigue and shortness of breath that makes his continued working very difficult. Upon taking a history it is determined he smoked all his adult life, the fatigue and shortness of breath first became troublesome about 6 months ago, and for the past several weeks he occasionally feels compelled to get up at night and open the window to get air. He also has noticed scattered wheezes when climbing his ladders to paint. Additionally, he gained some 10 to 15 lb during these 6 months and noticed a gradual swelling of his legs and ankles. He has been treated with hydrochlorothiazide and captopril for hypertension for the past 6 years and takes an 81-mg aspirin every night before going to bed. Otherwise, he has had no significant health problems or takes any other prescribed or over-the-counter medications. His vital signs are pulse, 110 beats/min and regular; respiration, 26 breaths/min; and blood pressure, 140/89 and he is afebrile. There is a 30° jugular venous distension (JVD) elevation, both lung fields demonstrate rales, and a positive hepatojugular reflux and moderate hepatic congestion are also found. Stethoscopic examination of the heart reveals an S_4 and atrial fibrillation. There is also 1+ pitting edema in both legs to his midcalves. An electrocardiogram shows sinus rhythm, no acute changes, but poor R-wave progression in the anterior leads. Chest radiography reveals cardiomegaly and pulmonary vascular congestion. Which of the following medications would be most appropriate to prescribe?

(A) Carvedilol
(B) Valsartan
(C) Nifedipine
(D) Pravastatin
(E) Metformin

10 A 32-year-old woman was in an automobile accident 2 days ago in which she suffered a fractured femur, fractured ribs, and lacerations. Examination conducted at admission showed no internal organ injuries. It was decided that to stabilize the femur it will be necessary to insert a rod. Consequently, an internist was called in to conduct a preoperative physical examination. Which test among those listed below must be performed?

(A) Serum glucose level
(B) Liver enzyme levels
(C) Hemoglobin level
(D) Coagulation times
(E) An electrocardiograph

11 A 36-year-old man with a 20-year history of alcoholism desperately wants to stop drinking. He has contraindications to disulfiram and stopped taking naltrexone after he became extremely dysphoric. He continues in a 12-step recovery program but describes a daily fight with the urge to drink. What should be the next step in his anticraving treatment?

(A) Start acamprosate therapy
(B) Reinitiate naltrexone therapy, combined with a low dose of paroxetine
(C) Explain that there are no other available agents that block alcohol craving and that he must work at the 12-step program more diligently
(D) Use low doses of lorazepam to block extreme alcohol craving
(E) Initiate lithium therapy

12 A 46-year-old man who belongs to a bicycle club and enjoyed long-distance biking on a regular basis for decades is suddenly afflicted with perineal pain while riding. Upon consulting a physician he reveals that he also needs to urinate frequently, has a burning pain upon urinating, and trouble voiding; he also has pain upon ejaculation with traces of blood in the ejaculate, erection problems, and vague lower back pains that worsen upon sitting, particularly when sitting on the small bicycle seat. Physical examination uncovers no abnormalities. His temperature is 98.9°F (37.2°C). Laboratory analysis of the urine demonstrates a mild hematuria but is otherwise normal. Expressed prostate fluid shows a few leukocytes. Microbiology cultures of urine and expressed prostatic secretions have negative results. The patient most likely suffers from which of the following disorders?

(A) Acute bacterial prostatitis
(B) Chronic bacterial prostatitis
(C) Prostatodynia
(D) Bladder carcinoma in situ
(E) Nonbacterial prostatitis

13 An afebrile 12-week-old infant is brought to the pediatrician by his mother because of a persistent cough. Upon physical examination the patient is found to have a temperature of 100°F (37.8°C) per rectum and is noted to have bilateral conjunctivitis. Other pertinent findings include tachypnea, inspiratory rales, and scattered expiratory wheezing. The rest of the physical examination is unremarkable. A complete blood count (CBC) reveals eosinophilia. The chest x-ray film shows hyperinflation and patchy interstitial infiltrates bilaterally. Which of the following is the most likely diagnosis?

(A) Respiratory syncytial viral pneumonia
(B) Bronchiolitis
(C) Chlamydial pneumonia
(D) Cystic fibrosis
(E) The larval phase of ascariasis

14 A 55-year-old medical director of a private hospital was admitted to the intensive care unit with a history of severe retrosternal chest pain associated with radiation to the jaw. Clinical examination and investigations confirmed an anterolateral myocardial infarction. A few hours later, his electrocardiogram revealed short runs of rapid rhythm, unsustained, wide-complex tachycardia. His vital signs were stable otherwise. Which of the following is the most appropriate antiarrhythmic drug to administer at this early time after his infarct?

(A) Cardioversion
(B) Amiodarone
(C) Flecainide
(D) Lidocaine
(E) Quinidine
(F) Verapamil

15 A recently discovered treatment for leukemia helps alleviate morbidity and consequently extends the life span of the patient; however, it does not prevent the disease nor does it provide a cure. In this scenario, this treatment for leukemia will have which of the following effects?

(A) Incidence will increase
(B) Prevalence will increase
(C) Incidence will decrease
(D) Prevalence will decrease
(E) Both incidence and prevalence will increase

16 A 45-year-old man with a history of alcohol abuse and chronic hepatitis C complains of skin lesions that develop whenever he is exposed to sunlight. He also states that the color of his urine has changed to a reddish color. Physical examination shows numerous fluid-filled vesicles and bullae over areas exposed to sunlight (e.g., face, neck, forearms, dorsum of the hands). The skin in these areas is friable and also shows thickening, scarring, and calcification. Hypertrichosis and hyperpigmentation are also present, particularly on the face. Results of the neurologic examination are normal. Laboratory studies including a complete blood cell count and electrolytes have normal results. Which of the following compounds is most likely responsible for the color change in the urine?

(A) Hemoglobin
(B) Myoglobin
(C) Porphobilin
(D) Urobilin
(E) Uroporphyrin I

17 A 29-year-old woman with a long history of impulsive behavior leading to adverse personal consequences has been in psychotherapy for 5 years. She has made several suicide attempts and has had many failed interpersonal relationships during the course of her therapy. Recently, she has come to believe that her therapist is both incompetent and uncaring. She has independently sought consultation with another psychotherapist, without informing her current psychotherapist. After the first session, she says that she is convinced that the new psychotherapist is markedly more competent, caring, and approachable, and asks him to take over treatment. Which of the following is the most appropriate next action for the new therapist to initiate?

(A) Immediately agree to take over the case
(B) Report the previous psychotherapist to the state licensing board for gross incompetence, thoroughly documenting his concerns by sending copies of his clinical notes
(C) Suggest to the patient that she thoroughly discuss with her current psychotherapist her plan to switch therapists and then return if she still wants to change therapists
(D) Call the current psychotherapist and inform him of the patient's actions
(E) Refuse to take over the case, explaining to the patient that her actions represent "splitting" and must be dealt with in treatment with the current therapist

18 A 6-month-old infant presents to the emergency department with his mother. The mother says that the patient was born via spontaneous vaginal delivery. He weighed 7 lb (3.2 kg) at birth and currently weighs 15 lb (6.8 kg). Immunizations are up to date. Upon physical examination the patient is noted to have

fever, intermittent inspiratory stridor, retraction of the intercostal muscles, and flaring of the nostrils. The mother states that the child has had an upper respiratory infection for the last 1 to 2 days. Which of the following diagnoses is most likely in this patient?

(A) Laryngotracheobronchitis (croup)
(B) Whooping cough
(C) Acute epiglottitis
(D) Bronchiolitis
(E) Acute bronchial asthma

19 A 55-year-old man in a primary care clinic requests a skin biopsy for a small nevus. He expresses worry that it is a malignant melanoma. Upon examination, the nevus does not have features suggestive of the malignancy. The patient has had two previous biopsies in the last year due to similar concerns, even though the dermatologists were doubtful that the lesions were malignant. Both biopsy specimens were negative. The patient's brother died of malignant melanoma approximately 2 years ago. Which of the following is the most likely psychiatric diagnosis?

(A) Body dysmorphic disorder
(B) Conversion disorder
(C) Delusional disorder, somatic type
(D) Hypochondriasis
(E) Somatization disorder

20 An infant is brought to the community clinic because the mother states that the baby has a rash that is composed of bullae and pustules, as well as wheals, papules, vesicles, and a superimposed eczematous dermatitis. The rash is located on the scalp, palms, and diaper area. The mother notes that this rash is extremely pruritic, and the infant has evidence of excoriation. Further questioning reveals that the mother also has a pruritic rash. The physician determines the diagnosis to be scabies. Which of the following best describes the manner in which infantile scabies differs from adult scabies?

(A) In infants it has bullae and pustules and no burrows
(B) In infants it does not affect the intertriginous areas
(C) In infants it often presents with red-brown nodules in the groin
(D) In infants it spares the face
(E) In infants it spares the soles

21 A 47-year-old man suffered a spontaneous spinal fracture and consequently was given a bone density scan, which demonstrated osteoporosis in his spinal column. When queried by his physician he revealed that for the last few years he has been having additional unusual symptoms. These included episodes characterized by the sudden but transient appearance of a cluster of symptoms, which include headache, acute lightheadedness to the point of syncope, nausea sometimes with vomiting, a crampy feeling in his stomach, flushing, itchiness, and palpitations. These attacks come on suddenly but symptoms subside within a period of minutes to hours; however, after suffering such an attack he is extremely lethargic. These attacks had been occurring intermittently for at least 2 to 3 years, and he could not point to one particular triggering event. The physician told him to come into his office the moment another attack occurs and he will draw blood and perform tests. He did so, and when the laboratory results returned, he was found to have hypercholesterolemia, a thrombocytopenic eosinophilia, elevated serum liver enzyme activities, elevated serum alkaline phosphatase activity, elevated serum tryptase activity, elevated histamine and elevated urinary N-methyl histamine and prostaglandin D_2 levels. His osteoporosis is most likely caused by which of the following conditions?

(A) Hyperparathyroidism
(B) Systemic mastocytosis
(C) Overactivity of the thyroid C-cells
(D) Underactivity of the thyroid C-cells
(E) Acute hypoparathyroidism

22 A third-year medical student who just finished his surgical clerkship is visiting the emergency room at his teaching hospital when the paramedics bring in a 14-year-old boy who accidentally pushed his arm through a glass window. He was very agitated, worrying he might bleed to death from two wounds on the arm. One was 2 inches (5.08 cm) long the other 1 inch (2.54 cm) long. Although both were deep enough to penetrate the dermal skin layer neither was deep enough to cause real trouble and neither cut an artery. The physician on duty calmed the patient down, anesthetized and cleaned up the wound, and prepared to close them. He then asked the medical student to select the proper type(s) of suture to use, which he did. Which of the following combination did he select?

(A) A multifilament one for the deep tissues and silk on the superficial ones
(B) Nylon for the deeper layers and catgut for the superficial ones
(C) Catgut for the deeper tissues and nylon for the superficial ones

(D) Silk for the deep wounds and a multifilament one for the superficial ones
(E) Nylon for both the deep and superficial layers

23 Results of test X for systemic lupus erythematosus (SLE) are positive in 60 of 100 patients with known SLE and negative in 80 of 100 normal controls. If results from test X return positive in a person who is randomly selected in this population under study, what is the percentage chance that the person has SLE?

(A) 60%
(B) 65%
(C) 70%
(D) 75%
(E) 80%

24 A 10-year-old boy has progressive ataxia and is brought to the pediatrician for evaluation. The parents state that the ataxia began approximately 1 month ago. Recently the patient has developed an explosive, dysarthric speech. The pediatrician observes that the patient appears apathetic. However, the parents note that the child's grades at school have not faltered. On physical examination the patient is noted to have nystagmus, pes cavus, and scoliosis. He has very poor proprioception and vibratory sensation and in addition is areflexic. The patient has a positive Romberg test result. Which of the following conditions might also be seen in this patient?

(A) Sick sinus syndrome
(B) Diabetes mellitus
(C) Mental retardation
(D) Progressive blindness
(E) Seizures

25 A 49-year-old woman presents with a complaint of urinary incontinence. In presenting her history she relates that in her early 20s she finished law school, passed the bar, and worked as an assistant district attorney for several years. She then married and worked as a stay-at-home mom for a decade, raising three children until they were well established in elementary school. At the age of 48 she reentered the law profession as an assistant to a prominent defense attorney. She says the job is very stressful and adding to that is the stress of still caring for her kids and husband. However, she adds that for the past 3 months her ultimate problem is sudden and uncontrollable urges to urinate, which are occurring more and more frequently. She states: "It is not only embarrassing but it forces me to interrupt presentations, leave social

occasions, and so on. What is my problem? Can you help me?" After concluding a physical examination that rules out cystitis, urethritis, tumors, stones, diverticulosis, and an outflow obstruction among other physical problems, which of the following is the proper response?

(A) Your problem is stress incontinence, and symptoms can be alleviated by reducing the stress you are under.
(B) Your problem is known as detrusor hyperreflexia incontinence, and symptoms can be alleviated by proper medication.
(C) Your problem is overflow incontinence, and symptoms can be alleviated by minor surgery.
(D) Your problem is functional incontinence, and symptoms can be alleviated by a set of exercises.
(E) Your problem is known as secondary incontinence and can be alleviated by curing the primary cause.

26 A 45-year-old male with a long history of paranoid schizophrenia, which is now in excellent remission comes in complaining of mild writhing movements of his extremities. He has been taking haloperidol 10 mg PO qd for 20 years. A review of systems indicates a family history of "sudden death" by heart attack in his father and uncle in their 50s, although neither was obese. The patient also has a history of unexplained syncopal episodes. Results of an electrocardiogram (ECG) are unremarkable. Which of the following changes in psychiatric medication would be most appropriate?

(A) Decrease the haloperidol to 5 mg PO qd
(B) Stop all antipsychotic medication unless psychotic symptoms return
(C) Start amantadine 100 mg PO tid
(D) Start ziprasidone 20 mg PO bid
(E) Start clozapine 25 mg PO tid

27 A 67-year-old woman presents with a complaint of severe muscle cramps. In taking her history it was determined that she has been an epileptic, and since her late teens, she has been taking phenytoin. Recently she also started taking alendronate for osteopenia; she rarely consumed alcohol. On further questioning it was determined that the muscle cramps were generally spontaneous but also could be initiated by pressure or use and that she also was troubled by dry skin, an occasional feeling of numbness, and/or a tingling sensation in her finger tips. In addition she said that her husband complained that her personality is changing; she is no longer always the cheerful upbeat person but has longer and longer periods of grumpiness and despair. Results of physical examination were not remarkable;

her thyroid function is normal, and she never had neck surgery. However positive Chvostek's and Trousseau's signs are elicited. Which of the following tests is most likely to be used to confirm the probable diagnosis?

(A) Serum albumin level
(B) Serum free calcium ion level
(C) Serum parathyroid level
(D) Serum total calcium level
(E) Serum calcitonin levels

28 A 6-year-old child comes to the pediatric clinic for the first time. The patient has renal disease that includes nephritis and a bilateral sensorineural hearing deficit. The mother reports that there are other family members with kidney disease who are deaf. The pediatrician suspects that the child has Alport's syndrome. Which of the following findings would support this diagnosis?

(A) Thrombocytosis
(B) Cataracts
(C) Papular lesions
(D) Hypotension
(E) Cardiomyopathy

29 A 21-year-old man with a diagnosis of schizoaffective disorder, bipolar type manic, is awaiting involuntary transfer to an inpatient unit from an emergency room. He was given risperidone 2 hours ago and was somewhat calmer until the last several minutes. He is now increasingly agitated and confrontative, demanding immediate transfer from the noise of the emergency room. He says that he refuses to take another dose of medication. Which of the following is the most appropriate next action?

(A) Rescind his involuntary detention and allow him to leave
(B) Place him in restraints
(C) Insist that he accept another dose of risperidone or give intramuscular (IM) antipsychotic medication
(D) Try to reassure him and calm him down
(E) Call security to arrest him

30 Annually there are some 134,000 new cases and 55,000 deaths from colorectal cancer, making it the second most prevalent cause of death from a malignancy in the Unites States. These statistics should be reducible because colorectal cancer is an ideal condition for screening. It affects 6% of the population, and if caught early, it is readily cured or actually prevented. Screening is now endorsed by the United Sates Preventative Task Force, the Agency for Health

Care Policy and Research, the American Cancer Society, and every relevant professional society. It will be paid for by Medicare and other third-party payers. Which of the following is part of a recommendation made for an average-risk individual by a recent multidisciplinary consensus panel?

(A) Begin screening at 60 years of age
(B) Begin screening at 50 years of age
(C) Begin screening at 40 years of age
(D) Begin screening at 30 years of age
(E) Begin screening at 10 years of age

31 A 12-year-old boy has a 5-year history of asthma with episodes of bronchospasm that have resulted in repeated hospitalizations. His respiratory symptoms occur daily, and he has been using a short–acting β$_2$-selective agonist drug via inhalation as needed and during exercise. He presents to the emergency department with severe respiratory distress, cyanosis, and tachycardia. The examination is consistent with severe bronchoconstriction and shows no other complicating factors. Which of the following statements about the treatment of this patient is accurate?

(A) The use of ipratropium via inhalation is likely to exacerbate his symptoms.
(B) Parenteral glucocorticoids should not be given until the bronchospasm is relieved.
(C) The present problem is due to excessive use of the inhaler.
(D) Cromolyn via inhalation should be given until the bronchospasm is relieved.
(E) Prophylactic corticosteroid therapy after recovery from this episode should be considered.

32 A 21-year-old military recruit's foot is x-rayed the day after he complains of intense pain in his right foot just behind the toes; the pain is accentuated by walking. No fracture is observed in the film. The pain continues, and 10 days later a second radiograph reveals new bone formation along the periosteum of the second and third metatarsals. Which of the following is the most likely diagnosis?

(A) Greenstick fracture
(B) Stress fracture
(C) Comminuted fracture
(D) Spiral fracture
(E) Compound fracture

33 A 19-year-old girl is brought into the emergency room by police after being taken into custody at a party, where she became highly agitated and assaultive after ingesting unknown drugs. She presents with pressured

speech, extreme suspiciousness that she is being stalked, tachycardia, and pupillary dilation. Her coordination appears unimpaired, and her mucous membranes are moist. Which of the following substances is the most likely cause?

(A) Amphetamine
(B) Cannabis
(C) Lysergic acid diethylamide (LSD)
(D) Phencyclidine
(E) Psilocybin

34 An investigator wishes to establish the efficacy of a new drug for treating acquired immune deficiency syndrome (AIDS). He proceeds to conduct a clinical trial. Which of the following is a key feature restricted to clinical trials?

(A) Use of blinding techniques
(B) Bias
(C) Random allocation
(D) Retrospective study
(E) Prospective study

35 A 31-year-old homeless man being examined in the medical emergency room complains that a nodule in his groin is in fact "an infrared camera" implanted surreptitiously during a herniography at another hospital several months ago. He believes that the device records his intimate activities. His is not mollified by reassurances from examining physicians and requests radiographic studies and surgical removal of the nodule. He refuses to leave the hospital. Which of the following is the most likely diagnosis?

(A) Body dysmorphic disorder
(B) Factitious disorder
(C) Hypochondriasis
(D) Schizophrenia
(E) Schizotypal personality disorder

36 A 62-year-old woman with a 30-year history of smoking cigarettes has had a "dragging" sensation in the right upper quadrant and a history of weight loss for the past several months. A computerized tomography (CT) scan of her liver shows multiple mass lesions. A liver biopsy specimen shows a low-grade adenocarcinoma. Which of the following is the most likely site of origin of this tumor?

(A) Distal esophagus
(B) Kidney
(C) Midesophagus
(D) Sigmoid colon
(E) Urinary bladder

37 Serum electrophoresis is performed on a sample obtained from a 56-year-old man who enjoyed his pint of whisky every day for the past few decades with no apparent adverse effect. However, for the past few months he has a greater need for a "nip" even while at work and actually appeared at work in an intoxicated condition. Consequently, he agreed to be admitted to a rehabilitation clinic. During his admission examination he confessed that recently he has lost his appetite, has been losing weight, and is suffering from weakness, fatigability, disturbed sleep, and muscle cramps. Abdominal palpation shows a firm enlarged liver with a sharp edge. His upper chest region shows spider nevi, and he has mild jaundice. Which of the following descriptions of serum electrophoretic patterns (SEPs) would be expected to be obtained from this patient?

(A) A polyclonal enlargement of the γ-globulin peak and decreased albumin level

(B) A deficient α-1 peak

(C) Increased IgG and IgA, decreased albumin

(D) A monoclonal gammopathy

(E) A reduction in albumin and a normal γ-globulin peak

38 During a medical assessment following a slip on a wet supermarket floor 4 months before, a 48-year-old woman complains of frequent episodes of sudden loss of consciousness since the accident. Initial examination at the time of the accident revealed no evidence of head trauma or other obvious physical injury. The patient states emphatically that with the exception of her fall and its sequela, her life is going very well. Results of extensive neurologic examination, routine laboratory studies, magnetic resonance imaging (MRI), and an electroencephalogram (EEG) are unremarkable. The patient says that she is unable to work and has initiated a lawsuit against the supermarket for large monetary damages. She spends her days at home, where she lives alone with a pet dog. Which of the following is the most likely diagnosis?

(A) Atonic seizure

(B) Conversion disorder

(C) Factitious disorder

(D) Hypochondriasis

(E) Malingering

Directions for Matching Questions (39 through 50): Each set of matching questions is preceded by a list of 4 to 26 lettered options followed by a brief explanation of the required task and then by a series of numbered statements. For each lettered statement you are to select ONE lettered option that best fulfills the task as it relates to that statement. Remember each of the listed options might be correctly selected once, more than once, or not at all.

Questions 39–45

Select one answer for each item in the set that is the most likely cause of the excess male pattern hair in the female described.

(A) Cushing syndrome

(B) Polycystic ovary syndrome (PCOS)

(C) Adrenal tumor

(D) Medication effect

(E) Congenital adrenal hyperplasia (CAH)

(F) Sertoli-Leydig ovarian tumor

(G) Idiopathic hair follicle sensitivity

39 A 28-year-old woman comes to the out patient office complaining of a sudden onset of excessive facial hair and body hair over the past 4 months. She has noticed that her breasts seem smaller and her libido is increased. On general examination she has a muscular body with obvious coarse, dark hair on her upper lip and chin as well as on her chest and back. There is thinning of hair on the frontal part of the head. Pelvic examination reveals male pubic hair distribution with enlargement of her clitoris. On bimanual examina-

tion you palpate a 5 × 6 cm nontender, mobile, left-sided adnexal mass.

40 A 28-year-old nulligravid woman complains of long-duration facial and body hair. She noticed it starting shortly after puberty. Her menses are irregular and unpredictable, but this has always been her menstrual pattern. Although she is married and sexually active without contraception, she has never been pregnant. Her older sister and aunt have similar complaints. Upon general examination she is observed to be an obese female appearing her stated age with obvious coarse, dark hair on her upper lip and chin as well as on her chest and back. She has normal female breasts and body contours. Pelvic examination reveals male pubic hair distribution with a normal sized clitoris. On bimanual examination you palpate bilaterally enlarged smooth, mobile, nontender ovaries.

41 A 32-year-old nulligravid woman presents to the office with gradual onset of body hair over the past 6 months. She states she has overwhelming fatigue with much less energy than she used to. Her menses, which used to be regular and predictable are now irregular and unpredictable. Her family history is negative for any similar complaints. Upon general examination her face appears round with increased upper body obesity especially around the neck and back. She has stretch marks on her abdomen, thighs, buttock, arms, and breasts. Pelvic examination reveals normal female external genitalia with a normal-sized clitoris. On bimanual examination you palpate a normal midline, mobile, nontender uterus with no adnexal masses.

42 A 28-year-old multiparous woman complains of long-duration facial and body hair. She noticed it starting shortly after puberty. Her menses are regular and predictable. Her two pregnancies were planned and were unremarkable, with normal-term vaginal deliveries. Her older sister and aunt have similar complaints. Upon general examination she is noted to be of average height and weight. She has coarse, dark hair on her upper lip and chin as well as on her chest and back. She has normal female breasts and body contours. Pelvic examination reveals male pubic hair distribution with a normal-sized clitoris, normal external genitalia, vagina, cervix, uterus, and adnexa.

43 A 32-year-old woman has noticed an increase in hair on her face, chest, abdomen, and back. In addition, her voice has become lower and coarser. She states the onset has been rapid over the past 6 months. She denies any family history of similar complaints. Her menstrual periods are now irregular. On physical examination you confirm the increased generalized body hair. On pelvic examination her escutcheon is male pattern with prominent enlargement of her clitoris. Bimanual pelvic examination reveals a normal vagina, uterus, and adnexa, without pelvic masses.

44 A 39-year-old woman presents to the outpatient clinic with a 12-month history of increasing coarse, darkly pigmented facial and body hair. She has a history of extensive endometriosis, with pain so severe and disabling that she underwent a total abdominal hysterectomy and bilateral oophorectomy. She was placed on estrogen therapy, which has been successful in treating vasomotor symptoms and vaginal atrophy. However, her libido markedly decreased after the surgery, so a year and a half ago she was placed on combination estrogen and testosterone therapy. Her libido has normalized since the added androgen therapy. On physical examination you find increased generalized body hair. Pelvic examination reveals a normal-sized clitoris and a normal vagina and uterus without adnexal masses.

45 A 21-year-old woman comes to the office with a long history of excessive dark hair on her upper lip, chin, chest, and proximal extremities. She first noticed these findings when she underwent puberty at age 13. Her menstrual periods have always been irregular. Two years ago she was placed on combination oral contraceptives for both contraception and cycle control. Many of her aunts and cousins have similar complaints. On physical examination she has normal female secondary sexual characteristics with normal breasts and body contours. You confirm male-pattern facial, chest, and extremity hair. On pelvic examination she has no clitorimegaly and a normal vagina and uterus. Her ovaries feel normal size without enlargement.

Questions 46–50

For each clinical description, select the ONE type of leukemia from the lettered list below that is best described in numbered questions below.

(A) Acute lymphoblastic leukemia
(B) Chronic lymphocytic leukemia
(C) Adult T-cell leukemia
(D) Hairy cell leukemia
(E) Acute myelogenous leukemia with maturation (M2)
(F) Chronic myelogenous leukemia (CML)
(G) Acute promyelocytic leukemia (M3)
(H) Acute monocytic leukemia (M5)

46 A 34-year-old man presents with epistaxis, generalized nontender lymphadenopathy, and hepatosplenomegaly. A complete blood count (CBC) reveals a normocytic anemia, a total white blood cell (WBC) count of 40,000 cells/mL with >30% blast cells present and thrombocytopenia. The illustration highlights some of the more typical histologic features.

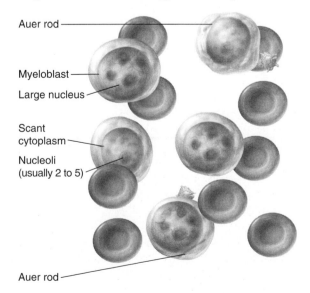

47 A 24-year-old man presents with ecchymoses, generalized lymphadenopathy, and hepatosplenomegaly. A CBC reveals a normocytic anemia, a total WBC count of 50,000 cells/mL, and thrombocytopenia. Hypergranular blast cells with numerous Auer rods are present. The prothrombin and partial thromboplastin times are prolonged, the serum fibrinogen level is reduced, and the d-dimer test result is positive. The hematologist treated with ATRA (all-*trans* retinoic acid).

48 A febrile 10-year-old girl complains of fatigue and has had frequent nosebleeds over the last few months. Physical examination shows sternal tenderness to percussion, generalized nontender lymphadenopathy, and hepatosplenomegaly. A CBC uncovers a moderately severe normocytic anemia, thrombocytopenia, and a WBC count of 35,000 cells/mm³. Occasional nucleated RBCs are present in the peripheral blood. The illustration illustrates the general histologic features that are present in the peripheral blood.

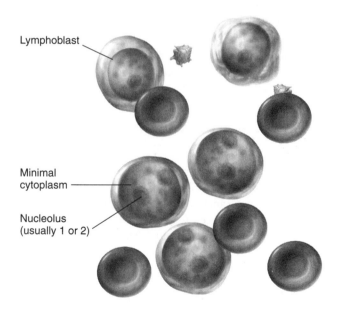

Lymphoblast

Minimal cytoplasm

Nucleolus (usually 1 or 2)

49 A 45-year-old man presents with fever, weight loss, sweating, epistaxis, generalized lymphadenopathy, and massive hepatosplenomegaly. A CBC exhibits a normocytic anemia, thrombocytopenia, and a WBC count of 125,000 cells/mL with 1% blast cells is present in the peripheral blood. The illustration highlights major histologic features.

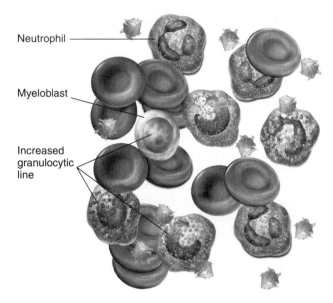

Neutrophil

Myeloblast

Increased granulocytic line

50 A 65-year-old man presents with fatigue, generalized lymphadenopathy, and hepatosplenomegaly. A CBC reveals a normocytic anemia, thrombocytopenia, and a WBC count of 80,000 cells/mL. Typical features are illustrated.

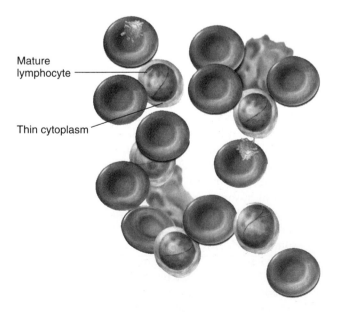

Mature lymphocyte

Thin cytoplasm

Answer Key

1	A	**11**	A	**21**	B	**31**	E	**41**	A
2	C	**12**	E	**22**	C	**32**	B	**42**	G
3	D	**13**	C	**23**	D	**33**	A	**43**	C
4	A	**14**	D	**24**	A	**34**	C	**44**	D
5	A	**15**	B	**25**	B	**35**	D	**45**	E
6	A	**16**	E	**26**	E	**36**	D	**46**	E
7	B	**17**	C	**27**	D	**37**	C	**47**	G
8	D	**18**	A	**28**	B	**38**	E	**48**	A
9	A	**19**	D	**29**	D	**39**	F	**49**	F
10	C	**20**	A	**30**	B	**40**	B	**50**	B

Answers and Explanations

1 **The answer is A** *Surgery*

Testicular cancer (choice **A**) represents only 1% of the cancers in men. However it is the most prevalent cancer in men between the ages of 15 and 34 years and an undescended testis at birth increases the risk. Cancer presents as a painless mass in the testes sometimes accompanied by a feeling of heaviness. Typically it is found by self-examination, which is recommended as a preventive technique for all males; however, unlike females who typically self-examine for breast cancer, relatively few males practice doing the same for testicular cancer and, as is the case with this patient, most wait 3 to 6 months after discovery to consult a physician. Scrotal ultrasound study is a noninvasive and critical procedure to assist in diagnosis, as it can readily distinguish between intra- and extratesticular masses; the former are almost always malignant and the latter benign. Serum markers may also help in the diagnosis.

Two basic testicular cancer types account for almost all cases. They are seminomas, which account for 35–40% and nonseminomas, which may be embryonal cell carcinomas (20%), teratomas (5%), choriocarcinoma (<1%), and mixed cell types (40%). Seminomas are derived from immature germ cells, tend to grow slowly, and only metastasize late; these cancers never cause an elevation of α-fetoprotein, and while they occasionally increase serum levels of human chronic gonadotropin (hCG), the increase is to a relatively low level. Nonseminomas are derived from more mature germ cells, are more aggressive, and produce α-fetoprotein and with less certainty hCG, which if present may induce development of gynomastia. Each type of tumor has its own staging system. Typically, treatment is orchiectomy achieved by an inguinal approach followed by chemotherapy, which varies somewhat depending upon tumor type; inclusion of cisplatin is particularly effective, and irradiation is sometimes used for retroperitoneal disease. Only a few decades ago a diagnosis of testicular cancer was tantamount to a death sentence but today the overall 5-year disease-free survival rate is 55 to 80%; that of course varies depending upon stage and type of tumor but is nearly 100% for early-stage seminomas.

Epididymitis (choice **B**) is accompanied by pain, swelling, and fever and thus is readily ruled out in the case described. A spermatocele (choice **C**) is a spermatic cyst that grows adjacent to the epididymis on top of the testicle. Although painless, it is readily distinguished from a testicular mass by a scrotal ultrasound study. A varicocele (choice **D**) is a painless scrotal swelling, usually on the left side, that can be distinguished readily from a tumor, since rather than feeling like a hard lump it feels like "a bag of worms" that tends to disappear when lying down. It is caused by problems with the venous valves. Normally, varicoceles cause no problem but might reduce fertility, in which case they are tied off surgically. A hydrocele (choice **E**) is a collection of clear fluid in the remnants of the processes vaginalis testis. It can be distinguished from a tumor by its softer, squishy feel and confirmed by ultrasound, which will show it to be extratesticular and not solid. They are more common in older men, usually not troublesome, but if they are they can be reduced by aspiration or excised. Orchitis (choice **F**) is an inflammation of the testis usually caused by infection, classically by the mumps. Orchitis causes a heavy feeling in the testis; however, it is painful and easily distinguished from a tumor, but must be distinguished from epididymis, which has similar symptoms.

2 **The answer is C** *Pediatrics*

Most cases of phenylketonuria (choice **C**) are caused by deficiency or absence of phenylalanine hydroxylase. A minority of cases is caused by deficiencies in either dihydropteridine reductase or dihydropteridine synthetase; these mutations cause a deficiency of dihydropteridine, an essential cofactor for phenylalanine hydroxylase as well as for tyrosine hydroxylase and tryptophane hydroxylase. In phenylketonuria, the accumulation of excess phenylalanine and toxic metabolites is responsible for brain damage. Infants are normal at birth, but after a few months, mental retardation becomes evident, and it is eventually severe.

Vomiting, often mistaken for pyloric stenosis, can occur. Physical examination shows these children to be fair, with blue eyes; some have a rash resembling eczema, which fades with age. They have a mousey or musty odor of phenylacetic acid. Hyperactive deep tendon reflexes are found. Treatment consists of early diagnosis and dietary management; however, patients whose phenylketonuria is caused by a deficiency of dihydropteridine have to be maintained on a more stringent diet than the more typical patient.

Patients with Down syndrome (trisomy 21) (choice **A**) have mental retardation and hypotonia. Other features associated with Down syndrome include a simian crease, epicanthic folds, a protruding tongue, and a gap between the first and second toes.

Characteristic features of tuberous sclerosis (choice **B**) include hypopigmented skin lesions ("ash leaf" spots), sebaceous adenomas, and a shagreen patch. Calcified tubers in the periventricular area may be seen on computed tomography (CT) scan of the head.

Children with cretinism (choice **D**) caused by congenital hypothyroidism have retardation of their physical and mental development. Growth is stunted, the extremities are short, and the skin is dry and scaly with little perspiration. Hypopigmentation is not a feature.

Children with galactosemia (choice **E**) may have jaundice, hepatomegaly, vomiting, hypoglycemia, hepatic cirrhosis, or mental retardation. Eczema and blue eyes are not features of this disease.

3 The answer is D *Surgery*

This patient has sustained a tear of the medial meniscus (choice **D**) of the left knee. A tear of the medial meniscus is one of the most common knee injuries observed because it is firmly tethered to the underlying tibia. Thus twisting the upper body while the foot is held immobile applies a large torsion force; this commonly happens in football. A tear is usually accompanied by a tearing or popping sound. Effusions result from injury to the synovium, capsule, or ligaments and not from tearing of the fibrocartilaginous meniscus; consequently, effusion accumulates slowly, and swelling is most severe on the second day. With other injuries excluded by radiography, a magnetic resonance imaging (MRI) study is used to confirm the diagnosis. Treatment is generally conservative, with application of ice packs, and compressive dressing and physical therapy after refraining from bearing weight for several days.

Tear of the medial collateral ligament (choice **A**) is associated with pain and swelling along the medial aspect of the knee. Distraction of the knee (valgus) will elicit pain. There is no pain along the joint line. An effusion may be present. Tear of the medial ligament alone does not lead to joint instability, which would result only if there was a concomitant tear of the anterior cruciate ligament. Results of both McMurray's test and Lachman's test will be negative, unless there is a concomitant tear of the anterior cruciate ligament. Tear of the anterior cruciate ligament (choice **B**) does not result in an inability to walk, and there is no pain along the joint line. It usually results in hemarthrosis and a positive Lachman's test result. Hyperextension will be noted. Tears of the anterior cruciate ligament result from sudden stopping and twisting. Patients will complain of a popping sound in the knee. Osteoarthritis of the knee (choice **C**) is a degenerative disease that may be idiopathic or secondary to a predisposing cause (e.g., infection, trauma, inflammatory or metabolic disease, old age). There is degeneration of the articular cartilage of the joint, osteophyte formation along the margins, and changes in the subchondral bone and bone marrow. The synovium undergoes fibrosis, and the capsule is thickened. In the early stages, the patient is asymptomatic. Once synovitis and effusion develop, the patient complains of joint stiffness. Capsular thickening and osteophyte formation cause further symptoms. The surrounding muscles go into spasm. This immobilizes the joint and prevents pain. Later in the process, valgus or varus could develop. Clinical examination will reveal pain on movement, and crepitus can often be elicited. Osteochondritis dissecans (choice **E**) is a painful condition of the knee in which a fragment of the articular cartilage along with some subchondral bone gets detached from the joint surface. The loose bit becomes a foreign body in the joint. It can occur in children, juveniles, and adults. Males are affected more often than females. The etiology includes trauma and heredity. The condition develops gradually, pain is diffuse and difficult to localize, and there may be a history of stiffness of the joint. In the presence of a loose body, locking of the knee can occur. However, most patients will have nonspecific or a paucity of physical findings. Atrophy of the quadriceps muscle may be present, and deep tenderness over the femoral condyle may be elicited. On rare occasions, a loose body may be felt.

4 **The answer is A** *Preventive Medicine and Public Health*

Mammography is most effective in detecting clinically occult, nonpalpable lesions in the breast (choice **A**). For women with palpable breast masses, however, it is less reliable as a diagnostic tool. In one study of patients with palpable breast cancer, the mammogram had a false-negative (FN) result in approximately 9% of cases. This is true particularly when the mass is in a background of dense tissue, as often occurs with fibrocystic change. This underscores the fact that a "normal" mammogram does not necessarily indicate that a mass is not present or that the mass is benign (choice **C**). Typically, malignant breast tumors have irregular, spiculated margins with fine-stippled calcifications within a radius of 1 cm. These findings, however, can also be seen in traumatic fat necrosis and fibrocystic change. One current recommendation for screening is a baseline mammogram between 35 and 40 years of age, a mammogram every 1–2 years between the ages of 40 and 49, and a yearly mammogram after the age of 50.

Mammography does not replace the use of fine-needle aspiration (choice **E**) or excisional biopsies (choice **D**). It is not used to assign a clinical stage for breast cancer (choice **B**).

5 **The answer is A** *Surgery*

The serum BUN-to-creatinine ratio is 20 (40/2), which is consistent with postrenal azotemia. Postrenal azotemia is most often due to urinary tract obstruction, a common finding in benign prostate hyperplasia due to obstruction of urine outflow through the urethra; this is the most likely cause of this patient's symptoms. In the initial stages of urinary tract obstruction, tubular function is intact, and there is a decrease in the glomerular filtration rate. However, after filtration, some of the urea is reabsorbed back into the blood by the proximal tubule, while creatinine is not reabsorbed. This causes a disproportionate increase in the serum BUN over that of serum creatinine, resulting in a BUN-to-creatinine ratio of >15. The $FENa^+$ is a sensitive indicator of tubular function. It represents the amount of sodium excreted in the urine divided by the amount of sodium that is filtered by the kidneys. The calculation is as follows: $FENa^+ = [(UNa^+ \times PCr) (PNa^+ \times UCr)] \times 100$, where UNa^+ is a random urine sodium, PNa^+ is serum sodium, UCr is random urine creatinine, and PCr is plasma creatinine level. Creatinine is used in the formula, because the amount of sodium filtered depends on the glomerular filtration rate (GFR), which closely approximates the creatinine clearance. $FENa^+$ values below 1% indicate intact tubular function, while those above 2% indicate tubular dysfunction. In prerenal azotemia, tubular function is intact, therefore, the $FENa^+$ is <1% (choice **A**).

Since tubular function is intact in this patient, reabsorption of sodium in the proximal and distal tubules is normal, and the random urine sodium level is <20 mEq/L (not >40 mEq/L [choice **B**]). A random urine sodium level above 40 mEq/L indicates tubular dysfunction. Furthermore, since tubular function is intact, renal concentration is normal, and the U_{Osm} is >500 mOsm/kg (not < 350 mOsm/kg [choice **C**]). A U_{Osm} below 350 mOsm/kg indicates a loss of urine concentration, which is the first sign of tubular dysfunction. In prerenal azotemia, there should be no casts in the urine (no renal tubular cell casts [choice **D**]) that indicate tubular dysfunction in renal failure.

6 **The answer is A** *Obstetrics and Gynecology*

Prenatal maternal serum analysis historically started with maternal serum α-fetoprotein (MS-AFP), which was directed at identifying open neural tube defects as indicated by an elevated MS-AFP value. When the MS-AFP levels were low, trisomy 21 was more likely, but the sensitivity for diagnosis was only 25%. By adding the two additional analytes (estriol and hCG), the sensitivity for diagnosis of trisomy 21 was increased to 65%. The findings of the analyte panel consistent with trisomy 21 are option **C** (MS-AFP levels decreased, estriol levels decreased, and hCG levels increased). The correct answer, however, for the diagnosis of trisomy 18 is option **A** in which all three analyte levels are low relative to normal. Even then only 50 to 65% of trisomy 18 fetuses are identified by this method. The three other options (**B, D,** and **E**) are incorrect and are not associated with any aneuploidy.

7 **The answer is B** *Medicine*

Orlistat (choice **B**) is a pancreatic lipase inhibitor that prevents the breakdown of triacylglycerides, thereby preventing their absorption. One pill taken with each meal containing fat brings about an approximate 30% reduction in lipid-related caloric intake. Since it does not interfere with metabolism, hormones, or neurotransmission, it is believed to be safe and is recommended for weight reduction in individuals with a BMI of

27 kg/m² or more who also have a weight-related health condition, such as diabetes or hypertension, and for anybody with a BMI exceeding 30 kg/m². However it does have drawbacks. The undigested lipids remaining in the gut promote defecation of greasy stools and production of gas (potentially a serious problem for a flight attendant), and absorption of fat-soluble vitamins is also inhibited. The physician pointed out the latter problem can be avoided by use of vitamin supplements, and the former one by avoiding use of orlistat before being scheduled for a flight.

Ephedra (choice **A**) has been used in Oriental medicine to treat bronchospasm and respiratory congestion as an extract of young stems of *Ephedra sinica*. Presently, it is widely marketed as a stimulant and appetite suppressor. Chemically and physiologically the ephedra alkaloids are similar to amphetamine. Clinical trials have shown that it does promote weight loss, but its use was also associated with a two- to threefold increased risk of psychiatric, gastrointestinal, and autonomic nervous system problems and/or heart palpitations. Fexofenadine (choice **C**) is a less cardiotoxic metabolite of terfenadine, which is not an appetite suppressor but is used as a nonsedating antihistamine. Dexfenfluramine (choice **D**) and fenfluramine (choice **E**) are serotonergic appetite suppressants once widely prescribed for obesity that were withdrawn from the market because of reports of causing heart valve complications (30% when gauged by echocardiography) as well as less commonly causing (1 per 17,000 cases) pulmonary hypertension.

8 The answer is D   *Pediatrics*

A child with severe asthma who is becoming sleepy and less responsive is most likely tiring and retaining carbon dioxide. In addition, if less wheezing is heard, it should not be assumed that the patient is improving. On the contrary, air exchange is diminished because of severe bronchospasm and decreased respiratory effort. Arterial blood gas (ABG) measurement (choice **D**) should be ordered to evaluate acid–base status and carbon dioxide content.

A chest x-ray film (choice **B**) and a complete blood count (CBC) (choice **E**) are not required at this stage. However, if the child continues to deteriorate, they may be ordered at a later time. The patient in this scenario is becoming sleepy and less responsive; we are not given any information to make us think that this patient is hypotensive or in shock or dehydrated. Therefore, choice **C** would not be the most appropriate action in the management of this patient. In this situation it is not appropriate to send the patient home (choice **A**).

9 The answer is A   *Medicine*

This patient suffers from systolic congestive heart failure. The first step in treatment is to reduce his edema by adjusting the dose of hydrochlorothiazide or changing to a loop diuretic since his present dose of hydrochlorothiazide is obviously not working. It is appropriate to follow this by addition of a β-blocker. Recent clinical trials have shown that careful addition of a β-blocker to a regimen including a diuretic and an angiotensin-converting enzyme (ACE) inhibitor reduces both mortality and morbidity. Carvedilol (choice **A**) is the first β-blocker specifically approved for treatment of congestive heart failure. It is a nonselective β_1 and β_2 receptor blocker with weak α-blocking activity, and several trials show that when used to treat congestive heart failure, it significantly reduces mortality. The drug must be slowly titrated and administered with great care because it is also a potent vasodilator, and marked hypotension and functional deterioration may occur.

ACE inhibitor drugs such as captopril, enalapril, or lisinopril have been shown to reduce both morbidity and mortality in patients with severe congestive heart failure, and this patient is already on captopril. Consequently, addition of an angiotensin-receptor blocker (ARB) such as valsartan (choice **B**) or losartan would be fruitless, since use of an ARB together with an ACE inhibitor offers no advantage. However, for patients who cannot tolerate ACE inhibitors ARBs are a reasonable alternative. Calcium-channel blockers have proved ineffective, and nifedipine (choice **C**) and other first-generation calcium-channel blockers may actually accelerate the progression of congestive heart disease. Although the statins are not used to treat congestive heart failure, it is well documented that use of pravastatin (choice **D**) as well as any of the other statin inhibitors of 3-hydroxy-3-methylglutaryl coenzyme A (HMG-CoA) reductase results in reduction of serum levels of low-density-lipoprotein (LDL) cholesterol and can increase high-density-lipoprotein (HDL) cholesterol. Recent data show use of pravastatin decreases the risk of first heart attacks in patients with hypercholesteremia, and simvastatin prevents second heart attacks in hypercholesterolemic patients. Although long-term efficacy has not been established for atorvastatin, the drug is the most effective agent available for the management of homozygous familial hypercholesterolemia. Other evidence also suggests that the statins may help prevent osteoporosis. Metformin (choice **E**) is an oral hypoglycemic agent and, since this patient shows no evidence of hyperglycemia, is irrelevant in this discussion.

10 The answer is C *Surgery*

A hemoglobin level (choice **C**) should be determined to uncover potential anemia that may become relevant during surgery and to establish a baseline for blood replacement should that become a necessity.

Unless the patient is a known diabetic or is over 45 years of age, it no longer is considered necessary to determine the serum glucose level (choice **A**). Liver enzyme levels (choice **B**) need only be determined if liver function is relevant to the surgery. Studies have shown that the yield of positive results for abnormal coagulation times (choice **D**) is too low to routinely test for them before surgery and if an abnormality were present it would rarely make a difference in management. The exception is a patient on anticoagulation therapy. An electrocardiograph (choice **E**) is only required if the patient is over 40 years of age or has a history of cardiac problems.

11 The answer is A *Psychiatry*

Acamprosate (choice **A**) is an anticraving medication approved by the Food and Drug Administration (FDA) in July 2004. It has been shown to significantly decrease relapse rates in alcoholic individuals who have been maintaining sobriety. The mechanism of action is unknown, but may involve modulation of γ-aminobutyric acid (GABA) receptors. Liver disease is not a contraindication, and it is not associated with dysphoria.

Naltrexone sometimes causes dysphoria and anhedonia, but there is no evidence that this is ameliorated by paroxetine (choice **B**) or other selective serotonin-reuptake inhibitors (SSRIs). While participating in the 12 steps of Alcoholics Anonymous is important in recovery, decreasing alcohol craving often can facilitate this work, and there are available agents, such as acamprosate, that block alcohol craving (choice **C**). Use of benzodiazepines to decrease alcohol intake is neither effective nor safe (choice **D**). Lithium has been described as having some efficacy in decreasing alcohol intake, but studies of efficacy in decreasing craving are inconclusive (choice **E**).

12 The answer is E *Medicine*

The most probable cause of the patient's symptoms is nonbacterial prostatitis (choice **E**). This is the most common urologic condition diagnosed in men between the ages of 35 and 50 years of age and the third most common after the age of 50, behind benign prostatic hypertrophy (BPH) and prostatic cancer. The symptoms are similar to those described in the vignette and bacteria cannot be cultured, making the cause obscure. As many as 50% may be due to occult infection by bacteria that are hard to culture, such as *Chlamydia trachomatis, Ureaplasma urealyticum,* or *Neisseria gonorrhoeae.* Viruses, fungi, or anaerobic bacteria may also be responsible. Most commonly, such occult bacterial infection is empirically demonstrated by a 4- to 6-week trial on various antibiotic combinations.

That still leaves some 50% with no known cause. Various hypotheses have been developed; none of which have been substantiated, including inflammatory irritation due to extended sitting as might occur with office workers or bicycle riders. If symptoms do not clear up with antibiotic treatment, there is no one best treatment. Symptoms may sometimes be alleviated with antiinflammatory agents, sitz baths, stress reduction, or dietary changes. Some urologists recommend frequent ejaculation. The prognosis is that most men in whom a specific cause cannot be found are left with a lifetime of annoying recurrent symptoms with no serious sequela. If a specific activity such as bicycle riding provokes symptoms, it may be necessary to change the activity in some way. For avid bicycle riders, it usually is recommended to use a seat that is designed not to irritate the prostate area.

Of all the men evaluated for prostatitis, only 5–10% are diagnosed with acute bacterial prostatitis (choice **A**). Symptoms are similar to those described for nonbacterial prostatitis except there is a higher temperature, and bacterial culture is positive, usually for *Escherichia coli* or *Pseudomonas aeruginosa* and less often by a gram-positive organism such as enterococci. Care must be taken in doing a rectal examination, as vigorous prostate manipulation may induce septicemia; for the same reason, prostate massage is contraindicated. Hospitalization is recommended with immediate parenteral administration of ampicillin and aminoglycosides until organism sensitivities are known. With effective treatment, chronic prostatitis rarely occurs. Chronic bacterial prostatitis (choice **B**) sometimes follows an acute case, but usually not. Symptoms again are similar to those of nonbacterial prostatitis, but bacteria can be isolated from expressed prostate fluid. These again are usually gram-negative rods that are sequestered within crypts in the prostate, making treatment difficult. Prostatodynia (choice **C**) is a noninflammatory disorder which, as in the other types of prostatitis, causes urinary retention and similar problems. Again the cause is obscure. Sometimes symptoms of bladder carcinoma in situ (choice **D**) can create symptoms similar to those of nonbacterial prostatitis and, therefore, if a firm diagnosis of nonbacterial prostatitis cannot be made, bladder cancer must be excluded, usually by cystoscopy.

13 The answer is C   *Pediatrics*

Chlamydial pneumonia (choice **C**) in infants presents at 3 to 16 weeks of age. Typically, the infants appear quite well, are afebrile, but have been ill with tachypnea and a repetitive staccato cough. Rales, and sometimes wheezing, can be heard. Conjunctivitis is present in approximately 50% of patients. Hyperinflation and patchy infiltrates are seen on chest x-ray films, and eosinophilia (>400 cells/mm^3) is apparent upon a complete blood count (CBC).

Respiratory syncytial virus (RSV) pneumonia (choice **A**) may present with temperature instability, respiratory distress, wheezing, apnea, clear nasal discharge, and poor feeding. Bronchiolitis (choice **B**) causes inflammation of the bronchioles with narrowing of the bronchial diameter. It is a viral disease caused by RSV in 50% of cases, but also by *Mycoplasma,* parainfluenza viruses, adenoviruses, and other viruses. It manifests with low-grade fever, tachypnea, nasal flaring, rales, and expiratory wheezing. Chest radiography shows hyperinflation or atelectasis without infiltration. Cystic fibrosis (choice **D**) commonly presents as respiratory insufficiency with cough, dyspnea, bronchiectasis, and pulmonary fibrosis. The child also shows signs of malabsorption and failure to thrive. The larval stage of ascariasis (choice **E**) is asymptomatic. However, if a large parasite load penetrates the lungs, it may manifest with cough, hematemesis, eosinophilia, and pulmonary infiltrates.

14 The answer is D   *Medicine*

Ventricular tachycardia is defined as three or more consecutive ventricular premature beats at a rate of 100–250. It can be sustained or nonsustained. A ventricular tachycardia that lasts more than 30 seconds or is associated with hemodynamic instability is classified as sustained, while an unsustained one is one that lasts less than 30 seconds and hemodynamic stability is maintained. In either event, the goal of therapy is to normalize the heart rate, ensure adequate cardiac output, and prevent death. This patient had short runs of rapid rhythm unsustained, wide complex, and tachycardia, and he was hemodynamically stable. In such cases, lidocaine (choice **D**) is the drug of choice. Furthermore, it is an excellent agent in a setting of post-myocardial infarction. Lidocaine is a class Ib antiarrhythmic agent that shortens repolarization. It is the least cardiodepressant of the drugs listed. Given intravenously, lidocaine has a rapid onset of action and reduces the incidence of ventricular fibrillation as well. However, high doses of lidocaine can depress myocardial contractility and may cause confusion, seizures, and respiratory arrest.

Cardioversion (choice **A**) would be the treatment of choice if: his systolic blood pressure were less than 90 mm Hg, he has mental status changes signifying poor cerebral circulation, he has congestive cardiac failure, or he has pulseless ventricular tachycardia. If he was hemodynamically unstable and the systolic pressure was over 90 mm Hg, amiodarone (choice **B**), a class III agent that prolongs the action potential, would be the drug of choice. Adverse cardiovascular actions to amiodarone include bradycardia, heart block, and sinus arrest. Procainamide is an alternative drug to amiodarone. The Cardiac Arrhythmia Suppression Trial (CAST) showed that flecainide (choice **C**), a class 1 agent, increased mortality when used prophylactically to suppress ventricular ectopy after a myocardial infarction. Neither is mortality reduced by other class I agents. Quinidine (choice **E**), a class Ia agent, is a sodium channel blocker that slows conduction and prolongs repolarization. It is a myocardial depressant, because it decreases myocardial excitability and conduction velocity and also may depress myocardial contractility. Since quinidine prolongs the duration of the cardiac action potential, there is an increased incidence of torsades de pointes (i.e., a twisting about the baseline into different QRS morphologies). Verapamil (choice **F**) is a class IV agent that is a slow calcium channel blocker. It is used to treat supraventricular tachycardias. It should never be administered to a patient with ventricular tachycardia, as death could ensue.

15 The answer is B   *Preventive Medicine and Public Health*

Prevalence (number of persons in a population with disease) approximates incidence (number of new cases over a period of time) times duration of a disease. Incidence remains a constant in this relationship. Because the new treatment increases the length of survival, the number of cases present at any point in time (prevalence) increases (choice **B**) (not decreases [choice **D**]). Incidence is based on the number of new cases; in this scenario it remains unchanged (choices **A, C,** and **E**).

16 The answer is E *Medicine*

The patient has porphyria cutanea tarda (PCT), the most common porphyria in the United States. PCT may be acquired (e.g., estrogens, alcoholic liver disease, hepatitis C) or inherited as an autosomal dominant disease. It is due to a deficiency of uroporphyrinogen decarboxylase, which converts uroporphyrinogen III to coproporphyrinogen III in heme synthesis. Deficiency of the enzyme causes a proximal accumulation of uroporphyrinogen III, which spontaneously converts to uroporphyrinogen I (choice **E**) and coproporphyrinogen I and their corresponding oxidation products, uroporphyrin I and coproporphyrin I. Uroporphyrin I colors the urine a red to brown hue in natural light and a pink to red tint in fluorescent light. Treatment includes chloroquine and repeated phlebotomies to reduce iron levels in the liver (iron is a precipitating factor for PCT, and in patients with liver disease, hemosiderosis is often present). Noninflammatory blisters form on sun-exposed skin, causing hypertrichosis and hyperpigmentation. The responsible UV wavelengths lie beyond that absorbed by most sunscreens, thus they offer little protection. Acquired cases generally clear up when the underlying condition is successfully treated.

Hemoglobinuria (choice **A**) occurs in patients who have intravascular hemolysis. The patient's hemoglobin level is normal, so a hemolytic anemia is not a likely diagnosis. Myoglobinuria (choice **B**) occurs when there is massive damage to skeletal muscle (e.g., severe exercise, trauma). There is no history of muscle pain or injury to muscle to suggest the presence of myoglobinuria. The porphobilin level (choice **C**) is increased in acute intermittent porphyria (AIP), which is an autosomal dominant disease caused by a deficiency of uroporphyrinogen I synthase (hydroxymethylbilane synthase). This enzyme converts porphobilinogen (PBG) to hydroxymethylbilane in heme synthesis. Deficiency of the enzyme leads to a proximal accumulation of PBG and δ-aminolevulinic acid, which are excreted in the urine. PBG is colorless unless it is exposed to light and is oxidized to porphobilin, which has a wine-red color. A characteristic feature of the disease is recurrent neurologically induced abdominal pain precipitated by drugs that induce the liver cytochrome P450 system (e.g., alcohol). Although there is a history of alcohol use in this patient, there is no recurrent history of abdominal pain. Furthermore, the wine-red color of urine in AIP only occurs after exposure to light. Urobilin (choice **D**) is the oxidation product of urobilinogen, which is normally present in trace amounts in urine. Urobilin is the pigment responsible for the yellow color of urine. If the urobilin concentration is increased in the urine (e.g., extravascular hemolytic anemia, hepatitis), the urine is a dark yellow color rather than a red-to-brown color.

17 The answer is C *Psychiatry*

The patient's symptoms are most suggestive of borderline personality disorder, characterized by impulsivity, self-destructiveness, suicide gestures, chaotic interpersonal relationships, and a fragile sense of identity. Such individuals frequently manage ambivalent feelings toward others by overidealizing some and denigrating others. Such behaviors may be improved through examination in psychotherapy, so choice **C** is the most appropriate action, since it combines a suggestion to do so, coupled with an offer to take over treatment.

Immediately agreeing to take over the case without a thorough analysis of the patient's behavior is a disservice (choice **A**). While psychotherapists are usually obligated to report harmful therapist behavior to licensing boards, there is little to suggest that such gross incompetence exists in this case. Further, one cannot release clinical records to a licensing board without patient consent (choice **B**). Likewise, one cannot violate confidentiality and call another treating psychotherapist, except in an emergency (choice **D**). Finally, while the behavior might represent splitting, it might just be that the patient reasonably wants a new therapist, and this desire should not be refused outright (choice **E**).

18 The answer is A *Pediatrics*

Croup, or laryngotracheobronchitis (choice **A**), is most common between 6 months and 3 years of age. Caused primarily by parainfluenza virus, it typically presents with prodromal symptoms of an upper respiratory infection. The child then develops fever and a brassy, barking, seallike cough, with intermittent inspiratory stridor. Acute respiratory distress can develop. The diagnosis of croup in a child older than 3 years should prompt suspicion of an underlying anatomic abnormality.

Pertussis (choice **B**) usually occurs in unimmunized infants and is usually preceded by a prodromal catarrhal stage with conjunctivitis. Spasms of coughing end with an inspiratory whoop. In younger infants, the whoop is not present and the signs are more subtle (e.g., apnea and cyanosis). Acute epiglottitis (choice **C**) is a rare disease among children in the United States because of the *Haemophilus influenzae* B vaccine. However, occasional cases of epiglottitis from *Haemophilus influenzae* B may occur in unimmunized children, and there are also some cases of epiglottitis caused by group A streptococci. In a previous age of greater prevalence of epiglottitis, the peak incidence was commonly seen in the 3- to 7-year-old age group; however infants and adults with epiglottitis have been well described. Drooling is usually present, but the barking cough is absent. Bronchiolitis (choice **D**) and asthma (choice **E**) can present with retractions of the intercostal muscles and nasal flaring, but wheezing is usually present.

19 The answer is D   *Psychiatry*

This man has been amply reassured that he does not have a malignant melanoma yet he continues to worry even to the extent of having repeated biopsies. Such behavior suggests hypochondriasis (choice **D**), which is characterized by worry about the meaning of a symptom that does not respond to physician reassurance after a thorough negative evaluation.

Body dysmorphic disorder (choice **A**) is characterized by excessive preoccupation with a defect in appearance that is in reality minor or nonexistent. In this case the patient's concern is with the meaning of the lesion, not its appearance per se. Conversion disorder (choice **B**) involves loss of sensory or motor function, related to psychologic stress. This patient may have stress related to his brother's death but does not have loss of sensory or motor function. Delusional disorder (choice **C**) may be difficult to distinguish from hypochondriasis and may become an additional diagnosis if the individual's preoccupation reaches delusional proportions. However, this patient's worry does not involve a preoccupation that is bizarre or overwhelmingly false. Somatization disorder (choice **E**) is characterized by multiple complaints from multiple organ systems, which does not appear in this patient.

20 The answer is A   *Pediatrics*

Scabies is caused by the mite *Sarcoptes scabiei* and is transmitted by direct contact with other infected individuals. Although burrows are demonstrable in 7 to 13% of adults with scabies, they are usually not present in infants. In infants with scabies, bullae and pustules predominate (choice **A**), and wheals, papules, vesicles, and superimposed eczema may also be present.

Although the face and scalp are spared in adults, they are common sites of infection in infants (choice **D**). Intertriginous areas are affected in infants (choice **B**), as well as the palms and soles (choice **E**). Red-brown nodules occasionally, not often (choice **C**), appear on the axillae, groin, and genitalia.

21 The answer is B   *Medicine*

Mastocytosis is a condition in which mast cells overreact; however, they rarely are malignant. There are several clinical subtypes and an overall prevalence of 1 case per 1000 to 8000 persons is distributed equally among the sexes and various ethnicities. In approximately 66% of these cases the symptoms are dermatologic, and the onset is at birth or during early infancy. The lesions are red-brown macules that first appear on the trunk and then spread to the extremities as small frecklelike spots that may evolve into papules, nodules, or plaques; this condition is also known as urticaria pigmentosa. As a rule there are no systemic problems, and the condition improves spontaneously as the child approaches adulthood. The diagnosis of urticaria pigmentosa is relatively easy, based upon the relatively unusual rash and a positive Darier's sign (a wheal and flair reaction when the skin is streaked).

The remaining third of patients first become symptomatic sometime during adulthood and exhibit internal symptoms. These cases are termed *systemic mastocytosis* (choice **B**); some 85% of these cases also have dermatologic symptoms. Typically among the 85% that do, patients frequently report intermittent brief spells of urticaria, flushing, pruritus, palpitations, headache, lightheadedness with possible syncope, rhinorrhea, nausea, and sometimes vomiting, diarrhea, and crampy abdominal pain; lethargy follows these attacks. The intermittent nature of these attacks makes the diagnosis difficult unless the urticaria lingers on and/or the physician pays careful attention to the history. Making a diagnosis is even more difficult if there are no dermatologic symptoms, as in the remaining 15% of systemic cases and the case described in the vignette. However, the presence of elevated mast cell markers will confirm a diagnosis provided the physician thinks about possible mastocytosis and asks for them. These tests may include serum tryptase activity, elevated histamine, and elevated urinary N-methyl histamine and prostaglandin D_2 levels. Of these, the tryptase assay is essentially 100% specific, since only mast cells express this protease. Although symptoms are intermittent, these repetitive attacks can lead to chronic conditions. Common ones include gastritis, esophageal and peptic ulcers, hematologic problems, and spinal osteoporosis, the latter as in the case described. Apparently the various substances released by the mast cells erode adjacent tissues, and symptoms vary depending upon which subpopulation of mast cells flares up. Although it would take an astute physician to make the correct diagnosis, in this case getting the correct answer simply depends upon recognizing some of the toxic substance released by mast cells.

Hyperparathyroidism (choice **A**) is the most common cause of hypercalcemia because the excess parathyroid hormone resorbs bone. However, in hyperparathyroidism the resorption of bone causes cystic bone lesions and osteitis fibrosa cystica, not osteoporosis. Calcitonin is synthesized by thyroid C-cells, which are also known as thyroid parafollicular cells. Overactivity of the thyroid C-cells (choice **C**) occurs in medullary thyroid cancer, which accounts for 5 to 8% of all thyroid cancers. About one third of these are sporadic, one third are familial with no other endocrine disorders, and one third are associated with MEN-2, primarily with MEN-2A (Sipple's syndrome). Most secrete calcitonin, which can be used as a serum tumor marker. About 30% cause flushing, diarrhea, and fatigue. Treatment is surgical removal, since C-cells do not take up radioactive iodine. There is no known clinical condition associated with underactivity of the thyroid C-cells (choice **D**). Acute hypoparathyroidism (choice **E**) causes hypocalcemia, which in turn causes tetany, with muscle cramps, irritability, carpopedal spasm, and convulsion. Chronic hypoparathyroidism is associated with lethargy, personality changes, anxiety, cataracts, and parkinsonism. In children, insufficient parathyroid also causes growth retardation.

22 The answer is C   *Surgery*

Catgut is used for deeper tissues because it self absorbs, and nylon is used for more superficial layers because of its strength (choice **C**). The nylon sutures can be removed with little trouble when the wound has healed sufficiently, in about a week.

Multifilament sutures (choice **A**) can harbor bacteria and have largely been replaced by monofilament types; this has significantly lowered the incidence of infection. Nylon for the deeper layers and catgut for the superficial ones (choice **B**) is incorrect; the nylon wouldn't self-absorb and the catgut might not be strong enough. Silk sutures are not suited for the deep wounds, as they will not self-absorb (choice **D**), and a multifilament suture for superficial use and nylon for both the deep and superficial layers (choice **E**) are both incorrect for reasons stated above.

23 The answer is D   *Preventive Medicine and Public Health*

When a test is performed on persons with a disease, a positive test result is called a true positive (TP), whereas a negative test result is called a false negative (FN). An FN misclassifies the patient as normal. Similarly, when a test is performed on a normal person, a negative test result is called true negative (TN), whereas a positive test result is called a false positive (FP). An FP misclassifies the person as having disease. The sensitivity of a disease represents the percentage of TPs. It is calculated with the following formula: Sensitivity = TP/(TP + FN) × 100. If a test has 100% sensitivity, there are no FNs. This result means that every person in the known disease population has a positive test result. Therefore, a negative test result means the person tested is a TN. Such a test qualifies as an ideal test for screening for disease, because it excludes disease. However, a positive test result also may be obtained for patients having other diseases; that is, the test may not be specific. Specificity is calculated with the following formula: Specificity = TN/(TN + FP) × 100. A test with 100% specificity has no FPs, meaning it only has positive results for patients having that specific disease. A test with 100% specificity qualifies as being useful to confirm disease, because a positive test result must be a TP and not an FP.

Once the sensitivity and specificity of a test are established, they remain the same because they are established under controlled conditions involving a known disease population and control population. However, when the test is applied in the clinical arena, the prevalence of disease in the general population or hospital setting does affect how the test is interpreted. In a low-prevalence situation, a negative test result is more likely to represent a TN than an FN, whereas a positive test result is more likely to represent an FP than a TP. In a high-prevalence situation, the reverse is true.

When a test result is positive, the question to ask is whether it represents a TP or an FP. This response is called the predictive value of a positive test (PV^{+test}) and is calculated as follows: PV^{+test} = TP/(TP + FP) × 100. *Note:* If the FP of the test is 0, as in a test with 100% specificity, the PV^{+test} indicating a TP is always 100%. This result underscores why tests with 100% (or at least a high) specificity are used to confirm disease. If the test result returns negative, then the question is whether it represents a TN or an FN. This determination is called the predictive value of a negative test (PV^{-test}). It is calculated with the following formula: PV^{-test} = TN/(TN + FN) × 100. *Note:* If the FN rate of the test is 0, as in a test with 100% sensitivity, then the PV^{-test} indicates that the TN value is 100%. This result underscores why tests with 100% sensitivity (or at least approaching 100%) are used to screen for disease.

The question asks for the predictive value of a positive test result when the prevalence of disease in the total population of 200 people studies is 50% (100 people with SLE in a population of 200). To simplify the calculation, the information is best placed into the following format.

	Patients with SLE	Control Population	Totals
Positive test result	TP 60	FP 20	80
Negative test result	FN 40	TN 80	120

The PV^{+test} is TP/(TP + FP) × 100 = 60/80 × 100 = 75% (choice **D**). That is, a random patient who tests positive will have a 75% chance of being a TP. Obviously, if choice **D** is correct, choices **A, B, C,** and **E** are not.

24 The answer is A *Pediatrics*

This patient has Friedreich's ataxia, which is inherited as an autosomal recessive trait. The onset of ataxia occurs somewhat later than that in ataxia-telangiectasia but usually manifests before the age of 10 years. The ataxia is slowly progressive, involving the lower extremities to a greater degree than the upper extremities. Patients with Friedreich's ataxia develop explosive, dysarthric speech, and most develop nystagmus. Although these patients may appear apathetic, their intelligence is preserved. There are also characteristic skeletal abnormalities seen in this condition that include high-arched feet (pes cavus) and hammer toes, as well as progressive kyphoscoliosis. Deep tendon reflexes are absent, and patients have poor proprioception and vibratory sensation. Cardiac abnormalities (e.g., sick sinus syndrome [choice **A**]) are often associated with Friedreich's ataxia, and myocarditis may be the eventual cause of death.

Diabetes (choice **B**), mental retardation (choice **C**), vision loss (choice **D**), and seizures (choice **E**) are not particularly associated with Friedreich's ataxia, but both diabetes and retardation can be associated with myotonic dystrophy, and any number of conditions have associated seizures.

25 The answer is B *Medicine*

Detrusor hyperreflexia incontinence, more commonly called urge incontinence, is the leakage, often of large volumes, of urine because of an inability to delay urination once the sensation of a full bladder occurs. It can be associated with several pathologies including: cystitis, urethritis, tumors, stones, diverticulosis, outflow obstructions, stroke, dementia, multiple sclerosis, Parkinson's disease, and suprasacral spinal cord injury. However, as in this case, most commonly the cause of detrusor hyperreflexia (urge) incontinence is idiopathic, and there are medications that can help (choice **B**). First-line treatment is usually tolterodine and extended-release oxybutynin.

The stress referred to in the condition known as stress incontinence (choice **A**) refers to physical stress such as sneezing, coughing, or lifting heavy objects, which causes an involuntary loss of urine. It results from weakness of the urinary sphincter. In women, this often is caused by pelvic floor muscle relaxation associated with multiparity, cystoceles, or advancing age. It less commonly occurs in men, and when it does, it is usually a residual effect of past prostate surgery. Overflow incontinence (choice **C**) is the leakage of small amounts of urine when the bladder becomes distended and the resultant pressure exceeds the urinary sphincter's ability to contain the urine. Causes include outlet obstruction from any of a host of possible factors. Often, hesitancy and incomplete voiding are reported by the patient, and postvoid residual volume usually exceeds 100 mL. Treatment involves alleviating the underlying condition. Functional incontinence (choice **D**) refers to urinary leakage associated with impaired cognitive or physical functional ability or psychologic unwillingness to try to control voiding. Such condition might include dementia, motor paralysis, regression, severe depression or anger, and hostility. Secondary incontinence (choice **E**) is not a medical designation.

26 **The answer is E** *Psychiatry*

The patient's writhing movements are highly suggestive choreoathetotic movements characteristic of tardive dyskinesia (TD). TD is often induced by prolonged exposure to older antipsychotic medications. Most of the newer antipsychotic medications are not associated with a significant incidence of TD. Clozapine (choice **E**), the model for the newer antipsychotic medications, is the best choice in this situation, because there are no obvious contraindications.

Ziprasidone (choice **D**) also is a newer antipsychotic medication, but it is contraindicated with a history suggestive of cardiac disease, because it prolongs the QTc interval. Decreasing the dose of haloperidol (choice **A**) is unlikely to stop the TD from worsening over time. Simply stopping haloperidol use (choice **B**) may precipitate an exacerbation of the patient's schizophrenia. Amantadine (choice **C**) is an antiviral medication that plays no role in treatment of TD.

27 **The answer is D** *Medicine*

Calcium is an underappreciated player in life's processes. Even when considered, attention tends to be focused on the 99% of the body's calcium stores found in bone and teeth rather than on the remaining 1% that also is essential for life. In fact, it can be argued that bone evolved to provide a reservoir to ensure that sufficient calcium would always be available to support its roles in intracellular metabolism, membrane stability, intracellular communication, and blood coagulation. In human physiology the importance of maintaining circulating calcium levels within a narrow range between 8.5 and 10.5 mg/dL (2.1–2.6 mM/L) is demonstrated by the complex homeostatic systems that have evolved. These involve parathyroid hormone, vitamin D, and calcitonin, and they control intestinal absorption, renal excretion, and turnover of labile calcium stores in bone. All these interactions are sensitive to the free calcium ion (Ca^{2+}) level, which represents about 50% of the 1% of calcium not associated with hard tissues. The remaining 50% of this 1% is complexed with albumin (about 43%) and citrate and other anions; these compounds act to buffer the free ion level by immediately releasing or binding Ca^{2+} as concentrations change.

Hypocalcemia is usually defined as a total serum calcium concentration of less than 8.5 mg/dL (2.1 mM/L), and symptoms of hypocalcemia include those described in the vignette plus other more severe ones (usually associated with total calcium levels of <7.0 mg/dL [<1.7 mM/L]) such as frank tetany, profound mental aberrations, laryngeal spasm, respiratory problems, generalized seizures, cardiac abnormalities, and smooth muscle contractures that cause gastrointestinal problems. The classical clinical methods for testing for hypocalcemia are Chvostek's sign (a light tapping over the facial nerve just anterior to the exterior auditor meatus causing an involuntary twitching of facial muscles) and Trousseau's sign (carpopedal spasm caused by reducing the blood supply to the hand by a blood pressure cuff inflated to 20 mm Hg higher than the systolic pressure). Although these tests provide a tentative diagnosis of hypocalcemia during an examination, direct calcium analysis is usually used to confirm this probable diagnosis (choice **D**). This is true because the ionized calcium level is generally reflected by the total value. However, remember that the critical factor is the ionized calcium level, and there may be cases in which the total level is within normal limits but Ca^{2+} concentration is not. If such a situation is suspected, the free calcium ion level can be measured (choice **B**) but because this is not a routine determination and is beset with potential technical difficulties it is not the most likely choice.

Serum albumin level (choice **A**) plays a role in regulating serum total calcium levels, since 43% of the circulating calcium is bound to albumin. Measuring albumin levels will not confirm a diagnosis of hypocalcemia, but a low serum albumin level can explain a low total calcium level. Low serum parathyroid levels (choice **C**) will cause hypocalcemia, but there is no hint of parathyroid malfunction in the vignette. Calcitonin levels that are above normal may be associated with medullary thyroid cancer and, in theory, that may lower circulating calcium levels, but that seems not to occur to a clinically significant extent and in addition, the vignette provides no suggestion that such a condition might exist in the case described (choice **E**).

28 **The answer is B** *Pediatrics*

Alport's syndrome is a progressive hereditary disorder. It is an X-linked dominant disorder, although autosomal dominant transmission has also been described. There is a familial association of hearing loss and nephritis.

Patients with Alport's syndrome usually present with microscopic or macroscopic hematuria. They can also present with deafness, hypertension (not hypotension [choice **D**]), proteinuria, thrombocytopenia, or renal failure. Ocular defects, such as cataracts (choice **B**), also may be found in individuals with Alport's syndrome. Patients with Alport's disease do not have problems with thrombocytosis (choice **A**). Papular lesions (choice **C**) would not be seen, because a rash is not associated with this syndrome.

29 The answer is D   *Psychiatry*

A principle of treatment, even in psychiatric emergencies, is to attempt less restrictive measures that may possibly be effective before other interventions are attempted. This patient may respond to reassurance (choice **D**), which should be tried before he is placed in restraints (choice **B**) or given medication against his will (choice **C**). Rescinding his involuntary detention (choice **A**) appears unwise, as he may likely remain dangerous or disabled in his present condition. Having him arrested (choice **E**) is likewise ill advised, as the evidence suggests that his behavior is the product of his illness, not criminal intent.

30 The answer is B   *Preventive Medicine and Public Health*

The recommendation is that those in the general public start one of the following protocols shortly after their 50th birthday (choice **B**): annual fecal occult blood testing, flexible sigmoidoscopy every 5 years, annual fecal occult blood testing and flexible sigmoidoscopy every 5 years, colonoscopy every 10 years or barium enema every 5 years. Annual fecal occult blood testing is relatively easy to self-perform and inexpensive; it also has both low sensitivity and specificity. Flexible sigmoidoscopy only permits examination of the rectosigmoid and the descending colon, and suspicious polyps have to be removed by colonoscopy. However, the risk of serious complication is less than 1 per 10,000 patients. Colonoscopy views the whole colon and polyps can be removed during the procedure. It is recommended as the procedure of choice by the American College of Gastroenterology. The estimated risk of serious complications is 0.3%

All organizations recommend that screening start before 60 years of age (choice **A**). Screening starting at 40 years of age (choice **C**) is recommended for patients with first-degree relatives diagnosed with colorectal cancer before or at the age of 60 years. The preferred method of screening is colonoscopy every 10 years if there is only one relative and every 5 years if there is more than one affected first-degree relative. An alternative recommendation in this latter case is to start screening 10 years before the age of the earliest diagnosed case. No group recommends screening the general public by 30 years of age (choice **D**). Persons with a family history of familial adenomatous polyposis or Ashkenazi Jews with a family history of colon cancers are recommended to have a genetic screen by the age of 10 years (choice **E**).

31 The answer is E   *Pediatrics*

Acute episodes of bronchial asthma represent one of the most common respiratory emergencies. Use of β_2-selective adrenoceptor agonists via aerosol plus oxygen and parenteral glucocorticoids (choice **B**) is appropriate for acute management in this situation. Maximal bronchodilation occurs within 30 minutes after use of albuterol or metaproterenol. Ipratropium (choice **A**), a muscarinic blocking agent used via inhalation, will not exacerbate the bronchoconstriction and is used in patients with acute severe asthma. Inhalers will not induce an asthma attack (choice **C**), but studies have reported that overuse of inhaler is associated with death or near-death episodes. Cromolyn plays no role in the treatment of acute asthma attacks (choice **D**). Because the current drug regimen appears to have limited prophylactic efficacy, consideration should be given to the daily use of aerosolic forms of a glucocorticoid (choice **E**) and either a long-acting β-agonist or a leukotriene modifier after recovery from the acute exacerbation.

32 The answer is B   *Surgery*

The patient has a stress fracture (choice **B**). These most commonly occur in the tibia and the second and third metatarsals. In the latter site, they are also called "march fractures," because they are associated with too much walking in ill-fitting shoes. Radiographs often fail to reveal a hairline crack immediately after the fracture but will show new bone formation (callus) along the lines of a microfracture in bone.

Greenstick fractures (choice **A**) primarily occur in children and refer to a break in the cortex on the convex side of the shaft but an intact concave side; this may cause the bone to bend. Comminuted fracture (choice **C**) refers to a fracture with many small fragments. Spiral fractures (choice **D**) are breaks that wind their way up the shaft of a bone in a spiral fashion. A compound fracture (choice **E**), also known as an open fracture, is one that breaks the skin.

33 The answer is A *Psychiatry*

The girl's symptoms suggest amphetamine intoxication (choice **A**), which can last for several hours. It is characterized by hypervigilance, insomnia, autonomic arousal, and occasionally bizarre ideas.

Cannabis intoxication (choice **B**) may have a similar presentation but is more likely to be accompanied by dry mouth, impaired coordination, time distortion, and perceptual disturbances. There is no evidence of perceptual disturbances, making lysergic acid diethylamide (LSD) (choice **C**), phencyclidine (choice **D**), psilocybin (choice **E**), and other hallucinogens less likely choices.

34 The answer is C *Preventive Medicine and Public Health*

Random allocation (choice **C**) is a hallmark of clinical trials in which the investigator manipulates or intervenes with one group and withholds interventions from the other; namely, the control group. Not only are the individuals selected randomly, they are also randomly assigned to the two groups. This provides the greatest confidence that the groups are similar at the beginning of the trial. If there are two groups of patients and each receives a different treatment, then one can establish a meaningful comparison of the outcome only if there is no extraneous factor in one group that influences the outcome. Random allocation achieves this.

Use of blinding techniques (choice **A**) is not exclusive to clinical trials. Bias (choice **B**) could occur and is minimized by double-blinding techniques. A clinical trial is not a retrospective study (choice **D**), but a prospective one. Prospective studies (choice **E**) can be conducted for other reasons.

35 The answer is D *Psychiatry*

The man's symptoms suggest schizophrenia (choice **D**), characterized by psychosis (delusions) and disintegration of the ability to think logically and maintain normal social behavior (e.g., maintaining shelter).

Body dysmorphic disorder (choice **A**) is characterized by a preoccupation with a minor physical defect but does not explain the presence of psychotic symptoms in this case. Factitious disorder (choice **B**) is characterized by the intentional production of physical or psychologic symptoms to assume the sick role. Although the patient refuses to leave the hospital, this behavior does not seem to be primarily motivated by a desire to assume the sick role. Hypochondriasis (choice **C**) is characterized by an intense concern over the meaning of symptoms but does not explain the presence of psychosis or social disintegration in this case. Schizotypal personality disorder (choice **E**) is characterized by social withdrawal and peculiar thinking, but does not present with psychosis.

36 The answer is D *Surgery*

Of the choices given, the sigmoid colon (choice **D**) is the most likely primary tumor site. Colorectal cancer is the second most common cancer and cancer killer in adults, and the CT scan shows metastatic disease in the liver, which is the most common site of metastasis from cancer of the colon because the sigmoid colon drains into the portal vein. Although smoking is not the major risk factor for colorectal cancer, it is a risk factor. If the lung were a choice in the question, it would be the most likely primary site, because adenocarcinomas are the most common primary cancer in the lung and lung cancer is the most common primary site for liver metastasis.

The distal esophagus (choice **A**) is the most common site for esophageal cancer. It is most often an adenocarcinoma arising from a Barrett's esophagus. The liver is a common site for metastasis; however, colorectal cancer is more common. Renal cell carcinoma (choice **B**) also is an adenocarcinoma; however, it most commonly metastasizes to the lungs and bone rather than the liver. A squamous cell carcinoma is the most common cancer of the midesophagus (choice **C**), it however is even less common than esophageal adenocarcinoma, and moreover the liver biopsy shows an adenocarcinoma. The most common cancer of the urinary bladder (choice **E**) is a transitional cell carcinoma, not an adenocarcinoma.

37 The answer is C *Medicine*

Serum protein electrophoresis (SPE) separates proteins on the basis of charge in the presence of an alkaline pH. Albumin moves the fastest to the anode (positive pole) because it has the most negative charges, whereas γ-globulins, with the fewest negative charges, remain at the cathode (negative pole). The five components of an SPE—in order of decreasing negative charge—are albumin, α_1-, α_2-, β-, and γ-globulins. The most common reason for ordering an SPE is to rule out a monoclonal gammopathy, as occurs in multiple myeloma. However, there are many other uses.

Cirrhosis is the end result of hepatocellular injury and is a serious, usually irreversible condition that is the 12th most common cause of death in the United States. The patient described in the vignette is suffering from symptoms associated with early alcohol-induced liver cirrhosis, which induces a very characteristic SPE pattern, called the beta–gamma bridge. This pattern is due to increased production of IgG, which migrates in the middle of the γ-globulin curve, and IgA, which migrates at the junction of the β and γ curves. Therefore, the increase in IgG produces a polyclonal peak. The increase in IgA fills in the valley between the β and γ curves, producing a beta–gamma bridge. In addition, the cirrhotic liver is unable to synthesize albumin, resulting in hypoalbuminemia. Thus, the correct answer is increased IgG and IgA, decreased albumin (choice **C**).

Sarcoidosis is a chronic granulomatous inflammatory disease of unknown cause that has a predilection for the African-American population. The diagnosis requires the demonstration of noncaseating granulomas plus the appropriate clinical picture. The lung is involved in 90% of patients. There is a restrictive type of lung disease with prominent perihilar adenopathy. Because it is a chronic inflammatory disease, there is polyclonal stimulation of B cells by unknown antigens, with subsequent formation of predominantly immunoglobulin G (IgG) antibodies (key immunoglobulin of chronic inflammation). These antibodies produce a diffuse enlargement of the γ-globulin curve, called a polyclonal peak; furthermore, albumin concentration is decreased (choice **A**). Such hypoalbuminemia occurs in any acute or chronic inflammatory state, because interleukin-1, produced by macrophages, decreases the synthesis of albumin in the liver in favor of synthesizing other proteins, called acute-phase reactants. Other causes of polyclonal gammopathy are tuberculosis, autoimmune disease, and cirrhosis of the liver. However in the latter case, as described above, the IgA peak is also increased causing the characteristic beta–gamma bridge.

An abnormally small α_1-peak is associated with one of the typical electrophoretic patterns found in association with α_1-antitrypsin deficiency. α_1-Antitrypsin deficiency has an autosomal recessive inheritance pattern and leads to a panacinar emphysema involving the lower lung lobes in a nonsmoking young adult and to cancer among those who do smoke. α_1-Antitrypsin (AAT) is the main globulin beneath the α_1-globulin curve. It is an antiprotease, synthesized by the liver, whose main function is to neutralize the elastases and collagenases emitted by neutrophils and other inflammatory cells, to prevent destruction of structural tissue in the lungs. Starch electrophoresis techniques have determined many different phenotypes. In one phenotype, AAT is not synthesized at all by the liver. These patients usually develop panacinar emphysema in early adult life. It is characterized by neutrophil destruction of the entire respiratory unit (i.e., respiratory bronchioles, alveolar duct, alveoli) in the lower lobes. In another phenotype, AAT is synthesized but cannot be secreted by the hepatocyte. It accumulates in the hepatocyte and produces neonatal hepatitis, cirrhosis, and hepatocellular carcinoma. The diagnosis of AAT causing panacinar emphysema is suggested by the absence of the α_1-peak on an SPE (choice **B**), which should be followed up by direct measurement of AAT. Once a deficiency has been established, the patient's and family members' phenotypes should be determined. Aerosol therapy with AAT is available for those patients with lung disease.

Monoclonal spikes (choice **D**) are the result of clonal proliferation of a neoplastic plasma cell, with production of its immunoglobulin and corresponding light chain (e.g., IgG kappa). Suppressor T cells prevent synthesis of immunoglobulins by the other plasma cells, so the uninvolved immunoglobulins are decreased. Multiple myeloma is an example of a malignant plasma cell disorder that produces monoclonal spikes due to IgG (most common), IgA, or light chains alone. Waldenström's macroglobulinemia is characterized by a monoclonal proliferation of lymphoplasmacytoid cells that produce IgM, which predisposes to the hyperviscosity syndrome. Monoclonal spikes that are unassociated with the preceding diseases are called monoclonal spikes of undetermined significance (MGUS), which is the overall most common cause of a monoclonal spike. Some of these patients later develop multiple myeloma or malignant lymphomas, so they should be carefully followed.

A reduction in albumin and a normal γ-globulin peak (choice **E**) is the SEP pattern that typifies acute inflammation. Inflammation causes reduced synthesis of albumin in favor of other proteins, called acute-phase reactants. These reactants include fibrinogen (nonspecific opsonin), C-reactive protein (opsonin, complement cascade activator), ferritin (storage form of iron), and the complement component C3 (opsonin). The primary immunoglobulin on first exposure to an antigen is IgM, which is not generated in sufficient amounts to alter the shape of the γ-globulin curve. This pattern is in contrast to the SPE patterns obtained in chronic inflammation, which are characterized by increased production of IgG.

38 The answer is E *Psychiatry*

The woman's symptoms suggest malingering (choice **E**), characterized by the production of physical or psychologic complaints for external incentives, often including monetary compensation. Atonic seizures (choice **A**) can present as sudden drop attacks (loss consciousness); however, the absence of electroencephalographic (EEG) abnormalities and the patient's lack of concern make this diagnosis less likely. Conversion disorder (choice **B**) is characterized by sensory or motor deficits without known physiologic bases that are associated with psychologic stress, but no obvious psychologic stress is present. Factitious disorder (choice **C**) is unlikely because the patient lives independently, cares for a pet, and does not seem to be assuming the sick role. In hypochondriasis (choice **D**) the patient is preoccupied with the fear of having an illness. This woman shows no sign of such preoccupation, such as seeking other physicians for treatment; she seems to be serenely waiting with her dog for settlement of her lawsuit.

39 The answer is F *Obstetrics and Gynecology*

It is important to determine if the patient has hirsutism (the presence of male pattern hair with an otherwise female body) or virilization (the presence of male pattern hair with loss of feminine body characteristics). This scenario includes many of the characteristics of virilization: loss of breast size and female body contours, clitorimegaly, and frontal balding. Virilization requires high levels of peripheral androgens, which most commonly result from an androgen-producing tumor. The rapid onset also strongly suggests a tumor. The anatomic sites of potentially high androgen production are the ovaries and the adrenals. The finding on physical examination of an adnexal mass suggests an ovarian tumor, most likely a Sertoli-Leydig tumor (choice **F**). Confirmation would be by pelvic imaging studies. One would expect to find high levels of serum testosterone. Management is surgical removal.

40 The answer is B *Obstetrics and Gynecology*

The history of long duration makes androgen-producing tumor unlikely. The physical findings are those of hirsutism not virilization. The positive family history would be consistent with PCOS (choice **B**), congenital adrenal hyperplasia (CAH), or idiopathic etiology. The history of irregular menses, infertility, and hirsutism suggests PCOS; the physical finding of bilaterally enlarged ovaries lends even more strength to the diagnosis. Pelvic imaging of polycystic ovaries and an elevated luteinizing hormone (LH)/follicle-stimulating hormone (FSH) ratio in the presence of a mildly elevated serum testosterone nails down the diagnosis. Oral contraceptives (OCs) are the preferred treatment. OCs decrease excess free testosterone by (1) suppressing the LH, which stimulates testosterone production, and (2) increasing bound testosterone by stimulating sex hormone–binding globulin.

41 The answer is A *Obstetrics and Gynecology*

The scenario is that of hirsutism not virilization, making androgen-producing tumor low on the differential diagnosis. The lack of family history leads away from PCOS, CAH, or idiopathic etiology. A number of otherwise unexplainable findings suggest Cushing syndrome (choice **A**): fatigue and weakness, upper body obesity, and stretch marks in a nulligravid woman. The mediating factor is excess production of adrenal cortisol. A 24-hour urinary test will measure for corticosteroid hormones. A dexamethasone suppression test will help differentiate whether the excess production of corticotropins is from the pituitary gland or tumors elsewhere. A corticotrophin-releasing hormone (CRH) stimulation test will differentiate a pituitary tumor from adrenal tumor. Management is directed at decreasing cortisol levels.

42 The answer is G *Obstetrics and Gynecology*

The description is of long-duration hirsutism. A positive family history of long duration is consistent with PCOS, CAH, or idiopathic etiology. The lack of obesity, infertility, and irregular menses tend to rule out PCOS and CAH. The scenario is far more consistent with idiopathic hair follicle sensitivity (choice **G**). In this condition, testing for free androgens shows normal levels of testosterone (elevated in PCOS and ovarian tumors), dehydroepiandrosterone sulfate (DHEAS) (elevated in adrenal tumors), and 17-hydroxyprogesterone (elevated in late-onset 21-hydroxylase deficiency, CAH). The underlying problem is increased 5-α-reductase enzyme activity in the hair follicles, which enhances conversion of androstenedione and testosterone to the very potent dihydrotestosterone. Management is by suppressing hair follicle 5-α-reductase activity with a spironolactone, a potassium-sparing diuretic.

43 The answer is C   *Obstetrics and Gynecology*

This patient has a history and physical findings of virilization similar to those of the patient with the ovarian tumor. Virilization can only occur in the presence of unusually high levels of peripheral androgens, most commonly the result of an androgen-producing tumor. With the pelvic examination showing no obvious ovarian mass, it would be appropriate to obtain a computerized tomography (CT) study of the adrenals to identify an adrenal tumor (choice **C**). Laboratory studies would probably show high levels of dehydroepiandrosterone sulfate, an androgen synthesized exclusively by the adrenal gland. If this was confirmed, management would be by surgical removal.

44 The answer is D   *Obstetrics and Gynecology*

The relationship is striking between the patient's increasing body hair and the androgen therapy she was given for treatment of decreased libido. It is most likely that the patient is taking a higher dose of androgen (choice **D**) for therapy than needed, resulting in the hirsutism. Ovarian production of testosterone is significant for providing the basis for female libido. When bilateral oophorectomy is performed not only is estrogen production markedly diminished, but testosterone production is also significantly decreased. Her physician was appropriate in providing her androgen as well as estrogen replacement, but monitoring of an optimal dose is also important.

45 The answer is E   *Obstetrics and Gynecology*

The finding of hirsutism, rather than virilization rules against an androgen-producing tumor. The irregular menses rule against a constitutional, idiopathic etiology with excessive dihydrotestosterone production from the hair follicle due to high 5-α-reductase enzyme activity. Idiopathic etiology is not associated with anovulation. The positive family history strongly suggests either polycystic ovarian syndrome (PCOS) or congenital adrenal hyperplasia. The absence of enlarged ovaries suggests this is a late-onset congenital adrenal hyperplasia (choice **E**), probably the 21-hydroxylase type. Laboratory studies would probably reveal an elevated 17-hydroxyprogesterone level, which is a cortisol precursor that is metabolized into androgen steroids. Treatment is glucocorticoid replacement therapy.

Answers 46–50

INTRODUCTION

Acute lymphoblastic leukemia (ALL) is most common in newborns and children up to 14 years of age, acute myelogenous leukemia (AML) from 15 to 39 years of age, acute and chronic myelogenous leukemia from 40 to 60 years of age, and chronic lymphocytic leukemia (CLL) after 60 years of age. Both acute and chronic leukemias are associated with anemia (usually normocytic), thrombocytopenia, and an elevated white blood cell (WBC) count (leukopenia in some cases). Relative to chronic leukemias, acute leukemias have a greater number of blast cells in the peripheral blood and bone marrow (>30%); contrariwise, chronic leukemias are associated with greater maturation of cells in the peripheral blood and bone marrow (blast cells, <30%).

46 The answer is E   *Medicine*

This 34-year-old man with epistaxis, generalized lymphadenopathy, and hepatosplenomegaly has acute myelogenous leukemia (AML) (choice **E**), also known as acute myeloid leukemia or as acute nonlymphocytic leukemia. The splinter-shaped inclusions called Auer rods are pathognomic for AML. AML is a bone marrow disease in which hemopoietic cells are arrested in a stage of early development. A distinctive feature in addition to Auer rods is the presence of more than 30% blast cells in the blood, bone marrow, or both. In AML, two disease processes are going on simultaneously. One is decreased numbers of blood cells causing anemia, thrombocytopenia, and a neutropenia. The anemia causes profound fatigue, which is often the presenting symptom. The second disease process is accumulation of blast cells, particularly in the liver and spleen. AML is actually a heterogeneous group of diseases that are categorized into eight subgroups on the basis of morphology and histochemistry. These eight subcategories are given an M designation from M0 to M7. The case pictured is M2, acute myeloblastic leukemia with differentiation. This is the most common type, accounting for some 25% of all cases. Some 10,000 new cases of all forms of ALL are diagnosed annually, almost all of which are in adults 24 years of age or older, but most patients are over 60 years of age. The disease is more common in whites than in blacks and in males than females. The mean 5-year survival is between 25 and 30% for patients younger than 60 years but is below 10% for older patients.

47 The answer is G *Medicine*

The 24-year-old man with ecchymoses, lymphadenopathy, hepatosplenomegaly, and hypergranular blast cells with numerous Auer rods most likely has acute myelogenous leukemia (M3), (choice **G**). The M3 variant is a promyelocytic leukemia and is the most common leukemia associated with disseminated intravascular coagulation (DIC), which is characterized by prolonged prothrombin and partial thromboplastin times, decreased fibrinogen, and a positive d-dimer test result (i.e., cross-linked dimers indicating fibrinolysis of fibrin clots). A t(15;17) translocation is a characteristic finding. AML M3 also has the best prognosis and is the only variant that can be treated with high doses of all-*trans* retinoic acid (ATRA). This drug induces a temporary maturation of the promyelocytes. Cases in which ATRA does not induce a remission often respond to arsenic trioxide.

48 The answer is A *Medicine*

The patient has acute lymphoblastic leukemia (ALL). The illustration shows lymphoblasts in the peripheral blood with prominent nucleoli and little cytoplasm. ALL is the most common cancer and leukemia in children (newborn to 14 years old). Subtypes include early pre-B (80%), pre-B, B, and pre-T cell ALL. The early pre-B cell type is the most common subtype of ALL. Positive marker studies for this subtype include presence of the common ALL antigen (CALLA-CD10) and terminal deoxynucleotidyltransferase (TdT). Presence of a t(12;21) translocation offers a favorable prognosis. In general, B-cell subtypes commonly metastasize to the central nervous system (CNS) and testicles, while T-cell subtypes present as an anterior mediastinal mass (malignant lymphoma) or as an acute leukemia. In early pre-B cell ALL, >90% achieve complete remission, and at least two thirds can be considered cured. Remission-induction therapy involves the use of prednisone, vincristine, and asparaginase. Consolidation uses the same drugs at lower doses. Maintenance therapy involves the use of 6-mercaptopurine and methotrexate. Common sites for residual blast cells include the bone marrow, CNS, and testes. Intrathecal administration of methotrexate and radiation of the neuraxis obliterate blast cells in the CNS.

49 The answer is F *Medicine*

The 45-year-old man with signs of a hypermetabolic state (i.e., fever, weight loss, sweating), epistaxis, generalized lymphadenopathy, and massive hepatosplenomegaly has chronic myelogenous leukemia (CML) (choice **F**). Myeloblasts account for less than 1% of the peripheral blood and bone marrow aspirate leukocytes. The illustration shows an increase in the granulocytic line of cells, and there are no Auer rods present in CML. Peripheral blood basophilia and eosinophilia are commonly present. Because all the neutrophils are neoplastic, they do not take up the leukocyte alkaline phosphatase (LAP) stain like normal mature neutrophils; therefore, the LAP score, which grades 100 cells on the intensity of the stain (0 to +4), is low. The Philadelphia (Ph) chromosome (chromosome 22 in the t[9;22]) is present in most cases. Most patients progress to a terminal blast crisis after 3 years, which may be associated with myeloblasts or lymphoblasts.

50 The answer is B *Medicine*

The 65-year-old man with generalized lymphadenopathy, hepatosplenomegaly, and an 80,000 cells/mm^3 leukocyte count has chronic lymphocytic leukemia (CLL, choice **B**). The illustration shows many small mature lymphocytes that cannot be distinguished from normal small lymphocytes. CLL is the most common cause of generalized lymphadenopathy and leukemia in adults over 60 years old. Traditionally, most patients with stage 0 or 1 disease could be told they would live their normal life span, while those with stage III or IV disease had a median survival time of 2 years. However, early results based on newer fludarabine-based combination therapies have reported 90% 2-year survivals.

CHOICES NOT USED

Adult T cell leukemia (choice **C**) is caused by the human T-cell leukemia virus (HTLV-1). It is a common leukemia in Japan. Clinical findings include hepatosplenomegaly, generalized lymphadenopathy, skin infiltration, and lytic bone lesions causing hypercalcemia.

Hairy cell leukemia (choice **D**) is a type of B-cell leukemia that occurs most commonly in middle-aged men. The neoplastic cells have hairlike projections and are positive for tartrate-resistant acid phosphatase stain (TRAP). Clinical findings include splenomegaly (90% of cases), absence of lymphadenopathy, hepatomegaly (20% of cases), and autoimmune vasculitis and arthritis. There is an excellent response to 2-chlorodeoxyadenosine (a purine nucleoside).

Acute monocytic leukemia (choice **H**) is the leukemia that is commonly associated with infiltration of the gums.

Questions

Single Best Choice Directions: This section consists of numbered statements or questions followed by a list of potential answers; you are to select the ONE best answer.

1 A 62-year-old woman presents with a complaint of a sore big toe on her right foot. She has been working for the past 35 years in an office that has a strict dress code, and consequently, she habitually wore high-heeled, narrow-toed shoes, similar to the pair she is wearing presently. Her medical history is significant for type-2 diabetes with peripheral circulatory compromise. An examination shows a painful bump on the first metatarsal joint and a distorted big toe. Which of the following conditions does this woman suffer from?

(A) Hallux valgus
(B) Metatarsalgia
(C) Morton's neuroma
(D) Hammer toe
(E) Plantar fasciitis

2 A young man started acting abnormally as a senior in high school, and by fall as he was preparing to leave home for college, he told his mother that he had started hearing voices who were trying to direct his behavior. The mother took him to a psychiatrist who prescribed medication. After the patient fails to respond to several trials of newer antipsychotic medications, he is started on clozapine therapy. Which of the following adverse effects is most likely to occur during his treatment with this drug?

(A) Seizures
(B) Renal failure
(C) Agranulocytosis
(D) Pigmentary retinopathy
(E) Anticholinergic delirium

3 A 3-year-old afebrile child develops unilateral, nontender anterior cervical nodes that have been enlarging over the past few weeks. A lymph node biopsy reveals microabscesses with neutrophils. Culture results are pending. A Mantoux test exhibits only 7-mm induration after 48 hours. The patient does not attend daycare, and there is no recent travel among family members. The patient has two pets, a goldfish and a turtle. Which of the following is the most likely diagnosis?

(A) *Mycobacterium tuberculosis* infection
(B) *Mycobacterium scrofulaceum* infection
(C) *Mycobacterium bovis* infection
(D) Cat-scratch disease
(E) Mononucleosis

4 A physician discovers that an 80-year-old woman with a serious heart condition has breast cancer. Her son asks the physician not to reveal the cancer finding to her because "it will kill her." With respect to the cancer finding, the physician should do which of the following?

(A) Tell her immediately
(B) Tell her son to tell her
(C) Get a member of a cancer support group to tell her
(D) Evaluate whether telling her will pose a risk to her health
(E) Tell her with her son in the room

5 A pediatrician is requested to attend the delivery of a term G3P2 female who is having a repeat cesarean section. On review of the mother's medical record, it is noted that she had good prenatal care, and although she smoked one pack of cigarettes per day, she denied the use of alcohol or drugs. The delivery is performed, and the patient's birthweight is 7 lb 13 oz (6.26 kg). The patient receives an Apgar score of 8 at 1 minute, derived from scores of 2 in each of the following parameters: heart rate, respiration, muscle tone, and reflex irritability to catheter in nostril. At 5 minutes of age, the infant has a heart rate of 140 beats/min and a vigorous cry. His arms and legs are well flexed, and when a catheter is placed in the nares, the infant grimaces. Which of the following parameters was not determined at 1 minute and therefore should be included when the patient's 5-minute Apgar score is assessed?

(A) Blood pressure
(B) Gestational age
(C) Muscle tone
(D) Color
(E) Respiratory effort

6 A 12-year-old female presents with a complaint of pain in the lower region of her back. In taking a history, it is determined that she has been competing in gymnastics since she was 6 years old and never has been injured. However some 4 weeks ago her back started to hurt for no apparent reason. The pain is localized to the lower back and is usually relieved with rest. On physical examination, the pain is aggravated with hyperextension of the lumbosacral spine. Sciatic tension tests and neurologic examination results are normal. Plain radiographs show lucency at the pars interarticular. Which of the following is the most likely diagnosis?

(A) Acute lumbar strain
(B) Scoliosis
(C) Herniated disk disease
(D) Sacroiliac sprain
(E) Spondylolysis

7   A 22-year-old woman with schizophrenia and a body mass index (BMI) of 23 is started on olanzapine 10 mg PO bid with excellent remission of her psychotic symptoms. Over the next 3 months, her BMI increases to 27. Results of laboratory studies, including hemoglobin A1c, are unremarkable. Which of the following would be the best next step in pharmacologic treatment?

(A) Add sibutramine
(B) Decrease olanzapine
(C) Switch to clozapine
(D) Switch to haloperidol
(E) Switch to aripiprazole

8   A 45-year-old woman receives a spinal anesthetic for lower back surgery. The surgery has a poor outcome, and she sues the anesthesiologist and the surgeon for malpractice. The lawsuit will be successful if she can prove which of the following?

(A) She has lost physical function because of the surgery.
(B) The physicians deviated from the accepted standard of medical practice.
(C) At least one of the doctors was not board certified in his specialty.
(D) She has lost income as a result of the surgery.
(E) She has constant pain as a result of the surgery.

9   A woman, gravida 1, para 0, has a seizure disorder that is controlled with phenytoin. The patient is married, and she is extremely compliant with prenatal care. She denies any tobacco, alcohol; or drug use. She tells her physician that she is concerned about harm to her fetus from the phenytoin. The obstetrician informs the patient that phenytoin taken by a pregnant woman can be teratogenic and cause the fetus to have which of the following?

(A) Microcephaly, spina bifida, and developmental delay

(B) Nail hypoplasia, growth retardation, and a "Cupid's bow" lip
(C) Brain malformations, thymic hypoplasia, and cardiac defects
(D) Vaginal carcinoma and adenosis
(E) Microcephaly, growth retardation, and stroke

10   An 18-year-old woman is found by police wandering partially clothed and disoriented in a public park in the early hours of the morning. The girl remembers only that she was taken to a party by a friend the previous evening and then went to continue the evening to a disco with people that she didn't know before meeting them at the party. She insists, however, that she only drank soft drinks. Mental status examination reveals a distressed and angry young woman who is alert and upset. Her speech is clear and coherent, her mood is labile, and her thoughts are logical. She says that she is unable to recall any events from the time she was at the disco around 12 PM until she awoke in the park around 6 AM. She believes that she may have been drugged and raped and demands police investigation. Physical examination is unremarkable except for evidence of recent sexual intercourse. Laboratory studies show no detectable blood alcohol. Which of the following is the most likely cause of her amnesia?

(A) Alcohol-induced amnestic disorder
(B) Dissociative amnesia
(C) Factitious disorder
(D) Nitrazepam intoxication
(E) Transient amnesia due to seizure

11   A heart murmur is heard during a routine physical examination being conducted on a 5-year-old female. It is a medium-pitched, ejection systolic murmur with a musical quality. It does not radiate to the apex, base, or back. The intensity of the murmur appears to change with respiration and position. Which of the following findings would also be characteristic of this type of murmur?

(A) It is best heard along the lower left and midsternal border
(B) It is common in infancy
(C) It is best heard with the patient lying on the left side
(D) It is indicative of a significant cardiac defect
(E) It is less intense with fever or excitement

12   A 21-year-old man was playing in a pick-up basketball game when he fell on his outstretched right arm with his wrist flexed dorsally. He felt a deep dull pain in his wrist and sat out for a while, but since there was no swelling he decided that it wasn't serious and joined in

the game again. However, the pain didn't let up, and he quit again after a short time. A week later there was minor swelling on the back of the hand over the thumb, and a persistent pain on the dorsum of his hand toward the base of the thumb. The pain became more intense when he tried to grip something. Consequently he consulted a physician who elicited sharp pain when he pressed on the "anatomical snuffbox". He then took an x-ray film (pictured). Which of the following bones is most likely fractured?

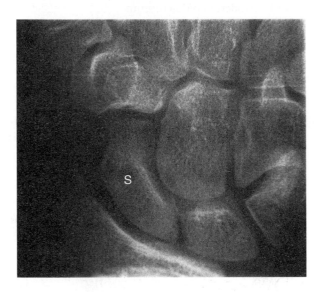

(A) Scaphoid
(B) Lunate
(C) Triquetrum
(D) Hamate
(E) Capitate

13 A 38-year-old homeless man with schizophrenia, hospitalized for 2 weeks on a psychiatric ward and facing discharge to a homeless shelter, is approached and asked by a researcher to consider participation in a research project regarding an investigational psychiatric medication. The investigation will take 2 weeks, during which time he will stay on the research unit and will receive a modest fee for participation. He carefully listens to the risks of the procedure and appears to understand them completely. He consents to participate. Which of the following is the most likely reason that the consent would not be considered invalid?

(A) Promising a research subject financial compensation is unethical.
(B) No formal testing of the patient's cognitive capacity was obtained.
(C) Schizophrenia precludes the ability to give informed consent.

(D) The informed consent was obtained by an individual directly involved in the research project.
(E) The patient will be discharged if he doesn't participate.

14 While bathing her 3-year-old daughter, a mother discovers an abdominal mass. The child has been asymptomatic, and her growth parameters have been within normal limits. A urinalysis is obtained and microscopic hematuria is seen. A flat plate of the abdomen and ultrasound are performed as well as a computed tomography (CT) scan. The presence of an intrarenal tumor consistent with Wilms' tumor is confirmed. This child may also have which of the following?

(A) Hypotension
(B) A propensity for bone metastasis
(C) Chromosome 6 abnormalities
(D) Less than a 5% 4-year survival rate
(E) Aniridia

15 A 47-year-old woman had a mass removed from the upper outer quadrant of her left breast. Upon biopsy, the pathologist reported the following findings: grade 2 infiltrating ductal adenocarcinoma; estrogen and progesterone assay, negative; tumor size, 1.0 cm. In addition, flow cytometric analysis revealed a diploid tumor with 4% of the cells in the S phase, and there is no amplification of the *erb-b2* oncogene. Which of the following prognostic results is of greatest concern for this patient?

(A) Flow cytometric analysis
(B) Location of tumor
(C) No amplification of *erb-b2*
(D) Estrogen and progesterone assay
(E) Tumor size

16 A 5-year-old boy is referred for psychiatric evaluation by a pediatrician because of severe distractibility, impulsivity, and a short attention span. The parents believe that they cannot manage his behavior at home, although they say they have had no similar problems with their other two children. Family counseling has not been successful in improving the situation. The child also has a history of stereotyped behaviors, including frequent hand washing. He also has numerous facial tics. Mental status examination reveals an alert, oriented, anxious and shy boy who is slightly depressed. His thought processes are logical, and there is no evidence of hallucinations or delusions. His memory appears intact. His impulse control during the examination is normal. Psychologic testing reveals a normal IQ. Which of the following choices, if any, is the best reason to avoid initiating atomoxetine therapy?

(A) It is not approved for this condition
(B) Preschool age
(C) Presence of obsessive–compulsive symptoms
(D) Presence of tics
(E) None of the choices is a reason to avoid initiation of atomoxetine therapy

17 A mother consults a dermatologist because she is concerned about a lesion on the left cheek of her 8-month-old daughter. The lesion is bright red, protuberant, compressible, and sharply demarcated. It first appeared when the child was 2 months old. The pediatrician told the mother not to worry because it would most likely resolve spontaneously. However, the lesion has grown rapidly over the past 6 months. Which of the following would be the most appropriate course of management?

(A) Treatment with cryotherapy
(B) Treatment with flashlamp-pumped pulsed-laser therapy
(C) Surgical excision of the lesion
(D) Radiation treatment
(E) Expectant observation

18 A recently retired 67-year-old man makes an appointment to see his physician because his hands are beginning to tremble in an uncontrollable manner. During the examination the physician notes that he does have an obvious resting tremor of both hands. However he had no difficulty in picking up a quarter, and during that process the tremor ceased. When asked to hold his hand out, palm up, his fingers underwent an involuntary movement as if he was rolling a pill across his palm. He states that although the tremor is annoying and sometimes embarrassing, it makes little difference in his lifestyle; it has not even interfered with playing golf. At this time which of the following is the best first step in treatment?

(A) Amantadine
(B) An anticholinergic drug
(C) Levodopa
(D) Carbidopa
(E) A dopamine agonist
(F) Selegiline
(G) Watchful waiting

19 An 8-year-old boy presents with squamous cell carcinoma. When born he appeared normal, but after his first exposure to sunlight he developed a severe erythema, as if he were severely sunburned, despite the fact his mother claims he was only exposed for a short time. The erythema did not heal, instead his skin became

scaly, and he developed hyperpigmented spots that looked like large freckles. By the age of 2 years his skin took on a poikilodermal appearance with skin atrophy, telangiectasis, and a mottled appearance with hyper- and hypopigmented areas. Now, at the age of 6 years, there are actinic changes, lesions that affect his left eye and now a lesion that is diagnosed as squamous cell carcinoma. His parents are first cousins. The boy most likely is suffering from which of the following conditions?

(A) Xeroderma pigmentosum
(B) Ataxia telangiectasia
(C) Bloom syndrome
(D) Cockayne syndrome
(E) Fanconi anemia
(F) Trichodystrophy

20 A 66-year-old male presents to the emergency department with extremely severe pain in his groin. He has not been engaged in any recent physical activity but does recollect feeling a bulge in the inguinal area. Because he had only minor discomfort, he dismissed it as being insignificant. Physical examination reveals the presence of a hernia. Which of the following is the most likely type of hernia present in this patient?

(A) Reducible hernia
(B) Incarcerated hernia
(C) Obstructed hernia
(D) Strangulated hernia
(E) Richter hernia

21 A 40-year-old woman is recently informed that she has renal failure. After disputing the accuracy of the laboratory testing, she then becomes angry and upset that she has "been cursed with a chronic illness." She struggles to determine how she can "build up her kidney function" with a proper diet and vitamins. When told this isn't really possible, she becomes despondent. A friend who is a registered nurse tells her that she is going through "Kübler-Ross stages" and must reach acceptance of her illness. After several weeks characterized by periods of anger, depression, hope, and doubt, she seeks counseling about her failure to "go through the grieving process" for her lost health. Which of the following is the most accurate statement about current understanding of Kübler-Ross stages?

(A) Environmental factors have little effect on the internal process of grieving.
(B) Kübler-Ross's insights no longer are valid and are no longer used to help provide help to people who are dealing with loss.
(C) People normally progress through the stages without becoming "stuck" in any particular stage.

(D) The stages may recur numerous times.

(E) The stages occur in a set order.

22 A 3-year-old child is brought to the emergency department by his parents with a temperature of 39°C (102.2°F). The parents describe a generalized seizure that lasted 5 minutes. The patient did not lose consciousness. The seizure was followed by a brief period of drowsiness. The patient is awake and alert on presentation to the emergency department. Physical examination reveals a right otitis media. It is determined that the patient had a febrile seizure. Which of the following statements about febrile seizures is true?

(A) They are focal in nature and can last from a few seconds to 10 minutes.

(B) They progress to epilepsy in 60% of patients.

(C) They are often associated with underlying neurologic problems.

(D) They are not associated with a family history of febrile seizures.

(E) They are rare before 9 months of age.

23 A pediatrician is the chief investigator in a study designed to determine if vitamin Q50 enhances the growth of children. The double-blind study matched children with respect to age, sex, and social status and divided them into two groups. Their heights were measured at the beginning and end of the study. One group received 250 units of vitamin Q50; the other group received a placebo, both for 3 months. Which of the following statistical tests would be most appropriate for assessing whether there were significant differences in mean height gain between the two groups?

(A) Logistic regression

(B) Analysis of variance

(C) Correlation coefficient

(D) Chi-square test

(E) Student's *t*-test

24 A mental health clinic decides to inaugurate state-of-the-art treatment for individuals with chronic schizophrenia by creating an Assertive Community Treatment (ACT) program. Which of the following features most closely describe ACT?

(A) Deviations by patients from acceptable social behaviors are corrected through a carefully constructed program of operant conditioning.

(B) Patients are court ordered to participate in outpatient treatment and can be rehospitalized if they are noncompliant.

(C) Services are available 24/7 from multiple individuals and include housing, vocational rehabilitation, and recreation.

(D) Services are centered in a highly structured community facility, with integrated laboratory, medication, and therapy services.

(E) Services are provided in the context of a "therapeutic community" that is composed of members with similar challenges who strive to help each other.

25 A 5-month-old male infant is taken to the pediatrician because of vomiting, tremors, and lethargy that began shortly after breast-feeding was discontinued and other nutrients were added to the diet. Physical examination shows scleral icterus and hepatomegaly. Laboratory studies reveal hypoglycemia, a mixed hyperbilirubinemia with an increase in both unconjugated and conjugated bilirubin, an increase in serum transaminases, and the presence of fructose in the urine. Which of the following should be restricted from the diet?

(A) Branched-chain amino acids

(B) Dairy products

(C) Phenylalanine

(D) Table sugar

(E) Tyrosine

26 A 38-year-old woman with a mass in her thyroid gland is being evaluated for paroxysmal hypertension and hypercalcemia. An abdominal computed tomography (CT) scan shows bilateral adrenal masses and multiple densities in both lobes of her liver. Her urine catecholamine levels are markedly increased. The organ of origin of the liver abnormality is most likely which of the following?

(A) Kidney

(B) Thyroid

(C) Parathyroid

(D) Ovary

(E) Adrenal

27 A 74-year-old man has been treated for essential hypertension for the past 15 years. His blood pressure has been under good control using the following medications: hydrochlorothiazide, enalapril, acebutolol, clonidine, and doxazosin mesylate. However, he recently flew back to visit relatives for Christmas in North Dakota. To save the hassle of counting pills, he simply packed his whole supply in his suitcase that was checked in. The trip to North Dakota was uneventful, but unfortunately, just as he was preparing to leave, a blizzard blew in and his flight was delayed, causing him to miss his connecting flight. This not only delayed his homecoming but for some reason, his suitcase, medications and all, got lost. After a day or so he notes his blood pressure is increasing, and then he develops chest and abdominal pain, a severe headache, and feels so anxious that he visits a local emergency department where they check his blood pressure and find it to be 245/122 mm Hg. However, despite his pains, an examination shows no evidence of end-organ damage. Which of the following statements concerning his condition is true?

(A) He is undergoing a hypertensive emergency due to sudden withdrawal of clonidine.

(B) He is undergoing a hypertensive crisis due to sudden withdrawal of hydrochlorothiazide.

(C) He is undergoing a hypertensive crisis due to sudden withdrawal of clonidine.

(D) His blood pressure must be reduced to normal levels with in minutes by administration IV nitroprusside.

(E) He should be provided with his usual medications and sent home.

28. A 16-year-old boy was undergoing emergency celiotomy because of fever, elevated white blood cell (WBC) count, and point tenderness in the right lower quadrant. The patient had no prior significant illness or surgical procedures. He was not receiving any medication and had no allergies. Induction of general anesthesia proceeded without difficulty. Prior to skin incision, the patient became tachycardic, and his end-tidal carbon dioxide level was elevated. Which of the following would be the most appropriate next step in the management of this patient?

(A) Rapidly complete the operation

(B) Perform a tracheotomy

(C) Administer dantrolene

(D) Increase the depth of anesthesia

(E) Administer third-generation cephalosporins

29. A 43-year-old man was diagnosed with insulin-dependent diabetes at the age of 5 years. He recently was divorced by his wife and as a result was living a somewhat careless and dissipated lifestyle, leading him to forget to stock up on his supply of insulin. Waking up one morning he realized he didn't take his usual dose before going to bed last night and that there was no insulin for his morning injection either. After eating a hearty breakfast, he goes outside and discovers it snowed heavily during the night and he would have to dig his car out. Which of the following is most likely to be true after he has been shoveling snow vigorously for an hour?

(A) His plasma glucose concentration will be lower after shoveling than it was before starting.

(B) His plasma glucose concentration will be higher after shoveling than it was before starting.

(C) His plasma ketone body concentration will be lower after shoveling than it was before starting.

(D) The exercise will promote recruitment of GLUT-5 in muscle cells thereby promoting glucose entry.

(E) The exercise will stimulate cortisol production, which will help mitigate his hyperglycemia.

30. A 14-year-old girl is started on antidepressant medication by a child psychiatrist. The mother becomes alarmed because she has heard that antidepressant medications cause suicide and have resulted in a "black box warning" for prescribers. Which of the following best describes the content of the black box warning relevant to this situation?

(A) Children who develop suicidal thoughts while taking certain antidepressants should be switched to different medications while under close observation.

(B) Children with suicidal thoughts should not be started on selective serotonin-reuptake inhibitors.

(C) Otherwise normal children with suicidal thoughts should not be started on any antidepressant medication.

(D) Children with psychosis should not be given antidepressants if suicidal thoughts are present.

(E) Families of children with suicidal thoughts should be advised by the caregiver of the need for close observation and communication with the prescriber.

31. A 34-year-old married woman who has two young children and does not work outside her home sees her physician because she is worried that she has a strange disease. As she explains to him, her hands intermittently get blotchy, turning white, blue, and then red. The phenomenon is always bilateral. In addition to these somewhat unpredictable color changes, there is some slight discomfort, marked by a prickly sensation or numbness, and sometimes her hands or fingers swell; the latter is most noticeable when she is putting on or taking off her rings. She further adds that these "attacks" are precipitated by cold but seem also to occur when she is under emotional stress. In taking a detailed history and running diagnostic serologic tests the physician rules out associated collagen-vascular diseases such as scleroderma, systemic lupus erythematosus, dermatomyositis, and rheumatoid arteritis, as well as cryoglobulinemia, neurogenic thoracic outlet syndrome, carpal tunnel syndrome, ergotamine

toxicity, use of any chemotherapeutic agents, smoking or any licit or illicit drug use. Which of the following is the most probable diagnosis?

(A) Raynaud's phenomenon
(B) Livedo reticularis
(C) Acrocyanosis
(D) Primary erythromelalgia
(E) Raynaud's disease

32 An enlarged, nontender right supraclavicular lymph node is surgically removed from a 29-year-old woman. Multiple histologic sections through the lymph node reveal nodular areas surrounded by connective tissue. Occasional multilobed cells with prominent nucleoli surrounded by a halo of clear nucleoplasm are present in spaces within the nodules. Results of a complete blood cell count, urinalysis, and biochemical tests are all normal. A chest radiograph shows a mass lesion in the anterior mediastinum. Which of the following is the most likely diagnosis?

(A) Burkitt's lymphoma
(B) Follicular B-cell lymphoma
(C) Hodgkin's lymphoma
(D) Metastatic cancer
(E) Reactive lymphadenitis

33 A 60-year-old woman with a history of coronary artery disease (CAD) presents to her physician for a regular examination. She had been hospitalized 2 years previously for an inferior myocardial infarction. Six months later, she was diagnosed with atrial fibrillation and was prescribed 325 mg of aspirin per day. A coronary angiogram revealed 70% obstruction in her right coronary artery. She is now very concerned because her neighbor, who has chronic atrial fibrillation, suddenly developed an embolic stroke that left him hemiplegic. The desire is to prescribe additional medication that will prevent atrial fibrillation from inducing a ventricular tachycardia. Prescription of which of the following drugs would generate the most criticism from the physician's colleagues?

(A) Digoxin
(B) Metoprolol
(C) Quinidine
(D) Verapamil
(E) Diltiazem

34 A 13-year-old girl presents to her pediatrician because she has developed a low-grade fever and rash. A maculopapular rash is present that began on the face and spread to the trunk. In addition, she has extremely painful postauricular and posterior occipital lymphadenopathy. She also complains of pain in both wrists and her right knee. Her mother states that the patient was in her usual state of good health until the previous day. Which of the following is the most likely diagnosis?

(A) Measles
(B) Infectious mononucleosis
(C) German measles
(D) Erythema infectiosum
(E) Roseola

35 A 63-year-old woman presents to the emergency department complaining of heart palpitations and shortness of breath. Upon taking a history she admitted that the prior evening she consumed more alcohol that she should have, but she also claims that is not her characteristic behavior. Examination revealed an irregular heart rate averaging 125 beats per minute. Her electrocardiogram (ECG) pattern is illustrated below. The most likely diagnosis is which of the following?

(A) Atrial flutter
(B) Chaotic atrial tachycardia
(C) Atrial fibrillation
(D) Atrial ventricular junctional rhythm
(E) Ventricular tachycardia

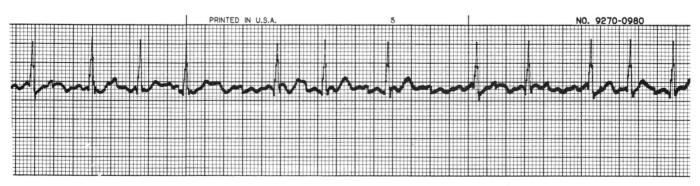

36 A 67-year-old woman had been suffering from an upper respiratory illness for which her physician prescribed penicillin V. He also administered the pneumococcal) vaccine. She apparently recovered fully; however, 2 months later she suffered a fracture of the neck of her left femur and was hospitalized. The fracture was repaired, but 62 hours after admission the duty nurse notices she is running a fever. When examined by the physician on call he notes her temperature is 100.5°F (38.1°C), her blood pressure is 98/75 mm Hg, pulse is 100 beats/min and regular, her respiratory rate is 26 breaths per minute, and her respiration is somewhat labored. The white blood cell count is 12,000 cells per mm^3 (normal, 4.3–10,000 cells/mm^3). A chest x-ray film shows right lower lobe consolidation. Which of the following organisms is the most likely cause of her infection?

(A) *Mycoplasma pneumoniae*
(B) *Klebsiella pneumoniae*
(C) *Streptococcus pneumoniae*
(D) *Legionella pneumophila*
(E) *Chlamydia pneumoniae*

37 A 7-year-old child presents to his physician with complaints of fever for the last few days. In addition, the parents state that the patient has been complaining of a generalized headache as well as a stiff neck. She further informs the physician that the child complains of nausea, has vomited, and has only been able to tolerate a small amount of fluids. Photophobia is also present on physical examination. The physician performs a lumbar puncture, and analysis of the cerebrospinal fluid (CSF) is done. Which of the following CSF findings characterizes a viral, rather than a bacterial, meningitis?

(A) Normal glucose level
(B) Substantially increased protein concentration
(C) Elevated lactate concentration
(D) Positive Gram's stain
(E) Polymorphonuclear predominance after 48 hours

Directions for Matching Questions (38 through 50): Each set of matching questions is preceded by a list of 4 to 26 lettered options followed by a brief explanation of the required task and then by a series of numbered statements. For each lettered statement you are to select ONE lettered option that best fulfills the task as it relates to that statement. Remember each of the listed options might be correctly selected once, more than once, or not at all.

Questions 38–41

For each disease described in questions 38 through 41, select the ONE microbial pathogen that most likely caused that disease.

(A) *Haemophilus ducreyi*
(B) *Bordetella pertussis*
(C) *Legionella pneumophila*
(D) *Pasteurella multocida*
(E) *Yersinia pestis*
(F) *Eikenella corrodens*
(G) *Borrelia burgdorferi*
(H) *Leptospira interrogans*
(I) *Bacteroides fragilis*

38 A 28-year-old man, who works in a summer camp in upstate New York, develops bilateral facial weakness involving both the upper and lower facial muscles. He also complains of joint pains in both knees. He has a history a few months ago of an erythematous rash on his right thigh that was circular, and had a central area of clearing.

39 A 28-year-old man that works in the grocery produce section of a supermarket develops a fever of 40°C (104°F) associated with a cough productive of bloody sputum, and malaise. Serum electrolytes show hyponatremia, hyperkalemia, and metabolic acidosis.

40 A 52-year-old man who is studying ancient Native American artifacts in the Sonoran desert in Arizona, develops fever and enlarged right inguinal lymph nodes that have sinus tracts draining pus to the surface of the skin. He recalls digging out pieces of pottery in the vicinity of a ground squirrel community.

41 A 22-year-old man was hiking on a hot, humid day in West Virginia when he came upon a pond. Neglecting the facts that much of it was algae covered and a herd of cattle was grazing nearby, he stripped down and plunged in to cool down. The following week he abruptly developed fever (39.5°C [103.1°F]), chills, abdominal pain, severe headache, and pain in his calf muscles. His fever only lasted 24 hours and by the third day he, felt fairly well. He then developed a severe case of uveitis in his left eye.

Questions 42–44

Spontaneous abortion occurs in 10–15% of pregnancies; they are divided into the 5 subtypes included as choices in these questions. For each numbered clinical presentation, select the ONE most appropriate diagnosis in reference to first-trimester loss.

(A) Threatened abortion
(B) Missed abortion
(C) Inevitable abortion
(D) Incomplete abortion
(E) Completed abortion

42 A 29-year-old woman comes to the emergency department complaining of cramping and bleeding. She states she had heavy bleeding since yesterday, which now is only minimal. She passed some tissues per vagina but flushed it down the toilet. She had initiated prenatal care 3 weeks ago with a local obstetrician. On that first visit an informal sonogram was performed showing a single embryo consistent with 7 weeks' gestation. Speculum examination shows a dilated cervical os, and endovaginal ultrasound reveals a normal endometrial stripe

43 A 21-year-old comes to the outpatient office for her first prenatal visit. This was a planned pregnancy. She has been taking prenatal vitamins and iron tablets. Pelvic examination reveals normal external genitalia and vagina. There are no cervical lesions. The cervix is closed and there is no evidence of bleeding. The uterus feels 10-week size on bimanual examination but no fetal heart tones are heard with Doppler stethoscope. An obstetric sonogram shows a nonviable embryo.

44 A 32-year-old woman comes to the outpatient office at 8 weeks' gestation by dates complaining of vaginal bleeding. She denies uterine cramping or passage of tissues. Results of a urine β-hCG test a week ago were positive. Speculum examination shows a closed cervical os. There are no vaginal or cervical lesions. An obstetric sonogram shows a normal gestational sac, fetal pole, and yolk sac.

Questions 45–47

The following are examples of glucose abnormalities encountered in type 1 diabetics on a split-dose, mixed-insulin regimen of neutral protamine Hagedorn (NPH) insulin and regular insulin, given 30 minutes before breakfast and dinner. For each numbered treatment option, select the lettered glucose abnormality that would benefit most from the change.

(A) 10 PM glucose concentration of 90 mg/dL, 3 AM glucose concentration of 40 mg/dL, and 7 AM glucose concentration of 200 mg/dL

(B) 10 PM glucose concentration of 110 mg/dL, 3 AM glucose concentration of 110 mg/dL, and 7 AM glucose concentration of 150 mg/dL

(C) 10 PM glucose concentration of 110 mg/dL, 3 AM glucose concentration of 160 mg/dL, and 7 AM glucose concentration of 220 mg/dL

(D) 12 PM glucose concentration of 200 mg/dL

(E) 5 PM glucose concentration of 220 mg/dL

(F) 9 PM glucose concentration of 200 mg/dL

45 Increase the morning dose of regular insulin

46 Decrease the NPH dose at dinner, give a portion of it at bedtime, or give more food at bedtime

47 Increase the NPH dose at dinner or give the dose at bedtime

Questions 48–50

Select the lettered pathogen most likely causing the skin lesions described in questions 48 through 50 below.

(A) Mycobacterium leprae
(B) Trichophyton tonsurans
(C) Trichophyton rubrum
(D) Microsporum canis
(E) Trichophyton schoenleinii
(F) Malassezia furfur
(G) Candida albicans

48 A 20-year-old homeless man has multiple circular areas of alopecia with erythema and scaling of the skin. In the areas of alopecia, a black dot remains where the hair shaft has broken off. A Wood's lamp examination is negative for fluorescence.

49 A 40-year-old man living in southern Texas presents with hypopigmented, macular skin lesions on both arms that are insensitive to pin prick.

50 A 23-year-old woman presents with a single circular lesion with an erythematous, scaling margin and central clearing. A Wood's lamp examination shows fluorescence of the lesion. A potassium hydroxide preparation reveals yeasts and hyphae.

Answer Key

1	A	**11**	A	**21**	D	**31**	E	**41**	H
2	A	**12**	A	**22**	E	**32**	C	**42**	E
3	B	**13**	E	**23**	E	**33**	C	**43**	B
4	D	**14**	E	**24**	C	**34**	C	**44**	A
5	D	**15**	D	**25**	D	**35**	C	**45**	D
6	E	**16**	E	**26**	B	**36**	B	**46**	A
7	E	**17**	E	**27**	C	**37**	A	**47**	C
8	B	**18**	G	**28**	C	**38**	G	**48**	B
9	B	**19**	A	**29**	B	**39**	C	**49**	A
10	D	**20**	D	**30**	E	**40**	E	**50**	C

Answers and Explanations

1 The answer is A   *Surgery*

Hallux valgus (choice **A**), also known as a bunion, is a common—sometimes painful but more often painless—condition in which the big toe (hallux) sits at an angle (valgus) that projects toward, sometimes under or over, the other toes. This creates a bump on the knuckle that projects outward, often projecting beyond the rest of foot, putting it at greater risk for pressure from shoes. The condition most often is caused by chronically wearing ill-fitting shoes and consequently is more common in females than in males. However, contributing factors also include a positive family history of bunions, hyperelastic syndromes, metatarsus varus, pes varus and a short first metatarsal joint. Symptoms usually are treated conservatively with wider shoes, bunion pads, and for acute pain, ice, rest, and nonsteroidal antiinflammatory drugs (NSAIDs). Surgery is usually required to straighten the toe and to remove the bunion and is sometimes done for cosmetic purposes as well as for more basic medical purposes. Patients referred for surgery typically have intermetatarsal angles greater than 10° or are those whose discomfort or pain does not respond to conservative treatment. Surgery is contraindicated in patients with vascular disease, as in the case described.

Metatarsalgia (choice **B**) is pain and/or a feeling of walking on pebbles in one of the metatarsal/phalangeal joints; it is usually due to chronic irritation caused by any of a host of factors including stress fractures, obesity, pregnancy, calluses, bunions, legs of different lengths, high-heeled shoes, or any other factor that puts excess pressure and/or use on one or more of the metatarsal/phalangeal joints; the condition may also be due to rheumatoid arthritis. Once diagnosed, the objective is to discover and remove the causative factor and treat symptoms conservatively, e.g., with NSAIDs. Morton's neuroma (choice **C**) is a benign growth that develops on a nerve at the base of a toe. It causes a burning sensation that radiates into the toes and is accompanied by sore feet. Conservative treatment consists of resting the feet with the shoes off; however, the neuromas often must be removed surgically. Hammer toe (choice **D**) is a bending or compressing of the distal end of a toe, most often the second toe; mallet toe is a similar condition in which the end of the toe is broadened. Both are caused by chronic pressure from shoes that are not long enough. These conditions again can be painful, are caused by ill-fitting shoes, and can usually be treated conservatively, but may also be treated surgically. It is particularly common among individuals in whom the second toe is longer than the big toe, an autosomal, dominantly inherited condition, which sometime is treated by surgically shortening the toe. Plantar fasciitis (choice **E**) is the most common cause of foot pain encountered in general practice. It results from constant strain on the plantar fascia at its insertion into the medial tubercle of the calcaneus. Most cases occur in patients with no associated disease, although certain inflammatory conditions may increase the risk. The pain is most severe upon arising and usually subsides upon walking. The diagnosis is confirmed by palpation; radiography is of no help. Treatment is a period of days without prolonged standing, arch supports to transfer more weight onto the arches, and NSAIDs. Rarely, injection of a corticosteroid is called for, and even less often, surgery to release the plantar fascia from its attachment at the os calcis is used.

2 The answer is A   *Psychiatry*

The incidence of seizures (choice **A**) with a daily dose of clozapine exceeding 600 mg is more than 5%. Agranulocytosis (choice **C**) is another serious adverse effect of clozapine treatment, but the incidence is about 1%. Renal failure (choice **B**), pigmentary retinopathy (choice **D**), and anticholinergic delirium (choice **E**) have rarely or never been associated with use of clozapine.

3 The answer is B   *Pediatrics*

Lymphadenitis is the most common presentation of atypical mycobacterial infection in children. The submandibular or anterior cervical nodes are most frequently involved. *Mycobacterium scrofulaceum* (choice **B**) and *M. avium-intracellulare* infections are the most common causes in the United States. Involvement is usually unilateral, and chest x-ray films are normal. Generally, there is no history of exposure to tuberculosis, and a Mantoux skin test result is usually negative or indeterminate.

Differential diagnosis includes other mycobacterial infections (e.g., *M. tuberculosis* [choice **A**], *M. bovis* [choice **C**]) as well as cat-scratch disease (choice **D**). Infectious mononucleosis (choice **E**) is not a likely choice; it is estimated to occur in 20 to 70 of 100,000 persons per year and is characterized by generalized lymphadenopathy, splenomegaly, and hepatomegaly. Most commonly, the cervical lymph nodes are affected, followed by the submandibular and axillary nodes. These signs are generally accompanied by pharyngitis and tonsillar enlargement.

4 The answer is D *Preventive Medicine and Public Health*

Ordinarily, patients must be provided with all of the information about their diagnosis to obtain informed consent for treatment. However, if the physician's medical opinion is that the patient's life or health will be at risk if he or she is informed, information can be withheld. Therefore, prior to telling this patient the diagnosis of breast cancer, the physician should first evaluate whether telling her will pose a risk to her health (choice **D**).

Telling her immediately would not be the correct course of action (choice **A**). The opinion of the patient's relative concerning this matter is not relevant to the physician's decision (choices **B** and **E**). A member of a cancer support group does not need to be involved (choice **C**).

5 The answer is D *Pediatrics*

The Apgar score is used as an immediate cardiorespiratory assessment of the newborn. A score of 0, 1, or 2 is given at 1 and 5 minutes after birth for each of five parameters. Scores can also be given at succeeding 5-minute intervals to aid in evaluating efforts at resuscitation. Parameters observed are heart rate, muscle tone (choice **C**), respiratory effort (choice **E**), response to a catheter in the nose, and color. In the scenario, color (choice **D**) was the only missing component. Blood pressure (choice **A**) and gestational age (choice **B**) are not a part of the Apgar score.

	Apgar Score		
	Assigned Points		
Signs	**0**	**1**	**2**
Heart rate	No heart rate	<100 beats/min	>100 beats/min
Respiration	None	Weak cry	Vigorous cry
Muscle tone	None	Some extremity flexion	Arms and legs well flexed
Reflex irritability to catheter in nostril	None	Grimace	Cough or sneeze
Color of body	Blue	Pink body, blue extremities	Pink

A good mnemonic to use when thinking about the APGAR score is A, appearance (color); P, pulse (heart rate); G, grimace; A, activity (muscle tone); and R, respirations.

6 The answer is E *Surgery*

Spondylolysis (choice **E**) is a nondisplaced stress or traumatic fracture of the pars interarticularis. Sports with hyperextension maneuvers, such as gymnastics, involve the greatest risk. Lumbar spine extension exacerbates symptoms. Oblique x-ray films of the lumbosacral spine may show sclerosis or "scotty dog" at the pars interarticularis.

Acute lumbar strain (choice **A**) is associated with nonradiating pain in the lower back due to mechanical stress on the lumbar spine. Plain radiographs are normal, and symptoms usually resolve within 1–3 weeks. Scoliosis (choice **B**) is a lateral curvature of the spine. Except in severe cases, patients with scoliosis usually do not have back pain. Patients with herniated disk disease (choice **C**) may present with back pain, leg pain, or both. Symptoms are usually worsened with prolonged sitting, Valsalva maneuvers, and forward flexion. Sciatic tension tests are positive. Plain films are usually normal but may show disk space narrowing. In sacroiliac sprain syndrome (choice **D**), there is tenderness over the sacroiliac joint. There is usually no pain with hyperextension of the lumbosacral spine, and plain radiographs are normal.

7 The answer is E *Psychiatry*

Some antipsychotics are associated with increased weight gain. When a patient's BMI increases above 25 while on such medication, switching to newer antipsychotics with a lower potential for weight gain is the most accepted strategy. Aripiprazole (choice **E**) has less associated weight gain than olanzapine or clozapine (choice **C**). Although haloperidol (choice **D**) is not associated with weight gain, it has other side effects that are less common with newer medications. There is limited experience for adding an appetite suppressant such as sibutramine (choice **A**) in cases of antipsychotic-induced weight gain, and it is not a first-choice treatment. Decreasing the olanzapine dosage (choice **B**) risks a clinical relapse, and olanzapine dose is not closely associated with weight gain.

8 The answer is B *Preventive Medicine and Public Health*

Medical malpractice is a physician's error caused by deviation from an accepted standard of medical practice that results in harm to a patient (choice **B**). An unfavorable outcome alone (i.e., loss of physical function [choice **A**] or constant pain [choice **E**]) does not constitute malpractice. Lack of specialty board certification by a doctor is not relevant to whether a doctor committed malpractice (choice **C**). Loss of income (as well as pain and suffering) can be important in deciding the amount of the award in a malpractice case if the doctor is found liable, but it is not important in deciding whether malpractice was committed (choice **D**).

9 The answer is B *Pediatrics*

Phenytoin taken by a pregnant woman can cause nail hypoplasia, growth retardation, and a "Cupid's bow" lip (choice **B**). Valproic acid taken by a pregnant woman can cause spina bifida, facial abnormalities, and developmental delay (choice **A**). Isotretinoin is most teratogenic in the first trimester, and effects include brain malformations, microtia, thymic hypoplasia, and cardiac defects (choice **C**). Diethylstilbestrol (DES) is responsible for vaginal carcinoma and adenosis (choice **D**) as well as genitourinary anomalies in exposed males. Cocaine can cause smaller head circumference, growth retardation, and cerebral infarction (stroke) (choice **E**) when taken during pregnancy.

10 The answer is D *Psychiatry*

Nitrazepam (choice **D**), a benzodiazepine "date-rape" drug, produces rapid sedation, disinhibition, and amnesia, making a victim vulnerable to sexual assault, and lasts up to 8 hours. The medication can be obtained illicitly and can be placed surreptitiously in a drink.

Alcohol-induced amnestic disorder (choice **A**) is less likely because the woman denies drinking, and no alcohol is detected in her blood after only a few hours. Dissociative amnestic disorder (choice **B**) is less likely because the woman seems angry but quite comfortable with discussing the situation and eager to pursue investigation. Factitious disorder (choice **C**) is unlikely because the young woman doesn't seem to assume a dependent attitude. A seizure episode (choice **E**) is less likely because it doesn't explain her state of dress, and there are no other significant physical findings.

11 The answer is A *Pediatrics*

This is an innocent murmur, which is best heard in the supine position, not on the side (choice **C**). Innocent murmurs occur only in systole, never diastole. They are grade 1 to 2 of a possible 6 and are commonly heard along the lower left midsternal border (choice **A**) in children 3 to 7 years of age (rarely in infants [choice **B**]). The murmur can intensify with fever or excitement (not become less intense [choice **E**]) or after exercise; sitting up can make the murmur less intense. Innocent murmurs are just that—they have no cardiac significance (not a significant cardiac defect [choice **D**]), and treatment consists of reassurance of the parents.

12 The answer is A *Surgery*

Scaphoid (choice **A**) bone fractures constitute 60% of all wrist fractures and are most common in men between the ages of 20 and 40. The usual cause is a fall with an outstretched arm with the wrist flexed dorsally. The second most common cause is in automobile accidents where the arm and hand assume the same position but up against the dashboard. The fractures leave little or no swelling and sometimes can be overlooked even on x-ray films. Clinically, pain elicited by applying pressure on the anatomic snuff box has 90% sensitivity but only 40% specificity, while tenderness over the scaphoid tubercle has 87% specificity and 57% specificity. Thus, these tests raise a high degree of suspicion even in the absence of radiologic confirmation, and the wrist and thumb should be immobilized at least until further tests can be conducted. These tests may be a second x-ray film about 2 weeks later when early healing should enhance signs of fracture, a bone scan, a computed tomography (CT) scan, or a magnetic resonance imagining (MRI) study. Proper treatment is critical because the blood enters the bone from the top, making supplying blood to fractures that occur in the middle or lower part of the bone tenuous, which makes this bone subject to avascular necrosis. Surgery, sometime involving bone grafts, is required in displaced fractures or in cases of nonunion. Depending on where the fracture is and whether it is displaced, the hand and lower arm will be in a cast for at least several weeks and sometimes up to 3 to 6 months. Traumatic arthritis may be a long-term complication.

The hamate bone (choice **D**) is infrequently fractured in golfers. The lunate bone (choice **B**) is more commonly dislocated than fractured. It can be associated with avascular necrosis (Kienböck's disease). The triquetrum (choice **C**) and capitate (choice **E**) bones are protected and are very infrequently fractured.

13 The answer is E   *Psychiatry*

Volunteerism, an essential feature of informed consent for research, may be compromised because the patient may feel coerced into participation because he faces discharge and homelessness if he declines (choice **E**). The other two essential features of informed consent are information sharing and decisional capacity, which is the ability to rationally think through the choices. Financial compensation for research (choice **A**) is common and not necessarily unethical. Formal testing of cognitive capacity for informed consent (choice **B**) is not required in most situations. Schizophrenia does not necessarily preclude the ability to give informed consent (choice **C**). Researchers who are not also treating the subject (choice **D**) can ethically obtain informed consent.

14 The answer is E   *Pediatrics*

Wilms' tumor is the most common renal neoplasm in children. Prognosis depends on staging; the 4-year relapse-free survival rate for all stages is approximately 60% (choice **D**). Stages I through III have a cure rate that fluctuates from 88 to 98%. Wilms' tumor is associated with congenital anomalies. Aniridia (choice **E**) occurs in 1.1% of patients; a deletion in chromosome 11 (not chromosome 6 [choice **C**]) was found in family members of children with aniridia and Wilms' tumor. Wilms' tumor usually presents as a unilateral abdominal mass, often discovered by the parent or during a routine physical examination. Diagnosis is usually made when the child is approximately 3 years of age. Hypertension (not hypotension [choice **A**]) is seen in approximately 60% of patients. Lung metastases (not bone metastases [choice **B**]) are seen in 5 to 10% of patients at the time of diagnosis. Treatment is surgical removal followed by chemotherapy and occasionally radiotherapy.

15 The answer is D   *Surgery*

Of the choices listed, negative results of estrogen and progesterone receptor assay (ERA/PRA, choice **D**) is the most important negative prognostic indicator for this patient. Patients with tumors that are ERA/PRA positive have a better remission rate (60–80% response rate) than those with ERA/PRA-negative neoplasms. Absence of steroid hormone receptors indicates a poor prognosis in addition to the fact that the patient will not be receptive to hormonal therapy (e.g., tamoxifen). The lack of a progesterone receptor has a more significant negative prognostic value than an absent estrogen receptor. However, overall, the stage of breast cancer is the single most reliable indicator of prognosis.

The generally accepted standard for staging is the TNM system. The *T* factor relates to the tumor (i.e., whether the tumor is in situ and its size), the *N* factor relates to potential lymph node involvement, and the *M* factor relates to distant metastasis. For example, stage I cases have a 92 to 96% 5-year survival rate, whereas the rate is 5 to 14% in stage IV cases. Lymph node status alone is an important prognostic index. For example, women with no nodal involvement have an 80% 5-year survival rate; with one to three nodes involved, a 50% rate; and with four or more nodes involved, a 20% rate.

Flow cytometric analysis (choice **A**) can be used to determine the S-phase fraction and the ploidy of the tumor. A high (>12%) S-phase fraction indicates high proliferative activity and a poorer prognosis. Aneuploidy is also a negative prognostic factor. This patient's tumor has only 4% of the cells in the S phase and is diploid, which are not negative prognostic indices. The location of the tumor (choice **B**) is also of some, but limited, prognostic value. The closer the tumor is located to an axillary lymph node, the greater the chance of lymph node involvement and the poorer the prognosis. This patient's tumor is located in the upper outer quadrant, where most breast tissue is normally located and consequently is of little prognostic value. No amplification (increased activity) of the *erb-b2* oncogene (choice **C**) is a good prognostic factor. Amplification of the oncogene is associated with a bad prognosis. Tumor size (choice **E**) is one of the components of the TNM staging system, and like lymph node involvement has great prognostic significance. This patient's tumor is relatively small; therefore, size is not a negative prognostic factor. A tumor larger than 2 cm would have been a very bad prognostic sign, because tumors of this size have usually invaded and metastasized.

16 The answer is E *Psychiatry*

None of the choices listed are reasons to avoid initiation of atomoxetine (choice **E**). The boy's symptoms strongly suggest attention-deficit/hyperactivity disorder (ADHD), an indication for which atomoxetine is specifically approved (choice **A**). Preschool children (choice **B**) are often started on medications for ADHD when symptoms are not manageable by other means. Anxiety symptoms (choice **C**) and tics (choice **D**) are not contraindications to atomoxetine or psychostimulants, another common treatment option.

17 The answer is E *Surgery*

The patient has a capillary hemangioma (strawberry nevus). Capillary hemangiomas occur more often in females than in males. They usually appear at 2 months of age and generally grow rapidly during the next 6 months. The lesion is bright red, protuberant, compressible, and sharply demarcated. Although the course of a particular lesion is unpredictable, 60% involute completely by the fifth year, and 90 to 95% by the ninth year. Therefore, except under unusual circumstances, treatment is not necessary (choice **E**). The physician's primary role is to provide reassurance.

Cryotherapy (choice **A**) has not been proved effective. Flashlamp-pumped pulsed-laser therapy (choice **B**) can be used to reduce growth and may be recommended therapy for ulcerated hemangioma but not the general case. Capillary hemangiomas should not be confused with nevus flammeus (port-wine stain), which is always present at birth, does not spontaneously involute, and may be associated with the Sturge-Weber syndrome or other syndromes. A port-wine stain is usually best treated with flashlamp-pumped pulsed-laser therapy. Surgical excision (choice **C**) is usually contraindicated, because it will leave a scar and more importantly may not completely remove the lesion, in which case it tends to reoccur. Radiation therapy (choice **D**) may also cause scarring and other complications and should be used only in life-threatening situations, which are rare.

18 The answer is G *Medicine*

This man is suffering from early parkinsonism. Most commonly this is due to Parkinson's disease, a condition of unknown etiology that generally starts between the ages of 45 and 65. Parkinson's disease is a heterogenous and progressive condition that has tremor, rigidity, bradykinesia, and postural instability as its cardinal features. Cases tend to fall into one of two major subtypes. In one group, tremor is the major symptom; in the other, postural instability and gait difficulty predominate. Even though symptoms do overlap, most patients clearly fall to the greatest extent into one or the other subcategory. Patients with predominantly tremor-type symptoms tend to have a slower progression of symptoms, have less trouble with bradykinesia, and less often develop severe mental symptoms. Other symptoms in more advanced cases include infrequent blinking, a blank stare, a shuffling gait with rapid acceleration and difficulty stopping once started, increased salivation, and severe depression or even dementia. No one patient needs to develop all symptoms, and patients who have early symptoms of gait disturbances progress more rapidly and are more apt to develop the more severe symptoms. The underlying pathology is dopamine depletion due to degeneration of the nigrostriatal system. This leads to an imbalance between acetylcholine and dopamine neurotransmission. The cornerstone of treatment is dopamine replacement coupled to blockage of the acetylcholine system. Unfortunately resistance to ceratin key drugs develops with use. Therefore, there is an attempt to refrain from using them as long as possible. Thus watchful waiting (choice **G**) is typically used until symptoms interfere with the patient's normal lifestyle. This patient clearly states that his tremor does not impinge upon his normal lifestyle.

Once it is decided some medical intervention will be of value, amantadine (choice **A**) is typically the first drug to be used while symptoms are still minimal. This antiviral drug helps to improve muscle control and reduce stiffness; its mode of action is not understood, but it is hypothesized to help release dopamine from nerve endings. Its effect is always less than profound, and the benefit further decreases with use. Anticholinergics (choice **B**) also are used to treat early parkinsonism, sometimes in conjunction with amantadine. Again, drug resistance develops, and these drugs are generally administered in increasing doses until the adverse effects outweigh the benefits. Thus eventually it becomes necessary to use the most effective treatment, namely, dopamine replacement. However, dopamine cannot cross the blood–brain barrier. Consequently, it is usually administered as Sinemet, a preparation that contains levodopa (choice **C**) and carbidopa (choice **D**) in fixed proportions. The levodopa is converted to dopamine in the body and the carbidopa inhibits the enzyme that converts levodopa to dopamine. But carbidopa cannot cross the blood–brain barrier; thus, by administering the two together there is both more levodopa available, and some of the adverse peripheral effects of dopamine—such as nausea, vomiting, hypotension, and cardiac irregularities—are avoided. Long-term administration of levodopa induces untoward CNS effects including dyskinesias, restlessness, confusion, and behavioral changes. Still later during therapy the so-called on–off phenomena may occur, in which severity of parkinsonism may quickly increase at any time of the day. Dopamine agonists (choice **E**) that act directly on dopamine receptors were once only used to reduce the symptoms associated with this on–off action associated with long-term levodopa use. However, with the advent of newer dopamine agonists that are not derived from ergot, such agonists are now used to help treat early Parkinson's disease and to keep the levodopa dose (via Sinemet) at a minimal level as long as possible. Selegiline (choice **F**) is an irreversible monoamine oxidase B (MAO-B) inhibitor. MAO-B selectively deaminates dopamine and phenethylamine (chocolate's amphetamine). Selegiline is sometimes used as an adjunct treatment with the idea of reducing symptom fluctuations associated with long-term levodopa therapy.

19 The answer is A *Medicine*

Xeroderma pigmentosum (choice **A**) is a relatively rare collection of mutations with an autosomal recessive mode of transmission that affect one of the seven *XP* genes, *XP-A* through *XP-G*. The normal products of these genes are enzymes that excise pyridine dimers (primarily thymine) formed by exposure to ultraviolet light and then repair the gap created. The overall prevalence in the United States and Europe is 1 case per 250,000 people. It is about 10 times more common among the Japanese. The normal repair process is started by the XP-A gene product, an endonuclease that identifies the problem, and nicks the DNA strand on the 5′ side of the dimer. This cut is followed by a series of reactions in which the nicked dimer is extended by polymerase activity on the 3′ side, another endonuclease then removes the dimer along with any excess DNA, and finally a DNA ligase seals the remaining gap. A defect in any step in this process can cause xeroderma pigmentosum; however, a mutation in the *XP-A* genes is the most common cause, and a mutation in the *XP-E* genes is the least common. Mutations in the *XP-G* gene cause the most severe cases, in the *XP-F* gene, the least severe. Historically, about 40% of affected individuals die before their 20th birthday. Some limited success in treatment with retinoids or gene therapy has been reported.

In ataxia telangiectasia (choice **B**) poor balance due to cerebellar degeneration becomes evident by the second year, and by their teen years, most are wheelchair dependent. Affected individuals also have serious immunologic problems resulting in recurrent infections, diabetes, and of course telangiectasia; about 10% develop premature cancer. The mutation is transmitted as an autosomal recessive trait and affects a gene product that normally blocks the cell cycle to provide time for DNA repair. In the Unites States the prevalence is 1 case per 40,000 to 100,000 persons.

Bloom syndrome (choice **C**) children have telangiectasia, are photosensitive, suffer from growth retardation starting prenatally, have a birdlike facies, have mental retardation, and develop early cancers, commonly leukemia by the age of 22 years. It is due to a mutation at 15q26.1 that can be transmitted as a recessive trait and which affects a DNA gyrase and leads to sister chromosome exchange and chromosomal instability. It is very rare; about 100 cases have been reported in the United States.

Cockayne syndrome (choice **D**) has two major criteria, growth retardation below the 5th percentile and delayed developmental milestones (walking, talking, etc.). These are accompanied by metal retardation and microcephaly. In addition there are sensory nerve defects (deafness), cataracts, bad teeth, "Mickey Mouse" ears, small chin, a sharp birdlike nose, lack of adipose tissue, sunken eyes, and a wizened appearance that looks like premature aging. They are hypersensitive to UV radiation but in most cases not to the extent exhibited in xeroderma nor are they prone to cancer. Most die of respiratory failure or some other complication before reaching their teens. About 25% of cases are type 1, which usually presents at about the first year and is caused by a mutation on a gene called *CS-A*. The remainder are type 2 (a congenital form) due to a mutation in *CS-B*. In a few cases, one of the xeroderma pigmentosum genes are also affected. Once again these mutations can be inherited as autosomal recessive traits that inhibit DNA repair, in this case transcriptionally coupled repair.

Fanconi anemia (choice **E**) (not to be confused with Fanconi syndrome) is due to a recessively transmitted mutation that affects any one of 11 different proteins that are part of a large complex involved with ubiquitination of D_2-protein, a factor involved in DNA repair. It results in fragile chromosomes that cause aplastic anemia and eventually bone marrow failure; death by the age of 30 years is common. The prevalence is about 1 case per 360,000 persons in the general U.S. population, but it is about ten times more prevalent among Ashkenazi Jews.

Trichodystrophy (choice **F**) is an extremely rare condition with some 25 known cases worldwide. It results in sulfur-deficient hair that is very brittle, delayed development, ataxia ichthyosis, stunted growth, and photosensitivity.

20 The answer is D *Surgery*

The patient has a strangulated indirect hernia (choice **D**). Extreme pain related to a hernia in the absence of vascular compromise is unusual; generally occurring only when the blood supply of the contents of the sac is compromised, and it becomes gangrenous. This is a medical emergency, and death is a common outcome if not operated upon within a short time after onset of symptoms.

A reducible hernia (choice **A**) is one in which the contents of the sac can be returned to the abdomen manually or even spontaneously. An incarcerated hernia (choice **B**), also called an irreducible hernia, is one in which the contents cannot be returned to the abdomen, generally because they are trapped by a narrow neck. An incarcerated hernia is not necessarily obstructed or strangulated; however, incarceration is required for obstruction or strangulation to occur. An obstructed hernia (choice **C**) is one in which the lumen of a segment of the bowel is compromised within the sac, but has not yet become strangulated. A Richter hernia (choice **E**) is a rare and dangerous type of hernia. It occurs when part of the circumference of the bowel becomes incarcerated or strangulated. This piece may easily be overlooked at operation and may subsequently perforate, causing peritonitis.

21 The answer is D *Psychiatry*

Clinical experience has shown that psychologic states do not necessary represent discretely ordered stages, but may be experienced repeatedly and in different orders during the coping process (choice **D**). Kübler-Ross described a stage theory of psychologic changes associated with coping with death. She believed that the stages occurred in a set order: denial/disbelief, anger, bargaining, depression, and acceptance. These stages have subsequently been widely applied to other situations characterized by grieving and loss. More recent work has shown that environmental factors heavily influence grieving stages (choice **A**). Nevertheless, Kübler-Ross's insights continue to assist caregiver in providing help to persons who are dealing with loss (choice **B**). There is no set timing for progressing through stages, and persons commonly have more trouble resolving one or another psychologic state (choice **C**). As noted above, the stages are no longer considered to be invariably experienced in a set order (choice **E**).

22 The answer is E *Pediatrics*

Febrile seizures rarely progress to epilepsy (choice **B**). They do, however, have a 50% chance of recurrence. Seizures are rare before 9 months (choice **E**) or after 5 years of age, with a peak onset between 14 and 18 months. There is usually a strong family history of febrile seizures (choice **D**). Seizures are generalized and tonic–clonic, not focal (choice **A**), and they usually last no longer than 15 minutes. The seizure is associated with a rapidly rising temperature, and often there is an associated viral infection or otitis media. Febrile seizures are not associated with underlying neurologic problems (choice **C**). Treatment consists of antipyretics.

23 The answer is E *Preventive Medicine and Public Health*

The question relates to assessing group differences between two groups of a continuous variable, which in this question is height. If the comparison were among three groups, analysis of variance (choice **B**) would be correct.

With two groups, it is necessary to use Student's *t*-test (choice **E**). A correlation coefficient (choice **C**) assesses the strength of association, not the differences between groups. The chi-squared test (choice **D**) assesses differences between groups of categorical variables. Logistic regression (choice **A**) is used to assess a categorical outcome for a continuous predictor.

24 The answer is C *Psychiatry*

Assertive Community Treatment (ACT) is an evidence-based treatment model characterized by 24/7 availability of mental health and social services delivered in the field and provided by a multidisciplinary clinical team (choice **C**). It has been shown to be effective in improving the integration of individuals with serious mental illness into the community.

The program is flexible and practical and is not characterized by operant conditioning (choice **A**). ACT is generally not court ordered and is often provided on a voluntary basis (choice **B**). Services are often provided outside traditional clinic settings (choice **D**). Individuals receiving ACT services are encouraged to fully integrate within the community and avoid reliance on a specific group of individuals with similar problems (choice **E**).

25 The answer is D *Pediatrics*

The patient has hereditary fructose intolerance. Table sugar (choice **D**) is sucrose, which is converted to glucose and fructose by sucrase, a brush border disaccharidase. Fructose is eliminated from the diet in patients with hereditary fructose intolerance, which is an autosomal recessive disorder associated with a deficiency of aldolase B. Aldolase B converts fructose 1-phosphate to glyceraldehyde 3-phosphate, which is used as a substrate for glycolysis in the fed state or a substrate for gluconeogenesis in the fasting state. A deficiency of aldolase B causes an increase in fructose 1-phosphate and fructose concentrations and a decrease in glyceraldehyde 3-phosphate. An increase in fructose 1-phosphate damages the liver (jaundice, cirrhosis) and kidneys (aminoaciduria). Fructose is excreted in the urine (fructosuria). Fasting hypoglycemia causes a decrease in glyceraldehyde 3-phosphate level. Products containing fructose must be eliminated from the diet (e.g., table sugar, corn syrup, fruits, fruit juices, and honey).

Branched-chain amino acids (leucine, isoleucine, valine) (choice **A**) should be excluded from the diet of patients with maple syrup urine disease, which is an autosomal recessive disease caused by a deficiency of branched-chain α-ketoacid dehydrogenase. Deficiency of the enzyme causes an increase in branched-chain amino acids and their corresponding ketoacids in the urine, the latter causing the urine to smell like maple syrup (not present in this patient). There is also a decrease in succinyl-CoA and acetyl-CoA. Feeding difficulties, vomiting, seizures (edema and demyelination in the brain), and hypoglycemia (deficiency of succinyl-CoA) occur in the first weeks of life. Dairy products (choice **B**) should be eliminated from the diet of patients with galactosemia, an autosomal recessive disease with a deficiency of galactose-1-phosphate uridyltransferase (GALT). Lactase converts lactose in dairy products to glucose and galactose. Galactose is converted by galactase to galactose-1-phosphate, which is further metabolized to glucose-1-phosphate by GALT. Glucose-1-phosphate is converted to glucose-6-phosphate, which is used as a substrate for glycolysis in the fasting state or gluconeogenesis in the fed state. Deficiency of GALT causes an increase in galactose-1-phosphate, galactose, and galactitol (sugar alcohol) and a decrease in glucose-1-phosphate. An increase in galactose-1-phosphate damages the brain (mental retardation) and the liver (cirrhosis). Excess galactose (not fructose) is excreted in the urine (galactosuria) and some is converted to galactitol by aldose reductase in the lens and causes cataracts. Phenylalanine (choice **C**) is increased in patients with phenylketonuria, which is caused by a deficiency of phenylalanine hydroxylase. This enzyme converts phenylalanine to tyrosine. Deficiency of the enzyme causes an increase in phenylalanine and neurotoxic phenyl-ketones and acids and a decrease in tyrosine. Patients usually have a mousey odor due to the phenylketones and their acids (not present in this patient). The treatment is to reduce dietary phenylalanine to a very low level and to replace it with tyrosine. Tyrosine (choice **E**) is eliminated from the diet of patients with tyrosinosis, an autosomal recessive disease caused by a deficiency of fumarylacetoacetate hydrolase. Deficiency of the enzyme causes an increase in tyrosine, which causes damage to the liver (cirrhosis, hepatocellular carcinoma) and kidneys (aminoaciduria). Tyrosine crystals are present in the urine (not present in this patient).

26 The answer is B *Surgery*

The available data suggest that this patient has bilateral adrenal pheochromocytomas. Multiple endocrine neoplasia type 2A (MEN-2A) is a triad of inherited neoplasms including medullary carcinoma of the thyroid, pheochromocytoma, and parathyroid hyperplasia/adenoma (accounting for the hypercalcemia). This rare syndrome has been reported in families of patients with medullary thyroid carcinoma and should be considered in all patients who have either a pheochromocytoma or medullary carcinoma of the thyroid. Patients with medullary carcinoma of the thyroid have a high incidence of pheochromocytomas, often bilateral. This trait is inherited in an autosomal dominant fashion and may result from a single defect or a combination of defects in the neural crest tissue. Any of the neoplasms making up the syndrome may produce the initial symptoms, but the thyroid tumor is present in 100% of those with MEN-2A. Approximately 40% of patients have pheochromocytomas, and 60% have parathyroid hyperplasia. The medullary thyroid carcinoma in this syndrome does not differ from a spontaneous carcinoma without associated endocrinopathies. The outcome of patients with MEN-2A depends on the course of the thyroid carcinoma. Medullary carcinoma of the thyroid is usually aggressive; it metastasizes to cervical lymph nodes, and it can exhibit rapid hematologic dissemination. The pheochromocytomas of MEN-2A are generally discovered in the second and third decades of life and have a bilateral incidence as high as 70%. The lesion is usually contained within the adrenal medulla and is almost always benign. In this patient, the metastatic lesions in the liver most likely represent widespread dissemination from an aggressive medullary carcinoma of the thyroid (choice **B**) rather than changes originating from the kidney (choice **A**), parathyroid (choice **C**), ovary (choice **D**), or adrenal (choice **E**).

27 **The answer is C** *Medicine*

Presently, some 60 million Americans are taking medication for hypertension, but less than 1% will undergo accelerated malignant hypertension, more simply known as a hypertensive crisis, defined as systolic pressure greater than 230 mm Hg and/or a diastolic pressure above 130 mm Hg. Hypertensive crises are divided into hypertensive emergencies associated with end-organ damage and hypertensive urgencies in the absence of evidence of end-organ damage. In a hypertensive emergency, the blood pressure must be brought down as quickly as possible, within minutes to hours by intravenous (IV) drug administration, usually in an intensive care unit. For hypertensive urgency, the pressure is usually brought down more slowly, often by oral administration of nitroprusside. Hypertensive crises can be generated by many mechanisms including an anxiety attack, pheochromocytoma, renal tumors, acute glomerulonephritis, preeclampsia, eclampsia, head injuries, licit drugs such as tricyclic antidepressants, illicit drugs such as cocaine, amphetamines, etc., and sudden withdrawal from antihypertensive agents, clonidine in particular. Normally some detective work is required to determine the triggering mechanism but in this case it clearly is sudden withdrawal from clonidine, with perhaps a concomitant effect of acebutolol withdrawal, since the simultaneous withdrawal of a β-blocker and clonidine acts synergistically. Thus, since in the case described, with no end-organ damage, there is withdrawal from clonidine, it is safe to conclude that he is in a hypertensive urgency condition due to sudden withdrawal of clonidine (choice **C**). In addition to treating him, he should be advised that when traveling by air, to always carry his medication with him.

He is undergoing a hypertensive emergency due to sudden withdrawal of clonidine (choice **A**) is not true because there is no evidence of end-organ damage. He is undergoing a hypertensive crisis due to sudden withdrawal of hydrochlorothiazide (choice **B**) is not likely, since hydrochlorothiazide withdrawal is not known to cause a crisis. His blood pressure must be reduced to normal levels within minutes by administration of IV nitroprusside (choice **D**) might be true if he were suffering from a hypertensive emergency, which he isn't. He should be provided with his usual medications and sent home (choice **E**) would be grounds for a malpractice suit; the longer his organs are exposed to such excess blood pressure, the more likely that damage will occur. Moreover, it is important to monitor his response to therapy closely, at least until the pressure falls to more acceptable levels.

28 **The answer is C** *Surgery*

Malignant hyperthermia may occur as a result of almost any anesthetic agent and can be triggered by stress alone. Early clinical signs are tachycardia, muscle rigidity, metabolic acidosis, and hypercarbia. However, the earliest manifestation of this hypermetabolic state is an elevation of the end-tidal carbon dioxide level. Fever may also occur. Once the diagnosis of acute malignant hyperthermia is made, anesthetics should be discontinued, the patient should be hyperventilated with 100% oxygen, cooled and dantrolene should be administered (choice **C**). The operation should not proceed (choice **A**). This patient with presumed appendicitis should be treated with antibiotics rather than risking additional exposure to anesthetic agents. Performing a tracheostomy (choice **B**) is unnecessary. Administering a third-generation cephalosporin (choice **E**) would not be an appropriate next step. Increasing the depth of anesthesia (choice **D**) would be fatal.

29 **The answer is B** *Medicine*

This man has had type 1 diabetes for decades, meaning he synthesizes no endogenous insulin at all. Furthermore, he has missed his normal insulin injections two consecutive times; meaning his plasma insulin levels are essentially depleted. The absence of insulin prohibits the entry of glucose into muscle or adipose cells. However, having just finished breakfast he will have ample liver glycogen stores. Accordingly, as he exercises liver glycogen will be converted to free plasma glucose that cannot be used by muscle, and the net result will be that his plasma glucose concentration will be higher after shoveling than it was before starting (choice **B**).

Obviously, for the reasons discussed above, under these conditions his plasma glucose concentration cannot be lower after shoveling than it was before starting (choice **A**). However, had there been a residual insulin reserve or if he were a type 2 diabetic, shoveling snow would lower plasma glucose levels, and he would be in danger of hypoglycemia. The difference being that the available insulin would permit glucose uptake by muscle cells. His plasma ketone body concentration would also increase not be lower (choice **C**) after shoveling snow, because free fatty acids would still be released from adipose tissue and be converted to ketones in the liver, but their metabolism would be inhibited since their metabolism requires pyruvate, a slight variation on the old theme of "fat burns in the flame of carbohydrate." Choice **D** is incorrect on two accounts: first, GLUT-5 promotes fructose not glucose transport, and second, recruitment of GLUT-4, the muscle cell's glucose transporter, requires insulin. Exercise may stimulate cortisol production, but cortisol is one of the "counterregulatory" glucogenic hormones, which act to increase not decrease glucose levels (choice **E**).

30 **The answer is E** *Psychiatry*

The FDA "black box warning" for antidepressants states that families of children with suicidal thoughts should be advised by the caregiver of the need for close observation and communication with the prescriber (choice **E**). This was because pooled analyses of short-term placebo-controlled trials of antidepressants in children and adolescents revealed a greater risk of suicidal thinking or behavior during the first few months of treatment in those receiving antidepressants. The average risk of such events on drug was 4%, twice the risk on placebo. The FDA did not recommend that children taking any particular antidepressants be switched to other antidepressants if suicidal thinking develops (choices **A** and **B**), nor did it recommend that otherwise normal children should not be started on antidepressants if suicidal thinking is initially present (choice **C**). The FDA did not recommend that antidepressants should be withheld from children with psychosis and suicidal thinking (choice **D**).

31 **The answer is E** *Medicine*

Both Raynaud's disease and Raynaud's phenomenon are characterized by intermittent attacks of pallor progressing to cyanosis and then to rubor upon recovery, and sometimes these color changes are accompanied by paresthesia, numbness, and mild swelling. In Raynaud's disease (choice **E**), the attacks are limited to the hands and fingers, and symptoms are symmetrical. To be diagnosed as Raynaud's disease the condition must be idiopathic and no other underlying condition, including those excluded in the vignette must be present or become present within a 3-year time span. The disease is estimated to affect 10% of the general population, usually first makes itself evident between 15 and 45 years of age, and affects women 80% of the time. Although annoying, the disease is usually benign and does not progress with time. As a rule, the extent of treatment required is to try to keep the hands warm.

Raynaud's phenomenon (choice **A**) is associated with similar symptoms usually affecting the hands but not necessarily symmetrically and sometimes affecting other parts of the anatomy such as the nose. The basic difference between the disease and the phenomenon is that the latter is always associated with one of the conditions excluded in the vignette. Since Raynaud's phenomenon may be the first symptom of any one of these often-serious conditions, the patient's concern is justified; nonetheless Raynaud's disease is relatively common, whereas most of the conditions associated with Raynaud's phenomenon are relatively rare. Because Raynaud's phenomenon is associated with an underlying condition, symptoms usually wax or wane depending upon progress of that condition. Treatment with vasodilators or other drugs may be required and, in extreme cases, even sympathectomy. Livedo reticularis (choice **B**) is a condition in many respects similar to Raynaud's disease; it too is a vasospastic disease of unknown etiology, but it results in a fishnet-like mottled pattern of discoloration covering large area of the extremities, particularly evident on the thighs. Usually there is a pale central core surrounded by reticulated cyanotic areas. It affects adult men and women equally and may present at any age. As a rule it is benign but in a minority of cases there is underlying pathology, including: malignancy, polyarteritis nodosa, atherosclerotic microemboli, or antiphospholipid antibody syndrome. Treatment again is protection from the cold. Acrocyanosis (choice **C**) is an uncommon condition characterized by vasospasms leading to cyanosis of the hands and feet and less commonly the arms and legs. It is associated with arterial constriction combined with dilation of the subpapillary venous plexus of the skin, through which deoxygenated blood slowly passes. Once again it is worsened by cold. It is most common in women in their teens and twenties and may improve with age or pregnancy. Disability does not occur. Primary erythromelalgia (choice **D**) is an idiopathic condition caused by vasodilation rather than constriction. Symptoms are induced by warm (not cold) environments or exercise and consist of erythema, a feeling of unusual warmth, and even a burning sensation that may last from minutes to hours. This most often occurs on the soles of the feet or palms of the hand but may extend into the limbs. Treatment consists of cooling and elevating the affected area. Aspirin, 650 mg every 4–6 hours, acts prophylactically and is in effect diagnostic. Secondary erythromelalgia is associated with an underlying condition such as polycythemia vera, hypertension, gout, or neurologic disease.

32 **The answer is C**   *Medicine*

The patient has nodular sclerosing Hodgkin's lymphoma (choice **C**), which is the most common subtype of Hodgkin's lymphoma and the type that is more common in women than men. The abnormal cells described in the histologic examination of the lymph node are Reed-Sternberg cells, which are the neoplastic cells found in Hodgkin's lymphoma. It is a large, multilobed cell with prominent nucleoli surrounded by a halo of clear nucleoplasm. They are essential for diagnosing Hodgkin's lymphoma. The classic presentation of nodular sclerosing Hodgkin's lymphoma is nodal involvement of the anterior mediastinum plus one other lymph node group above the diaphragm (e.g., right supraclavicular node, cervical node). The prognosis in Hodgkin's lymphoma correlates with the stage of the disease and the type of Hodgkin's lymphoma. This patient has stage IIA, in which two or more lymph node regions are involved on the same side of the diaphragm. The upper case letter A indicates absence of fever above 38°C (100.4°F), drenching night sweats, and weight loss above 10% of body weight within the preceding 6 months. An upper case letter B indicates presence of the above findings. The treatment involves the use of combination chemotherapy (e.g., doxorubicin, bleomycin, vincristine, dacarbazine) and radiation to the nodal areas. Complications related to this therapy include second malignancies (e.g., acute nonlymphocytic leukemia, B cell non-Hodgkin's lymphoma).

Burkitt's lymphoma (choice **A**) is characterized by a diffuse infiltrate of small, round B lymphocytes interspersed with pale-staining macrophages and apoptotic bodies. Follicular B-cell lymphoma (choice **B**) is a common non-Hodgkin's lymphoma in adults, which is characterized by a nodular or diffuse pattern of nodal involvement. The neoplastic cells, which arise from the germinal follicle, are primarily small and cleaved. Metastatic cancer (choice **D**) is the most common malignancy of the lymph nodes, but it is an uncommon cause of nodal enlargement in patients younger than 30 years. Reactive lymphadenitis (choice **E**) is associated with painful lymphadenopathy, but the enlarged lymph node in this patient was painless (indicating a malignant process). Reactive lymphadenitis is caused by an inflammatory condition (e.g., tonsillitis or rheumatoid arthritis). Nodal enlargement is caused by hyperplasia of B cells, T cells, histiocytes, or a combination of these.

33 **The answer is C**   *Medicine*

Quinidine (choice **C**) is a group IA antiarrhythmic drug. It prolongs the action potential and mainly acts on the sodium channels. However, it can enhance conduction through the atrioventricular (AV) node because of its vagolytic effects and, therefore, could actually increase ventricular response during atrial fibrillation.

Digoxin (choice **A**), by means of its parasympathomimetic action, decreases AV conduction velocity and also slows ventricular rate by increasing the refractory period at the AV node. Metoprolol (choice **B**) induces β blockade, thus reducing cyclic adenosine monophosphate (cAMP) levels; this decreases sodium and calcium currents. As a result, conduction through the AV node is slowed, and ventricular response is decreased. Verapamil (choice **D**) and diltiazem (choice **E**) are first-generation calcium channel blockers that induce depression of calcium currents in tissues (such as those generated in the AV node) that require the participation of calcium channels (L-type). As a result, the refractory period is increased, and conduction velocity is decreased.

34 **The answer is C**   *Pediatrics*

This girl has rubella also known as 3-day or German measles (choice **C**). This condition can present with joint manifestations in older children, particularly in older girls and women; recently, most new cases have been in teenagers and young adults. The joints of the hand and wrist are most commonly involved. The prodromal catarrhal stage is shorter than that of measles (rubeola) (choice **A**). Lymphadenopathy is the most characteristic sign, specifically of the posterior occipital, retroauricular, and posterior cervical lymph nodes. The rash begins on the face and spreads quickly but also disappears quickly, usually within 3 days. Desquamation is minimal compared to that of rubeola.

Infectious mononucleosis (choice **B**) may manifest with fever, myalgia, generalized lymphadenopathy (most commonly cervical), and sore throat. A generalized maculopapular rash appears in patients taking ampicillin. Arthralgia is not seen in infectious mononucleosis. The rash of erythema infectiosum (choice **D**) is characteristic. Initially it has a "slapped face" appearance. It spreads to the trunk and arms as a macular rash that later develops a central clearing and finally appears fine and reticulated. The arthropathy of erythema infectiosum can range from diffuse arthralgias with morning stiffness to frank arthritis. Children infected with human herpesvirus (HHV) 6 or 7 have roseola (exanthema subitum) (choice **E**) and present with fever followed by a rash. The lesion is maculopapular, starting on the trunk and spreading to the extremities and neck (mildly affecting the face and legs). Lymphadenopathy, respiratory symptoms, or mild diarrhea may appear, but arthralgias do not occur.

35 The answer is C *Medicine*

Electrocardiogram (ECG) traces obtained from patients with atrial fibrillation (choice **C**) include the absence of an obvious P wave and an irregular response of QRS complexes, as illustrated. Intraatrial contractions are very rapid, many in the 300–600 beats per minute (bpm) range. Typically, the intraventricular rate ranges irregularly between 80 and 180 bpm, the final rate depending on the number of atrial beats blocked by the atrioventricular node. Atrial fibrillation is the most common chronic arrhythmia, with a prevalence that increases with age; there is 10% prevalence among individuals in their 80s. The cause is often idiopathic; although it can also be initiated by valvular diseases, dilated cardiomyopathy, atrial septal defect, hypertension, or coronary artery disease, it also may be the presenting sign in thyrotoxicosis, be associated with pulmonary disease, be caused by chest trauma, or by administration of theophyline or β-adrenergic agonists, and, most relevant for the case presented, by acute alcohol excess and withdrawal. This latter presentation is sometimes termed "holiday heart"; once stabilized it usually is transient and self-limiting. The most serious complication of chronic atrial fibrillation is thrombus formation due to blood stasis in the atria and consequent embolization, with the most drastic consequence being a stroke.

Atrial flutter (choice **A**) is accompanied by 250 to 350 atrial impulses per minute. Only every second, third or fourth beat is transmitted to the ventricle, resulting in a heart rate of some 150 bpm. ECG traces show characteristic saw-toothed flutter waves. Atrial flutter is less common than atrial fibrillation and most often is found in association with chronic obstructive pulmonary disease (COPD). Although it too increases the risk of embolus formation, the risk is considerably lower than that for atrial fibrillation, because of the persistence of atrial contraction. Chaotic atrial tachycardia (choice **B**) is a disease associated with severe COPD. It is marked by varying P wave morphology and very irregular PP intervals. The rate is usually between 100 and 140 bpm. Atrial ventricular junctional rhythm (choice **D**) refers to conditions in which the atrial–nodal junction or the nodal–His bundle junctions assume a pacemaker function. Usually they maintain a rate of 40 to 60 bpm, and the rate responds normally to exercise. Ventricular tachycardia (choice **E**) is defined as three or more consecutive premature ventricular beats. ECG changes show wide QRS complexes with no discernible P waves. The pulse rate is greater than 120 bpm, and the patient may report palpitations and dizziness. Syncope or circulatory collapse may occur, and hypotensive ventricular tachycardia must be treated immediately with synchronized direct current shock and lidocaine. This can potentially be a life-threatening event and should be treated. However, ventricular tachycardia may also be nonsymptomatic, in which case it may not need to be treated.

36 The answer is B *Medicine*

Pneumonia is the most common serious infection among elders living in the community or in nursing homes and the second most common among hospitalized elderly patients (urinary tract infections are more common in the hospital setting). This woman has acquired a case of pneumonia while in the hospital (defined as pneumonia that develops 48 or more hours after admission), an all-too-common sequela to a broken hip. The mortality rate for hospital-acquired pneumonia among seniors is between 20 and 50%, making it the leading cause of death from nosocomial infections. Hospital-acquired cases are apt to differ from community-acquired ones in several respects: the patient is liable to be in poorer health; the responsible organism is more likely to be antibiotic resistant since it developed in an environment where antibiotics are frequently used; and the organism is less likely to be *Streptococcus pneumoniae* the organism that accounts for 60–80% of all community-acquired cases of bacterial pneumonias in the general population, for some 40–60% of cases among community-based elderly persons, and a still smaller percentage among hospitalized seniors. This is because bacterial species that are rarely found in the community are more commonly encountered in a hospital setting. Consequently, when treating a hospitalized patient, in particular an elderly one, it is necessary to think beyond *S. pneumoniae* (choice **C**) and in fact it can essentially be excluded in patients such as the one described who received the pneumococcal vaccine more than 3 weeks and less than 5 years earlier. *Haemophilus influenzae* and *Klebsiella pneumoniae* infection follow as the organisms most commonly causing pneumonia in the hospitalized patient. Since *S. pneumoniae* is unlikely and *H. influenzae* is not listed among the choices, *K. pneumoniae* represents the most likely cause of her infection among those listed (choice **B**).

Mycoplasma pneumoniae (choice **A**), *Legionella pneumophila* (choice **D**), and *Chlamydia pneumoniae* (choice **E**) are organisms that also cause pneumonia in hospitalized patients. Although not as common as *S. pneumoniae*, *H. influenzae*, and *K. pneumoniae*, they still must be considered. Consequently, antibiotic treatment is initiated with antibiotics that will effectively inhibit growth of a wide spectrum of organisms.

37 The answer is A *Pediatrics*

Viral or aseptic meningitis usually presents with a normal to slightly elevated (not substantially increased [choice **B**]) protein concentration. The lactate concentration is not elevated (choice **C**). Rather, glucose (choice **A**) and lactate concentrations are usually both normal. In contrast, they are decreased in bacterial meningitis. No organisms are seen on Gram's stain (choice **D**) or routine cultures. White blood cell (WBC) count in the cerebrospinal fluid (CSF) is usually 100 to 700/µL, with polymorphonuclears during the first 48 hours, after which lymphocytes predominate (choice **E**). Pressures are normal.

38 The answer is G *Medicine*

The patient has Lyme disease caused by the spirochete *Borrelia burgdorferi* (choice **G**). The disease is named after the town of Old Lyme, Connecticut. It is transmitted to humans by the bite of the tick *Ixodides dammini* (scapularis) in the northeastern, north central, and mid-Atlantic regions and by *I. pacificus* on the west coast. The reservoir for the spirochete when transmitted by *I. dammini* is the white-footed mouse and the white-tailed deer, which are obligatory hosts in the tick's life cycle. The nymphal stage of the tick transmits disease during the summer. It must feed 24–48 hours to transmit the infection. In the west, *I. pacificus* prefers to feed on lizards, making them the primary reservoir. Lyme disease is the most common vector-borne disease in the United States. Stage 1 of the disease is heralded by a rash called erythema chronicum migrans (ECM), and flulike symptoms. The rash develops at the bite site and is characterized by a spreading, circular, erythematous, nonpruritic rash. Stage 2 disease is associated with myocarditis (first-degree heart block is common), meningitis, peripheral neuropathy, and Bell's palsy, which is often bilateral, as in this patient. Stage 3 (late disease) is characterized by potentially disabling arthritis (e.g., knees) and progressive central nervous system disease. The diagnosis is made with serologic tests. Routine cultures are usually negative. The treatment is varied depending on the stage and complication. Common drugs that are used include doxycycline (to treat ECM, Bell's palsy, arthritis), amoxicillin (to treat ECM, Bell's palsy, arthritis), cefuroxime axetil (to treat ECM), doxycycline or ceftriaxone (to treat myocarditis), or erythromycin (to treat ECM). Most patients respond well to therapy, and the long-term outcome is generally favorable.

39 The answer is C *Medicine*

The patient has pneumonia and tubulointerstitial nephritis due to *Legionella pneumophila* (choice **C**). It is transmitted by aerosol from water coolers and mists (e.g., grocery stores, restaurants, rain forests). It stains weakly with Gram's stain and is best visualized with a Dieterle silver stain or by direct immunofluorescent stains. The pneumonia of Legionnaires' disease is characterized by high fevers, cough productive of bloody sputum, malaise, and flulike symptoms. Renal complications include an interstitial nephritis with destruction of the juxtaglomerular apparatus causing a hyporeninemic hypoaldosteronism with hyponatremia, hyperkalemia, and normal anion-gap metabolic acidosis type IV. (Type IV is the most common type of renal tubular acidosis found in clinical practice. The defect is caused by aldosterone deficiency or antagonism [induced by any of several factors including some infections], which impairs distal nephron Na$^+$ reabsorption and K$^+$ and H$^+$ excretion.) The diagnosis is made with a sputum silver stain, detection of urinary antigen (rapid diagnosis), and culture. Fluoroquinolones or azithromycin can be used for treatment.

40 **The answer is E** *Medicine*

The patient has bubonic plague caused by *Yersinia pestis* (choice **E**). In the United States the primary vector for transmission of plague is the bite of a rat flea that has bitten an infected ground squirrel, the primary reservoir for the bacteria. Most cases have been reported in the Southwest, particularly the desert regions with a large population of ground squirrels. In bubonic plague, the infected lymph nodes (usually in the groin) enlarge (70% of cases), mat together, and drain to the surface (buboes). The treatment is streptomycin, gentamicin, or tobramycin.

41 **The answer is H** *Medicine*

Leptospira interrogans (choice **H**) is a tightly wound spirochete with a crook at the end that resembles a shepherd's staff, and it causes leptospirosis. Reservoirs for the pathogen include, dogs (most common in the United States), cattle, and rats (each of which is infected by a species-specific substrain of *L. interrogans*). The organisms are excreted in urine. Transmission to humans is by ingestion of urine-contaminated food and drinks or through recreational swimming in pools or ponds contaminated with urine from an infected animal; in this latter case, the organism may again be ingested or absorbed though the conjunctiva or via minor breaks in the skin. Persons who work with raw sewage are also at risk for infection. Leptospirosis is a biphasic disease that is subdivided into a septicemic phase and an immune phase. The septicemic phase is characterized by fever, chills, abdominal pain, severe headache, and myalgia. This phase lasts 1 to 3 days, during which the fever subsides, and the patient feels better. In the subsequent immune phase, specific antibodies appear, and the organism has disappeared from the blood and cerebrospinal fluid but may still be found in the kidneys and other tissues. The disease then tends to flare up, exhibiting symptoms similar to those exhibited in the septicemic phase. As a rule these symptoms are self-limiting, and complete recovery occurs in 4 to 30 days. Sometimes complications occur; these may include uveitis, iridocyclitis, myocarditis, aseptic meningitis, renal failure, and pulmonary infiltrates with hemorrhage. The most severe manifestations of the disease occur in Weil's syndrome (icteric leptospirosis), characterized by impaired renal and hepatic function, jaundice, hemorrhagic pneumonia, hypotension, mental aberrations, and a 5 to 40% death rate.

CHOICES NOT USED

Haemophilus ducreyi (choice **A**) is the cause of chancroid. It is transmitted by sexual contact. The disease is characterized by a painful chancre with suppurative inguinal nodes. The treatment is azithromycin or ceftriaxone.

Bordetella pertussis (choice **B**) is the cause of whooping cough. It produces a toxin that causes a profound absolute lymphocytosis with normal-appearing lymphocytes. The disease is transmitted by respiratory droplets. Children older than 1 year have no protection from the mother's immunoglobulins; hence the importance of immunization. Whooping cough is subdivided into three phases. The catarrhal phase lasts 1–2 weeks and is characterized by mild coughing, rhinorrhea, vomiting, and conjunctivitis. The paroxysmal coughing phase lasts 2–4 weeks. Characteristically there are four to five coughs in succession on expiration followed by an inspiratory whoop. A complete blood cell count shows an absolute lymphocytosis (20,000–50,000 cells/µL) composed of mature lymphocytes. The convalescence phase lasts 1–2 weeks and shows a slow decline in the whoop and lymphocyte count over the ensuing 3–4 weeks. Complications of whooping cough include hemorrhage (e.g., dermal, subconjunctival, bronchial, intracerebral) from the paroxysmal coughing; otitis media; meningoencephalitis (10% of cases); rectal prolapse from coughing; and pneumonia, which is the most common cause of death in children under 3 years old. The diagnosis is made by obtaining material from the posterior nasopharynx and plating it onto Bordet-Gengou medium (cough plate) or by direct immunofluorescent stains of material smeared on slides. The treatment of choice is erythromycin. Prevention is accomplished with acellular vaccine made from proteins of the organism, not killed organisms.

Pasteurella multocida (choice **D**) is present in the mouth of cats and dogs. It is transmitted to humans by the bite of a cat (most common) or dog. A rapid onset of cellulitis in the bite site is a characteristic finding. Complications include tendinitis, arthritis, and osteomyelitis. The treatment choices include penicillin G, amoxicillin, or ampicillin.

Eikenella corrodens (choice **F**) is a common pathogen in human bites, soft tissue infections in immunocompromised patients, and head and neck soft tissue infections in intravenous drug abusers who lick needles prior to injection. The treatment choices include penicillin G, ampicillin, or amoxicillin clavulanate.

Bacteroides fragilis (choice **I**) is an anaerobe that is the predominant organism in the human colon. Infections typically have vessel thrombosis due to the elaboration of heparinase by the organisms. It is involved primarily with infections below the diaphragm, such as peritonitis, subdiaphragmatic abscesses, and septicemia. The treatment of choice is metronidazole.

42 The answer is E   *Obstetrics and Gynecology*

A completed abortion (choice **E**) is characterized by a history of first-trimester bleeding, cramping, and passage of tissue. However, the bleeding and cramping subside, and a transvaginal sonogram shows an empty uterus with a normal endometrial stripe. Management is conservative. If previous sonographic confirmation of an intrauterine pregnancy was not available, the clinical picture of an empty uterus with positive pregnancy test could not be distinguished from an ectopic pregnancy.

43 The answer is B   *Obstetrics and Gynecology*

A missed abortion (choice **B**) is characterized by sonographic evidence of a nonviable pregnancy, including an abnormal gestational sac, an absent or amorphous embryo, and a lack of cardiac activity. Bleeding and cramping with resulting cervical dilation are absent. Management is either scheduled dilation and curettage or awaiting spontaneous expulsion of the products of conception. The most common cause of a missed abortion is embryonic aneuploidy with a chromosomal complement so severely abnormal that the embryo undergoes developmental arrest.

44 The answer is A   *Obstetrics and Gynecology*

A threatened abortion (choice **A**) is characterized by minimal vaginal bleeding, with or without mild cramping, and a closed internal cervical os. A key element is sonographic findings of a normal gestational sac, yolk sac, and trophoblastic reaction and an embryo with cardiac activity. Most pregnancies with threatened abortions have successful outcomes.

CHOICES NOT USED

Inevitable abortion (choice **C**) is characterized by bleeding of intrauterine origin with continuous and progressive dilation.

Incomplete abortion (choice **D**) by definition is the partial expulsion of fetal material.

INTRODUCTION TO ANSWERS 45–47

Most insulin-dependent type 1 diabetic patients are best managed on a split-dose, mixed-insulin regimen using neutral protamine Hagedorn (NPH) and regular insulin. The total dose of insulin is calculated with the following formula—0.7 units/kg body weight. Two thirds of this dose is given in the AM and one third in the PM. Two thirds of the AM dose is NPH and one third is regular insulin, and the PM dose is divided into one-half to two-thirds NPH and one-third to one-half regular insulin. Insulin is given 30 minutes before breakfast and dinner. The following example is a calculation for a 68-kg (150-lb) insulin-dependent diabetic:

$$\text{Total dose} = 68 \text{ kg} \times 0.7\,\text{unit/kg} = 48 \text{ units/day}$$
$$\text{AM dose} = 2/3 \times 48 = 32 \text{ units} : \text{NPH } 2/3 \times 32 = 22 \text{ units; regular} = 10 \text{ units}$$
$$\text{PM dose} = 1/3 \times 48 = 16 \text{ units} : \text{NPH } 2/3 \times 16 = 10 \text{ units; regular} = 6 \text{ units}$$

Interpretation of the blood sugar values at different time intervals uses:

• 7 AM glucose correlates with the PM NPH insulin
• 12 PM glucose correlates with the AM regular insulin
• 5 PM glucose correlates with the AM NPH insulin
• 10 PM glucose correlates with the PM regular insulin.

Two- to 5-unit increments should be used when changing the doses of insulin.

45 **The answer is D**   *Medicine*

In patient **D,** who shows a 12 PM glucose concentration of 200 mg/dL, the dose of regular insulin should be increased in the morning.

46 **The answer is A**   *Medicine*

Patient **A,** with a 10 PM glucose value of 90 mg/dL, a 3 AM glucose level of 40 mg/dL, and a 7 AM glucose value of 200 mg/dL, is demonstrating the "Somogyi effect." The nocturnal hypoglycemia at 3 AM is a reactive hypoglycemia precipitated by too much NPH at dinnertime. The treatment is to decrease the NPH dose at dinnertime, give a portion of it at bedtime, or give more food at bedtime.

47 **The answer is C**   *Medicine*

Patient **C,** with a 10 PM glucose level of 110 mg/dL, a 3 AM glucose concentration of 160 mg/dL, and a 7 AM glucose level of 220 mg/dL, has the "waning effect." This patient does not take enough NPH insulin at dinnertime. The treatment is to increase the NPH at dinnertime or to give the NPH at bedtime.

CHOICES NOT USED

Patient **B,** with a 10 PM glucose concentration of 110 mg/dL, a 3 AM glucose concentration of 110 mg/dL, and a 7 AM glucose concentration of 150 mg/dL, is demonstrating the "dawn phenomenon." This phenomenon is secondary to increased growth hormone (GH) release between 5 AM and 8 AM. GH antagonizes insulin, thus causing the early AM hyperglycemia. The treatment is to divide the NPH dose between dinner and bedtime.

Patient **E,** with a 5 PM glucose concentration of 220 mg/dL, requires an increase in the AM dose of NPH.

Patient **F,** with a 9 PM glucose concentration of 200 mg/dL, requires an increase in regular insulin at dinnertime.

48 **The answer is B**   *Medicine*

The patient has tinea capitis due to *Trichophyton tonsurans* (choice **B**). The superficial dermatophytes are a group of fungi that are confined to the outermost layers of the skin (stratum corneum) or its appendages. Dermatophytoses infect skin, nails, and/or hair. There are three genera: *Trichophyton* spp. infect hair, skin, or nails; *Microsporum* spp. infect hair and skin; and *Epidermophyton* spp. infect the skin alone. Transmission is by direct contact with skin scales, contact with animals (e.g., *Microsporum canis,* dogs), and soil. Diagnosis is made by culture of skin scrapings secured from the leading edge of the lesion, use of a Wood's lamp to check for fluorescent metabolites, and direct potassium hydroxide (KOH) preparations of the scraped material. *Trichophyton tonsurans* is the most common cause of tinea capitis followed by *Microsporum canis* (choice **D**). Both fungi produce circular or ring-shaped patches ("ringworm") of alopecia (hair loss) with erythema and scaling. There is a black dot where the hair breaks off. *T. tonsurans* has negative Wood's lamp examination results, because the fungus infects the inner hair shaft (endoprix), where fungal metabolites cannot be identified. *M. canis,* however, infects the outer hair shaft exoprex, producing a positive Wood's lamp result. The treatment of choice is terbinafine (an allylimine) by mouth.

49 **The answer is A**   *Medicine*

The patient has tuberculoid leprosy due to *Mycobacterium leprae* (choice **A**). Organisms have low infectivity; therefore, transmission of infection to humans is by prolonged contact (nasal secretions, skin lesions) with patients with lepromatous leprosy.

Tuberculoid leprosy is characterized by intact cellular immunity, which means that granulomas are produced, very few organisms are present, and patients have a positive lepromin skin test result (similar to PPD). The skin lesions are hypopigmented, macular lesions that are insensitive to pain. As the disease progresses, the superficial nerves become thickened, and there is autoamputation of the digits. Lepromatous leprosy, on the other hand, is characterized by a lack of cellular immunity, the presence of numerous organisms, and a negative lepromin skin test result. Multiple nodular skin lesions are produced that cause a leonine facies. Dapsone is the treatment of choice. Male patients should be screened for glucose-6-phosphate dehydrogenase deficiency before starting the drug, since it is an oxidant drug that can result in hemolytic anemia.

50 **The answer is C**   *Medicine*

The patient has tinea corporis (ringworm), which is most often caused by *Trichophyton rubrum* (choice **C**). Tinea corporis affects the skin, not a hair shaft and is recognized as a circular lesion with erythematous, scaling margins and central clearing. The treatment for dermatophytic skin infections is a topical imidazole compound such as ketoconazole.

CHOICES NOT USED

Trichophyton schoenleinii (choice **E**) produces favus, which is a variant of tinea capitis that is associated with the formation of crusted lesions.

Malassezia furfur (choice **F**) is the cause of tinea versicolor and seborrheic dermatitis. Tinea versicolor is recognized by the presence of hyperpigmented and hypopigmented skin. The fungus produces an acid that inhibits melanin transfer to keratinocytes. A KOH preparation reveals "spaghetti" (hyphae) and "meatball" (yeasts) fungal morphology. The treatment of choice is a single oral dose of ketoconazole.

Cutaneous *Candida albicans* (choice **G**) produces intertrigo, an erythematous rash in body folds (e.g., diaper rash) and paronychial infections (nail-fold infection). A KOH preparation shows yeast and pseudohyphae (extended yeast). The presence of pseudohyphae indicates active infection. The treatment for skin infections includes topical application of amphotericin B, clotrimazole, miconazole, or nystatin.

test **16**

Questions

Single Best Choice Directions: This section consists of numbered statements or questions followed by a list of potential answers; you are to select the ONE best answer.

1 A 76-year-old man was diagnosed with type 2 diabetes at the age of 62-years and now complains to his primary care physician that his urogenital problems have increased during the past 6 months. He reiterates that as the physician knows he had been having erection problems that were adequately controlled by "Viagra", but for the past half year or so, Viagra no longer worked and in addition he cannot ejaculate, even if he tries to masturbate. He also states that on the good side of the coin, his need to urinate has decreased to a remarkable degree, although sometimes that results in a prevoiding dribble because by the time the urge hits him, the pressure has built up to an almost uncontrollable level. These symptoms suggest which of the following?

(A) Peripheral neuropathy
(B) Autonomic neuropathy
(C) Mononeuropathy
(D) Nephropathy
(E) Macrovascular disease

2 A 62-year-old woman who had no specific complaint asked her physician for a complete checkup. Upon physical examination he found her blood pressure to be 145/75 mm Hg and uncovered no other significant abnormality. A routine chemistry panel provided the following results:

Parameter Measured	Value	Units	Reference Range
Glucose	102	mg/dL	65–109
Na⁺	140	mEq/L	135–147
K⁺	4.3	mEq/L	3.5–45
Cl⁻	101	mEq/L	96–108
CO₂	26	mEq/L	22–29
Anion gap	13	mEq/L	5–14
BUN^a	23	mg/dL	8–23
Creatine	1.1	mg/dL	0.4–1.1
Urea/creatine	21	Ratio	10–22
Osmolarity	283	mos/kg	268–292
Total protein	7.3	g/dL	6.3–8.3
Albumin (A)	4.5	g/dL	3.6–5.0
Globulin (G)	2.8	g/dL	2.4–4.4
A/G ratio	1.6	Ratio	0.7–2.5
Total bilirubin	0.4	mg/dL	0.2–1.2

Parameter Measured	Value	Units	Reference Range
SGOT (AST)^b	25	Units/L	0–39
GPT (ALT)^c	27	Units/L	0–39
Alkaline phosphatase	73	Units/L	40–129
Total calcium	11.8	Units/L	8.4–10.5

^{a}Blood urea nitrogen.
^{b}SGOT (AST), serum glutamate-oxaloacetate transaminase (aspartate aminotransaminase).
^{c}GPT (ALT) = glutamate-pyruvate transaminase (alanine amino transferase).

Which of the following choices is the best next step in the course of treating this patient?

(A) Congratulate her on being so healthy and send her home
(B) Subject her to a mammography because of suspect metastatic breast cancer
(C) Add a thiazide diuretic to treat hypertension
(D) Measure her circulating parathyroid level
(E) Subject her to a chest radiographic study because of suspected sarcoidosis

3 A 6-year-old child was in the school cafeteria when his eyes rolled back suddenly, and his entire body musculature had tonic–clonic retractions. This lasted a few minutes and came to an abrupt stop. The school nurse calls 911 emergency services to transport the child to the local emergency department. She notes that the child had urinary incontinence as well as a small laceration of the tongue. Which of the following is a common characteristic of this type of seizure?

(A) Flaccidity of all extremities, followed by 15 to 30 seconds of tremors
(B) Urinary retention
(C) Tongue and/or cheek biting
(D) Clonic jerking for 1 to 2 minutes, followed by normal consciousness
(E) Localized onset in the primary form of the disease

4 An 11-year-old boy with extremely easy distractibility is started on methylphenidate therapy with good control of his symptoms. However, he complains of anorexia and nervousness that are not ameliorated with a decrease to the minimal effective dose. Which one of the following medications would be the most appropriate choice for the next medication trial?

(A) Bupropion 150 mg PO qAM
(B) Olanzapine 5 mg PO qAM
(C) Clonidine .1 mg PO qAM
(D) Topiramate 25 mg PO qd
(E) Desipramine 25 mg PO qAM

5 A 2-year-old boy is brought via ambulance to the emergency department because of bleeding from the mouth and gastrointestinal tract. The mother states that they are visiting the child's grandfather, who takes warfarin for chronic atrial fibrillation. A few days ago the patient's grandfather noticed that some of his pills were missing. The patient's mother now suspects that the child may have accidentally ingested the warfarin. Which of the following coagulation test results is expected?

	Platelet Count	Bleeding Time	PT	APTT
(A)	↓	↑	N	N
(B)	N	N	N	↑
(C)	N	N	↑	↑
(D)	N	↑	N	N
(E)	N	↑	N	↑

N, normal; ↓, decreased relative to normal; ↑, increased relative to normal; PT, prothrombin time; APTT, activated partial thromboplastin time.

6 A 34-year-old woman complains of chronic low back pain, intermittent abdominal cramps, headaches, migratory joint pain, bloating, heavy menses, and anxiety. These symptoms have resulted in many work absences and resultant losses of multiple employments. She has had many previous extensive medical workups, but no significant physical findings were discovered. The patient feels that her physicians were generally uncaring and dismissive. There are some entries in her medical records that suggest possible benzodiazepine abuse and hesitancy to prescribe opioid medication for pain. Which of the following is the most likely psychiatric diagnosis?

(A) Factitious disorder
(B) Hypochondriasis
(C) Malingering
(D) Pain disorder
(E) Somatization disorder

7 A 10-year-old female complains of generalized headaches for the last month. The headaches are present on awakening and worsen when the patient sneezes or defecates. She also complains of diplopia, and physical examination of the eyes shows papilledema. The physician suspects a brain tumor. Based on her age, what type of brain tumor is most likely present in this patient?

(A) Medulloblastoma
(B) Pilocytic astrocytoma of the cerebellum
(C) Ependymoma
(D) Neuroblastoma
(E) Oligodendroglioma

8 A 26-year-old female was going down a ski slope and decided to suddenly change direction. She heard a sudden pop and felt pain in the left knee. The emergency department physician notes a fluctuant swelling of the left knee. Which of the following was most likely injured when this patient suddenly changed direction?

(A) Lateral collateral ligament
(B) Medial collateral ligament
(C) Anterior cruciate ligament
(D) Posterior cruciate ligament
(E) Patella dislocation

9 A 68-year-old female with Alzheimer's dementia is increasingly agitated and combative. She is resistant to attempts to help her with eating, personal hygiene, or ambulation. She sleeps poorly and shouts out whenever she hears any noise. There is no evidence of psychosis. Results of her physical examination are unremarkable, as are her laboratory indices. Which of the following would be the best choice for initial treatment of her symptoms?

(A) Chlorpromazine 25 mg PO bid
(B) Clozaril 12.5 mg PO qd
(C) Haloperidol 2 mg PO hs
(D) Olanzapine 5 mg PO hs
(E) Ziprasidone 20 mg PO bid

10 A 66-year-old Caucasian woman, who was born, raised, and still lives in Phoenix, Arizona, loves to play golf. She started playing at the age of 5 years and was the star of her high school and college teams. She also is proud of the fact that she could play 18 holes even in the heat of a 100°F (37°C) summer day in Phoenix. Moreover, she did not wear makeup or apply sunscreen until she was well into her 30s. About a year ago she noted a newly formed frecklelike spot on her left cheek. Recently she became increasingly concerned as this freckle seemed to spread, turning into a more highly and irregularly pigmented area. By the time its diameter reached 2 cm she made an appointment to see a dermatologist. This spot was most likely diagnosed as which of the following conditions?

(A) Lentigo malignant melanoma
(B) Superficial spreading melanoma

(C) Nodular melanoma

(D) Acral lentiginous melanoma

(E) Mucosal lentiginous melanoma

11 A 46-year-old acquired immune deficiency syndrome (AIDS) patient is being treated with zidovudine (AZT). His CD4+ lymphocyte count has remained unchanged for the past 8 weeks and is currently 145/mm³. Recently he has been treated with nystatin and now for the past 2 weeks has developed almost daily temperature spikes above 37.7°C (100°F), suggesting he is at risk for *Pneumocystis carinii* pneumonia (PCP). Which of the following would most likely be the most effective prophylactic drugs for preventing development of PCP?

(A) Pentamidine

(B) Trimethoprim–sulfamethoxazole (TMP-SMX)

(C) Primaquine

(D) Dapsone

(E) Pyrimethamine–sulfadiazine

12 A 20-year-old woman progressed through an unremarkable pregnancy with the only abnormality being a fundal height greater than expected. An obstetric sonogram revealed a 4-quadrant amniotic fluid index of 30 cm, consistent with polyhydramnios. She underwent spontaneous onset of contractions at 39 weeks' gestation and progressed normally through labor. When the fetal membranes were ruptured, a copious amount of amniotic fluid was seen. Her male fetus weighed 9 lb 8 oz (4.3 kg). After the placenta was delivered, her uterus did not contract well, resulting in postpartum hemorrhage and an estimated blood loss of 2000 mL. She was administered intravenous oxytocin, intramuscular ergotamine, and intramuscular prostaglandin $F_{2\alpha}$. During the heavy bleeding she experienced hypotension and tachycardia. Which one of the following hormone levels would most likely be altered if significant end-organ hypoperfusion has taken place?

(A) Luteinizing hormone (LH)

(B) Thyroid-stimulating hormone (TSH)

(C) Adrenocorticotropic hormone (ACTH)

(D) Follicle-stimulating hormone (FSH)

(E) Prolactin

13 Despite a good appetite, a 32-year-old woman complains of weight loss. She also complains of an overawareness of her heart beating at night with palpitations, excessive sweating, heat intolerance, emotional liability, weakness, fatigue, diarrhea, and irregular menstrual periods. Physical examination reveals exophthalmos and lid retraction. Which of the following additional findings would you expect?

(A) Decreased thyroid binding globulin (TBG) level

(B) Decreased serum T_3

(C) Decreased iodine-123 uptake (^{123}I)

(D) Decreased serum thyroid-stimulating hormone (TSH) level

(E) Decreased free thyroxine (T_4) level

14 A 3-year-old girl with no previous psychiatric symptoms is taken with her family to a refugee center following a local battle 2 weeks ago in which she saw several relatives killed and shops and dwellings burned. She reportedly sleeps poorly and appears frightened and hypervigilant, even though she is not in immediate danger. Her attention span is very short, and she fidgets constantly. She is extremely frightened by strangers and spends hours hiding under her cot. On assessment, she seems distracted and confused. Her thought processes appear disjointed. Physical assessment is unremarkable. Which of the following diagnoses is most likely?

(A) Acute stress disorder

(B) Attention-deficit/hyperactivity disorder

(C) Brief psychotic disorder, with marked stressors

(D) Panic disorder

(E) Posttraumatic stress disorder

15 A 7-year-old child is brought to the hospital because of a severe headache. He had been in his usual state of good health until this morning when he developed nausea and vomiting. A computed tomography (CT) scan of the head is performed that shows an intracranial hemorrhage. The patient has no family history of migraines, no contact with ill persons, no recent travel, and no pets. Which of the following conditions is the most likely cause of his intracranial hemorrhage?

(A) Hypertension

(B) Ruptured berry aneurysm

(C) Arteriovenous malformation

(D) Trauma

(E) Brain abscess

16 A 27-year-old man is involved in an automobile accident and is brought into the emergency department unconscious and bleeding from several lacerations. His "Medic-Alert" bracelet shows that he has hemophilia A. He is stabilized, but the bleeding cannot be stopped. Which of the following could be used at the least volume to stop the bleeding?

(A) Fresh frozen plasma

(B) Packed platelets

(C) Whole blood

(D Packed red blood cells

(E) Cryoprecipitated blood

17 A 53-year-old woman had a complete blood count as part of a routine physical examination. The results came back as shown in the tables below.

Cell Counts	Observed	Normal Range
White blood cells (WBCs)	$28.0 \times 10^3/\mu L$	$4.3–10.8 \times 10^3/\mu L$
Hemoglobin (Hgb)	13.0 g/dL	11.5–15.0 g/dL
Hematocrit (Hct)	39.1%	35.0–47.0%
Mean corpuscular volume (MCV)	93 fL	80–98 fL
Red blood cells (RBCs)	$4.22 \times 10^6/\mu L$	$3.90–5.20 \times 10^6/\mu L$
Mean corpuscular hemoglobin (MCH)	30.8 pg	27.0–34.0 pg
Mean corpuscular hemoglobin concentration (MCHC)	32.2 g/dL	32.0–36.0 g/dL
RBC distribution width index	13.8%	0.0–15.5%
Platelets	$325 \times 10^4/dL$	$150–450 \times 10^3/dL$

Differential	%	Absolute Differential	Number	Normal Range
Neutrophil	58	Neutrophil	$4.7 \times 10^3/\mu L$	$1.8–.57 \times 10^3/\mu L$
Lymphocyte	31	Lymphocyte	$2.57 \times 10^3/\mu L$	$0.8–4.57 \times 10^3/\mu L$
Monocyte	7	Monocyte	$0.67 \times 10^3/\mu L$	$0.1–1.57 \times 10^3/\mu L$
Eosinophil	4	Eosinophil	$0.37 \times 10^3/\mu L$	$0–0.47 \times 10^3/\mu L$
Basophil	1	Basophil	$0.17 \times 10^3/\mu L$	$0–0.57 \times 10^3/\mu L$

This patient is most likely in the early stages of which one the following myeloproliferative disorders?

(A) Chronic myelogenous leukemia (CML)
(B) Polycythemia vera (PV)
(C) Chronic idiopathic myelofibrosis
(D) Essential thrombocytopenia (ET)

18 A 63-year-old white male is brought into the emergency department by the police who found him staggering on the street and stopping passing individuals by asking inane questions. He has a strong smell of alcohol on his breath. When examined he is found to be drowsy, wanting to be let alone so he could sleep; he also is disoriented. He can no longer ambulate because of his unsteady gait and has vomited twice since being admitted. His vital signs are: temperature, 37.5°C (99.5°F); pulse, 100 beats/min; respirations, 16/min; blood pressure, 114/75 mm Hg. Ophthalmo-logic examination shows horizontal nystagmus and 6th nerve ophthalmoplegia. This man most likely has a deficiency of which of the following nutrients?

(A) Ascorbic acid (vitamin C)
(B) Thiamine (vitamin B_1)
(C) Riboflavin (vitamin B_2)
(D) Niacin (vitamin B_3)
(E) Pyridoxine (vitamin B_6)

19 A 4-year-old child presents with fever and conjunctivitis. The mother states that the child had been in his usual state of good health until 2 days ago when he developed upper respiratory tract symptoms. She also states that the patient has had photophobia and cervical adenopathy. On physical examination the pediatrician notes that red lesions with a white center are present on the buccal mucosa. A generalized, blanching, erythematous rash is also noted. Which of the following is the most likely diagnosis?

(A) Kawasaki disease
(B) Rubella
(C) Adenovirus infection
(D) Rubeola
(E) Still's disease

20 A 35-year-old woman presents to the outpatient department with a history of a painless, bloody discharge from the right nipple that she noticed that morning. She reports that until this time she has been in good health. She exercises regularly, does not smoke, and has a healthy lifestyle. She is nulliparous and denies a history of bleeding disorder, allergies, or medications. Clinical examination of the right breast reveals no palpable mass, but blood is expressed from the nipple. The left breast is normal. Examination of both axillae reveals no lymphadenopathy. Which of the following is the most likely diagnosis?

(A) Intraductal papillomatosis
(B) Breast abscess
(C) Intraductal papilloma
(D) Infiltrating ductal carcinoma
(E) Fibrocystic change

21 A 36-year-old pregnant woman in the last stages of labor is brought to the emergency department by her boyfriend, who informs the admitting nurse that he is seropositive for the human immunodeficiency virus (HIV). The woman is a prostitute, takes drugs intravenously along with her boyfriend, and has had no prenatal care. A normal-appearing 3.2-kg (7-lb) girl is born 5 minutes after the woman's arrival. Which of the following represents the best next medical response possible under these circumstances?

(A) Conduct an enzyme-linked immunosorbent assay (ELISA) on the newborn child
(B) Conduct an ELISA on the mother
(C) Immediately start the child on antiviral drug therapy
(D) Do not administer antiviral drugs unless the infant shows a mucocutaneous candidiasis infection
(E) Do not administer antiviral drugs unless the infant shows signs of developing Kaposi's sarcoma

22 A 41-year-old male heroin addict has been unable to successfully maintain recovery despite participation in many sobriety-centered treatments. He is functioning well occupationally and socially and lives with his wife and 3 young children. He fears that it is only a matter of time before he is arrested for heroin possession, develops medical complications associated with impure heroin, or wastes all his money on drugs. There are no methadone maintenance clinics in his area. Which of the following pharmacologic interventions would be the most reasonable next step?

(A) Acamprosate
(B) Buprenorphine
(C) Codeine
(D) Disulfiram
(E) Naltrexone

23 A febrile 35-year-old woman has a 4-day history of precordial chest pain that increases when she inhales and decreases when she leans forward. She now complains of progressively worsening dyspnea. Physical examination shows muffled heart sounds and neck vein distention during inspiration. Blood pressure and pulse amplitude both decrease during inspiration. Which of the following is the most likely diagnosis?

(A) Aortic dissection
(B) Congestive cardiomyopathy
(C) Constrictive pericarditis
(D) Pericarditis with effusion
(E) Restrictive cardiomyopathy

24 A 50-year-old woman in seemingly good health has a routine screening mammogram. The mammogram of the right breast shows microcalcification in the upper outer quadrant of the breast. Clinical examination reveals no mass lesion on palpation. What is the most likely diagnosis?

(A) Ductal carcinoma *in situ*
(B) Phyllodes tumor
(C) Medullary carcinoma

(D) Lobular carcinoma *in situ*
(E) Fibroadenoma

25 A 19-year-old man presents for an armed forces induction physical and is noted to have severely chapped hands. He admits only reluctantly and after much questioning that he scrubs his hands at least 25 times a day, mostly surreptitiously. He says that he fears that germs are everywhere and can't stop thinking that he may be contaminated. His thoughts are disturbing to him, and he sometimes tries to avoid washing but finally gives in to the impulse to do so. There is no other evidence of peculiar thoughts or behavior. His mood is somewhat anxious. Which of the following is the most likely diagnosis?

(A) Delusional disorder
(B) Generalized anxiety disorder
(C) Malingering
(D) Obsessive–compulsive disorder
(E) Posttraumatic stress disorder

26 A 25-year-old man has fever, fatigue, difficulty breathing, and substernal chest pain while walking or at rest. Physical examination shows bibasilar inspiratory crackles, distention of the jugular neck vein, hepatomegaly, and dependent pitting edema. A chest radiograph shows generalized enlargement of the atria and ventricles. Laboratory studies show an increase in cardiac-specific troponins and an ejection fraction of 0.20 (normal, >0.55). An antistreptolysin O titer is negative. An electrocardiogram shows low-voltage QRS complexes, and echocardiography shows global myocardial dysfunction. What is the most likely diagnosis?

(A) Congestive cardiomyopathy
(B) Coronary artery thrombosis
(C) Ischemic heart disease
(D) Restrictive cardiomyopathy
(E) Rheumatic fever

27 Utopiaville is a midsize urban center with a large population of homeless individuals. This disturbs many of the upstanding citizens who feel that they are not only a visual blight, but they upset people by panhandling and might even be a threat. An individual with political ambitions who is running for city council makes removing all homeless persons from within city limits the focus of his platform. According to him, almost all the homeless are simply too lazy to work and are making a good living from government programs and/or panhandling. His opponent claims this is not true but rather most are ill, suffering from persistent mental illness. According to many studies, the percentage of the homeless population with severe and persistent mental illness is closest to which of the following?

(A) 15%
(B) 30%
(C) 50%
(D) 60%
(E) 90%

28 A 9-year-old boy presents with his parents to his pediatrician because of confusion and decreased school performance. The parents also state that he has developed a spastic gait with dysarthria and dysphagia. In addition, the patient's teacher has noted that the child appears to have visual loss. A magnetic resonance imaging (MRI) scan shows massive demyelination of the white matter in the posterior areas of the hemispheres. Which of the following is the most likely diagnosis?

(A) Multiple sclerosis
(B) Metachromatic leukodystrophy
(C) Adrenoleukodystrophy
(D) Subacute sclerosing panencephalitis
(E) Creutzfeldt-Jakob disease

29 A 32-year-old man sees his physician because of a rash on his elbows. He states that the lesion becomes more prominent during periods of physical stress. Examination of the rash shows multiple well-defined erythematous scaling plaques as shown in the accompanying figure. When viewed in person these plaques are salmon-colored and covered by loosely adherent silver-white scales. Which of the following dermatologic conditions does this man most likely have?

(A) Herpes zoster
(B) Acne rosacea

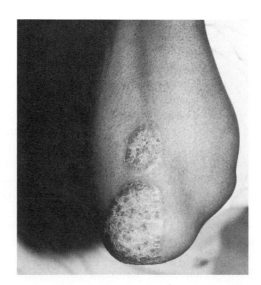

(C) Solar lentigo
(D) Actinic keratosis
(E) Xerosis
(F) Psoriasis

30 A couple, married for 5 years has four children from three separate pregnancies with one set of twins, decides that they can't afford to have any more children. The wife is very religious and feels that she cannot practice any form of birth control. Consequently, the husband decides to get a vasectomy, which he does after discussing the pros and cons with his surgeon. After the operation, the surgeon told him the operation was a success. However a little less than 2 months after the surgery the wife announces she is pregnant again. The most likely reason for this pregnancy is which of the following?

(A) The surgeon used the newer "no-scalpel method" and did not completely tie off the vas deferens.
(B) The man ejaculated twice before the couple resumed sexual relations.
(C) The wife was unfaithful.
(D) The vas deferens recanalized.
(E) The patient had epididymitis causing the procedure to fail.

31 A 41-year-old woman is brought to the emergency department after she threatened to commit suicide during a 911 call. She is agitated and emotionally labile. However, she now states that she is no longer suicidal. Which of the following most significantly increases her risk for completing suicide?

(A) A history of childhood sexual abuse
(B) Dissatisfaction with her job
(C) Marriage to an abusive spouse
(D) Recent sexual conflicts
(E) Schizophrenia

32 A 73-year-old woman is watching television when suddenly she has a sudden headache followed by numbness on the right side of her face and in her right arm and leg. She also feels confused and has vision problems. Although she has right-sided numbness, her limbs remain functional and she manages to get to a telephone and dial 911. However, when she tries to tell the operator what the problem is she is only able to barely, and laboriously, mumble "sick–help." This lady's language difficulty is most likely an example of which of the following?

(A) Agnosia
(B) Apraxia
(C) Astereognosis
(D) Wernicke's aphasia

(E) Agraphia

(F) Alexia

(G) Broca's aphasia

33. An 82-year-old, physically active woman who has a committed interest in local and national social and political events, trips on a throw rug in her living room, falls, and breaks her hip. The fracture is repaired surgically; however, she never fully recovers and now, a year later, she lives in a nursing home and shows little interest in the world around her. Which of the following is true concerning falls in the over-65 population?

(A) A single risk factor is generally involved.

(B) Medication is rarely a factor.

(C) Several factors operating in conjunction generally contribute to risk of a fall.

(D) Uncontrolled hypertension is a common cause.

(E) There is little a physician can do to help prevent falls among elderly patients.

34. A 22-year-old woman is distressed by inflamed pimples that she has on her face. She started to get them at the age of 15 years and has been self-treating them ever since by scrubbing her face with strong soap every night before going to bed. She also has been "popping them" in an attempt to clear out the accumulated pus. She believes that the number of "pimples" increases monthly with initiation of her menses. Which of the following dermatologic condition is this woman suffering from?

(A) Acne vulgaris

(B) Erysipelas

(C) Seborrheic keratosis

(D) Junctional nevus

(E) Dysplastic nevus

35. Test X has a 60% sensitivity and 80% specificity for systemic lupus erythematosus (SLE), and it is being used to determine the possibility that a patient has SLE in a population in which SLE has a prevalence of 10%. The patient is randomly selected from this population, and the test result is positive. What is the percentage chance that this person has SLE?

(A) 25%

(B) 50%

(C) 60%

(D) 75%

(E) 80%

36. A 3-month-old infant is brought to the emergency department by his mother because of a firm inguinal bulge. For the past 2 weeks the mother had noted this bulge when he cried, but it always disappeared when she calmed him. The bulge has now remained for 3 hours. The infant is crying and has a firm inguinal mass that is not discolored. The infant's temperature is 37.5°C (99.3°F). Which of the following is the most appropriate initial step in the management of this patient?

(A) Resuscitation in preparation for operation

(B) Administration of pancuronium bromide, intubation, and placement in the Trendelenburg position

(C) Injection of local anesthesia into the bulge followed by manual pressure

(D) Application of ice and manual compression

(E) Administration of a muscle relaxant and barbiturate and placement in the Trendelenburg position

37. A 68-year-old woman is on a picnic with her husband and friends and is visibly upset when she is told distressing news about a mutual friend. Shortly afterward, she wants to pour coffee for everybody. However, her hands shake so badly that she spills a great deal; so much so that her husband takes over. At that time she rapidly consumes a glass of wine that had been poured earlier. Within a few minutes her tremor is reduced to a less conspicuous level. After she and her husband left, the friends speculate about the cause of her tremor and present the following ideas. Which one is correct?

(A) Parkinsonism-associated tremor

(B) Drug-induced tremor

(C) Essential tremor

(D) Pheochromocytoma-associated tremor

(E) Alcohol withdrawal-induced tremor

38. A soldier was injured when his Humvee hit a land mine. His fellow officers risked their lives to rescue him from the burning vehicle, and the army medics did a miraculous job to save his life. However his spinal cord was severed at C-4. After stabilization, he was transferred to a rehabilitation center where they tried to help him cope with his paralysis. However, while there he developed a pressure sore that became infected by an organism that was refractory to the usual antibiotics. They finally found one that worked. This was most likely which one of the following drugs?

(A) Oxacillin

(B) Ceftazidime

(C) Penicillin G

(D) Nafcillin

(E) Linezolid

(F) Methicillin

39. A 61-year-old postmenopausal woman comes to the outpatient office with complaints of vaginal bleeding

for the past 5 days. Her last menstrual period was 7 years ago. She has not taken any hormone replacement therapy. Her height is 61 in (1.54 m) and she weighs 210 lb (95.25 kg). An endometrial biopsy shows simple hyperplasia without atypia. Hysteroscopy shows no polyps or submucosal leiomyomas. Which of the following is most likely responsible for her endometrial biopsy findings?

(A) Estriol
(B) Ethynyl estradiol
(C) Estrone
(D) Phytoestrogen
(E) Estradiol

40 A 20-year-old football player is tackled during a game by a member of the opposing team. During the event,

his knee is subjected to a valgus stress. He complains of severe pain and falls to the ground. When seen in the emergency department, he has a swollen left knee, which is fluctuant. Which of the following sets of injuries is most likely present?

(A) Rupture of the lateral meniscus, lateral collateral ligament, and anterior cruciate ligament
(B) Rupture of the lateral meniscus, lateral collateral ligament, and posterior cruciate ligament
(C) Rupture of the medial meniscus, medial collateral ligament, and posterior cruciate ligament
(D) Rupture of the medial and lateral menisci, medial collateral ligament, and anterior and posterior cruciate ligaments
(E) Rupture of the medial meniscus, medial collateral ligament, and anterior cruciate ligament

Directions for Matching Questions (41 through 50): *Each set of matching questions is preceded by a list of 4 to 26 lettered options followed by a brief explanation of the required task and then by a series of numbered statements. For each lettered statement you are to select ONE lettered option that best fulfills the task as it relates to that statement. Remember each of the listed options might be correctly selected once, more than once, or not at all.*

Questions 41–45

You will be required to select one letter choice from the list below that represents the most likely cause of the female involuntary loss of urine that is described in the clinical condition described in questions 41 through 45.

(A) Bypass or fistula
(B) Overflow
(C) Urge
(D) Genuine stress
(E) Pregnancy

41 A 58-year-old postmenopausal nulliparous woman comes to the outpatient office complaining of intermittent, sudden onset of urinary urgency which she cannot suppress. This results in loss of significant amounts of urine that wet her underpants and clothes. She has resorted to wearing adult diapers to function in her daily activities. The loss of urine occurs day and night, and she has a feeling that her bladder is almost always full. These symptoms started approximately 5 years ago when she underwent menopause. Surgical history is negative. Upon physical examination she has no evidence of uterine or vaginal prolapse. Results of urinalysis and urine culture are negative.

42 A 25-year-old primigravida woman is seen at the prenatal obstetric clinic at 37 weeks' gestation complain-

ing of pelvic pressure. She states her underpants are frequently moist, especially when she coughs and sneezes. She is concerned regarding possible rupture of membranes and uterine infection. Her uterine fundus measures 39 cm from her pubic symphysis. Fetal heart tones are 145/min in the left lower quadrant. A speculum examination shows no pooling of fluid in the posterior fornix. Nitrazine paper placed in the vaginal vault remains yellow.

43 A 35-year-old woman underwent a spontaneous labor requiring prolonged oxytocin augmentation resulting in a subsequent vaginal delivery under epidural analgesia 12 hours ago. Her 3600 g (7 lb, 6 oz) daughter (with Apgar scores of 8 and 9 at 1 and 5 minutes, respectively) is doing well and is beginning breastfeeding. The mother's lochia is normal, and her vital signs are stable. Her uterus is firm to palpation but is deviated to the right above her umbilicus. She unpredictably dribbles small amounts of urine but has no sensation of fullness. She has no pain on urination. On placement of a Foley catheter she is found to have a residual bladder volume of 800 mL.

44 A 48-year-old multiparous woman complains of involuntary loss of urine with coughing and sneezing. She notices that she does not lose any urine when she is sleeping at night. She denies any burning, urgency, or pain on urination. She has five children, each of whom she delivered vaginally. Her largest baby weighed 10 lb (4.5 kg). Pelvic examination reveals second-degree uterine prolapse along with a prominent cystocele and rectoceles. She has a normal anal wink.

45 A 39-year-old woman underwent radical hysterectomy and pelvic lymphadenectomy 3 weeks ago for invasive cervical cancer. The surgery appeared uncomplicated, but she now complains of continual involuntary loss of urine day and night. She denies any burning, urgency, or pain on urination. On pelvic examination the vaginal cuff is healing well, but there is clear fluid in the vagina. She has a normal anal wink.

Questions 46–50

Match the following clinical scenarios with the correct direction of change in serum calcium and/or serum parathyroid hormone (PTH) levels. (The square *represents the normal range values, and the* arrows *represent increasing magnitude of concentration of calcium and/or PTH. Thus, as an example, point E represents a condition that raises serum calcium concentrations but lowers serum PTH levels, relative to the normal range of values indicated by the square.)*

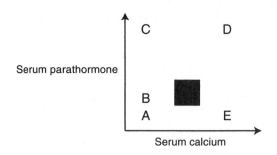

46 A 60-year-old man has hypoalbuminemia and a normal ionized calcium level.

47 A 30-year-old woman has long-standing, untreated celiac disease.

48 A 65-year-old woman has a renal cell carcinoma and a short QT interval on an electrocardiogram (ECG).

49 A 13-year-old boy diagnosed with Addison's disease at 12 years of age, presents with tetany, a prolonged QT interval on an ECG, and mucocutaneous candidiasis.

50 A 68-year-old woman has epigastric pain with radiation into the back, a positive stool guaiac test result, and a long history of renal stone formation.

Answer Key

1 B		**11** B		**21** C		**31** E		**41** C	
2 D		**12** E		**22** B		**32** G		**42** E	
3 C		**13** D		**23** D		**33** C		**43** B	
4 A		**14** A		**24** A		**34** A		**44** D	
5 C		**15** D		**25** D		**35** A		**45** A	
6 E		**16** E		**26** A		**36** E		**46** B	
7 B		**17** D		**27** B		**37** C		**47** C	
8 C		**18** B		**28** C		**38** E		**48** E	
9 C		**19** D		**29** F		**39** C		**49** A	
10 A		**20** C		**30** B		**40** E		**50** D	

Answers and Explanations

1 **The answer is B** *Medicine*

Autonomic neuropathy is a relatively common potential complication of long-term diabetes. It often accompanies peripheral neuropathy but affects the nerves that supply the small blood vessels in an autonomic neural system. Signs and symptoms vary, depending upon the system primarily affected. In the cardiovascular system it primarily affects the vagus nerve and may result in resting sinus tachycardia without sinus arrhythmia, exercise intolerance, a tendency for orthostatic hypotension, and symptomless myocardial infarction, which may lead to death. Gastrointestinal autonomic neuropathy may cause esophageal dysfunction and gastroparesis, which may be manifested in several ways, such as diarrhea, or constipation, and fecal incontinence. Sudomotor neuropathy may cause facial sweating and heat intolerance. In men, genitourinary autonomic neuropathy is a common cause of impotence accompanied by normal libido; in addition it may lead to retrograde ejaculation (inability to ejaculate) and bladder problems (choice **B**). In the early stages, neurogenic bladder dysfunction is characterized by diminished sensation of bladder fullness and a decreased urge to urinate. As the disease progresses, overflow incontinence may develop as well as difficulty in voiding completely. This latter problem may cause urinary tract infection. In women, autonomic neuropathy of the urogenital symptom may cause dyspareunia due to vaginal dryness and an inability to achieve an orgasm.

Peripheral neuropathy (choice **A**) is the most common form of diabetes-induced neuropathy. Initial symptoms are altered sensations in the toes and fingers that progress proximally in a "stocking-glove" manner, leading to the alternative name of *distal symmetrical polyneuropathy*. Early symptoms are usually mild, but as the disease progresses, symptoms may include numbness, tingling, coldness or alternatively a burning sensation, a dull ache, and/or cramping. Often the proprioceptor nerve endings are affected, causing problems with walking because locating the position of the feet is no longer an unconscious automatic function. Symptoms may advance to sensory loss leading to foot ulcers, unbalanced gait, muscle weakness, foot drop, and loss of fine motor skills. Diabetic mononeuropathy (choice **C**) involves single nerves or a group of nerves that are chronically exposed to pressure. Nondiabetics may be prone to similar problems, but the diabetic person is more sensitive to such precipitating factors. Examples are carpal tunnel syndrome, radiculopathy, 3rd cranial nerve palsy-ptosis, and footdrop. After 10 to 25 years of diabetes, 25% of patients with diabetes, types 1 or 2, develop end-stage renal disease. The earliest sign of nephropathy (choice **D**) is albumin in the urine. Macrovascular disease (choice **E**) involves changes in medium- to large-sized blood vessels. These lead to coronary artery disease, cerebrovascular disease, and occlusive peripheral arterial disease.

2 **The answer is D** *Surgery*

The chemistry panel shows hypercalcemia; no other abnormalities are evident. In an asymptomatic woman with a normal examination and no history of bone pain, hypercalcemia is most likely due to primary hyperparathyroidism. About 1 in 1000 adult patients are found to have hyperparathyroidism. Most commonly it occurs in patients over 52 years old and three times more often in females than in males. The presenting symptom is usually hypercalcemia, often picked up accidentally during a routine laboratory analysis. In 80% of cases the disease is caused by hypersecretion by one of the inferior parathyroid glands; in almost all remaining cases two or more parathyroid glands have undergone a benign hyperplasia. Parathyroid carcinoma is exceedingly rare and usually causes severe hypercalcemia. In addition to increasing serum calcium levels, hyperparathyroidism also lowers serum phosphate concentration. However, the most direct way of confirming the clinical suspicion of hyperparathyroidism is by measuring parathyroid levels (choice **D**). Although early mild hyperparathyroidism seems innocuous, over the long run it is anything but. Eventually it is likely to become symptomatic, as succinctly described in the classic rhyme "bones, stones, abdominal groans, psychic moans with fatigue overtones." Commonly a renal stone is the first physical presentation, but skeletal abnormalities and psychic manifestation are liable to be not far behind. Treatment is surgical removal of the offending gland.

Congratulating her on being so healthy and sending her home (choice **A**) would be tantamount to malpractice because the probable outcome would development of one or more of the many symptoms associated with hypercalcemia. Metastatic breast cancer could result in hypercalcemia, but subjecting her to mammography because of suspect metastatic breast cancer (choice **B**) when the only symptom is hypercalcemia is not a very logical first step to take. Adding a thiazide diuretic to treat her hypertension (choice **C**) could be acceptable treatment provided hypertension is confirmed, dietary intervention is found to be unsuccessful, and the patient does not have hypercalcemia; thiazides are liable to acerbate hypercalcemia because they decrease renal calcium excretion. This tends to raise serum calcium levels and probably accounts for their antiosteoporotic action. Laboratory findings in sarcoidosis may include hypercalcemia, and chest radiography may show mediastinal lymphadenopathy, a hallmark finding in 90% of cases. But this woman shows no symptoms of sarcoidosis other than hypercalcemia, so conducting a radiographic study because of suspected sarcoidosis (choice **E**) would mark the physician as a poor diagnostician.

3 **The answer is C** *Pediatrics*

These symptoms are characteristic of a generalized tonic (grand mal) seizure. The postictal phase of generalized tonic–clonic seizures lasts approximately 30 minutes to 2 hours (not 1 to 2 minutes [choice **D**]). The actual seizure consists of loss of consciousness, followed by the eyes rolling back and tonic contractions, not flaccidity (choice **A**). The clonic phase then ensues. Urinary incontinence, not retention (choice **B**), is common. These children may also bite their tongue and or cheek (choice **C**) during the seizure but rarely vomit. In the primary form of the disease, the generalized tonic–clonic seizure occurs de novo (choice **E**); however, a generalized seizure may follow a partial seizure with focal onset (secondary generalization).

4 **The answer is A** *Psychiatry*

The boy's symptoms and initial treatment regimen strongly suggest that he has attention-deficit/hyperactivity disorder (ADHD), with predominantly inattentive type. In this subtype of ADHD, impulsivity and hyperactivity are less prominent. While psychostimulants are often the initial treatment of choice for ADHD, anorexia and nervousness are sometimes intolerable adverse effects. Bupropion (choice **A**) and certain other antidepressant medications are often effective for symptoms of ADHD when psychostimulants are not tolerated.

Antipsychotic medication such as olanzapine (choice **B**) and anticonvulsant mood stabilizing medications such as topiramate (choice **D**) play no role in treatment of ADHD. Clonidine (choice **C**) and guanfacine, α_2 auto-receptor blockers, may have some usefulness in treatment of ADHD, but are usually considered only after psychostimulants and antidepressants have proved ineffective or are contraindicated. Desipramine (choice **E**) has been shown to be an effective antidepressant medication for treatment of ADHD but is not used in children because of concerns about causing cardiac arrhythmias.

5 **The answer is C** *Pediatrics*

Warfarin is an anticoagulant that inhibits epoxide reductase, which normally converts inactive vitamin K to active vitamin K_1. Active vitamin K_1 γ-carboxylates the vitamin K-dependent coagulation factors (prothrombin [factor II] and factors VII, IX, and X) that are produced in a nonfunctional state in the liver. γ-Carboxylation allows calcium to bind to these factors so that they can be used to form a fibrin clot. Deficiency of vitamin K_1 renders the vitamin K-dependent coagulation factors nonfunctional; therefore, the patient is anticoagulated. Bleeding from the mouth and gastrointestinal tract is a common sign of overanticoagulation. Since warfarin does not affect platelet production or function, the platelet count and bleeding time (test of platelet function) are normal. The prothrombin time (PT) evaluates the activity of coagulation factors in the extrinsic system (factor VII) to the formation of a fibrin clot in the final common pathway (factors X, V, II, and fibrinogen [factor I]). The activated partial thromboplastin time (APTT) evaluates the activity of the coagulation factors in the intrinsic system (factors XII, XI, IX, and VIII) to the formation of a fibrin clot. Both the PT and APTT are prolonged in warfarin overanticoagulation, because factors X and prothrombin (factor II) are present in the final common pathway. In summary, a patient taking warfarin has a normal platelet count, normal bleeding time (test of platelet function), and increased PT and APTT (choice **C**).

The laboratory findings in choice **A** (decreased platelet count, increased bleeding time, normal PT and APTT) are found in any patient with thrombocytopenia. The bleeding time is increased because the end of the bleeding time correlates with the formation of a temporary platelet plug composed of aggregated platelets held together by fibrinogen. Signs of thrombocytopenia include petechiae and ecchymoses. Bleeding from the gastrointestinal tract is uncommon unless thrombocytopenia is very severe. Thrombocytopenia does not affect the PT and APTT. Warfarin does not affect the platelet count and bleeding time, but it increases the PT and APTT.

The laboratory finding in choice **B** (normal platelet count, bleeding time, and PT; increased APTT) indicates a factor deficiency in the intrinsic coagulation system, usually a factor VIII deficiency (hemophilia A). A normal PT indicates that there are no coagulation factor deficiencies in the extrinsic system or in the final common pathway. Warfarin increases the PT and APTT.

The laboratory findings in choice **D** (normal platelet count, increased bleeding time, normal PT and APTT) indicate a defect in platelet function. The most common cause of increased bleeding time is aspirin or another nonsteroidal antiinflammatory drug, since they inhibit the aggregation of platelets and the formation of a temporary hemostatic plug. Warfarin does not affect platelet production or function, so the bleeding time and platelet count are normal.

The laboratory findings in choice **E** (normal platelet count, increased bleeding time, normal PT, increased APTT) are present in von Willebrand's disease. In von Willebrand's disease, the absence of von Willebrand factor decreases platelet adhesion, which increases the bleeding time. Von Willebrand factor also forms a complex with factor VIII coagulant in the intrinsic system and activates factor VIII. Therefore, a decrease in von Willebrand factor automatically decreases factor VIII activity, causing an increase in the APTT. Warfarin does not affect the bleeding time and increases the PT and the aPTT.

	Platelet Count	Bleeding Time	PT	APTT	
(A)	↓	↑	N	N	Autoimmune thrombocytopenia
(B)	N	N	N	↑	Factor XII, XI, IX, or VIII deficiency
(C)	N	N	↑	↑	Heparin or warfarin therapy
(D)	N	↑	N	N	Aspirin or other nonsteroidal drug
(E)	N	↑	N	↑	Von Willebrand's disease

6 The answer is E *Psychiatry*

This is a case characterized by multiple complaints about multiple organ systems over a long period of time, with unproductive medical assessments and interventions. Since there are no obvious external incentives, and the patient does not appear to relish the sick role and in fact does not get along with medical personnel, malingering (choice **C**) and factitious (choice **A**) disorder are unlikely. Consequently, the symptoms are most suggestive of somatization disorder (choice **E**)

Hypochondriasis (choice **B**) is characterized by misinterpretation of physical symptoms, but this patient is much more concerned with the discomfort itself. Pain disorder (choice **D**) is characterized by pain that is strongly influenced by psychologic factors, but the disorder is not diagnosed when criteria for somatization disorder are present.

7 The answer is B *Pediatrics*

Brain tumors are the most common solid tumors in childhood and are second only to leukemia as the most prevalent malignancy. Infratentorial tumors are the most common in childhood; supratentorial are the most common in adults. Infants less than 2 years of age and adolescents approximate adults in location of tumors. Tumors can further be broken down into those of glial cells and those of primitive neuroectodermal origin. Astrocytomas, ependymomas, and glioblastoma multiforme make up the glial tumors. Neuroectodermal tumors include medulloblastoma and pineoblastoma. Cerebellar astrocytomas (choice **B**) constitute the most common posterior fossa tumors of childhood. They also have the best prognosis, with a 90% 5-year survival rate.

Medulloblastomas (choice **A**) are the second most common posterior fossa tumors of childhood. Ependymomas (choice **C**) are responsible for about 10% of tumors of the posterior fossa. Neuroblastoma (choice **D**) is the most common extracranial solid tumor of childhood. Patients with oligodendrogliomas (choice **E**) may have a long-term history of complex partial epilepsy, especially if the location of the tumor is in the temporal lobe.

8 **The answer is C** *Surgery*

Because the anterior cruciate ligament (ACL) (choice **C**) is thinner and weaker, it is more prone to rupture than the posterior cruciate ligament (choice **D**). In addition, it remains taut in extension. The ACL limits hyperextension at the knee and external rotation of the tibia. ACL tears also may occur when a jogger stops suddenly or a tennis player twists his knee. Hearing a popping sound is pathognomonic. Hemarthrosis is noted, because the artery to the anterior cruciate ligament runs along the ligament. The most common cause of hemarthrosis in an otherwise stable knee is rupture of the ACL (see below). Treatment is surgical repair.

The Lachman test is the most sensitive and the best test used to evaluate the ACL. The posterior drawer test is used to evaluate the posterior cruciate ligament (PCL).

Tears of the medial collateral ligament (choice **B**) or the lateral collateral ligament (choice **A**) usually present with tenderness along the ligament. Distraction aggravates pain. Dislocation of the patella (choice **E**) usually occurs due to a tear of the lateral expansion of the quadriceps and most often reduces spontaneously. A patient with a dislocated patella cannot straight leg raise, and a defect is noticeable over the anterior aspect of the knee.

9 **The answer is C** *Psychiatry*

The patient's symptoms suggest dementia with behavioral symptoms. Antipsychotic medications have been shown to be effective for this indication and should be started in low doses in elderly individuals because of greater sensitivity to their effects. Haloperidol (choice **C**) has been used for this indication for many years because it causes minimal sedation and relatively fewer anticholinergic and cardiovascular adverse effects than less potent older antipsychotic medications like chlorpromazine (choice **A**).

Recent studies have demonstrated a significant increase in deaths in older adults treated with newer (atypical) antipsychotic medications for behavioral problems associated with dementia. Consequently, pending further data, atypical antipsychotic medications (choices **B, D,** and **E**) should not be used for initial treatment of this condition, unless specific contraindications to other agents exist.

10 **The answer is A** *Surgery*

The prevalence of malignant melanoma is estimated to be increasing worldwide at an annual 6% rate. Lightly pigmented individuals are at a higher risk. The ABCD signs of melanoma are *A*symmetry, *B*orders irregular, *C*olor changes, *D*iameter increasing. Types of melanoma include superficial spreading melanoma (about 70% of cases of melanoma), lentigo maligna melanoma (10–15%), nodular melanoma 10–15%), acral lentiginous melanoma (<10%), and mucosal lentiginous melanoma (3%). The depth of invasion best determines biologic behavior. Lesions with <0.76 mm invasion do not metastasize. Lesions with >1.7 mm invasion have the potential for lymph node metastasis. Treatment for melanomas is excision with wide margins. The survival rate for whites diagnosed with melanoma rose from 60% in 1960–1963 to 85% in 1983–1990 primarily because better surveillance caused earlier detection.

The patient has a lentigo malignant melanoma (choice **A**), which most commonly affects sun-exposed, fair-skinned whites, who are 60 to 80 years old on the face, head, and neck. These lesions usually show variegated colors ranging from black, to brown, to reddish and are relatively large, 2 to 60 cm in diameter. They also have a prolonged radial phase, during which the malignant melanocytes proliferate laterally within the epidermis, along the dermoepidermal junction, or within the papillary dermis. There is no metastasis in this phase; thus surgical removal results in a high cure rate. The vertical phase, in which invasion extends deeper into the reticular dermis and subcutaneous fat is heralded by the development of raised areas that often reach several centimeters in diameter. Metastasis commonly occurs in the vertical phase.

Superficial spreading melanoma (choice **B**) is the most common malignant melanoma in lightly pigmented individuals and most commonly develops on the lower extremities and trunk from a pigmented dysplastic nevus. In the process of malignant transformation the nevus will show early changes, which might include ulceration, enlargement, or color change. Some sort of undefined irritative change is the most probable triggering factor; suspect factors include sunburn (not so much long-term sun exposure) or irritating clothing. Superficial spreading melanoma, as the name implies also spreads laterally along the epidermal line before penetrating deeper tissues. These lesions are generally smaller, 2 to 3 cm in diameter, and most often affect people in their 50s and 60s. Nodular melanoma (choice **C**) appears as uniformly colored, dark brown to black, relatively small, symmetric nodules on patients 30 to 50 years old. They truly deserve the name malignant since they directly invade the dermis without a radial growth phase and have a poor prognosis. Acral lentiginous melanoma (choice **D**) is not related to excess ultraviolet light exposure as indicated by the fact it is located on the palms, soles, beneath the nail, or in the inguinal region. It is at least as common in African Americans as in whites, is very aggressive, and has a poor prognosis. Mucosal lentiginous melanoma (choice **E**) arises in mucosal epithelial lining of the respiratory tract, gastrointestinal tract, and genitourinary tract and has a very poor prognosis, primarily because it is diagnosed too late.

11 The answer is B *Medicine*

Because this patient with AIDS was recently treated with nystatin, he is presumed to have suffered from oropharyngeal candidiasis, which puts him at greater risk for the development of pneumonia due to *Pneumocystis carinii* (PCP). This is especially likely to occur given the daily spikes of body temperature that are occurring. Trimethoprim–sulfamethoxazole (TMP-SMX) (choice **B**) is normally considered the drug of choice in both prophylaxis and treatment of PCP.

Pentamidine (choice **A**) (via aerosol) or dapsone (choice **D**) given individually is a reasonable alternative for prophylaxis in patients who are unable to tolerate TMP-SMX or who are allergic to sulfonamides. AIDS patients are treated with pyrimethamine–sulfadiazine (choice **E**) for prevention of toxoplasmosis. However, this drug will also serve as prophylaxis against PCP. Note that patients on TMP-SMX are adequately protected against infections due to *Toxoplasma gondii*. The antimalarial drug primaquine (choice **C**), given alone, does not afford adequate protection against PCP. However, primaquine given together with clindamycin can be effective.

12 The answer is E *Obstetrics and Gynecology*

The concern in this question has to do with Sheehan syndrome, which results from anterior pituitary insufficiency due to severe postpartum hemorrhage. The impact on the anterior pituitary tropic hormones can vary from only partial deficit of one hormone to complete loss of all hormones. The syndrome can have rapid onset or gradual onset over many months. The answer is option **E,** prolactin, which is the hormone most commonly affected. The clinical finding will be failure to lactate because of lack of breast engorgement.

The other options would be less likely to be affected. If the damage is more severe, it can involve the gonadotropins (option **D**, FSH, and option **A**, LH). The most severe forms of Sheehan syndrome will involve option **B**, TSH, and option **C**, ACTH.

13 The answer is D *Medicine*

A patient with exophthalmos and lid retraction has Graves' disease, which is the most common cause of hyperthyroidism. It is a female-dominant autoimmune disease seen predominantly between the ages of 20 and 40 years, and it has a characteristic triad of symptoms—exophthalmos, a diffuse goiter, and hyperthyroidism. Other features that are unique to Graves' disease are pretibial myxedema (nonpitting) and immunoglobulin G (IgG) thyroid-stimulating autoantibodies against the thyroid-stimulating hormone (TSH) receptor. These autoantibodies continually stimulate the gland without any negative feedback. Nodular toxic goiters also produce hyperthyroidism but do not have the features unique to Graves' disease. Laboratory findings in Graves' disease include a normal thyroid-binding globulin level (not decreased [choice **A**]), increased serum triiodothyronine (T_3) and thyroxine (T_4) levels (not decreased [choices **B** and **E**], increased ^{123}I uptake (not decreased [choice **C**]), and decreased serum TSH level (choice **D**).

The treatment of Graves' disease is varied. β-Blocking agents are useful for blocking adrenergic symptoms associated with the disease. Antithyroid medications (e.g., methimazole and propylthiouracil) are used to block hormone synthesis, but there are problems with rashes, agranulocytosis, and recurrent disease. Radioactive iodine (^{123}I) is used to ablate the gland if oral medications are unsuccessful. A subtotal thyroidectomy has a high success rate but carries a risk for hypoparathyroidism.

14 The answer is A *Psychiatry*

The usual triad of symptoms following severe emotional trauma is intrusive recollections and reexperiencing, emotional numbness, and anxiety. Young children in such circumstances often present with nightmares with disorganized behavior. The time frame in this case is too short for diagnosis of posttraumatic stress disorder (PTSD) (choice **E**), which requires duration of symptoms more than one month. Acute stress disorder (choice **A**) is therefore more likely. Attention-deficit/hyperactivity disorder (choice **B**) involves short attention span, impulsivity, and hyperactivity, but the rapid onset of these symptoms in the face of significant emotional trauma makes this a less likely diagnosis for this child. Brief psychotic disorder with marked stressors (choice **C**) involves the sudden onset of psychosis after emotional trauma, but in this case there is no clear evidence of hallucinations, delusions, or disorganized thinking. Panic disorder (choice **D**) involves attacks of anxiety, but the diagnosis is not made when the anxiety is better accounted for by another disorder, as is the case here.

15 The answer is D   *Pediatrics*

Trauma (choice **D**) is the most common cause of intracranial hemorrhage in children and consequently must be viewed with a high degree of suspicion in this child. In infants, intracranial hemorrhage can result from trauma or asphyxia. Aneurysms (choice **B**) and arteriovenous malformations (choice **C**) are less common causes of hemorrhage in children. Hypertension (choice **A**) is rarely involved. A brain abscess (choice **E**) may cause coma and death. Brain abscesses are rare in children of any age. Causes include meningitis, orbital cellulitis, dental infection, and embolization due to congenital heart disease with right-to-left shunts.

16 The answer is E   *Surgery*

Cryoprecipitated blood (choice **E**) has a high concentration of proteins including factor VIII, the missing coagulation factor in hemophilia A; consequently, a small volume can be used to treat the patient's deficiency and stop the bleeding. It can also be used to treat other coagulation factor deficiencies such as von Willebrand's factor, or factor IX deficiency (hemophilia B).

Fresh frozen plasma (choice **A**) also contains the coagulation factors, but in such limited amounts that a very large volume would be required; hence, it is not the best choice. Packed platelets (choice **B**) would not contain coagulation factors but could be used to treat thrombocytopenia or platelet dysfunction. Whole blood (choice **C**), like fresh frozen plasma, contains the coagulation factors in very low concentration but, because storage is inefficient, most blood banks do not store it, and it likely would not be readily available. Packed red blood cells (choice **D**) can be stored for up to 35 days. They lose platelets, factor V, and factor VII activity but retain factor VIII activity and could thus be used to stop the bleeding in this patient in a practical way but, once again, a larger volume would be required.

17 The answer is D   *Medicine*

The myeloproliferate disorders are a group of disease states that arise from hyperproliferation of hemapoietic precursor stem cells. Since normally these stem cells give rise to mature erythroid, myeloid, and platelet cells, a myeloproliferative disorder results in a qualitative and/or quantitative aberration in one or more of these cell types. On the basis of well-defined clinical and laboratory features, most clinicians recognize four distinct myeloproliferative disease states: chronic myelogenous leukemia (CML), polycythemia vera (PV), chronic idiopathic myelofibrosis, and essential thrombocytopenia (ET). This patient's platelet count, which is almost an order of magnitude higher than the high normal range, clearly points to ET (choice **D**).

ET is a myeloproliferative disorder characterized by overproduction of megakaryocytes, the platelet precursor cells. In this condition, the blood white cell count is either high normal or as in this case slightly elevated, and the hematocrit and red cell count and morphology are normal. Bone marrow shows a megakaryocytic hyperplasia, and the life span of the mature platelets is normal, confirming it is a disease of hyperproliferation. The median age at presentation is 50 to 60 years, and females are affected slightly more often than males. Although it is an acquired condition, the cause is unknown. A southern Minnesota study estimates the incidence to be 2.38 cases per 100,000 persons. A quarter to a third of cases is discovered during a routine examination before there are any symptoms other than a high platelet count. The progress of the disease is rather indolent, but symptoms associated with thromboses will develop; these may be minor or life threatening, and they often respond to aspirin. Paradoxically abnormal bleeding, usually mucosal, is another common symptom in more advanced cases. Some 0.6 to 5% of cases will convert to acute myelogenous leukemia; this transformation appears to be enhanced by chemotherapeutic agents. There is a 64 to 80% 10-year survival rate that, taken in conjunction with the relatively advanced age at inception means that normal life spans are, on average, not greatly decreased.

Chronic myelogenous leukemia (CML) (choice **A**) is a myeloproliferative disorder characterized by overproduction of myeloid cells, and it accounts for about 50% of all the myeloproliferative disorders. These myeloid cells retain the capacity to differentiate normally for years, and normal bone marrow function is retained for years (the primary differentiating feature is a lower-than-normal alkaline phosphatase level). Eventually, a malignant transformation occurs. In 95% of cases the initiating event to the accelerated growth phase is a reciprocal translocation between the long arms of chromosomes 9 and 22. A larger piece of 22q is translocated to 9q, and a smaller piece of 9q goes to 22q, forming the Philadelphia chromosome in which the smaller 9q segment contains the *abl* protooncogene that now is placed in juxtaposition to the *bcr* gene, which possesses tyrosine kinase activity. This new *bcr/abl* gene leads to the leukemia. The tyrosine kinase activity of the *bcr* sequence is inhibited by imatinib, which provides effective treatment.

Polycythemia vera (choice **B**) (sometimes called polycythemia rubra vera) is a myeloproliferative disorder characterized by overproduction of all three hematopoietic cell lines but most prominently the red cell line. The hallmark of polycythemia vera (PV) is a hematocrit above normal, sometimes over 60%. The disease is most commonly diagnosed in the 60-year-old age group, with a male-to-female ratio of 1.4 to 1; the prevalence is 5–17 cases per 10^6 persons. The white cell and platelet counts are also elevated but to a lesser degree. PV needs to be differentiated from spurious polycythemia caused by blood volume contraction and from secondary polycythemia. In PV, erythroid progenitor cells grow in vitro in the absence of erythropoietin, and the bone marrow is hypercellular with panhyperplasia of all hemopoietic elements. The excessive rate of red cell production can deplete the marrow of iron stores. Vitamin B_{12} levels are elevated because of increased levels of transcobalamin III secreted by leukocytes. In uncontrolled PV, there is a high incidence of thrombosis and paradoxically increased bleeding, particularly gastrointestinal. This bleeding may lower the red cell count and confuse diagnosis. Treatment is phlebotomy to lower the hematocrit below 45%. Occasionally, myelosuppressive therapy is required, and hydroxyurea is the drug of choice. Daily consumption of a low-dose aspirin reduces the risk of thrombosis and is generally recommended as a prophylactic agent. PV is an indolent disease with a median survival of 11–15 years. The major cause of morbidly is arterial thrombosis. Over time, PV may convert to myelofibrosis or chronic myelogenous leukemia, and in about 5% of cases the disease progresses to a form of acute myelogenous leukemia that resists therapy.

Chronic idiopathic myelofibrosis (choice **C**), also known as agnogenic myeloid metaplasia, is a myeloproliferative disease that causes fibrosis in the bone marrow and severe splenomegaly and results in a leukoerythroblastic peripheral blood smear with teardrop poikilocytosis. Patients usually present after the age of 50 years with anemia. In response to marrow fibrosis, fetal hematopoiesis in the liver, spleen, and lymph nodes can be reactivated. Eventually liver and spleen enlargement may lead to portal hypertension and splenetic rupture, respectively. The median lifetime survival after diagnosis is 5 years; however, several new treatment modalities are presently in clinical trials.

18 **The answer is B** *Preventive Medicine and Public Health*

This man shows signs of Wernicke syndrome, which is caused by a deficiency of thiamine (vitamin B_1) (choice **B**) and is associated with alcoholism. This deficiency leads to neurologic deficits and, in 80% of cases, is associated with Korsakoff syndrome characterized by short-term memory deficits. The combination of Wernicke's encephalopathy and Korsakoff's psychosis is the familiar Wernicke-Korsakoff syndrome. Wernicke's encephalopathy is a medical emergency that can cause permanent brain damage because thiamine in the form of thiamine pyrophosphate is the cofactor for pyruvate dehydrogenase and α-ketoglutarate dehydrogenase, two key energy-generating reactions of critical importance for neurologic function. Thus, when Wernicke syndrome is suspected, intravenous thiamine should be administered immediately. This should be done before glucose is administered because glucose catabolism can deplete the body of any residual thiamine. Wernicke-Korsakoff syndrome is the primary symptom of thiamine deficiency in the United States and is due to a combination of poor nutrition and impaired intestinal absorption. Worldwide, thiamine deficiency is called beriberi and is typically caused by a diet in which polished white rice constitutes a substantial part. Infant beriberi can have a rapid onset in nursing infants whose mothers are thiamine deficient. It is characterized by tachycardia, vomiting, convulsions, and, if not treated, death. Adult beriberi is characterized by dry skin, confusion, irritability, and progressive neuropathy, which may lead to paralysis.

Ascorbic acid (vitamin C) (choice **A**) is a cofactor for the hydroxylation of lysine and proline residues during collagen synthesis. Hydroxylation sites are where cross-bridges anchor strands and increase the tensile strength of collagen. The vitamin is also important as an antioxidant and in preventing nitrosylation (it inhibits amides from combining with nitrites present in food preservatives). Nitrosamines and nitrosamides are carcinogens that have been implicated in stomach cancer. Vitamin C deficiency (scurvy) is most often caused by diets that are lacking in fruits and vegetables (e.g., elderly patients on "tea and toast" diet). Clinical findings in vitamin C deficiency are due primarily to weak collagen in tissue leading to skin and perifollicular hemorrhages, hemarthroses, bleeding gums, glossitis, and poor wound healing. Riboflavin (vitamin B₂) deficiency (choice **C**) causes dermatitis, cheilosis, and glossitis but is not associated with any major diseases. Niacin (vitamin B₃) in the form of nicotine adenine dinucleotide (NAD⁺) and nicotine adenine dinucleotide phosphate (NADP⁺) is a cofactor in catabolic reactions (e.g., glycolysis) and anabolic reactions (e.g., cholesterol synthesis) throughout the body. Niacin deficiency (choice **D**), known as pellagra, is generally caused by diets that are deficient in niacin and tryptophan (an amino acid that can be used to synthesize niacin). Corn-based diets are deficient in both tryptophan and niacin. Clinical findings of niacin deficiency include the 3 D's—diarrhea, dermatitis (hyperpigmentation in sun-exposed areas), and dementia. Pyridoxine (vitamin B₆) deficiency (choice **E**) is rare except in individuals being treated for tuberculosis with isoniazid, since isoniazid forms an inactive derivative with pyridoxal phosphate, the active form of vitamin B₆.

19. The answer is D *Pediatrics*

The lesions described in the mouth are known as Koplik's spots, which are pathognomonic of rubeola (choice **D**), aka measles. Koplik's spots occur during the prodromal stage, which also presents with fever, dry cough, coryza, conjunctivitis, photophobia, and cervical lymphadenopathy. The temperature rises with the advent of the rash. Koplik's spots are transient, lasting approximately 12 to 18 hours. They are best seen opposite the lower molars.

Kawasaki disease (choice **A**) is a febrile disease affecting children. It is associated with fever, conjunctival infection, and infection of the oral mucosa, strawberry tongue, nonvesicular polymorphous rash, and cervical lymphadenopathy. Rubella, aka German measles (choice **B**), is a viral exanthematous disease of children and adults with worldwide distribution. The signs and symptoms include adenopathy (posterior auricular), low-grade fever, arthralgias, coryza, and conjunctivitis. The exanthem is descending, beginning on the face or neck and spreading in hours to the trunk and extremities. Adenovirus infection (choice **C**) is the cause of a wide array of syndromes. It may manifest as pharyngoconjunctival fever. More importantly, it is a cause of acute respiratory disease in children. Still's disease (choice **E**) is a subset of juvenile rheumatoid arthritis in which the main manifestations are systemic. Fever, rash, leukocytosis, lymphadenopathy, pericarditis, pharyngitis, and hepatosplenomegaly are common in association with the arthritis.

20. The answer is C *Surgery*

A bloody nipple discharge in a woman under 50 years of age is most commonly caused by an intraductal papilloma (choice **C**) located in the lactiferous duct. In most cases, a mass is not palpable. Applying pressure circumferentially around the nipple to see which lactiferous duct is emptying blood identifies the involved duct. Cytology should be performed on the bloody material. Intraductal papillomas may be multicentric (involve other ducts) or can involve the contralateral breast (25% of cases). A segmental resection of the lactiferous duct is recommended.

A bloody nipple discharge in a woman older than 50 years of age is most commonly associated with malignancy, an infiltrating ductal carcinoma (choice **D**). Any bloody discharge from an adult male nipple is usually due to malignancy. Intraductal papillomatosis (choice **A**) refers to ductal hyperplasia in fibrocystic change (choice **E**). It is nonpalpable. A subareolar abscess (choice **B**), most commonly due to *Staphylococcus aureus*, produces a purulent nipple discharge. Subareolar abscesses are usually associated with breast-feeding.

21. The answer is C *Pediatrics*

The primary risk factors for acquiring the human immunodeficiency virus (HIV) are intravenous drug use, prostitution, and sexual relations with a seropositive individual. Contaminated blood transfusion is currently a lesser risk. This woman has all of the primary risk factors; therefore, she is most likely seropositive. Although perinatal treatment of HIV-infected mothers with antiretroviral drugs has dramatically decreased transmission rates, the risk of perinatal transmission of the virus approaches 12 to 30% in the United States and 25 to 52% in Haiti and Africa without treatment. Hence, in this case, there is a very good chance that the newborn has also acquired the virus. The ideal treatment is to administer oral zidovudine (AZT) during pregnancy and intravenously during delivery, and then immediately start the newborn on oral drug therapy (choice **C**); obviously in this case, only the last aspect can be carried out. Such a regimen has been shown to reduce the risk of infection in the newborn by 67.5%. To be effective, treatment has to be started within 24 hours, before the virus has a chance to start replication. Therefore, waiting to treat the infant until symptoms appear (choices **D** and **E**) would not be the most appropriate response. Candidiasis infection is a relatively early and common symptom of HIV infection in infants, whereas development of Kaposi's sarcoma is a relatively rare manifestation in children.

Conducting an enzyme-linked immunosorbent assay (ELISA) on the newborn (choice **A**) has diagnostic value provided the mother is not infected by the virus. However, if she is infected, the test result would be positive whatever the status of the child because of the passive transmission of maternal antibodies. From 60 to 80% of antibody-positive cases in infants are just that—the test result reverts to negative with time, and the children show no sign of infection. However, withholding treatment on the chance that the child will test negative would deny the chance of reducing the risk of disease. Withholding treatment until the mother is tested (choice **B**) would not be the best course of action for the same reason.

22 The answer is B *Psychiatry*

Buprenorphine (choice **B**) is used alone or in combination with naltrexone for prevention of relapse into heroin abuse. Buprenorphine, like methadone, is an opioid agonist that decreases craving for illicit opioids such as heroin and thus makes relapse less likely. Unlike methadone, it can be prescribed outside of specialized methadone maintenance programs. Because it acts as an antagonist at higher doses, there is a ceiling effect. As an additional safeguard against misuse, it is sometimes combined with naloxone (Suboxone). Naloxone is poorly absorbed orally, but if an inappropriately high dose of buprenorphine is ingested, the naloxone blocks opioid receptors.

Acamprosate (choice **A**) is a GABA modulator that has efficacy in preventing alcohol relapse. Codeine (choice **C**) is an opioid analgesic and antitussive that has no use in prevention of heroin relapse. Disulfiram (Antabuse) (choice **D**) inhibits aldehyde dehydrogenase and makes alcohol relapse more difficult. Naltrexone (choice **E**) is an opioid agonist related to naloxone that is sometimes given to make severe heroin relapse less likely but has not been shown to be as effective as buprenorphine.

23 The answer is D *Medicine*

The patient has pericarditis complicated by a pericardial effusion (choice **D**). It is most likely due to a coxsackievirus infection; however, a serum antinuclear antibody test should be ordered to rule out systemic lupus erythematosus (SLE), in which pericardial and pleural effusions are common presenting diseases. Inflammation of the pericardium causes increased vessel permeability and leakage of a fibrinous exudate onto the serosal surface. The exudate produces a friction rub heard over the precordium during filling and emptying of the heart. Fluid accumulates in the pericardial sac, produces muffled heart sounds, and prevents filling of the right side of the heart during inspiration. During inspiration, venous blood is normally drawn into the right side of the heart by the increasing negative intrathoracic pressure; this causes the observed neck vein distention, called Kussmaul's sign. Decreased right-sided filling causes a decrease in cardiac output, resulting in decreased pulse amplitude and blood pressure during inspiration (pulsus paradoxus). The pain caused by inflammation of the pericardium is aggravated by inspiration and is relieved by leaning forward. Chest radiography reveals a "water-bottle"–shaped heart, and an electrocardiogram (ECG) shows ST wave elevation. The first step in management is to order an echocardiogram to confirm the presence of an effusion. Fluid must then be removed from the pericardial sac by paracentesis or death will occur.

Aortic dissections (choice **A**) most often occur in elderly men with hypertension or younger individuals with defects in collagen (Ehlers-Danlos syndrome) or elastic tissue (Marfan syndrome). Blood enters an intimal tear causing dissection proximally and/or distally through the weakened media of the aorta. Pain radiates into the back and is often associated with absent upper extremity pulses. These findings are not present in the patient. Congestive (dilated) cardiomyopathy (choice **B**) is associated with an enlarged heart with dilation of atria and ventricles as well as biventricular congestive heart failure. Signs of right-sided heart failure (e.g., dependent pitting edema) or left-sided heart failure (e.g., pulmonary edema) are not present in this patient. Constrictive pericarditis (choice **C**) is most often idiopathic or a complication of tuberculosis. Thickening of the parietal pericardium causes incomplete filling of the cardiac chambers. Pericardial effusions are not present. Restrictive cardiomyopathy (choice **E**) is characterized by decreased ventricular compliance (decreased filling of the heart) caused by an infiltrative disease of the myocardium (e.g., amyloid). Pericardial effusions are not usually present.

24 **The answer is A** *Surgery*

Ductal carcinoma in situ (DCIS) (choice **A**) is a nonpalpable malignancy that commonly contains foci of microcalcifications in areas of necrosis in the duct. One third of low-grade DCIS will eventually invade.

A phyllodes tumor (choice **B**) is a bulky tumor (often reaches massive size) that is derived from stromal cells. It is most often benign; however, it is considered a low-grade malignancy when there is hypercellular stroma with an increased number of mitoses. Grossly, it is a lobulated tumor that has cystic spaces with leaflike extensions. It does not have calcifications. A medullary carcinoma (choice **C**) is a bulky, soft tumor with large cells and a lymphoid infiltrate. It does not have calcifications. A lobular carcinoma in situ (choice **D**) is the most common cancer involving the terminal lobules. The tumor is nonpalpable and does not calcify. The lobules are distended with bland neoplastic cells. There is an increased incidence of cancer in the opposite breast (any type of cancer). One third will eventually develop into an invasive lobular cancer. A fibroadenoma (choice **E**) is the most common breast mass in women less than 35 years old. It is a benign tumor that is derived from the stroma (similar to a phyllodes tumor except the stroma is not hypercellular). The stroma proliferates and compresses the ducts giving them a "Chinese letter" appearance. Clinically, it is a discreet, movable, painless or painful mass that may increase in size during the menstrual cycle or pregnancy (estrogen-sensitive). It rarely becomes malignant and does not calcify.

25 **The answer is D** *Psychiatry*

The symptoms suggest a hand washing compulsion, a common presentation of obsessive–compulsive disorder (OCD) (choice **D**). The disorder is characterized by obsessions (repetitive thoughts) and/or compulsions (irresistible impulses, often without logic).

Delusional disorder (choice **A**) is less likely because the individual seems to recognize that the compulsion is peculiar and tries to resist it. Generalized anxiety disorder (choice **B**) is excessive worry about several things. Although OCD is an anxiety condition, in this case his anxiety is focused on dirty hands and the anxiety is controlled by his obsessive hand washing. Malingering (choice **C**) is the deliberate production of symptoms for some external gain. While individuals sometimes engage in malingering to avoid armed service, this symptom was difficult to elicit and is unlikely to result in a medical service deferment, making malingering less likely. Posttraumatic stress disorder (choice **E**) sometimes presents with anxiety, but there is no evidence of past emotional trauma or reexperiencing in this case.

26 **The answer is A** *Medicine*

The patient has cardiomyopathy as shown by the increased level of cardiac-specific troponins, indicating myocardial necrosis. In this young man this may well be due to a myocarditis arising as a complication of a coxsackievirus infection. Clinical findings include left-sided heart failure (dyspnea, bibasilar inspiratory crackles); right-sided heart failure (neck vein distention, hepatomegaly, dependent pitting edema); and myocardial damage (increased cardiac troponin levels), all suggestive of congestive (dilated) cardiomyopathy (choice **A**). The chest x-ray film shows generalized cardiac enlargement, which is compatible with a congestive (dilated) type of cardiomyopathy due to the myocarditis. Echocardiography shows global myocardial dysfunction, the ejection fraction (stoke volume/left ventricular end-diastolic volume) is 0.20, and an electrocardiogram (ECG) reveals a low-voltage QRS. Again, these findings are compatible with a diagnosis of congestive (dilated) type of cardiomyopathy due to the myocarditis. The treatment is to the underlying cause, if it is clearly defined, and to manage the biventricular heart failure. Patients are usually anticoagulated because of the high incidence of left mural thrombi developing in the left atrium. A partial left ventriculotomy may be indicated in some cases. Cardiac transplantation is required in medically resistant cases.

Coronary artery thrombosis (choice **B**) producing an acute myocardial infarction is unlikely because the ECG does not reveal new Q waves and ST elevations. Ischemic heart disease (choice **C**) is unlikely because of the patient's age and the lack of an antecedent history of angina. It is associated with replacement of myocardial tissue by collagen. Restrictive cardiomyopathy (choice **D**) is associated with systolic dysfunction due to reduced contractility (decreased ejection fraction) and diastolic dysfunction owing to reduced compliance of the ventricles because of amyloid deposition, glycogen deposition, or fibrous tissue. The ECG will reveal a low-voltage pattern and conduction disturbances. Unlike congestive cardiomyopathy, chest radiography does not show generalized enlargement of the atria and ventricles. A patient with rheumatic fever (choice **E**) would have a history of group A streptococcal infection. Since the antistreptolysin O titers are normal, the diagnosis of acute rheumatic fever is unlikely.

27 The answer is B   *Psychiatry*

Studies of the homeless population suggest that approximately one third (choice **B**) have severe and persistent mental illness; therefore, choices **A** (15%), **C** (50%), **D** (60%), and **E** (90%) are incorrect. Common pathologies include schizophrenia and severe mood disorders. The prevalence of substance abuse in the homeless population is even higher and includes a substantial percentage of the mentally ill homeless population.

28 The answer is C   *Pediatrics*

Adrenoleukodystrophy (choice **C**) is an X-linked disease that affects young males, usually beginning at 7 or 8 years of age. It is characterized by demyelination of the central nervous system (CNS), adrenal insufficiency, mental deterioration, aphasia, apraxia, and dysarthria. Approximately one third of patients with this disease also have vision loss.

   Although multiple sclerosis (choice **A**) is also a CNS-demyelinating disease, the clinical scenario with posterior hemisphere predominance and age of onset best fits adrenoleukodystrophy. Metachromatic leukodystrophy (choice **B**) generally presents with weakness and decreased reflexes instead of spasticity and with symmetric CNS demyelination. Subacute sclerosing panencephalitis (choice **D**) is a slow viral disease caused by the measles virus. Creutzfeldt-Jakob disease (choice **E**) is a spongiform encephalopathy caused by proteinaceous infectious particles called *prions*. It occurs in adults and produces dementia.

29 The answer is F   *Medicine*

The patient has psoriasis (choice **F**). Psoriasis is a chronic inflammatory dermatosis with unregulated proliferation of keratinocytes (epithelial hyperplasia). Genetic factors and infection (e.g., streptococcal pharyngitis) are implicated in its pathogenesis. The lesions are well-demarcated, flat, elevated salmon-colored papules and/or plaques that are covered by adherent white to silver-colored scales. Pinpoint areas of bleeding occur when the scales are scraped off (Auspitz sign). Common skin sites include the scalp (simulates seborrheic dermatitis) and pressure areas such as the elbows and lower back. The lesions commonly develop in areas of trauma, which is called Koebner's phenomenon. Pitting of the nails is present in 80% of cases. Treatment of limited disease includes topical steroids, calcipotriene (vitamin D analogue), tar products, and retinoids (e.g., tazarotene). More extensive disease is treated with ultraviolet B (UVB) light exposure, psoralen plus UVA light (PUVA), methotrexate, cyclosporine, or alefacept (recombinant protein that selectively targets T cells). There may be associated arthritis that resembles the rheumatoid type, but affected persons test negative for the rheumatoid factor.

   Herpes zoster (shingles) (choice **A**) is due to reactivation of a latent varicella-zoster virus in the sensory dorsal root ganglia. It tends to occur in older persons and also may occur in immunoincompetent or immunosuppressed patients. Pain along the affected nerve is the first symptom, followed by a rash characterized by an eruption of painful vesicles that follows a dermatomal distribution. The treatment involves pain control (e.g., nonsteroidal antiinflammatory drugs, or aspirin with codeine in severe cases) and oral administration of valacyclovir or famciclovir. Acne rosacea (choice **B**) is an inflammatory reaction involving the pilosebaceous units of facial skin, which most commonly affects middle-aged or older persons. The lesion simulates the malar rash of systemic lupus erythematosus, except there is erythema accompanied by papules, pustules, cysts, nodules, and telangiectasia. Although the condition itself affects women more often that men, hyperplasia of sebaceous glands and soft tissue of the nose (rhinophyma) is commonly seen in men. Topical antibiotics (e.g., metronidazole cream, sodium sulfacetamide), topical benzoyl peroxide, or systemic antibiotics (e.g., tetracycline or doxycycline) are used for therapy. Solar lentigo (choice **C**) is a skin change related to ultraviolet light damage. It is characterized by pigmented areas commonly called "liver spots" and common in elderly persons. They are not precancerous and do not require therapy. Actinic keratosis (choice **D**) also is associated with excessive ultraviolet light exposure but presents as slightly raised, rough, hyperkeratotic areas commonly found on sun-exposed sites such as the dorsum of hands and forearms, the cheeks, and the back of the neck. These may appear as an isolated spot or spread over an extensive area. They are a precursor lesion (i.e., squamous dysplasia) for squamous cell carcinoma, which occurs in 2 to 5% of cases. They are treated with either liquid nitrogen or topical 5-fluorouracil. Highly suspicious lesions or lesions that do not clear up with such treatment are removed by curettage and biopsied for pathologic confirmation. Xerosis (choice **E**) is a common inflammatory disorder in elderly patients that is characterized by severe dryness and pruritus of the skin. It may be generalized or localized, especially on the arms, legs, or hands. The lesions are coin-shaped with scaling and erythema, the latter from constant scratching. Topical steroid creams are used for treatment.

30 The answer is B   *Surgery*

Pregnancy after a vasectomy occurs about 0.3% of the time. The most common reason for it is that the couple resumed unprotected sexual relations before azoospermia was complete; it takes about 15 to 20 ejaculations to clear the sperm, not two (choice **B**). After the patient has cleared himself of sperm he still is not considered sterile until two sperm-free ejaculations are obtained on different days.

The classical method of performing a vasectomy is to make a small incision resecting a small piece of the vas and then ligating both ends. The newer "no-scalpel" method involves finding and obliberating the vas without making an incision; this method is less traumatic and just as successful. A competent surgeon should rarely, if ever, fail to completely tie off the vas deferens (choice **A**). There is no way to be sure that the wife is faithful; however, considering the seemingly stable family situation and the fact she is religious, this seems an unlikely possibility. Recanalization of the vas deferens (choice **D**) also is rare, and if it does happen it is a later occurrence. Sperm granulomas are the typical risk factor. Such patients should have semen samples checked for sperm periodically.

31 The answer is E   *Psychiatry*

Schizophrenia (choice **E**) is a very significant risk factor for suicide. Other serious risk factors include feelings of hopelessness, substance abuse, social isolation, and old age. A history of sexual abuse (choice **A**), job dissatisfaction (choice **B**), abusive relationships (choice **C**), and sexual conflicts (choice **D**) are not as closely associated with an increased risk for suicide.

32 The answer is G   *Medicine*

This woman just suffered a stroke. It is fortunate that she is able to get to a phone and utter anything, because the 911 operator should have the wherewithal to get help, and she has a good chance to get to a stroke treatment center within 3 hours; the critical time period in which stroke can most often be successfully treated. Among other symptoms being demonstrated, this woman cannot talk properly, and she has aphasia. Aphasia can be subdivided into several types. One of the more common ones is Broca's aphasia (choice **G**) caused by a lesion in the left frontal area (areas 44 and 45) of the cerebrum and characterized by an inability to speak more than a few words, usually fewer than four, and these are generally enunciated with great difficulty. Such patients retain the ability to understand spoken and written language but may have a problem with writing as well as speaking.

Agnosia (choice **A**) is characterized by an inability to recognize sensory input, which may be visual, auditory, tactile, gustatory, or olfactory. Apraxia (choice **B**) is the inability to carry out movement despite the absence of paralysis or inhibited sensory input. An example is a patient with asphasia who is unable to express thoughts by motion or pantomime/gestures as well as by speech. Astereognosis (choice **C**) refers to the inability to recognize objects via the sense of touch. Wernicke's asphasia (choice **D**) is caused by a lesion in the temporal lobe. The affected person speaks fluently in long convoluted sentences that make little sense. The patient's ability to comprehend the meaning of the spoken or written word is also affected. Agraphia (choice **E**) and alexia (choice **F**), respectively, are defined as the inability to write and read.

33 The answer is C   *Preventive Medicine and Public Health*

In the United States some 30% of community-dwelling individuals over the age of 65 have serious falls each year. The percentage increases to about 50% among those over 80 years old, and about 25% of these have serious injuries, making falls the sixth leading cause of death in the older age group. In addition, older persons have greater difficulty in fully recovering; consequently, 40% of those with serious injuries end up in a nursing home, often for the remainder of their lives. In general, it is difficult to pinpoint a single factor responsible for a fall, but even a seemingly healthy aged person has some impairment of gait control, balance (choice **C**), muscle tone, vision, or cognition. While blame may be placed on any one of these factors, generally several of these factors acting in concert cause a fall (choice **A**) when a person encounters an environmental risk factor (such as the throw rug in the vignette) that would be of minimal concern for a younger person.

Unfortunately, overmedication is commonly a factor (choice **B** is incorrect). Benzodiazepines, sedative–hypnotics, antidepressants, neuroleptics, and the use of four or more medications have been singled out as major risk factors. Whereas uncontrolled hypertension is not a common cause (choice **D**), overcontrol may be. A problem of particular concern is postural hypotension (>20 mm Hg drop in systolic pressure or a systolic pressure <90 mm Hg). While physicians are generally isolated from a patient's home environment they can play an important role in reducing the risk of falls among elderly patients (choice **E,** is incorrect). Among these are: reviewing the list of medications on a regular basis, including nonprescribed, over-the-counter drugs the patient may be taking; checking the change in blood pressure readings when the patient moves from a supine to a standing position; checking gait and balance and recommending gait training, balance or strengthening exercises (perhaps via a physical therapist), or use of an aid such as a cane if appropriate; checking for nutritional deficiencies and educating and/or arranging for nutritional assistance if appropriate; and educating the patient about proper sleeping habits with the goal of eliminating benzodiazepines or sedative–hypnotic sleeping aids. It also may be possible to have a visiting healthcare provider visit the home to check for and arrange for the correction of environmental hazards.

34 The answer is A   *Medicine*

Acne vulgaris (choice **A**) is a condition in which numerous papules and pustules develop at various stages. Acne vulgaris is caused by sebaceous glands, with androgen receptors having increased sensitivity to androgen; this causes androgen stimulation of sebaceous glands and leads to follicular hyperkeratosis and increased sebum secretion. *Propionibacterium acnes* infect these hair follicles and releases chemotactic factors that attract leukocytes and secrete lipases that break down fat in the sebum; this releases fatty acids, promoting further bacterial growth and acting synergistically with the invading leukocytes to cause an inflammatory reaction. Treatment depends on the severity of the condition. In general, initial treatment is simple, gentle face washing twice daily with warm water and mild soap (not scrubbing the face with strong soap or "popping" the pustules; mechanical trauma can exacerbate acne) and application of benzoyl peroxide. Women also should be instructed to use oil-free, noncomedogenic cosmetics and to expect worsening of the acne the week before menses. If the condition persists, topical or systemic antibiotics and/or topical tretinoin may be prescribed. For still more severe, persistent acne in which nodules and cysts predominate, oral isotretinoin is recommended. Females must have a pregnancy test before this medication is started and have contraception during the time the drug is taken, because isotretinoin is extremely teratogenic.

Erysipelas (choice **B**) is a cellulitis caused by group A *Streptococcus pyogenes*. The cellulitis is slightly raised, erythematous, and warm to the touch. Hyaluronidase produced by the pathogen causes the infection to spread through the subcutaneous tissue. Enlarged, tender cervical lymph nodes indicate an inflammatory reaction secondary to the infection. The treatment of choice is an intramuscular injection of benzathine penicillin G. Seborrheic keratosis (choice **C**) is a benign pigmented epidermal tumor that usually occurs in individuals who are over 50 years of age. These tumors are pigmented, warty lesions that have a "stuck on" appearance. When such lesions develop suddenly, especially in the setting of epigastric pain and weight loss, they indicate the presence of an underlying gastric adenocarcinoma (Leser-Trélat sign). The treatment for isolated lesions is liquid nitrogen therapy with or without curettage. A junctional nevus (choice **D**) is a benign tumor of neural crest-derived nevus cells (modified melanocytes). It begins in early childhood as a flat, pigmented lesion with nests of nevus cells along the basal cell layer. They later evolve into a compound nevus in which nevus cells extend into the superficial dermis (containing both junctional and intradermal components) and finally into an intradermal nevus in adults. When more than 100 nevi are present on the body surface, the patient most likely has the dysplastic nevus syndrome, which is an autosomal dominant disorder. There is an increased risk for developing a malignant melanoma, hence the need to visit a dermatologist at least once a year. A dysplastic nevus (choice **E**) arises sporadically or in association with dysplastic nevus syndrome. Characteristic findings include a >5-mm diameter growth with irregular borders and irregular distribution of melanin pigments. Treatment is excision.

35 **The answer is A**   *Preventive Medicine and Public Health*

In this question the prevalence of SLE is 10%, and the question asks for percentage probability of a positive test result indicating the patient has SLE. First, the prevalence must be converted to the number of diseased and normal persons in the relevant population. Using 1000 persons as an arbitrary population, a prevalence of 10% means that 100 persons have SLE and 900 persons are normal. Because the sensitivity of test X is 60%, then 60 of the 100 persons in this population will have a true-positive (TP) and 40 a false-negative (FN) test result. Because the specificity of test X is 80%, then 720 of the 900 people will have a true-negative (TN) and 180 a false-positive (FP) test result.

	Positive Test Result	**Negative Test Result**
Patients with SLE	60 = TPs	40 = FNs
Control population	180 = FPs	720 = TNs
Totals	240	760

The predictive value (PV) for a positive test result being a true positive predictive value (PV^{+test}) result is only 25% (choice **A**) [60/(60 + 180) × 100], because FPs outnumber TPs. The predictive value for a negative test (PV^{-test}) result being a TN is 95% [720/(720 + 40) × 100], because TNs outnumber FNs. In summary, the PV^{+test} result is highest when the prevalence of disease is highest, because TPs outnumber FPs; and the PV^{-test} result is highest when the prevalence of disease is lowest, because TNs outnumber FNs. Hence choices **B, C, D,** and **E** are incorrect.

36 **The answer is E**   *Pediatrics*

This question is directed at the management of an incarcerated inguinal hernia in the child. From the first description of the child in the emergency department, an attempt at reduction is appropriate. Resuscitation, especially in preparation for an operation, is not necessary as an initial step (choice **A**). Injection of a local anesthetic into the bulge is contraindicated (choice **C**). Application of ice in combination with manual pressure is usually not effective (choice **D**). Although total muscle relaxation and intubation (choice **B**) would probably accomplish reduction, administration of a barbiturate for sedation and muscle relaxant is simpler, less invasive, and usually effective (choice **E**). If incarceration occurs, operation is mandatory. The only issue is timing. The accepted practice is to operate on the patient after a brief period of observation (usually less than 24 hours). An immediate operation is not indicated, and any lengthy delay is inappropriate. Because there were no signs of strangulation on presentation, and assuming the patient remains well during the brief period of observation, then visualization of the bowel is not necessary during repair. It would have been necessary if an immediate operation had been undertaken.

37 **The answer is C**   *Medicine*

Essential tremor (choice **C**) is a relatively common trait that may present at any adult age. The etiology is unknown, although in some families it is inherited as an autosomal dominant trait. It tends to become more conspicuous with age, and it worsens in times of emotional stress. For some unknown reason a small amount of alcohol commonly alleviates the tremor for a brief period. The tremor usually is in a hand or hands but sometimes involves the head, tongue or larynx (voice), and legs. It is a fine, rapid tremor that is less conspicuous when at rest and is worsened by maintenance of a sustained position. As an affected person ages, the tremor usually becomes more apparent, may affect more body parts, and even persist to some degree when at rest. Although annoying and possibly embarrassing, it rarely is debilitating. It commonly interferes with letter writing. If treatment is required, the condition is most often treated with propranolol or primidone. If the tremor is not controlled by one of these agents, alprazolam, clozapine, mirtazapine, or topiramate may be tried. In a small minority of very severe, resistant cases, contralateral thalamotomy or unilateral high-frequency thalamic stimulation may be used.

Parkinsonism-associated tremor (choice **A**) may be distinguished from benign essential tremor by the pronounced "pill rolling" tremor present at rest typical of parkinsonism. Parkinson syndrome patients may be further recognized by rigidity that may lead to resistance to passive moment, causing bradykinesis, a flexed position, and a masklike face. A parkinsonism-like tremor may be induced by drugs (choice **B**) including phenothiazines and butyrophenones. These same drugs may also induce other abnormal movement disorders including motor restlessness (akathisia), acute dystonia, chorea, and tardive dyskinesia. Typical parkinsonism may also be caused by 1-methyl-4-phenyl-1,2,5,6-tetrahydropyridine (MPTP), a recreational drug. Some 40% of patients with pheochromocytoma have an associated tremor (choice **D**) in addition to more characteristic pheochromocytoma-associated symptoms that may include: hypertension (90%), headache (80%), perspiration (70%), palpitations (50%), anxiety (50%), and a sense of impending doom (40%). Tremor is a typical early symptom of alcohol withdrawal (choice **E**). Since persons with benign essential tremor may also imbibe to treat their tremors, the casual observer my conclude that they are alcoholics.

38 The answer is E *Medicine*

This man has a methicillin-resistant *Staphylococcus aureus* (MRSA) infection. At one time methicillin was used as the standard treatment for *S. aureus* infections. However, many strains of *S. aureus* became resistant, and the term *MRSA strains* was born. The name persists even though methicillin was replaced as the drug of choice several times over as *S. aureus* strains quickly became resistant to a greater number of antibiotics, generating what the press called "super bugs." This problem is particularly acute in nursing homes, rehabilitation units, and hospitals, where there is a population who on the whole use a greater number of antibiotics, and there are a greater number of infectious agents circulating in a circumscribed area. At this time, vancomycin is still regarded as the drug of choice to treat MRSA and could have been selected as a correct choice had it been on the list. However, vancomycin-resistant MRSA strains are becoming more common, and newer antibiotics have been introduced to treat vancomycin-resistant strains. These are linezolid (choice **E**) and quinupristin/dalfopristin. It is hoped that by restricting their use, evolution of *S. aureus* strains that are resistant to them will be inhibited. In addition, linezolid is a synthetic product, making the presence of bacterial strains that developed resistance to the natural antibiotic very unlikely.

Oxacillin (choice **A**), ceftazidime (choice **B**), penicillin G (choice **C**), nafcillin (choice **D**), and methicillin (choice **F**) are all antibiotics to which a large number of MRSA strains have become resistant.

39 The answer is C *Obstetrics and Gynecology*

This patient has the mildest form of endometrial hyperplasia without atypia. This results from unopposed estrogen, which in the postmenopausal woman is predominately estrone (choice **C**). Estrone is formed via conversion in the peripheral adipose tissue from adrenal androgens. With a high body mass index, this patient has plenty of peripheral conversion.

Choice **A,** estriol, is incorrect because it is the most dominant estrogen during, not after, menopause. Choice **B,** ethynyl estradiol, is incorrect because it is the synthetic estrogen used in combination oral contraceptive pills. Choice **D,** phytoestrogen, is incorrect because this is an estrogen-like substance found in plant products such as soy and tofu. Choice **E** estradiol is incorrect because it is the dominant estrogen seen during the reproductive years, not after menopause.

40 The answer is E *Surgery*

This patient has the classic triad of injuries known as the *unhappy triad*. The injuries typically follow a sudden valgus stress to the knee, a stress commonly encountered during American football. Distraction of the medial collateral ligament results in it being torn, and because the medial meniscus is intimately attached to the medial collateral ligament, it tears as well. Finally, the anterior cruciate ligament tears (choice **E**).

The lateral collateral ligament (choices **A** and **B**) does not tear, because the distracting force is medial. In lateral collateral ligament tears, the lateral meniscus (choices **A, B,** and **D**) is not involved because the lateral collateral ligament is attached to the head of the fibula, not to the lateral meniscus. The anterior cruciate ligament is weaker and tears more easily than the posterior cruciate ligament (choices **B, C,** and **D**). The posterior cruciate ligament is composed of two bands, one thick and one thin.

41 **The answer is C** *Obstetrics and Gynecology*

They key elements of this scenario that suggest urge incontinence (choice **C**) is the patient's age and sudden, uncontrollable urinary urgency day and night. The key finding is involuntary detrusor contractions. Synonyms include hyperactive bladder, detrusor dyssynergia, and unstable bladder. Postmenopausal women are at higher risk for this condition. Because the urgency and loss of urine is so uncontrollable, the patient's daily activities are rearranged to allow easy access to toilet facilities. The lack of pelvic prolapse and sensation of an "itty-bitty" bladder are also frequently seen. Management involves suppression of detrusor contractions with anticholinergic medications.

42 **The answer is E** *Obstetrics and Gynecology*

Loss of urine in the latter part of the pregnancy (choice **E**) is a common complaint. As the uterus grows in size and exerts increasing pressure on the bladder and lower reproductive tract, loss of urine becomes more frequent. The resulting moistness of undergarments can be confused with spontaneous membrane rupture, so a speculum examination is in order, looking for positive pooling, positive Nitrazine, and positive ferning. Management is conservative after ruling out bladder infection with urinalysis and urine culture if indicated.

43 **The answer is B** *Obstetrics and Gynecology*

The bladder is attached to the anterior lower uterine segment and is often affected by labor and delivery, particularly if the labor is long and protracted. Regional analgesia or anesthesia can affect the innervation of both the lower urinary tract and the reproductive tract. Prolonged lack of sensation to the bladder can lead to overflow incontinence (choice **B**). Since the patient does not sense a need to void, her bladder continues to fill until the intravesical pressure exceeds the urethral pressure, at which time a dribbling of urine continues until the intravesical pressure falls below the urethral pressure and the urine leakage stops. However, the bladder never contracts. The classic finding is a high residual volume. Management involves cholinergic agents to stimulate detrusor contractions or an indwelling Foley catheter to allow return of normal bladder sensation.

44 **The answer is D** *Obstetrics and Gynecology*

The most common type of involuntary female urinary loss is genuine stress (choice **D**) incontinence. It is associated with coughing or sneezing. The key historical finding is that it does not occur at night, whereas all other kinds of incontinence do. The underlying pathophysiology is an anatomic one, with loss of support of the pelvic floor and the bladder neck. With loss of support to the bladder neck and the proximal urethra, increases in intraabdominal pressure are transmitted to the bladder but not to the urethra. Therefore, whenever intravesical pressure rises above urethral pressure (e.g., coughing, sneezing), urine is lost. However, the detrusor muscle never contracts. Management involves strengthening the pelvic floor muscles with Kegel exercises or estrogen (for postmenopausal women) or a surgical sling procedure to support the bladder neck.

45 **The answer is A** *Obstetrics and Gynecology*

The characteristic presenting symptom of a fistular cause (choice **A**) of urinary incontinence is continual loss of urine day and night. The most common risk factor is either radical pelvic surgery (e.g., colorectal resection for carcinoma or radical hysterectomy for cervical carcinoma) or pelvic radiation (e.g., advanced cervical or uterine cancer). The diagnosis and location of the fistula is confirmed by performing an intravenous pyelogram and observing for dye leakage. Management involves surgical repair.

46 **The answer is B** *Medicine*

The laboratory measurement of total serum calcium includes calcium bound to albumin (40%), calcium bound to other anions (10%), and free ionized calcium (50%); the latter represents the physiologically active form. Thus, the total calcium concentration must decrease in a patient with hypoalbuminemia, but this does not decrease the free ionized calcium level. This is for two reasons: (1) because of the law of mass action, as the total concentration of albumin drops, more Ca^{2+} will dissociate, and (2) because of physiologic homeostatic mechanisms, the calcium-sensing protein of the parathyroid gland and kidney only senses Ca^{2+}, and these organs will initiate compensating mechanism the moment Ca^{2+} levels decline. (These compensating mechanisms will involve increased secretion of parathyroid hormone, but the increase will be miniscule and not measurable). Thus, total serum calcium will decline along with the albumin, and parathyroid hormone (PTH) concentration will remain in the normal range (choice **B**). To estimate how the serum calcium concentration would compare to levels obtained when albumin levels are in the normal range (corrected serum calcium) the following formula may be used: Corrected serum calcium = measured calcium (mg/dL) + 0.8 × [4 − (albumin in g/dL)].

47 **The answer is C** *Medicine*

A patient with long-standing, untreated celiac disease would be expected to have steatorrhea and multiple fat- and water-soluble vitamin deficiencies. Hypovitaminosis D results in hypocalcemia, which is a stimulus for the release of PTH and development of secondary hyperparathyroidism (choice **C**).

48 **The answer is E** *Medicine*

A short QT interval on an electrocardiogram (ECG) indicates hypercalcemia, which most likely is caused by ectopic secretion of a PTH-related peptide. The peptide increases the renal reabsorption of calcium and decreases phosphate reabsorption. Hypercalcemia suppresses the patient's endogenous PTH production. Therefore, the calcium level is increased, and the PTH concentration is decreased (choice **E**).

49 **The answer is A** *Medicine*

Both tetany and a prolonged QT interval indicate hypocalcemia. This plus mucocutaneous candidiasis in a patient with Addison's disease indicates that this patient has autoimmune hypoparathyroidism. In hypoparathyroidism, the serum calcium and serum PTH are decreased (choice **A**).

50 **The answer is D** *Medicine*

A patient with epigastric pain with radiation into the back, a positive stool guaiac test result, and a long history of renal stone formation most likely has a posterior penetrating duodenal ulcer with extension into the pancreas or acute pancreatitis. This constellation of findings is most consistent with primary hyperparathyroidism. Hypercalcemia is a stimulus for gastrin release, which in turn increases gastric acidity and thus the potential for peptic ulcer disease and bleeding. Hypercalcemia also activates pancreatic lipase, causing acute pancreatitis, which (unlike peptic ulcer disease) causes pain to radiate into the back. The presence of recurrent renal stones is another finding that is highly predictive for primary hyperparathyroidism, the most common cause of which is a parathyroid adenoma. Laboratory findings are increased serum calcium and serum PTH levels (choice **D**).

test **17**

Questions

Single Best Choice Directions: This section consists of numbered statements or questions followed by a list of potential answers; you are to select the ONE best answer.

1 A 78-year-old woman is dying from lung cancer that has metastasized to various sites including bone. She has had surgery to remove the primary cancer in the lung as well as a secondary tumor from her pelvis and has been subjected to extensive chemotherapy. She now is in pain. Which of the following is a phenomenon is that the clinician should respond to while treating a patient for end-of-life pain?

(A) Tolerance
(B) Dependence
(C) Addiction
(D) Pseudoaddiction
(E) Legal repercussions for overprescription of opioids

2 A 36-year-old man develops fever, headache, and pain when moving his neck. He complains that he cannot think clearly. No petechial lesions are noted on the skin or mucous membranes. A Gram's stain of the cerebrospinal fluid will most likely show which one of the following types of bacterial morphology?

(A) Gram-negative diplococcus
(B) Gram-negative rod
(C) Gram-positive coccus
(D) Gram-positive diplococcus
(E) Gram-positive rod

3 A 25-year-old woman comes to the outpatient clinic with early-pregnancy bleeding. Speculum examination shows no vaginal or cervical lesions. She undergoes an endovaginal ultrasound examination, which reveals a normal-appearing viable embryo with crown–rump length consistent with 8 weeks' gestation. The embryo size is appropriate for the weeks expected based on her last menstrual period. However, a repeat sonogram at 19 weeks' gestation shows a fetus with all biometric measurements (including the head, abdomen, and femur) symmetrically less than expected, with an estimated fetal weight at the 5th percentile. These findings are most consistent with:

(A) Edward syndrome
(B) Klinefelter syndrome

(C) Turner syndrome
(D) Down syndrome
(E) Patau syndrome

4 A 48-year-old man with postnecrotic cirrhosis due to chronic hepatitis B requires surgery to reduce portal vein pressures. If the surgeon decides to use a shunt that reduces the risk for developing hepatic encephalopathy, the most likely shunt is which one of the following?

(A) Mesocaval shunt
(B) Side-to-side portacaval shunt
(C) End-to-side portacaval shunt
(D) Distal splenorenal shunt

5 It has been estimated that about 10 million Americans over the age of 50 have osteoporosis and another 34 million, osteopenia. Four of 10 Caucasian women will break a hip, spine, or wrist during their lives, and 20% of hip fracture patients end up in a nursing home within a year, and many of these die. According to recent studies, which of the following choices is currently being recommended to help protect the elderly from pathologic fractures?

(A) A daily intake of no more than 400 IU vitamin D if over the age of 70 years
(B) A daily intake of at least 150 µg of vitamin K
(C) A daily intake of no more than 1000 mg calcium if over 50 years of age
(D) A daily intake of at least 10,000 IU of retinol
(E) A daily intake of less than 25 g of protein

6 A 34-year-old man is moving logs on his woodpile when he is bitten by a shiny black spider with a red hourglass on the ventral aspect of the abdomen. He feels a sharp pain in his right index finger soon after being bitten. Which of the following is the most probable clinical outcome of this bite?

(A) Ascending paralysis and hypertension
(B) Disseminated intravascular coagulation
(C) Muscle cramping and severe abdominal pain
(D) Mydriasis and muscle paralysis
(E) Ulceration with extensive necrosis

7 Cocaine's mode of action involves increased release of norepinephrine and blockage of its reuptake, and it is often abused. With crack cocaine, stimulatory effects start within 10 seconds; other forms of cocaine initiate early effects in 3 to 5 minutes and have their peak effect in some 10 to 20 minutes. The quick passage of the euphoric feeling leads to trying more, and addiction is common. Which of the following drugs or drug combinations has provided the best results for treating cocaine addiction?

(A) Methadone with buprenorphine
(B) Naloxone with disulfiram
(C) Lithium with an antidepressant
(D) Disulfiram with methadone
(E) Phenytoin with methadone
(F) Buprenorphine with naloxone
(G) Carbamazepine with buprenorphine

8 A 41-year-old African-American man has cancer involving the lungs, brain, liver, spleen, and kidneys. He has a 20-year history of smoking cigarettes. Physical examination shows a dark lesion under the nail of the middle finger of the right hand. Which of the following is the most likely cause of this metastatic disease?

(A) Glioblastoma multiforme
(B) Hepatocellular carcinoma
(C) Malignant melanoma
(D) Primary lung cancer
(E) Renal cell carcinoma

9 A 23-year-old man presents with problems involving his teeth, bones, and vision. There is a family history of adenomatous polyps involving the colon, colorectal cancer, and tumors of the thyroid and adrenal glands. Clinical examination reveals supernumerary teeth, long-bone osteomas, and increased retinal pigmentation. Which of the following conditions would most likely be associated with these findings?

(A) Gardner syndrome
(B) Villous adenoma
(C) Familial adenomatous polyposis syndrome
(D) Turcot syndrome (also known as Turcot-Després, or Turcot-Després-St. Pierre syndrome)
(E) Tubular adenomas

10 A 49-year-old man has been having progressively more severe hearing problems for the past two decades. He fears he will soon be completely deaf, a fear compounded by the fact that his 78-year-old mother is deaf. Consequently, he finally consults an otorhinolaryngologist who observes normal-appearing tympanic membranes. The physician also conducts a Weber and Rinne test. The Weber test lateralized to the right ear,

and the Rinne's test showed bone conduction to be greater than air conduction. His hearing loss is most likely due to which of the following?

(A) Presbycusis
(B) Chronic otitis media
(C) Otosclerosis
(D) Cholesteatoma
(E) Ménière's disease

11 A 29-year-old woman, gravida 3, para 2, aborta 0, is being seen for prenatal care and is currently at 28 weeks by dates confirmed by an 11-week sonogram. An obstetric sonogram performed a few days ago reveals a normal-appearing single female fetus with size appropriate for known gestational age. The fetal anatomy is unremarkable, with no evidence of ascites, effusions, or edema. The amniotic fluid volume is normal, with a 4-quadrant amniotic fluid index of 15 cm. Her blood type is O with rhesus positive. Her indirect Coombs test results are positive. The blood bank identifies the atypical antibody as anti-Lewis. The antibody titer is 1:32. The blood type of her husband and father of this pregnancy is AB with rhesus negative. The postdelivery course of her two previous neonates was characterized by only mild hyperbilirubinemia, successfully treated with short-term phototherapy. Which one of the following factors from this case is reassuring that this fetus is not at risk for hemolytic disease of the newborn?

(A) Maternal blood type and Rh
(B) Paternal blood type and Rh
(C) Atypical antibody type
(D) Atypical antibody titer
(E) Previous baby outcomes

12 Autosomal dominant polycystic kidney disease has an incidence of 1 in 800 births, making it one of the most common hereditary diseases in the United States, affecting some half million individuals. Fifty percent of affected persons will have end-stage renal disease (ESRD) by the age of 60 years. A 62-year-old woman with autosomal dominant polycystic kidney disease is on hemodialysis. Which of the following laboratory findings would most likely be reported?

(A) Decreased serum parathyroid hormone
(B) Decreased serum phosphorus
(C) Increased serum calcium
(D) Increased urine-specific gravity >1.020
(E) Serum blood urea nitrogen (BUN):creatinine ratio <10

13 A 19-year-old blue-eyed blonde woman was brought to the emergency room with a history of having come down heavily on the right leg while getting off a curb.

The paramedics reported that she had vomited once during the trip to the emergency department. The patient states that she has had a dull ache in the right thigh for the past few weeks and had noticed a "boil" there. She had made an appointment to see her primary care physician for this. The emergency physician notes that she is in moderate distress. Her blood pressure is 90/60 mm Hg; pulse, 98/min, regular and thready; respirations, 22/min; and temperature, 37.5°C (99.5°F). She has no cyanosis but has pallor of the mucosa. Cardiovascular examination is unremarkable except for a sinus tachycardia and a capillary circulation of more than 2 seconds. Examination of the respiratory system reveals normal breath sounds bilaterally. Her right thigh is swollen, and she has lateral rotation and shortening of the leg due to the fact the femur torpedoed up toward her pelvis. The right groin is tender to palpation, and movement of the leg induces severe pain. There is a raised papular lesion over the anterior midthigh, surrounded by inflammation. The pelvis and the left leg are normal. Which of the following conditions most likely predisposed her to this pathologic fracture?

(A) Osteosarcoma
(B) Osteoporosis
(C) Stress fracture
(D) Osteogenesis imperfecta
(E) Chronic osteomyelitis
(F) Metastatic bone disease

14 A pediatrician notes that a neonatal male has a small penis (micropenis) and urinates through an opening in the perineum. Testes are not present in the scrotal sac but are present in the inguinal canals. Laboratory studies reveal a decrease in serum dihydrotestosterone and normal serum testosterone level. A random urine sodium level is normal. Which of the following enzymes is deficient?

(A) Aromatase
(B) 11-Hydroxylase
(C) 21-Hydroxylase
(D) Oxidoreductase
(E) 5-α-Reductase

15 A 57-year old woman presents at the emergency department because of a severe and steady pain localized to the epigastrum. While being checked in she vomited twice and reported that the vomiting relieved the pain but only for a short time. In taking a history the physician on duty determines that by her own admission the woman ate too much of a rather heavy, fatty meal a few hours before the attack started. Physical examination shows that she is 62 in (1.57 m) tall, weighs 148 lb (67.1 kg), her blood pressure is 145/82 mm Hg, pulse is 78/min and regular, her respirations are 24/min, and her temperature is 37.9°C (100.2°F). Her white cell count is 14,000/μL (normal, 4.8–10.8 × 10³/μL). Her total serum bilirubin is 2.0 mg/dL (normal, 0.1–1.2 mg/dL), and her serum aminotransferase and alkaline phosphatase levels are elevated. Why should morphine not be used to relieve the pain in this patient?

(A) It may cause addiction.
(B) It may cause the sphincter of Oddi to spasm.
(C) It may cause angle-closure glaucoma by widening the pupils.
(D) It may cause tachycardia.
(E) It may cause death by pulmonary aspiration of gastric contents.

16 A 31-year-old man with many past suicide gestures, fleeting and unsatisfactory interpersonal relationships, mood lability, and a lack of goals or convictions says that he wants some sort of medication to help him get his life together. He has been in Dialectic Behavioral Therapy for about 1 year. He denies any periods of severe depression or periods in which he sleeps little and feels full of energy. However, he describes times in which "everything becomes overwhelming and difficult to track." This usually occurs during stressful situations, and these feelings are accompanied by the sensation of "floating outside of his body." There is no history of hallucinations, delusions, or grossly disorganized thinking. The patient says that he drinks socially but denies any significant problems with alcohol or other drugs. He has no known general medical problems. Mental status reveals an alert, oriented, moderately anxious, and depressed man, with no evidence of psychosis. He denies current suicidal ideation. Which of the following is the most appropriate next step in treatment?

(A) Explain to the patient that intensive psychotherapy takes more than 1 year for the kind of problems that he presents with, and that medication is not effective for them
(B) Start the patient on low-dose diazepam therapy
(C) Start the patient on sertraline therapy
(D) Start the patient on aripiprazole therapy
(E) Start the patient on gabapentin therapy

17 A premature, small-for-gestational-age infant is born to a 16-year-old primigravida by spontaneous vaginal delivery. The mother did not have any prenatal care but denies using drugs, alcohol, or tobacco. Except for the prematurity, the delivery was unremarkable. Apgar scores were 7 at 1 minute and 8 at 5 minutes. Eight hours after birth, the infant has a serum glucose level of 20 mg/dL. Which of the following disorders is the most likely cause of this infant's hypoglycemia?

(A) Leucine sensitivity
(B) Nesidioblastosis
(C) Inadequate fat and glycogen stores
(D) Immature pituitary–hypothalamic axis
(E) Mother with diabetes

18 A 37-year-old woman, gravida 3, para 3, comes to the outpatient office for an annual examination. She has no complaints and has regular menstrual periods every 30 days. Her last Pap smear was a year ago and was reported as negative for intraepithelial lesion or malignancy. On bimanual pelvic examination her uterus is found to be mobile, nontender, firm, and asymmetrically enlarged to 8 weeks' gestation size. A pelvic sonogram confirms an asymmetrically enlarged uterus with multiple subserosal leiomyomas; the largest have dimensions of 4 × 4 cm. Which of the following is the most appropriate management?

(A) Embolization
(B) Leuprolide shrinkage
(C) Hysterectomy
(D) Myomectomy
(E) Observation

19 A 63-year-old man who was retired as an airline pilot at the age of 60 and has not seen a physician since then makes an appointment in October for a general examination. He enjoys general good health and an examination can find no problems. However, he is interested in updating any preventive steps he might take to help him avoid the "diseases of old age," as he expressed it. He says that as a pilot who flies to "exotic" countries, the company doctor vaccinated him against pneumonia and tetanus the year before he retired, and a decade or so earlier, he was given a two-dose vaccination treatment against hepatitis A. He also has had a colonoscopy performed as part of his retirement physical. Which of the following is a preventive action relevant at this time for this man?

(A) Influenza vaccination
(B) Pneumococcal vaccine booster
(C) Hepatitis A booster
(D) Chest radiography
(E) A colonoscopy

20 A 36-year-old woman with a history of heavy polydrug abuse is incarcerated for suspected erratic driving. One day after incarceration, she becomes increasingly agitated and has a grand mal seizure. Which of the following substances is most likely responsible for her symptoms?

(A) Methamphetamine
(B) Cocaine
(C) Cannabis
(D) Diazepam
(E) Pentazocine

21 A grammar school teacher who is 3 months' pregnant visits her obstetrician. She is concerned because there is an outbreak of parvovirus B19 in her class. One of her students with sickle cell disease developed aplastic crisis after exposure to the parvovirus and is hospitalized. She fears that her exposure to the virus may harm her fetus. The obstetrician informs her that there is less than a 5% chance that her fetus will contract which of the following anomalies?

(A) Chorioretinitis
(B) Hydrops fetalis
(C) Rhagades
(D) Microcephaly
(E) Hutchinson's teeth

22 A 16-year-old boy complains that he suddenly developed blindness. He has recently been under emotional distress. He reportedly had an episode of conversion disorder 6 months ago in which he had paralysis. Physical examination reveals pupils that react to light and accommodation. A nurse reports that she observed him reading the note in his medical record when left alone in the examination room. Which of the following is the most likely diagnosis?

(A) Relapse of his conversion disorder
(B) Factitious disorder
(C) Malingering
(D) Hypochondriasis
(E) Somatization disorder

23 A parent reports that 12 hours after her 6-month-old daughter received the diphtheria–tetanus–acellular pertussis (DTaP) vaccine, she developed a seizure that lasted approximately 3 minutes. The child had previously been in her usual state of good health. The mother describes the seizure as generalized in nature. The child has not had any more seizures since the immunizations and appears to be developmentally appropriate for her age. Which procedure is recommended for future immunizations?

(A) Leave out the diphtheria component of the vaccine, and give pertussis and tetanus during the course of the next immunization
(B) Leave out the tetanus component of the vaccine, and give diphtheria and pertussis during the course of the next immunization

(C) Leave out the tetanus and pertussis components of the vaccine, and give diphtheria toxoid alone during the course of the next immunization

(D) Leave out the pertussis component of the vaccine, and give diphtheria and tetanus toxoids during the course of the next immunization

(E) Give DTaP again on the next immunization

24 A 19-year-old nulligravid woman comes to the emergency department with complaints of unilateral lower-abdominal pelvic pain and vaginal bleeding. Her last menstrual period was 8 weeks ago. She is sexually active with multiple sexual partners. She uses a condom for contraception. Her blood pressure is 80/40 with a pulse of 130/min. Which of the following is the most appropriate management?

(A) Observation
(B) Laparotomy
(C) Methotrexate
(D) Laparoscopy
(E) Serial β-hCG titers

25 A 74-year old man sees his physician for a routine checkup. His blood pressure is 200/75 mm Hg; during the previous visit 4 months earlier it was measured at 185/72 mm Hg, and when measured at home, the systolic pressure often exceeds 160 mm Hg, although the diastolic pressure commonly is below 80 mm Hg. Relevant aspects of his history are that he takes metformin to treat diabetes and his hemoglobin A1c values are always under 7%. He also has no signs of renal malfunction. He also takes multiple drugs to treat his hypertension. His present medication regimen prescribed for hypertension is hydrochlorothiazide (HCTZ) 25 mg qd; enalapril 20 mg bid; doxazosin mesylate, 2 mg bid; acebutolol, 200 mg bid; and clonidine 0.3 mg tid. Which is the next best step to lower his systolic pressure?

(A) Add furosemide
(B) Add eprosartan
(C) Add reserpine
(D) Add nifedipine.
(E) Add nitroprusside

26 A 5-year-old male comes to the pediatric clinic for the first time with choreoathetoid movements. According to the mother, the patient had been in his usual state of good health until 2 weeks ago when he developed a sore throat that was thought to be viral. The mother states that the child has become clumsier over the past few weeks, and there has been marked deterioration in his handwriting. The physician suspects that the patient has rheumatic fever. In addition to Syden-

ham's chorea, which of the following is another major criterion for the diagnosis of acute rheumatic fever?

(A) Increased antistreptolysin O (ASO) titer
(B) Arthralgia
(C) Erythema migrans
(D) Elevated erythrocyte sedimentation rate (ESR)
(E) Subcutaneous nodules

27 A 32-year-old woman underwent routine cervical Pap smear screening using the thin-layer liquid-based cytology. The report was returned as consistent with a high-grade squamous intraepithelial lesion. She underwent colposcopy which was satisfactory, and no lesion was seen entering the endocervical canal. However, an area of white epithelium and mosaicism was seen at 6 o'clock on the ectocervix and was biopsied. The histology was reported as consistent with severe dysplasia or CIN 2 (cervical intraepithelial neoplasia 2). Which of the following is the appropriate next step in management?

(A) Observation
(B) Cryotherapy
(C) HPV-DNA testing
(D) Repeat Pap smear in 6 months
(E) Simple hysterectomy

28 There are both preventable and nonpreventable risk factors for the development of diabetic macrovascular disease. The nonpreventable ones are age, genetic composition, and in particular for the type 1 diabetic, duration of diabetes. (The onset of type 2 diabetes may be delayed and even prevented by lifestyle changes). One of the several factors that encourage development of diabetic macrovascular disease does so by causing arterial spasms, increasing the amount of low-density lipoprotein, decreasing the level of high-density lipoprotein, increasing platelet aggregation, increasing fibrinogen concentration, and decreasing red blood cell flexibility. All these actions are caused by which one of the risk factors listed below?

(A) Smoking
(B) Visceral obesity
(C) Hypertension
(D) Hyperglycemia
(E) Hyperinsulinemia

29 A 51-year-old pig farmer complains of sudden jerking movements in his extremities and a constant headache. Physical examination shows no focal neurologic deficits; however, calcified nodular masses within the muscles of his extremities and chest are palpated. A complete blood cell count (CBC) shows a marked peripheral blood eosinophilia. A magnetic resonance

imaging (MRI) study of his head shows multiple cysts with focal areas of calcification located at the junction of the gray and white matter. Which of the following is the most likely diagnosis?

(A) Cerebral infarctions
(B) Cysticercosis
(C) Echinococcosis
(D) Metastatic lung carcinoma
(E) Trichinosis

30 A 57-year old single mother of two immigrated from Mexico to the United States 32 years ago. She presently supports herself and her children by working as a cleaning woman. During these 32 years she has never visited a physician because she entered the country illegally and is afraid that if she surfaces she might be deported. In addition, she has no health insurance and feared the expense. However one night she develops a fever and is violently ill; her eldest daughter, fearing the worst, takes her to the nearest emergency department. It turns out that her present symptoms are due to an enteric infection and are not serious. However, while she was there, the physicians gave her a thorough physical examination and discovered that she is a probable diabetic. The intraocular pressure and found it to be 24 mm Hg in the right eye and 21 mm Hg in the left eye. The physician in charge of the emergency clinic was community oriented and arranges to send the woman to a local free clinic where an ophthalmologist examines her eyes further and discovers that the ratio of the diameter of the optic cup to the optic disc is 0.8 in the right eye and 0.5 in the left eye. The most probable diagnosis of this woman's eye problems is which one of the following?

(A) Angle-closure glaucoma
(B) Diabetic retinopathy
(C) Macular degeneration
(D) Open-angle glaucoma
(E) Cataracts

31 A 34-year-old woman was seen in the prenatal diagnosis center at 18 weeks' gestation for counseling and fetal evaluation regarding a positive triple marker screen result that revealed an elevated maternal serum α-fetoprotein (MS-AFP). A sonogram shows a single viable fetus with size appropriate for dates. The anatomic survey reveals concave frontal bones of the fetal cranial vault ("lemon" sign) and an abnormal configuration of the cerebellum ("banana" sign) as well as a lumbosacral spina bifida. Which of the following medications the patient had been taking could cause this teratogenic injury?

(A) Thalidomide
(B) Lithium

(C) Diethylstilbestrol
(D) Valproic acid
(E) Isotretinoin

32 A 61-year-old man with ischemic heart disease has shortness of breath even at rest, consistent fatigue, no tolerance for exercise, a nonproductive cough when lying down, edema, nocturia due to excretion of fluid retained during the day, and increased renal perfusion in the recumbent position. In short he has signs of both left- and right-sided heart failure. Which of the following is a finding shared by both left and right heart failure?

(A) Bibasilar inspiratory crackles
(B) Decreased cardiac output
(C) Dependent pitting edema
(D) Paroxysmal nocturnal dyspnea
(E) Passive congestion in the liver

33 A 2-year-old child presents to the pediatrician with a bloody vaginal discharge. The parents deny any significant past medical history. However, for the past month they say that the patient has had a grapelike mass bulging through the vaginal vault as shown in the accompanying figure. Which of the following is the most likely diagnosis?

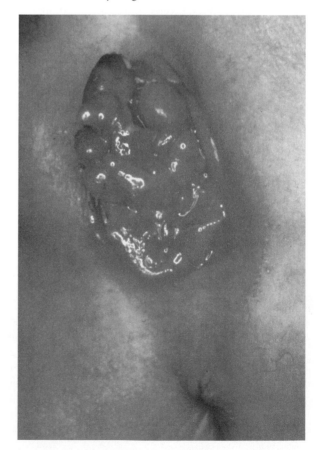

(A) Clear cell adenocarcinoma of the vagina
(B) Embryonal rhabdomyosarcoma
(C) Leiomyosarcoma
(D) Granular cell myoblastoma
(E) Squamous cell carcinoma of the genital tract

34 A 57-year-old male complains of insomnia of 5 years' duration. Attempts to determine a causal general medical condition or psychiatric condition have been unsuccessful. Training in sleep hygiene also has been ineffective. He is unable to tolerate trials of sedating antidepressants, and he develops tolerance with benzodiazepines. When benzodiazepines are tapered, his insomnia invariably returns. Which of the following pharmacologic interventions would be the next best step?

(A) Zolpidem
(B) Quetiapine
(C) Eszopiclone
(D) Alcohol in moderation
(E) Diphenhydramine

35 A patient with Albright's hereditary osteodystrophy (pseudohypoparathyroidism) sees his physician for an upper respiratory tract infection. The patient has a stocky build with a round face, short stature, and brachydactyly of the fourth and fifth metacarpals. There is dimpling of the dorsum of the hand. Lenticular cataracts are also present. Which of the following conditions is also associated with pseudohypoparathyroidism in such a patient?

(A) Mental retardation
(B) Decreased serum parathormone
(C) Increased serum calcium
(D) Decreased serum phosphorus
(E) Retinoblastoma

36 A 25-year-old man who had his left cryptorchid testis removed as a child develops painless enlargement of the right testicle. The enlarged testicle does not transilluminate. Serum human chorionic gonadotropin

and α-fetoprotein are absent. Which of the following is the most likely diagnosis?

(A) Choriocarcinoma
(B) Hydrocele
(C) Seminoma
(D) Varicocele
(E) Yolk sac tumor

37 A full-term newborn, with blood group A, Rh negative, develops jaundice in the first 24 hours of life. The infant's mother is blood group O and Rh negative. Result of a direct Coombs' test of cord blood red blood cells (RBCs) is positive. The infant's total bilirubin levels continue to increase, and the physician orders phototherapy with blue fluorescent light. After 24 hours of phototherapy, the intensity of the jaundice decreases, and blood total bilirubin levels show a drop of 3 mg/dL over the previous day's levels. What is the mechanism for lowering of bilirubin with phototherapy?

(A) Conjugated bilirubin (CB) in skin is converted into unconjugated bilirubin (UCB) and excreted in urine.
(B) CB is mobilized out of the skin and excreted in the urine.
(C) UCB is converted into CB and excreted in urine.
(D) UCB is mobilized out of the skin and excreted in urine.
(E) UCB in skin is converted into water-soluble dipyrroles called lumirubin.

38 A 46-year-old afebrile man with chronic pancreatitis has a tender abdomen, a palpable abdominal mass, and persistently elevated serum and urine amylase levels. He has had a 22-year history of alcohol abuse. Which of the following is the most likely diagnosis?

(A) Pancreatic cystadenoma
(B) Pancreatic pseudocyst
(C) Pancreatic carcinoma
(D) Pancreatic abscess
(E) Macroamylasemia

Directions for Matching Questions (39 through 50): *Each set of matching questions is preceded by a list of 4 to 26 lettered options followed by a brief explanation of the required task and then by a series of numbered statements. For each lettered statement you are to select ONE lettered option that best fulfills the task as it relates to that statement. Remember each of the listed options might be correctly selected once, more than once, or not at all.*

Questions 39–40

Match each substance with the ONE corresponding bar in the figure, derived from the National Institute on Drug Abuse (NIDA) 2004 data.

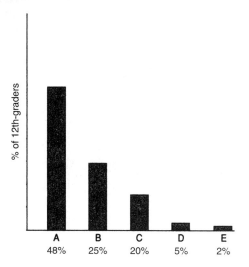

39 Cocaine use within the last month

40 Tobacco use within the last month

Questions 41 and 42

Match each disorder with the ONE best-associated graph shown.

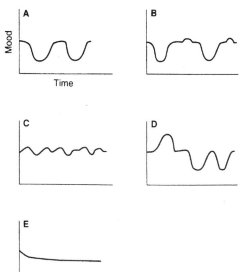

41 Cyclothymic disorder

42 Bipolar II disorder

Questions 43–46

For each clinical description in questions 43 through 46 select the ONE most appropriate location of the causative lesion from the lettered (A–E) list below.
(A) Dominant frontal lobe
(B) Nondominant temporal lobe
(C) Dominant parietal lobe
(D) Occipital lobe
(E) Temporal–occipital–parietal junction

43 A 65-year-old patient cannot tell his right hand from his left hand.

44 A 45-year-old stroke patient clearly understands what someone is saying to him but is unable to respond verbally to that person.

45 Although he can repeat phrases, the speech of a 52-year-old stroke patient is impaired, and he has difficulty understanding what someone says to him.

46 Although the patient can read, write, and speak lucidly she cannot add 2 plus 2.

Questions 47–50

For questions 47 through 50 select the ONE most appropriate lettered disease from the list (A–E) below.
(A) Leopard syndrome
(B) Pendred syndrome
(C) Usher syndrome
(D) Alport syndrome
(E) Waardenburg syndrome

47 An autosomal recessive disorder characterized by congenital deafness due to middle ear aberrations and goiter. The goiter appears at puberty, and although most patients are euthyroid, hypothyroidism can occur.

48 An autosomal dominant condition that has variable expression. Individuals have mild-to-profound hearing problems and often have a white forelock. Sometimes their hair becomes completely grey before puberty, and patches of hyperpigmentation are common, as is unusual eye pigmentation. Often one eye is blue and other brown; sometimes a single eye is two toned. A broad base of the nose causes a lateral displacement of the inner canthi.

49 An autosomal recessive condition characterized by deafness and retinitis pigmentosa. Deafness and blindness develop at different ages, depending upon the variant form present.

50 This is the most common of the hereditary nephritides. Although males are more severely affected than females, cases are transmitted in a dominant X-linked fashion. Male patients develop glomerulonephritis that progresses to end-stage renal failure. Some patients develop hearing loss. Approximately 10% have eye abnormalities such as cataracts.

Answer Key

1 A	**11** C	**21** B	**31** D	**41** C
2 D	**12** E	**22** B	**32** B	**42** B
3 B	**13** E	**23** D	**33** B	**43** C
4 D	**14** E	**24** B	**34** C	**44** A
5 B	**15** B	**25** D	**35** A	**45** E
6 C	**16** D	**26** E	**36** C	**46** C
7 F	**17** C	**27** B	**37** E	**47** B
8 C	**18** E	**28** A	**38** B	**48** E
9 A	**19** A	**29** B	**39** E	**49** C
10 C	**20** D	**30** D	**40** B	**50** D

Answers and Explanations

1 The answer is A *Medicine*

Pain is often undertreated; it has been estimated that up to 50% of severely ill hospitalized patients spend half their time in moderate-to-severe pain during the last 3 days of their lives. This is due in part to the fear of some physicians to overprescribe opioids and in part to the absence of social, psychologic, and spiritual support in a hospital setting. It has been estimated that intensity at which pain is felt is due in equal measure to physical, social, psychologic, and spiritual factors. The physician obviously has the greatest aspect of control regarding the physical aspect and consequently should provide whatever analgesic at whatever dose he or she feels is required to make the patient comfortable short of potentially killing the patient. Use of narcotic drugs will be expected to create tolerance and induce dependency. The physician should respond to tolerance by either increasing the dose or providing an equianalgesic dose of a different drug (choice **A**).

Dependency, the required use of a drug to prevent withdrawal symptoms, doesn't require a physician's response in the treatment of the end-of-life patient (choice **B**). If the drug still alleviates the pain, it can be administered until the patient dies; if because of tolerance another drug must administered, it can still be administered as long as the combination can be tolerated physiologically. The risk of psychologic or physical addiction (choice **C**) is irrelevant for a dying individual. Pseudoaddiction (choice **D**) demonstrated by demanding a drug, irritability, anger, disturbed interpersonal relations, or any of the other symptoms sometimes associated with the addicted person who cannot get a "fix," is caused by untreated pain, not addiction. Legal repercussions for overprescription of opioids (choice **E**) are feared by some clinicians. However, government and professional organizations clearly state that it is the clinician's duty to adequately treat pain and law suits have been initiated by relatives who claim their "loved one's" pain was not adequately treated. Physicians also have the option of referring patients to a pain management specialist.

2 The answer is D *Medicine*

The patient most likely has bacterial meningitis caused by *Streptococcus pneumoniae,* a gram-positive diplococcus (choice **D**). This pathogen is the most common cause of bacterial meningitis in individuals over 18 years of age. It is generally advised to start treatment with ceftriaxone as soon as the diagnosis is suspected and then add vancomycin when gram-positive organisms are found. This regimen should be continued until it is confirmed that the organism is not penicillin resistant. Once susceptibility is confirmed, the treatment of choice is aqueous penicillin G.

Bacterial meningitis caused by *Neisseria meningitidis* (gram-negative diplococcus, choice **A**) most often occurs in individuals between 1 month and 18 years of age. It commonly produces disseminated intravascular coagulation leading to bilateral hemorrhagic infarctions of the adrenal glands (Waterhouse-Friderichsen syndrome). Petechial hemorrhages are invariably present (absent in this patient) and are due to a combination of thrombocytopenia and fibrin clots obstructing the lumen of small vessels. The treatment of choice is aqueous penicillin G. Meningitis caused by gram-negative rods (choice **B**) is most commonly due to *Escherichia coli.* It usually occurs in newborns and in individuals older than 50 years of age. The treatment of choice is ampicillin plus cefotaxime. Meningitis due to *Haemophilus influenzae,* a gram-negative rod, used to be the most common meningitis in children; however, it is now uncommon due to immunization. A notable feature of this type of meningitis is the presence of sterile subdural effusions that commonly cause persistence of fever in meningitis being treated appropriately. The treatment of choice is cefotaxime or ceftriaxone. Meningitis caused by *Staphylococcus aureus,* a gram-positive coccus (choice **C**), usually occurs in postsurgical patients, patients with penetrating trauma to the brain, and intravenous drug abusers. Treatment is based on whether or not it is a methicillin-resistant *S. aureus* (MRSA) strain. Meningitis caused by *Streptococcus agalactiae,* which is also a gram-positive coccus (group B streptococcus), is the most common cause of meningitis in newborns. The treatment of choice is ampicillin plus cefotaxime. Bacterial meningitis caused by gram-positive rods

517

(choice **E**) is most often due to *Listeria monocytogenes.* It causes bacterial meningitis in newborns and in immunocompromised patients, particularly those with AIDS. The treatment of choice is ampicillin.

3 | The answer is B   *Obstetrics and Gynecology*

In this scenario the gestational dating of the 8-week sonogram is highly reliable, with an accuracy of plus or minus 5 days. With the repeat sonogram showing a falling off of the growth curve, the diagnosis is consistent with intrauterine growth restriction (IUGR). IUGR is asymmetric if the head is larger than the abdomen (due to head sparing). This is usually from inadequate placental perfusion of nutritional substrates due to maternal factors such as hypertension (chronic hypertension or preeclampsia) or small-vessel disease (long-standing type 1 diabetes mellitus, systemic lupus erythematosus). IUGR is symmetric if all biometric measurements are small, such as in this case. This usually indicates that the decreased growth potential is attributable to fetal problems (aneuploidy, early intrauterine fetal infection, gross fetal anatomic defects). All of the five options to this question are cytogenic abnormalities with aneuploidy. Four of them ([**A**] trisomy 18, [**C**] monosomy X, [**D**] trisomy 21, and [**E**] trisomy 13) are associated with asymmetric IUGR and short stature. Thus, the correct answer is choice **B**, Klinefelter syndrome, which is associated with normal or even tall stature.

4 | The answer is D   *Surgery*

The surgical treatment for portal hypertension encompasses a variety of shunt operations. Shunt types include a portocaval shunt, mesocaval shunt, and the distal splenorenal shunt. Since the portal vein is formed by the superior mesenteric vein and the splenic vein, a distal splenorenal shunt (choice **D**) reduces portal vein pressure (splenic vein blood is shunted into the renal vein) without bypassing the liver. Therefore, portal vein blood containing ammonia produced by colon bacteria is partially metabolized in the liver by the urea cycle; this reduces the risk for inducing hepatic encephalopathy. In contradistinction, portosystemic shunts reduce portal pressure but deprive the liver of portal blood flow, thus exacerbating hepatic encephalopathy by increasing serum ammonia levels.

The side-to-side (portal vein–inferior vena cava) (choice **B**) and the end-to-side (portal vein–inferior vena cava) (choice **C**) shunts decompress sinusoidal pressure in the liver and relieve ascites in most patients by redirecting portal vein blood into the vena cava. Mesocaval shunts (choice **A**) are anastomoses between the superior mesenteric vein and vena cava, the portal vein and vena cava, and the mesenteric vein and renal vein. These are most often performed as an emergency procedure for active esophageal bleeding that is resistant to therapy. In general, these shunts decompress esophageal veins, control ascites, and have a high rate of patency.

5 | The answer is B   *Preventive Medicine and Public Health*

One recent, controlled study has shown that supplementation with a daily dose of 254 µg of vitamin K reduced fracture risk by 65%, while another noted that 1000 µg daily slowed bone loss significantly. The theory is that vitamin K-induced γ-carboxylation of the osteocalcin of bone matrix promotes calcium retention and new bone development. The optimal intake of vitamin K has not yet been established, but there are presently two large clinical trials under way with results expected by 2006–2007. In the meantime, it is clear that the present recommended daily allowance (RDA) of 90 µg for women and 120 µg for men, while adequate for blood clotting, is too little for optimal bone health, at least among the elderly. Present evidence shows 100 µg is not enough and 200 µg is better; consequently, it is suggested that the daily intake should be between 150 and 250 µg (choice **B**). Because of bacterial synthesis and the wide distribution of vitamin K, particularly in green leafy vegetables, this amount can easily be reached without further supplementation. However, unfortunately among the elderly, intake of these vegetables often is inadequate, particularly if a person has a problem with alcohol.

Whereas a daily intake of 400 IU of vitamin D is recommended for persons between the ages of 50 and 70 years, over the age of 70 years an intake of 1000 IU is recommended (choice **A**). A daily intake of 1000 mg of calcium is recommended between the ages of 19 and 50 years, and over 50 years the daily recommended allowance is 1200 mg (choice **C**). Of all the vitamins, when consumed as a retinoid, retinol, or retinal, vitamin A is the most toxic; however, when consumed as a carotinoid it has little toxicity. A 2002 study of 72,000 postmenopausal women found that those who consumed 6600 IU or more of retinol daily had almost twice the risk of hip fractures compared with a control group with a daily intake of less than 1700 IU daily. Clearly, an intake of at least 10,000 IU of retinol (choice **D**) will not help prevent fractures. Unfortunately, many vitamin supplements have a relatively high level of retinol and many foods are also supplemented. Good bone health also depends upon an adequate intake of protein; 25 g/day clearly is too little (choice **E**). The present recommendation is at least 46 g/day for women and 56 g/day for men.

6 The answer is C *Medicine*

Muscle cramping and abdominal pain (choice **C**) are due to a neurotoxin produced by the black widow spider *(Latrodectus mactans)*. It is a glossy black spider with a red hourglass on the ventral aspect of the abdomen. They can inject a very potent toxin, but fortunately in quantities too small to mortally affect any but the very young and very old, in whom paralysis and death may occur unless treated with antitoxin. Diazepam or calcium gluconate are useful in controlling pain from muscle spasms. Tetanus prevention is recommended.

Ascending paralysis and hypertension (choice **A**) are due to a neurotoxin produced by the scorpion (*Centruroides* species). Antivenom therapy is recommended. Disseminated intravascular coagulation (choice **B**) is associated with activation of the intrinsic and extrinsic coagulation system. It is a common complication of crotalid bites (e.g., rattlesnake). The venom has cytotoxic, hemotoxic, and neurotoxic components. Antivenom therapy is recommended. Mydriasis and muscle paralysis (choice **D**) are due to a neurotoxin produced by the coral snake. The neurotoxin binds to presynaptic nerve terminals and acetylcholine receptors. Antivenom therapy is recommended. Ulceration with necrosis (choice **E**) is characteristic of the necrolytic toxin produced by the brown recluse spider *(Loxosceles reclusa)*. Initial symptoms from the bite are usually minimal and are followed within a few hours by severe pain and swelling and erythema in the area of the bite. A central area of vesiculation usually is followed by extensive ulceration and necrosis of the skin and subcutaneous tissue. Excisions of the wound, intravenous corticosteroids, and dapsone have been used for treatment.

7 The answer is F *Preventive Medicine and Public Health*

Buprenorphine with naloxone (choice **F**) or buprenorphine alone have the potential of ameliorating signs and symptoms of cocaine withdrawal, making psychologic treatment of addiction easier.

Methadone with buprenorphine (choice **A**) also makes withdrawal symptoms less severe, but most of the time patients convert to heroin addiction, which users must then be weaned from. Naloxone alone or with disulfiram (choice **B**) has not proved to help alleviate withdrawal symptoms and neither have lithium with an antidepressant (choice **C**), disulfiram with methadone (choice **D**), phenytoin with methadone (choice **E**), or carbamazepine with buprenorphine (choice **G**).

8 The answer is C *Surgery*

The pigmented lesion under the nail is consistent with acral lentiginous melanoma, a form of malignant melanoma (choice **C**). This variant of melanoma is extremely aggressive and commonly causes widespread metastatic disease. It is the only type of malignant melanoma that occurs in African Americans at least as often as in less pigmented individuals. Smoking is not a risk factor for malignant melanoma. The nail bed is not a common location for metastasis; thus melanoma in the nail bed is almost assuredly a primary lesion of acral lentiginous melanoma.

A glioblastoma multiforme (choice **A**) is the most common primary cancer of the brain in adults. It does not metastasize outside the central nervous system. Hepatocellular carcinoma (choice **B**), primary lung cancer (choice **D**), and renal cell carcinoma (choice **E**) do not metastasize to the nail bed.

9 The answer is A *Medicine*

All five of the syndromes listed as potential choices are associated with colonic polyps and are risks for adenocarcinoma of the colon. However, each has different characteristics. Gardner syndrome (choice **A**) is associated with adenomatous polyps involving the colon (terminal ileum and proximal small bowel are rarely involved), and 95% of these patients develop colorectal cancer. Extraintestinal manifestations include congenital hypertrophy of the retinal pigment; osteomas of the mandible, skull, and long bones; supernumerary teeth; epidermoid and sebaceous teeth; soft tissue tumors; and thyroid and adrenal tumors. Colectomy should be performed in all patients before malignancy develops.

Adenomas represent 75% of all colonic polyps and are divided into tubular, villous, and tubulovillous types on the basis of histology. Once they grow beyond 2 cm, they have a 20% chance of becoming cancerous because of accumulation of oncogenes. Villous adenomas (choice **B**) represent 5–10% of all adenomatous polyps. They are usually sessile, are larger than tubular adenomas, tend to be found in the more distal parts of the colon and have a 20–30% chance of becoming malignant. Familial adenomatous polyposis syndrome (choice **C**) is an autosomal dominant disease in which there is a 100% risk of adenocarcinoma in the colon because of the large number of polyps, each with a finite chance of transforming. There are no extraintestinal manifestations, and colectomy should be performed in all patients. In Turcot-Després syndrome (choice **D**), adenomatous polyps of the colon are associated with malignant gliomas and brain tumors. The inheritance is autosomal recessive. Tubular adenomas (choice **E**) represent 80–86% of all adenomas, are pedunculate rather than sessile, and although less likely percentage wise to transform into a cancerous growth, because of their greater numbers, are responsible for cancer more often, particularly when they grow larger than 2 cm.

10 The answer is C *Medicine*

The Weber test and Rinne test are used to distinguish conductive from sensorineural hearing loss. In conductive hearing loss, the Weber test lateralizes to the affected ear, and bone conduction is greater than air conduction (Rinne's test). In sensorineural hearing loss, the Weber test lateralizes to the normal ear (contralateral ear is affected), and air conduction is greater than bone conduction in both the normal and affected ear. The results of these tests when conducted on the patient described, as well as his normal tympanic membranes, point to conductive loss, particularly in the right ear. In other words, the patient most likely has otosclerosis (choice **C**), which refers to sclerosis and fixation of the middle ear ossicles, associated with a conductive type of hearing loss and possible deafness. It may be bilateral and has a strong autosomal dominant inheritance pattern. It is the most common cause of conductive hearing loss in adults. Impaction of the ear canal can also produce findings of the conductive hearing loss type. This is easily excluded by examining the canal with an otoscope.

Presbycusis (choice **A**) is the most common cause of sensorineural deafness in adults. It is associated with a progressive, predominantly symmetric, high-frequency hearing loss. There is loss of speech discrimination, particularly in noisy places. There is a genetic predisposition. Chronic otitis media (choice **B**) can be associated with the ingrowth of keratinizing squamous epithelium, which is called a cholesteatoma (choice **D**). The tympanic membrane would be thickened in chronic otitis media and it is normal in this patient. Ménière's disease (choice **E**) causes sensorineural hearing loss, tinnitus (ringing in the ears), and vertigo (room spins around). It is due to an increase in endolymph in the inner ear and a loss of cochlear hairs.

11 The answer is C *Obstetrics and Gynecology*

For a fetus to be at risk of hemolytic disease of the newborn (HDN), the following five requisites must be met: (1) the mother must be negative for the antibody; (2) the father must be positive for the antibody; (3) results of the indirect Coombs' test or atypical antibody test must be positive; (4) the identified antibody must be associated with severe HDN; and (5) the antibody titer must be over 1:8. In this case of anti-Lewis isoimmunization, choices **A** and **B** are irrelevant since they have nothing to do with anti-Lewis antibodies. We can assume that the mother is negative for the antigen, but we do not know what the father is, since none of the options relate to paternal status. The correct answer (choice **C**, atypical antibody type) is the critical factor, since anti-Lewis antibodies are NOT associated with HDN. Therefore, choice **D**, atypical antibody titer, is irrelevant because no matter how high the titer, anti-Lewis antibodies do NOT cross the placenta. Choice **E**, previous baby outcomes, is incorrect since past history is no guarantee regarding the current pregnancy.

12 The answer is E *Medicine*

Tubular dysfunction is present in chronic renal failure (CRF) that typically leads to end-stage renal disease (ESRD). This tubular dysfunction results in decreased clearance of both creatinine and urea by the kidneys and a proportionate increase in both the serum BUN and serum creatinine level. Normally, the ratio of serum BUN (~10 mg/dL) to creatinine (~1 mg/dL) is 10. In CRF, the ratio is <10:1 (choice **E**), because urea is resorbed.

In CRF, the second hydroxylation of vitamin D is impaired because of the loss of 1α-hydroxylase in the renal tubules. Hypovitaminosis D occurs with development of hypocalcemia (not hypercalcemia) (choice **C**), which is a stimulus for the synthesis and release of parathyroid hormone (secondary hyperparathyroidism) (not decreased parathyroid hormone) (choice **A**). Phosphorus is normally is reabsorbed in the proximal tubule. In CRF, the decrease in the glomerular filtration rate causes accumulation of phosphorus in the blood, leading to hyperphosphatemia (not hypophosphatemia) (choice **B**). An increase in urine-specific gravity (urine density, >1.021) indicates that the urine is concentrated, a sign of intact tubular function. In CRF, neither concentration nor dilution occurs; therefore, the urine specific gravity is essentially the same as the glomerular filtrate, which is about 1.010 (not increased >1.021) (choice **D**). In CRF, this specific gravity remains unchanged, regardless of time of day and fluid intake (fixed specific gravity).

13 The answer is E *Surgery*

This patient has sustained a spontaneous fracture of the shaft of the femur and as a result is in hemorrhagic shock. Among the choices presented, osteosarcoma (choice **A**) is the most logical choice of a factor predisposing her to a pathologic (spontaneous) fracture. Osteosarcoma is the most common of the primary malignancies of bone. It is most common in adolescents, commonly affects the femur, and is often first recognized by a spontaneous fracture, which is preceded by several weeks of pain. The cancer weakens the bone by creating lytic lesions. Lytic lesions are also found in various other primary bone diseases including multiple myeloma, which is the most common primary hematologic malignancy of bone. Nonmalignant diseases causing pathologic fractures include bone cysts, Paget's disease of bone, (in which the fractures are usually transverse and usually involve the femur or the tibia), osteogenesis imperfecta, and osteoporosis.

More often than arising in situ, bone cancers are derived secondarily as metastases from primary tumors arising in several tissue types, including: breast carcinoma, small cell carcinoma of the lung, follicular carcinoma of the thyroid, and, in men, prostate carcinoma. Nonetheless, metastatic bone disease (choice **F**) is less likely to have predisposed this young lady to this pathologic fracture than an osteosarcoma because of her age and because one would expect symptoms of the primary malignancy to be more obvious.

Chronic osteomyelitis (choice **E**) results from acute hematogenous infection to the bone. The condition is usually quiescent for several months or even years before it flares up. The patient with chronic osteomyelitis has fever, prostration, local inflammation, and a draining sinus. This patient had a furuncle on her thigh, not a draining sinus; also, fractures are unusual in a setting of chronic osteomyelitis. Treatment is surgical, and cure is difficult. The goal is to remove the sequestrum (dead bone), which is a continual nidus for infection. Heavy antibiotic use is only used to treat acute (not chronic) osteomyelitis.

Osteoporosis (choice **B**) is unlikely. Not withstanding the hot flushes that she has been experiencing recently, the patient is still premenopausal. In women, bone density usually starts to gradually decrease shortly after menopause, and frank osteoporosis is rare before the age of 65. Colles' fracture, fracture of the proximal humerus, neck of the femur, and collapse of the vertebra are the most common fractures associated with osteoporosis, and only femoral neck fracture and vertebral collapse are not preceded by a history of fall.

Stress fractures (choice **C**) are caused by repetitive excessive load on the bones. This can involve the second and third metatarsals (march fracture), which was initially noted in infantrymen during long marches, and femoral neck in the case of young soldiers who have to march for great distances carrying a full, heavily loaded backpack. Stress fractures can also involve the tibiae in runners, especially when they run over uneven surfaces. Physical examination usually reveals localized tenderness without deformity. An x-ray film may not show the fracture, especially in the early stages. A bone scan using ^{99m}Tc-labeled diphosphonate will clinch the diagnosis, by demonstrating increased uptake at the site. Most stress fractures resolve with rest.

Osteogenesis imperfecta (choice **D**), also known as brittle bone disease, presents itself in four forms, of varying severity. Type I is the most common form and is associated with a blue sclera 98% of the time (not blue irises, as in this woman); typically, fractures are not excessive and primarily occur before puberty. Type II manifests in utero or in infancy and is lethal. Type III is rare; fractures abound, causing bone deformities such as scoliosis and deformed limbs and result in dwarfism. Type IV is similar to type I but much rarer and differs in that blue sclera are not seen. Both types I and IV are associated with fractures in childhood after minimal trauma and are easily mistaken for child abuse, particularly type IV, in which blue sclera are not present. Although in types I, III, and IV, fractures become rarer after growth ceases, the bone structure remains less dense than normal making, then susceptible to fractures throughout life and to osteoporosis as they age. Types I and IV are transmitted as autosomal dominant traits, and commonly cases can be traced back several generations. In contrast, type II and III cases lack a family history but most likely are either autosomal recessive conditions or new mutations.

14 The answer is E *Pediatrics*

The patient is a male newborn with ambiguous genitalia caused by a 5-α-reductase deficiency (choice **E**); 5-α-reductase is an enzyme that converts testosterone to dihydrotestosterone (DHT). DHT is important in the male fetus for converting female-appearing genitalia to male genitalia; thus, deficiency of the enzyme leads to ambiguous genitalia. In this case, the patient has a micropenis and hypospadias with the urine meatus located on the perineum. The testicles are undescended (cryptorchidism) and are located in the inguinal canal.

Aromatase (choice **A**) converts androgens to estrogens (e.g., testosterone to estradiol) and not androgens to androgens. In males, this reaction occurs in the Leydig cells, where small amounts of testosterone are converted to estradiol. Aromatase deficiency is extremely rare and does not produce ambiguous genitalia in a male.

11-Hydroxylase deficiency (choice **B**) is part of the adrenogenital syndrome, which represents a group of autosomal recessive disorders, each characterized by a hereditary defect in an enzyme involved in cortisol synthesis. In these conditions, a decrease in cortisol results in a compensatory increase in ACTH secretion, which not only stimulates the adrenal cortex but also stimulates melanocytes to produce diffuse skin pigmentation (not present in this patient). Depending on the enzyme that is lacking, the resultant adrenal hyperplasia may or may not cause increased production of androgens, glucocorticoids, and mineralocorticoids. In 11-hydroxylase deficiency, 11-deoxycortisol level is increased, deoxycorticosterone is increased, and androgens are increased (androstenedione, dehydroepiandrosterone, testosterone, and testosterone). Since DHT is present, there is normal development of the male external genitalia, and the child is at risk for developing precocious puberty because of an increase in androgens. 21-Hydroxylase deficiency (choice **C**) is the most common cause of the adrenogenital syndrome. Cortisol level is decreased, mineralocorticoids are decreased, and androgens are increased; thus there is normal development of the male external genitalia. Furthermore, the random urine sodium level is normal in this patient. In 21-hydroxylase deficiency, the loss of mineralocorticoids causes sodium wasting in the urine. Oxidoreductase (choice **D**) normally converts androstenedione to testosterone. Deficiency of this enzyme results in a decrease in testosterone as well as DHT. The testosterone level is normal in this patient.

15 The answer is B *Surgery*

This woman has acute cholecystitis in which an attack is commonly precipitated by a large meal, particularly a fatty meal. It is characterized by the sudden appearance of steady pain localized to the epigastrium or right hypochondrium, leukocytosis, and elevated total bilirubin and hepatic enzymes. Meperidine is preferable to morphine to treat the pain, because morphine has a tendency to cause the sphincter of Oddi to spasm (choice **B**).

While morphine is addictive, addiction caused by treatment of an acute condition under a physician's supervision is extremely unlikely (choice **A**). Opioids including morphine constrict, not widen, the pupils (choice **C**) and cause bradycardia, not tachycardia (choice **D**). Whereas death by pulmonary aspiration of gastric contents (choice **E**) is not an uncommon consequence of opioid overdose, it would be gross medical malpractice if that happened when morphine is prescribed to counteract pain.

16 The answer is D *Psychiatry*

The patient's symptoms are characterized by mood instability, impulsivity, self-destructive behavior, difficult interpersonal relationships, and identity disturbance, suggesting borderline personality disorder. Dialectic Behavioral Therapy is specifically designed to improve this condition. In this case, however, the patient remains troubled by episodes of confusion and vaguely psychotic-like symptoms, a relatively common associated feature with borderline personality disorder. Consequently, supplementation of this psychotherapy with medication is in order (not ineffective) (choice **A**). Low doses of antipsychotic medications, such as aripiprazole (choice **D**) are frequently prescribed for such an individual. Aripiprazole is the first neuroleptic drug that is a dopamine stabilizer. Diazepam (choice **B**) and other benzodiazepines should usually be avoided in persons with personality disorder because of the increased danger of substance abuse. There are no clear indications in this case for sertraline (an antidepressant) (choice **C**) or gabapentin (choice **E**), an anticonvulsant and mood stabilizer sometimes used to treat bipolar disorder.

17 The answer is C *Pediatrics*

Premature or low-birth-weight infants have inadequate stores of fat and glycogen; consequently, they are at high risk for hypoglycemia (choice **C**). Early, frequent feedings help avoid this problem.

Infants of diabetic mothers tend to be macrosomic (choice **E**). Their hypoglycemia is caused by relative hyperinsulinism. Beta cell endocrine tumors are usually seen in the form of nesidioblastosis (choice **B**). Leucine-sensitive hypoglycemia is associated with excessive insulin secretion after leucine administration (choice **A**). Although the gluconeogenic enzymes may not be fully developed in small-for-gestational-age and premature infants, most neonates have functional, normal hormonal systems (choice **D**).

18 The answer is E   *Obstetrics and Gynecology*

Uterine leiomyomas are benign smooth muscle tumors that have no malignant potential. Since the myomas in this scenario are small and the patient is asymptomatic, the correct option is **E,** observation and follow-up with regular pelvic examinations. All other options are incorrect.

Choice **A,** embolization, is only appropriate for symptomatic, large myomas in a patient who has completed childbearing but chooses not to have a hysterectomy. This invasive radiologic procedure selectively injects polyvinyl microspheres into the uterine arteries, resulting in ischemia and shrinkage. Choice **B,** leuprolide shrinkage, is only used for large myomas interfering with fertility but must be followed by surgical myomectomy or the myomas will enlarge once the leuprolide is discontinued. Choice **C,** hysterectomy, is only appropriate for management of symptomatic large myomas when childbearing is completed. Choice **D,** myomectomy, is used for large myomas interfering with fertility, often in conjunction with preoperative leuprolide shrinkage.

19 The answer is A   *Preventive Medicine and Public Health*

Annual vaccination against the flu strains expected to predominate is recommended every fall for persons who are 50 years of age or older (choice **A**) as well as health care workers, pregnant women, and immunocompromised persons. The pneumococcal vaccine is generally thought to provide life-long immunity, although some experts recommend giving a booster after 5 years to persons who might be immunocompromised because of age or disease. It has only been 4 years since this man was vaccinated, and there is no reason to think he is immunocompromised; consequently, there is no reason to give him a pneumococcal vaccine booster (choice **B**). Vaccination against hepatitis A is recommended for individuals who might be exposed to the virus because of their employment and to persons who travel to places where the disease is endemic. However, the two-dose immunization process should provide life-long immunity; hence, this man does not need a booster shot (choice **C**). Chest radiographic screening is not recommended for asymptomatic patients (choice **D**). For the average at-risk person, colon cancer screening should start at the age of 50 years and should consist of an occult fecal blood test annually plus either a flexible sigmoidoscopy or a barium enema every 5 years or a colonoscopy every 10 years. Since this man had a colonoscopy 4 years ago, he does not need another now (choice **E**).

20 The answer is D   *Psychiatry*

Persons who abuse drugs heavily sometimes have involuntary withdrawal syndromes after hospitalization or incarceration. Alcohol and benzodiazepines, including diazepam, are associated with anxiety and occasional generalized seizures during withdrawal (choice **D**).

Although methamphetamine (choice **A**), cocaine (choice **B**), cannabis (choice **C**), and pentazocine (choice **E**) produce a variety of unpleasant symptoms during withdrawal, they are not commonly associated with seizures.

21 The answer is B   *Pediatrics*

Pregnant women infected by parvovirus may be asymptomatic or have nonspecific symptoms. However, fetal infection may occur via transplacental passage of the virus, which results in stillbirth and nonimmune hydrops fetalis in less than 5% of cases (choice **B**). The fetus is most sensitive to infection during the second trimester. Parvovirus is not considered a teratogen and is not associated with a typical syndrome.

Chorioretinitis (choice **A**) and microcephaly (choice **D**) are seen in congenital toxoplasmosis. Rhagades (choice **C**) and Hutchinson's teeth (choice **E**) are typical findings of congenital syphilis.

22 The answer is B   *Psychiatry*

The presentation is most consistent with factitious disorder (choice **B**). The blindness is clearly being feigned, as the patient is capable of reading. His earlier paralysis likely was also feigned.

Conversion disorder (choice **A**) involves an involuntary loss of function. In the case described there is no apparent external incentive to produce his symptoms, as would be present in malingering (choice **C**). Hypochondriasis (choice **D**) involves misinterpretation of a physical symptom. Somatization disorder (choice **E**) involves multiple physical complaints.

23 **The answer is D** *Pediatrics*

Although adverse events associated with DTaP are less significant than with the administration of whole-cell pertussis (i.e., DTP), most of the reactivity of the diphtheria–tetanus–acellular pertussis (DTaP) vaccine is still due to the pertussis component. Most seizures occurring after immunization with DTaP are self-limited and generalized and are usually associated with fever. They do not result in the development of epilepsy or other neurologic sequelae. The same special considerations, contraindications, precautions, and reporting requirements for serious adverse events that apply for DTP vaccination also apply to DTaP vaccination. Serious reactions, such as seizures, contraindicate further use of the pertussis vaccine (choice **D**). This reaction, however, does not contraindicate further use of the tetanus and diphtheria toxoids.

Choices **A, B,** and **E** all include pertussis as part of future vaccines. Choice **C** excludes both the tetanus and pertussis components of any future vaccines, which is not necessary; only the pertussis component should be left out.

24 **The answer is B** *Obstetrics and Gynecology*

This patient has the classic historical triad of ectopic pregnancy—unilateral pain, bleeding, and amenorrhea. With the patient exhibiting unstable vital signs, the diagnosis must be assumed to be ruptured ectopic pregnancy with massive hemoperitoneum. This calls for rapid emergency surgery to stop the internal bleeding (choice **B**, laparotomy).

Choice **A,** observation is never appropriate for an ectopic pregnancy. Choice **C,** methotrexate, is used in a stable patient with an early unruptured ectopic pregnancy, typically with a serum β-hCG titer below 5000–6000 mIU. Choice **D,** laparoscopy, is used in a stable patient with an advanced unruptured ectopic pregnancy, typically with serum β-hCG titer above 5000–6000 mIU. Choice **E,** serial β-hCG titers, is only used if the β-hCG titer is less than 1500 mIU and no intrauterine pregnancy is seen on a transvaginal sonogram.

25 **The answer is D** *Medicine*

The man described has isolated systolic hypertension, a condition common among the elderly because of age-related loss of arterial elasticity. His condition is made more complex by the fact that he is also diabetic. Isolated systolic hypertension, particularly in conjunction with diabetes or renal nephropathy, is particularly hard to treat, and use of three, four, or more drugs, as in this case, is not unusual. The drugs are generally chosen so that they affect different systems, with the hope that their effects will be additive. This patient is already taking HCTZ (a thiazide diuretic), enalapril (an ACE inhibitor), doxazosin mesylate (a blocker of postsynaptic α-receptors), acebutolol (a β₁-blocker), and clonidine (a central α-adrenergic receptor stimulator). Consequently, it makes sense to add a calcium channel blocker such as nifedipine (choice **D**).

Adding furosemide (choice **A**), a loop diuretic, makes little sense, since a thiazide diuretic is already in use. Moreover, loop diuretics lead to electrolyte and volume depletion more readily that the thiazide diuretics and have a short half-life, factors that generally limit their use to cases involving renal dysfunction (serum creatinine above 2.5 mg/dL). Eprosartan is an angiotensin II receptor blocker (ARB), so its effects should be similar to those of an ACE inhibitor. At this time, the consensus is that because of limited experience, high cost, and unproved benefits ARBs should only be prescribed when a patient is intolerant to ACE inhibitors, for example, because of cough or rash (choice **B**). Reserpine is a peripheral sympathetic inhibitor and one of the earliest antihypertensive agents developed. However, most physicians hesitate to use it (choice **C**) because of its tendency to induce depression, sedation, nasal stuffiness, sleep disturbances, and peptic ulcer. Moreover, there is little experience concerning its use in a poly-drug environment. Nitroprusside is rarely, if ever, used to treat chronic hypertension (choice **E**). IV nitroprusside is particularly effective in hypertensive emergencies, in which its use causes direct arterial and venous dilation and lowers blood pressure within seconds after administration.

26 **The answer is E** *Pediatrics*

Discriminating clinical findings (Jones criteria) are used to make the diagnosis of acute rheumatic fever. The major criteria are carditis, polyarthritis, chorea, subcutaneous nodules (choice **E**), and rash (erythema marginatum). Minor criteria include fever; arthralgia (choice **B**); previous rheumatic fever; elevated acute phase reactants, such as erythrocyte sedimentation rate (ESR) (choice **D**) and C-reactive protein (CRP); and a prolonged time between the P wave and QRS complex (P-R interval) in an electrocardiogram (ECG). Previously, two major or one major and two minor criteria plus evidence of a recent streptococcal infection, such as an elevated anti-streptolysin O (ASO) titer (choice **A**), were required to consider the diagnosis of acute rheumatic fever. Because Sydenham's chorea may be the only symptom of rheumatic fever, the World Health Organization (WHO) now suggests that this symptom alone satisfies the Jones criteria. Chorea rarely, if ever, leads to permanent neurologic sequelae.

Erythema migrans (choice **C**) is pathognomonic of Lyme disease.

27 The answer is B *Obstetrics and Gynecology*

This patient has progression of cervical dysplasia to CIN 2, in which the basal cells of the cervical epithelium involve 50% of the thickness. CIN 2 or CIN 3 must be treated with an ablative modality (cryotherapy, laser vaporization, or electrofulguration) or an excisional procedure (loop electrosurgical excision procedure [LEEP] or cold-knife conization). The only one of these procedures listed in the options is choice **B**, cryotherapy. Choices **A** (observation), **C** (HPV-DNA testing), and **D** (repeat Pap smear in 6 months) are only appropriate for CIN 1, never for CIN 2 or 3. Option **E** (simple hysterectomy) is only indicated with biopsy-confirmed recurrent CIN 2 or 3.

28 The answer is A *Preventive Medicine and Public Health*

If not the most critical factor, smoking is the easiest risk factor to modify. It contributes to development of macrovascular disease by inducing vascular spasms that last for about an hour after a cigarette is smoked. This narrows the passage through which blood must flow. To further encourage disease development, smoking raises total cholesterol level, including low-density lipoprotein (LDL) levels and lowers high-density (HDL) levels. Thus this increased concentration of LDL has less HDL to pass the LDL lipid load to; this promotes dumping of lipid into the intima of the arterial walls. To add further insult to injury, smoking also increases platelet aggregation and the level of fibrinogen and decreases red cell flexibility. Consequently, the not-so-lithe red cells are now asked to pass through narrower-than-normal orifices in the presence of higher-than-normal levels of clotting factors in an environment that is abnormally hydrophobic. In short, smoking causes arterial spasms, increases the level of LDL, decreases the level of HDL, increases platelet aggregation, increases fibrinogen concentration, and decreases red blood cell flexibility (choice **A**); thereby, promoting plaque formation and macrovascular disease.

Visceral obesity (choice **B**) promotes insulin resistance in nearly 100% of Pima Indians, and some Pacific Islanders, in 60–70% of individuals of European or African ancestry, but in only about 30% of people with a Japanese heritage. Other than obviously having a strong genetic component, the mechanism is not understood, although altered levels of one or more adipokines, including leptin, adiponectin, tumor necrosis factor-α, and resistin, are suspect. From a clinical perspective, the important point is that by reducing visceral fat the insulin requirements may be reduced, and in some cases hypoglycemic therapy can be dispensed with. Naturally, this also reduces risk of diabetic complications.

Hypertension (choice **C**) obviously increases the risk of complications associated with any of the macrovascular diseases by putting added stress on the vascular system. Type 2 diabetes and even the prediabetic metabolic syndrome (syndrome X) that often precedes frank type 2 diabetes promote hypertension; the prevalence of hypertension among type 2 diabetics is 60%, versus 20% in the age-matched general population.

Hyperglycemia (choice **D**) is an important contributor to several complications associated with diabetes. These are best demonstrated in the microvascular disease states in which excess glucose activates the sorbitol pathway by serving as substrate for aldose reductase. In the complete pathway, formation of sorbitol is followed by its rereduction to form fructose in a reaction catalyzed by sorbitol dehydrogenase. In early embryogenesis this pathway was used to provide fructose as the primary fuel for fetal development, and it is still used by the seminal vesicle to meet primary nutritional requirements of sperm, and for less understood reasons, the complete pathway also is expressed by liver cells and ovaries. However, in the adult, some tissues retain aldose reductase activity but have lost sorbitol dehydrogenase activity. These tissues include lens, retina, Schwann cells, kidney, and red blood cells; thus in these cells the sorbitol formed by the aldose reductase reaction is trapped within the cells and creates an osmotic gradient that plays an important role in development of diabetic cataracts, retinopathy, neuropathies, and nephropathy. Excess protein glycosylation caused by hyperglycemia plays a contributing role in plaque formation associated with both microvascular and macrovascular disease.

Hyperinsulinemia (choice **E**) has been shown in nondiabetics to increase the risk of coronary artery disease (CAD). Since hyperinsulinemia is a known component of pre–type 2 diabetes as well as frank type 2 diabetes, very likely hyperinsulinemia per se contributes to CAD.

29 The answer is B   *Medicine*

The patient has cysticercosis (choice **B**), which is caused by the larval form of the pork tapeworm *Taenia solium*. The patient likely ingested improperly cooked pork contaminated with feces containing eggs of the adult *T. solium*, which developed into larvae (cysticerci) in the intestinal tract. From this location, the larvae gain access to the systemic circulation, resulting in lesions in the muscle and brain. In the brain, the cysts are located at the junction of the gray and white matter. The cysts contain the scolex of the immature worm. Cysts frequently undergo calcification and also cause focal or generalized seizures. There is no benefit in treating the patient with an antiparasitic drug (e.g., albendazole).

A cerebral infarction (choice **A**) is most often due to atherosclerosis involving the middle cerebral artery or internal carotid artery. The infarction usually is pale and occurs at the periphery of the brain. The brain undergoes liquefactive necrosis, resulting in the formation of a cystic space. Multiple cerebral infarctions are uncommon. Echinococcosis (option **C**) is caused by the tapeworm *Echinococcus granulosus* or *E. multilocularis*, which infects sheep. It is transmitted to humans via contact with a dog that harbors the adult worms and eggs of the *Echinococcus*. The eggs are ingested by humans and develop into larvae that enter the liver, where they form cysts. The patient need not have any contact with sheep, just the dog. Metastatic lung carcinoma foci (choice **D**) also are usually located at the junction of gray and white matter but are more likely to show hemorrhage and necrosis rather than cystic structures with calcifications. Trichinosis (choice **E**) is caused by the nematode *Trichinella spiralis*, which is present in its larval form in pigs (the intermediate host). Ingestion of improperly cooked pork results in the formation of adult worms in the human host (the definitive host). The adult worms produce larvae that gain access to the systemic circulation where they encyst in skeletal muscle. The cysts frequently calcify and produce muscle pain. Although larvae can enter the central nervous system, this is extremely uncommon.

30 The answer is D   *Surgery*

Open-angle glaucoma (choice **D**) is characterized by a slow but progressive excavation ("cupping") of the optic disc accompanied by degeneration of the outer layers of the optic nerve. This causes a gradual loss of peripheral vision. There are no acute symptoms (thus the alternative name *chronic glaucoma*), and because loss of peripheral vision occurs slowly, patients are not likely to notice the loss until they are significantly visually impaired. Open-angle glaucoma provides no other symptoms, such as pain, red eye, or blurred vision. Open-angle glaucoma may be associated with either elevated intraocular pressure (>21 mm Hg) or normal ocular pressure (10–21 mm Hg). Pressure elevation is due to reduced drainage of the aqueous humor through the trabecular network. Normal-tension chronic glaucoma is thought to be due to vascular insufficiency. The pattern of nerve damage in both types of open-angle glaucoma is similar, as is the treatment. Obviously, elevated pressure is a risk factor but is not diagnostic; indeed some individuals with elevated pressure do not have glaucoma. Upon examination, glaucoma may be diagnosed by a cup-to-disc ratio above 0.5 or asymmetry between the eyes in the cup-to-disc ratio greater than 0.2 (both present in the patient described) and observed changes in the retinal fiber layer. Actual loss of peripheral vision is measured by a visual field test. Treatment is typically with a topical β-blocking agent such as timolol, carteolol, levobunolol, or metipranolol; however, use of prostaglandin analogues, such as latanoprost, bimatoprost, and travoprost, is becoming more popular. Other agents are available for patients with special needs.

Angle-closure glaucoma (aka *acute glaucoma*) (choice **A**) occurs with closure of a preexisting narrow anterior chamber angle. A narrow anterior chamber angle predominantly preexists in farsighted persons (hyperopes) and in eastern Asians. Angle closure can then be precipitated by various factors. Aging further sets the stage for an acute attack due to enlargement of the lens in association with developing cataracts. In such susceptible persons angle closure may be precipitated by pupillary dilation and thus may occur upon entering any darkened area such as a subway or theater, at times of stress, or from pharmacologic mydriasis or anticholinergic or sympathomimetic agents. Secondary glaucoma may also be caused by anterior uveitis, lens dislocation, or topiramate therapy. An "attack" of angle-closure glaucoma comes on suddenly and is accompanied by severe pain, profound visual loss with halos around lights, red eye, steamy cornea, dilated pupil, and an eye hard to palpitate. Unlike chronic glaucoma, which is bilateral, acute glaucoma usually only affects one eye. Because of the obvious discomfort, affected individuals usually seek medical attention as soon as possible. Angle-closure glaucoma accounts for about 10% of all cases of glaucoma; the remaining 90% are of the open-angle variety.

In the United States, diabetic retinopathy (choice **B**) is the leading cause of blindness between the ages of 20 and 65 years. Cases are classified as being either proliferative or nonproliferative. The latter is more common and is characterized by vein dilation, microaneurysms, retinal hemorrhages, retinal edema, and hard exudates and is sometimes diagnosed in pre–type 2 diabetes. The best treatment is control of the diabetes. Proliferative retinopathy is typified by neovascularization, often resulting in vitreous hemorrhage. Without treatment the visual prognosis is more serious than in nonproliferative retinopathy. Treatment is by panretinal laser photocoagulation or vitrectomy.

Macular degeneration (choice **C**) is the leading cause of blindness after the age of 65. It is more common in whites, has a slight female predominance, and tends to run in families. A history of smoking is a major risk factor. The macula is in the center of the retina, and contrariwise from glaucoma, blindness starts centrally and peripheral vision is spared. The only therapy is laser therapy to coagulate leaking blood vessels.

Cataracts (choice **E**) are very common among the elderly. They are characterized by clouding of the lens that causes blurred vision, halos around lights, and decreased ability to see in dim light. They usually are bilateral, although one eye is generally affected before the other. Once a major cause of blindness, 95% of cases today are effectively treated by surgical removal and implantation of an artificial lens. Each year over a million such operations are performed in this country.

31 **The answer is D** *Obstetrics and Gynecology*

A teratogen is any agent that disturbs normal fetal development and affects subsequent function. The gestational window in which teratogenesis can occur is from 3 to 8 postconceptional weeks. Choice **D**, valproic acid, which is frequently used as an anticonvulsant, is the correct answer to this question because it is associated with an increased risk of spina bifida, one of the anomalies described in the scenario.

The other options are incorrect. Choice **A**, thalidomide, is associated with phocomelia, limb reduction defects. Choice **B**, lithium, is associated with Ebstein anomaly, a right heart defect in which the tricuspid valve is displaced downward. Choice **C**, diethylstilbestrol, is associated with a T-shaped uterus, vaginal adenosis, and vaginal clear cell carcinoma. Choice **E**, isotretinoin, is associated with microtia, congenital deafness, and cardiac defects.

32 **The answer is B** *Medicine*

The heart fails when it cannot pump blood delivered to it by the venous system. By definition, heart failure occurs when cardiac output is decreased (choice **B**), no matter if heart failure is left-sided or right-sided.

Bibasilar inspiratory crackles (choice **A**) are a sign of left-sided heart failure, which is "forward" heart failure, causing decreased cardiac output and backup of blood in the left ventricle, left atrium, and pulmonary capillaries. Increased pulmonary capillary hydrostatic pressure causes fluid to enter the interstitium of the lung and eventually the alveoli (pulmonary edema). Air entering alveoli containing fluid produces inspiratory crackles that are best heard at the base of both lungs. A chest x-ray film shows congestion of blood in the upper lobes and patchy interstitial and alveolar infiltrates. Kerley's lines in radiographs are due to fluid in the interstitium.

Paroxysmal nocturnal dyspnea (choice **D**) is also a sign of left-sided heart failure. It occurs primarily at night when the patient is supine in bed. At this time, gravity does not impede blood flow to the right side of the heart, and fluid from the interstitial space enters the venous system. Excess blood enters the failed left ventricle and backs up into the lungs, causing pulmonary edema and dyspnea, which awaken the patient. Because increased gravity decreases venous return to the right side of the heart, symptoms resolve when patients stand up or place pillows under their heads (pillow orthopnea). Left-ventricular heart failure (LVF) is subdivided into systolic and diastolic types. Systolic dysfunction is a type of LVF in which there is a problem with left ventricular contractility (e.g., ischemic heart disease). The left ventricle loses its ability to eject blood into the aorta, causing a decrease in the ejection fraction (EF). The EF equals stroke volume/left ventricular end-diastolic volume (LVEDV). The normal stroke volume is 80 mL, and the normal LVEDV is 120; thus the normal EF is 0.66 (0.55–0.80). In systolic dysfunction, the EF is <0.40. Therapy is directed at improving performance of the failed left ventricle by using positive inotropic agents (e.g., digoxin; dobutamine), reducing afterload (angiotensin-converting enzyme

[ACE] inhibitors that inhibit angiotensin II synthesis; angiotensin II receptor blockers; direct vasodilating drugs, e.g., hydralazine), and reducing preload (ACE inhibitors plus aldosterone blockers, which inhibit aldosterone; diuretics). β-Blockers are also a mainstay of treatment of systolic dysfunction since they reduce excessive sympathetic stimulation, which normally produces tachycardia, increased myocardial oxygen demand, cardiac hypertrophy, and impaired myocyte function. Nonpharmacologic treatment includes restriction of sodium and fluid intake. Diastolic dysfunction is a type of LVF that is due to noncompliance of the left ventricle with decreased filling ("stiff heart"; e.g., concentric hypertrophy in essential hypertension). The EF is normal or high, because of increased contraction by the left atrium. Dyspnea from pulmonary edema is a common symptom. Treatment is directed at correcting hypertension (cause of left ventricular hypertrophy), if present, and increasing preload by slowing the heart rate, which prolongs left ventricular filling at low pressures (β-blockers, calcium channel blockers, ACE inhibitors).

Dependent pitting edema (choice **C**) and passive congestion in the liver (choice **E**) are both signs of right-ventricular heart failure, a "backward" heart failure causing systemic venous congestion. The increase in hydrostatic pressure in the venous system causes fluid (transudate) to leak into the interstitial space through the venules, leading to dependent pitting edema. The hepatic vein empties into the inferior vena cava, and blood backs up into the central veins, leading to passive congestion in the liver.

33 The answer is B *Pediatrics*

Rhabdomyosarcomas account for half of the soft tissue sarcomas. Those occurring before 5 years of age have a predilection for the neck, head, prostate, bladder, and vagina. A second peak occurs at 15 to 19 years of age, involving primarily the genitourinary tract. Embryonal rhabdomyosarcomas account for 60% of all rhabdomyosarcomas. Sarcoma botryoides is a form of embryonal rhabdomyosarcoma (choice **B**) and accounts for 6% of the embryonal type. It occurs in the vagina, uterus, bladder, nasopharynx, and middle ear, and it looks like a bunch of grapes.

Clear cell adenocarcinoma of the vagina (choice **A**) is a rare complication of diethylstilbestrol (DES) exposure in utero. Leiomyosarcoma (choice **C**) is a tumor of the smooth muscle. It is the most common pediatric retroperitoneal soft tissue tumor. Granular cell myoblastomas (choice **D**) are benign tumors derived from Schwann cells and are found in the mediastinum. Squamous cell carcinoma of the genital tract (choice **E**) is rarely seen in this age group.

34 The answer is C *Psychiatry*

Based upon the negative work-up for other disorders, the man likely suffers from primary insomnia, defined as an inability to initiate or maintain sleep or a lack of satisfying sleep. Primary insomnia increases in prevalence in older individuals and is sometimes not responsive to sleep hygiene (e.g., setting regular sleep periods and refraining from caffeine). Eszopiclone (choice **C**) is approved as a long-term hypnotic for use in this condition.

Most hypnotic medications, including zolpidem (choice **A**) are either ineffective or contraindicated for long-term use. Quetiapine (choice **B**), a sedating antipsychotic medication, should be reserved for individuals with psychotic disorders. Alcohol (choice **D**) often is used by patients but causes mid-night or early morning awakening and may lead to addiction. Antihistamines such as diphenhydramine (choice **E**) are found in over-the-counter formulations and often cause persistent daytime drowsiness or impairment.

35 The answer is A *Pediatrics*

Patients with pseudohypoparathyroidism have normal or hyperplastic parathyroid glands that can synthesize and secrete parathormone. The disorder is associated with low (not increased [choice **C**]) calcium levels and high (not decreased [choice **D**]) phosphate levels. When calcium levels are low, parathormone levels are high (not decreased [choice **B**]). However, in Albright's hereditary osteodystrophy there seems to be unresponsiveness to parathormone at the receptor level, leading to symptoms of hypoparathyroidism (pseudohypoparathyroidism), and neither endogenous nor administered parathormone increases the calcium level. By contrast, patients with true hypoparathyroidism have a deficiency of parathormone. If pseudohypoparathyroidism is diagnosed late, the patient may have lenticular cataracts, calcification of the basal ganglia, and mental retardation (choice **A**). Although retinoblastoma (choice **E**) may occur as a "13q syndrome" characterized by growth delay and mental retardation with facial and other anomalies, it is not related to Albright's hereditary osteodystrophy.

36 The answer is C *Surgery*

A painless testicular mass that does not transilluminate is highly predictive of testicular cancer. Adults with a cryptorchid testis are at risk for seminoma in the undescended testis (if still present) and descended testis (choice **C**).

A choriocarcinoma of the testicle (choice **A**) typically is small and does not cause enlargement of the entire testicle. The syncytiotrophoblast component of the tumor produces human chorionic gonadotropin, which is absent in this patient. A hydrocele (choice **B**) is an accumulation of serous fluid in the tunica vaginalis, thus causing scrotal enlargement, and the mass of fluid transilluminates, unlike in this patient. A varicocele (choice **D**) is the tortuous dilation of the veins of the spermatic cord that is often described as a "bag of worms." A varicocele typically occurs on the left side, because the left spermatic vein empties into the left renal vein rather than into the inferior vena cava. It does not present as a painless mass lesion. Yolk sac tumors (choice **E**) typically occur in infants and children and are not associated with cryptorchidism. They secrete α-fetoprotein, which is absent in this patient.

37 The answer is E *Pediatrics*

The child has ABO hemolytic disease of the newborn (HDN), which is a common cause of jaundice in the first 24 hours of birth. ABO HDN occurs when blood group O mothers carry blood group A (this case) or B babies. Blood group O individuals have anti-A IgM, anti-B IgM, and, in most cases, anti-AB IgG antibodies. Anti-AB IgG antibodies in the mother cross the placenta and attach to the blood group A or B fetal red blood cells (RBCs). Fetal macrophages in the spleen have IgG receptors and phagocytose IgG-coated fetal RBCs, causing a normocytic anemia. The end product of macrophage destruction of RBCs is unconjugated bilirubin (UCB), which is a lipid-soluble compound. The maternal liver removes UCB. After delivery, the amount of UCB produced in the baby overwhelms the conjugating enzymes in the newborn's liver, causing jaundice in the first 24 hours. Fetal RBCs with IgG on the surface are detected with a direct Coombs' test. A positive direct Coombs' test result confirms that immune destruction is responsible for the anemia and unconjugated hyperbilirubinemia. UCB in skin absorbs light energy from blue fluorescent light, which by photoisomerization converts it into a nontoxic, unconjugated water-soluble dipyrrole called lumirubin (choice **E**), that is excreted in either bile or urine.

Photoisomerization of conjugated bilirubin (choices **A** and **B**) in the skin causes grayish brown discoloration of the skin ("bronze baby" syndrome). The bilirubin that is increased in ABO HDN is unconjugated bilirubin. Phototherapy does not convert UCB to CB (choice **C**) but converts it into an unconjugated water-soluble dipyrrole for excretion in the urine. UCB is lipid soluble and cannot be filtered by the kidneys (choice **D**).

38 The answer is B *Surgery*

The patient has a pancreatic pseudocyst (choice **B**), which is a cystic collection of tissue, fluid, and necrotic debris surrounding the pancreas. Pancreatic pseudocysts do not have a true epithelial lining and are most commonly associated with chronic pancreatitis but may also be seen following acute pancreatitis. They present as an abdominal mass with persistent hyperamylasemia, because enzyme-rich fluids continue to leak into the circulation. Computed tomography (CT) scan is the best test for identifying pseudocysts. If the pseudocyst persists beyond 4 to 6 weeks or continues to enlarge, surgical decompression is indicated. The cyst fluid is drained into the stomach or bowel (not to the skin surface).

Pancreatic cystadenomas (choice **A**) are rare and are not associated with chronic pancreatitis. They do not cause a persistent increase in amylase. Pancreatic carcinoma (choice **C**) can be associated with chronic pancreatitis but rarely present as a palpable mass with persistent hyperamylasemia. Pancreatic abscesses (choice **D**) are a feature of acute pancreatitis. Macroamylasemia (choice **E**) is a cause of increased serum amylase and negative urine amylase (patient has a positive urine amylase). It is an immune complex of amylase with circulating antibodies.

39 The answer is E *Psychiatry*

Approximately 2% of 12th graders have used cocaine within the last month. This percentage has held fairly constant over the last few years.

40 **The answer is B** *Psychiatry*

Approximately 25% of 12th graders have used cigarettes within the last month. This percentage has gradually declined over the last few years.

CHOICES NOT USED

Approximately 48% of 12th graders have used alcohol within the last month (choice **A**); approximately 20% of 12th graders have used marijuana/hashish within the last month (choice **C**); and approximately 5% of 12th graders have used amphetamines within the last month (choice **D**).

41 **The answer is C** *Psychiatry*

The clinical course of cyclothymic disorder (graph **C**) is characterized by numerous periods of hypomanic symptoms and numerous periods of depressive symptoms. During none of these episodes do patients have full manic or depressive episodes. Cycling is often rapid.

42 **The answer is B** *Psychiatry*

The clinical course of bipolar II disorder (graph **B**) is characterized by depressive episodes and one or more hypomanic episodes.

CHOICES NOT USED

Graph **D** represents bipolar I disorder, which includes both manic and depressive episodes. Graph **A** represents the clinical course of major depressive disorder, recurrent type. Graph **E** represents the clinical course of dysthymic disorder.

43 **The answer is C** *Medicine*

Right–left disorientation is seen with damage to the dominant parietal lobe (choice **C**).

44 **The answer is A** *Medicine*

In Broca's (expressive) aphasia, caused by damage to the dominant frontal lobe (choice **A**), patients can understand speech but cannot speak themselves.

45 **The answer is E** *Medicine*

This patient is probably suffering from transcortical aphasia, because both speech and comprehension are impaired. This condition is caused by damage to the temporal–occipital–parietal junction (choice **E**).

46 **The answer is C** *Medicine*

Dyscalculia (i.e., problems doing mathematical calculations) is caused by damage to the dominant parietal lobe (choice **C**).

CHOICES NOT USED

A lesion in the nondominant temporal lobe (choice **B**) can interfere with recovery of newly learned names and recognition of faces. One of the functions of the occipital lobe (choice **D**) is organization of visual perception. This lobe is tucked in toward the back of the brain and is somewhat protected from injury, but damage to this lobe can cause visual distortions, hallucinations, and illusions.

47 **The answer is B** *Medicine*

Pendred syndrome (choice **B**) is due to any one of several mutations in the *PDS* gene that affect a protein called pendrin, which functions as an iodide/chloride ion transporter, resulting in incomplete oxidation and inability to organify iodide in the thyroid. This goes a long way toward explaining the basis of goiter development in this condition, but pendrin's role in inner ear development remains obscure.

48 **The answer is E** *Medicine*

The condition describes Waardenburg syndrome (choice **E**). The variability in expression has recently been partially explained by the discovery that mutation in any one of four different genes can cause the syndrome. The commonality among these genes is that they affect aspects of development of the face and inner ear.

49 **The answer is C** *Medicine*

Infants with type I Usher syndrome (choice **C**) are born deaf and have trouble balancing. These conditions retard their development. They slowly start going blind about the age of 10 because of retinitis pigmentosa. Type II Usher children are born with moderate-to-severe hearing loss but can usually function normally in the speaking world with hearing aids throughout their teen years. At this time their vision starts to slowly deteriorate, and they become both blind and deaf after puberty. Individuals with type III Usher syndrome have essentially normal hearing and sight at birth, but these begin to deteriorate at variable rates, even within the same family, and by middle age most are deaf and blind.

50 **The answer is D** *Medicine*

Alport syndrome (choice **D**) includes kidney disease, sensorial deafness, and eye abnormalities. It is caused by a mutation in any one of six genes, *COL4A1* through *COL4A6*, that code for type IV collagen, the major structural component of basement membranes. About 85% of these mutations are in *COL4A5*, located on the X-chromosome. As a consequence males with such a mutation are more severely affected and often present with hematuria in infancy and die from end-stage renal disease by the 2nd or 3rd decade. Females with similar mutations show only mild symptoms and generally have a normal life span, but because they do have symptoms, Alport syndrome is classified as an autosomal dominant.

INCORRECT CHOICES

Leopard syndrome (choice **A**) is also known as *multiple lentigines syndrome*. (Lentigines are dark freckles thought to look like a leopard's spots). It is an extremely rare condition, and most cases are sporadic. When found in families, it appears to be an autosomal dominant condition; however males seem to be more severely affected. Although leopard describes the character of the spots the name was created as a mnemonic that was coined to describe the prevalent signs and symptoms, namely, **L**entigines, **E**lectrocardiogram (ECG) abnormalities, **O**cular hypertelorism (wide spread eyes), **P**ulmonary stenosis, **A**bnormal genitalia, **R**etarded growth, and **D**eafness (sensory).

Questions

Single Best Choice Directions: This section consists of numbered statements or questions followed by a list of potential answers; you are to select the ONE best answer.

1 A 26-year-old man is troubled with reddish patches of skin that flare up periodically on his face, neck, and upper trunk, but most commonly and most severely, behind the knees, and in the folds of the elbow. He says that these patches of skin itch so badly that it takes all his will power to refrain from scratching until they bleed. In addition to the itch and reddish coloration, the skin in these areas tends to be dry, leathery, and thickened, with more prominent skin markings. His mother tells him he had terrible diaper rash as a baby and itchy skin as a child. He also is troubled with seasonal hay fever as are a brother and his mother. A first cousin has asthma. This man is most likely troubled by which one of the following conditions?

(A) Molluscum contagiosum
(B) Atopic dermatitis
(C) Impetigo
(D) Pemphigus vulgaris
(E) Bullous pemphigoid

2 At 24 hours of life, a newborn infant is noted to have a pink conjunctivitis with a nonpurulent eye discharge. The baby was born by normal spontaneous vaginal delivery to a 21-year-old primigravida who had no prenatal care. The birth was uncomplicated, and the patient weighed 7 lb 6 oz (3.3 kg). Apgar scores were 8 at 1 minute and 9 at 5 minutes. Except for the eye discharge, the physical examination is unremarkable. Which of the following is the most likely cause of the conjunctival irritation in this newborn?

(A) Gonococcal ophthalmia
(B) Chlamydial conjunctivitis
(C) *Staphylococcus aureus* conjunctivitis
(D) Chemical conjunctivitis
(E) Lacrimal duct obstruction

3 Asthma is one of the more critical health problems in the United States, affecting about 5% of the population. Each year there are close to one-half million hospital admissions and 5000 deaths due to asthma. Most cases are suspected of being caused by a predisposition for atopy (a genetic tendency to develop classical allergic diseases), and most cases of asthma have an underlying allergic reaction; nonspecific, seemingly not allergy-related triggers of asthma attacks are also known. These include exercise, breathing dry cold air, upper respiratory infection, rhinitis, sinusitis, postnasal drip, aspiration, gastroesophageal reflux, weather changes, and stress. Asthma prevalence, hospital admissions, and deaths due to asthma have been increasing steadily for more than two decades. Fortunately, the number of agents available to treat asthma has also been increasing. Of the drugs listed below, which one specifically acts to block the IgE activation of mast cells?

(A) Inhaled corticosteroids
(B) Long-acting β_2-agonists
(C) Leukotriene antagonists
(D) Cromolyn
(E) Theophylline
(F) Omalizumab

4 A 36-year-old female presents with a history of a lump in her right breast. She noted it after being hit on the breast by a ball thrown by her 6-year-old son. She has localized pain and tenderness. There is no family history of breast cancer. The patient does not smoke, and she takes birth control pills. Clinical examination reveals a moderate-sized, tender, mobile mass in the right breast, without axillary lymphadenopathy. No nipple discharge or skin retraction is noted. The left breast and axilla are normal. A fine-needle biopsy of the mass reveals fat necrosis. Which of the following is the most appropriate next step in the management of this patient?

(A) Excise the mass
(B) Observe the patient and excise the mass if it causes pain or enlarges
(C) Repeat the biopsy after 1 month
(D) Reassure the patient, prescribe antiinflammatories, and follow up in 2 weeks
(E) Refer her for mammography

5 A 92-year-old man, who is vigorous for his age and the primary caregiver for his 76-year-old wife who has multiple sclerosis, fell from a ladder while changing a bulb and broke his femur. He was taken to a local hospital where his fracture was repaired under general anesthesia. After the operation he was semidelirious for 2 days, when his kidneys also failed. The resident on duty felt renal dialysis might be the next logical step in therapy. The physician should base her decision as to whether he will receive dialysis on which of the following?

(A) The patient's quality of life
(B) The wishes of the patient's children
(C) The patient's other medical conditions
(D) Medicare reimbursement
(E) The cost of dialysis

6 A 39-year-old man presents to his physician with a complaint of chronic fatigue. On the basis of elevated liver enzyme levels, circulating antibody levels, and a liver biopsy, the physician concludes that the man has early cirrhosis. The patient is religious and has not consumed alcohol since he turned 20; that plus the antibody studies led to the conclusion that the cirrhosis arose from a viral infection. The patient has kept a diary since childhood and let his physician read it to see if he could discover the source of the infection. He focused on a flulike illness the patient had when he was 18-years old. The symptoms mentioned in the diary included headache, nausea, vomiting, abdominal pain, and jaundice, with weakness and fatigue; pale, white-ash colored feces, and dark tealike urine. The physician concluded that this incident was most likely an attack of acute hepatitis. In looking for a potential cause of the hepatitis he found a brief notation saying the patient had unprotected sex with a prostitute 6 weeks earlier. The patient most likely has a chronic form of which of the following conditions?

(A) Hepatitis A
(B) Hepatitis B
(C) Hepatitis C
(D) Hepatitis D
(E) Hepatitis E
(F) Hepatitis F
(G) Hepatitis G

7 A 62-year-old man with intermittent, cramping abdominal pain also has difficulty defecating. He manages a bowel movement every third or fourth day only with a great deal of straining and then only passes small hard feces with a lot of mucous and sometimes fresh blood. His physician suspects obstipation and orders a barium enema that reveals a massively dilated sigmoid colon with a column of barium resembling a "bird's beak." Which of the following is the most likely diagnosis?

(A) Intussusception
(B) Volvulus of the sigmoid colon
(C) Toxic megacolon

(D) Ogilvie's syndrome
(E) Impacted stool

8 A 56-year-old woman who has given birth to three healthy children by vaginal delivery and who is presently perimenopausal is concerned because of a recent strange bilateral discharge from her nipples. The serous discharge appears just before menstruation and has a greenish brown color. The most likely cause of the discharge is which of the following?

(A) Ductal carcinoma
(B) Ductal papilloma
(C) Prolactinoma
(D) Chronic manual stimulation
(E) Ductal ectasia
(F) Hypothyroidism
(G) Oral contraceptives

9 After visiting a friend who lives on the third story of a walk-up apartment, a 7 months' pregnant woman who does not take vitamins or other nutritional supplements walks out into a brightly lit hallway that leads to the stairway where the light bulb has burned out, leaving the steps dimly lit. Rather than stepping carefully down the first few steps the woman continues walking as if she were continuing on the landing. Consequently, she misses the first two steps, injures her ankle, and has to be helped back into the apartment. When asked what happened she replies: "For some reason as I stepped out of the bright hallway into darker area I could see very little and didn't realize the steps were there." The underlying cause of this woman's accident is most likely a deficiency of which one of the following nutrients?

(A) Vitamin E
(B) Pantothenic acid
(C) Biotin
(D) Folate
(E) Vitamin B_{12}
(F) Vitamin A

10 A 23-year-old male was having vigorous intercourse with his wife when he felt sudden, severe pain in the scrotal area. Soon afterward he was retching and vomiting. He was rushed to the emergency department, where his vital signs were as follows: pulse, 100/min; respirations, 24/min; blood pressure, 130/90 mm Hg; temperature, 38°C (100.4°F). The scrotum was swollen and tender, especially on the right side, and the testis appeared to be drawn up into the inguinal canal. There is an absent cremasteric reflex when stroking the inner right thigh with a tongue blade. Transillumination

showed no abnormality. Which of the following is the most likely diagnosis?

(A) Torsion of the appendix of the testis
(B) Idiopathic scrotal edema
(C) Acute epididymitis
(D) Trauma to the testis
(E) Torsion of the testis

11 A 10-year-old presents to the pediatrician with sore throat and fever for the past 2 days. Physical examination is pertinent for a temperature of 39°C (102.2° F) and an erythematous throat with 3+ tonsils and exudates. A Rapid Strep antigen detection test is performed and the result is positive. The patient then was given an intramuscular (IM) injection of benzathine penicillin G 600,000 units; the IM route is chosen because his mother states that he has been complaining when he swallows and she feared he would not take oral medication. Approximately 20 minutes after the injection the patient becomes flushed and starts to have a pruritic rash consisting of wheals over the chest and extremities. He also begins to have shortness of breath and difficulty breathing, with lip swelling. Auscultation of the lungs is pertinent for wheezing. Oxygen saturation is 97% saturation via pulse oximetry. Which of the following is the appropriate next step?

(A) Intubation
(B) Oral diphenhydramine
(C) Epinephrine injection
(D) Intravenous (IV) corticosteroids
(E) Histamine blockers
(F) No specific therapy is indicated

12 The diagram below represents the four main sites (cardiac, site 1; arterial, site 2; renal, site 3; and venous, site 4) at which the actions of antihypertensive drugs can be expressed.

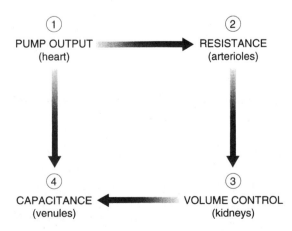

Among the drugs listed below is one whose action is primarily expressed at site 1. When it is used long-term in mild-to-moderate hypertension, the drug decreases morbidity and mortality. Which one of the drugs listed below best fits this description?

(A) Clonidine
(B) Furosemide
(C) Acebutolol
(D) Trimethaphan
(E) Nitroprusside
(F) Hydrochlorothiazide
(G) Phentolamine
(H) Captopril
(I) Verapamil

13 A 39-year-old, never-married man is considered somewhat eccentric by his friends and acquaintances because of strange behaviors. For example, when he walks on the sidewalk he religiously avoids stepping on the cracks; when he sees a digital clock report a number 13, he stands at attention until 14 appears; and he washes his hands incessantly. He knows these actions are irrational and that they have a negative affect on his relationships, particularly with women. Consequently, he tries to resist but almost always yields to the impulse to carry them out. There is no other evidence of peculiar thoughts or behavior. His mood is somewhat anxious. Which of the following is the best initial treatment?

(A) Clomipramine 25 mg PO tid
(B) Counseling regarding proper behaviors
(C) Fluvoxamine 50 mg PO bid
(D) Risperidone 2 mg PO bid
(E) Suggest gloves to reduce need for washing

14 A 19-year-old man presents to an emergency facility with a 48-hour history of extreme anxiety, tremulousness, diaphoresis, persecutory ideation, and suspiciousness. He admits to recent cessation of extensive substance abuse but will not reveal which substance he used. Before a diagnosis is made and treatment can be started, he has a generalized tonic–clonic seizure. Assuming these symptoms are due to drug withdrawal, which of the following drugs had he most likely been abusing?

(A) Benzodiazepine
(B) Cocaine
(C) Heroin
(D) Lysergic acid diethylamide (LSD)
(E) Cannabis

15 A 77-year-old woman is brought to the emergency department with a history of having lost large quantities of blood while having a bowel movement. She presents with hypotension; cold, clammy skin; and a rapid pulse when lying down. Results of an abdominal examination are normal. Which of the following is the most likely cause of this patient's condition?

(A) Meckel's diverticulum
(B) Small bowel infarction
(C) Angiodysplasia
(D) Internal hemorrhoids
(E) Ulcerative colitis

16 A 42-year-old man worries about so many things in his life that he has become "paralyzed" at work and feels "nervous" all the time. He has been taking diazepam for 2 weeks, with mild but incomplete relief. However, he now complains of feeling "mentally dulled" and does not want to take it anymore. Which of the following would be the best pharmacologic intervention at this point?

(A) Lower the dose of diazepam
(B) Taper off medication entirely over several weeks while concentrating on relaxation training
(C) Switch to alprazolam, a shorter-acting benzodiazepine
(D) Switch to buspirone
(E) Switch to propranolol

17 A 2-year-old, symptomatic human immunodeficiency virus (HIV)-infected child presents to his physician because he was exposed to measles. The child is up to date on all immunizations, including his measles–mumps–rubella (MMR) combination vaccine. The child received immunoglobulin (IG) 6 weeks ago. All household occupants have been immunized against measles. Which of the following is the most appropriate first step in the management of this patient?

(A) Administer monovalent measles vaccine
(B) Administer another MMR combination vaccine
(C) Administer immunoglobulin (Ig)
(D) Administer vitamin C
(E) Do nothing, because the child is already immunized for measles

18 A 62-year-old man who has been treated for asthma for the past 50 years develops nasal polyps and allergic rhinitis; at about the same time his asthma symptoms flare up. His erythrocyte sedimentation rate (ESR) and C-reactive protein value are elevated, and a complete blood count (CBC) finds the white cells are 55% eosinophils (normal, <5%). Before a diagnosis can be made he develops a fever and severe pain and weakness in his arms and legs so extensive that he can

no longer walk without help. He also has severe breathing difficulties. Chest radiography shows pulmonary infiltrates and multiple nodules. The physician starts him on a high dosage (60 mg/day) of prednisone, with added cyclophosphamide. His symptoms quickly improve, but the extensor muscles on his arms are left paralyzed, with his hands frozen in a clawlike position. This man most likely is afflicted with which one of the following conditions?

(A) Polyarteritis nodosa
(B) Kawasaki disease (aka mucocutaneous lymph node syndrome)
(C) Wegener's granulomatosis
(D) Churg-Strauss syndrome (aka allergic granulomatosis angiitis)
(E) Takayasu's arteritis
(F) Hypersensitivity vasculitis
(G) Temporal (giant cell) arteritis
(H) Polymyalgia rheumatica
(I) Behçet syndrome
(J) Buerger's disease (aka thromboangiitis obliterans)
(K) Henoch-Schönlein purpura
(L) Microscopic polyangiitis
(M) Rheumatoid vasculitis
(N) Granulomatis angiitis of the central nervous system

19 A 67-year-old woman with a history of coronary artery disease complains of severe substernal chest pain for the past 12 hours. She states that the pain radiates down the left arm. A blood sample is drawn for analysis of serum electrolytes and troponins (I and T). Owing to technical difficulties in collecting the blood, the sample is visibly hemolyzed. An electrocardiogram (ECG) pattern shows Q waves and an ST elevation in a manner consistent with an infarct; however, it does not show peaked T waves. Which of the following choices correctly describes the results of the serum potassium and serum troponin tests?

	Serum Potassium	Serum Troponins
(A)	False negative	True positive
(B)	False positive	False positive
(C)	False positive	True positive
(D)	True positive	False positive
(E)	True positive	True positive

20 A young man was thrown from his motorcycle. The paramedics took him to the nearest trauma center, where physical examination showed no life-threatening injury. However, he has pain and swelling on the lateral side of his right leg just beneath the knee. X-ray

films showed no fractures; however, he could not evert his foot, and he had impaired sensation on the lateral dorsum of the foot. Dorsiflexion and inversion of the foot were not adversely affected. This patient most likely experienced trauma to which of the following nerves?

(A) Deep peroneal nerve (also known as the anterior tibial nerve)

(B) Tibial nerve (also known as the posterior tibial nerve)

(C) Sciatic nerve

(D) Obturator nerve

(E) Superficial peroneal nerve (also known as the fibular nerve)

21 A 5-year-old child presents to the pediatrician with her mother because of headaches for the last 2 weeks. The mother, who is a nurse, is concerned because the child awakens each morning with a headache. The mother has been giving the child over-the-counter analgesics, but they have not helped very much to relieve the pain. Suspecting a brain tumor the pediatrician orders a magnetic resonance imaging (MRI) scan of the head. Results confirm that the patient has a posterior fossa tumor. Additionally, the patient also complains of diplopia. On examination of eye movements, the child is noted to have strabismus. Which extraocular palsy is most likely to be found in this patient?

(A) Superior oblique palsy

(B) Lateral rectus palsy

(C) Inferior oblique palsy

(D) Medial rectus palsy

(E) Superior rectus palsy

22 About 90% of the energy expenditure by muscles for normal individuals in the resting state is derived from the oxidation of fatty acids. However, for the first 10 minutes of exercise the primary source of fuel switches to muscle glycogen. Simultaneously, the uptake of glucose from the blood increases, up to 20-fold. Consequently, as the muscle glycogen stores become depleted, about three quarters of the glucose consumed by the exercising muscle is derived from liver glycogen and the remainder from gluconeogenesis, and this glucose is removed from the circulating blood by the increased rate of uptake. As liver glycogen is depleted, gluconeogenic production becomes more important, eventually accounting for about 50% of muscle fuel consumption; the remainder is from fatty acid oxidation and eventually from ketones. After 2 hours of low- to moderate-intensity exercise, stored fat is the main source of energy. Although the same systems operate in the exercising diabetic, diabetes

establishes some special considerations. Which of the following factors is such a consideration?

(A) Exercise increases the amount of insulin required by the type 1 diabetic.

(B) Running for extended periods as in a marathon, promotes healthy feet in persons with diabetic peripheral neuropathy.

(C) A type 1 diabetic should refrain from eating before exercising.

(D) Vigorous exercise is recommended to help lower circulation glucose levels in persons with serum glucose values above 300 mg/dL.

(E) Blood glucose concentration monitoring is essential for a type 1 diabetic who engages in exercise.

23 A 57-year-old postmenopausal woman notices a lump in her left breast. She is concerned about the possibility of it being malignant and schedules an appointment with her gynecologist. Physical examination reveals a nontender breast mass in the left upper outer quadrant. The mass is fixed and causes the skin to indent with movement of the arm. Which of the following is the most appropriate next step in the management of this patient?

(A) Perform a fine-needle aspiration of the mass with cytologic evaluation

(B) Schedule the patient for a modified radical mastectomy

(C) Order a mammogram to define whether the mass is malignant or benign

(D) Send the patient home and reevaluate in 3 months

(E) Start treatment immediately without further diagnostic evaluation because the nontender nature of the mass and the skin dimpling are such strong clinical evidence of malignancy

24 A 7-year-old presents to the pediatric clinic with painless bilateral swelling of his knees for the past 3 days. Synovial fluid is obtained by arthrocentesis, and the fluid is sterile. The patient is thought to have a synovitis. On physical examination, the child is noted to have a saddle nose, peg-shaped upper central incisors, and saber shins. The physician suspects that the child has late congenital syphilis. Which of the following is an associated physical finding also found at this time?

(A) Snuffles

(B) Maculopapular rash

(C) Failure to thrive

(D) Rhagades

(E) Pseudoparalysis of Parrot

25 A middle-aged man went to visit his mother who was recently placed in a nursing home upon being discharged from the hospital after repair of a fractured femur. He was greatly distressed by seeing several old persons, mainly women, sitting in wheelchairs staring vacantly into space. He asked the attendant what was wrong with them and was told, "Oh they have no real physical problems; they are only depressed, real old people get that way." The prevalence of severe major depressive disorder in the general population of elderly individuals is closest to which of the following?

(A) 10%
(B) 33%
(C) 66%
(D) 75%
(E) Over 90%

26 A 64-year-old man with carcinoma of the tongue was hospitalized and received chemotherapy. He was brought to the operating room for radical neck dissection and received 2 g of cefoxitin intravenously. Within 10 minutes the patient was wheezing and had developed an urticarial rash. His systolic blood pressure had dropped to 45 mm Hg. The operation was postponed; and the patient was given intravenous (IV) epinephrine, dexamethasone, diphenhydramine, and fluids. Blood pressure was restored and maintained by intravenous (IV) dopamine. In the intensive care unit (ICU), the electrocardiogram (ECG) reveals myocardial injury, and a subsequent x-ray film shows bilateral pulmonary edema, which responds to supportive care over the next 5 days. Which of the following statements regarding the use of an antibiotic in this patient is the most accurate?

(A) Cefoxitin is not appropriate in a patient who is markedly immunosuppressed.
(B) The prophylactic use of an antibiotic during surgery is valid in this patient.
(C) The reaction could have been avoided with a lower dose of cefoxitin.
(D) In this patient, erythromycin would have provided more effective coverage against postoperative infection.
(E) A prophylactic antibiotic should have been administered for at least 24 hours before the surgical procedure.

27 An overweight but not obese (body mass index [BMI] 27 kg/m^2) 43-year-old man who jogged 2 or 3 miles daily in an attempt to lose weight develops severe pain in his right knee with no swelling. The pain not only has curtailed his jogging but is so bad that he hesitates to walk; it even keeps him awake during the night. His

primary care physician prescribed a nonsteroidal antiinflammatory drug (NSAID) and refers him to an orthopedist who, after examining him and performing suitable imaging studies, informs him that he has developed severe osteoarthritis limited to the medial compartment. He recommends surgery. Which of the following procedures is most likely recommended?

(A) Total knee arthroplasty
(B) Unicompartmental arthroplasty
(C) Osteotomy
(D) Arthrodesis
(E) Synovectomy

28 A 47-year-old woman who had been working for the same company for the past 16 years slowly rose up through the ranks of employees and last year was appointed executive vice president in charge of sales. This promotion added stress to her life and required her to travel fairly often to visit company branches located throughout the country. It also required her to look fit. However she has been gaining weight at an average rate of 1 lb (0.4536 kg) per month. Trying to mitigate this gain in weight she watches her diet carefully and exercises faithfully, but nothing helps. In desperation she consults a physician who specializes in weight control. One of his questions concerns the number of hours of sleep she gets each night. Which one of the following choices best describes the relationship between weight gain and hours spent sleeping in a 24-hour period?

(A) Sleeping fewer than 7–8 hours in a 24-hour period results in weight gain partially due to a decrease in leptin levels.
(B) Sleeping fewer than 7–8 hours in a 24-hour period results in weight loss because more calories are burned while awake than while sleeping.
(C) Sleeping fewer than 7–8 hours in a 24-hour period results in weight loss because leptin levels are increased.
(D) Sleeping fewer than 7–8 hours in a 24-hour period results in weight gain in part due to decreased levels of ghrelin.
(E) Sleeping fewer than 7–8 hours in a 24-hour period increases insulin sensitivity.

29 A 16-year-old female presents to the adolescent health clinic for a physical examination. The patient tells the triage nurse that for the past week she has had a mucoid whitish discharge from her vagina. In addition the patient states that she has some burning when she urinates. She has no fever, vomiting, or abdominal pain. Her last menstrual period was 2 weeks ago. The patient says that her parents do not know that she is being evaluated at the clinic. She came alone because she is sexually active and she does not want her parents to know this. After obtaining a complete history, the physician performs a physical examination including pelvic examination. The physician suspects that the patient has a chlamydial infection. Which of the following is the most appropriate next step?

(A) Inform her sexual partner(s)
(B) Inform her parents
(C) Get permission from her parents to treat her
(D) Inform her school guidance counselor
(E) Obtain informed consent for treatment from the patient

30 A 61-year-old woman has been undergoing treatment for hypertension and type 2 diabetes. Her hemoglobin A1c values have been in the 7 to 7.5% range, and typically her systolic blood pressure has been between 135 and 145 mm Hg, but on occasion it has been measured at 180 mm Hg or even higher. One evening while watching television with her husband, she suddenly notices onset of right arm and leg weakness, with normal sensation and speech. Her husband, fearing a stroke, calls 911, and she is taken to a nearby trauma center. By the time she arrives she says normal strength is returning to her affected limbs, and she apologizes for causing so much trouble. However upon her arrival at the emergency center she was immediately subjected to a computed tomography (CT) scan, an electrocardiogram (ECG), and had blood drawn with a request to run a complete blood count (CBC) with platelet count, prothrombin time, International Normalized Ratio, partial thromboplastin time, and electrolyte and glucose values. The CT scan shows no bleeding or pathology, and all other measured parameters are within normal limits. Which of the following is likely to be the best long-term treatment?

(A) Send her home with a pat on the back and tell her to forget about the incident, it was just one those inexplicable things of no consequence.
(B) Put her on insulin to better control her diabetes
(C) Left carotid endarterectomy
(D) Treatment of underlying heart disease
(E) Watchful waiting in conjunction with treatment to better control her hypertension and diabetes

31 An 18-year-old female has just graduated from high school and has applied for admittance into a local college, which has implemented the American College Health Association (ACHA) recommendations for prematriculation immunization. Her immunizations are current for mumps, rubella, diphtheria, tetanus, and polio. Consequently, she must also be immunized against which of the following diseases?

(A) Hepatitis B, varicella, and meningococcal infection
(B) Pertussis, measles, and meningococcal infection
(C) *Haemophilus influenzae* type B, varicella, and measles
(D) Influenza, hepatitis B, and measles
(E) Measles, varicella, and hepatitis B

32 A 46-year-old woman presents with an irrational belief that her food is being poisoned by unknown individuals who are conspiring to steal her body. She says that she can see some of these people hiding behind trees as she walks near her apartment. Further, she can detect a strange taste in her food, which she ascribes to poison. Mental status examination reveals severe anxiety and a markedly impaired recent memory. Which of the following of this patient's symptoms most specifically suggests a cognitive disorder?

(A) Elaborate delusions
(B) Severe anxiety
(C) Significant memory loss
(D) Olfactory hallucinations
(E) Visual hallucinations

33 A 27-year-old Caucasian woman has been bothered by sinusitis all her life and had minor surgery as a child resulting in blood loss that was treated by giving her a unit of blood. She otherwise has been in good health and now accepts a ride on the back of a friend's motorcycle. Unfortunately, the motorcycle skids on an oil slick, and she is thrown to the ground. She suffers lacerations, which are bleeding profusely. The paramedics control the obvious bleeding and transport her to an emergency facility where her blood pressure is determined to be 65/40 mm Hg. After a quick cross-match of her blood she is transfused with 2 units of blood plasma. Her blood pressure quickly improves but about 10 minutes later she has an anaphylactic reaction. The patient most likely has which of the following conditions?

(A) Common variable immunodeficiency (CVID)
(B) Selective immunoglobulin A deficiency
(C) X-linked agammaglobulinemia (Burton's syndrome)
(D) Adenosine deaminase
(E) Monoclonal gammopathy of uncertain significance (MGUS)

34 A 28-year-old man with a 4-year history of heroin abuse and two previous drug rehabilitation failures is started on methadone maintenance. Which of the following statements about the management of this patient is true?

- (A) He may receive maintenance methadone only through a federally licensed program.
- (B) He must agree to random drug testing.
- (C) He must be warned that concurrent use of heroin may result in severe physical distress.
- (D) His social or occupational function is less likely to improve with methadone treatment than with nonpharmacologically based heroin rehabilitation programs.
- (E) If he resumes regular heroin abuse, methadone maintenance must be discontinued.

35 A 78-year-old man signs a living will in which he states that if he is in a persistent vegetative state he does not want heroic measures taken to resuscitate him. One week later he has a stroke and is in a coma on life support. His daughter, who lives in another city, asks the physician to remove life support. His son, with whom he lives, asks the physician to keep his father on life support. The physician should do which of the following?

- (A) Listen to the son and keep the patient on life support
- (B) Listen to the daughter and remove life support
- (C) Evaluate whether the patient has a reasonable chance of recovery
- (D) Ask for a decision from the hospital ethics committee
- (E) Get a court order to turn off life support

36 An 81-year-old woman inpatient recovering from surgical hip replacement has the onset of confusion, anxi-

ety, suspiciousness, and disorientation. She has received several doses of meperidine (Demerol) for pain control over the past 24 hours. She is afebrile, and her lungs are clear to auscultation. Her electrolytes, complete blood count (CBC), blood urea nitrogen (BUN), and urinalysis are all unremarkable. Her chest x-ray film is clear. Magnetic resonance imaging (MRI) scan reveals mild cortical atrophy. Which of the following is the most likely diagnosis?

- (A) Alzheimer's dementia
- (B) Delirium due to occult infection
- (C) Generalized anxiety disorder
- (D) Opioid-induced delirium
- (E) Posttraumatic stress disorder

37 A patient is brought to the pediatrician's office for a well-child visit. According to the parents, the patient has been in his usual state of good health and they have no complaints. Growth parameters for the patient are at the 25% for age level for head circumference, height, and weight. The vital signs are normal, and the physical examination is unremarkable. The developmental assessment shows that the child can transfer an object from hand to hand, maintain a seated position, and imitate speech sounds, and he has a neat pincer grasp. Which of the following is the most likely age of this child?

- (A) 2 months
- (B) 4 months
- (C) 6 months
- (D) 8 months
- (E) 10 months

Directions for Matching Questions (38 through 50): Each set of matching questions is preceded by a list of 4 to 26 lettered options followed by a brief explanation of the required task and then by a series of numbered statements. For each lettered statement you are to select ONE lettered option that best fulfills the task as it relates to that statement. Remember each of the listed options might be correctly selected once, more than once, or not at all.

Questions 38–42

The response options for questions 38–42 require selection of the one most likely cause of hypertension in pregnancy (from choices A–H) as described in the numbered clinical vignettes.

- (A) HELLP syndrome
- (B) Mild preeclampsia
- (C) Chronic hypertension
- (D) Transient hypertension
- (E) Superimposed preeclampsia
- (F) Gestational hypertension
- (G) Malignant hypertension
- (H) Severe preeclampsia

38 A 38-year-old gravida 5, para 4, abortus 0 woman comes to the outpatient office for her initial prenatal visit. Her previous pregnancies were uncomplicated with spontaneous term vaginal deliveries of healthy babies. Her last menstrual period was 10 weeks ago. She has no complaints other than mild nausea in the morning resolving as the day goes on. Her blood pressure is 150/95 and remains so 15 minutes later. Her other vital signs are normal. A urine dipstick test reveals no glucose or protein. Pelvic examination shows an enlarged uterus consistent with 10 weeks' gestation.

39 A 25-year-old prima gravida woman is seen at the prenatal obstetric clinic at 28 weeks' gestation for a routine visit. She has no headache, epigastric pain, or visual disturbances. Her prenatal course has been unremarkable except for gestational diabetes with home glucose values in the target range on diet therapy alone. An obstetric sonogram at 19 weeks' gestational showed a single fetus with grossly normal anatomy. Fundal height on each of her visits has been appropriate for dates. Today, 2 weeks later, her fundal height is 27 cm with fetal heart tones at 130/min in the right upper quadrant. Her blood pressure on her previous visits has been in the normal range, but now it is 148/92 and remains so 15 minutes later. Her urine dipstick test result is negative for protein but shows 1+ glucose.

40 A 19-year-old primigravida is seen at the prenatal obstetric clinic at 32 weeks' gestation confirmed by a 22-week sonogram. She has no headache, epigastric pain, or visual disturbances. Her prenatal course has been complicated by iron deficiency anemia, which is being treated with oral iron tablets. Today her fundal height is 30 cm, with fetal heart tones in the normal range in the left lower quadrant. Her blood pressure is 150/95 mm Hg and remains elevated on a repeat measurement 15 minutes later. Her urine dipstick test result is 2+ positive for protein but negative for glucose.

41 A 42-year-old gravida 4, para 2, abortus 1 woman comes to the outpatient clinic for a routine prenatal visit. Her pregnancy has been complicated by chronic hypertension diagnosed 3 years prior to her pregnancy. Throughout the pregnancy she had been treated with oral methyldopa, which has maintained her blood pressure (BP) at 150/95 mm Hg. Her urine dipstick test results have been negative for protein. Today her blood pressure is 165/115 mm Hg and remains so on repeat measurement 15 minutes later. Her urine dipstick test result is 3+ for protein today. She states she has had a mild occipital headache for the past 24 hours.

42 A 32-year-old gravida 2, para 1 woman comes to the office for a prenatal visit. Her pregnancy is complicated by sonographically confirmed dizygotic twins. She complains of occipital headache, midepigastric pain, and seeing spots before her eyes. Her blood pressure on all prior visits has been in the 130/75 mm Hg

range but today is 160/115 mm Hg. Repeat measurement 15 minutes later is the same. Her urine dipstick test result is 3+ positive for protein.

Questions 43–45

For questions 43–45 you are required to select the ONE drug in the lettered set (A–L) that best matches the description.

(A) Carvedilol
(B) Cefepime
(C) Cidofovir
(D) Dexfenfluramine
(E) Donepezil
(F) Fexofenadine
(G) Meropenem
(H) Mirtazapine
(I) Olanzapine
(J) Pravastatin
(K) Valsartan
(L) Zileuton

43 This drug is a vasodilator and, in patients with congestive heart failure, can improve left ventricular function by blocking excessive adrenergic stimulation.

44 A blocker of serotonin receptors, this drug improves both positive and negative symptoms of schizophrenia.

45 This drug reduces the risk of heart attacks in patients with hypercholesteremia.

Questions 46–50

You are required to select the one answer for each item in the lettered set (A–G) that is the most likely cause of postpartum hemorrhage as described in question 46–50 below.

(A) Disseminated intravascular coagulation (DIC)
(B) Genital lacerations
(C) Unexplained postpartum hemorrhage
(D) Uterine inversion
(E) Retained placental fragments
(F) Vaginal prolapse
(G) Uterine atony

46 A 22-year-old gravida 2, now para 2 woman is experiencing excessive vaginal bleeding after undergoing a term spontaneous vaginal delivery 1 hour ago of a 3500 g (7 lb, 11 oz) female neonate with Apgar scores of 8 and 9. Her prenatal course was unremarkable. Onset of labor was spontaneous, and her cervical dilatation progressed at a rate of 2 cm per hour. On abdominal palpation, the uterine fundus cannot be palpated. On pelvic examination, a beefy bleeding mass is seen at the vaginal introitus.

47 A 32-year-old gravida 5, now para 5 woman is experiencing excessive vaginal bleeding after undergoing a emergency primary cesarean section 1 hour ago at 33 weeks' gestation for a nonreassuring fetal monitor tracing. The patient has a history of substance abuse including cocaine. She came to the maternity unit complaining of painful vaginal bleeding associated with an electronic fetal monitor tracing showing minimal variability and repetitive late decelerations. The uterine fundus is firm to palpation below the umbilicus. Examination of the patient reveals diffuse skin petechiae.

48 An 18-year-old gravida 1, now para 1 woman is experiencing excessive vaginal bleeding after undergoing a spontaneous vaginal delivery 1 hour ago of a 4250 g (9 lb, 6 oz) male neonate with Apgar scores of 7 and 9. She underwent prolonged induction of labor at 41½ weeks with an unfavorable cervix. She initially

was administered vaginal prostaglandin with subsequently 18 hours of intravenous oxytocin. The second state of labor lasted 45 minutes. The uterine fundus is above the umbilicus and is soft and boggy on palpation.

49 A 45-year-old gravida 2, now para 2 woman is experiencing excessive vaginal bleeding after undergoing a term outlet forceps vaginal delivery 1 hour ago of a 4100 g (9 lb, 6 oz) female neonate with Apgar scores of 6 and 7. Her prenatal course was complicated by gestational diabetes. Onset of labor was spontaneous, and she was 5 cm dilated on admission. She progressed to complete dilation in 2 hours. She pushed for 3 hours but was unable to deliver the fetus spontaneously, thus requiring the assistance of obstetrics forceps.

50 A 25-year-old gravida 3, now para 3, woman is experiencing excessive vaginal bleeding after undergoing a term spontaneous vaginal delivery 1 hour ago of a 2900 g (5 lb, 14 oz) male neonate with Apgar scores of 4 and 8. The neonate requires deep suctioning after delivery because of thick meconium. The first and second stages of labor were unremarkable. The third stage of labor lasted 40 minutes, requiring manual placental removal.

Answer Key

1	B	**11**	C	**21**	B	**31**	E	**41**	E
2	D	**12**	C	**22**	E	**32**	C	**42**	H
3	F	**13**	C	**23**	A	**33**	B	**43**	A
4	A	**14**	A	**24**	D	**34**	A	**44**	I
5	C	**15**	C	**25**	A	**35**	C	**45**	J
6	B	**16**	D	**26**	B	**36**	D	**46**	D
7	B	**17**	C	**27**	C	**37**	E	**47**	A
8	E	**18**	D	**28**	A	**38**	C	**48**	G
9	F	**19**	C	**29**	E	**39**	F	**49**	B
10	E	**20**	E	**30**	E	**40**	B	**50**	E

Answers and Explanations

1 **The answer is B** *Medicine*

Atopic dermatitis (commonly known as eczema) (choice **B**) is an IgE-mediated disease that is often associated with a family history of atopic disease such as asthma, allergic rhinitis (hay fever), or atopic dermatitis. It is intermittent and can appear at any age but commonly starts in infancy. When it does, it tends to follow the classic three-stage pattern as follows: stage 1: a rash that begins at 2 to 3 months and lasts until about the 18th month; stage 2: childhood eczema marked by patches of itchy rash at various sites; and stage 3: postpuberty adolescent/adult form only present in some 30% of cases. Although in most cases eczema does not persist into adulthood, in some cases eczema first appears in adulthood. The diaper rash this man had likely was mild stage 1 atopic dermatis. Acute eczema has a variable presentation ranging from only thickened skin, with more prominent skin markings (lichenification), to patches covered by scales with edematous vesicles and bullae. Pruritus is always present. Typically, the pigmentary alterations are characterized by a pink/reddish coloration; however, other darker hues also occur, typically in more heavily pigmented individuals. The rash most commonly occurs on the extensor surfaces and face in infants and flexural areas in children and adults. However, atopic patients have hyperirritable skin, and any irritation is liable to precipitate dermatitis. They should try to avoid dry skin by limiting application of soap to sensitive areas, limiting bathing, avoiding woolen and acrylic clothing, using lubricating skin creams, and when necessary treating with topical steroids. Some cases are caused by food sensitivities. Dairy products and wheat are the most the most common offending foods. Itching typically occurs within minutes to hours after an offending food is ingested, permitting a patient to omit one food at a time for several months to monitor occurrence and/or severity of the disease.

Molluscum contagiosum (choice **A**) is due to a poxvirus. The lesions are bowl-shaped, with a central depression filled with keratin (containing viral particles called molluscum bodies). They commonly occur in children or in adults as a pre-AIDS skin lesion. In children, the options are to allow the lesions to spontaneously resolve or to apply topical salicylic acid, cantharidin, or tretinoin gel. Older patients can be treated with liquid nitrogen therapy in combination with curettage.

Impetigo (choice **C**) is most commonly caused by group A β-hemolytic streptococci. The rash usually begins on the face with vesicles and pustules that rupture to form honey-colored crusted lesions that cover shallow ulcerations of the skin. If the lesion has a bullous component, *Staphylococcus aureus* is the most probable causative agent. Impetigo is highly contagious; towels used by the affected person should be segregated. The treatment is topical application of mupirocin ointment or oral antibiotics (e.g., dicloxacillin) in severe cases.

Pemphigus vulgaris (choice **D**) is an autoimmune skin disease with IgG antibodies that are directed against intercellular attachment sites between keratinocytes. Vesicles and bullae develop on the skin and oral mucosa. The skin overlying the bullae slips with pressure (positive Nikolsky sign). Systemic steroids are often required for treatment. Bullous pemphigoid (choice **E**) is an autoimmune disease with IgG antibodies that are directed against the basement membrane. Vesicles and bullae develop on the skin. Oral mucosal lesions are less common than in pemphigus vulgaris. There is a negative Nikolsky sign (skin does not slough off with pressure). Systemic steroids are used for treatment.

2 **The answer is D** *Pediatrics*

Chemical irritation (e.g., AgNO₃ or an antibiotic) (choice **D**) is a common cause of a nonpurulent and transient conjunctivitis in the first 24 hours after birth. All 50 states require prophylactic application of eye drops shortly after birth to reduce the chance of neonatal infection. For many years the standard treatment was a couple of drops of an AgNO₃ solution; however, most states now use an antibiotic, often erythromycin. Consequently, the incidence of chemically induced conjunctivitises is less common, although some babies are sensitive to antibiotic treatment. In either case, chemical irritation (or even antibiotic allergy) almost always produces mild conjunctivitis that becomes evident within a few hours after the drops are administered, which then spontaneously clears up in a matter of hours.

Gonococcal ophthalmia (choice **A**) presents as a purulent conjunctivitis approximately 2 to 4 days after birth—or up to 21 days after if prophylaxis is given. The conjunctivas are very red, there is a thick purulent drainage, and there is swelling of the eyelids. Chlamydial conjunctivitis (choice **B**) occurs 5 to 23 days after birth and is the most common infectious cause of ophthalmia neonatorum (i.e., conjunctivitis of the new-born); it is about 10 times more common than gonococcal conjunctivitis. *Staphylococcus aureus* conjunctivitis (choice **C**) is uncommon. Congenital lacrimal duct obstruction (choice **E**) appears days to weeks after birth, is usually unilateral, and generally resolves over time with gentle massage of the duct.

3 The answer is F *Preventive Medicine and Public Health*

Omalizumab (choice **F**) is a humanized, recombinant murine monoclonal antibody that binds to mast cell Fc-receptor binding domains on human circulating IgE. This inhibits IgE activation of mast cells and basophils, making them less capable of releasing their contents. In this way omalizumab suppresses both early- and late-phase allergic reactions and effectively controls symptoms and improves pulmonary function and quality of life in patients with allergic asthma and allergic rhinitides. However, improvement does not continue after cessation of treatment, which requires daily subcutaneous injection.

The primary mediatory of the inflammatory reactions causing asthma attacks are the release of inflammatory mast cell products, including the leukotriene eicosanoids. Cortisol is a powerful inhibitor of phospholipase A_2, and consequently it inhibits synthesis of both arms of eicosanoid syntheses (i.e., all of the prostaglandins, thromboxanes, and leukotrienes), leading to a broad range of systemic effects. Because inhaled corticosteroids (choice **A**) are the most potent antiinflammatory agents available, they are generally considered the first-line agents for the long-term control of asthma in patients with persistent asthma. Although inhalation reduces systemic effects, these effects are still a problem. In children they retard growth, and in adults they inhibit adrenal function and promote the development of osteoporosis; thus, it is important to use steroids as conservatively as possible.

Long-acting β_2-agonists (choice **B**) relieve potential asthma attacks by providing bronchodilation for up to 12 hours. However they are not effective against sudden bronchoconstriction because they have a slow onset of action, and instead they are used for long-term prevention of asthma attacks, particularly nocturnal and exercise-induced attacks. They are not recommended for use in place of antiinflammatory agents (e.g., corticosteroids). However, when used in conjunction with corticosteroids, the required dose of both can generally be reduced.

There are two types of leukotriene antagonists (choice **C**). One type (e.g., zileuton) are specific inhibitors of 5-lipoxygenase, which converts arachidonic acid to 5-hydroxy-6,8,11,14-eicosapentaenoic acid (5-HPETE) the precursor of the leukotrienes. The other type (montelukast and zafirlukast) are leukotriene receptor antagonists. These agents can substitute for low-dose corticosteroids in mild cases of asthma but in general cannot substitute for corticosteroids. Zileuton may cause reversible elevation in serum aminotransferase activity, and patients who have taken montelukast or zafirlukast have subsequently been diagnosed with Churg-Strauss syndrome.

Cromolyn (choice **D**) and its newer analogue nedocromil are mast cell stabilizers; they inhibit the breakdown of mast cell granules and release of the inflammatory mediators. They are used as long-term medications that help alleviate symptoms in patients with mild persistent asthma and can be used prophylactically to avoid an exercise- or cold air–induced asthma attack.

Theophylline (choice **E**) is a phosphodiesterase inhibitor (increases c-AMP levels) that provides mild bronchodilation in asthmatics. It may also have mild antiinflammatory activity, and it increases clearance of mucous and strengthens diaphragmatic contractility. It must be used judiciously because of the narrow window between the therapeutic and toxic doses.

4 The answer is A *Surgery*

Based on the history and the biopsy, this patient has fat necrosis, in which some 50% of affected women give a positive history of trauma and pain to the breast. In addition to a palpable mass, there may be nipple retraction suggesting malignancy. Rarely, there may be ecchymosis in the region of the mass. Even if fine-needle aspiration determines that the problem is fat necrosis, the mass must be excised in its entirety (choice **A**), because there may be an underlying malignancy. If the mass is not excised, it may resolve over a period of time. However, the most judicious approach is to remove the entire mass.

Observation of the patient (choice **B**), repeat biopsy after 1 month (choice **C**), reassurance and prescription of antiinflammatories (choice **D**), and referring her for mammographic examination (choice **E**) are not appropriate in view of a possible underlying malignancy.

5 **The answer is C** *Preventive Medicine and Public Health*

The physician should base her decision as to whether the 92-year-old, now bed bound, delirious man should receive dialysis on the patient's overall medical condition. If he has a condition that renders dialysis physically dangerous, then dialysis should be withheld (choice **C**).

   The physician's decision should not be based on the patient's quality of life (choice **A**) or on the cost of (choice **E**) or payment method for the treatment (e.g., Medicare [choice **D**]). Likewise, the patient's children have no role in the physician's ultimate decision (choice **B**).

6 **The answer is B** *Medicine*

Hepatitis B virus (HBV) is a DNA hepadnavirus that is usually transmitted sexually, by blood, or by blood products and is particularly common in intravenous drug users and patients with AIDS. It is diagnosed by finding an elevation of liver transaminases and by vital antigens and/or antibodies in the serum. It is estimated that in the United States during 1999 the disease killed over 5000 persons. Most cases in the United States are in adults, and since the 1980s with the advent of a test for the virus in donated blood, the incidence has dropped 75%. At this time the greatest risk of infection is via heterosexual relations with a chronic carrier. However, the disease is also prevalent among men who have sex with men and IV drug users. Health care workers are also at higher-than-average risk, but this risk has been greatly reduced with the advent of the HBV vaccine. HBV has a partially double-stranded DNA genome, an inner core protein (the HBV core antigen [HBcAg]), and an outer surface coat protein (the HBV surface antigen [HBsAg]). There are eight different genotypes (A–H), and the course of infection may be influenced by the genetic variant involved. In about 35% of cases infection results in symptoms of acute hepatitis with a flulike disease similar to the one described in the diary; another 65% of infected individuals go into a transient state with subclinical symptoms. Essentially all of the latter group will recover completely and become noninfective. Among the 35% with early acute hepatitis, some 70–80% become asymptomatic carriers of chronic hepatitis capable of transmitting the disease, and 2–8% of these recover spontaneously every year. However, among this group with chronic hepatitis, another 10–30% go on to develop cirrhosis (as in the case described [choice **B**]) and eventually may develop hepatocellular carcinoma. Less than 1% of those with acute symptomatic cases develop fulminating hepatitis, and about 60% of these die as a result. These relationships are summarized in the following diagram.

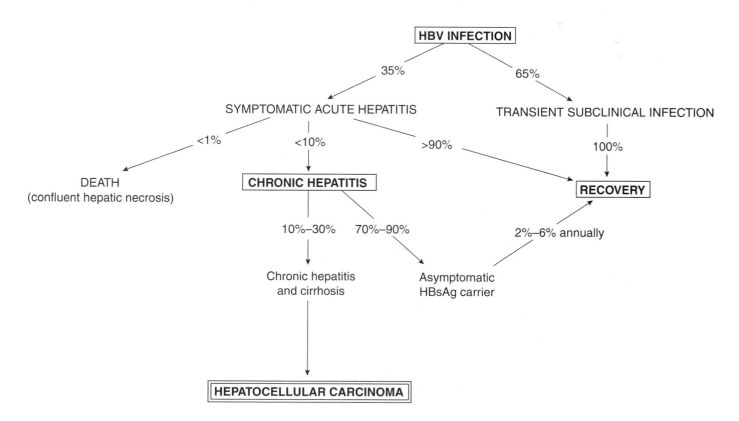

The appearance of HBsAg in the serum is the first evidence of infection, and persistence of HBsAg after an acute illness suggests chronic infection; on the other hand, replacement of HBsAg with anti-HBsAg indicates recovery. HBeAg is a secreted soluble protein related to the presence of the core protein and is only found in the presence of HBsAg. It is a marker of viral replicative activity and is present in chronic infective hepatitis. Disappearance of the HBeAg from the serum indicates cure, and as mentioned, such recovery is spontaneous to the tune of 2–8% of cases per year. The goal of treatment is to accelerate this conversion.

Treatment typically consists of a parenteral injection of recombinant alfa-2b interferon three times a week for 4 months. Some 40 to 60% of the time the HBeAg will convert to anti-HBeAg, signifying a cure. Injection of alfa-2b interferon per se will make the patient sick, and since the chronically infected person has few symptoms, the cure often seems worse than the disease. Lamivudine, a nucleoside analogue that can be taken orally, is much better tolerated than alfa-2b interferon and may be used instead. However only 20% of users seroconvert to anti-HBeAg status and 15–30% relapse as a result of a mutation in the polymerase gene. Such relapse can be avoided by continued use of the drug. Adefovir dipivoxil, another nucleoside analogue, can be used with similar results to treat patients who have become lamivudine resistant.

Hepatitis A (choice **A**) is an RNA virus spread by the fecal–oral route. The primary symptoms are anorexia, nausea, vomiting, malaise, and aversion to smoking; the clinical signs are fever, enlarged tender liver, and jaundice; and the relevant laboratory findings are normal-to-low white blood cell count and abnormally elevated alanine aminotransferase (ALT), aspartate aminotransferase (AST), bilirubin, and alkaline phosphatase values. The definitive diagnostic test is the presence of serum IgM anti-HAV. The only treatment required is symptomatic, namely rest; it is rarely fulminating and does not become chronic. Prevention is meticulous hand washing because the oral–fecal route is the main route of spread. Although meticulous hand washing is important for all, it is essential for food handlers. Hepatitis A vaccine is now available for persons at risk.

The hepatitis C virus (HCV) causes hepatitis C (choice **C**). HCV is a single-stranded RNA virus first discovered in 1989. Six basic genotypes, 15 subtypes, and more than 100 strains are recognized. As is the case with the human immunodeficiency virus (HIV), also an RNA virus, its high mutation rate makes production of a vaccine difficult, and one does not exist. The derivation of a test for the virus in the blood supply reduced the risk of transfusion-associated HCV from 1 in every 10 units of blood in 1990 to the present rate about 1 infected unit per 2×10^6 units of blood. Accordingly, the incidence of new cases has decreased from about 240,000 annually, to 30,000. Even though at this time HCV is the leading cause of cirrhosis and end-stage liver disease in the United States, surpassing alcoholism, it is still an underpublicized "sleeper" disease. There is about a 6- to 7-week postexposure incubation period during which no symptoms are found, and when symptoms first make themselves apparent, they are generally very mild, similar to mild flu. While 30 to 50% of these patients spontaneously recover, a larger proportion, some 50 to 70%, convert to a chronic but still infective version, of which 20 to 30% will eventually produce cirrhosis, and 2 to 5% transform into a hepatocellular carcinoma each year. This progression is summarized in the illustration on the following page.

Typically, cases are first discovered because of elevated liver enzyme activities noted during routine examination or by antibodies discovered in donated blood samples. Often infected persons remain symptomless but infective for decades, but eventually 80% develop cirrhosis or cancer. Luckily, the risk of sexual and maternal to neonate transfer is low. At this time more than 50% of new cases are caused by needle sharing among intravenous drug users. Other risk factors include sharing straws while snorting cocaine (the virus can be transmitted via oral fluids), being a health care worker (there is no vaccine to protect them), being in the military, being an alcoholic, and being incarcerated (a survey in Californian prisons found very high rates of infection on some institutions). In the general population, infection is higher among lower socioeconomic groups and among new immigrants. As with HBV, the aim is to cure the chronically infected. The typical treatment is a combination of peg-interferon (a slow release form) and virazole. Cure rates with HCV genotypes 2 or 3 are particularly good.

Hepatitis D (HDV) (choice **D**), also called the delta agent, is a defective RNA viroid that is only infective in the presence of active hepatitis B. Once HBsAg is cleared from the blood so is HDV. Coinfection with HDV has little effect on symptoms of acute HBV infection but tends to convert chronic HBV infection to the fulminating type or to severe hepatitis that quickly progresses to cirrhosis. For some reason, in recent years coinfection with HDV is becoming increasing rare. Hepatitis E (choice **E**) is rare in the United States but should be considered in travelers who return from endemic regions such as India, Burma, Afghanistan, Algeria, and

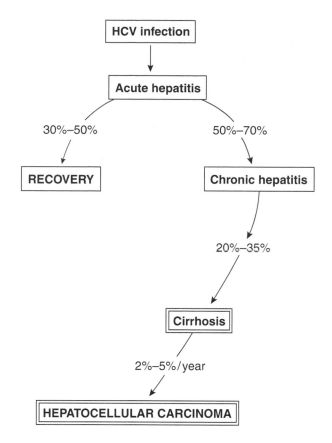

Mexico. It is a waterborne disease with no chronic carrier state, similar to HAV. It is generally self-limiting but kills some 10–20% of pregnant women. In 1994, a group of investigators reported a case they called non-A, B, C, D, E hepatitis and named it hepatitis F (choice **F**). The existence of hepatitis F as a separate entity has not been confirmed, but at least for the time being, the name slot is occupied. Hepatitis G (choice **G**) is a flavivirus associated with a chronic viremia; the virus is found in 50% of IV drug users, 30% of hemodialysis patients, 20% of hemophiliacs, 15% of patients with chronic hepatitis B or C, and 1.5% of blood donors. It seems to have little if any adverse effect and actually may contribute to the survival of HIV patients.

7 **The answer is B** *Surgery*

The patient has volvulus of the sigmoid colon (choice **B**). Volvulus is a twisting of the bowel around the mesenteric root. It is most common in the sigmoid colon (65%) and is most often seen in the elderly population. Obstruction and strangulation with infarction are potential sequelae. Clinical signs include colicky abdominal pain, abdominal distention, and vomiting. In sigmoid volvulus, there is a single dilated loop of bowel resembling a "coffee bean" rising up out of the pelvis. The concavity of the coffee bean points toward the left lower quadrant. Barium studies reveal a "bird's beak" or "ace of spades" appearance, with the lumen of the bowel tapering toward the volvulus. A volvulus can frequently be decompressed with a flexible colonoscope, but it often recurs. If it cannot be decompressed, then surgery should be performed with resection of the redundant bowel.

Intussusception (choice **A**) is uncommon in adults. It refers to the telescoping of one segment of proximal bowel into the distal bowel. In adults, it commonly results from an underlying mucosal lesion that serves as the nidus for the intussusception, producing obstruction and strangulation of the bowel. Bloody diarrhea and a palpable mass are usually present. Toxic megacolon (choice **C**) is associated primarily with ulcerative colitis. The diameter of the descending colon exceeds 6 cm. Perforation is a common complication. The patient does not have a history compatible with ulcerative colitis (e.g., intermittent bouts of bloody diarrhea). Ogilvie's syndrome (choice **D**) is a pseudoobstruction of the ascending colon in elderly persons. There is a sudden, massive distention of the colon without pain or tenderness. The right colon is distended with a cutoff at the splenic flexure. Barium studies are negative for obstruction. An impacted stool (choice **E**) would not likely result in complete obstruction.

8 **The answer is E** *Surgery*

Nipple discharge is the third most common medical complaint voiced by women. It follows breast lumps and breast pain. Green-brown nipple discharge in a premenopausal woman just before menstruation is usually due to mammary duct ectasia (plasma cell mastitis) (choice **E**). Ductal ectasia is a widening and hardening of ducts associated with aging or injury. The material discharged is debris that collects in the dilated lactiferous ducts, which are surrounded by a heavy plasma cell infiltrate.

Ductal carcinoma (choice **A**) is of course the most serious but is also the least prevalent cause of nipple discharge. It however becomes more prevalent as a woman ages and is almost the exclusive cause of nipple discharge in men. It is almost always a unilateral condition, whereas the condition described in the vignette is bilateral. Ductal papillomas (choice **B**) are the most common cause of abnormal breast discharge, accounting for some 50%. A papilloma is a benign wartlike growth with roots that extent into a duct, usually a large duct near the nipple, but occasionally several smaller ones more distant from the nipple. Like ductal carcinomas, they produce a bloody discharge and tend to be unilateral. They usually are not palpable and should be excised surgically. Prolactinoma (choice **C**) is the most common pituitary tumor. These tumors are located in the anterior pituitary and produce prolactin, which induces lactation; the discharge is bilateral and is milk. Chronic manual stimulation (choice **D**) can also stimulate milk production and produce a milky discharge (galactorrhea) in a nonlactating woman. Abnormal secretion of milk can also be due to primary hypothyroidism (choice **F**), which is associated with decreased levels of thyroxine (T_4); this causes an increase in thyrotropin-releasing hormone (TRH), a potent stimulator of lactation (a prolactin). Clear, serous, or milky discharges may also be caused by various drugs, including oral contraceptives (choice **G**) and several antipsychotic medications, particularly before onset of menses. Newborns often have a nipple discharge at birth ("witches' milk") caused by the mother's hormones.

9 **The answer is F** *Preventive Medicine and Public Health*

The earliest symptom of vitamin A deficiency is night blindness, and the earliest symptom of night blindness is an inability to adapt from a bright to a dim environment, a condition called nyctanopia or nyctalopia. (Other causes of night blindness are cataracts and retinitis pigmentosa.) Pregnancy increases the requirement for vitamin A and in the absence of sufficient intake can cause vitamin A deficiency (VAD), as in the case described (choice **F**). In America, VAD is rarely caused by insufficient intake, and a borderline deficiency resulting only in nyctalopia would most likely not be recognized clinically; consequently, frank VAD is generally recognized only in association with malabsorption conditions such as celiac disease, sprue, cystic fibrosis, pancreatic disease, duodenal bypass surgery, bile duct obstruction, giardiasis, and cirrhosis and in the newborn with congenital jejunum obstruction. Worldwide, however, VAD is the leading cause of blindness, and prevention is a goal of the World Health Organization (WHO). The progression of deficiency symptoms is poor dark adaption, night blindness, xerosis of the conjunctiva and cornea, xerophthalmia, keratomalecia. Keratinization of the lung, gastrointestinal tract, and urinary tract epithelia can also occur. In addition, there is increased susceptibility to infection and follicular hyperkeratosis of the skin. Vitamin A is also required for bone growth and remodeling; thus in the very young VAD also causes neurologic problems because nerves get squeezed as they try to pass through foramina that become too small because nerve diameters continue to increase but the diameter of the foramina do not keep pace. Vitamin A is also the most toxic of the vitamins. Until 2001, levels up to 10,000 IU (3,000 µg) were considered safe. Recent work has shown that retinoic acid, a vitamin A derivative, promotes osteoclastic activity in adults, and intake of as little as 4000–5000 IU per day of vitamin A as retinol or retinal (precursors of retinoic acid) promotes osteoporosis in an aging population. Consequently, the current recommended maximal daily intake is 3000 IU (900 µg) for men and 2330 IU (700 µg) for women over the age of 65. Another nutritional source of vitamin A are the carotenes, particularly β-carotene. These are converted to the active derivatives in the body at a rate that depends upon the need; hence they are not toxic even when consumed at high levels. However, supplementation with β-carotene was found to increases the risk of lung cancer in smokers by 18%.

Vitamin E is an antioxidant. A clinical deficiency (choice **A**) is almost entirely limited to premature babies. In adults, low circulating levels are recognized by abnormal sensitivity of red blood cells to hydrogen peroxide. Recent clinical studies suggest that high levels of ingested α-tocopherol do not protect against coronary artery disease (CAD) or lung cancer, as once believed, and may increase the risk of hemolytic stroke. On the other hand, at least one clinical trial found that α-tocopherol helps protect against prostate cancer. Several new clinical trials are presently being conducted. Pantothenic acid is a component of coenzyme A; however, a deficiency syndrome (choice **B**) is not recognized in humans. A nutritionally induced biotin deficiency (choice **C**) normally does not occur in humans because it is so widely distributed and is synthesized by intestinal bacteria. However, it is bound by avidin, a component of egg white; thus, a diet of some 40 raw eggs per day can cause a biotin deficiency, not a likely occurrence. A deficiency of either folate (choice **D**) or vitamin B_{12} (cobalamin) (choice **E**) will cause a macrocytic anemia. If the anemia is caused by a vitamin B_{12} deficiency, it can be masked by folate, and the underlying vitamin B_{12} deficiency will cause a neuropathy. Folate supplementation during pregnancy will reduce the risk of spina bifida, and both these vitamins along with vitamin B_6 (pyridoxine) are required for normal homocysteine metabolism.

10 The answer is E   *Surgery*

This patient has torsion of the testis (choice **E**), which involves rotation of the testis and twisting of the spermatic cord. Blood flow to and from the testis is impeded and, if left unattended, leads to gangrene. It usually affects males between the ages of 13 and 24, and generally there is no history of trauma. It can occur during sleep, straining at stool, or intercourse. The mechanism is sudden contraction of abdominal muscles and concomitant contraction of the cremasters. The affected testis lies horizontally (bell clapper deformity) and is drawn up into the inguinal canal. The scrotum is swollen and tender. There is an absent cremasteric reflex on the affected side. Elevation of the testis does not relieve pain. Treatment involves immediate manual detorsion followed by surgical fixation of the affected and normal testes. Differential diagnoses include orchitis, torsion of the appendix of the testis, epididymitis, and idiopathic scrotal edema.

Torsion of the appendix of the testis (choice **A**) presents like torsion of the testis. There may be a small hydrocele. Transillumination of the scrotum reveals a blue dot. Treatment is surgical excision. The opposite testis does not require exploration. Idiopathic scrotal edema (choice **B**) is a condition in which the scrotum swells suddenly. It is painless, and the testis is not tender. The cause is believed to be allergy. Epididymitis (choice **C**) is usually seen in men over 25 years of age. A history of urinary tract infection, previous attacks of pain, fever, and localized tenderness are additional features. Elevation of the testis relieves pain (Prehn's sign). Treatment involves antibiotics, scrotal elevation, and analgesics. Trauma to the testis (choice **D**), while a possibility, is unusual during consensual intercourse.

11 The answer is C   *Pediatrics*

The patient is having a systemic anaphylactic reaction to penicillin. Anaphylaxis is a clinical condition resulting from activation of mast cells and basophils via cell-bound allergen-specific IgE molecules. This causes skin (urticaria, angioedema, flushing), respiratory (bronchospasm, laryngeal edema), cardiovascular (hypotension, myocardial ischemia, dysrhythmia), and gastrointestinal symptoms (emesis, diarrhea, abdominal colic). Treatment of the reaction depends on the severity of the patient's symptoms, but an anaphylactic reaction as seen in this patient with compromised airway must be managed aggressively. Epinephrine injection (choice **C**) either intramuscularly or subcutaneously is the best first step in management of this patient. Epinephrine given promptly will rapidly reverse an anaphylactic reaction.

Intubation (choice **A**) is not initially indicated in this case, as epinephrine should reverse any airway edema quickly. The oxygen saturation in this patient is good, and epinephrine should be given an opportunity to work. Should the patient begin to desaturate significantly as indicated by pulse oximetry or should the patient have respiratory arrest, intubation would be indicated. Oral diphenhydramine (choice **B**) would not be a good option in this case because the patient is already in distress and an intervention that works more rapidly such as intramuscular or subcutaneous epinephrine is required. Intravenous (IV) corticosteroids (choice **D**) and histamine blockers (choice **E**) are sometimes given AFTER epinephrine in severe cases of anaphylaxis. No specific therapy is indicated (choice **F**) is incorrect, since untreated anaphylaxis can result in death.

12 The answer is C   *Medicine*

The three groups of antihypertensive drugs documented to decrease both morbidity and mortality when used clinically in the management of hypertension are β-blockers, thiazide diuretics, and angiotensin-converting enzyme (ACE) inhibitors. Acebutolol is a selective $β_1$-antagonist. There are three types of β receptors—$β_1$, $β_2$, and $β_3$. The $β_1$ receptors are cardiac specific, the $β_2$ receptors have a wide distribution, and the $β_3$ receptors are poorly understood but are found in adipocytes. Most β-blockers are nonselective; that is, they inhibit binding of sympathetic agonists to cells having either a β_1 or β_2 receptor. However at lower concentrations, acebutolol is a selective β_1-blocker, limiting its action to the heart, site 1 on the diagram (choice **C**). It lowers hypertension by limiting cardiac output.

Clonidine (choice **A**) is thought to modify sympathetic output from the central nervous system (CNS) via its agonist action on α_2-adrenergic receptors, which inhibit norepinephrine action. It is used for chronic management of mild-to-moderate hypertension and for withdrawal in drug-dependency states. Since it is a sympatholytic drug and it acts at levels above the neuroeffector junction (prejunctional), it decreases activity at all sites innervated by the sympathetic nervous system, including the heart (site 1), kidneys (renin release) (site 3), and vasculature (site 2).

Furosemide (choice **B**) and hydrochlorothiazide (choice **F**) are diuretics, and accordingly their site of action is site 3, the kidney tubules; however their mode of action is to reduce peripheral vascular resistance by decreasing the volume load (site 4); they reduce capacitance. A thiazide diuretic is often the first antihypertensive drug prescribed, usually at a dose of 12.5 or 25 mg/day. As initial monotherapy, thiazide diuretics are more potent antihypertension agents for the treatment of hypertension in blacks, aged individuals, and the obese than are the β-blockers or ACE inhibitors. Furosemide and other loop diuretics lead to electrolyte and volume depletion more readily than the thiazides and have a short half-life; consequently, they are rarely used except in cases of renal dysfunction.

Trimethaphan (choice **D**) is a ganglionic blocking drug that, because it acts at levels above the neuroeffector junction, causes marked hypotensive effects by decreasing activity at all sites innervated by the sympathetic nervous system (sites 1, 2, and 3). It has been used in hypertensive urgencies and emergencies for quick reduction of blood pressure but has largely been replaced by nitroprusside (choice **E**). Nitroprusside is metabolized to nitric oxide (NO). NO activates a soluble cyclic guanylate cyclase in the vascular epithelium, and the resultant increase in cGMP concentration causes muscle relaxation (site 2) via the action of protein kinase 3, which phosphorylates and inhibits myosin light-chain kinase, causing vasodilation. Both trimethaphan and nitroprusside are used to treat aortic dissection.

Phentolamine (choice **G**), a nonselective α-blocker, acts primarily at the arteriolar level (site 2) to decrease peripheral vascular resistance. Captopril (choice **H**) is an ACE inhibitor. Renin is synthesized by the kidney and acts in the circulation to proteolytically convert a plasma globulin to angiotensin I; the angiotensin-converting enzyme located in the vascular endothelium then converts angiotensin I to angiotensin II, a potent vasoconstrictor and stimulator of aldosterone secretion. Angiotensin II formation is limited by the presence of an ACE inhibitor. This reduces resistance (site 2) by inhibiting contraction (causing vasodilation) and promotes capacitance (site 4) by reducing aldosterone effects in the kidney tubule to decrease Na^+ and water retention (site 3). ACE inhibitors slow the development of diabetic nephropathy. This salutary action is not shared by thiazide diuretics or β-blockers, the other antihypertensive agents documented to decrease both morbidity and mortality when used to manage hypertension. The ACE inhibitors also are being used increasingly in congestive heart failure. Their tendency to cause repetitive coughing may be alleviated by the use of baclofen, cromolyn, or methylxanthines or by substituting an angiotensin II-receptor blocker which, although not as well studied, is thought to have clinical properties similar to those of the ACE inhibitors. Captopril is classified as a pregnancy risk factor category D because there is positive evidence of human fetal risk. Verapamil (choice **I**) is a calcium channel blocker; calcium channel blockers act as peripheral vasodilators (site 2); they have less reflex tachycardia and fluid retention properties than do other vasodilators.

13 The answer is C *Psychiatry*

This man suffers from obsessive–compulsive disorder (OCD), which is characterized by peculiar behaviors used to reduce anxiety-provoking intrusive thoughts. Treatment of choice for OCD involves use of selective serotonin inhibitors (SSRIs). Fluvoxamine is an SSRI commonly used for this purpose. Behavioral techniques such as thought stopping used in conjunction with an SSRI are also helpful.

Clomipramine (choice **A**) is a tricyclic antidepressant that is also used for this condition, but is generally used only when SSRIs are ineffective or contraindicated, because of its more limiting side-effect profile (anticholinergic effects, hypotension, lowered seizure threshold, sedation). Interventions such as counseling regarding proper behaviors (choice **B**) or suggestions to use gloves (choice **E**) are unlikely to be effective, as the individual already knows that his behaviors are irrational. Risperidone (choice **D**), an antipsychotic medication, is not indicated for OCD.

14 The answer is A *Psychiatry*

Symptoms of benzodiazepine withdrawal include anxiety, insomnia, psychosis, and seizures (choice **A**). Seizures are not commonly associated with withdrawal from opioids (e.g., heroin [choice **C**]), cocaine (choice **B**), lysergic acid diethylamide (LSD) (choice **D**), or cannabis (choice **E**). Opioid withdrawal is characterized by anxiety, malaise, pain, diarrhea, rhinorrhea, yawning, piloerection, and sleep disturbance. Cocaine withdrawal is characterized by anxiety, sleep disturbance, and depression. LSD and cannabis are not associated with specific withdrawal symptoms.

15 The answer is C *Surgery*

The patient most likely has angiodysplasia (choice **A**) that, next to sigmoid diverticulosis (not a choice), is the most common cause of massive lower gastrointestinal (GI) bleeding (hematochezia) in elderly patients. Angiodysplasia is characterized by the presence of dilated submucosal vessels (vascular ectasias) located in the cecum and ascending colon. Vascular ectasias increase with age and are caused by increased wall stress. Submucosal venules on the antimesenteric border of the right colon dilate and may rupture, causing massive blood loss. The initial step in management is nasogastric suction to rule out upper GI bleeding. If this is negative, colonoscopy is performed to identify and cauterize the lesions. Angiography helps localize the disease. A right hemicolectomy is performed if the site is documented to be the source of bleeding.

Meckel's diverticulum (choice **A**) is persistence of the omphalomesenteric duct. It is located approximately 2 feet from the terminal ileum, is about 2 inches long, and is present in approximately 2% of the population. In 20% of cases, it contains heterotopic epithelium (gastric, colonic, or sometimes pancreatic tissue). Rectal bleeding is seen in the presence of ectopic tissue, and may mimic a bleeding duodenal ulcer. Bleeding is seen in young individuals, 50% of whom are below the age of 2. In this age bracket, it is the most common cause of iron deficiency anemia. Bleeding from a Meckel's diverticulum can be determined by technetium (Tc) 99m-pertechnetate scan, in the presence of gastric mucosa. Rarely is bleeding significant enough to produce hypovolemic shock as in this patient. A small bowel infarction (choice **B**) is associated with severe, diffuse abdominal pain and bloody diarrhea. The patient does not have abdominal pain. Internal hemorrhoids (choice **D**) cause painless rectal bleeding; however, the bleeding is not significant enough to produce hypovolemic shock. Ulcerative colitis (choice **E**) usually presents in younger individuals, mainly women. It is a chronic disease characterized by relapses and remissions. Patients usually have bloody or watery diarrhea. Severe hemorrhage is very rare.

16 The answer is D *Psychiatry*

This patient's symptoms are most suggestive of generalized anxiety disorder. Buspirone (choice **D**) is often helpful for patients with this disorder who cannot tolerate benzodiazepine-induced cognitive changes. Other reasonable choices of medication would include venlafaxine and other newer antidepressants with anxiolytic effects.

Lowering the diazepam dose (choice **A**) would be less likely to help because the patient's residual anxiety would probably worsen. Alprazolam (choice **C**) is less sedating than diazepam, but its very short half-life and high potential for dependence make its use problematic for generalized anxiety disorder. Propranolol (choice **E**) and other β-blockers are sometimes useful in treating situational panic (e.g., stage fright) but are not useful for treating generalized anxiety disorder. Relaxation training may be most valuable in the long run but is less likely to be successful while tapering the patient from benzodiazepines (choice **B**).

17 The answer is C *Pediatrics*

Symptomatic human immunodeficiency virus (HIV)-infected children exposed to measles should receive immunoglobulin (IG) (choice **C**) prophylaxis at a recommended dose of 0.50 mL/kg (maximum, 15 mL) regardless of vaccination status. Asymptomatic HIV-infected children exposed to measles should also receive IG, at a recommended dose of 0.25 mL/kg. If a child received IG within 2 weeks of exposure, no additional IG is required. Generally, children with symptomatic HIV infection have poor immunologic response to vaccines. Therefore, when these children are exposed to a vaccine-preventable disease (e.g., measles), passive immunoprophylaxis is indicated regardless of the history of vaccination (choices **A, B,** and **E**). Low serum concentrations of vitamin A, not vitamin C (choice **D**), have been found in children with more severe measles.

18 **The answer is D** *Medicine*

Vasculitis, sometimes known as angiitis, is an inflammation of vascular vessels that may cause hardening, clotting and occlusion, and even rupture of affected vessels. In large part symptoms relate to the organ(s) deprived of blood. Although each type of vasculitis is a rare entity, collectively they represent significant numbers, and since many require rapid treatment to reduce long-term effects and even death, it behooves practitioners to be aware of their existence. Vasculitis may be caused by many conditions but is generally part of an immune syndrome, often autoimmune. Each of the choices listed is a form of vasculitis.

Whereas there may be confusing similarities among some types of vasiculitises, there are also distinct differences. Churg-Strauss syndrome (choice **D**) presents in a manner similar to that described in the vignette. The American College of Rheumatology lists six signs/symptoms and specifies that a diagnosis may be made on the presence of four or more of these. The six are (1) asthma; (2) eosinophilia (>10%, often up to 60%); (3) mononeuropathy multiplex (causing severe tingling shooting pains, numbness, muscle wasting, and power loss in the hands and/or feet); (4) transient pulmonary infiltrates observed on chest x-ray films; (5) paranasal and sinus abnormalities; and (6) extravascular eosinophils observed upon biopsy. It may affect other organs not included in the vignette, including the kidneys and skin. Prior to the advent of prednisone, the disease was fatal. Now with aggressive treatment with prednisone plus a cytotoxic drug, improvement is rapid, and after a month or two, it is usually possible to taper the dose down, but treatment is usually continued for 1–2 years or more. Progress is often monitored by the erythrocyte sedimentation rate and eosinophil count. However, even after the vasculitis is in remission, end-organ damage may remain, an example being the loss of extensor function of muscles in the hands in the case described.

Polyarteritis nodosa (choice **A**) is a systemic vasculitis that affects small-to-medium sized muscle arteries; it causes purpura, skin ulcers, muscle and joint pain, abdominal pain, and hypertension, and about 10% of cases are found in association with hepatitis B. Kawasaki disease (aka mucocutaneous lymph node syndrome) (choice **B**) is a pediatric disease that primarily affects children under the age of 5 years and presents with fever, rash, and eye inflammation.

Wegener's granulomatosis (WG) (choice **C**) is a systemic disease usually affecting arteries, venules, arterioles, and capillaries and occasionally large arteries. It is thought to be an autoimmune reaction to an antineutrophilic cytoplastic antibody (ANCA), either one found on the surface of the cells, called C-ANCA, or a perinuclear serine protease 3 which is then called P-ANCA. The prevalence of WG is estimated to be 3 cases per 100,000 persons; it affects men and women equally, most often during their 4th or 5th decade of life. The mnemonic ELK is sometimes used to designate the most common symptoms: *E,* ears, nose, and throat (middle ear hearing loss, nasal obstruction with serosanguinous discharge, chronic sinusitis, deep central facial pain, and hoarseness); *L,* lungs (initially asymptomatic cough, progressing to cough with hemoptysis, to dyspnea and respiratory failure with hemorrhage); and *K,* kidney (inially asymptomatic but possibly progressing to end-stage kidney failure). Left untreated, there is a 90% mortality rate within 2 years. If treated aggressively in a manner similar to that described for Churg-Strauss syndrome, most recover, but residual end-organ damage is common (hearing loss, 35%; nervous system damage, 30%; nasal deformation, 28%; rash, 14%; tracheal stenosis, 13%; visual loss, 8%).

Takayasu's arteritis (choice **E**) affects the largest arteries, with a special predilection for the branches of the aorta. It primarily is a disease of Asian women under 40 years of age. Blood flow through affected arteries may be impeded by occlusion, stenosis, or aneurysms. Typically, pulse from the affected artery is lost, leading to an alternative name, the "pulseless disease." Stroke may occur if the carotic artery is affected, and hypertension occurs in over 25% of patients due to proximal renal artery stenosis or aortic coarctation.

Hypersensitivity vasculitis (choice **F**) affects the small arteries of the skin causing rashes and is caused by allergy, most often to a new medication or disease. Temporal (giant cell) arteritis (choice **G**) and polymyalgia rheumatica (choice **H**) are considered to be extreme manifestations of the same disease. Both conditions are most common in persons over 50 years of age, and vasculitis occurs in medium- and large-sized arteries throughout the body. Giant cell arteritis has the greatest propensity to involve arteries of the head and particularly the temporal artery, while polymyalgia rheumatica primarily affects the shoulder and pelvic girdle areas, causing a variety of aches and pains. If not treated quickly and aggressively, temporal arteritis may cause blindness. Behçet's syndrome (choice **I**) causes inflamed arteries and veins primarily in persons in the 20–35 age range. It is very rare in the United States and primarily affects persons of Middle-Asian (e.g., Afghanistan and neighboring countries) descent. It also causes acnelike skin lesions or mouth and genital ulcers and eye inflammation. Buerger's disease (choice **J**), also known as thromboangiitis obliterans (and not to be confused with Berger's disease—an IgA-related nephropathy), causes inflammation and clots in the arms and legs; it is particularly prevalent among cigarette-smoking men 20–40 years of age and is more common among those of Middle-Asian descent. It, or at least a very similar condition, is also caused by arsenic poisoning. Henoch-Schönlein purpura (choice **K**) is a pediatric vasculitis that primarily affects children between the ages of 4 and 6 years. It causes bleeding into skin, resulting in purpura and is induced by infection with group A streptococci, varicella, parvovirus, or hepatis B virus or by sensitivity to antibiotics, antihistamines, thiazide diuretics, insect bites, or inoculations. The condition is generally self-limiting. Microscopic polyangiitis (choice **L**) primarily affects small blood vessels in the kidney, skin, and lung, resulting in glomerulonephritis, purpura, and pulmonary hemorrhage. It is often associated with antineutrophil cytoplasmic antibody (ANCA) directed against myeloperoxidase found in neutrophil granules. Because it sometimes affects larger vessels, its spectrum of symptoms may overlap with that of polyarteritis nodosa or Wegener's granulomas. Rheumatoid vasculitis (choice **M**) may complicate severe rheumatoid arthritis. Granulomatis angiitis of the central nervous system (choice **N**) is a recently recognized, poorly understood, and difficult-to-study condition marked by vasculitis in the brain.

19 **The answer is C** *Preventative Medicine and Public Health*

A hemolyzed blood sample will falsely increase the serum potassium level because potassium, the major intracellular cation, will escape into the sample. Thus this represents a false-positive result, not a false negative (choice **A**) or true positive (choices **D** and **E**). In addition, the absence of peaked T waves in the ECG, a sign of pathologic hyperkalemia, indicates hyperkalemia is absent.

The clinical symptoms indicate that the patient has an acute myocardial infarction (chest pain for 12 hours and radiation of the pain down the arm and into the jaw), and the electrocardiogram (ECG) pattern is consistent with an infarct. Because this woman is almost certainly having a myocardial infarct that started about 12 hours ago and serum troponin values begin to increase in 3–6 hours, peak in 24 hours, and disappear in 7–14 days after a heart attack, the increase in serum troponins I and T are a most probably true-positive results (not a false positive, choices **B** and **D**). Moreover, the troponins are essentially cardiac specific, and consequently, serum values are not affected by hemolysis of red cells. Thus, in summary, the elevated serum potassium value represents a false-positive result, and the elevated serum troponin level is a true-positive result (choice **C**).

Determination of troponin levels is now the gold-standard test for diagnosing an acute myocardial infarction; however, their long-term elevation limits their use as markers for reinfarction. Renal failure may also elevate serum troponin T levels somewhat; however, the patient does not have renal failure.

20 **The answer is E** *Surgery*

The common peritoneal nerve is composed of fibers from L4, L5, S1, and S2 of the sciatic nerve. As it courses down the thigh it supplies the posterior head of the biceps femoris, crosses laterally to the head of the gastrocnemius, becomes subcutaneous behind the head of the fibula, and then penetrates the posterior intermuscular septum and becomes associated with the periosteum of the proximal fibula. It then divides into the superficial and the deep peroneal nerve. Because the superficial peroneal nerve (SPN) passes down the lateral side of the fibula, it is also known as the fibular nerve. Because of its close affiliation with the fibula, it is easily traumatized when that bone is fractured, and because it runs through the lateral compartment between the underlying muscles, the peroneus longus and brevis, and the overlaying fascia, it can be entrapped when only soft tissue injury occurs in that area. Because the SPN enervates these muscles and because these muscles cause eversion of the foot, injury to the SPN inhibits eversion. Moreover, the SPN also supplies sensory nervation to the lateral dorsum of the foot. Consequently, the patient's inability to evert his foot and impaired sensation on the lateral dorsum of the foot indicate that the SPN has been traumatized (choice **E**). In entrapment, immediate surgical reduction of compartmental pressure is usually called for to avoid permanent injury to the nerve.

Whereas the SPN branch of the common peroneal nerve innervates the lateral compartment, the deep peroneal nerve branch (aka the anterior tibial nerve) (choice **A**) passes anteriorly over the fibula into the anterior compartment, where it enervates the six muscles contained within this compartment. Among other functions, these muscles permit dorsiflexion and inversion of the foot, functions found not to be affected. The tibial nerve (aka the posterior tibial nerve) (choice **B**), another branch of the sciatic nerve, innervates the six muscles of the posterior compartment, four of which are responsible for plantar flexion and two of which flex the toes. Before it branches going into the leg, the sciatic nerve (choice **C**) supplies the posterior muscles of the thigh, while the obturator nerve (choice **D**) supplies the adductors of the thigh.

21 **The answer is B** *Pediatrics*

In the pediatric population, lateral rectus palsy (choice **B**), not superior oblique palsy (choice **A**), inferior oblique palsy (choice **C**), medial rectus palsy (choice **D**), or superior rectus palsy (choice **E**), is most commonly associated with brain tumors. Thus, it is the extraocular palsy most likely responsible for this patient's symptoms. Children rarely complain of diplopia (double vision) because they suppress the image of the affected eye. With brain tumors, diplopia is a sign of increased intracranial pressure. Eye examination may reveal strabismus from palsy of the lateral rectus secondary to involvement of the abducent nerve. Many children tilt their heads in an effort to compensate for the diplopia. Other affected nerves are the oculomotor and, rarely, the trochlear.

22 **The answer is E** *Medicine*

In the diabetic patient, as in the normal individual, as long as sufficient insulin is available, exercise depletes serum glucose levels. Since in the type 1 diabetic the availability of insulin depends solely on the amount and type of insulin administered and cannot be altered once administered, such glucose depletion can readily lead to hypoglycemia. Type 2 diabetics can face a similar problem but to a lesser extent because they still depend somewhat upon endogenous insulin production, which, as in the normal individual, will tend to decrease in response to lower glucose levels. However, this normal physiologic response can be overridden by the effects of certain oral hypoglycemic agents, in particular by the sulfonylureas and to a lesser extent by the meglitinides. By monitoring blood glucose concentrations prior to engaging in exercise, the type 1 diabetic can determine the risk of hypoglycemia (choice **E**). If the value is near 100 mg/dL it is advisable to consume a small quantity of carbohydrate before engaging in the exercise program and, at the least, to be aware of a greater potential for hypoglycemia. In addition, by monitoring the level after exercise, the type 1 diabetic can estimate what effect that exercise has with respect to lowering the blood glucose level and, assuming the exercise program is continued on a regular basis, eventually determine by how much the insulin dosage can be decreased.

Exercise decreases (not increases) the amount of insulin required by the type 1 diabetic (choice **A**). Running for extended periods as in a marathon increases the risk of further damaging feet of persons with diabetic peripheral neuropathy (not promote healthy feet; choice **B**). This is because persons with peripheral neuropathy may be less aware of pain and other signs of what normally would be minor foot inconveniences, which may then bloom into more serious problems, particularly in a diabetic foot whose circulation is already compromised. A type 1 diabetic should refrain from eating before exercising (choice **C**) is not necessarily so; eating a light carbohydrate snack may prevent exercise-induced hypoglycemia. Although counterintuitive, vigorous exercise is not recommended for persons with serum glucose values above 300 mg/dL (choice **D**). Under such conditions of obvious poor metabolic control, functional insulin levels are already insufficient. Consequently, exercise can activate the earlier aspects of the normal physiologic response, namely, muscle glycogenolysis and release of glucose from the liver, which is controlled at both the substrate and the hormonal level. This will result in a further increase of serum glucose levels that cannot be countered by a sufficient increase in uptake by muscle because the recruitment of GLUT 4 glucose transporters is 100% insulin dependent. Furthermore, there may also be an increase in ketone production, increasing the probability of ketoacidosis.

23 **The answer is A** *Surgery*

The patient very likely has breast cancer and requires fine-needle aspiration (FNA) (choice **A**) with cytologic evaluation to establish the histologic diagnosis of the breast mass. The sensitivity of FNA in correctly diagnosing breast cancer is in the range of 95%.

A diagnosis of breast cancer must be established before surgery is scheduled (choice **B**). The age of the patient, the location of the mass (upper outer quadrant is the most common site for cancer), and the nontender nature of the mass and skin dimpling strongly suggest that it is malignant, but cytologic conformation is still required (choice **E**). Sending the patient home and reevaluating in 3 months (choice **D**) is not acceptable. The combination of physical examination, mammography, and FNA is highly accurate in diagnosing breast cancer when all of the tests give the same result. The combination increases overall specificity, thus decreasing false-positive results. The purpose of mammography (choice **C**) is to evaluate the breasts for clinically occult lesions. If the mass is palpable, then FNA is the first step in management, not mammography.

Mammography has a sensitivity approaching 90% in diagnosing breast cancer, with a false-negative rate of approximately 10 to 50% in some studies. These percentages reflect the deficits in mammography in detecting breast cancer in general and in distinguishing benign from malignant tumors. The sensitivity of correctly diagnosing breast cancer by physical examination is between 60 and 85%. A suggested management plan of a palpable breast mass is to perform FNA first. If the mass is cystic and results of the mammogram are negative, the patient should be observed. If the mass is cystic and the mammogram results are positive or if the mass persists, the fluid is bloody, or there are multiple recurrences, an outpatient biopsy is recommended. If the mass is solid, the FNA is positive for malignancy, and the mammogram is positive or negative, an intraoperative biopsy is performed with frozen section before definitive surgery is performed.

24 The answer is D   *Pediatrics*

Manifestations of congenital syphilis are divided into early and late. Early manifestations present during the first 2 years of life and include fever, anemia, snuffles (choice **A**), a maculopapular rash (choice **B**), failure to thrive (choice **C**), and hepatomegaly. Osteochondritis may be so painful that the infant refuses to move the involved extremity. This is known as pseudoparalysis of Parrot (choice **E**). Manifestations later in childhood are primarily skeletal and include Clutton joints (symmetric, painless swelling of the knees), saber shins, saddle nose, Hutchinson's teeth (peg-shaped, notched central incisors), and rhagades (perioral fissures or cracks in the skin) (choice **D**). Some sequelae of intrauterine infection may not become apparent until many years after birth, such as interstitial keratitis (5–20 years of age) and eighth cranial nerve deafness (10–40 years of age).

25 The answer is A   *Psychiatry*

The vast majority of older persons in the general population are not depressed; however, the risk increases with the development of chronic illnesses and the death of loved ones, friends, and acquaintances. The prevalence of severe major depressive disorder in the over-65 population is estimated to be below 10%, no higher than in the general population; (choice **A**); therefore, choices **B** (33%), **C** (66%), **D** (75%), and **E** (over 90%) are incorrect. Including a broader spectrum of depressive symptoms increases the prevalence to approximately 20%. Unfortunately, the prevalence in nursing homes is a great deal higher, over 25%. It is also unfortunate that most depressed elderly persons receive no treatment for the condition. It is estimated that only about 10% of clinically depressed elders receive treatment for depression.

26 The answer is B   *Medicine*

Antimicrobial prophylaxis is indicated in surgery when the postoperative infection rate is 5% or more under optimal conditions. In this case, the patient may be immunosuppressed from cancer chemotherapy and thus may be at special risk. Consequently, the prophylactic use of an antibiotic during surgery is valid in this patient (choice **B**). First- or second-generation cephalosporins (bacteriocidal) are the most frequently used antibiotics in this setting.

Cefoxitin is slightly less active against gram-positive cocci than are first-generation drugs, but cefoxitin is more active against strains of *Proteus, Serratia,* and other penicillinase-producing gram-negative rods, and there is no reason not to use it in an immunosuppressed patient (choice **A**). Since the anaphylactic reaction is a relatively unusual and unfortunate response, it is very unlikely that this reaction would have been avoided with a lower dose of cefoxitin (choice **C**), but it might have been less severe. Erythromycin, which is usually bacteriostatic, would not have provided adequate coverage in this patient (choice **D**). Antimicrobial prophylaxis in surgical situations should be instituted immediately before the procedure, not 24 hours prior (choice **E**), and should not normally be continued for longer than 12 hours postsurgically.

Regarding the skin reaction, it is a classic type I (IgE-mediated) allergic reaction, which commonly includes urticaria, anaphylaxis, and angioedema. Such reactions are more likely with penicillins than with cephalosporins. However, partial cross-allergenicity (<10%) exists between these two groups of β-lactam antibiotics. Hypoxia due to bronchoconstriction is likely to have been responsible for the cardiopulmonary dysfunction, especially if the patient had ischemic heart disease.

27 The answer is C   *Surgery*

This patient is only 43 years old and on the heavy side. As a result he will likely put a lot more wear and tear on his knee before he dies. A total knee arthroplasty (replacement) (choice **A**) would most likely have been the recommended surgery had this man been over 60 years old. However, since the prosthetic knee replacement can be expected to loosen or break down within 10 to 20 years, this 43-year-old can expect to need more than one additional replacement during his lifetime, and the procedure becomes more difficult and more prone to complications with each subsequent replacement attempt. Osteotomy (choice **C**) is a procedure in which either the tibia or the femur is shaved so that the bones line up in a way that shifts the body's weight to a compartment with normal cartilage, which is possible in this case since the damage is limited to the medial compartment. Although the knee is not as functional as it could be if a total knee replacement were successfully performed, this eliminates, or at least eases, the pain and also retains the basic bone structure intact, permitting total knee arthroplasty in the future, should that become necessary.

Unicompartmental arthroplasty (choice **B**) is, as the name implies, replacement of the worn out cartilage in a single compartment with a prosthetic device. If the patient were older, he could be a candidate, since this procedure is limited to knees with single-compartment damage. However, it is not suitable for him because it is not compatible with heavy or long-term wear and is only recommended for light-weight persons over 60 years of age. Its advantage is that it requires less extensive surgery than total knee replacement, so that recovery time is very short, permitting a person to return to a moderately active lifestyle within a short time. In addition, it retains the basic knee structure so that total replacement surgery can be done at a later time. Arthrodesis (choice **D**) involves bone fusion and fixes a joint. This too will relieve pain but obviously leaves a nonfunctional joint. Not too many years ago it was the recommended procedure for the more complicated joints, such as the ankle. However, total joint replacement is now available for most joints, including ankle, elbow, fingers, shoulder, and, of course, hip and knee; consequently, this procedure is used less often. Synovectomy is the removal of the synovium in an attempt to relieve inflammation. In this case there was no swelling, thus no inflammation. In addition to making synovectomy (choice **E**) unnecessary, the absence of inflammation makes this patient a better candidate for osteotomy.

28. The answer is A *Medicine*

Although it is counterintuitive, several studies show that both children and adults who do not get the optimal number of hours of sleep in a 24-hour period tend to gain weight. The optimal number is not rigorously defined and likely varies somewhat from person to person, but it is generally taken to be about 8 hours and is almost certainly at least 7 hours for the vast majority of persons. It may also be that naps can mitigate the effects of too little night sleep; hence, the question is written to cover a 24-hour period. One such study gauging the relationship between hours slept and weight found that relative to a control group who slept between 7 and 9 hours a night, those who got only 6 hours sleep are 23% more likely to be obese, those who slept for 5 hours are 50% more likely to be obese, and those who slept for 4 or fewer hours are 73% more likely to be obese. It has also been found that sleeping less than 7–8 hours lowers serum leptin levels and increases serum ghrelin concentrations. Leptin is a hormone released by adipose cells that signals the brain to stop eating, while ghrelin is a hormone synthesized in the stomach, that increases appetite. Consequently, the working hypothesis is that by lowering leptin and increasing ghrelin levels (choice **A**), sleep deprivation increases appetite, causing weight gain.

Although intuitively it would seem that sleeping fewer than 7–8 hours in a 24 hour period results in weight loss because more calories are burned while awake than while sleeping (choice **B**), experimental evidence has shown this not to be true. Presumably, the increased appetite caused by sleep deprivation coupled to the greater number of hours available for eating when not sleeping, unconsciously leads to a greater caloric intake. In addition, a drop in leptin levels changes metabolism so that the basal number of calories burned is decreased; thus, weight gain will occur even if caloric intake is not increased. Sleeping fewer than 7–8 hours in a 24-hour period results in weight gain (not loss) because leptin levels are increased (choice **C**). Sleeping fewer than 7–8 hours in a 24-hour period results in weight gain in part due to increased (not decreased) levels of ghrelin (choice **D**). Sleeping fewer than 7–8 hours in a 24-hour period decreases (not increases) insulin sensitivity (choice **E**). In fact, sleep deprivation studies have shown that lack of sleep raises the serum glucose level and decreases insulin sensitivity. In effect, insufficient sleep tilts the body toward the prediabetic insulin-resistant syndrome (syndrome X) marked by increased weight, glucose, total cholesterol, and low-density cholesterol (LDL) levels and decreased high-density cholesterol (HDL) levels.

29. The answer is E *Pediatrics*

The physician must obtain informed consent (choice **E**) from the patient and treat her infection. Although parental consent generally must be obtained before a minor (person under the age of 18 years) can receive medical treatment, most state laws create an exception whereby a minor can be treated for a sexually transmitted disease (STD) without obtaining parental consent (choice **C**). Neither her sexual partner(s) (choice **A**) nor her parents (choice **B**) need to be informed before treating the patient. The school guidance counselor (choice **D**) should not be informed by the physician regarding the patient's potential sexually transmitted disease.

30 The answer is E *Medicine*

A transient ischemic attack (TIA) is defined as a brief interlude (less than 24 hours and usually less than 1 hour) of neurologic dysfunction caused by focal brain or retinal ischemia with clinical symptoms and is in effect a ministroke that may be the forerunner of major problems. Some 200,000 to 500,000 TIAs are treated annually in the United States, and an unknown number are never brought to the attention of the medical establishment. The transient nature of the symptoms plus obtaining only normal findings in all of the tests conducted suggests that this woman had a TIA. The pure motor hemiparesis in the case described would most likely be associated with a small lacunar infarct of the left internal capsule. In the absence of signs of bleeding or risk of bleeding, TIAs are commonly given thrombolytic therapy, very likely with tissue-type plasminogen activator t-PA. However, provision of t-PA is short-term therapy, and the question asks for long-term therapy. Moreover, in this case symptoms are so mild and so transient that thrombolytic therapy likely would be limited to prescribing a baby aspirin nightly. However, both a TIA and hypertension are risk factors for a future full-fledged stroke, and diabetes is a particularly strong risk factor for small vessel disease, also possibly leading to stroke. Consequently, watchful waiting (which might include additional imagining studies) in conjunction with treatment to better control her hypertension and diabetes is likely to be the best long-term treatment (choice **E**).

To send her home with a pat on the back and tell her to forget about the incident (choice **A**) is irresponsible. A TIA is no longer considered a benign event. Statistics show that 10% will be followed by a major stroke within 90 days, and half of these will occur within 4 days of the TIA. True her diabetes could be under better control, but putting her on insulin to better control her diabetes would be a radical move, particularly without further data (choice **B**). The symptoms most likely did not derive from large-vessel disease of the carotid artery because that would cause a wider range of symptoms including aphasia; thus, left carotid enterectomy would not be an appropriate treatment (choice **C**). No evidence is presented to suggest that the patient has underlying heart disease; thus, treatment of underlying heart disease (choice **D**) is not correct.

31 The answer is E *Pediatrics*

The American College Health Association (ACHA) recommendations for prematriculation immunization require protection from mumps, rubella, diphtheria, tetanus, polio, measles, varicella, and hepatitis B; thus this young lady must be immunized for measles, varicella, and hepatitis B (choice **E**) to meet the ACHA recommendations. As a result of outbreaks of measles on college campuses in recent years, the ACHA recommendations mandate that colleges and universities require either two doses of measles vaccine or proof of immunity to measles (rubeola) as a condition for matriculation for students born after 1956.

Meningococcal vaccine (part of choice **A** and choice **B**) is recommended by some colleges and universities and required by law for college students in many states but is not included in the ACHA recommendations. Vaccination against influenza (part of choice **D**) is not mandated, although health-care providers should consider administering influenza vaccine to students living in dormitories or to students who are members of athletic teams. Pertussis (part of choice **B**) and *Haemophilus influenzae* type B (part of choice **C**) are not required prematriculation immunizations.

32 The answer is C *Psychiatry*

Memory impairment (choice **C**) suggests the presence of a cognitive disorder such as delirium or dementia. Other psychotic disorders do not often present with significant memory impairment.

Hallucinations and delusions (choice **A**) are common in delirium and dementia but are also present in many other psychotic disorders, such as schizophrenia. While olfactory and visual hallucinations (choice **D** and **E**) should alert one to the possibility of a general medical condition that may account for these symptoms, similarly, hallucinations can also occur with schizophrenia and other psychotic disorders. Compared with memory loss, severe anxiety (choice **B**) is not more closely associated with cognitive disorders.

33 The answer is B *Medicine*

Immunoglobulin A (IgA) is normally found in mucosal secretion and on mucosal surfaces, where it binds to, and leads to the destruction of, toxins and pathogens. Selective IgA deficiency (choice **B**) is a surprisingly common condition in which IgA is not expressed because B cells cannot finish differentiating into IgA-synthesizing plasma cells. Typically, affected persons appear to be asymptomatic or near asymptomatic (some 5–10 % of affected individuals, as in the case described, have frequent and recurrent infections such as sinusitis, otitis, and bronchitis). Affected persons also are in danger of developing an allergic reaction to IgA, as in the case described. In this case, exposure to IgA as a child probably developed antibodies, and infusion of more IgA after the motorcycle accident triggered an anaphylactic response. It has been suggested that persons with known selective IgA deficiency wear a "Med Alert" bracelet to avoid such situations; anaphylactic-type reactions have even been reported in persons never known to have been previously exposed to IgA-containing blood.

In the Western world, the prevalence of selective IgA deficiency has been reported to be as high as 1 per 142 in Arabia and 1 per 170 in Spain and as low (relatively speaking) as 1 per 875 among the English and is estimated to be about 1 per 500 among Caucasians in general. It has also been reported to be 1 per 255 among eastern Nigerians, suggesting that African Americans also have a high prevalence. However, among the Chinese and Japanese it is much less common. It was found to be 1 per 2600 among Han Chinese, 0 per 5300 among Zhuang Chinese, and about 1 per 15,000–20,000 among Japanese. This variation among different ethnic groups suggests a genetic basis, but one has not yet been elucidated. Present suspicion centers on some type of mutation that involves a region in the major histocompatability complex type III (MCH III) gene that codes for cytokines involved in immunoglobulin production. If true, this still leaves many questions open, including how is the disease induced or transmitted? (While there is a familial tendency, it is not inherited in a mendelian fashion except in syndromes involving other features such as mental retardation.) How can it sometimes improve or conversely become more serious as a person ages? (If it presents before the age of 5 years it generally clears up with age; on the other hand, some cases transform into common variable immunodeficiency, a more serious condition.) Why is the prevalence of a variety of autoimmune diseases and food allergies so high among persons with selective IgA deficiency? (A rational hypothesis for this is that IgA normally clears away undigested polypeptide sequences before they can be absorbed in the gut, and in the absence of IgA, such peptides are absorbed and establish antigenic sensitivity that cross-reacts with one or another endogenous constituent or with some ingested food.) Finally, why is the prevalence so high in so many ethic groups? Can it enhance reproduction in some mysterious fashion? While it does not per se promote mortality, it certainly encourages morbidity and should logically decrease reproductive potential.

Common variable immunodeficiency (CVID) (choice **A**) is the most common panhypogammaglobulinemia, with a prevalence of about 1 case per 50,000–80,000 persons in the United States. The three basic features characterizing CVID are (1) levels of most members of the IgG class of antibodies as well as those of the IgA class approach null values, and IgM levels are approximately halved; (2) patients lack functional B lymphocytes or plasma cells; and (3) affected persons suffer frequent bacterial infections. The initial presentation may be any time from infancy to middle age or older, with peak presentations between the ages of 1 and 5 years and between the ages of 16 and 20 years. A relation between CVID and selective IgA deficiency is suggested by the following— approximately 20% of persons with CVID have a relative with selective IgA deficiency; some cases of selective IgA deficiency evolve into CVID, and both diseases have their roots in the MHC III area of the genome. CVID is treated aggressively with antibiotics at the first sign of infection and with intravenous infusions of immunoglobulin, which is used prophylactically. Most affected individuals lead near-normal productive lives.

Choice **C**, X-linked agammaglobulinemia (XLA) is also known as Burton syndrome or Burton's agammaglobulinemia. It is inherited according to mendelian principles in a sex-linked manner and only affects boys. The mutation is located at Xq21.3, a large gene with 19 exons that is sometimes called Burton's tyrosine kinase gene. Mutations at different sites create some clinical heterogeneity, and in some cases, growth hormone levels are also negatively affected. XLA first presents after 2 months of age as the levels of IgG acquired from the mother decline, and presenting symptoms are respiratory infections, often pneumonias, and rashes. The prevalence in the United States is about 1 case per 100,000 live male births. It too is treated with antibiotics and γ-globulin with some success. All told, almost 100 different aglobulinemias have been described; the three described above are the most common. Adenosine deaminase (ADA) deficiency (choice **D**), a so-called severe combined immunodeficiency (SCID), is quite rare—fewer than 100 cases have been authenticated. However, it accounts for 15% of all SCIDs and a third of all recessive SCIDs, indicating how rare some of the others are. ADA deficiency deserves special mention because it was made famous by the highly publicized story of the "bubble-boy" who was kept in isolation (a bubble) for many years until the inevitable happened and he caught a disease and died and because it has been the focus of avant-garde therapies. The adenosine deaminase (ADA) gene is located on chromosome 20, and ADA deficiency is inherited in an autosomal recessive fashion. Because it seems that enzyme, gene replacement, or stem cell therapy should be relatively straightforward, it has been the subject of several experimental therapies. Although some limited success has been obtained, no clear modality of treatment has emerged. Monoclonal gammopathy of uncertain significance (MGUS) (choice **E**) is a gammopathy characterized by overproduction of γ-globulin. The incidence increases with age and approaches 3% by the age of 70. No clinical symptoms are found upon presentation, but a monoclonal spike is observed on protein electrophoresis. MGUS patients should be periodically monitored for changes in serum M-globulins, urinary Bence Jones proteins, evidence of renal failure, anemia, hypercalcemia, lytic bone lesions, or bone marrow plasma cytosis because the risk of developing a malignancy is 12% within 10 years, 25% within 20 years, and 30% in 25 years. However, since the initial presentation is usually in older persons, they commonly die from other causes before such malignant transformations occur.

34 The answer is A *Psychiatry*

Maintenance methadone can be used to treat heroin addiction only in federally licensed programs that are mandated to provide a range of rehabilitative services (choice **A**). It can be administered only to patients who have a well-documented history of heroin addiction.

Such programs have been demonstrated to be effective in improving psychosocial function in many patients who have not responded to nonpharmacologically based heroin rehabilitation programs (choice **D**). Concurrent use of heroin is quite common and is unlikely to cause severe physical distress (choice **C**). Methadone maintenance does not have to be discontinued if the patient resumes regular heroin abuse (choice **E**). He does not have to agree to random drug testing because there is no mandated requirement for random drug testing in methadone maintenance programs (choice **B**).

35 The answer is C *Preventive Medicine and Public Health*

The decision of whether to keep this patient on life support is a medical one. Although the patient has stated in his living will that if he is in a persistent vegetative state he does not want heroic measures taken to resuscitate him, his medical condition is not yet known. The opinions of the son (choice **A**), daughter (choice **B**), ethics committee (choice **D**), or court (choice **E**) are not relevant to this decision. The correct choice is to evaluate whether the patient has a reasonable chance of recovery (choice **C**). If he does, life support should be maintained. If he does not have a reasonable chance of recovery, life support should be discontinued, per his living will.

36 The answer is D *Psychiatry*

Opioid-induced delirium (choice **D**) is fairly common in hospitalized, elderly individuals. Opioid-induced delirium usually develops rapidly and has a short clinical course (usually less than 1 month).

Alzheimer's dementia (choice **A**) has a relatively lengthy course of development, and it is unlikely that a significantly demented individual would receive a hip replacement. An occult infection is not likely to be causing her delirium because the rather extensive laboratory assessment is unremarkable (choice **B**). Generalized anxiety disorder (choice **C**) and posttraumatic stress disorder (choice **E**) are unlikely to be responsible for disorientation and confusion.

37 The answer is E *Pediatrics*

Transferring objects from hand to hand occurs at $4\frac{1}{2}$ to $7\frac{1}{2}$ months of age. Most infants are able to sit without support between 5 and 7 months of age. Speech sounds can be imitated between $5\frac{1}{2}$ and $11\frac{1}{2}$ months of age. A neat pincer grasp is not seen until approximately $9\frac{1}{2}$ months of age and may be seen as late as 15 months of age. Therefore, the child described must be at least $9\frac{1}{2}$ months of age (choice **E**).

The abilities of this child would not all be present in a child at 4 months (choice **B**), 6 months (choice **C**), or 8 months (choice **D**) of age. A 2-month-old child (choice **A**) smiles responsively, follows to midline, and regards a face but cannot imitate speech sounds, cannot transfer an object from hand-to-hand, does not have a neat pincer grasp, and cannot maintain a seated position.

38 The answer is C *Obstetrics and Gynecology*

Chronic hypertension (choice **C**) in pregnancy is diagnosed by either a prepregnancy diagnosis of chronic hypertension or development of hypertension (defined as sustained elevation of blood pressure >140/90) prior to 20 weeks' gestation. Proteinuria may or may not be present. Often patients with chronic hypertension diagnosed before the pregnancy will present for prenatal care with blood pressures in the normotensive range due to the normal physiologic fall in both systolic and diastolic pressures. In this scenario, the diagnosis is based on onset of hypertension prior to 20 weeks. Management is conservative, using methyldopa as the primary anti-hypertensive agent because of its record of safety in pregnancy.

39 The answer is F *Obstetrics and Gynecology*

Gestational hypertension (choice **F**) is diagnosed with the development of any sustained elevation of blood pressure after 20 weeks' gestation in the absence of significant proteinuria (defined as >300 mg in a 24-hour urine collection). The absence of proteinuria distinguishes it from preeclampsia. Management is conservative but watching carefully for development of proteinuria. If the patient had true gestational hypertension, her blood pressure will return to the normal range after the pregnancy is over. In retrospect, it would be defined as transient hypertension (choice **D**), which occurs late in pregnancy, causes no problems, and subsides after birth but is a risk factor for the development of hypertension later in life. On the other hand, if after delivery the blood pressure remains elevated, in retrospect the diagnosis is chronic hypertension (choice **C**) that had its onset during the pregnancy.

40 The answer is B *Obstetrics and Gynecology*

Mild preeclampsia (choice **B**) is diagnosed with the development of mild sustained elevation of blood pressure (defined as >140/90 but <160/110) after 20 weeks' gestation in the presence of significant proteinuria (defined as >300 mg in a 24-hour urine collection or 1–2+ protein on a urine dipstick test). The presence of proteinuria distinguishes it from gestational hypertension. Temporizing management is conservative in preterm gestations, often with in-hospital admission. The only definitive management is delivery. This should be accomplished in term patients using intravenous (IV) magnesium sulfate for seizure prophylaxis.

41 The answer is E *Obstetrics and Gynecology*

Chronic hypertension with superimposed preeclampsia (choice **E**) is diagnosed with documented chronic hypertension in the presence of worsening hypertension and increasing proteinuria. Maternal cerebral vessels, which have been weakened by the chronic hypertension, are placed at a higher risk of hemorrhage by the effects of preeclampsia. Superimposed preeclampsia has such an adverse effect on both mother and fetus that delivery must be expedited at any gestational age using magnesium sulfate for seizure prophylaxis. In addition, the diastolic BP should be lowered to between 90 and 100 mm Hg using either labetalol or hydralazine.

42 The answer is H *Obstetrics and Gynecology*

Severe preeclampsia (choice **H**) is diagnosed with sustained blood pressure elevation and proteinuria in the presence of severe end-organ effects on either mother or fetus. The following criteria alone will constitute severe preeclampsia: (1) sustained severe blood pressure elevation (defined as >160/110) or (2) severe proteinuria (defined as >5 g in a 24-hour urine collection or 3–4+ protein on a urine dipstick test). However, even mild BP elevation and mild proteinuria will constitute severe preeclampsia if accompanied by any one of the following: persistent unexplained headache, epigastric pain, or visual disturbances; disseminated intravascular coagulation; elevated liver enzymes; pulmonary edema; cyanosis; oliguria. Management is to lower the diastolic BP to between 90 and 100 mm Hg, use IV magnesium sulfate to prevent convulsions, and expedite delivery at any gestational age.

INCORRECT CHOICES

The HELLP syndrome (choice **A**) is an uncommon phenomenon that may be a variant of preeclampsia. It is often misdiagnosed and if not treated can lead to poor outcomes. It is characterized by hemolysis, elevated liver enzymes, and a low platelet count, the latter being the most specific indicator. HELLP is a mnemonic standing for **h**emolysis, **e**levated **l**iver enzyme **l**evels, **l**ow **p**latelet count. Malignant hypertension (choice **G**) refers to rapidly developing, very high blood pressure values that cause end-organ damage. It is a medical emergency.

43 The answer is A *Medicine*

Carvedilol (choice **A**) is the first drug approved for congestive heart failure that has β-adrenoceptor-blocking actions. The drug is also a potent vasodilator, and marked hypotension may occur, even at low initial doses.

Carvedilol significantly slows the progression of the disease and improves survival in patients with left ventricular failure. In some patients, the drug may be an alternative to the use of angiotensin-converting enzyme (ACE) inhibitors and digitalis.

44 The answer is I *Psychiatry*

Olanzapine (choice **I**) is an atypical antipsychotic agent with minimal activity as a dopamine receptor-blocking agent. Consequently, the drug is less likely to cause hyperprolactinemia or extrapyramidal dysfunction than conventional drugs used in the management of schizophrenia. The use of olanzapine, like clozapine, does not appear to result in tardive dyskinesias. Olanzapine may exert its effects by acting as an antagonist at serotonin receptor subtypes in the central nervous system (CNS). Adverse effects of the drug include hypotension, somnolence, and weight gain.

45 The answer is J *Medicine*

The use of pravastatin (choice **J**) or other "statin" inhibitors of 3-hydroxy-3-methylglutaryl coenzyme A (HMG-CoA) reductase in patients with hypercholesterolemia is well documented to result in the reduction of most plasma lipids, especially low-density lipoprotein (LDL) cholesterol, and can increase high-density lipoprotein (HDL) cholesterol. Recently, data have become available regarding the long-term efficacy of "statins" in patients at risk for atherosclerotic disease. The use of pravastatin decreases the risk of first heart attacks in patients with hypercholesteremia, and simvastatin has been demonstrated to prevent second heart attacks in hypercholesterolemic patients. Although long-term efficacy has not been established for atorvastatin, the drug is the most effective agent available for the management of homozygous familial hypercholesterolemia.

INCORRECT CHOICES

Cefepime (choice **B**) is a 4th-generation cephalosporin. Cidofovir (choice **C**) is an antiviral drug used as a backup to foscarnet and ganciclovir in the treatment of cytomegalovirus (CMV) retinitis in acquired immune deficiency syndrome (AIDS). Dexfenfluramine (choice **D**) is a serotonergic appetite suppressant used for treatment of obesity. Donepezil (choice **E**) is an acetylcholinesterase inhibitor used to treat Alzheimer's disease. Fexofenadine (choice **F**) is a nonsedating antihistamine that is a less cardiotoxic metabolite of terfenadine. Meropenem (choice **G**) is a newer "imipenem" that does not require cilastatin and is less likely to cause seizures in renal dysfunction. Valsartan (choice **K**) blocks binding of angiotensin II to receptor sites and acts similarly to losartan. Zileuton (choice **L**) is an antiasthmatic that is a lipoxygenase inhibitor. Mirtazapine (choice **H**) is an antidepressant.

46 The answer is D *Obstetrics and Gynecology*

Uterine inversion (choice **D**) occurs when the fundus of the uterus develops a dimple that becomes a depression that deepens to where the endometrial lining of the fundus descends through the cervix and protrudes at the introitus. The classic description is a "beefy bleeding mass" in the vagina or at the introitus. This is the appearance of the endometrial lining, and a beefy bleeding mass is the key phrase in the scenario that identifies the bleeding cause. Risk factors include myometrial weakness. Management is uterine replacement by elevating the vaginal fornices and lifting the uterus by replacing the inverted fundus through the cervix into its normal anatomic position. Intravenous (IV) oxytocin helps by contracting the uterus.

47 The answer is A *Obstetrics and Gynecology*

This scenario describes placental abruption, which is the most common obstetric cause of disseminated intravascular coagulation (DIC) (choice **A**). Other obstetric causes of DIC include severe preeclampsia, prolonged retention of a dead fetus, and amniotic fluid embolus. The key phrase in this scenario is the finding of diffuse skin petechiae. Management includes removal of all products of conception, intensive care support, and selected blood product replacement until the patient generates her own clotting factors, platelets, and red blood cells.

48 The answer is G *Obstetrics and Gynecology*

The most common overall cause of postpartum hemorrhage is uterine atony (choice **G**). The key phrase in this scenario is a soft and boggy uterine fundus above the umbilicus. Risk factors in this scenario include an overdistended uterus (from a macrosomic fetus) and prolonged labor. Other risk factors are an infected uterus and tocolytic agents (such as magnesium sulfate). Management includes initial uterine massage, then administration of uterotonic agents (IV oxytocin, IM methylergonovine, and IM carboprost).

49 The answer is B   *Obstetrics and Gynecology*

This scenario suggests that genital laceration (choice **B**) has occurred, and the most common cause of genital lacerations is uncontrolled vaginal delivery. Risk factors in this scenario include macrosomic infant and operative forceps vaginal delivery. It is imperative to inspect the perineum, vagina, and cervix following every vaginal delivery. Management is surgical repair.

50 The answer is E   *Obstetrics and Gynecology*

The most common reason why placental fragments may be retained (choice **E**) is inadequate uterine contractions required to shear the placental anchoring villi and thereby enable normal placental separation. An accessory or succenturiate placental lobe may remain unnoticed in the uterus, resulting in hemorrhage. The maternal surface of the placenta must always be examined to ensure that all placental cotyledons are accounted for. The fetal surface of the placenta must be inspected to ensure that no vessels disappear across the placental membranes, suggesting the presence of an accessory lobe. Management is manual uterine exploration to remove the remaining fragments. If this is unsuccessful, ultrasound-guided uterine curettage must be performed.

INCORRECT CHOICES

Unexplained postpartum hemorrhage (choice **C**) is a leading cause of maternal death, usually in births not taking place in a medical facility. The usual cause is uterine atony (see question 48), but it may also be due to any one of a host of possible coagulopathies. A drop in blood pressure is usually the presenting symptom.

Vaginal prolapse (choice **F**) refers to the weakening of supportive structures that permits collapse of the uterus, bladder, or rectum into the vaginal vault. It is a common condition that may develop gradually or occur suddenly. It most commonly occurs in postmenopausal women but can also happen during the birthing process. It is treated by either Kegel exercises or surgery.

Questions

Single Best Choice Directions: This section consists of numbered statements or questions followed by a list of potential answers; you are to select the ONE best answer.

1 A 48-year-old patient presents to the emergency room with a history of tiredness, vomiting, and abdominal pain. He has a long history of hypertension, diabetes mellitus, and hyperlipidemia, and during this past year he developed end-stage renal disease. He admits to being depressed of late and has not kept his appointment with the nephrologist for renal dialysis, which he used to go to three times a week. The patient is on medications for hypertension, diabetes, and hyperlipidemia in addition to medications for renal failure. Which of the following is the initial medication that should be administered to reverse the clinical condition reflected by the accompanying electrocardiogram pattern?

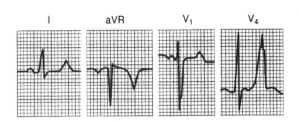
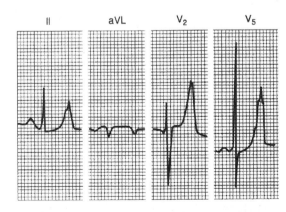
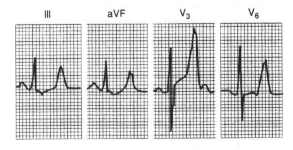

(A) Sodium bicarbonate
(B) Furosemide
(C) Calcium gluconate
(D) Glucose plus insulin
(E) Cation-exchange resin

2 A 63-year-old woman underwent an emergency laparotomy and bowel resection for volvulus of the large bowel. She presented with severe abdominal pain, distention, nausea and vomiting, and obstipation. Radiologic examination confirmed the presence of a volvulus of the sigmoid colon. During the postoperative period, she was administered high doses of analgesics and a benzodiazepine. As a result, she developed mild confusion, disorientation, and anxiety. Which of the following is best used in the management of her behavioral symptoms?

(A) Attempts at guided imagery
(B) Soft restraints to a stationary bed
(C) A well-lighted room with frequent interaction
(D) Adequate doses of benzodiazepines for sedation
(E) A darkened room with decreased sensory stimulation

3 An 18-year-old high school student who is due to graduate in a few months is sluggish during the day and has had two motor vehicle accidents related to falling asleep at the wheel. She also has abrupt sleeplike attacks during which she collapses to the ground briefly without loss of consciousness, and on several occasions she has had episodes of terrifying hallucinations just as she is falling asleep. She was referred to a sleep clinic for evaluation. Which condition of the following would be observed during the study?

(A) Delayed sleep phase disorder
(B) Sleep-onset rapid eye movement (REM)
(C) Episodic obstructive sleep apnea
(D) Periodic leg movement disorder
(E) Non–rapid eye movement (non-REM)
(F) Advanced sleep phase disorder

4 A 45-year-old man who is a manager at a local super market comes to his family physician for a physical. The patient has no prior history of medical illness, and his family history is noncontributory. He does not use any tobacco products but drinks an occasional glass of red wine with dinner. He does not take any prescription or over-the-counter medications. His vital signs are stable: blood pressure, 110/78 mm Hg; pulse, 78/min regular; respirations, regular at 16/min; and his temperature is normal. He is well nourished, moderately built, has no pallor, cyanosis, clubbing, or peripheral edema. Cardiovascular system examination is unremarkable as are also examinations of the respiratory, abdominal, and neurologic systems. Routine blood tests are run. The only abnormality noted is a serum low-density lipoprotein (LDL) level of 160 mg/dL (normal, <130 mg/dL). Which of the following is the most important initial step in lowering the serum LDL?

(A) Drug therapy
(B) Decreasing intake of carbohydrates
(C) A low total-fat and saturated-fat diet
(D) Decreasing stress
(E) Increasing exercise

5 A 3-year-old child is brought to the family doctor by a concerned parent. She states that the child has been irritable over the last month and has had some trouble with defecation. There were occasions when the child would wet the bed and even cry at night. Following a careful examination, the family physician decides to use a perianal cellophane-type preparation to establish the diagnosis. The condition he was concerned about is which of the following?

(A) Rectal bleeding
(B) Pain on defecation
(C) Constipation
(D) Anal pruritus
(E) Increased mucus in the stool

6 A 42-year-old woman is arrested for making terrorist threats. During the last 2 years, she had been repeatedly telephoning various physicians and health systems administrators to bitterly complain of negligent and abusive care and indifferent management. Numerous internal and external investigations could find no basis for her claims. Starting about 6 months ago, her calls became increasingly hostile and threatening, culminating in a voicemail that made veiled references to "taking out the leaders of the cover-up." The woman's public defender enters a plea of not guilty by reason of insanity. Psychiatric testimony indicates that the woman suffers from delusional disorder, persecutory type. Which of the following facts is the most critical for the defense to establish to successfully pursue this course?

(A) Her mental illness involved delusions that she was in danger.

(B) Her mental illness makes it impossible for her to understand the charges.
(C) Because of her mental illness, she could not recognize that she needed treatment.
(D) Because of her mental illness, she did not have access to competent treatment.
(E) Because of her mental illness, she could not have legally intended to commit the crime.

7 A 6-month-old infant, born to a 22-year-old female with a history of alcohol and drug abuse, sees a physician at the community clinic. Physical examination shows the infant to have short palpebral fissures, epicanthal folds, a thin upper lip, and developmental delay. The physician makes the diagnosis of fetal alcohol syndrome. Which of the following would also likely be found in this infant?

(A) Maxillary hyperplasia
(B) Hydrocephalus
(C) Cardiac defects
(D) Macrognathia
(E) Alopecia

8 A 54-year-old male presents to his doctor's office with a history of a change in his voice that began a few months ago. At first he thought that this was a touch of "sore throat" and tried taking cough drops and other remedies, but it did not go away. Recently he has started getting "winded" when he tries to walk too fast. He has never been to a doctor before and has not had regular physicals. He has no history of hypertension, diabetes mellitus, or other major illness. The only reason he is here he said is because his wife insisted that he gets checked up. He has worked at a local factory, turning out machined parts. He has been a cigarette smoker for the last 15 years, consuming a pack a day. He drinks a six pack of beer during the weekends and spends free time tending to the garden or watching football or other sports on TV. The most likely specific anatomic location for this patient's problem would be which of the following?

(A) Supraglottic
(B) Subglottic
(C) Larynx
(D) Glottic
(E) Hypopharynx
(F) Superior mediastinum

9 A 19-year-old mentally retarded man was brought to the emergency room of a local hospital after having developed severe abdominal pain, nausea, vomiting, and bloody diarrhea. The patient complains of severe thirst and a burning sensation in the throat. Following repeated questioning, he admits to consuming an unknown liquid, which he thought was alcohol. The liquid most likely contained which one of the following metallic elements?

(A) Arsenic
(B) Lead
(C) Mercury
(D) Iron
(E) Selenium

10 A 22-year-old woman immigrant, born and raised in Kiev, Ukraine, was exposed to radiation while residing there. She went to her family physician because she noted a lump in the neck while putting on a necklace. She does not have a history of difficulty swallowing, breathing, or talking. There is no history of change in voice or irradiation to the neck. Clinical examination reveals a hard, painless, fixed solitary nodule within the thyroid gland. Cervical lymph nodes are not palpable. She has no symptoms or signs suggestive of hyperthyroidism. Which of the following choices is the most likely diagnosis?

(A) Medullary carcinoma
(B) Undifferentiated carcinoma
(C) Papillary carcinoma
(D) Follicular carcinoma
(E) Primary malignant lymphoma

11 A mother brings her 1-year-old male child for a checkup because she is not sure if the child is "growing up right." Physical examination reveals severe mental retardation, flat occiput, epicanthal folds, and a flat nasal bridge. There is a simian crease in both palms. Chromosome analysis shows 46 chromosomes. Which of the following types of genetic mutation is responsible for this condition?

(A) Balanced translocation
(B) Frameshift mutation
(C) Microdeletion
(D) Nondisjunction
(E) Point mutation

12 A 28-year-old woman with a long history of anxiety attacks and bowel problems presents to her family physician with a recent history of pain on defecation. She also noticed bright red blood in the stool and was very alarmed by it. Physical examination reveals a petite frail young woman, who is obviously very anxious. She has some tenderness in the abdomen along the left lower quadrant, and a small tag of skin is noted in the perianal area. A digital examination can not be done due to pain. Which of the following is the most likely diagnosis?

(A) Internal hemorrhoids
(B) External hemorrhoids
(C) Fissure in ano
(D) Solitary rectal ulcer
(E) Proctitis due to ulcerative colitis
(F) Fistula in ano

13 A woman brings a 68-year-old man to the physician's office. She states that her husband has been having problems with his memory. She has noticed that he seems to forget words and faces, cannot remember things that she asks him to do, but somehow remembers things from the past. Other problems include difficulty with paying the bills, and that he just sits there, doing almost nothing. He also gets irritated very easily. He has no history of head trauma, has not consumed tobacco, and drinks alcohol only on special occasions. He has not had any illness and has not been on any medications. Clinical examination reveals loss of short-term memory and a positive grasp reflex. The neurologic examination was normal otherwise. As part of the workup, a Mini-Mental Status Examination was conducted. Based on the above, you would expect his score to be between which of the following sets of values?

(A) 0 to 10
(B) 11 to 20
(C) 21 to 30
(D) 31 to 40
(E) Above 40

14 A 24-year-old married male patient is brought to the emergency department by the paramedics after an automobile accident. After emergency surgery he was transferred to the intensive care unit where he succumbed the following morning. The physician in charge declares him to be brain dead. Which of the following is the most appropriate next step in the management of this patient?

(A) Keep him on life support until his organs can be harvested
(B) Turn off life support
(C) Ask his wife's permission to keep him on life support until his organs can be harvested
(D) Get a court order to keep him on life support until his organs can be harvested
(E) Keep him on life support indefinitely

15 A 45-year-old male is taken to the emergency room of a local hospital with a history of sudden onset of difficulty breathing. The patient states that he had been suffering from shortness of breath, difficulty climbing stairs, headaches and recently noticed swelling of his feet. He also complains of nonradiating chest pain, mainly in the precordial area. He has not been on any medications. Physical examination reveals a man in acute distress, who is orthopneic, has a blood pressure of 150/110 mm Hg, pulse of 89 beats per minute with dropped beats, and a respiratory rate of 20 breaths per minute with some audible wheezes. His temperature is 37°C (98.6°F). The nail beds are bluish, and no clubbing is noted. His accessory muscles of respiration are active, and rales and crepitations are heard in both lungs, the latter mainly at the base. Auscultation of his heart will reveal which of the following sounds?

(A) A loud S_1
(B) A fixed splitting of S_2
(C) A soft A_2
(D) A loud P_2
(E) An S_3
(F) Widened splitting of S_2
(G) An absent S_4

16. A 35-year-old woman is referred to you for a complete physical examination. She asks you what tests or examinations should be performed to reduce her risk for developing cancer. Which of the following screening tests has most reduced the incidence of cancer in women in the United States?

(A) Cervical Pap smear
(B) Clinical breast examination
(C) Flexible sigmoidoscopy
(D) Mammography
(E) Stool guaiac

17. A 42-year-old man, who delivers mail for a living, is applying for health insurance. He is asked by the insurance company to submit another urine sample, because the previous sample had a positive reading using a reagent strip for protein determination. All the other urinalysis reagent strip tests and sediment examination were negative. The patient is specifically asked to submit the first AM urine for repeat analysis. It returns negative for protein. Which of the following types of proteinuria is most likely present?

(A) Functional
(B) Glomerular
(C) Overflow
(D) Tubular
(E) None, it was a laboratory error

18. A newborn male infant with Down syndrome fails to pass meconium within the first 24 hours after birth. A rectal examination shows a narrow anal canal and absence of stool in the rectal vault. An abdominal radiograph shows distended loops of colon. Which of the following is the most likely diagnosis?

(A) Anorectal malformation
(B) Enterocolitis
(C) Functional constipation
(D) Hirschsprung's disease
(E) Malrotation

19. A febrile 43-year-old man has pain and swelling in the metatarsophalangeal joint of the great toe. He has a 15-year history of alcohol abuse. A complete blood cell count shows an absolute neutrophilic leukocytosis with >10% band neutrophils. Which of the following microscopic findings is most likely to be present in the synovial fluid?

(A) Neutrophils with phagocytosed gram-negative diplococci
(B) Neutrophils with phagocytosed gram-positive cocci
(C) Neutrophils with phagocytosed negative birefringent crystals
(D) Neutrophils with phagocytosed positive birefringent crystals
(E) Neutrophils with phagocytosed rheumatoid factor immunocomplexes

20. A 38-year-old man presents with bouts of severe, right retro-orbital pain lasting one-half hour or more, up to several times a day. The pain often occurs at night and is associated with nasal congestion on the right side and right conjunctival injection. Which of the following would be an effective short-term treatment in this patient?

(A) Sublingual nitroglycerin
(B) An alcoholic beverage
(C) Vigorous exercise
(D) Nasal oxygen
(E) A warm pack over the eye

21. An 8-year-old boy resists going to school because he wants to remain with his mother. He becomes terrified whenever his parents leave the house. During the day, he worries that his family will be kidnapped and that he will never see them again. Which of the following disorders in adulthood is the most closely associated sequel to these symptoms?

(A) Dysthymic disorder
(B) Obsessive–compulsive personality disorder
(C) Panic disorder
(D) Schizophrenia
(E) Pain disorder

22 A 47-year-old, medium-build schoolteacher presents with a history of numbness and a burning sensation followed by tingling of the thumb, index finger, and middle finger of the right hand. These symptoms occur at night and are present when she awakens. She states that at times the pain seems to "rise up my arm." Shaking the hand, elevating it, or even immersing the hand in hot water tends to relieve the symptoms. On one occasion the fingers turned blue. Apart from a "whiplash" injury to the neck 1 year ago, she has no positive medical history. Clinical examination reveals impaired sensation over the index and middle fingers, but not over the thumb. However, she can perceive light touch when tested with a wisp of cotton wool. Sensations of position, vibration, and temperature can be perceived normally. Muscle power in the hand is unaffected, and there is no evidence of wasting or atrophy. There is no tenderness in the elbow region. The radial pulse is normal and unaffected by position of the arm. Movements of the neck are not painful. Which of the following is the most likely diagnosis?

(A) Cervical radiculopathy
(B) Thoracic outlet syndrome
(C) Carpal tunnel syndrome
(D) Pronator teres syndrome
(E) Raynaud's phenomenon

23 A 67-year-old female presents to her doctor's office with a history of sudden severe backache. The patient states that she was working in the garden and tried to lift a sack of fertilizer, when her "back gave out." She states that the pain was very intense, was stabbing in nature, and went across her abdomen, like a belt. She has a history of hypertension and diabetes mellitus and some urinary problems. Her vital signs are as follows: blood pressure, 130/100 mm Hg; pulse, 86 beats/min, regular; respirations, 18/min; and temperature, 37°C (98.6°F). Physical examination reveals tenderness to deep palpation in the lower thoracic spine, paraspinal spasm, and a restricted straight leg raise on both lower extremities. The deep tendon reflexes are normal in the knees, but are absent in both ankles. There are a few beats of clonus that were not sustained. She also has decreased touch in both legs below the knees. The most likely diagnosis is which of the following?

(A) Spinal cord tumor
(B) Epidural abscess
(C) Fractured vertebra
(D) Posterolateral lumbar disk herniation
(E) Central lumbar disk herniation

24 A 72-year-old woman has been receiving an aminoglycoside for sepsis caused by a gram-negative organ-

ism found to be resistant to other antibiotics. After a week of treatment she develops adduction of the thumb into the palm whenever her blood pressure is taken. In addition, tapping of the facial nerve causes contraction of the muscles around the mouth. Most likely these clinical findings result from a functional deficiency of which of the following mineral ions?

(A) Chloride
(B) Magnesium
(C) Phosphate
(D) Potassium
(E) Sodium

25 During a psychotherapy session, a clinician says to a 32-year-old woman, "Let us explore the unconscious psychological conflicts that interactions with other people might awaken in you." Which of the following conditions is most likely to be successfully treated with this technique?

(A) Bipolar disorder
(B) Dysthymic disorder
(C) Enuresis
(D) Obsessive–compulsive disorder
(E) Schizophrenia

26 A 17-year-old male plays varsity football for his high school. While running for a touchdown, he is tackled. The team physician ascertains that the player is confused but without amnesia or loss of consciousness. There is no evidence of broken bones, sprains, or bruising. This is the first time that this football player has ever sustained a head injury. The football player says that he is ready to go back in the game. What should the recommendation for return to play be for this football player?

(A) If the patient remains asymptomatic, he may return to contact sports in 20 minutes.
(B) If the patient remains asymptomatic for 1 week, he may return to contact sports in 1 week.
(C) If the patient remains asymptomatic for 1 week, he may return to contact sports in 1 month.
(D) If the patient remains asymptomatic for 1 week, he may return to contact sports in 2 weeks.
(E) The patient may not return to contact sports this season.

27 A married 16-year-old male supports himself and his wife, who is 7 months' pregnant, by working as a roofer. Last night he was out with some old high school buddies and was talked into participating in a drag race. He lost control of his car and crashed into a tree. As a result, he requires surgery to set a badly fractured leg. Consent for the surgery must be given by which of the following?

(A) One parent
(B) The spouse
(C) Both parents
(D) A court-appointed legal guardian
(E) The 16-year-old male himself

28 A 73-year old woman sees her primary care physician because she has pain and discomfort behind the knee while walking; she is particularly concerned because she is no longer able to play golf. The pain is increased when she squats to line up a putt, to place the tee, to pick up the golf ball, or to do work about the house and garden; however, the pain is relieved by rest. Swelling can be felt when she stands, but pitting edema is absent. Sometimes when she swings the knee it clicks. Which of the following is the most likely diagnosis?

(A) Right sciatic radiculopathy
(B) Calf muscle hematoma
(C) Superficial thrombophlebitis
(D) Deep venous thrombosis
(E) Baker's cyst

29 A star 19-year-old high school football player graduated last June and is granted an athletic scholarship to a college. He moves from his home to the town in which the college is situated just before Labor Day. At that time of year the average temperature in his home town is 78°F (25.6°C), while in the town in which college is located, the temperature is 98°F (36.7°C). Because he is anxious to be accepted onto the college football team, he starts conditioning himself by running 5 miles each morning. While running the day after moving he suddenly collapses and is comatose. The paramedics take him to the local emergency facility where physical examination shows the following data: blood pressure, 88/58 mm Hg; pulse, 130 beats/min; respiratory rate, 47 breaths/min; and temperature, 107.6°F (42°C). Which of the following statements is true?

(A) The first line of treatment is intravenous fluids with electrolytes.
(B) The first line of treatment is lowering body temperature by placing him in a cool environment, spraying him with tepid water, and cooling him with fans.
(C) The first line of treatment is to assess and treat if necessary the airways, breathing, and circulation.
(D) This person exhibits clinical signs typically attributed to heat exhaustion.
(E) This person has heat cramps.

30 A 68-year-old man who had been treated for leukemia is admitted to the hospital with malaise, chills, and high fever. His chest is clear to percussion and auscultation, with no heart murmurs. His abdomen is free of masses and tenderness. Extensive erythematous lesions are present on his trunk and extremities, some of which have progressed to the hemorrhagic stage with necrosis. Skin scrapings and blood samples are obtained for Gram's staining and microbiologic culture. Which of the following actions is most appropriate?

(A) Withhold antibiotics until all microbiologic results are available
(B) Start treatment with intravenous (IV) ampicillin
(C) Treat patient with azithromycin perorally
(D) Start treatment with cilastatin–imipenem
(E) Treat patient with IV ciprofloxacin

31 A 35-year-old female from San Luis Obispo, California went camping in the woods while she was visiting relatives in Connecticut. Upon her return home, she developed a rash that appeared to have a ring around it, and she also developed mild fever and fatigue. However, she quickly recovered and thought no more of it. A month later, upon awakening one morning she noticed difficulty speaking and closing her right eye, and the right side of her mouth drooped. In addition, food would stay on the right side of the mouth and did not seem to taste right. Loud sounds bothered her as well, and her smile was "twisted." Fearing she had suffered a stroke, she rushed to the nearest emergency facility. Which of the following types of tests would best confirm the cause of her condition?

(A) Examination of the urine
(B) Electromyography
(C) Nerve conduction study
(D) Magnetic resonance imaging of the brain
(E) Examination of the cerebrospinal fluid
(F) Examination of the serum

32 A 54-year-old woman with a 30-year history of schizophrenia and multiple past hospitalizations for psychosis and aggressive behavior has been treated with risperidone 4 mg PO qd and is newly enrolled in a multidisciplinary outpatient treatment program. She lives in a homeless shelter and is unemployed. There are no close friends or family. She has a history of past domestic abuse, lack of motivation for treatment, difficulty tolerating medication regimens, and intermittent binge drinking. Mental status examination reveals a mildly withdrawn woman with moderate anxiety, blunted affect, and slightly tangential thought processes. The treatment team is considering referral to

a peer support (self-help) group. It was decided that she should not be referred to a peer support group because she demonstrated which of the following symptoms?

(A) Aggressive symptoms
(B) Anxiety
(C) Psychotic symptoms
(D) Social withdrawal
(E) Substance abuse

33 A 19-year-old man was given a physical examination after enlisting in the marines. The examination reveals a systolic murmur that decreases in intensity when the patient lies down and increases in intensity when he stands up. An echocardiogram shows abnormal movement of the anterior mitral valve leaflet against an asymmetrically thickened interventricular septum (IVS). In taking a history the physician finds out that his older brother died from a heart attack at the age of 22. What is the most likely diagnosis?

(A) Aortic regurgitation
(B) Aortic stenosis
(C) Hypertrophic cardiomyopathy
(D) Mitral stenosis
(E) Mitral valve prolapse

34 A 66-year-old male moved in with his daughter after his wife of 44 years died of breast cancer a year ago. His daughter now insists he visit his family physician and accompanies him when he does. She tells the physician that her father has been behaving in a rather odd manner over the last few months. He seems to be losing his memory, is unable to recall names, dates, and places, and has been getting lost at times at home. He used to be very good at mathematics, which he taught at a local junior college, but now he has difficulty doing simple calculations. In fact, he got angry and yelled at her one day when she stated that he had written a check for the wrong amount. Sometimes she noticed that he would kick his legs and he jerks his arms in a weird way while resting. The most likely diagnosis in this patient is which of the following?

(A) Multiinfarct dementia
(B) Chronic subdural hematoma
(C) Pseudodementia
(D) Alzheimer's disease
(E) Creutzfeldt-Jakob disease

35 A 23-year-old man is arrested for attempted embezzlement. He has previously been arrested for burglary and battery but has been let go because of insufficient evidence. He has had several relationships with women during which he managed to talk them in to lending him money that he never repaid, and he also left three of them pregnant and never gave the mother or child a second thought. Which of the following statements about this man's antisocial behavior also is true?

(A) It probably had its onset after age 15.
(B) It is associated with rigid family upbringing.
(C) It tends to fluctuate in intensity over a short period of time.
(D) It is often accompanied by periods of extreme remorse.
(E) It is likely to decrease markedly after age 40.

36 Colonoscopic studies show a 3.5-cm annular mass in the sigmoid colon of a 66-year-old woman. Multiple biopsies show a poorly differentiated adenocarcinoma. A colectomy is performed, and a few nodular lesions on the surface of the liver are apparent. A frozen section shows a poorly differentiated adenocarcinoma. Gross and microscopic findings of the colectomy specimen show a mucosally derived cancer that has invaded through the muscle wall and out into the serosal fat. There is metastasis in 6 of 20 mesenteric lymph nodes directly beneath the tumor. Which of the following most influences the patient's prognosis?

(A) Differentiation of the tumor
(B) Extent of local invasion
(C) Liver involvement
(D) Lymph node involvement
(E) Size of the tumor

37 A 26-year-old woman complains of headaches and double vision. She is 5 ft 7 in tall (26.4 cm) and weighs 230 lb (104.3 kg). Her physician suspects that she has benign intracranial hypertension (pseudotumor cerebri). Which of the following is the most feared complication of this condition?

(A) Visual loss
(B) Sixth nerve palsy
(C) Herniation syndrome
(D) Migraine headache
(E) Hemiplegia

38 A 32-year-old man with AIDS has chronic nonbloody, watery diarrhea. A stool sample shows partially acid-fast–positive oocysts. Which of the following pathogens is most likely present?

(A) *Balantidium coli*
(B) *Cryptosporidium parvum*
(C) *Entamoeba histolytica*
(D) *Giardia lamblia*
(E) *Strongyloides stercoralis*

39 A father is brought in to a counseling session at his 7-year old son's elementary school. The teacher says that his son is a generally good student and a joy to work with, but she complains that the boy does not pay attention during reading sessions and as a consequence is falling further and further behind expected first-grade reading norms. She adds that he also cannot spell. The father, a successful orthopedic surgeon, has immediate empathy with his son because he had similar problems, and he realizes that the boy's problem is difficulty in decoding some single words and, rather than struggling to comprehend what he perceives as gibberish, allows his attention to wander. Which of the following is the most likely diagnosis of the son's problem?

(A) A low IQ
(B) Attention deficit disorder (ADD)
(C) Poor vision
(D) A hearing disorder
(E) Dyslexia

40 A 32-year-old woman comes to her family physician with increasing fatigue. She states that a few months ago, she had an episode of double vision that went away spontaneously. During the past few days she has noticed tingling in the fingers of her right hand, which comes and goes. Her past medical history is non-contributory, as is her family history. She does not use tobacco, drugs, or alcohol but is on birth control pills. Physical examination reveals normal vital signs, and a neurologic examination has normal findings. The physician suspects multiple sclerosis. The best way to follow-up this patient would be which of the following?

(A) Spinal fluid examination in 6 months
(B) Physical examination in 6 months
(C) Magnetic resonance imaging in 6 months
(D) Computerized tomography scan in 6 months
(E) Physical examination on a monthly basis

Directions for Matching Question (41 through 50): *Each set of matching questions is preceded by a list of 4 to 26 lettered options followed by a brief explanation of the required task and then by a series of numbered statements. For each lettered statement you are to select ONE lettered option that best fulfills the task as it relates to that statement. Remember each of the listed options might be correctly selected once, more than once, or not at all.*

Questions 41–43

Match each numbered case or description below with the lettered test that is the most useful for the case or best fits the description.

(A) Halstead-Reitan Battery (HRB)
(B) Minnesota Multiphase Personality Inventory (MMPI)
(C) Rorschach test
(D) Sentence Completion Test (SCT)
(E) Stanford-Binet Scale
(F) Thematic Apperception Test (TAT)
(G) Wide-Range Achievement Test (WRAT)

41 The first developed projective personality test that uses a patient's interpretation of a set of standard images. A psychoanalyst interprets the patient's response to probe his or her subconscious feelings.

42 The projective personality test that is most likely to be given to a 29-year-old sailor undergoing evaluation for suitability for submarine service.

43 The test likely to be given to a 42-year-old woman with a traumatic brain injury who is being evaluated for cognitive impairment

Questions 44–50

For questions 44–50 you will be required to select ONE ANSWER of the lettered organism or disease in the set that most likely causes the sexually transmitted disease in females numbered below.

(A) Herpes simplex virus-2 (HSV-2)
(B) *Neisseria gonorrhea*
(C) *Haemophilus ducreyi*
(D) *Chlamydia trachomatis* immunotypes D–K
(E) *Treponema pallidum*
(F) Granuloma inguinale
(G) Lymphogranuloma venereum (LGV)

44 A 28-year-old woman presents to the outpatient clinic with enlarged, mildly painful left inguinal lymph nodes. This was preceded two weeks ago by a painless, round vulvar ulcer that spontaneously disappeared. Examination reveals that she has a unilateral left-sided double genitocrural fold known as a "groove sign." These lymph nodes are tender to palpation with pus found on aspiration.

45 An 18-year-old female college student comes to the student health service complaining of diffuse, exquisitely painful vulvar lesions along with malaise and fever. She has one current boyfriend but she has a history of multiple sexual partners. Her temperature is 103.0°F (34.4°C). She has bilaterally enlarged and painful inguinal lymph nodes. Inspection of the external genitalia reveals multiple shallow, painful ulcers with smooth raised edges. They are diffusely located, involving her urethra, labia major, and labia minora as well as perineal body.

46 A 31-year-old woman presents to the outpatient office with a painless vulvar ulcer that has been present for 1 week. She is sexually active with a single male partner. She has been treated in the past for both gonorrhea and *Chlamydia* infections. For the past 5 years she has used combination oral contraceptive pills. Her temperature is normal, and her vital signs are stable. Examination reveals painless ulcers on her right labia majora as well as her right vaginal wall and cervix. The lesions are shallow, with sharply defined borders and slightly raised edges that are firm to the touch.

47 A 26-year-old woman presents to the out-patient clinic with painless right vulvar ulcerative lesions. She says that they started as small reddened "bumps" which developed into ulcers that bleed easily when they are touched. Examination reveals a group of elevated, "beefy red," coalescing, velvety nodules on her right labia that extend upward to the inguinal folds.

48 A 33-year-old woman presents to the emergency department with a painful right vulvar ulcerative le-

sion. It started as small flat lesion that elevated within 3–4 days to become a boil that broke and became a painful ulcer. The lesion is associated with pain with intercourse as well as pain with urination. Examination reveals a shallow, nonindurated, soft, painful ulcer with a "ragged" edge on the right vulva. She also has tender right inguinal lymph nodes.

49 A 22-year-old woman comes to the emergency department saying she feels feverish and for the past 1 to 2 days has had severe lower abdominal pain with nausea and vomiting. Her temperature upon admittance is 103.3°F (39.6°C). Examination reveals adnexal tenderness, a mucopurulent cervical discharge, and tenderness upon cervical motion. She says she has had unprotected intercourse with at least a dozen men since she left home at the age of 18 but never has contracted a sexually transmitted disease, a fact she attributes to her instinctive ability to only have relations with "clean" men.

50 A 16-year-old girl presents with frequent need to urinate, a burning sensation upon urinating, and the accompaniment of a purulent, mildly odorous urethral discharge. The symptoms started during her last menstrual period. She said that in her whole life she has only had sex once with the captain of her high school football team after he led the team to the conference championship. That event took place about the week before her period.

Answer Key

1	C	**11**	A	**21**	C	**31**	F	**41**	C
2	C	**12**	C	**22**	C	**32**	A	**42**	B
3	B	**13**	C	**23**	C	**33**	C	**43**	A
4	C	**14**	B	**24**	B	**34**	E	**44**	G
5	D	**15**	E	**25**	B	**35**	E	**45**	A
6	E	**16**	A	**26**	A	**36**	C	**46**	E
7	C	**17**	A	**27**	E	**37**	A	**47**	F
8	D	**18**	D	**28**	E	**38**	B	**48**	C
9	C	**19**	C	**29**	C	**39**	E	**49**	D
10	C	**20**	D	**30**	D	**40**	C	**50**	B

Answers and Explanations

1 **The answer is C** *Medicine*

The electrocardiogram (ECG) pattern shown indicates that this patient has hyperkalemia. It reveals tall, slender, tented T waves in leads I, II, aVF, and V_2 through V_6. Other findings suggesting hyperkalemia include a widened QRS complex and even biphasic QRS-T complexes. Although hyperkalemia produces these characteristic patterns, the ECG not a sensitive indicator of hyperkalemia, as almost 50% of patients with serum potassium levels above 6.5 mEq/L do not show any changes in the ECG pattern. This is because atrial cells are more sensitive to elevated levels of potassium than ventricular cells, permitting normal conduction even if atrial depolarization is inhibited; as a result, a junctional rhythm can result. To avoid dangerous arrhythmias and asystole, hyperkalemia above 6.5 mEq/L warrants immediate correction. In this case hyperkalemia also is suspected clinically because the patient has end-stage renal disease, has not been undergoing dialysis, and has a history of tiredness, vomiting, and abdominal pain. Hyperkalemia could, in addition, have caused motor paralysis. Calcium gluconate 10% (choice **C**) or 5% calcium chloride is the initial drug of choice. Approximately 5–30 mL of either administered intravenously provides calcium ion, which acts within minutes to antagonize cardiac conduction abnormalities; the effect lasts approximately an hour. In patients who are on digoxin, one must ensure that they do not have digoxin toxicity; if that were the case, calcium would only increase its toxic effects on the myocardium.

While administering calcium has a rapid effect, it does not promote the shift of potassium into the cells, consequently its effect is transitory. To secure a more permanent effect, one usually follows up with insulin and glucose (choice **D**). This drives potassium into the cells, thereby lowering serum potassium levels. Regular insulin (5–10 units) combined with 25 g of 50% glucose is administered intravenously. Insulin takes about 15 minutes to an hour to act, and the action lasts anywhere from 4 to 6 hours. Use of sodium bicarbonate (choice **A**) is an alternative to insulin plus glucose. It creates a metabolic alkalosis causing potassium ion to enter the cells in exchange for hydrogen ions. One or two ampules of sodium bicarbonate (approximately 44 mEq each) can be administered intravenously. Its effects begin in approximately 15–30 minutes and last anywhere from 1 to 2 hours. Thus, it is not as long lasting as insulin. The use of furosemide (choice **B**) is inappropriate in an emergency situation because it takes anywhere from 30 minutes to 2 hours to lower potassium levels, and one may very well not have the luxury of time. It is a loop diuretic that exchanges sodium for potassium, expelling the latter in the urine. Like loop diuretics, sodium polystyrene sulfonate in 20% sorbitol, a cation-exchange resin (choice **E**), may be used in nonemergency situations; 15–30 mL is administered orally or rectally. Potassium ions bind to the resin, lowering serum potassium levels. Due to the mode of administration, it takes much longer to act; its action lasts approximately 3 hours.

2 **The answer is C** *Psychiatry*

This patient's condition is most suggestive of delirium, possibly caused by analgesics or hypnotic medications. This reaction is relatively common in hospitalized older adults. In addition to treatment for the underlying cause, she should receive supportive measures, such as frequent interaction in a well-lighted room and help with orientation (choice **C**).

Darkness (choice **E**) and restraint (choice **B**) often further agitate delirious patients. Benzodiazepines (choice **D**) also can increase confusion, especially in the elderly. Guided imagery (choice **A**) or other cognitive tasks usually are nonproductive in treating delirium.

3 **The answer is B** *Medicine*

This patient has narcolepsy, a disorder in which there is excessive daytime sleepiness manifested as "sleep attacks" that can last from minutes to hours. It usually begins in the teens, and the severity plateaus by the time the patient is in the third decade of life, but unfortunately, this is a life-long disorder. It can be mistaken for epilepsy. Sometimes, children at school with this pathology are deemed "inattentive" and labeled as such. Four symptoms characterize narcolepsy:

First are sudden attacks of sleep that occur during any kind of activity (as manifested in this patient while she was driving).

Second, cataplexy, which is the sudden loss of skeletal muscle tone, either selective or generalized. This may lead to transient paralysis of arms, legs, and even the face and are often triggered by emotions such as sadness, fear, sexual desire, anger, or happiness.

Third, sleep paralysis, which is a flaccidity of muscle while the patient is fully conscious that occurs just before falling asleep or while the patient is waking up. This is the most terrifying symptom of all because the patient gets a feeling of sudden impending death.

Fourth; episodes of vivid visual or auditory hallucinations that manifest while falling asleep (hypnagogic) or at the time of awakening (hypnopompic). Visual hallucinations are usually described as someone coming into the room or having an out-of-body experience.

Hypnagogic hallucinations result from REM sleep that encroaches into the patient while still awake. Normally REM sleep does not occur until 90 minutes after initially falling asleep.

It is believed that patients with narcolepsy have a deficiency in the neurotransmitter hypocretin (aka orexin) that is essential for the waking state and is secreted by hypothalamic neurons. Diagnosis is confirmed by polysomnography that demonstrates shortened daytime sleep latency and a rapid transition to REM sleep (choice **B**).

Delayed sleep phase disorder (choice **A**) is common in teenagers and young adults who remain awake for longer hours during the night and compensate for this by getting up late. If they have to get up early, as for school, they may have episodes of somnolence. Delayed sleep phase disorder usually resolves with age. Advanced sleep phase disorder (choice **F**) occurs in the elderly, who sleep early and wake up early; the length of REM sleep also decreases with age. Episodic obstructive sleep apnea (choice **C**) leads to periods of apnea during sleep. As a result, the patient has increased sleepiness during the daytime. Obstruction is exacerbated by obesity, nasal obstruction, supine posture, hypothyroidism, alcoholism, and use of sedatives. It can result in hypertension, heart attack, congestive cardiac failure, and even a stroke. Periodic leg movement disorder (choice **D**), causes the limbs to jerk every 20 seconds or longer for several minutes or hours. It may be idiopathic or related to metabolic disorders, emphysema, rheumatoid arthritis, or medications. Most often the patient's bed partner is the first to notice this. The patient will complain of daytime drowsiness due to disturbed sleep. Non-rapid eye movement (REM) (choice **E**) is incorrect. There are two types of normal sleep. Non-REM, which has four levels based on EEG patterns and named I to IV, where I corresponds to the lightest and IV to the deepest level of sleep. During non-REM sleep, body tone is maintained, (unlike in REM sleep in which there is lack of tone in all muscles except the extraocular muscles and some muscles of the nasopharynx). It is during REM sleep that dreaming occurs, as if the eyes were following the visual images. Under normal circumstances, a person goes through at least one cycle of non-REM sleep (stages I to IV) before entering REM sleep. EEG recordings of REM sleep and stage I non-REM sleep are similar, and the only way in which these two can be distinguished is by placing EMG (electromyography) and ENG (electronystagmograph) leads—the latter to record the presence or absence of rapid conjugate ocular movements.

4 **The answer is C** *Medicine*

Dietary management is the initial step in lowering the serum LDL. LDL is the primary vehicle for carrying cholesterol. The recommended distribution of total caloric intake in a cholesterol-lowering diet is as follows: 50–60% carbohydrates; ≤30% fats (ideal is <25% with 10% monounsaturated fats), 10% polyunsaturated fats, 10% saturated fats), and 10–20% proteins (choice **C**). Cholesterol intake should be less than 300 mg/day, and fiber intake should be 20–30 g/day. Increasing the intake of soluble fiber (e.g., psyllium, oatmeal) is useful in lowering the cholesterol level. In addition to diet, the patient should exercise (e.g., fast walking). The patient does not have any major risk factors (i.e., history of ischemic heart disease, diabetes mellitus, or hypertension); therefore, the goal is to lower the serum LDL below 130 mg/dL. If any of the above risk factors are present, then the goal would an LDL below 100 mg/dL and, in some cases, below 70 mg/dL.

Restricting carbohydrate intake (choice **B**) decreases the synthesis of very-low-density lipoproteins (VLDLs) by the liver; therefore, decreasing the level of carbohydrate will not lower the patient's LDL. Drugs (choice **A**) are reserved for persons who do not reach their ideal LDL level by diet and exercise after a minimum of 6 months. Reducing stress (choice **D**) has no significant effect in lowering the LDL level. Exercise (choice **E**) is an important adjunct to a low-fat, high-fiber diet.

5 The answer is D   *Pediatrics*

A cellophane-tape preparation from the perianal area is used to detect the eggs of *Enterobius vermicularis* (pinworm) in a patient with complaints of anal pruritus (choice **D**). Enterobiasis is the most common worm infection in the gastrointestinal tract. Patients acquire the infection by ingestion of the embryonated eggs. Larvae develop in the lumen of the small intestine. The adult worms have a superficial attachment to the cecum and appendix. Because the attachment is superficial, there is no peripheral blood eosinophilia. At night, the females lay eggs in the perianal area, which causes intense itching (pruritus ani) and restless sleep. Pyrantel pamoate or mebendazole are the treatment options. All members of the family should be treated with the drug.

A cellophane-tape preparation is not used to diagnose rectal bleeding (e.g., internal hemorrhoids, choice **A**), pain on defecation (e.g., anal fissures, choice **B**), constipation (choice **C**), or increased mucus in the stool (e.g., irritable bowel syndrome, choice **E**).

6 The answer is E   *Psychiatry*

The insanity defense is based upon the legal principle that an individual commits a crime only when the action was intentional. The defense must prove that as a result of a mental illness, the defendant did not have an intention to commit the crime (choice **E**). There are three generally recognized ways a mental illness could interfere with intention: (1) it prevents the defendant from understanding that the action was illegal, (2) it prevents the defendant from being aware of his or her actions, and (3) it irresistibly forces the person to commit the crime. In this case, the defense would likely argue that the woman was irresistibly pushed by her delusions into making these threats.

Delusions (choice **A**) or other symptoms of mental illness alone do not establish lack of guilt. Inability to understand charges (choice **B**) may prevent an individual from standing trial but doesn't establish innocence. Ability to recognize the need for treatment (choice **C**) or not having access to treatment (choice **D**) might influence the severity of penalties but does not directly pertain to the issue of guilt.

7 The answer is C   *Pediatrics*

Alcohol is the most common major teratogen to which a fetus may be exposed. Even consumption of moderate levels of alcohol during early pregnancy may affect the growth and development of the fetus. However, the severity of fetal alcohol syndrome seems to correlate with the amount of alcohol ingested (i.e., the greater the intake, the more severe the signs). The prognosis and the pattern of malformation is predicted by the severity of maternal alcoholism. Findings include microcephaly, short palpebral fissures, maxillary hypoplasia (not hyperplasia [choice **A**]), early tremors from hypoglycemia, smooth upper lip, smooth philtrum, and cardiac defects (choice **C**) such as ventricular or atrial septal defects. These patients also have an average IQ of 63.

Hydrocephalus (choice **B**), macrognathia (choice **D**), and alopecia (choice **E**) are not associated with fetal alcohol syndrome.

8 The answer is D   *Surgery*

Laryngeal carcinomas are usually squamous celled and are most often seen in men. Some 70% of carcinomas of the larynx involve the glottic region, namely, the true vocal cords. Carcinomas involving the glottic fold (choice **D**) usually arise in the anterior half of one of the vocal cords. They are usually papillary and rarely ulcerative. Because of the paucity of lymphatics in this area, the tumor tends to be locally malignant for a long time, improving the prognosis. Such cancers usually occur in the fourth to sixth decades of life, and while cigarette smoking is a definite contributory factor, alcohol consumption is the most important risk. The initial and most frequent symptom is a change in voice—a huskiness that becomes progressive. Thereafter, the patient can barely whisper, until finally aphonia develops as the vocal cord becomes fixed.

Some 20% of laryngeal carcinomas involve the supraglottic region (choice **A**). Supraglottic carcinomas involve the false cords, laryngeal ventricles, or the base of the epiglottis. The first symptom is a sense of discomfort in the larynx. Pain and hoarseness of the voice are late features. In fact, the pain may be referred to the ears. These cancers metastasize early to the cervical lymph nodes, in fact, 60% of patients with supraglottic carcinoma have cervical lymphadenopathy at the time of presentation. Subglottic (choice **B**) laryngeal carcinomas together with carcinoma involving the hypopharynx (choice **E**) are the least common and consequently not the most likely location. Laryngeal carcinomas involving the subglottic area occur beneath the vocal folds, and the patient presents with difficulty in breathing. Metastasis occurs to the paratracheal and lower deep cervical nodes and even to the thyroid gland. The larynx (choice **C**) comprises the glottic, supraglottic, and infraglottic areas. Laryngeal carcinoma could be located in any one of these three regions. Hence, it does not describe a specific location, and choice **C** is not the best answer. Movement of the vocal cord can be visualized by indirect laryngoscopy, and endoscopic examination of the larynx can help diagnose the specific problem. Indirect laryngoscopy should be done in any patient who has hoarseness of the voice lasting more than 2 weeks. Laryngeal carcinomas involving the hypopharynx (choice **E**) affect the pyriform sinus, postcricoid area, and posterior pharyngeal wall. Postcricoid carcinoma has a female predominance. Women with Plummer-Vinson syndrome have a predilection for this condition. The patient presents with pain on swallowing and dysphagia. Metastasis to the cervical nodes bilaterally is usually noted. Treatment of laryngeal carcinoma ranges from irradiation to total laryngectomy. The latter is performed when the vocal cord is fixed, when irradiation has failed, or if there is a recurrence following irradiation and in patients with subglottic carcinoma or carcinoma involving the hypopharynx. Pathology within the superior mediastinum (choice **F**) can cause hoarseness of the voice due to pressure on the recurrent laryngeal nerve, as from an aneurysm of the arch of the aorta, around which the recurrent laryngeal nerve loops. However, there is no cervical lymphadenopathy.

9 | The answer is C *Medicine*

The patient has acute mercury poisoning (choice **C**). Mercury is still widely used today in a variety of compounds (e.g., thimerosal is used in merthiolate and in contact-lens cleaning solutions). Acute poisoning causes predominantly gastrointestinal and renal symptoms. Oral intake of mercury can cause stomatitis, abdominal pain, nausea and vomiting, and explosive, bloody diarrhea. Nephrotoxicity can lead to renal failure and death. Central nervous system (CNS) symptoms include ataxia, slurred speech, and visual and hearing impairment and are usually features of chronic mercury poisoning. Exposure to organic mercury derivatives such as dimethylmercury from contaminated fish or fungicides used on seeds also leads to CNS problems. Inhalation of mercury vapors can lead to acute fulminant chemical pneumonia. Treatment of acute mercury poisoning consists of correction of fluid and electrolyte imbalance and removal of mercury by gastric lavage. British antilewisite (BAL, dimercaprol) is the best therapy for mercury poisoning unless the patient has severe gastroenteritis, in which case succimer (DMSA) is preferred.

The features of iron poisoning (choice **D**) will depend on the amount that has been consumed. Ingestion of less than 30 mg/kg of elemental iron usually produces mild gastrointestinal symptoms. On the other hand, ingestion of iron above this—up to 60 mg/kg results in vomiting, hematemesis, diarrhea, hypotension, and metabolic acidosis. The hypotension results from its direct depressive effects on the myocardium and peripheral vascular resistance. Peritonitis due to intestinal perforation, and fulminant hepatitis could be fatal. Nephrotoxicity is not a feature of iron poisoning. Treatment includes aggressive management of hypotension, whole-bowel irrigation to remove unabsorbed iron tablets, and administration of polyethylene glycol-electrolyte solution via gastric tube until the rectal effluent is clear, and deferoxamine is used to treat symptomatic toxicity in which serum iron levels exceed 800 μg/dL. Activated charcoal does not help in the treatment of iron poisoning.

The effects of acute arsenic poisoning (choice **A**) usually occur about an hour after ingestion of the agent. Symptoms include skeletal muscle cramps, abdominal pain, watery diarrhea, and vomiting. Treatment includes gastric lavage and administration of activated charcoal. In those who have overdosed massively, BAL followed by oral penicillamine is useful.

Acute lead poisoning (choice **B**) usually presents with headache, abdominal pain, constipation, and, in severe cases, coma and convulsions. Chronic lead poisoning is usually seen in children, who develop learning disabilities or develop wrist drop. While lead-based paints are no longer used, lead poisoning can still occur in children if they were to swallow curtain weights or lead fishing weights. Treatment for acute lead poisoning is administration of activated charcoal. For severe intoxication manifested by encephalopathy or lead levels over 80 μg/dL, ethylenediaminetetraacetic acid (EDTA) and British antilewisite (BAL) are used in combination. For values below 80 μg/dL, EDTA alone would suffice. In children who have swallowed lead weights, removal by cathartics, endoscopy, or surgery may be required.

Selenium (choice **E**) is a required trace element but is toxic when ingested at too-high levels (the RDA for adults is 50–200 µg). Its demonstrated function is as a cofactor for glutathione reductase, consequently it contributes to a wide range of antioxidant functions including anticancer activity and protection against poisoning by several metals including mercury. Intake of toxic quantities causes the breath to have a garlicky odor in the absences of garlic ingestion, hair loss, skin depigmentation, abnormal nail growth, and profound fatigue.

10 The answer is C   *Surgery*

The patient most likely has a papillary carcinoma (choice **C**) of the thyroid secondary to radiation exposure. Thyroid carcinoma represents approximately 1% of all malignancies. Females are twice as likely as males to develop the disease. It is rare in children and frequency increases with age. Carcinoma of the thyroid is rarely detectable clinically. Papillary adenocarcinoma is the most common malignant tumor of the thyroid gland (85% of all thyroid malignancies). It usually affects young individuals and presents as a firm-to-hard, non-tender, solitary nodule that contains psammoma bodies. Thyroid-stimulating hormone (TSH) tends to promote its growth. Spread is via lymphatics to the regional nodes. Most patients have palpable nodes at the time of initial presentation. Distant metastasis usually strikes the lungs or bone. Fine-needle aspiration is the most accurate diagnostic screening procedure available to distinguish between a benign and malignant thyroid nodule. It is the preliminary diagnostic step in the investigation of a thyroid nodule. Results of fine-needle biopsy are usually reported as benign, suspicious, or malignant. The surgical treatment for papillary adenocarcinoma that is greater than 1.5 cm in size is total thyroidectomy followed by ablation with radioactive iodine. Use of radioactive iodine after surgery permits identification and treatment of occult or apparent local or distant metastasis. It is important to perform a total thyroidectomy, because residual normal thyroid tissue has a greater avidity for radioactive iodine than do metastatic deposits. The recurrence rate after total thyroidectomy is half that of subtotal thyroidectomy (10% as opposed to 20%). For tumors that are less than 1.5 cm, lobectomy or near-total thyroidectomy (ipsilateral total lobectomy and contralateral subtotal lobectomy) are available options. However, after lobectomy there is a recurrence rate of 7%, which is unacceptable because 50% of patients with recurrent thyroid carcinoma die as a result of the illness.

Medullary carcinoma (choice **A**) is rare (5–10% of thyroid malignancies). The tumor is hard and nodular, and it contains amyloid-like material. It secretes calcitonin, corticotropin, prostaglandins, melanin, and serotonin. While 80% of the tumors are solitary and sporadic, 20% are familial and associated with bilateral pheochromocytoma and hyperparathyroidism; namely, multiple endocrine neoplasia (MEN) types 2A and 2B. Familial forms are bilateral and usually precede the onset of associated pathology. Patients with metastatic medullary carcinoma of the thyroid have increased levels of carcinoembryonic antigen (CEA). There is no association with previous radiation exposure. Undifferentiated carcinoma (choice **B**) is even less common than medullary carcinoma (<5% of thyroid malignancies). It is usually seen in older individuals (about 70 years of age) and is especially common in areas where iodine deficiency is prevalent. In addition, patients may have a history of a goiter. It is the most rapidly growing of all thyroid malignancies, and it is undifferentiated (i.e., anaplastic). The tumor may be painful and tender. It invades the trachea and neurovascular structures early in its course, necessitating a tracheostomy in some cases. In most cases, metastasis is to the regional lymph nodes, while in a minority of cases, it is distant, particularly to the lungs. This tumor should be differentiated from primary malignant lymphoma. There is no association with radiation exposure. Follicular carcinoma (choice **D**) represents approximately 10% of malignant tumors of the thyroid gland. The incidence of this tumor is decreasing in the United States because of adequate intake of iodine in the diet (e.g., iodized salt). The tumor usually occurs after the fifth decade. It presents as a solitary nodule, varying in consistency from soft to rubbery. It is usually encapsulated and histologically may be mistaken for normal tissue because of the presence of colloid. Unlike a follicular adenoma, which is benign, follicular adenocarcinoma invades vascular structures. Unlike other malignant tumors of the thyroid gland that favor lymphatic spread, metastases from a primary follicular adenocarcinoma preferentially use the hematogenous route; consequently, they spread to the lungs, liver, central nervous system, and bones. Metastases may appear two decades later. The incidence for distant metastasis is greater than 30%, while that for lymphatic spread is less than 10%. Because of its propensity to disseminate by blood, the prognosis is not as good as that of papillary adenocarcinomas. There is no association with radiation exposure. Primary malignant lymphoma (choice **E**) is an extremely rare tumor. It usually occurs in older women and grows rapidly. The tumor is nontender and firm to touch. There is usually a history of chronic lymphocytic thyroiditis. It has to be differentiated from undifferentiated thyroid carcinoma, because the prognosis after treatment is better for primary malignant lymphomas than for undifferentiated thyroid carcinomas. There is no association with radiation exposure.

11 The answer is A *Pediatrics*

The child has Down syndrome (epicanthal folds, flat nasal bridge, simian creases). The presence of 46 chromosomes in the child indicates that a translocated chromosome (choice **A**), inherited from one of the parents, is responsible. Translocation occurs when one part of a chromosome is transferred to a nonhomologous chromosome. In balanced (robertsonian) translocation, the translocated fragment is functional. In this case, the long arm of chromosome 21 was translocated onto chromosome 14 in the mother, creating one long chromosome (14:21 chromosome). The translocated chromosome was inherited by the child as a second chromosome 14 that functions as a third chromosome 21.

In a frameshift mutation (choice **B**), nucleotides are inserted into or deleted from a DNA strand, resulting in synthesis of an abnormal protein product (e.g., Tay-Sachs disease). Frameshift mutations do not produce chromosomal alterations. Microdeletion (choice **C**) involves the loss of a small portion of one chromosome, which can be detected only by high-resolution techniques. It is not a cause of Down syndrome. Nondisjunction (choice **D**) refers to unequal separation of chromosomes in the first meiotic phase, resulting in an egg or a sperm with 22 or 24 chromosomes. Nondisjunction is responsible for most numeric chromosome disorders (e.g., trisomy 21), but because this patient has 46 chromosomes, a different type of mutation (a balanced translocation) is responsible. A point mutation (choice **E**) involves the substitution of a single nucleotide base. It is not a cause of Down syndrome.

12 The answer is C *Surgery*

The patient has a fissure in ano (choice **C**). Anal fissures are due to trauma from hard, large-caliber stool. These patients usually complain of severe pain while defecating, with specks of bright red blood in the stool. Pain lasts for some time after defecation. Most anal fissures are located in the posterior aspect of the anal canal. In women, they may be located anteriorly instead. Tear of the squamous epithelium that is rich in pain fibers, results in painful defecation. A tear of the anal sphincter causes it to go into spasm, and digital examination is very painful. Furthermore, fear of pain leads to further constipation, as the patient tries to avoid defecation. In such cases, there may be tenderness on abdominal palpation in the left lower flank due to a loaded distended colon, as was the case in this patient. A skin tag or sentinel pile may be associated with it. The presence of a fissure in ano should prompt one to exclude the presence of sexually transmitted diseases, hidradenitis suppurativa, and Crohn's disease. Treatment includes stool softeners, high-fiber diet including fruits and vegetables, psyllium powder, emollient suppositories, and sitz baths. In refractory cases, lateral internal sphincterotomy should be carried out. Any fissure that fails to heal should have a biopsy.

Hemorrhoids are dilated venous plexuses in the mucosa and submucosa. Internal hemorrhoids (choice **A**) are due to dilatation of the superior hemorrhoidal veins, are located proximal to the dentate line, and are covered by mucosa. They result from straining at stool, pregnancy, or portal hypertension. Patients usually complain of pruritus in the anal area, discomfort, and painless rectal bleeding that is bright red. The blood comes out in spurts and may be very alarming to the patient. As time progresses, the hemorrhoid may prolapse to the exterior and regress spontaneously or may have to be pushed back. Internal hemorrhoids cannot be palpated on digital examination unless they are thrombosed. They can be observed on anoscopy. Pain occurs in the event that the hemorrhoid gets thrombosed. Initial management involves a high-fiber diet and use of hydrophilic colloids. Surgical options include rubber band ligation, infrared coagulation, sclerotherapy, and, if the hemorrhoid has prolapsed or cannot be reduced, hemorrhoidectomy.

External hemorrhoids (choice **B**) are of differing kinds. An external hemorrhoid could be thrombosed, it could be associated with internal hemorrhoids, or it could be a sentinel pile that is usually associated with an anal fissure as described above. A thrombosed external hemorrhoid is also known as a perianal hematoma. It appears suddenly and is exceedingly painful. Examination reveals a tense, dark bluish, tender swelling in the perianal area. If seen early, it can be incised and drained; otherwise, it resolves spontaneously or undergoes fibrosis. An external hemorrhoid that is associated with an internal hemorrhoid is basically a hemorrhoid that is located between the dentate line and anal margin. It is covered by skin instead of mucosa. Through the skin, blue superior hemorrhoidal veins can be seen. Very rarely, instead of a vein, the skin may cover a branch of the superior rectal artery, in which case it is known as an arterial pile and could lead to rather alarming bleeding at surgery.

Solitary rectal ulcer (choice **D**) is being diagnosed more often nowadays. It is usually located on the anterior wall of the rectum and should be differentiated from carcinoma of the rectum or inflammatory bowel disease such as Crohn's. The ulcer may not be solitary in some cases. It has been associated with internal intussusception and anterior rectal wall prolapse. Pain occurs on defecation, and massive lower gastrointestinal bleeding may be an added feature. A sentinel pile is absent. Internal prolapse can be prevented by abdominal rectopexy.

Proctitis due to ulcerative colitis (choice **E**) is usually an ulcerative proctocolitis in which the rectal mucosa is inflamed in addition to that of the colon. The inflammation could be acute or chronic. In acute cases, the patient will have fever and swelling and tenderness on digital examination of the rectal mucosa. Patients usually have tenesmus, accompanied by blood and mucus in their stool. Sometimes pus is present as well. Other causes of proctitis include infection due to *Clostridium difficile*, bacillary dysentery, amebic dysentery, gonococcal infection following anal intercourse, and primary syphilis (in which the patient has a painless anal fissure). Proctitis due to Crohn's disease is extremely rare. It is not associated with a skin tag/sentinel pile.

A fistula in ano (choice **F**) usually presents as an acute abscess or a draining sinus that irritates the perineal skin. Subcutaneous induration may be felt from the draining sinus to the anal margin. Digital examination is not painful and usually reveals a palpable nodule in the anal wall. An external skin tag is not found, nor is rectal bleeding a feature.

13 The answer is C   *Medicine*

This patient has mild Alzheimer's dementia. Neuropsychologic testing with the Mini-Mental Status Examination (MMSE) is the most sensitive generally available tool for the early diagnosis of Alzheimer's disease. Recently, positron emission tomography (PET) scan has been found to be more sensitive as a predictor of Alzheimer's disease but still is not widely used. The MMSE detects difficulties that the patient may encounter with memory, orientation, language, visuospatial dexterity, and problem-solving ability. The score ranges from 0 to 30. As the disease progresses, new difficulties are added onto the older ones, as will be apparent from the explanation below. A person with mild Alzheimer's dementia will have disorientation to date only, some difficulty naming objects, impaired recall, irritability, apathy, and problems with paying bills or doing simple math. The scores in these patients will fall between 21 and 30 (choice **C**).

A person with moderate Alzheimer's dementia will score between 11 and 20 (choice **B**). These patients will additionally develop disorientation to time and place, trouble with comprehension, and get lost in areas that they are familiar with (e.g., within the confines of their own home). Other features include Wernicke's aphasia, poor judgment and recall, and difficulty with activities of daily living such as shopping and cooking. Behavioral problems such as aggression and problems with sleep are other features. Patients with severe Alzheimer's dementia will score between 1 and 10 (choice **A**). They cannot use the language in a fitting manner. They get lost easily and have problems with activities of daily living such as bathing, dressing, and using the toilet, requiring assistance for these. It is important to emphasize that these patients do not have motor paralysis or weakness; they have apraxia, that is, an inability to perform motor functions in the absence of motor paralysis or paresis. As time goes on, the patient's behavior deteriorates further. In addition, fecal and urinary incontinence ensue, and the patient becomes mute. Choices **D** and **E** are incorrect because the MMSE score ranges only from 0 to 30.

14 The answer is B   *Preventive Medicine and Public Health*

Historically, cessation of discernible cardiac function was considered the legal definition of death. However, as newer techniques of resuscitation were developed, more and more persons came back to life after death as defined by cardiac function, a remote possibility that had been found worrisome during earlier times. Accordingly, in 1965 the term "brain death," was coined and has become the legal definition of death in the United States. Therefore, this patient is legally dead, and life support can be removed (choice **B**) not continued indefinitely (choice **E**).

Unless the physician has documentation (written or verbal) that this patient wished to donate his organs after death (there is a form on the back of driver's licenses in some states), his organs cannot be harvested (choice **A** and **D**). No individual without a durable power of attorney, including a wife, can give permission for donation of the organs of another adult (choice **C**). A family member or friend can, however, relay verbally that the patient stated that he did or did not want to donate his organs after death (the substituted judgment standard).

15 The answer is E   *Medicine*

This patient has acute left ventricular failure secondary to untreated hypertension. As a result he has pulmonary edema, which explains the respiratory findings. Normally in adults, only two heart sounds are heard, S_1 and S_2. The S_3 sound (choice **E**) is an added low-pitched sound that is normal in children, but in adults over the age of 30, it signifies left ventricular failure or volume overload.

A loud first heart sound, namely S_1 (choice **A**), is usually heard in mitral stenosis. The second heart sound, S_2 is composed of two sounds—aortic (A_2) and pulmonary (P_2). A fixed splitting of S_2 (choice **B**) is usually heard in atrial septal defects. A soft A_2 (choice **C**) is usually found in aortic stenosis, while a loud P_2 (choice **D**) is found in pulmonary arterial hypertension. A widened splitting of the S_2 (choice **F**) is usually found in right bundle-branch block, pulmonary stenosis, and mitral valve regurgitation. A fourth heart sound, S_4 (choice **G**), is an extra sound usually present in patients with hypertension, hypertrophic cardiomyopathy, aortic stenosis, and coronary artery disease. In view of the hypertension that this patient has, it is likely that he has an S_4, (not an absent one) and a loud A_2 (not soft) in addition to an S_3.

16 The answer is A   *Preventive Medicine and Public Health*

The incidence of cervical carcinoma has markedly decreased because of the increased use of the cervical Pap smear (choice **A**). This screening test can detect squamous dysplasia, the precursor lesion for squamous cell carcinoma. Colposcopy is used to identify the dysplastic site, which is then surgically removed. Cervical cancer is the least common of the gynecologic cancers (endometrial, ovarian, cervical, in order of decreasing incidence).

There has been a slight decline in the incidence of breast cancer because of annual clinical breast examinations (choice **B**) and mammography (choice **D**). However, breast cancer remains the most common cancer in women. There has been a slight decline in the incidence of colorectal cancer because of screening with stool guaiac (detects blood in stool; choice **E**) and flexible sigmoidoscopy (choice **C**). However, colorectal carcinoma remains the second most common cancer in adults.

17 The answer is A   *Medicine*

The patient has orthostatic (postural) proteinuria, which is a type of functional proteinuria (choice **A**) that is not associated with an underlying renal disease. In orthostatic proteinuria, proteinuria occurs after standing or walking and is absent after having been in the recumbent state (e.g., first morning void). It occurs in 15–20% of healthy young male adults. Glomerular proteinuria (choice **B**) is associated with a loss of protein ranging from 150 mg/24 hours to more than 3 g/24 hours. It is subdivided into selective and nonselective proteinuria. Selective proteinuria refers to a loss of albumin and not globulins. It is due to loss of the negative charge in the glomerular basement membrane (e.g., nephrotic syndrome caused by lipoid nephrosis). Nonselective proteinuria refers to the loss of plasma proteins (e.g., albumin and globulins) in urine. It is due to damage of the glomerular basement membrane (e.g., poststreptococcal glomerulonephritis). Glomerular proteinuria is unlikely in this patient, because his proteinuria disappeared after reclining, and no abnormal casts are present in the urine (e.g., RBC or fatty casts). In overflow proteinuria (choice **C**), the protein loss is variable (0.2 to >10g/24 hours). It is a low-molecular-weight proteinuria in which the amount filtered exceeds the tubular capacity to reabsorb it (e.g., Bence Jones proteinuria, hemoglobinuria, myoglobinuria). Overflow proteinuria is unlikely in this patient, because the proteinuria disappeared after reclining. Tubular proteinuria (choice **D**) is associated with a protein loss < 2 g/24 hours. It is due to a defect in proximal tubule reabsorption of low molecular weight proteins (e.g., microglobulin, amino acids) at normal filtered loads (e.g., heavy metal poisoning, Hartnup's disease). Tubular proteinuria is unlikely in this patient, because proteinuria disappeared after reclining. A laboratory error (choice **E**) is incorrect. The several samples of urine that were tested turned out to be negative for protein because they were taken in the morning. On the other hand, one test with positive results was obviously from a sample of urine taken later during the day. If it were a laboratory error, the morning sample of urine tested the second time around would have had positive, not negative, results, as it did the first time on several samples.

18 **The answer is D** *Pediatrics*

The patient has Hirschsprung's disease (congenital megacolon, choice **D**), which is the most common cause of lower intestinal obstruction in neonates. The most common manifestation is failure to pass meconium within the first 24 hours after birth. There are no ganglion cells in both the Meissner submucosal and the Auerbach myenteric plexuses. In 75% of cases, the rectosigmoid is aganglionic. Characteristic findings include a narrow anal canal, absence of stool in the rectal vault, and an abdominal radiograph showing distended loops of colon. Peristalsis occurs in segments of colon that do contain ganglion cells. In 3% of cases, there is an association with Down syndrome.

Anorectal malformations (choice **A**) are uncommon in newborns. Malformations include imperforate anal membrane, anal stenosis, anal agenesis (association with tracheoesophageal fistulas), rectal agenesis, and rectal atresia. There is a high association with vertebral and genitourinary abnormalities and no association with Down syndrome. Enterocolitis (choice **B**), which is the most common complication of Hirschsprung's disease, is a type of ischemic necrosis related to increased intraluminal pressure and decreased intramural capillary blood flow. Presenting signs include fever and bloody diarrhea. These findings are not present in this patient. Functional constipation (choice **C**) is a type of chronic retentive constipation. Meconium passes within the first 24 hours of life, the anal canal is dilated, and palpable stool is present in the rectal vault. Most congenital malrotations (choice **E**) involve the small intestine and present with bloody stools.

19 **The answer is C** *Medicine*

The patient has acute gouty arthritis (inflamed metatarsophalangeal joint in the great toe). In gout, there is deposition of needle-shaped monosodium urate (MSU) crystals in the joint. Negatively birefringent MSU crystals are phagocytosed by neutrophils (choice **C**), which causes them to release inflammatory mediators, leading to inflammation of synovial tissue. Negative birefringence is defined by color changes in the crystals that occur when they are examined under a microscope with compensated polarized light. MSU crystals are yellow when they are aligned parallel to the slow ray of the compensator in the microscope. A synovial tap must be performed to confirm the diagnosis of gout, because hyperuricemia is not always present in acute attacks. Excess alcohol intake frequently precipitates acute gouty arthritis, because products of alcohol metabolism lead to underexcretion of uric acid by the kidneys. Most cases of gout are due to underexcretion of uric acid rather than overproduction of uric acid; hence, uricosuric agents like probenecid are more likely to be used in the treatment of gout once the inflammation in the joint is relieved by indomethacin.

Septic arthritis due to *Neisseria gonorrhoeae*, a gram-negative diplococcus (choice **A**), usually involves the knee. In addition, tenosynovitis and pustules involving the wrists and ankles may also occur. Disseminated gonococcemia is more likely to occur in patients who are deficient in complement components C6 to C9. These components are necessary to phagocytose the organism. *Staphylococcus aureus*, a gram-positive coccus (choice **B**), is the most common nongonococcal cause of septic arthritis. Both the history of alcohol abuse and the location of the inflammatory arthritis in the great toe exclude the diagnosis of septic arthritis. Calcium pyrophosphate crystals have positive birefringence (choice **D**). The crystals are either needle shaped or rhomboid. Under compensated polarized light, the crystals are blue when aligned parallel to the slow ray of the compensator. Arthropathy associated with these crystals usually involves the knee. Neutrophils with phagocytosed rheumatoid factor immunocomplexes (choice **E**) are called ragocytes. Rheumatoid arthritis does not specifically involve the metatarsophalangeal joint of the great toe.

20 **The answer is D** *Medicine*

This patient is suffering from cluster headaches, which often strike young men in the nocturnal hours. Oxygen in a high concentration is a vasoconstrictor and can abort many cluster headaches (choice **D**). Both nitroglycerin (choice **A**) and alcohol (choice **B**) are vasodilators and may worsen vascular headaches. Exercise (choice **C**) and a warm pack (choice **E**) may distract the sufferer but do nothing to end the underlying cluster attacks.

21 **The answer is C** *Psychiatry*

This case is most suggestive of separation anxiety disorder. Separation anxiety disorder is characterized by worry about being separated, resistance to impending separation, and anxiety after separation. School avoidance is often present in children with this disorder. A history of this disorder in childhood is common in adult patients with panic disorder (choice **C**).

Schizophrenia (choice **D**) is sometimes associated with a history of emotional withdrawal during childhood. Dysthymic disorder (choice **A**), obsessive–compulsive personality disorder (choice **B**), and pain disorder (choice **E**) are not clearly associated with a childhood history of separation disorder.

22 The answer is C *Surgery*

Compression of the median nerve can take place at various sites en route to the hand. The most common location for compression is at the wrist as the nerve traverses under the transverse carpal ligament together with the tendons of the flexor muscles. The resulting condition is known as carpal tunnel syndrome (choice **C**). It most commonly affects women between the fourth and sixth decades of life. It is often unilateral but may be bilateral. It can result from repeated local trauma, displaced Colles' fracture, dislocated lunate, conditions that promote fluid retention (e.g., myxedema, renal failure, pregnancy), and amyloidosis or Raynaud's phenomenon. In young, active individuals, the most common cause for carpal tunnel syndrome is compression of the median nerve by aberrantly placed muscle bellies of the palmaris longus or flexor digitorum profundus during repetitive movement. In the initial stages, carpal tunnel syndrome causes numbness and a burning sensation in the hand. This is followed by paresthesias (sensation of pins and needles) of the thumb, index finger, and middle finger. In the initial stages, the thumb is spared. The symptoms usually occur during the night or in the early hours of the morning, and they awaken the patient. All of these symptoms are intermittent. Shaking the hand, elevating it, or even immersing it in hot water often relieves pain. Sometimes the pain ascends up the arm, suggesting proximal pathology (e.g., cervical radiculopathy). Weakness of the muscles of the thumb and the first two lumbricals results in clumsiness of the hand. The first muscle to be weakened is the abductor pollicis brevis, as the median nerve innervates it exclusively. Cyanosis is surprisingly common in patients with carpal tunnel syndrome. In the initial stages, there are no physical signs to support the patient's complaints. In such cases, they may be misdiagnosed as suffering from anxiety neurosis. The diagnosis of carpal tunnel syndrome is made by the typical history of nocturnal paresthesias, painful numbness and tingling, reproduction of symptoms by sustained flexion or extension of the wrist, relief of symptoms by neutralizing the wrist in a neutral position, objective sensory and motor loss, and delayed nerve conduction on electromyogram (EMG) studies. Tinel's sign, in which symptoms are reproduced when the median nerve is percussed at the wrist, is unreliable because it is infrequently positive in patients with carpal tunnel syndrome. One should not wait for the development of objective sensory and motor dysfunction before making a diagnosis. Although sensory symptoms can be relieved, recovery of motor function is variable.

Cervical radiculopathy (choice **A**) is usually seen in patients between 40 and 70 years of age and is most often due to degenerative disease involving the cervical vertebrae, intervertebral canals, or the disk. The onset of pain is insidious, although the patient may give a history of antecedent trauma or periods of neck stiffness. The patient will complain of neck pain and soreness that extends to the scapular and interscapular area. Paresthesias may accompany the pain and may be described as tingling, coldness, burning, or the limb "going to sleep." Physical examination reveals limited cervical spine movement.

Thoracic outlet syndrome (choice **B**) is most commonly seen in young to middle-aged women, especially those who are obese. The term includes outlet narrowing due to a cervical rib, compression due to aberration in the scalene muscles, fractures of the first rib or clavicle with deformity or callus formation narrowing the thoracic outlet, and tumors at the outlet (rare). Symptoms are variable, and the condition can cause compression of the neural or vascular structures, or both. Compression of the lower cord results in paresthesias of the ring and little fingers, weakness of the hypothenar muscles, or even atrophy. Compression of the upper cord results in pain in the chest, neck, mandible, face, and temporal and occipital areas of the head. Compression of the subclavian artery could result in poststenotic dilatation and aneurysmal formation.

Pronator teres syndrome (choice **D**) is an important differential diagnosis to carpal tunnel syndrome. The median nerve traverses between the two heads of the pronator teres muscle, at which point it can be compressed and simulate carpal tunnel syndrome. A key differentiating physical finding between the two conditions is that sensations are impaired in the thenar eminence in the case of pronator teres syndrome, whereas they are diminished on the flexor surface of the thumb, index finger, and middle finger in carpal tunnel syndrome.

The hallmark of Raynaud's phenomenon (choice **E**) is episodic vasospasm, which constricts the small arteries and arterioles in the distal parts of the extremities in response to exposure to cold or emotional stress. The patient's fingers become blue for short periods of time. A variety of disorders are associated with Raynaud's phenomenon, including scleroderma, systemic lupus erythematosus, rheumatoid arthritis, dermatomyositis, and Sjögren's syndrome. Almost 20% of patients with carpal tunnel syndrome have associated Raynaud's phenomenon.

23 **The answer is C** *Medicine*

This patient has developed a compression fracture of the vertebra (choice **C**). She probably has osteoporosis, which makes it possible for a compression fracture to occur. Sudden onset of pain that radiates to the front of the abdomen like a belt is a characteristic presentation. This, together with tenderness in the vertebra to palpation, should suggest the diagnosis. Additional features include neurologic deficits secondary to spinal cord compression. The sensory deficits in the legs of this patient and the absent ankle jerks are due to diabetic neuropathy.

A spinal cord tumor (choice **A**) is usually associated with chronic pain, and there may be tenderness on palpation of the vertebra. Clonus has to be sustained to be pathologic and signifies involvement of the corticospinal pathway. Thus, there are no neurologic findings in this patient to support a spinal cord tumor. An epidural abscess (choice **B**) can present with pain over a few days and tenderness in the spine, together with pyrexia, which is absent in this patient. Furthermore, the patient may have neurologic deficits as well. A posterolateral lumbar disk herniation (choice **D**) is associated with radicular pain (i.e., pain going down one lower extremity) together with sensory loss over the distribution of the appropriate dermatome in the leg. There may be motor weakness, either weak dorsiflexion or weak plantar flexion of the appropriate foot, depending on which nerve root is involved. No spinal tenderness will be elicited. A central lumbar disk herniation (choice **E**) is associated with saddle anesthesia and an absent or weakened anal wink reflex, or weakness of the lower extremity with partial saddle anesthesia. The former is due to involvement of the conus medullaris, while the latter is due to involvement of the cauda equina. In neither case will there be tenderness of the vertebral spine.

24 **The answer is B** *Medicine*

The aminoglycosides are large family of bactericidal antibiotics with a similar spectrum of antimicrobial activities and analogous pharmaceutical and toxic characteristics. They act by binding to the 30S ribosomal subunit of sensitive bacteria, inhibiting protein synthesis. Because they cannot be administered orally and because of their toxicity, their use is generally reserved for treatment of gram-negative bacteria resistant to other antibiotics or they are used in low concentration with other antibiotics to create a synergistic effect. Use of an aminoglycoside is associated with potential ototoxicity and nephrotoxicity. The nephrotoxicity causes tubular wasting of Mg^{2+} (choice **B**) into the urine, leading to a functional hypomagnesemia. Loss in the feces caused by overgrowth with *Clostridium difficile* also may contribute to the deficiency of Mg^{2+}. Like K^+, only a small fraction of the total body stores of magnesium is found in the serum, thus measurement of serum levels can be misleading. Approximately 60% of the body's total magnesium store is associated with bone, 38% is intracellular, and the remainder is in the extracellular compartment. That remaining 1–2% is equal to 1.8–3.0 mEq/L, and about one third of this is bound to protein, mainly albumin. It has been estimated that the prevalence of magnesium depletion in the general public is about 2% but may be as high as 60% in hospitalized patients in whom depletion may not show up as hypomagnesemia because such a small fraction is normally found in the extracellular fluid (ECF). Although normally there is very little of it, free Mg^{2+} is a required cofactor for hundreds if not thousands of reactions, including all the kinase reactions, as well as many hormonal, transport, and other functions. Magnesium depletion may be expressed clinically by weakness, muscle cramps, tremor, neuromuscular and central nervous system hyperirritability, with tremors, jerking, nystagmus, and a positive Babinski response. There also may be hypertension, tachycardia, and ventricular arrhythmias as well as confusion and disorientation. This patient's primary symptoms (e.g., thumb adduction into the palm with blood pressure measurements [Trousseau's sign]) and contraction of the muscles around the mouth caused by tapping of the facial nerve (Chvostek sign) suggest hypocalcemia (not provided as a potential choice). This is due to the involvement of magnesium ion in calcium metabolism, where it is required for the activation, synthesis, and release of parathyroid hormone (PTH). Magnesium depletion may then produce hypoparathyroidism with a concomitant decrease in the total serum calcium concentration including the metabolically active ionized calcium concentration. This produces tetany by lowering the threshold potential (Et) for muscle and nerves so that it is closer to the resting membrane potential (Em). Therefore, the muscles and nerves are hyperirritable in a partially depolarized state and are subject to the clinical findings of tetany.

Chloride (choice **A**) is involved in neuromuscular excitability; however, deficiency does not result in tetany. Phosphate (choice **C**) is an important component of ATP. Hypophosphatemia results in muscle weakness, often leading to paralysis and rhabdomyolysis (rupture of muscle), but does not induce tetany. Potassium (choice **D**) is involved in neuromuscular excitability; however, when it is decreased, patients develop muscle weakness rather than signs of tetany. Sodium (choice **E**) is involved in neuromuscular excitability; however, when it is decreased, muscle cramping results rather than signs of tetany.

25 The answer is B   *Psychiatry*

The psychotherapeutic exploration of unconscious conflict is a component of psychodynamic psychotherapy, a form of treatment that is often effective for patients with the chronic depression seen in dysthymic disorder (choice **B**). The response rate for antidepressants in this disorder is only about 30%.

Enuresis (choice **C**) and obsessive–compulsive disorder (choice **D**) respond best to behavioral therapies combined with antidepressant medications. Successful treatment of bipolar disorder (choice **A**) necessitates mood-stabilizing medication. Treatment of schizophrenia (choice **E**) usually necessitates antipsychotic medication and social therapies.

26 The answer is A   *Pediatrics*

Cerebral concussion is a common head injury seen in children. The patient gives a history of brief (seconds to minutes) unconsciousness, then normal arousal. Disturbance of vision and equilibrium may occur with cerebral concussion. There are three grades of concussion:

Grade I—the patient has confusion, but no amnesia, and no loss of consciousness
Grade II—the patient has confusion and amnesia, but no loss of consciousness
Grade III—the patient has confusion, amnesia, and loss of consciousness

The patient in this scenario has a grade I concussion. He has confusion but no amnesia and no loss of consciousness. Recommendations for returning to play in contact sports (including practice) after a concussion are as follows: a patient with grade I concussion, if asymptomatic, may return to contact sports in 20 minutes (choice **A**). A patient with grade II concussion, if asymptomatic for 1 week may return to contact sports in 1 week (choice **B**). A patient with grade III concussion if asymptomatic for 1 week may return to contact sports in 1 month (choice **C**). A patient with a second-time grade I concussion may return to play contact sports in 2 weeks after being asymptomatic for 1 week (choice **D**). A patient with a second-time grade II concussion may return to play contact sports in 1 month after being asymptomatic for 1 week. However, if the patient has repeated concussions after contact sports, grade I (×3), grade II (×2), grade III (×2), then it should be recommended that the season is over (choice **E**).

27 The answer is E   *Preventive Medicine and Public Health*

Most states have laws that emancipate minors over the age if 14 years from parental control provided they meet certain criteria. These criteria include marriage, demonstration that they are fully self-supporting, or demonstration that they are members of an armed service. Such emancipation permits self-consent for medical procedures as well as the ability to engage in various legal transactions. Despite his immature engagement in drag racing, this 16-year-old has earned adult rights including the legal right to give consent for a medical procedure himself (choice **E**) because he is married and self-supporting.

Consequently, the approval of one (choice **A**) or both parents (choice **C**) is not required. A spouse never can give consent (choice **B**). A court-appointed guardian can give consent for an incompetent person as decided by the court (choice **D**).

28 The answer is E   *Surgery*

Baker's cyst (choice **E**) is usually an inflammation involving the posterior bursa of the knee. Typically, the patient has pain and discomfort behind the knee while walking, because contraction of the quadriceps muscle squeezes the suprapatellar bursa, forcing the synovial fluid posteriorly into the cyst. The pain also increases during activities such as repetitive squatting and is relieved by rest. A tender cystic swelling can be palpated when the patient is standing. It is differentiated from a popliteal artery aneurysm by its nonpulsatile nature. Pretibial pitting edema is usually absent, but in the presence of large cysts, such pitting may result from compression of the popliteal vein. Most Baker's cysts (85%) communicate directly with the knee joint. In most patients there is an underlying disease of the knee (e.g., degenerative arthritis, rheumatoid arthritis, tears of the menisci or cruciate ligaments). Thus, resolution of the problem requires addressing the primary cause.

In sciatic radiculopathy (choice **A**), there is usually a history of previous back pain or injury. The pain is not localized and radiates from the posterior thigh down to the knee or foot. The patient may have weakness on dorsiflexion or plantar flexion, depending on the nerve root involved, and the deep tendon reflexes may be depressed or absent at the ankle. Calf muscle hematoma (choice **B**) is usually preceded by a history of trauma due to excessive muscular strain (e.g., during running). There is localized swelling and tenderness. Ecchymosis may be present over the skin. Superficial thrombophlebitis (choice **C**) is usually associated with varicose veins, local bacterial infection, or catheter placement. Features of this condition are pain in the leg, erythema, and induration along the route of the long saphenous vein, which is tender and may be felt like a cord. Embolization of the clot is unlikely, because it adheres firmly to the vessel wall because of the infective process. Deep venous thrombosis (choice **D**) can result from problems involving the walls of the veins (varicosity, prior thrombophlebitis), a decreased rate of blood flow (prolonged bed rest or sitting, as in a prolonged airplane trip, immobilization of the leg in a cast, pressure behind the knee, congestive cardiac failure), and problems inherent in the blood (hypercoagulable states, trauma, polycythemia, oral contraceptives, malignancy). Manner of presentation depends on the location of the thrombus. The most frequent site of thrombus formation is in the venous sinuses of the calf muscles, resulting in swelling of the ankle and foot. The patient may also complain of pain, especially on dorsiflexion of the foot (Homans' sign). Tenderness can be elicited by compressing the calf muscle against the tibia, which is a very sensitive sign, and pretibial pitting edema may also be present. However, pain, tenderness, and pitting edema may also be absent. Thrombosis of the femoral vein, which is frequently associated with thrombosis of the calf, involves the thigh and knee. Clinical examination provides the diagnosis of deep venous thrombosis in only 50% of cases; thus, further investigation is required.

[29] **The answer is C**   *Preventive Medicine and Public Health*

Heat-related ailments are public health problems as demonstrated by reports of athletes collapsing and dying on the field and elderly persons without access to air conditioning dying in their homes during heat waves. There are three stages of heat-related ailments all connected to high environmental temperatures. They are heat cramps, heat exhaustion, and heat stroke. Heat cramps are usually also associated with strenuous physical activity, and symptoms include painful spasms of skeletal muscles, weakness, fatigue, nausea, vomiting, and tachycardia. The symptoms are caused by depletion of sodium chloride, and the core body temperature remains within the normal range. Treatment is by mild cooling and oral electrolyte replacement. In heat exhaustion there is both volume and electrolyte depletion due to sweating. Symptoms are profuse sweating, fatigue, lightheadedness, nausea and/or vomiting, headache, tachycardia, hyperventilation, and hypotension. The body temperature is usually normal or only slightly elevated. The treatment is intravenous replacement of fluid with electrolytes, removal to a cool environment, removal of excess clothing, spraying with tepid water (40°C, 104°F), and cooling with fans. Heat stroke is a medical emergency that usually presents abruptly, with the rapid onset of neurologic dysfunction including loss of consciousness with hyperpyrexia (>104°F [40°C]).

In the elderly, heat stroke typically is characterized by altered mental status and absence of sweating, while in exertional heat stroke, usually seen in younger persons undergoing rigorous exercise, as in the case described, there commonly is profuse sweating. All patients with heat stroke have tachycardia and hyperventilation. Risk factors for heat stroke include (1) the extremes of age, infants and the elderly; (2) preexisting cardiovascular disease; (3) high environmental temperature and humidity; (4) engagement in vigorous activities during hot weather, as might be done by professional or amateur athletes, laborers, and military recruits; and (5) ingestion of certain pharmacologic agents, including anticholinergic drugs, phenothiazines, tricyclic antidepressants, monoamine oxidase inhibitors, and antihistamines.

Heat stroke is a medical emergency, and as in all medical emergencies, the first line of treatment is always the classic ABCs, assess and treat if necessary the airways, breathing, and circulation (choice **C**). Following that, heat stroke is treated by removing all clothing, applying cool water to the entire skin prior to reaching the emergency facility, followed by treatment in the emergency room consisting of spraying with a mist of tepid water while using a high-volume fan, ice packs applied to the groin and axillae, ice water gastric lavage, and iced peritoneal lavage. As indicated, the ABCs are always the first line of treatment; therefore, the first line of treatment cannot be intravenous fluids with electrolytes (choice **A**). Moreover, since unlike in heat exhaustion, dehydration and volume depletion may not occur in heat stroke, vigorous fluid replacement may result in pulmonary edema. Choice **B,** lowering body temperature by placing him in a cool environment, spraying him with tepid water and cooling him with fans, will suffice to reverse the effects of heat exhaustion, but more vigorous methods of cooling should be used in heat stroke. The person described exhibits clinical signs typically attributed to heat stroke not heat exhaustion (choice **D**) or heat cramps (choice **E**).

30 The answer is D *Medicine*

The clinical picture suggests bacteremia in this patient, who may still be immunosuppressed as a consequence of chemotherapy. The likely causative organisms include gram-positive cocci and gram-negative rods. To possibly avoid further deterioration of his condition, antibiotic treatment must be initiated before the results of culture and susceptibility are available; treatment must not be withheld (choice **A**). (*Note:* The present infection may be nosocomial, in which case knowledge of the hospital pathogens and their drug susceptibility would be helpful in decisions concerning drug treatment.) Ampicillin (without sulbactam) (choice **B**) would not cover staphylococci, which are overwhelmingly penicillinase producing. Although it is somewhat more active than erythromycin against streptococci, azithromycin (choice **C**) would provide minimal coverage for gram-negative rods. Its oral administration would not be appropriate in this case. Ciprofloxacin (choice **E**) has a wide spectrum of activity and, given intravenously, might be a possible choice in this case; however, it has minimal activity against anaerobes. Moreover, resistance of gram-positive cocci to fluoroquinolones is increasing rapidly, and streptococcal superinfections during treatment with such drugs have been reported. Overall, the best choice here is intravenous (IV) cilastatin–imipenem (choice **D**). A carbapenem antibiotic, imipenem is active against gram-positive cocci, including penicillinase-producing and some methicillin-resistant staphylococci. Imipenem is also active against a wide range of gram-negative rods, including many anaerobes.

31 The answer is F *Medicine*

This patient contracted Lyme disease caused by a bite from an infected *Ixodes dammini* deer tick during her visit to Connecticut. The secondary disseminated phase of this condition has affected lower motor neurons of the right facial nerve causing Bell's palsy. As this is a lower motor neuron lesion, the entire right half of the face has been involved. Serologic testing of the serum (choice **F**) for antibodies to *Borrelia burgdorferi* will confirm the infection and provide the probable cause of the palsy. Antibodies to *B. burgdorferi* are commonly found in patients with Bell's palsy who reside in areas where Lyme disease is endemic, strongly suggesting a direct cause and effect. The *B. burgdorferi* infection can be cured with doxycycline, and the Bell's palsy will most likely clear up spontaneously.

Examination of urine (choice **A**) is noncontributory. Electromyography (choice **B**) may show delayed response but is not diagnostic. Slowing may be noted on nerve conduction study (choice **C**), but once again, it does not contribute to determining the cause of the paralysis. Results of magnetic resonance imaging of the brain (choice **D**) will be normal and not helpful in establishing the cause. Examination of the cerebrospinal fluid (choice **E**) is more difficult and less sensitive than examining the serum.

32 The answer is A *Psychiatry*

Aggressive symptoms (choice **A**), characterized by violence with poor impulse control, are a contraindication to referral to peer support groups. However, a history of violence, without current evidence of poor impulse control, is not an absolute contraindication. Peer support groups, also referred to as self-help groups, are peer-led groups characterized by sharing and social interaction. The purpose of such groups is to pursue personal and or social growth and change. Peer support groups have open membership, rotated leadership, and nominal or absent membership fees and are independent of any particular individual. They may be part of larger programs with established structures and policies, such as Alcoholic Anonymous, other "12-step" programs, and Recovery Inc. Properly selected peer support groups can help members to manage problems with anxiety (choice **B**), psychotic symptoms (choice **C**), social withdrawal (choice **D**), and substance abuse (choice **E**). Therefore, none of these problems are contraindications to referral. Aside from aggressiveness, the only other clear contraindication is refusal to attend, although this is unlikely with adequate explanation by an informed clinician and an introduction to someone who already attends the group.

33 The answer is C *Medicine*

Hypertrophic cardiomyopathy (choice **C**) is the most common cause of sudden cardiac death in young people. Most cases have an autosomal dominant inheritance pattern with variable penetrance. The condition can be caused by mutations in a number of genes, most of which code for myosin heavy chains or proteins regulating calcium metabolism involved in regulation of conduction. Clinical outcome is determined by the gene affected; some lead to an early death, as in the case described, others permit a nearly normal life span. Aberrant myofibers in the asymmetrically thickened interventricular septum (IVS) or abnormalities in the conduction system are responsible for precipitating a fatal ventricular arrhythmia and sudden death. The asymmetrically hypertrophied IVS bulges into the outflow tract, causing the anterior leaflet of the mitral valve to be closer to the septum than normal. This significantly narrows the outlet tract for blood flow to the aortic valve. When systole occurs, the anterior leaflet of the mitral valve is drawn against the IVS and obstructs blood flow, producing a systolic ejection murmur that is commonly confused with aortic stenosis. Unlike aortic stenosis, the obstruction to blood flow is below the aortic valve, while in aortic stenosis, the obstruction is at the level of the aortic valve. Whenever left ventricular volume (preload) is increased, the intensity of the murmur of hypertrophic cardiomyopathy decreases, indicating decreased obstruction to blood flow. Lying down (increasing venous return to the right side of the heart) or using drugs that decrease cardiac contractility and heart rate (e.g., β-blockers, calcium channel blockers) also decrease murmur intensity. Standing reduces venous return to the heart (decreases preload) and intensifies the murmur, indicating increased obstruction. A Valsalva maneuver (holding the breath against a closed glottis) also decreases venous return to the heart and intensifies the murmur.

The murmur of aortic regurgitation (choice **A**) is an early diastolic murmur that occurs directly after the second heart sound. The murmur of aortic stenosis (choice **B**) is a systolic ejection murmur that is similar to the murmur of hypertrophic cardiomyopathy. In contradistinction to hypertrophic cardiomyopathy, the intensity of the murmur of aortic stenosis either remains constant or increases when the patient is lying down. In mitral stenosis (choice **D**), there is an opening snap after the second heart sound followed by a middiastolic rumble. It is the most common complication of recurrent rheumatic fever. In mitral valve prolapse (choice **E**), there is a midsystolic click followed by a murmur of mitral regurgitation. It does not cause sudden cardiac death except when associated with Marfan syndrome.

34 The answer is E *Medicine*

This patient has moderate dementia stemming from Creutzfeldt-Jakob disease (choice **E**). Creutzfeldt-Jakob disease is due to a prion, and takes many years to manifest. Although it is a dementia in many ways similar to Alzheimer's disease, patients with Creutzfeldt-Jakob disease also suffer from myoclonus. These are sudden jerky movements of the limbs that are not patterned. There is no treatment for this disease.

Multiinfarct dementia (choice **A**) is seen in patients who have hypertension and develop stroke. The dementia in these individuals has a stepladder pattern of deterioration. Treatment involves control of hypertension and prevention of stroke. Chronic subdural hematoma (choice **B**) is generally associated with fluctuating signs and symptoms such as hemiparesis, memory problems, and bizarre behavior. There may be a history of direct head trauma, and it is confirmed on computerized tomography scan. Treatment is evacuation of the hematoma through burr holes. Pseudodementia (choice **C**) is usually found in depression and generally lasts no longer than 6 months. Thereafter, the patient recovers fully. Myoclonus is not a feature, and this patient lost his wife a year ago. Alzheimer's disease (choice **D**) is the most common cause of dementia, it is progressive, and motor function is not impaired. Myoclonus is not a feature of Alzheimer's disease.

35 The answer is E *Psychiatry*

This man has antisocial behavior disorder, which is define by the DSM IV as a condition in which a person older than 18 years of age and who is neither schizophrenic nor manic demonstrates at least three of the following traits:

- A failure to conform to social norms as reflected by acts that are grounds for arrest
- Chronic acts of lying and deceitfulness, conning others for profit or pleasure
- Impulsivity—failure to plan ahead and consider the consequences of an action
- Irritability/aggressiveness—frequently engaging in fights and/or assaults
- Reckless disregard for the safety of self or others
- Consistent irresponsibility—can't keep a job, fails to meet financial obligations
- Lack of remorse if his actions hurt others

In short, such a person consistently neglects the rights of others. Although symptoms of impending antisocial behavior disorder begin in childhood and are most prevalent in young men (and women), antisocial behavior tends to decreases greatly after age 40 (choice **E**). Antisocial behavior disorder is more commonly recognized in men because aggressive behavior makes them more conspicuous. However, the trait is also recognized in women, who tend to be more conniving.

The onset of antisocial behavior is more often before, not after (choice **A**), midadolescence. It is associated with chaotic family settings rather than rigid family upbringing (choice **B**). It does not fluctuate in intensity over a short period (choice **C**) but tends to remain as a constant personality trait for a prolonged period. It is characterized by a lack of guilt not extreme remorse (choice **D**).

36 The answer is C *Surgery*

The tumor-node-metastasis (TNM) system is used to stage cancers arising from epithelial tissues. **T** refers to the size and nuclear features of the tumor; **N** refers to the presence or absence of lymph node metastasis; and M refers to the presence or absence of metastasis to sites other than lymph nodes, such as the liver. M is the most important prognostic factor. The presence of distant metastases to the liver (choice **C**) implies that the cancer has already infiltrated through regional lymph nodes (choice **D**) draining the cancer and has entered the bloodstream. Although tumor size (choice **E**) is a staging criterion, it is not as important as N or M in the staging system.

Differentiation or grade of the tumor (choice **A**) describes the histologic appearance of the tumor. If the tumor has recognizable features, such as keratin in squamous cells or glands, then the tumor is well-differentiated or low grade. If the tumor has no histologic features with characteristics identifying the tissue of origin, then the tumor is poorly differentiated, anaplastic, or high grade. The degree of differentiation and extent of local invasion of the tumor (choice **B**) are less important prognostic factors than the M of the TNM system.

37 The answer is A *Medicine*

Pseudotumor cerebri (benign intracranial hypertension) is defined as intracranial hypertension in the absence of tumor or obstruction to cerebrospinal fluid (CSF) flow. It is most commonly noted in young, obese females. Results of computerized tomography and magnetic resonance imaging studies are usually normal. Lumbar puncture shows elevation of intracranial pressure (usually >200 mm Hg); however all other CSF values are normal. The disorder can cause progressive visual loss (choice **A**) due to transmission of elevated intracranial pressure through the optic nerve sheath to the optic disc. An early finding might be an enlarged blind spot on visual field testing. Benign intracranial hypertension is often self-limited but usually needs to be treated with diuretics, acetazolamide, spinal taps, steroids, or even cerebrospinal fluid (CSF) shunting via a lumboperitoneal shunt. To avoid visual loss, optic nerve sheath fenestration can be carried out.

Sixth nerve palsy (choice **B**) may be unilateral or bilateral and is usually transient, reverting when the cerebrospinal pressure is normalized. Herniation syndrome is not usually a consequence of an unrecognized mass lesion in the middle cranial fossa and is not usually associated with benign intracranial hypertension (choice **C**). Migraine headaches (choice **D**) are not associated with benign intracranial hypertension. Hemiplegia (choice **E**) is not a complication that is usually seen with pseudotumor cerebri.

38 The answer is B *Medicine*

The patient has infectious diarrhea caused by *Cryptosporidium parvum* (choice **B**). It is a sporozoan that is contracted by ingesting the oocysts. *C. parvum* is one of the most common pathogens causing diarrhea and biliary tract disease in AIDS patients. The oocysts, which are partially acid fast–positive, attach to the brush border of the mucosal cells of the small intestine. The treatment is nitazoxanide or paromomycin plus azithromycin.

Balantidium coli (choice **A**) is a ciliate protozoan that produces colonic ulcers, causing bloody diarrhea; *B. coli* is not partially acid fast. Tetracycline is the treatment of choice. *Entamoeba histolytica* (choice **C**) is an ameba with trophozoites that produce flask-shaped ulcers in the cecum, causing bloody diarrhea. The trophozoites and cysts are not partially acid fast. Metronidazole is the treatment of choice. *Giardia lamblia* (choice **D**) is a flagellate protozoan with cysts that attach to the small intestine mucosa, causing acute and chronic diarrhea with malabsorption. The cysts are not partially acid fast. Metronidazole is the treatment of choice. *Strongyloides stercoralis* (choice **E**) is the most common helminthic infection causing diarrhea in AIDS patients. Adult worms lay eggs, not oocysts, in the bowel mucosa that develop into rhabditiform larvae, which are excreted in the feces. The treatment of choice is ivermectin.

39 The answer is E *Psychiatry*

This boy has dyslexia (choice **E**). Dyslexic individuals have problems determining which letters in words normally follow each other and confuse similar-looking letters. Thus, *girl* might be read as *gril* and the letter *b* might be confused with *d* or *p*. The cause of dyslexia is unknown, but most experts believe it is left hemisphere-linked and is associated with dysfunctions in Wernicke's area for language association and/or Broca's area dealing with sound and speech production or the interconnections between these areas. Involvement of Broca's area helps explains why dyslexic persons often have delayed development of speech. Dyslexia has been blamed on cerebrovascular accidents, prematurity, and intrauterine problems; however, as in the case described, there is as strong genetic link, suggesting that the brain is wired differently due to genetic causes. There is variation in the degree and character of dyslexia as well as in the IQ of the dyslexic person. However dyslexic persons are often highly intelligent and can often compensate for the disadvantage by having excellent memories and talents in other areas, often those involving spatial orientation. Consequently, dyslexic adults are often found in professions such as dentistry or orthopedic surgery. Most dyslexic adults reach their level of achievement, professional or otherwise, without the benefit of any special education or training. However, for the past few decades there have been special educational programs designed to help dyslexic children improve their reading, writing, and in some cases speaking proficiency.

A low IQ (choice **A**) or attention deficit disorder (ADD) (choice **B**) are improbable because of the teacher's comment that the boy is a generally good student and a joy to work with. One would expect that poor vision (choice **C**) or a hearing disorder (choice **D**) would have been identified by the school nurse or a parent.

40 The answer is C *Medicine*

A magnetic resonance imaging (MRI) (choice **C**) study is the best way to follow the patient. As multiple sclerosis tends to affect the white matter randomly, an MRI of the brain and spinal cord should be done. It will reveal the presence of plaques confirming the diagnosis and the appearance of new plaques if the disease has progressed.

Note that additional plaque formation does not necessarily cause physical findings. Hence, repeating a physical examination on a monthly basis (choice **E**) or after 6 months (choice **B**) is not helpful. Examination of the spinal fluid (choice **A**) will not confirm or exclude the presence of lesions. A computerized tomography scan (choice **D**) is not as sensitive as an MRI in the diagnosis of multiple sclerosis.

41 The answer is C *Psychiatry*

The Rorschach test was first developed by Dr. Rorschach in 1918 and published in 1921. As ultimately developed, it uses a set of 10 standard ink blots, and as patients are shown each one, they are asked what they observe. The idea is that in doing so, they project facets of their thoughts, attitudes, and personality that the analyst is trained interpret and to use as an aid in diagnosis and ultimately in treatment. As the first developed "projective personality test," (i.e., a test used to probe the subconscious by interpreting a person's reaction to ambiguous test materials), it became very popular, reaching its zenith of use in the 1950s. Since then, it has lost much credibility in scientific circles because of its subjective nature. However, the concept of projective personality testing has been used in the development of other tests that have the goal of being less subjective. These include the Sentence Completion Test (SCT) (choice **D**), the Thematic Apperception Test (TAT) (choice **F**), and the Minnesota Multiphase Personality Inventory (MMPI) (choice **B**). In the SCT, the psychoanalyst asks a patient to complete a sentence that has been started; the analyst probes the subconscious by interpreting the response. (A nonpsychiatric variant of the sentence completion test is used to test a person vocabulary. In this use the person being tested is provided with a sentence missing one word and is given a choice of 5 words to finish the sentence. This permits computerized grading and is used by standardized test makers as in the PSAT, SAT, and GRE). The TAT was developed in the 1930s at Harvard and consists of 31 illustrations, each with a standardized interpretation that is used in a manner analogous to the Rorschach test. Although it too uses illustrations, it is not the first such test to be developed and thus is an incorrect choice.

42 The answer is B *Psychiatry*

The Minnesota Multiphase Personality Inventory (MMPI) (choice **B**) was developed in the 1930s and was completely revamped in 1989; the newer version is called MMPI-2. Among projective personality tests it is unique in that it has normative national standards and it had 10 clinical scales designed to make the test less subjective; in addition, it has a large number of subscales and validity sales designed to help uncover test subjects who "cheat" by providing answers they think will please the tester. Because of this greater use of normative standards and internal checks, it has garnered greater acceptability and is widely used by psychologists and psychiatrists to assess a wide range of psychologic characteristics in individuals. Consequently, it is used to help predict responses to stressful situations such as service in a submarine. In addition, the results of a MMPI test are often accepted as evidence in court. Sometimes computerized versions are used; however, because at their core a projective personality test depends upon a subjective interpretation for the test results to be valid, it still needs to be administered and evaluated by a trained professional.

43 The answer is A   *Psychiatry*

The Halstead-Reitan Battery (HRB) is a neuropsychologic test used to detect and to localize brain lesions.

CHOICES NOT USED

Choice **G,** the Wide-Range Achievement Test (WRAT), is used to evaluate achievement in areas in which an individual has been instructed (e.g., spelling, reading, and arithmetic). Choice **E,** the Stanford-Binet Scale is a measure of the intelligence quotient (IQ).

44 The answer is G   *Obstetrics and Gynecology*

The lack of pain with this genital ulcer is an important finding because it helps narrow the differential diagnosis to syphilis, granuloma inguinale, and lymphogranuloma venereum (LGV). While syphilis is the most common painless genital ulcer in the United States, the presence of lymphadenopathy in this scenario strongly suggests LGV. The positive "groove sign," a depression between groups of tender, inflamed inguinal nodes, confirms a diagnosis of LGV. LGV is a sexually transmitted disease that is relatively rare in the United States. In women, the lymphatic drainage is to the perirectal glands where it may initially cause proctitis with tenesmus and a bloody purulent discharge, which if left untreated can lead to obstipation and rectal stricture. Similar conditions may develop in homosexual men. The diagnosis is established by a culture of pus aspirated from the node. The causative agent is *Chlamydia trachomatis* immunotypes L1–L3. Management is with doxycycline or erythromycin for 21 days.

45 The answer is A   *Obstetrics and Gynecology*

The most common cause of painful genital ulcers in the United States is genital herpes caused by herpes simplex virus-2 (HSV-2) (choice **A**); this is an infection shared by about 25% of the adult population. The primary lesion consists of clear vesicles developing at the site of mucocutaneous genital contact that spontaneously rupture, forming the typical shallow, painful ulcers. The case described, with systemic and diffuse involvement, is typical for primary herpes. Recurrent herpes has no systemic symptoms, may be activated by stress or menses, and is preceded by prodromal paresthesias. The diagnosis is established by culture of vesicular fluid or the base of the ulcer. Management is with antiviral therapy using acyclovir, famciclovir, or valacyclovir. Because of changing patterns of sexual behavior, genital herpes is becoming more commonly caused by herpes simplex virus-1 (HSV-1), which is now estimated to be the infectious agent in as many as 25% of the cases of genital herpes.

46 The answer is E   *Obstetrics and Gynecology*

The most common cause of painless genital ulcers in the United States is a *Treponema pallidum* (choice **E**) infection, commonly referred to as syphilis. The primary lesion is the chancre, which if untreated resolves spontaneously within 4–6 weeks. Systemic spread of the spirochete now takes place, resulting in the classical genital lesion of a condyloma lata (fused weeping papules on moist areas of the skin and mucous membranes) and rash. This secondary stage also spontaneously clears. Two thirds of patients develop asymptomatic latent syphilis, while a third will go on to develop tertiary syphilis with its classical lesion of the gumma. Darkfield microscopy is the most specific technique for diagnosing syphilis when an active chancre or condyloma lata is present. Guidelines from the Centers for Disease Control and Prevention (CDC) recommend parenterally administered penicillin G for the treatment of all stages of syphilis.

47 The answer is F *Obstetrics and Gynecology*

The differential diagnosis for painless genital ulcers includes syphilis, granuloma inguinale, and lymphogranuloma venereum. While syphilis is the most common painless genital ulcer in the United States, "beefy red" lesions specifically point to the granulation tissue of granuloma inguinale (choice **F**). The disease gradually eats away the skin and forms elevated, beefy-red, velvety nodules, which can coalesce, spread, and destroy genital tissue. This sexually transmitted disease is rare in the United States. The diagnosis is established by identification of Donovan bodies in smears and ulcer specimens. Management is 21 days of oral doxycycline.

48 The answer is C *Obstetrics and Gynecology*

The differential diagnosis for painful genital ulcers includes genital herpes and chancroid. While herpes is the most common painful genital ulcer in the United States, a "ragged-edge" lesion specifically points to the granulation tissue of chancroid caused by *Haemophilus ducreyi* (choice **C**). This sexually transmitted disease is rare in the United States, with only a few hundred cases reported annually. The organism is difficult to culture, so often the diagnosis is made by excluding syphilis and herpes. Management is a single dose of oral azithromycin.

49 The answer is D *Obstetrics and Gynecology*

This young woman most likely has acute pelvic inflammatory disease (PID) caused by *Chlamydia trachomatis* immunotypes D–K (choice **D**). *C. trachomatis* infection in females may be asymptomatic, but seemingly dormant infection may bloom into cervicitis, salpingitis, or as in this case, PID. Historically, diagnosis has been clinical, but the newly developed ligase chain reaction has high sensitivity (90–95%) and is likely to become the diagnostic method of choice. Treatment is usually azithromycin or doxycycline.

50 The answer is B *Obstetrics and Gynecology*

This young woman most likely has gonorrhea caused by *Neisseria gonorrhea* (choice **B**). Diagnosis can be confirmed by a Gram's stain of a smear, culture, or DNA analysis based on the ligase chain reaction. Although culture is the classic "gold standard," DNA analysis is quicker, is more sensitive, and also identifies chlamydial coinfection. Although the annual incidence has decreased since the 1970s, in 2002 it was estimated to be about 700,000 cases, 75% of which occurred in females between the ages of 15 and 19 years or in males between the ages of 20 and 24 years. Females are first infected in the cervix and can remain symptomless. Symptoms are sometimes provoked by the onset of a period, but they can also be very mild and be overlooked. Infection can then spread from the cervix into the uterus and upward into the fallopian tubes causing pelvic inflammatory disease (PID). The patient with PID has crampy or constant pelvic pain and menorrhagia or intermenstrual irregular bleeding and may have fever and nausea. Ectopic pregnancy can result because of a blocked fallopian tube, and infertility is the usual outcome. Treatment with penicillin or tetracycline is no longer recommended because of microbial resistance. Instead, oral cefixime, ceftriaxone, ciprofloxacin, or ofloxacin is used, generally with doxycycline or azithromycin to treat possible coinfection with chlamydia.

Questions

Single Best Choice Directions: This section consists of numbered statements or questions followed by a list of potential answers; you are to select the ONE best answer.

1 An 18-year-old woman presents to the emergency department with a swollen left eye and respiratory difficulty. She provides a history of falling asleep while sunbathing on the grass in her backyard, then waking up suddenly with pain and swelling in her face and trouble breathing. Physical examination reveals expiratory wheezes. There is no inspiratory stridor or swelling of the oropharyngeal mucosa. Which of the following is the most appropriate first step in the management of this patient?

(A) Administer intravenous hydrocortisone
(B) Treat the patient with nebulized albuterol sulfate
(C) Administer intravenous aminophylline
(D) Administer intramuscular aqueous epinephrine 1:1000
(E) Administer intravenous aqueous epinephrine 1:10,000

2 A 46-year-old Chinese woman immigrated to the United States some 5 years previously. She is in relatively good health, doesn't smoke, and has two teenage children who attend school. Her husband has a thriving store in the same area where she works part time. One day while in the shower she noticed a small lump located on the right side of the neck, near the throat. Consequently, she made an appointment to see her family physician who notes a smooth, nontender mobile lump in the right anterior cervical triangle of the neck. Otherwise, she finds no abnormalities in the area of the nose, throat, ears, and neck. Results of chest radiography and indirect laryngoscopy are normal. Results of a complete blood count and complete chemistry panel also are normal. Which of the following is the most appropriate next step in the management of this patient?

(A) Sputum cytology
(B) Biopsy of the nasopharynx
(C) Biopsy of the lymph node
(D) Iodine-123 (^{123}I) scan of the thyroid
(E) Bronchoscopy

3 A 36-year-old man suffered a fracture of his vertebrae in a motorcycle accident. As a consequence, his spinal cord was severed, and he was paralyzed from the waist down and confined to a wheelchair. He also was depressed and started drinking alcohol as an escape mechanism and spent much time wheeling from his residence to various bars. Consequently, he did not practice optimum hygiene and self-care and developed a pressure sore (aka a decubitus ulcer) on his sacrum that became infected. He eventually sought help at an emergency facility. Upon examination, the attending physician found his blood pressure to be 108/80 mm Hg; pulse, 76 beats/min and regular; and temperature, 39.5°C (103.1°F). He found an 8 cm × 6 cm pressure ulcer on his sacrum that emitted a purulent and foul-smelling discharge. Which of the following is true concerning pressure ulcers?

(A) Pressure sores are more likely to occur in bedridden patients than in patients whose mobility is compromised in any other way.
(B) Erythema may progress to ulceration quickly.
(C) A pressure ulcer is unlikely to ever be located on the heel.
(D) Pressure sore infections are almost always caused by *Staphylococcus aureus.*
(E) An infected pressure ulcer should be treated with a topical antiseptic such as hypochlorite solutions, povidone–iodine, acetic acid iodophor, or hydrogen peroxide.

4 A 66-year-old Italian-American male sees his primary care physician with a history of recurrent attacks of "sore throat." He states that over the years he has been active in outdoor sports but of late has been getting tired, which he states because of getting old. The patient does not smoke, drinks a glass of wine with dinner, and indulges in pasta and cheese. He takes no medications other than multivitamins and an aspirin a day to "maintain a healthy heart." Other than surgery for a right inguinal hernia 20 years ago, his past medical history is noncontributory. Both his parents lived to a ripe old age and died of natural causes. There is no family history of medical illness. His exercise routine includes biking, hiking, trekking, and water sports. Physical examination reveals a muscular 186 cm (6 ft 1 in) tall male, weighing 75 kg (165 lb, 6 oz), with normal vital signs. He has no pallor of the conjunctival mucosa, no icterus, and no clubbing or cyanosis. He has a solitary mobile, nontender lymph node in the left anterior triangle of the neck. On examination, the throat is normal; there is no thyromegaly. Cardiovascular and respiratory systems are normal. The abdomen is soft and nontender. The liver and spleen are just palpable. No masses are felt, and bowel sounds are present. His white cell count is 120,000/μL (normal range, 4.8 to 10.8×10^3/μL), 80% of which are lymphocytes. The hematocrit and platelet counts are normal. The bone marrow is filled with small lymphocytes, and this is reflected in the lymph node biopsy as well. Based on the clinical findings his condition is best treated by which of the following?

(A) Alemtuzumab

(B) Chlorambucil

(C) Prednisone

(D) Intravenous infusion of fludarabine

(E) A combination of fludarabine and prednisone

(F) Intravenous infusion of a combination of fludarabine and rituximab or of fludarabine and cyclophosphamide

(G) Intravenous infusion of a combination of fludarabine, rituximab, and cyclophosphamide

5 A 24-year-old woman, gravida 4, para 1, aborta 2, is at 28 weeks' gestation as estimated by her admittedly uncertain date of last menstrual event. She admits to intravenous (IV) drug use and having sex in exchange for drugs and is unsure who the father of this pregnancy is. She has recently undergone treatment for syphilis identified by a positive venereal disease research laboratory (VDRL) test and confirmed with a positive fluorescent treponemal antibody (FTA) test. On her last prenatal visit she underwent human immunodeficiency virus (HIV) testing by enzyme-linked immunosorbent assay (ELISA), which had positive results confirmed with a positive Western blot assay result. She inquires as to the significance of this finding for herself as well as her baby. Which of the following statements best summarizes what you will say?

(A) Pregnancy accelerates maternal progression from HIV positive to acquired immune deficiency syndrome (AIDS).

(B) Mode of delivery has a significant impact on maternal–neonatal transmission of HIV.

(C) Breast-feeding does not increase neonatal risk of becoming HIV positive.

(D) Neonates can be protected from HIV by passive immunization at birth.

(E) Rapidity of disease progression is the same in mother and neonate.

6 A 23-year-old single woman presents to her doctor's office with a history of bleeding from the nose that occurs spontaneously and frequently. She is sexually active on and off and has started using a contraceptive pill. She has also noticed an increased amount of flow during her periods, which decreases when she takes oral contraceptives but worsens if she stops taking it. She has no history of substance abuse but does give a history of recent admission to a hospital and treatment with intravenous antibiotics for a severe respiratory infection that turned out to be pneumonia. Laboratory studies show a normal prothrombin time (PT), prolonged activated partial thromboplastin time (APTT), prolonged bleeding time, and a normal platelet count. Which of the following is the most likely diagnosis?

(A) Hemophilia A

(B) Hemophilia B

(C) Disseminated intravascular coagulation (DIC)

(D) Qualitative platelet defect due to aspirin

(E) Von Willebrand's disease

(F) Factor VII deficiency

7 A 58-year-old-man, is seen in the emergency room for chest pains. The pain is of a crushing nature, retrosternal, and radiating to the left jaw. It is associated with increased sweating, nausea, and dizziness. His past history is significant for cigarette smoking over a 40-year period, and he admits to a past history of chest pains, especially when he exercises. However, prior to this episode he chose to ignore it. An electrocardiogram confirms acute myocardial infarction, and the patient is admitted to the intensive care unit. Angiography confirms coronary artery occlusion for which a coronary artery bypass graft is being considered. Which of the following is the best preoperative screen of pulmonary function for this patient?

(A) Arterial pH

(B) Arterial carbon dioxide tension (PCO_2)

(C) Arterial oxygen tension (PO_2)

(D) Forced expiratory volume in 1 second/forced vital capacity (FEV_1/FVC) ratio

(E) Oxygen saturation

8 A 25-year-old woman, gravida 2, para 2, was brought to the emergency room with spontaneous premature rupture of membranes. Labor was induced, and a 7 lb 1 oz (3200 g) male neonate was spontaneously delivered vaginally. Unfortunately, the third stage of labor was prolonged and required manual removal of a retained placenta. On the first postpartum day, she underwent bilateral tubal sterilization. She returns to the emergency department on the fourth postpartum day complaining of midlower abdominal pain, fever, and foul-smelling lochia. Her vital signs are as follows: temperature, 39.2°C (102.5°F); pulse, 110/min; respiration, 22/min; blood pressure, 120/80 mm Hg. Examination reveals her uterus to be boggy, located 4 cm above her umbilicus, and exquisitely tender to palpation. She is breast-feeding, and both breasts are engorged. Which of the following obstetric events is likely to be the most significant for her peripartum course?

(A) Manual removal of a retained placenta
(B) Postpartum tubal sterilization
(C) Retained products of conception
(D) Spontaneous vaginal delivery
(E) Prolonged premature rupture of membranes (PROM)

9 A 64-year-old African-American male has a long history of coronary artery disease for which he underwent a triple bypass 5 years previously. Approximately 3 years ago he developed difficulty passing urine and was found to have an enlarged prostate. His prostate-specific antigen level was raised, and a biopsy confirmed prostate cancer, which was treated by radiotherapy. The patient also has moderate hypertension and type 2 diabetes mellitus and is on an ACE inhibitor and a diuretic for his hypertension, and metformin for diabetes. Two weeks ago he starts to complain about low back pain but rationalized that it was from back strain caused by working in his yard. However, he has now developed weakness in his legs and problems with urination and consequently presents himself to a local emergency department. Neurologic examination reveals paraparesis with a sensory level below T10 and a distended urinary bladder. There is tenderness over the thoracic spine in that area. Which of the following is the proper next step in diagnosis?

(A) Order an emergency computed tomography (CT) myelogram after an intravenous (IV) bolus of steroids
(B) Order magnetic resonance imaging with contrast after an IV bolus of steroids
(C) Order radiography of the thoracic spine after an IV bolus of steroids
(D) Order electromyography (EMG) after an IV bolus of steroids
(E) Send for radiation therapy over the lumbar and sacral areas after an IV bolus of steroids

10 A 47-year-old male is admitted to the hospital with complaints of shortness of breath, swelling of the feet, and tiredness. He suffered a myocardial infarction a year ago. His vital signs are as follows: temperature, 37.5°C (99.3°F); pulse, 88 beats/min (regular); respirations, 22/min (regular); and blood pressure 110/90 mm Hg. The patient is orthopneic and has mild cyanosis, raised jugular venous pressure, and inspiratory crackles in the bases of both lungs. Pitting edema is present over both feet. The electrocardiogram shows sinus tachycardia with left axis deviation, evidence of an old inferior myocardial infarction, a right bundle-branch block, and occasional premature ventricular contractions. A chest x-ray film reveals patchy haziness of the lungs. A diagnosis of acute left ventricular failure with pulmonary edema is made, and a rapid bolus dose of furosemide is administered intravenously. A complication that could arise from this intervention would affect or cause which of the following?

(A) Gastrointestinal tract
(B) Sense of taste
(C) Hearing
(D) Sense of smell
(E) Transient loss of vision

11 A 26-year-old female was presented to a class of medical students during a rotation. The patient had a lump in the neck that turned out to be Hodgkin's lymphoma. After listening to this presentation, a 23-year-old second-year female medical student discovers a similar lump in her neck and becomes so concerned that it may be due to Hodgkin's disease that she consults an oncologist on staff. A routine workup is completely negative for the disease, but the student says that she cannot stop worrying about it. Which of the following is the most likely diagnosis?

(A) Conversion disorder
(B) Hypochondriasis
(C) Delusional disorder, somatic type
(D) Somatization disorder
(E) Factitious disorder

12 An intern on the pediatric service frequently smells alcohol on the breath of a pediatric resident. Although the resident appears to be giving good patient care and he is able to function adequately as a team member, the intern is concerned about patient safety. The intern discusses this with him, but the resident denies that he has been drinking. The intern is concerned by the response and feels strongly that she must share her suspicions with someone in authority. At this point, the intern should inform which of the following?

(A) Law enforcement
(B) The medical ethics committee of the hospital
(C) The director of the residency program
(D) The dean of the medical school
(E) Chief of the medical staff

13 A 61-year-old alcoholic male left a bar during the early hours of the morning but could not make it home. He decided to spend the rest of the night in the hallway of an abandoned building in a nearby area. On his way to his resting place he stumbled over some garbage strewn on the alley and fell to the ground. Upon waking up the following midmorning, he noticed that his right hand was not moving in a normal way. Concerned, he managed to go to the local emergency facility. Physical examination reveals a rather disheveled male who is unkempt, reeks of alcohol, and slurs his words. He has bruises over his face and body, presumably due to the fall. The intern on duty cannot clearly understand him, so the patient points to his right hand. He is unable to move it. Which of the following is most likely reason for this problem?

(A) Entrapment of the median nerve
(B) Entrapment of the ulnar nerve
(C) Entrapment of the musculocutaneous nerve
(D) Entrapment of the axillary nerve
(E) Entrapment of the radial nerve
(F) Fracture of the scaphoid bone
(G) Fracture of the radius
(H) Fracture of the shaft of the humerus

14 A 42-year-old man, who recently has become unemployed due to downsizing of his factory, comes to see his physician with a history of having burnt his chest accidentally with hot water while in the shower; he didn't realize how hot the water was. He stated that he had also noticed some weakness of his hands and had dropped things on and off. He did not make much of it, as he stated that his wife said he had "butter fingers" anyway. He also felt that he has some problem with writing but thinks it may be psychologic; he says his wife thinks he subconsciously is just finding an excuse not to get another job. He denies a history of trauma, diabetes mellitus, or other neurologic disease. He does have long-standing scoliosis and, as a child, he contracted meningitis, after which, he said his "mind worked kinda slow-like." Clinical examination did confirm rather slowed thinking, and he did not seem to grasp the potential gravity of the problem. There is definite wasting of the thenar eminence in both hands and loss of pinprick sensation in the hands, arms, and shoulders, but pinprick sensation is preserved in the lower extremities. He is able to discern the position of his fingers and toes with his eyes closed, and appreciates vibration sense as well. Deep tendon jerks are equal and diminished in the upper extremities but increased in the lower. The plantar reflexes are equivocal. He has a 5° scoliosis of the thoracic spine with the convexity to the right. A magnetic

resonance imaging (MRI) scan of the cervical and thoracic spine would show which of the following?

(A) No abnormality
(B) Stenosis of the cervical spine
(C) Herniated cervical disk(s)
(D) Plaques in the spinal cord
(E) A dilated central canal
(F) Motor neuron disease (amyotrophic lateral sclerosis)

15 Some months ago a 37-year-old male went to see his primary care physician with a complaint of increasing fatigue and recurrent attacks of upper respiratory tract infection. Physical examination revealed pallor of the skin, evidence of petechiae, and hepatosplenomegaly, and histologic studies confirmed a diagnosis of acute myelogenous leukemia, for which he received allogeneic bone marrow transplantation. Thirty days later, the patient returns to the hospital with a history of fever and difficulty breathing. His temperature is 38.5°C (101.3°F), pulse is 92 beats/min and regular, respirations are 22 per minute, and the blood pressure is 130/78 mm Hg. An electrocardiogram (ECG) reveals a sinus tachycardia, but is otherwise normal. A chest x-ray film shows a predominantly interstitial pattern. A hematoxylin–eosin–stained lung biopsy specimen reveals basophilic-staining intranuclear inclusions in alveolar cells. Which of the following is the most likely pathogen?

(A) *Pneumocystis carinii*
(B) Cytomegalovirus (CMV)
(C) *Cryptococcus neoformans*
(D) *Blastomyces dermatitidis*
(E) *Candida albicans*

16 A 59-year-old Caucasian woman presents to her family physician with a history of pain in the chest and back. The chest pain is constant, midline, nonradiating, and increased by coughing or taking a deep breath. The pain in the back is constant, increases with activity, and is worse at night. She has also been complaining of increasing tiredness and is unable to function like before. She has always exercised and has been taking vitamin supplements including calcium regularly. Physical examination reveals a slender woman who is in apparent distress. She has mild pyrexia, moderate tachycardia, and normal respirations and blood pressure. Pallor of the mucous membrane is noted. She has no icterus or cervical lymphadenopathy, nor does she have jugular venous distention. Cardiovascular examination reveals a precordial soft systolic murmur with no thrill. Air entry is equal in both lungs, and she has no adventitious sounds. Results of

an abdominal examination are unremarkable, and the neurologic examination is nonfocal. She has exquisite tenderness over the sternum and along the iliac crests. A skeletal survey reveals radiolucent areas in the sternum, ribs, and pelvic bones. Her complete blood count (CBC) shows a hemoglobin level (Hgb) of 8.0 g/dL (normal, 12–16 g/dL), normal red blood cell (RBC) indices, and normal leukocyte and platelet counts. The peripheral smear shows prominent rouleaux formation. The accompanying figure shows the findings of a bone marrow aspirate taken from the left posterior iliac crest. Which of the following would be expected in this patient?

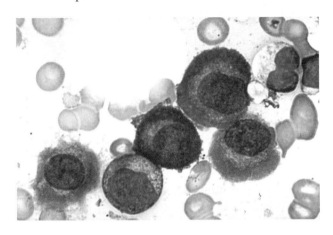

(A) Estrogen and progesterone receptor–positive cells in the bone marrow
(B) A normal erythrocyte sedimentation rate
(C) Decreased serum calcium concentration
(D) A monoclonal spike on serum protein electrophoresis
(E) A decrease in bone pain with tamoxifen therapy

17 A mother takes her 16-year-old daughter to the primary care physician. The daughter is a high school student in Los Angeles. She is very conscious of her body and looks. She has been an avid reader of fashion magazines and follows the life and times of her favorite actress. In fact, she aspires to become a Hollywood actress herself. To keep in shape she has taken up running, but her mother states that her daughter has been secretly inducing vomiting as a form of weight control. The daughter will not confirm this behavior. Which of the following best supports the mother's contention?

(A) Amenorrhea
(B) Binge eating
(C) Erosion of tooth enamel and abraded fingers
(D) Normochromic microcytic anemia
(E) Weight loss
(F) Gaunt features

18 A 22-year-old woman, gravida 2, para 1, is seen for her first prenatal visit at the outpatient clinic. This is a planned pregnancy, and she took prepregnancy folic acid supplementation. Her last menstrual period was 8 weeks ago. Her previous pregnancy prenatal course was uncomplicated, but after undergoing spontaneous labor and a vaginal delivery, her first child was found to have a lumbar spina bifida. During a pelvic examination on her current visit, the physician noted a mobile, soft, nontender left adnexal mass approximately 5 cm in size. A pelvic sonogram shows it to be a thin-walled, round, fluid-filled simple cyst without loculations or calcifications. Which of the following is the most likely diagnosis and course for this adnexal mass?

(A) It is benign and will gradually enlarge
(B) It is benign and will remain the same size
(C) It is benign and will spontaneously regress
(D) It is malignant but will remain encapsulated
(E) It is malignant and will metastasize

19 A 67-year-old male comes to the office for a checkup because of a recent, worrisome incident in which he had a sudden onset of visual loss in the right eye followed by tingling and numbness in the left upper extremity. The problem lasted for approximately 5 minutes, after which time he recovered fully. This was the first time he ever experienced this type of incident. On examination his higher functions and speech were normal. The visual fields were normal to confrontation. Results of funduscopy were normal. He had no diplopia nor did he have nystagmus or other cranial nerve abnormalities. There was no pronator drift, and the tone and deep tendon reflexes were normal. The plantar reflexes were flexor, and he had no sensory deficits. Cerebellar function was normal. A carotid bruit was present over the right side of the neck. Duplex ultrasonography confirmed stenosis of the internal carotid artery. Initial treatment with medications did not ameliorate the bruit; therefore, surgery was advised. He underwent carotid endarterectomy under general anesthesia. Twenty-four hours after surgery, the patient died. Which of the following is the most likely cause of his death?

(A) Embolic stroke
(B) Pulmonary embolism
(C) Air embolism
(D) Acute myocardial infarction
(E) Atherosclerotic stroke

20 A 24-year-old man was admitted to the hospital with a history of fatigue and confusion. A few days previously he developed an infection in his foot, which has become worse. The patient is a diabetic who takes insulin. His temperature is 38.5°C (101.3°F); pulse, 96 beats/min regular; respirations 20/min; and blood pressure, 90/60 mm Hg. His tongue is dry, and he has poor skin turgor. Apart from confusion, his neurologic examination is nonfocal. Cardiovascular examination is normal except for a sinus tachycardia. Respiratory system examination is unremarkable with the exception of a fruity odor in his breath. He has diffuse abdominal tenderness, but no masses or organomegaly are noted. Bowel sounds are present. He has cellulitis of his right leg, as a result of the infection in his foot. Serum glucose level is 700 mg/dL. The appropriate diagnosis was made, and he received intravenous fluids, antibiotics, and human insulin. During therapy, the patient develops respiratory paralysis requiring intubation and assisted ventilation. Which of the following is the cause for the patient's respiratory failure?

(A) An anaphylactic reaction due to insulin
(B) Glucose toxicity
(C) Ketoacidosis
(D) Hypophosphatemia
(E) Hyperkalemia
(F) Bacteremia

21 A male patient was taken by a family member to see their family's primary care physician for problems that the patient had been having for some time. His family was most concerned about this because the problem seemed to be getting worse. After a careful history and physical and mental status examinations, the physician decides that cognitive psychotherapy would be the best therapeutic option for him. Which particular problem among those listed did the primary care physician think that this would address?

(A) Dementia caused by neurodegenerative disease
(B) Developmental reading disorder
(C) Major depressive disorder, single episode, without psychosis
(D) Dissociative amnesia
(E) Substance intoxication

22 A 22-year-old woman, para 0, gravida 1, presents to her obstetrician for a routine examination. Physical examination reveals normal vital signs. Results of examinations of the cardiovascular and respiratory systems are normal. Examination of the abdomen suggests that the uterus is at 30 weeks. Based on the history and examination of this patient, which of the following laboratory test results is a normal finding at this stage of her pregnancy?

(A) Decreased arterial pH
(B) Decreased creatinine clearance
(C) Decreased plasma hemoglobin concentration
(D) Decreased serum cortisol level
(E) Increased serum blood urea nitrogen concentration
(F) Increased serum thyroxine level.

23 A 24-year-old woman, gravida 1, now para 1, underwent induction of labor with intravenous oxytocin. Her gestational age was 42 weeks. Serial uterine measurements showed a decreasing fundal height. Obstetric ultrasound showed decreasing amniotic fluid. Her labor progresses normally, but the electronic fetal monitor tracing shows intermittently repetitive fetal heart rate (FHR) decelerations characterized by a sudden drop of 40 beats a minute, lasting 30 seconds then rapidly returning to baseline. These decelerations disappear after normal saline is infused into the uterus through an intrauterine catheter. After a spontaneous vaginal delivery, the 2850-g (6 lb 4.5 oz) neonate is noted to have decreased subcutaneous tissue; meconium-stained, peeling skin; and long fingernails. Which of the following is the most likely diagnosis?

(A) Dysmaturity syndrome
(B) Immaturity syndrome
(C) Small-for-gestational-age syndrome
(D) Beckwith-Wiedemann syndrome
(E) Meckel-Gruber syndrome

24 A 34-year-old female with known acquired immune deficiency syndrome (AIDS) is admitted to the hospital with a history of fatigue and difficulty swallowing. She has a temperature of 39.0°C (102.2°F); pulse, 88 beats/min regular; respiratory rate, 18/min; and a blood pressure of 108/89 mm Hg. She lost 20 lb during the last 3 weeks and has evidence of candidiasis in the throat. Her CD4+ cell count is 25/mm³. She is being treated with fluconazole, ganciclovir, indinavir, lamivudine (3TC), and zidovudine (AZT). Which of the following statements is most accurate regarding this combination of drugs?

(A) Because this patient is on AZT and indinavir, higher than normal doses of AZT should be used.
(B) Indinavir is included in the drug regimen for prophylaxis against herpes simplex virus (HSV).
(C) Human immunodeficiency virus (HIV) viral RNA titers in this patient will be less than 100 copies/mL
(D) Fluconazole is the drug of choice for treatment of cryptosporidiosis.
(E) The effects of lamivudine (3TC) are additive to those of zidovudine (AZT) against HIV.

25 A 56-year-old woman, gravida 0, para 0, underwent a cone biopsy for carcinoma in situ of the cervix at age 29. She experienced spontaneous menopause at age 51. Although she has a history of endometriosis, she has been on unopposed estrogen replacement therapy since menopause. She is 165 cm (65 in) tall and weighs 57 kg (125 lb). Her temperature is normal, pulse is 80 beats/min, and respirations are 16 per min. Her blood pressure is 110/65 mm Hg, and she has no systemic diseases. Which of the following is a risk factor for this woman relative to her development of endometrial carcinoma?

(A) Cervical carcinoma in situ
(B) Body mass index
(C) Blood pressure
(D) Estrogen replacement therapy
(E) Endometriosis

26 A 37-year-old man has been in an automobile accident and hit his head on the dashboard, knocking him unconscious. However, by the time the paramedics arrived he regained consciousness and was quite lucid. He then lapsed back into an unconscious state and went into a deep coma. An epidermal hematoma was diagnosed, identified by computed tomography (CT) as a bright-white, lens-shaped (lentiform) mass on the side of the hematoma. A burr hole is made to evacuate the hematoma, but 24 hours later the patient remains in a deep coma, although he does move his head intermittently and seems to try to mouth words. Initially his nutritional requirements will most likely be met by which one of the following routes?

(A) Per os
(B) Enterally via small-bore feeding tube placed via the nose into the stomach
(C) Parenterally via a central vein
(D) Parenterally via a peripheral vein
(E) Anally via a suppository

27 A 23-year-old man, who recently came to the United States from Southeast Asia, makes an appointment to see his family physician for a physical. He is concerned that he may die of liver cancer. The patient smokes 10 cigarettes per day and has been doing so for the past 5 years. He does not consume alcohol but likes to consume carbonated sodas. He states that his father and two uncles recently died in China province of liver cancer. The patient is slender and has normal vital signs. He has no icterus or pallor and no thyromegaly or lymphadenopathy. Examination of the cardiovascular, respiratory, and abdominal systems is unremarkable. Which of the following preventive measures is most likely to reduce the incidence of hepatocellular carcinoma?

(A) Immunization against hepatitis B
(B) Increase in dietary fiber
(C) Control of disease sexually transmitted by the human papillomavirus (HPV)
(D) Smoking cessation
(E) Immunization against hepatitis A

28 A 33-year-old anxious, gravida 3, para 1, aborta 1, woman is seen for her first prenatal visit at 10 weeks' gestation by dates. This was a planned pregnancy, and she discontinued the transdermal contraceptive patch 4 months ago. She is taking prenatal vitamins including iron and folic acid. First-trimester bleeding that progressed to hemorrhage complicated her first pregnancy, necessitating a suction dilatation and curettage at 8 weeks' gestation. Her last pregnancy was uncomplicated prenatally. She went into spontaneous labor at 39 weeks' gestation, progressing normally during labor with a reassuring electronic fetal heart rate monitor pattern. However, after an uncomplicated spontaneous vaginal delivery with neonatal Apgar scores of 8 and 9 at 1 and 5 minutes, respectively, her female neonate died on the second day of life from overwhelming group B β-hemolytic streptococcal infection. Which of the following statements best expresses what you will tell her about her current pregnancy?

(A) Most women with a positive vaginal culture will have uninfected infants.
(B) A negative vaginal culture means the fetus will not be at risk at delivery.
(C) Appropriate treatment for a positive vaginal culture can eradicate the organism.
(D) The organism is a pathologic bacterium in the female genital tract.
(E) Rapid nonculture assay tests are highly specific for the organism.

29 A 51-year-old obese female was admitted to the hospital for recurrent pain in the right upper quadrant of her abdomen that radiated to the back. She also complained of occasional nausea and vomiting but revealed no other relevant medical history. At that time, her vital signs were normal, and she had no icterus, pallor, or cyanosis. Tenderness was present to palpation in the right upper abdominal quadrant; there was no guarding or rigidity. No organomegaly was noted, and no masses were felt. Bowel sounds were normal. Findings of examinations of the cardiovascular and respiratory systems were normal. Her electrolytes and serum chemistries were normal except for a mild leukocytosis. Ultrasound confirmed cholelithiasis for which she underwent laparoscopic cholecystectomy under general anesthesia. She now has an intravenous line in place, together with an indwelling urinary catheter and a nasogastric tube. Twenty-four hours after the procedure she develops fever, tachycardia, sudden difficulty breathing, and pain in the chest. The most likely cause for this patient's current condition is which of the following?

(A) Pulmonary embolus
(B) Postoperative wound infection
(C) Atelectasis
(D) Intravenous (IV) catheter-related sepsis
(E) Spontaneous pneumothorax
(F) Aspiration pneumonitis

30 Following a recent marital separation, a 35-year-old woman who had been a cheerful, outgoing working mother develops insomnia, weight loss, irritability, hypervigilance, and feelings of worthlessness. These feelings become so strong and worrisome to her that she consults a clinical psychologist who diagnosed an adjustment disorder. Which of the following would indicate that these symptoms are caused by an adjustment disorder?

(A) Her reaction is not part of a pattern of overreaction to stress.
(B) She has a history of difficulty in adjusting to new situations and is often anxious and depressed.
(C) She has a pattern of anxiolytic medication abuse.
(D) She was involved in an abusive relationship with her spouse.
(E) The stressor is beyond the range of normal human experience.

31 A 36-year-old male presents at an emergency department with his wife of 2 years. She explains that while they were watching television at home, the patient said that he felt funny and dropped to the ground. He then started shaking violently, and became unconscious but recovered after a few minutes. The patient adds that he had been a long-term seizure patient and had been taking 300 mg of phenytoin daily and was compliant with the medication. However, during the past decade his seizures became less frequent, and he had none for at least 3 years. His serum phenytoin level is 11 mg/dL (therapeutic range is 10–20 mg/dL). Which of the following is the best therapeutic maneuver?

(A) Order another electroencephalogram (EEG)
(B) Raise the phenytoin dosage
(C) Add phenobarbital
(D) Substitute with carbamazepine
(E) Order a magnetic resonance imaging (MRI) study

32 A 17-year-old female has had disturbing auditory hallucinations for the past year in which voices utter derogatory statements to her. For the first 2 to 3 months, she perceived the voices only on occasion, and they perplexed and frightened her. During this period, she sought constant reassurance from her family and friends. However, the voices have continued to become more frequent. As she has become more accepting of the voices, she has withdrawn more from social contact. Which of the following statements about her case is most accurate?

(A) No genetic predisposition has been established for her most likely diagnosis.
(B) There is a clear pattern of predisposing family psychodynamics for her symptoms.
(C) She is very likely to have a progressive downhill course.
(D) There is evidence that early use of antipsychotic medication alters the course of her illness.
(E) There is likely to be no benefit to her from social rehabilitation therapies.

33 A 47-year-old woman has the onset of severe anxiety and tremulousness after forgetting to take her midday dose of medication. The early onset of these severe withdrawal symptoms suggests that she is most likely taking which one of the following medications?

(A) Alprazolam
(B) Diazepam
(C) Fluoxetine
(D) Imipramine
(E) Paroxetine

34 A 44-year-old man complains of back and joint pains. He states that his urine turns black if left standing. Physical examination reveals increased pigmentation in the sclera and ears. There is restriction to forward flexion of the spine and swelling and pain in both knees. Which of the following enzymes is most likely deficient?

(A) Arylsulfatase A
(B) α_1-Antitrypsin
(C) β-Glucocerebrosidase
(D) Homogentisate oxidase
(E) Phenylalanine hydroxylase

35 A 24-year-old medical student accidentally sticks his finger after drawing blood from a woman who is having elective surgery for removal of a benign breast mass. As part of the normal routine in handling accidental needle sticks, a baseline liver profile is routinely conducted on all employees at risk. The profile consists of a total bilirubin, serum aspartate aminotransferase (AST), serum alanine aminotransferase (ALT), serum alkaline phosphatase, and serum γ-glutamyltransferase. What is the approximate percentage chance of one of these five tests having had a value outside the normal reference interval for that test at the time the baseline test values were determined?

(A) 5%
(B) 10%
(C) 15%
(D) 20%
(E) 25%

36 A 27-year-old man makes an appointment to see a physician because he and his wife have been trying to get pregnant for the past year with no success. His wife previously consulted her gynecologist, and no problem was found that might suggest she was not fertile. Examination of the patient disclosed that he was of normal height but had disproportionally long arms and legs, a female pattern of pubic hair distribution, gynecomastia, and small testicles. Which of the following laboratory findings is most likely present?

(A) Decreased concentration of follicle-stimulating hormone (FSH)
(B) Decreased concentration of luteinizing hormone (LH)
(C) Increased concentration of serum estradiol
(D) Normal concentration of serum testosterone
(E) Normal sperm count

37 A 32-year-old woman, gravida 2, para 1, aborta 1, has recurrent gestational trophoblastic disease with metastasis to the liver. She was diagnosed with a benign complete molar pregnancy 3 months previously and was managed with monitoring of serial quantitative β-human chorionic gonadotropin (β-hCG) titers. Chemotherapy was not used. Her serum β-hCG titers initially fell to very low levels from a peak of 200,000 mIU/mL, but it has started to rise again and now is 30,000 mIU/mL. Which of the following criteria place her in the poor-prognosis category?

(A) Her chronologic age
(B) Time since antecedent pregnancy

(C) Current β-hCG level
(D) Parity
(E) Location of metastasis

38 A 23-year-old man seeks counseling because he is extremely angry with his coworkers. He believes that they deliberately torment him by exposing his lack of skill and experience. He also believes that his family may be conspiring with them to have him fired. During the first counseling session, he describes fantasies of taking a gun to work and shooting everyone in his office. Which of the following is the most ominous sign that he might take action?

(A) A history of alcohol abuse
(B) A history of violence toward others
(C) A lack of anxiety associated with his statements
(D) The presence of persecutory delusions
(E) The presence of temporal lobe epilepsy

39 A 49-year-old man complains of a 6-month history of worrying about his health, increased desire to sleep, demoralization, and difficulty focusing attention on tasks. Which of the following is the most likely diagnosis?

(A) A manic episode
(B) Somatization disorder
(C) Generalized anxiety disorder
(D) A depressive episode
(E) Delirium

40 A 33-year-old man presents to the emergency department with an acute onset of severe, colicky left flank pain, with radiation of the pain down the abdomen into the groin. He has increased frequency of urination and dysuria. Urinalysis shows a dipstick result positive for blood; urinary pH is 5.85. Sediment examination confirms the presence of hematuria and shows the presence of calcium oxalate crystals. Which of the following is the most common metabolic abnormality associated with this patient's disease?

(A) Hypercalciuria
(B) Increased urine citrate
(C) Hyperuricemia
(D) Alkaline urine pH
(E) Distal renal tubular acidosis

Directions for Matching Questions (41 through 50): *Each set of matching questions is preceded by a list of 4 to 26 lettered options followed by a brief explanation of the required task and then by a series of numbered statements. For each lettered statement you are to select ONE lettered option that best fulfills the task as it relates to that statement. Remember that each of the listed options might be correctly selected once, more than once, or not at all.*

Questions 41–50

Match the ONE lettered choice that is best associated with the numbered (41–50) condition described below.

(A) Substitution of valine for glycine in the β-chain of hemoglobin

(B) Hydrops fetalis

(C) Hemoglobin H disease

(D) Tetrahydrobiopterin (TH4B) deficiency

(E) Branched-chain α-keto acid dehydrogenase deficiency

(F) Deficiency of cystathionine β-synthetase

(G) Abnormal or deficient type I collagen

(H) Abnormal or deficient type II collagen

(I) Abnormal or deficient type III collagen

(J) Glucose-6-phosphatase deficiency

(K) Lysyl hydroxylase deficiency

(L) Williams syndrome

41 A 6-month-old infant has a hematocrit of 26%. Electrophoresis of a red cell homogenate shows the presence of a β-globin tetramer.

42 A baby girl is born with unusually blue sclera and numerous fractures.

43 A 3-month-old infant has been thriving poorly and has a prominent belly, hypotonia, hepatomegaly, and hypoglycemia. The infant's parents are first cousins who are non-Ashkenazi Jews who immigrated to the United States from Tunisia via France.

44 A newborn's fetal membranes broke 34 hours prior to birth. At birth the boy was unusually limp; he had flexible kyphosis, very loose joints, and hematomas of the conjunctivae and eyelids. By the age of 3 years his scoliosis is even more evident, as are his hyperflexable joints and hyperelastic skin; in addition, he has retinal detachment. His parents are third cousins.

45 A first-grade boy with unusual elflinlike features is referred to a pediatric psychologist to determine if he has attention deficit disorder (ADD) because he is inattentive at school and has obvious learning difficulties. He is also characterized as being outgoing and socially adept.

46 A fussy neonate's diapers have a sweet order.

47 A 6-year-old boy presents with a head having a bulging forehead. His head also seems large for his body size, and his arms, legs, and digits are extremely short. In addition, his legs are bowed and he has lordosis.

48 A mentally retarded 12-year old boy also suffers from dislocated lens and has had deep vein thrombolic events in both legs.

49 A 12-month-old African-American girl has been beset with bone pain accompanied by low-grade fever for the past 2 months and yesterday was rushed to the emergency department because of a hemolytic crisis.

50 A newborn child tests positive after being screened for high serum phenylalanine levels. However, she does not respond as expected to the reduced phenylalanine formula used to treat phenylketonuria (PKU).

Answer Key

1	D	**11**	B	**21**	C	**31**	B	**41**	C
2	B	**12**	C	**22**	C	**32**	D	**42**	G
3	B	**13**	E	**23**	A	**33**	A	**43**	J
4	D	**14**	E	**24**	E	**34**	D	**44**	K
5	B	**15**	B	**25**	D	**35**	E	**45**	L
6	E	**16**	D	**26**	D	**36**	C	**46**	E
7	D	**17**	C	**27**	A	**37**	E	**47**	H
8	E	**18**	C	**28**	A	**38**	B	**48**	F
9	B	**19**	D	**29**	C	**39**	D	**49**	A
10	C	**20**	D	**30**	A	**40**	A	**50**	D

Answers and Explanations

1 The answer is D   *Medicine*

Pain in the face followed by swelling of the face and respiratory difficulties while resting outdoors is most likely due to an anaphylactic reaction caused by a bee sting. Bee stings are the most common cause of death from venomous animal bites in the United States. Most systemic reactions to insect stings are type I hypersensitivity reactions that occur in previously sensitized patients who have produced high titers of immunoglobulin E (IgE) antibodies against venom from that insect. These antibodies attach to mast cells and basophils and are distributed throughout the body. The release of histamine and other mediators that are vasodilators and bronchoconstrictors results from reexposure to antigen, with the bridging of two subjacent IgE antibodies by antigen on the surface of mast cells and basophils. The predominant clinical findings involve the skin and the respiratory and cardiovascular systems. Clinical findings in mildly sensitized persons include a local wheal-and-flare reaction at the site of the bite, pain, hives, flushing, wheezing, rhinitis, conjunctivitis, and fever. A severely sensitized patient often presents with hypotension, diffuse urticaria, laryngeal edema, bronchospasm, diarrhea with abdominal cramping, and arrhythmia. Laryngeal obstruction is the most common cause of death in these patients, followed by cardiovascular collapse. Initially, anaphylaxis is treated with intramuscular administration of aqueous epinephrine 1:1000 (choice **D**). The dose is 0.2–2.5 mL. This can be repeated every 5–15 minutes or so as needed. If there is no response to this therapy or if the patient is in profound shock, a 1:10,000 dose of aqueous epinephrine is given intravenously (choice **E**). Intravenous fluids such as lactated Ringer's and plasma expanders may be necessary as well to redress the loss of intravascular plasma into the tissue spaces. If orofacial swelling is present, the patient is intubated before laryngeal edema sets in.

Other options in less severe envenomations include the use of diphenhydramine hydrochloride (1 mg/kg) either by mouth or parenterally. A nebulized β₂-agonist, such as albuterol (choice **B**), or intravenous aminophylline (choice **C**) is useful in the treatment of bronchospasm. Intravenous administration of hydrocortisone (choice **A**) is sometimes used in moderation to treat severe envenomations but does not appear to prevent recurrent waves of anaphylaxis.

The sting site should be examined and the stinger removed by scraping it off with a knife rather than using tweezers, which can introduce more venom into the wound. Patients who have demonstrated exaggerated local cutaneous, respiratory, or cardiovascular reactions to insect stings should be prescribed an emergency epinephrine kit with syringe and should be taught how to use it. They should carry this with them at all times. Venom immunotherapy is 95% effective in preventing anaphylaxis on subsequent exposures. Children with only localized cutaneous reactions are at low risk (<10%) for developing systemic reactions; therefore, immunotherapy is not recommended in them.

2 The answer is B   *Surgery*

This patient has carcinoma of the nasopharynx. It usually occurs in younger individuals, and there is a high incidence among those of Chinese ethnicity. In early stages, almost 50% of patients have elevated anti–Epstein-Barr virus antibodies, while in the late stages, it goes up to 100%. It would be interesting to see if the development of an Epstein-Barr virus vaccine in Britain would help in eradicating this disease. In adults, most cases turn out to be squamous cell carcinoma, while among children, lymphoma is most common. Initial management is to biopsy the nasopharynx (choice **B**) to confirm the diagnosis.

Sputum cytology (choice **A**) is not going to contribute to the diagnosis, given that this patient has had no respiratory symptoms such as cough, hemoptysis, or a history of smoking and weight loss. Biopsy of the lymph node (choice **C**) should not be performed. Doing so will affect block dissection of the neck later on, or it may lead to implantation of tumor cells in the subcutaneous tissues. A thyroid tumor would most likely be evident on physical examination, and since it was not noted, an iodine-123 (^{123}I) scan of the thyroid (choice **D**) would be noncontributory. Bronchoscopy (choice **E**) will not be helpful for the same reasons that sputum cytology would be futile.

3 **The answer is B** *Surgery*

Pressure sores, also known as decubitus ulcers and commonly called bed sores, are generally associated with bedridden elderly individuals. However, they occur whenever there is prolonged pressure of the skin against an external object in persons of any age. However, persons who are aged, debilitated, paralyzed, or unconscious are more susceptible. To avoid ulcer formation, prolonged pressure on any given area of the skin must be avoided. This requires frequent rotation of immobilized bedridden patients and changing the position of wheelchair-bound individuals. Friction must also be avoided, since friction is liable to occur on the sacrum, buttocks, and upper legs of patients in wheelchairs who drive around, as in the patient described. Once erythema develops it may progress to ulceration quickly, and a small ulcer can progress to a large ulcer within 24 to 48 hours (choice **B**). The progression is caused by local edema or infection. Severe infection must be recognized and treated with appropriate therapy before it leads to more generalized problems.

Although pressure sores are commonly thought of as a problem unique to bedridden patients (as demonstrated by the alternative name of bed sores), persons who sit in a given position are just as prone to develop an ulcer as one who lies still in bed (choice **A**). The most common sites for pressure sores to develop are the sacrum, the trochanters, the heels (choice **C** is incorrect), the lateral malleoli, and the buttocks over the ischium. The heel is susceptible in bed because it may press upon the mattress, in wheelchairs because it may press upon the back of the footrest, and a distinctive type of ulcer may develop on the heels of diabetic individuals with neuropathy who do not realize that their shoes are rubbing on the back of their heels.

Gram-positive cocci are found in fewer than 40% of infected ulcers; consequently, pressure ulcer infections are not almost always caused by *Staphylococcus aureus* (choice **D** is incorrect). Other organisms commonly found in such infections include *Pseudomonas aeruginosa*, *Providencia* species, *Proteus* species, and *Bacteroides fragilis* and other anaerobic species. The best combination of antibiotics, therefore, is one that will treat gram-positive aerobic cocci, gram-negative aerobic rods, and anaerobic bacteria. A recommended drug combination is clindamycin and gentamicin, with the warning to monitor renal function carefully while the patient is on gentamicin.

In addition to using systemic antibiotics, the ulcer must be treated. An infected pressure sore should not be treated with topical antiseptics that may irritate the wound, because this might inhibit healing; thus choice **E** is incorrect. However, clearing up the infection is critical, since otherwise septicemia, bacterial cellulitis, osteomyelitis, or septic arthritis may develop. The first step in treatment is cleaning and débridement. Cleaning is best done by rinsing with a sterile isotonic saline solution. The débridement may be facilitated by use of enzymatic agents such as collagenase, fibrinolysin, deoxyribonuclease, streptokinase, and streptodornase, augmented by using hydrophilic polymers such as dextranomer. Once an ulcer is clean and granulation or epithelialization begins to occur, then a moist wound environment should be maintained without disturbing the healing tissue.

4 **The answer is D** *Medicine*

Chronic lymphocytic leukemia (CLL) usually affects individuals older than 50 years of age and his symptoms and the lymphocystosis indicated that this man has developed this disease. Intravenous infusion of fludarabine (choice **D**), an antimetabolite, is the first line of treatment. The treatment is given 5 days a week once a month for up to 6 months. As the patient has a normal hematocrit and no evidence of autoimmune hemolytic anemia, this medication can be given safely. Administering it to patients with autoimmune hemolytic anemia will only exacerbate that condition. Although an oral form of fludarabine is available in other countries, at the time of writing it is not available in the United States.

Alemtuzumab (choice **A**) is used only for refractory cases of CLL and is administered intravenously. It is a monoclonal antibody that binds to the CD52 antigen, which is a glycoprotein found on the surface of both normal and malignant B and T lymphocytes. In binding to this antigen it destroys both malignant and normal cells; however, the latter recover. Alemtuzumab is very effective in clearing malignant lymphocytes from both the peripheral blood and bone marrow. Chlorambucil (choice **B**) is an alkylating agent that is no longer the first choice in the treatment of CLL. In the United States, it is reserved for the very elderly, as this is the only available oral antineoplastic agent for this disease in the United States at this time. The drug is given for 3 weeks in a month for a total of 6 months and is often combined with prednisone. Prednisone (choice **C**) is used if the patient has an associated immune thrombocytopenia or autoimmune hemolytic anemia. If this patient had an associated autoimmune hemolytic anemia or immune thrombocytopenia, then a combination of fludarabine and prednisone (choice **E**) would be appropriate. Intravenous infusion of a combination of fludarabine and rituximab or of fludarabine and cyclophosphamide (choice **F**) does produce a better response rate; however, it is not the first line of treatment. (Rituximab is a monoclonal antibody that is directed against the CD20 antigen found on the surface of normal and malignant B lymphocytes. Cyclophosphamide is an alkylating agent that prevents cell division by cross-linking DNA strands.) Intravenous infusion of a combination of fludarabine, rituximab, and cyclophosphamide—three agents (choice **G**)—can be used sometimes if the two-agent combination does not provide desired results. However, once again, this is not a first-line therapy.

5 **The answer is B** *Obstetrics and Gynecology*

Infection with the human immunodeficiency virus (HIV) results in development of the acquired immune deficiency syndrome (AIDS), which has been a recognized disease in the United States since 1981. All pregnant HIV-positive women regardless of HIV RNA viral load and CD4 count should be placed on AZT at 14 weeks and continued on it throughout pregnancy and labor. Mode of delivery is one of the most significant factors that affect maternal–neonatal transmission (choice **B**). Current recommendations are that HIV-positive women should be offered elective cesarean section at 38 weeks to minimize vertical HIV transmission.

Pregnancy does not appear to accelerate progression of HIV to AIDS (choice **A**). Neonates can be infected from HIV-positive breast-feeding mothers (choice **C**). There is no current effective immunization for neonates (choice **D**). Disease progression of HIV to AIDS in neonates and infants is more rapid than in adults, probably because of their immature immune status (choice **E**).

6 **The answer is E** *Medicine*

This patient has von Willebrand's disease (VWD) (choice **E**), a condition characterized by defective hemostasis. There are several subtypes of the disease. Types I, IIA, and IIb are autosomal dominant, while type III is autosomal recessive. VWD also can be acquired because of formation of autoantibodies, for example in myeloproliferative disorders. Abnormal hemostasis is due to defective or absent von Willebrand's factor (VWF), a high-molecular-weight plasma protein that arbitrates adherence of platelets to injured endothelium. VWF is essential for normal platelet function and to maintain adequate levels of factor VIII:coagulant (VIII:C). In the absence of adequate functional VWF, bruising transpires readily, and bleeding can occur from the nasal and oral mucosa, and genital, renal, or gastrointestinal tract. In addition, increased bleeding could occur during menstruation and following surgical procedures or tooth extraction. Type I VWD is the most common variant, constituting about 80% of cases. In types I and III VWD there is a quantitative defect; decreased amounts of normal factor are synthesized, and bleeding tends to be mild or moderate. On the other hand, in types IIa and IIb a defective VWF is produced (qualitative defect) that cannot form the normal multimeric quaternary structures essential for activity. In these patients, severe mucocutaneous and deep tissue bleeding can result. In all types of VWD, laboratory studies will reveal a normal platelet count, normal prothrombin time (PT), prolonged bleeding time (BT), and prolonged activated partial thromboplastin time (APTT). VWF level is decreased, and factor VIII:C is decreased as well. The ristocetin agglutination assay is decreased in types I, IIa, and III but increased in type IIb. In type I, IIa, and III disorders, platelet aggregation is defective. This is confirmed by the ristocetin induced platelet aggregation (RIPA) test, in which platelet aggregation is reduced. In type IIb disorder on the other hand, the RIPA result is increased. The epistaxis in this patient is due to platelet dysfunction. The menorrhagia, on the other hand, is due to deficiency in factor VIII:C, which improved when she took estrogens.

The treatment for VWD depends on the type and severity of bleeding. Mild bleeding in type 1 is treated with desmopressin, which acts by releasing endogenous factor VIII from plasma storage sites. Desmopressin is ineffective in type IIa and harmful in type IIb VMD, where it could lead to thrombocytopenia. Factor VIIII concentrate is used in severe bleeding and when desmopressin is contraindicated or ineffective. Prophylaxis prior to dental extraction is achieved by using ε-aminocaproic acid, which inhibits fibrinolysis.

Hemophilia A (choice **A**) is a sex-linked recessive disease; consequently, it occurs in males only. In the vignette, the patient is a female. The disease results from a deficiency of factor VIII:C, leading to a prolonged APTT, but the BT and PT are normal. The decrease in factor VIII:C levels distinguishes hemophilia A from prolonged APTT due to other causes. Hemophilia B (choice **B**) is also known as Christmas disease and is characterized by low levels of factor IX coagulant activity. Like hemophilia A, this disease is a sex-linked recessive disorder that affects males only. Also as in hemophilia A, the APTT is prolonged and the PT and BT are normal.

The distinction between hemophilias A and B is made by determining which coagulation factor level is deficient. Disseminated intravascular coagulation (DIC) (choice **C**) is due to in vivo activation of the coagulation system causing formation of fibrin thrombi throughout the microcirculation. Major risk factors for the development of DIC are gram-negative sepsis and trauma. In the process of forming fibrin thrombi, factors I, II, V, and VIII are consumed, resulting in low concentrations of these in plasma. This makes the patient anticoagulated, as manifested by bleeding from all orifices and puncture sites along with prolongation of the APTT and PT. In addition, small vessels are occluded by fibrin thrombi. Platelets are trapped within fibrin thrombi, resulting in thrombocytopenia and a prolonged bleeding time. Secondary activation of the fibrinolytic system leads to release of plasmin, which breaks down fibrin clots into fibrin degradation products that are readily detected in the blood. Qualitative platelet defects are most commonly due to aspirin (choice **D**). Aspirin prolongs the BT but has no effect on the coagulation tests; thus, the PT and the APTT are normal. Factor VII deficiency (choice **F**) is an autosomal recessive disease. Deficiency of factor VII prolongs the PT because factor VII is in the extrinsic system. Both the APTT and BT are normal.

7 The answer is D   *Surgery*

This patient has a long history of smoking, which leads to chronic obstructive pulmonary disease (COPD). This increases the risk for atelectasis, pneumonia, and even hypoxemia following surgery. While chest x-ray films, electrocardiograms (ECGs), and arterial blood gases (ABGs) are all useful preoperative screens, pulmonary function tests provide the best preoperative screen, because they reflect dynamic measurements of pulmonary function in the patient. The forced expiratory volume in 1 second (FEV_1) indicates how much air can be expelled from the lungs in 1 second after a maximal inspiration (normally, 4 L). The forced vital capacity (FVC) represents the entire amount of air that can be expelled (normally 5 L). The ratio of the FEV_1 to the FVC (normally 80%) is considered the best overall screen (choice **D**). Values less than 50% of the predicted outcome correlate with a high risk for postoperative pulmonary complications.

Arterial blood gas (ABG) measurements include arterial pH (choice **A**), arterial carbon dioxide tension (P_{CO_2}) (choice **B**), P_{O_2} (choice **C**), and oxygen saturation (choice **E**). These measurements reflect primary acid–base disorders (e.g., acidosis or alkalosis), but they do not predict pulmonary complications in the postoperative state. Respiratory acidosis secondary to retention of carbon dioxide is the main reason for evaluating ABGs, because respiratory acidosis is always associated with hypoxemia and low oxygen saturation.

8 The answer is E   *Obstetrics and Gynecology*

The scenario is consistent with postpartum endometritis. Puerperal infection and sepsis account for significant postpartum maternal morbidity and mortality. The most significant obstetric event of those listed in the peripartum course is prolonged premature rupture of membranes (PROM) (choice **E**), by far the most common cause of postpartum infection. The diagnosis is based on clinical findings, and an exquisitely tender uterus is diagnostic. Lochial cultures are not done because the cause is polymicrobial normal flora from the genital tract. Management is with in-hospital parenteral broad-spectrum antibiotics.

Manual placental removal (choice **A**) is appropriate when the third stage of labor exceeds 30 minutes and is not a likely risk factor for infection. Postpartum tubal sterilization (choice **B**) is typically an elective procedure performed through a clean, refined incision and is not a risk factor. Retained products of conception (choice **C**) can get infected, but they are more likely to cause postpartum hemorrhage. Spontaneous vaginal delivery (choice **D**) is an unlikely risk factor for puerperal genital tract infection.

9 The answer is B   *Medicine*

This patient has metastatic deposits causing spinal cord compression. The most sensitive test is magnetic resonance imaging (MRI) with gadolinium contrast (choice **B**). This will demonstrate the location and extent of the deposit. Administering intravenous steroids is a temporizing measure to deal with cord edema.

An emergency CT myelogram (choice **A**) would not be as helpful as MRI in establishing the exact location and extent of the lesion. Radiography of the thoracic spine (choice **C**) would only show bony erosion or collapse of the vertebra; it would not define the location or extent of the metastatic mass. An electromyograph (EMG) (choice **D**) would not be diagnostic and would not be expected to show abnormalities for approximately 3 weeks after the onset of weakness. Once the MRI is done, further treatment could be decided. This could entail a further course of radiotherapy (choice **E**) or a combination of surgery followed by radiotherapy.

10 The answer is C *Medicine*

Rapid intravenous administration of furosemide (choice **C**) could lead to transient hearing loss. It would be judicious to ascertain that there is no hearing loss before administering a rapid intravenous dose of furosemide to avoid being accused of inducing it if there was evidence for it in the first place. Other adverse effects include dizziness and vertigo.

Furosemide can affect the gastrointestinal tract (choice **A**) but usually not after rapid intravenous administration. Gastrointestinal effects include nausea and vomiting, constipation, anorexia, abdominal pain, and pancreatitis. The sense of taste (choice **B**) is not affected, nor is the sense of smell (choice **D**). Transient loss of vision (choice **E**) does not occur after rapid intravenous administration of furosemide; however, transient blurring of vision does.

11 The answer is B *Psychiatry*

Hypochondriasis (choice **B**) is characterized by misinterpretation of the meaning of symptoms that does not respond to physician reassurance even after medical assessment. Its incidence is unknown in the general population but is about 5% in the medical community and affects both sexes equally. The psychodynamic explanation is displaced anxiety, and it is generally brought about by stress. To be diagnosed, the condition must last at least 6 months and not be of delusional intensity. The onset is variable, but often it first occurs during early adulthood, and if the onset was sudden, complete remission often occurs. Otherwise, treatment consists of psychotherapy, often with concomitant treatment of anxiety and depression.

Conversion disorder (choice **A**) involves a loss of sensory or motor function. Delusional disorder, somatic type (choice **C**) is characterized by more irrational somatic beliefs, such as believing that diamonds are in the muscles or a "force field" is emanating from a limb. Somatization disorder (choice **D**) is characterized by multiple, simultaneous complaints, including pain symptoms. In factitious disorder (choice **E**), individuals deliberately produce symptoms.

12 The answer is C *Preventive Medicine and Public Health*

Since the potentially impaired individual is a pediatric resident, the problem should be reported to the director of the residency program (choice **C**). Informing law enforcement (choice **A**), or the medical ethics committee of the hospital, (choice **B**) is incorrect. Were he a medical student, he should be reported to the dean of student affairs in the medical school (choice **D**). On the other hand, if he was an attending physician, he should be reported to the chief of medical staff (choice **E**).

13 The answer is E *Surgery*

This patient has typical "Saturday night palsy" as a result of entrapment of the radial nerve (choice **E**). This leads to weakness and paralysis of all muscles supplied by this nerve. It occurs when a person rests his arm over an object that compresses the radial nerve in the spiral groove. On arising, the patient notices a wrist drop and is unable to dorsiflex it. Sensations are usually minimally affected by problems at this level; sensory loss is limited to a small area on the back of the hand, between the thumb and index finger. Axial radial nerve entrapment also commonly occurs in patient on crutches or even by hanging the arm over the back of a chair. The radial nerve may also be entrapped or injured more distally, for example at the elbow, affecting the extensors of the wrist and fingers, or immediately below the elbow (the interosseous branch), only affecting the finger extensors. Finally, the superficial radial nerve may be compressed at the wrist by binding the hands, wearing handcuffs that are too tight, and even by bracelets or wrist watch straps that are too tight and not promptly removed.

Entrapment of the median nerve (choice **A**) results in carpal tunnel syndrome. This is a progressive condition that usually follows repetitive stress injury. The patient complains of pain over the flexor aspect of the wrist, and hypesthesia may be noted over the sensory distribution of the median nerve in the hand. Phalen's sign will be positive. Entrapment of the ulnar nerve (choice **B**) results in hypesthesia over the little finger and the medial half of the ring finger. Paralysis of the small muscles of the hand (with the exception of the thenar group of muscles and the radial two lumbricals) leads to inability to abduct and adduct the fingers. Entrapment of the ulnar nerve often follows adhesions that result from osteoarthritis at the elbow. Treatment involves transposition of the nerve. Sometimes fractures at the elbow can change the carrying angle, resulting in stretching of the ulnar nerve. In such cases, surgical transposition is carried out as well. Entrapment of the musculocutaneous nerve (choice **C**) is incorrect; this nerve does not usually get entrapped and is rarely injured. The musculocutaneous nerve is a motor nerve supplying the biceps and the brachialis muscles, and it is sensory to the lateral aspect of the forearm. Entrapment of the axillary nerve (choice **D**) is incorrect. However, this nerve can be injured in fractures of the surgical neck of the humerus. It is motor to the deltoid and teres minor muscles and sensory to the shoulder joint and the skin overlying the lateral aspect of the shoulder. Fracture of the scaphoid bone (choice **F**) results from a fall on the outstretched hand. It does not cause a wrist drop or inability to move the hand or wrist. Nor does it damage a nerve. Movements of the wrist are possible but painful, and tenderness is elicited in the anatomic snuffbox. Fracture of the radius (choice **G**) is usually due to a fall or direct blow to it. It is associated with pain and deformity. Radial nerve paralysis is unlikely; however, paralysis of the posterior interosseous nerve could result. In approximately 8% of cases, fracture of the shaft of the humerus (choice **H**) causes injury to the radial nerve with subsequent paralysis. In such an injury, there is pain, swelling, and deformity of the arm, which this patient clearly does not have.

14. The answer is E   *Medicine*

This patient has syringomyelia, in which there is a syrinx in the cervical spinal cord. As a result, the central canal is dilated (choice **E**), and is demonstrable on MRI with contrast enhancement. The term *syrinx* refers to an abnormal collection of fluid within the spinal cord. Syringomyelia is often congenital and most commonly located in the cervical spinal cord. It may also sometimes be seen in patients with diastematomyelia, spinal cord tumors, Arnold Chiari malformation, and following spinal cord trauma. The lesion grows slowly. Hence, it may be years before the patient actually seeks attention. The syrinx expands anteriorly, causing pressure on the anterior commissure through which the second order neurons of the spinothalamic tract (anterolateral tract) cross to the contralateral side. The resulting pressure leads to selective loss of pain and temperature sensation only. It is called dissociative anesthesia, as the loss spares the sensations of touch, vibration, and proprioception that are carried in the dorsal columns. The loss of pain and temperature in the upper extremities and the chest has been described as having a "capelike distribution." Further expansion of the syrinx in an anterolateral direction leads to loss of anterior horn cells, with resultant atrophy of the small muscles of the hand. The patient may have spasticity in the lower extremities and weakness in the upper.

Normal MRI (choice **A**) results would be unlikely given the extensive neurologic deficits noted in this patient. In cervical spinal canal stenosis (choice **B**) the cervical canal is narrowed. This can be due to hypertrophy of the ligamentum flavum. The patient may have weakness of his upper extremities and difficulty walking due to spasticity in the lower extremities. Pain and temperature sensation is preserved. Herniated cervical disks (choice **C**) can result in neck pain or pain going down one or both shoulders. The patient may have decreased sensations and, as the disease progresses, weakness in one or the other hand, and even problems with walking due to spasticity. Pain and temperature sensations are not usually affected. Plaques in the spinal cord are usually seen in multiple sclerosis (MS) (choice **D**), a demyelinating disease that targets the oligodendrocytes; each oligodendrocyte myelinates between 20 and 60 axons. Involvement of the anterior horn cells and corticospinal pathways can occur, but selective loss of pain and temperature sensation is unusual. MS patients usually present with a history of diplopia that resolves, visual disturbance, and fatigue and may have fecal and urinary incontinence. Clinical examination would demonstrate optic atrophy and internuclear ophthalmoplegia among other features. Motor neuron disease (choice **F**), also known as amyotrophic sclerosis, is a progressive disorder that primarily targets the corticospinal tract and the anterior motor neurons. Thus, the patient will have a combination of upper and lower motor neuron signs. Fasciculations are an early feature. There is no sensory involvement in this disease.

15. The answer is B   *Medicine*

The patient has the basophilic intranuclear inclusion of cytomegalovirus (CMV) (choice **B**), which will have the classic "owl's eye" pattern. CMV pneumonitis is particularly common in organ transplantation patients, especially in bone marrow allograft recipients (10–15%), and in those with acquired immune deficiency syndrome (AIDS); the mortality rate is 85%. CMV hyperimmune globulin given to seronegative bone marrow recipients provides some protection from contracting the infection. Ganciclovir, a synthetic purine nucleoside analogue of guanine, is used in the prevention of CMV disease in transplant recipients. The drug is administered intravenously for up to 10 days prior to transplantation and taken orally thereafter.

Pneumocystis carinii (choice **A**) is not visualized with standard hematoxylin–eosin stains. Methenamine silver, Giemsa stains, and direct immunofluorescent stains are useful in identifying organisms in bronchial lavage specimens or lung biopsy specimens. The organisms look like crushed ping-pong balls. *Cryptococcus neoformans* (choice **C**) is the most common systemic fungal infection in the immunocompromised host. In tissue, it is an encapsulated yeast with narrow-based buds. *Blastomyces dermatitidis* (choice **D**) causes systemic fungal infection and in tissue is a yeast with broad-based buds. *Candida albicans* (choice **E**) causes a systemic fungal infection with yeast forms and pseudohyphae, the latter indicating the invasiveness of the organism. *Pneumocystis*, *Cryptococcus*, *Blastomyces*, and *Candida* do not produce intranuclear inclusions.

16 The answer is D *Medicine*

This patient has multiple myeloma, a malignant disorder of plasma cells, in which a serum protein electrophoresis (SPE) frequently exhibits a monoclonal spike (choice **D**) owing to a malignant clone of plasma cells that synthesize a single immunoglobulin (most commonly IgG) and its light chain (most commonly a κ light chain). There is T-cell suppression for synthesis of other immunoglobulins by B cells. Excess light chains are filtered into the urine, where they are identified as Bence Jones protein by urine electrophoresis. Hematologic findings include a normocytic anemia (60% of cases) and pancytopenia in advanced cases. The bleeding time may be prolonged because of qualitative platelet defects. Rouleaux (stack-of-coins effect) of the red blood cells (RBCs) occur due to an increase in fibrinogen, an acute phase reactant synthesized in the liver. Thus, the erythrocyte sedimentation rate (ESR) is increased and is frequently over 100 mm/hour. As a consequence, the ESR is increased in multiple myeloma, not normal (choice **B**). The bone marrow aspirate in the photograph shows a cluster of malignant plasma cells with eccentric nuclei, prominent nucleoli, and vacuoles in the cytoplasm. Bone pain is the initial manifestation in 70% of patients with multiple myeloma, and because osteoclast-activating factor is released by the neoplastic plasma cells, osteolytic lesions occur in 70% of cases; therefore, in approximately 20% of cases the serum calcium level is increased, not decreased (choice **C**).

In malignant breast cancer, stains are frequently positive for carcinoembryonic antigen (CEA) and estrogen and progesterone receptors (ERA and PRA, respectively) (choice **A**). These cells are glandular in appearance. Neither ERA nor PRA receptors are present in malignant plasma cells. Treatment with tamoxifen (choice **E**), an antiestrogen agent, is effective along with radiation in relieving bone pain in metastasis due to breast cancer, which also produces lytic lesions in the bone. It has no role to play in the management of multiple myeloma. Treatment of multiple myeloma, on the other hand, involves alkylating agents.

17 The answer is C *Psychiatry*

Frequent self-induced vomiting is a form of purging and can cause caries and erosion of tooth enamel owing to gastric acid, and fingers can be abraded by insertion of fingers into the pharynx, resulting in scratches from the teeth (choice **C**). Purging may occur as an isolated behavior or it may be part of an eating disorder such as bulimia nervosa or anorexia nervosa.

Amenorrhea (choice **A**) is a component of anorexia nervosa. Binge eating (choice **B**) is a component of bulimia nervosa, and normochromic microcytic anemia (choice **D**), weight loss (choice **E**) and gaunt features (choice **F**) may result from self-starvation in either anorexia nervosa or bulimia nervosa, but these factors, in isolation, do not demonstrate that the daughter is secretly inducing vomiting.

18 The answer is C *Obstetrics and Gynecology*

Adnexal disease can coexist with pregnancy. Neoplastic ovarian masses must be considered. However, for this young patient in the first trimester with a unilateral simple cystic adnexal mass, a benign corpus luteum cyst is the most likely diagnosis. After the placenta can produce adequate progesterone to maintain the pregnancy, the corpus luteum cyst will spontaneously regress (choice **C**).

Thus options suggesting a prognosis of gradual enlargement (choice **A**) and remaining the same size (choice **B**) are incorrect. Malignant adnexal masses are rare in this age group; thus, choices **D** and **E** are incorrect.

19 The answer is D *Surgery*

The most common complication after a carotid endarterectomy is an acute myocardial infarction (MI) (choice **D**). Endarterectomy is the standard treatment for symptomatic internal carotid artery stenosis greater than 70%. During the procedure, great care is taken to ensure that circulation to the hemisphere on the ipsilateral side is not compromised, which could result in a hemispheric infarction. Overall, there is approximately a 4% incidence of complications after this procedure.

In addition to acute MI, complications include stroke (uncommon) (choices **A** and **E**), numbness beneath the chin, and damage to the descending branch of the hypoglossal nerve. A pulmonary embolus (choice **B**) is not a common complication of carotid endarterectomy. Air embolism (choice **C**) is a potential problem in surgery or trauma in the head and neck area. Venous injury can result in air being sucked into the right atrium from the negative intrathoracic pressure associated with inspiration.

20 The answer is D *Medicine*

This patient has diabetic ketoacidosis (DKA), most likely due to the increased insulin requirement generated by the infection, a common problem. In DKA, glucosuria results in the loss of significant amounts of sodium, potassium, and phosphorus in the urine. When insulin is used in the treatment of DKA, phosphate is normally transported along with glucose into muscle and adipose cells; this permits phosphorylation of glucose, allowing further metabolism. Insulin treatment also enhances glycolysis, which further depletes the already decreased concentration of phosphate in the blood, leading to hypophosphatemia (choice **D**). Depletion of phosphate results in a corresponding decrease in adenosine triphosphate (ATP) within the muscle, leading to paralysis of the respiratory muscles and respiratory failure in the patient. This sequence of events is the rationale for providing phosphate supplementation in the treatment of DKA when phosphate levels begin to decline during insulin therapy.

Human insulin does not produce anaphylactic reactions (choice **A**). Glucose toxicity (choice **B**) refers to the effect of hyperglycemia in reducing the sensitivity of tissues to insulin therapy in both type 1 and type 2 diabetes mellitus. Ketoacidosis (choice **C**) is not a cause of muscle weakness resulting in respiratory problems. Although hyperkalemia (choice **E**) is commonly seen in the setting of DKA, it is not due to an excess of potassium stores, but is the result of a transcellular shift of potassium out of cells as excess hydrogen ions in ketoacidosis are buffered intracellularly. This transcellular shift often disguises the marked deficits in total body potassium that these patients have because of urinary potassium loss due to the osmotic effect of glucosuria. Severe hypokalemia can also cause muscle paralysis by preventing muscle repolarization. Therefore, potassium supplementation is extremely important in the treatment of DKA and can be given as potassium phosphate rather than potassium chloride. Bacteremia (choice **F**) is a feature of septic shock, in which the cardiovascular system is the target. Endotoxins, especially those due to gram-negative sepsis lead to hypotension, tachycardia, and tachypnea but not to paralysis of the respiratory muscles.

21 The answer is C *Psychiatry*

Much literature suggests that positive outcomes using cognitive psychotherapy approach use of antidepressant medication in efficacy for treatment of a single episode of major depressive disorder without psychosis (choice **C**). The task in cognitive psychotherapy is to define and change the thoughts and beliefs that lead to depressive mood.

The effectiveness of this technique is not well documented for dementia (choice **A**), developmental reading disorders (choice **B**), dissociative amnesia (choice **D**), or substance intoxication (choice **E**).

22 The answer is C *Medicine*

In a normal pregnancy the plasma volume is disproportionately increased relative to an increase in red blood cell mass (absolute increase in the number of red blood cells). This has a dilutional effect, causing a decrease in the concentration of hemoglobin (choice **C**), hematocrit, and red blood cell count (number of RBCs/mm³). Whereas the concentration (or level) of these factors are decreased, the amount need not be.

In pregnancy, estrogen and progesterone stimulate the central nervous system's respiratory center causing respiratory alkalosis (increase in arterial pH) (not decreased arterial pH; choice **A**). The increase in plasma volume increases the glomerular filtration rate, causing an increase in the creatinine clearance (not decreased; choice **B**) and a decrease in the serum blood urea nitrogen (not increased; choice **E**) because of a dilutional effect and increased clearance of urea in the urine. In pregnancy, the increase in estrogen causes increased synthesis of transcortin, the binding protein for cortisol. Since serum cortisol represents the cortisol that is bound to transcortin plus free cortisol (metabolically active), the serum cortisol is increased (not decreased; choice **D**). Serum adrenocorticotropic hormone levels are normal, because the free cortisol levels are normal. There are no signs of hypercortisolism. Estrogen also increases the synthesis of thyroid-binding globulin, causing an increase in serum thyroxine level (choice **F**) without increasing the free thyroxine level.

23 The answer is A   *Obstetrics and Gynecology*

Dysmaturity syndrome (choice **A**) is the correct answer. It occurs in 20–30% of postterm pregnancies and is characterized by aging of the placenta, "dehydration" of the fetoplacental unit, and meconium staining in utero. Oligohydramnios is frequently seen. The variable decelerations described in the scenario are a consequence of umbilical cord compressions due to the decreased amniotic fluid. Saline amnioinfusion creates a pseudoamniotic fluid that protects against cord compression.

Beckwith-Wiedemann syndrome (choice **D**) refers to macrosomic fetuses with hypoglycemia and macroglossia. Meckel-Gruber syndrome (choice **E**) is associated with a variety of anomalies, including encephalocele. Immaturity syndrome (choice **B**) and small-for-gestational-age syndrome (choice **C**) are spurious distractors.

24 The answer is E   *Medicine*

Combinations of drugs are commonly used in the management of patients with acquired immune deficiency syndrome (AIDS). This is partly due to the susceptibility of the immunocompromised patient, necessitating prophylaxis against, and treatment of, infections caused by opportunistic viral, bacterial, parasitic, and fungal pathogens. In addition, combinations of drugs with activity against human immunodeficiency virus (HIV) often exert additive effects and may also delay the emergence of resistant forms of the virus. Though they are both nucleoside reverse transcriptase inhibitors, lamivudine (3TC) and zidovudine (AZT) together have additive actions against HIV that can be seen at the clinical level (choice **E**).

Higher-than-normal doses of AZT (choice **A**) are not used in patients taking indinavir, as this may precipitate severe bone marrow suppression with resultant anemia, agranulocytosis, and thrombocytopenia. Indinavir has no activity against herpes (choice **B**) but does inhibit the hepatic metabolism of AZT and many other drugs. Nonetheless, synergistic actions occur with drug regimens that combine reverse transcriptase inhibitors with protease inhibitors (e.g., indinavir). In some patients treated with such anti-HIV drug combinations, viral RNA titers have fallen below detectable levels. However, this is not always the case, and there is no a priori reason to conclude that the viral RNA titer in this patient is below 100 copies/mL (choice **C**). Fluconazole is the drug of choice for treatment of esophageal candidiasis, and the patient has been prescribed this for candidiasis. It is also used very effectively in AIDS patients to prevent cryptococcal meningitis. There is no effective drug against cryptosporidiosis (choice **D**).

25 The answer is D   *Obstetrics and Gynecology*

The risk of developing endometrial carcinoma is related largely to conditions associated with anovulatory states or unopposed estrogen. Clearly, this patient's 5 years of unopposed estrogen replacement therapy (choice **D**) is her greatest risk factor.

While breast, colon, and ovarian carcinomas are risk factors for endometrial carcinoma, cervical carcinoma in situ (choice **A**) is not. Obesity and hypertension increase the risk of endometrial cancer, but this patient's normal body mass index (choice **B**) and normal blood pressure (choice **C**) show that these are not issues. Endometriosis (choice **E**) is not related to endometrial cancer risk.

26 The answer is D   *Surgery*

This unconscious man obviously needs nutritional support, not only to survive, but also to heal. A variety of oral diets and solutions have been made to meet the special needs of very ill patients. However, an unconscious person cannot take in food by mouth without choking (choice **A** is incorrect). Patients who cannot meet their nutritional requirements the usual way may have their nutritional requirements delivered enterally by nasogastric or nasoduodenal feeding tubes or by tubal enterostomies. Nutrition may also be obtained parenterally by lines into either a peripheral or a central vein. There are commercially available special solutions for each route of administration; these solutions provide all required nutrients and may be supplemented, if required, by substances that meet special needs. The route chosen for administration will depend upon the condition of the patient. Parenteral routes are chosen for persons whose gastrointestinal tract is nonfunctional or who cannot protect their airway. The latter is obviously true of this unconscious person who still moves his mouth and head (thus, choice **B** is incorrect). Parenteral administration via a central vein (choice **C**), usually the subclavian or sometimes the superior vena cava, is preferred over the peripheral route for any patient who will be on support for more than a few weeks, because a more concentrated solution can be administered. On the other hand, nutrients can be administered via standard lines peripherally, which is more convenient and carries less risk. Thus, this is the most logical route to use initially (choice **D**); particularly with the hope that this man will recover consciousness within 2 weeks or so. A tubal enterostomy could also deliver nutrients directly to the stomach, avoiding airway complications, but it is more complicated than the peripheral vein route and has a greater chance of complications; also it is not provided as a potential choice. Nutritional requirements cannot be administered anally (choice **E**).

27 The answer is A *Preventive Medicine and Public Health*

Hepatocellular carcinoma commonly develops from postnecrotic cirrhosis caused by chronic hepatitis B. Liver cancer is very common in Southeast Asia, as demonstrated by the death of the patient's father and uncles; the carcinoma usually is associated with chronic hepatitis B. Consequently, immunization of the patient with hepatitis B vaccine (choice **A**) will prevent the development of hepatitis B and is likely to help prevent hepatic cancer in the future.

Infection by the sexually transmitted human papillomavirus (HPV) (choice **C**) is a risk factor for squamous cell carcinoma of the vulva, vagina, and cervix. HPV is not a risk factor for hepatocellular carcinoma. Increasing dietary fiber (choice **B**) reduces the risk of colorectal cancer. It does not reduce the risk of hepatocellular carcinoma. Smoking cessation (choice **D**) reduces the risk of cancer in the lung, oropharynx, esophagus, kidney, and urinary bladder. It does not reduce the risk of hepatocellular carcinoma. Immunization against hepatitis A (choice **E**) is incorrect. There is no association between hepatitis A and hepatocellular carcinoma.

28 The answer is A *Obstetrics and Gynecology*

The group B β-hemolytic streptococcus (GBS) has potential for significant adverse impact on the fetus, neonate, or both. The GBS neonatal attack rate is only 1–2 cases per thousand; however, if neonatal sepsis does occur, the mortality rate approaches 50%. This is why screening for GBS is now recommended by the Centers for Disease Control and Prevention (CDC) for all women at 36 weeks' gestation, with intrapartum penicillin prophylaxis if culture results are positive. Even though most infants born to women with a positive GBS culture are not infected (choice **A**), a negative culture does not rule out the organism being present at delivery, because most GBS carriers only test positive intermittently or transiently, thus a negative vaginal culture does not mean the fetus will not be at risk at delivery (choice **B**).

Treating carriers is ineffective for eradicating the organism (choice **C**). Up to 30% of reproductive age women will have colonization with GBS; the organism is part of the normal female genital tract flora (the organism is not a pathologic bacterium in the female genital tract, choice **D** is not true). Current nonculture assay tests are specific but not very sensitive; thus, the diagnostic modality of choice is culture, not a rapid nonculture assay (choice **E**).

29 The answer is C *Surgery*

The word *atelectasis* (choice **C**) implies that there has been no expansion of the lung tissue. Nevertheless, it is the term used to describe the postoperative condition in which small airways and alveoli lose their patency and collapse. It is the most common complication following general anesthesia. Patients with nasogastric tubes are at higher risk to develop this. Under normal circumstances alveoli do collapse but expand thereafter because of release of surfactant. Taking deep breaths stimulates release of surfactant in the normal individual. As a result of pain following surgery, the patient cannot take deep breaths, and the tidal volumes are also low. This inhibits the release of surfactant, leading to collapse of the alveoli. If the patient has tenacious sputum, this in turn will aggravate the situation further. Clinically, rales, diminished breath sounds, tachycardia, and fever, all point to this diagnosis. Pain may or may not be a feature. Chest radiography may demonstrate atelectasis even in the absence of clinical signs. Most often, atelectasis is patchy and does not involve large segments of the lung.

Treatment involves clearing the secretions and promoting expansion of the lungs. Physiotherapy, nebulized mucolytic agents, deep breathing exercises, and early ambulation are helpful.

Pulmonary embolus (choice **A**) is a sudden event that usually occurs several days after surgery and is usually due to venous stasis in the calf secondary to deep venous thrombosis. Breakage of the clot leads to a shower of emboli that commonly enter the pulmonary circulation. A massive embolus could be fatal immediately. It has even been known to happen so rapidly that a patient stops talking in midsentence. In other cases, the patient will complain of sudden chest pain and shortness of breath and have hemoptysis. Tachycardia and hypotension also occur. Dyspnea and tachycardia are the most frequent clinical features, and there will be an audible split pulmonary second sound on auscultation. Some patients will have gallop rhythm and cyanosis. Postoperative wound infections (choice **B**) are more common in the 5- to 10-day postsurgical period. Intravenous (IV) catheter-related sepsis (choice **D**) usually results in thrombophlebitis at the site of cannulation. Its frequency is much greater if it is done in the lower extremities. Hence this route is reserved only if no venous access is available elsewhere. Fever due to phlebitis usually occurs on the third postoperative day. The local area is inflamed and tender. If it leads to a suppurative phlebitis, the patient looks very ill. Tachycardia and hypotension may ensue together with tachypnea. Chest pain is unusual. Removing and relocating the intravenous catheter is essential. Blood samples should be drawn and sent for culture and sensitivity together with the tip of the catheter, and antibiotics started. A spontaneous pneumothorax (choice **E**) is a cause of atelectasis. It is associated with chest pain, difficulty breathing, and tachycardia. Fever is not a feature. Aspiration pneumonitis (choice **F**) is associated with dyspnea, cyanosis, and tachycardia. It usually occurs within half an hour after aspiration. Clinical examination will reveal wheezes and rales. Respiratory failure could ensue.

30 The answer is A   *Psychiatry*

The patient's complaints suggest anxiety and depression, which may be caused by an adjustment disorder with mixed anxiety and depressed mood. An adjustment disorder is diagnosed when the presenting pathology in response to a discrete stressor is not simply an exacerbation of another preexisting mental disorder (choice **A**).

The duration of an adjustment disorder is often quite brief, and it resolves when the stressor goes away or the patient learns to live with it; consequently, in adjustment disorder usually there is not a history of difficulty in adjusting to new situations (choice **B**). A pattern of anxiolytic medication abuse (choice **C**) also suggests a longer-term problem. Abusive relationships (choice **D**) often suggest preexisting psychopathology in one or both partners. Situations and stressors that cause adjustment disorder vary greatly from individual to individual and are not necessarily catastrophic (choice **E**).

31 The answer is B   *Medicine*

The patient had been doing well for 3 years on phenytoin monotherapy, and raising the dosage slightly is likely to take care of the small risk of additional seizures (choice **B**).

Ordering another electroencephalogram (EEG) (choice **A**) adds little to the long-term management, because the seizure disorder is already diagnosed. Adding phenobarbital (choice **C**) is less preferable because of the sedative properties and the increased risk of adverse effects and interactions with anticonvulsant polypharmacy. Carbamazepine (choice **D**) is another excellent anticonvulsant, but in a patient who has a single breakthrough seizure while in the low therapeutic range, substitution is less preferable than optimizing the dose of a proved medication. Finally, an imaging study (choice **E**) adds little to the management in a patient with longstanding epilepsy unless there are new neurologic deficits or additional breakthrough seizures not explained by low medication levels.

32 The answer is D   *Psychiatry*

The symptoms are most suggestive of schizophrenia. Several studies suggest that a better outcome for schizophrenia is correlated with early use of antipsychotic medication (choice **D**); maintenance of social skills via interaction with others also helps mitigate the course of the disease. This provides a strong rationale for early treatment with both antipsychotic medication and social rehabilitation therapies (choice **E** is incorrect).

Adoptive studies indicate that there is a genetic predisposition for the disease (choice **A**). These studies show that for individuals who are adopted at birth, the probability of developing schizophrenia is determined entirely by the prevalence of schizophrenia in the biologic family, not the adoptive family. There is also a 50% concordance rate in identical twins and a 10% chance of getting the disease if a first-degree relative has it.

There is no pattern of predisposing family psychodynamics for schizophrenia (choice **B**). A sizable number of individuals with schizophrenia have amelioration of symptomatology in later decades of life (choice **C**), which contradicts earlier views that a downhill course is prevalent.

33 **The answer is A** *Psychiatry*

The symptoms are most suggestive of benzodiazepine withdrawal. Alprazolam (choice **A**) is the benzodiazepine most commonly associated with early, severe withdrawal symptoms. This may be related to its high potency and short half-life. For this reason, it is used less commonly for adjustment disorders or generalized anxiety disorder and is usually reserved for treatment of panic disorder.

Diazepam (choice **B**), fluoxetine (choice **C**), imipramine (choice **D**), and paroxetine (choice **E**) are also used in the treatment of panic disorder. However, none of these medications would be expected to produce the early onset of severe withdrawal symptoms present in this case.

34 **The answer is D** *Medicine*

The patient has alkaptonuria, which is an autosomal recessive disease caused by a deficiency of homogentisate oxidase (choice **D**). The enzyme normally converts homogentisate to maleylacetoacetate. Deficiency of the enzyme causes an increase in homogentisate in articular cartilage in the spine, hip, and knee and an increase in homogentisate in the urine. Homogentisate is oxidized to a black pigment, whether it is in the urine or in cartilage. Deposition in the articular cartilage leads to degenerative joint disease. Increased pigmentation is also seen in the sclera, ears, and anterior thorax.

Arylsulfatase A (choice **A**) is deficient in metachromatic leukodystrophy, an autosomal recessive lysosomal storage disease. Deficiency of this enzyme results in accumulation of sulfatides, causing demyelination and neurodegenerative disease in the brain and peripheral nerves. Death usually occurs in the first decade of life, which excludes this diagnosis in this patient. α_1-Antitrypsin (choice **B**) is a serine protease inhibitor that makes up 90% of the total α_1-globulin in the blood and whose primary function is to inhibit the action of elastase elaborated by neutrophils in the lung. The α_1-antitrypsin protein is highly polymorphic, and several mutant forms with decreased activity are found in relatively high frequency, particularly among Europeans and their decendents. Individuals homozygous for a defective enzyme are generally asymptomatic until late in life when they develop emphysema (due to destruction of lung tissue by uninhibited elastase) or cirrhosis of the liver (thought to be due to accumulation of mutant protein aggregates in the rough endoplasmic reticulum). Moreover, individuals who have inherited this recessively transmitted condition are extremely sensitive to cigarette smoking, making this condition a prime example of the interaction between environment and genetics. A deficiency of β-glucocerebrosidase (choice **C**) causes Gaucher's disease, an autosomal recessive condition leading to the accumulation of sphingolipids throughout the body. Over 200 genetic variants have been uncovered; however, clinically, the disease is generally divided into three subtypes. Type I commonly causes anemia and thrombocytopenia due to hypersplenism and infiltration of the bone marrow by "Gaucher cells," which usually results in erosion of cortical bone. This form of the disease is particularly prevalent among Ashkenazi Jews, in whom the carrier frequency is 1 in 15. In fact, a pathologic fracture in an Ashkenazi Jew with a palpable spleen is almost diagnostic for Gaucher's disease. Types II and III occur less commonly, and neurologic problems predominate. Type II has an infantile onset and a particular poor prognosis. A deficiency of phenylalanine hydroxylase (choice **E**) causes phenylketonuria, an autosomal recessive disease. This enzyme converts phenylalanine to tyrosine. Deficiency of the enzyme causes increases in phenylalanine, neurotoxic phenylketones, and acids, causing demyelination in the brain leading to mental retardation, vomiting, and a peculiar mousy odor in the urine.

35 **The answer is E** *Preventive Medicine and Public Health*

Most normal ranges are established by adding and subtracting 2 standard deviations (SD) from the mean of the test, which encompasses 95% of the normal population. Therefore, out-of-normal range test results (outliers) may occur in 5% of normal persons. The likelihood of an outlier increases as the number of tests ordered increases. The likelihood of an outlier = $100 - (0.95 \times 100)n$, where n is the number of tests ordered. In this patient, five tests were ordered; thus, outliners = $(100 - 0.95 \times 100) \times 5 = 25\%$ chance of an outlier in one of the five tests (choice **E**). The other choices (**A, B, C,** and **D**) are incorrect.

36 The answer is C   *Medicine*

The patient has Klinefelter's syndrome, which is a sex-chromosomal disorder associated with an XXY genotype and one Barr body, due to the random inactivation of one of the two X chromosomes. The testicles in Klinefelter's syndrome show fibrosis of the seminiferous tubules and hyperplasia of the Leydig cells. Destruction of the seminiferous tubules leads to complete absence of spermatogenesis (not normal; choice **E**), infertility, and loss of Sertoli cells, which normally secrete inhibin. Inhibin has negative feedback with respect to FSH; therefore, FSH levels are markedly increased (not decreased; choice **A**). Since FSH normally increases the synthesis of aromatase in the Leydig cells, the excess FSH causes greater aromatization of testosterone, forming increased levels of estradiol (choice **C**) and producing signs of hyperestrinism, namely gynecomastia and a female pattern of pubic hair distribution. Serum testosterone is decreased (not normal; choice **D**), which causes a corresponding increase in serum luteinizing hormone (not decreased; choice **B**).

37 The answer is E   *Obstetrics and Gynecology*

The outcome of malignant gestational trophoblastic disease can be predicted by whether the findings fall into the good-prognosis or poor-prognosis group. Whereas 95 to 100% of the former group of patients can be cured with chemotherapy, only 50 to 70% of the latter are cured. Criteria for the poor-prognosis category include β-human chorionic gonadotropin (β-hCG) titers at onset of therapy above 40,000 mIU/mL (not a current level of 30,000 mlU/mol; choice **C**) for longer than 4 months (not 3 months; choice **B**) since antecedent pregnancy, metastasis to the brain or liver, failed response to previous single-agent chemotherapy, and choriocarcinoma following full-term delivery. In this case, the liver metastasis (choice **E**) placed this patient in the poor-prognosis category. Her chronologic age (choice **A**) and parity (choice **D**) are not criteria.

38 The answer is B   *Psychiatry*

A history of violence (choice **B**) is the strongest predictor of future violence. Alcohol abuse (choice **A**) and persecutory delusions (choice **D**) are not as strongly associated with violence. Temporal lobe epilepsy (choice **E**) is rarely associated with premeditated violence. A lack of anxiety associated with violent ideation (choice **C**) is not associated with a higher likelihood of actual violence. If the counselor believes that there is a reasonable likelihood that this man might carry out such a plan, the Tarasoff rulings impose on the counselor the duties to warn and protect any identifiable potential victims.

39 The answer is D   *Psychiatry*

A depressive episode (choice **D**) is characterized by a depressed mood, coupled with rumination and demoralization, trouble concentrating, and changes in circadian rhythms. Hypersomnia and hyposomnia are both fairly common.

Mania (choice **A**) and anxiety (choice **C**) might both be associated with decreased sleep, but concurrent demoralization would be unusual. Somatization disorder (choice **B**) involves complaints concerning multiple organ systems, with a long clinical course starting before age 30. Delirium (choice **E**) usually has a shorter course with less clearly defined worries.

40 The answer is A   *Medicine*

The patient has renal colic secondary to a renal stone, which is most likely composed of calcium oxalate, because calcium oxalate crystals are present in the urine sediment. Renal colic characteristically has an abrupt onset of colicky pain in the flank, with radiation of the pain toward the abdomen and into the groin. It is associated with urinary frequency, dysuria, and hematuria. Men are more frequently affected than women. The most common metabolic abnormality in stone-formers is idiopathic hypercalciuria (choice **A**) not hyperuricemia (choice **C**); this most likely is due to increased reabsorption of calcium from the gastrointestinal tract. Calcium oxalate stones account for most renal stones (60% of cases). There is an increased incidence of these stones in Crohn's disease because of increased reabsorption of oxalate in the damaged mucosa of the terminal ileum. Other factors that predispose to stones are low urine citrate levels (not increased levels [choice **B**]), because citrate chelates calcium and effectively reduces its functional concentrations, and reduced urine volume. Incomplete distal renal tubular acidosis causes calcium phosphate stones in children (choice **E**); the recurrence rate for stone-formers is 75%. Only stones that contain calcium, such as calcium oxalate or calcium phosphate, are radiopaque. However, uric acid, xanthine, and magnesium ammonium phosphate stones are radiolucent on x-ray films and show up as a filling defect. Urinary tract infections caused by urease-producing uropathogens (e.g., *Proteus* species) produce an alkaline urine pH due to the presence of ammonia (not present in this patient); thus choice **D** is not correct. Magnesium ammonium phosphate stones (i.e., staghorn calculi) may develop under such conditions. Crystals associated with these stones are called triple phosphate stones. They are rectangular and look like a coffin lid.

41 The answer is C *Pediatrics*

In the fetus, the synthesis of α- and γ-globin chains are synchronized to form the normal fetal hemoglobin (Hb), $\alpha_2\gamma_2$. Similarly, after about the third month, synthesis of the α and β chains of Hb A is normally synchronized so that two of each type are always available to produce the normal adult type A tetramer, $\alpha_2\beta_2$. This synchrony is upset in the thalassemias. Each chromosome 16 has two α-globin genes. Thus normally from about the fourth month of fetal development there are four functional α genes. In α-thalassemia, one or more of these genes is nonfunctional. Individuals with one aberrant α gene are called silent carriers because physiologically they are normal; however, their descendants may inherit the bad gene, which can result in more severe disease if they also inherit additional nonfunctional α-globin genes from the other parent. Individuals with two nonfunctional α-globin genes are said to have α-thalassemia trait because they have mild clinical symptoms. Three defective α genes cause a condition called hemoglobin H (Hb H) disease (choice **C**); this results in clinically moderate-to-severe symptoms. In this condition after the third postbirth month, the circulating Hb is a mixture of Hb forms, usually with a predominance of a β tetramer called Hb H; hence the name Hb H disease (choice **C**) for this condition.

If all four α genes are defective, the α-globin chain cannot be synthesized at all so that during most of fetal development and at birth the only circulating Hb is a tetramer consisting of four γ chains. This tetramer, called Hb Bart, is associated with hydrops fetalis (choice **B**), a fatal condition. Hydrops fetalis is so named because of the presence of edema in fetal tissues together with serous effusion in one or more body cavities. Hydrops fetalis occurs more commonly in the countries of Southeast Asia, such as Thailand and among inhabitants of Mediterranean countries.

42 The answer is G *Pediatrics*

Type I collagen (choice **G**) is the main structural protein in bone and tendon and also contributes to sclera structure. As a consequence, mutations in either the α_1 or α_2 genes of type I collagen cause conditions characterized by brittle bones, weak tendons, and blue sclera. These conditions are called osteogenesis imperfecta (OGI), or brittle bone disease, and the child described with multiple fractures at birth most likely has either type II or type III OGI.

43 The answer is J *Pediatrics*

This infant most likely has type I glycogen storage disease, also known as von Gierke's disease. It is caused by glucose 6-phosphatase (G6Pase) deficiency (choice **J**). G6Pase deficiency is inherited as an autosomal recessive trait and has an incidence of about 1 case per 100,000 births in the general population. However, the prevalence is at least 5 times greater among North African non-Ashkenazi Jews. G6Pase is only found in the gluconeogenic organs—liver, kidney, and intestine—and it serves to dephosphorylate glucose 6-phosphate (G6P) formed from the glucokinase reaction, glycogenolysis, or gluconeogenesis, thereby permitting free glucose to enter the bloodstream. Not surprisingly, two of the primary symptoms of G6Pase deficiency are postabsorptive hypoglycemia and hepatomegaly due to hepatic accumulation of glycogen. At least 17 different mutant variations have been discovered; however, they fall into one of two major clinical variants, types 1a and 1b, and the respective genes have been localized to chromosomes 17 and 11. Type 1b mutation is largely distinguished by causing susceptibility to infections. At one time infants with G6Pase deficiency were doomed to an early death. However now with early diagnosis and treatment, mainly by frequent feeding and provision of slowly digested uncooked complex carbohydrates, extended bouts of extreme hypoglycemia are avoided, and children grow into adults only to be beset by additional problems. These include: retarded growth, delayed puberty, chronic hepatomegaly, hyperlipemia, lactic acidemia, fatty liver, gout, and osteopenia.

44 The answer is K   *Pediatrics*

This boy has Ehlers-Danlos (ED) syndrome type VI, which is caused by an aberrant lysyl hydroxylase (choice **K**) due to a mutation in the *PLOD* gene. There are a host of ED syndrome variants, with several different associated and confusing nomenclatures not worth trying to memorize. However, all share decreased tensile strength and integrity of skin, joints, and other tissues. In large part, the various members of the ED family are distinguished clinically by which tissues, and how severely the tissues, are affected. ED type VI is clinically characterized by severe but flexible kyphosis and ocular fragility, and because the mutant protein is an enzyme, it is inherited as an autosomal recessive trait, as suggested by the fact the boy's parents were third cousins.

These facts distinguish it from ED type IV, due to an abnormal type III collagen (choice **I**). Type III collagen is particularly abundant in blood vessels, and ED type IV is sometimes called *vascular type ED*. Affected persons bruise easily, and unlike patients bearing the other types of ED, type IV individuals tend to have a shortened life span. Typically they die in their 50s from an aortic dissection or some type of aneurism. In keeping with the fact that type III collagen is a structural component, ED type IV is inherited as an autosomal dominant trait.

45 The answer is L   *Pediatrics*

Williams syndrome (choice **L**) can be inherited as an autosomal dominant trait or may appear as a new mutation. It affects about 1 in 20,000 individuals and is usually due to a deletion on chromosome 7 that removes or makes the elastin gene nonfunctional. However, a clinically indistinguishable syndrome sometimes called Williams-like syndrome is due to the insertion of this elastin gene in the reverse order. The genetic aberration can be uncovered using the fluorescent in situ hybridization (FISH) technique with elastin probes. Individuals with Williams syndrome can be recognized by their characteristic facial appearance that is described as cheerful and elfinlike. Affected children also have characteristic mental capacities and psychologic behaviors. They are friendly, outgoing, and social and are often thought to suffer from attention deficit disorder. They may excel in the arts but are regarded as retarded when it comes to fine motor function and spatial function and have problems with the basic academic disciplines. As might be expected because of the wide distribution of elastin-containing tissues they also may have any of a variety of physical problems. These include: low birth weight, slow physical development, feeding problems, problems with the heart and blood vessels, kidney problems, dental problems, hernias, and muscular weakness. Commonly their sense of hearing is abnormally acute.

46 The answer is E   *Pediatrics*

Branched-chain α-keto acid dehydrogenase deficiency (choice **E**) is an autosomal recessive disease commonly called *maple sugar urine disease* because of the sweet smell of the diapers of affected individuals. Normally the first step in the catabolism of the three branched-chain amino acids (valine, leucine, and isoleucine) is transamination to the corresponding α-keto acids. This reaction is followed by oxidative decarboxylation using the same branched-chain α-ketoacid dehydrogenase for all three ketoacids. When this enzyme is deficient, these ketoacids accumulate and are excreted in the urine, imparting the characteristic sweet smell. Unless it is diagnosed early and the infant is put on a diet restricting the intake of these three amino acids, ketosis, convulsions, coma, and death ensue, often within a few days. Countrywide, the incidence is about 1 case per 120,000 live births, and in Mennonite communities it is about 1 in 760 births. Twenty-four states have obligatory screening of newborns for this condition.

47 The answer is H   *Pediatrics*

Type II collagen is primarily found in cartilage, intervertebral disks, and the vitreous body. A heterogeneous group of inherited disorders collectively called chondrodysplasia results from mutations in the *COL2A1* gene, which codes for type II collagen (choice **H**). These mutations include deletions, insertions, or glycine substitutions. Clinically, these conditions are characterized by dwarfism, joint disorders, and a variety of skeletal abnormalities. A typical chondrodysplastic dwarf looks like the dwarfs included in many pictures of nobility painted with their dwarfed court jester. Typically a chondrodysplastic dwarf is intelligent and has a sharp wit.

The condition is inherited as an autosomal dominant trait. The homozygous state is fatal in utero and is called achondroplasia.

48 The answer is F *Pediatrics*

Homocystinuria is an autosomal recessive condition affecting about 1 per 100,000 newborns. It is caused by mutations affecting cystathionine β-synthase (choice **F**) or, in a minority of cases, *N*-5,10-methylenetetrahydrofolate reductase (MTHR). The symptoms of congenital cystathionine β-synthase deficiency include dislocated lenses, cataracts, glaucoma, osteoporosis, muscle weakness with a shuffling gait, and early thromboembolic events. Mental retardation occurs in almost all cases, even with early intervention. The occurrence of multiple thrombotic events in a child is essentially diagnostic. The three critical reactions in homocysteine metabolism are catalyzed by cystathionine β-synthase, MTHR, and methionine synthase (aka homocysteine methyltransferase). Cystathionine β-synthase uses pyridoxal phosphate (vitamin B_6) as a cofactor and catalysis the condensation of serine with homocysteine to form cystathionine, which then is converted to cysteine and α-ketobutyrate. Normally this is the end part of the major pathway in methionine catabolism, and hypoactivity of cystathionine β-synthase results in accumulation of methionine and homocysteine and makes cysteine an essential amino acid required in the diet. Approximately 50% of patients respond positively to high doses of vitamin B_6, suggesting that in these individuals, the mutation causing homocystinuria reduced the affinity of the enzyme for this cofactor. MTHR and methionine synthase work in tandem to reverse this process by synthesizing methionine from homocysteine; both of these reactions require folate and vitamin B_{12} as cofactors. MTHR catalyses the conversion of *N*-5,10-methyltetrahydrofolate to *N*-5-methyltetrahydrofolate, and methionine synthase catalyses the transfer of the methyl group from *N*-5-methyltetrahydrofolate to homocysteine, forming methionine and plain tetrahydrofolate. These reactions also decrease homocysteine levels. (Although not relevant to this discussion, the return of tetrahydrofolic acid to the functional folate pool plays a critical role in DNA synthesis.) Recently, it has been recognized that some cases of congenital homocystinuria are caused by mutations affecting MTHR.

The normal fasting range of serum homocysteine is from 5 to 14 μmol/L in males and is a little lower in premenopausal women. Individuals with congenital homocystinuria have levels exceeding 100 μmol/L, and about 10% of the adult population has intermediate levels and consequently experiences noncongenital homocystinemia. An increasing body of evidence suggests that by their fourth or fifth decade these more moderately hyperhomocystinemic persons are at greater risk than average for a thrombolic event such as a myocardial infarction or a stroke. In many cases, supplementation with three relevant vitamin cofactors, folate, B_{12}, and B_6, lowers circulating homocystine levels in these individuals. However, it remains to be proved that this will reduce morbidly or mortality.

49 The answer is A *Pediatrics*

Sickle cell disease is inherited as an autosomal recessive disease with a prevalence of about 289 cases/100,000 African Americans (incidence of 1 per 357 births), 36 cases/100,000 Native Americans, 7.6 cases/100,000 Asian Americans, 5.3 cases/100,00 Hispanic Americans, and 1.7 cases/100,000 Caucasian Americans (incidence of 1 case per 58,000 births). It is due to a mutation in the β-globin gene resulting in a substitution of valine for glycine at position 6 (choice **A**). The disorder makes itself evident during the first year after birth when the γ subunit of hemoglobin F has been largely substituted by the β subunit of hemoglobin A. In this disease acute painful episodes occur due to occlusions in the microvascular systems of various organs caused by clusters of sickled red cells. Hemolytic crises related to splenic sequestering of sickled cells primarily occur in childhood before the spleen has become infarcted due to repeated episodes of sequestering. Similar occluding events occur in all organ systems, and death eventually occurs due to failure of a vital organ. At this time, with good supportive care, average life expectancy is between 40 and 50 years of age.

50 The answer is D *Pediatrics*

Tetrahydrobiopterin (TH4B) (choice **D**) is an essential cofactor for phenylalanine hydroxylase, tyrosine hydroxylase, tryptophan hydroxylase, nitric oxide synthase, and glycerol-ether monooxygenase. Normally TH4B is synthesized starting with GTP in a series of four enzymatic steps using three different enzymes. As might be expected, mutations in any one of these enzymes result in reduced levels of TH4B, which in turn inhibits the activity of all enzymes using TH4B as a cofactor. Since one of these enzymes is phenylalanine hydroxylase, newborns with a defect in one of the enzymes used to synthesize TH4B will test positive for phenylketonuria (PKU) (i.e., the phenylalanine concentration will exceed 4 mg/mL [0.060 mM]). Some babies with a TH4B deficiency have a relatively small elevation, with values between 4 and 10 mg/dL (0.061 to 0.605 mM) and are said to have benign hyperphenylalaninemia. However, others have phenylalanine concentrations into the range found in classic PKU (>20 mg/mL [1.21 mM]). If these babies are placed on the typical low-phenylalanine diet used to treat PKU they will continue to deteriorate, primarily because tyrosine hydroxylase and tryptophan hydroxylase activities are also affected. These babies are said to have malignant PKU. Once such infants are diagnosed, they have to be put on an even more stringent regimen than the classic PKU patient. Tyrosine and tryptophan intake must be restricted as well as phenylalanine, and serotonin and the catecholamines replaced. To some extent the latter is accomplish by use of monoamine oxidase inhibitors. In the United States some 1–3% of PKU babies have the malignant variant. However there is great variation among different ethnicities; Taiwanese have been reported to have 2–30%; Turks, 15%; and Saudi Arabians, a whopping 66%. One of the diagnostic tests for TH4B-deficient variant PKU is a TH4B loading test. The serum phenylalanine concentration is lowered (often to normal values) within 4 to 8 hours after oral administration of a standard amount of TH4B. Consequently, TH4B supplementation has been used as an adjunct to treatment with some success.

Test 12: (0)
Test 13: 8, 12, 18, 38
Test 14: 4, 15, 23, 30, 34
Test 15: 4, 8, 23
Test 16: 18, 33, 35
Test 17: 5, 7, 19, 28
Test 18: 3, 5, 9, 19, 35
Test 19: 14, 16, 27, 29
Test 20: 12, 27, 35

Psychiatry

Test 1: 1, 3, 5, 21, 24, 36, 47, 48
Test 2: 6, 13, 15, 21, 49, 50
Test 3: 6, 17, 33, 38, 39, 45, 46
Test 4: 2, 11, 15, 36, 44, 45, 49, 50
Test 5: 1, 14, 16, 22, 31, 33, 37
Test 6: 5, 6, 11, 14, 17, 23, 34, 38
Test 7: 4, 6, 12, 16, 20, 27, 31, 37
Test 8: 3, 5, 9, 5, 12, 17, 18, 25, 33, 39
Test 9: 2, 8, 9, 11, 19, 27, 29, 39
Test 10: 7, 13, 21, 15, 26, 31, 32, 34
Test 11: 4, 12, 13, 16, 20, 26, 27, 30, 34
Test 12: 20, 21, 32, 38, 47, 48, 49, 50
Test 13: 1, 4, 10, 13, 20, 21, 28, 40
Test 14: 11, 17, 19, 26, 29, 33, 35, 38
Test 15: 2, 7, 10, 13, 16, 21, 24, 30
Test 16: 4, 6, 9, 14, 22, 25, 27, 31

Test 17: 16, 20, 22, 34, 39, 40, 41, 42
Test 18: 13, 14, 16, 25, 32, 34, 36, 44
Test 19: 2, 6, 21, 25, 32, 35, 39, 41, 42, 43
Test 20: 11, 17, 21, 30, 32, 33, 38, 39

Surgery

Test 1: 6, 8, 10, 16, 26, 32, 37
Test 2: 5, 10, 16, 20, 33, 37, 40, 41, 42
Test 3: 7, 9, 26, 29, 34, 35, 40
Test 4: 1, 6, 12, 14, 24, 26, 27, 35, 39
Test 5: 4, 9, 15, 24, 28, 30
Test 6: 2, 7, 16, 25, 26, 28, 33, 46, 47, 48, 49, 50
Test 7: 10, 19, 24, 32, 36
Test 8: 41, 42, 43, 44, 45, 46, 47
Test 9: 3, 6, 12, 20, 32, 34, 37
Test 10: 1, 5, 10, 12, 16, 18, 23, 33
Test 11: 14, 33, 35, 36
Test 12: 1, 7, 10, 12, 14, 15, 26, 29, 35, 36
Test 13: 6, 7, 14, 17, 35, 36
Test 14: 1, 3, 5, 10, 22, 32, 36
Test 15: 1, 6, 12, 15, 17, 20, 26, 28
Test 16: 2, 8, 10, 16, 20, 24, 30, 40
Test 17: 4, 8, 13, 15, 30, 36, 38
Test 18: 4, 7, 8, 10, 15, 20, 23, 27
Test 19: 8, 10, 12, 22, 28, 36
Test 20: 2, 3, 7, 13, 19, 26, 29

Discipline Index

Medicine

Test 1: 2, 4, 11, 13, 14, 15, 17, 20, 27, 30, 31, 33, 35, 49, 50

Test 2: 1, 4, 8, 14, 18, 22, 25, 27, 28, 38, 43, 44, 45, 46, 47, 48

Test 3: 8, 12, 16, 18, 20, 22, 24, 27, 32, 41, 42, 43, 44, 47, 48, 49, 50

Test 4: 13, 17, 20, 23, 25, 28, 29, 31, 34, 37, 41, 42, 43, 46, 47, 48

Test 5: 2, 3, 5, 7, 8, 11, 19, 20, 21, 25, 26, 32, 36, 39

Test 6: 1, 3, 8, 9, 10, 12, 13, 15, 18, 20, 22, 27, 29, 30, 31, 32, 35

Test 7: 3, 5, 7, 8, 14, 15, 18, 29, 30, 33, 35, 45, 46, 47, 48, 49, 50

Test 8: 4, 6, 7, 10, 11, 14, 15, 16, 20, 21, 27, 30, 31, 34, 35, 40

Test 9: 1, 4, 5, 10, 13, 14, 15, 16, 21, 22, 23, 24, 28, 30, 31, 48, 49, 50

Test 10: 3, 8, 9, 17, 19, 22, 27, 28, 29, 35, 36, 37, 38, 39, 40

Test 11: 3, 5, 6, 9, 10, 11, 15, 18, 19, 21, 22, 31, 32, 37, 38, 40

Test 12: 2, 4, 6, 8, 9, 11, 13, 16, 17, 18, 19, 22, 25, 27, 28, 30, 37

Test 13: 2, 11, 16, 22, 25, 27, 29, 41, 42, 43, 44, 45, 46, 47, 48, 49, 50

Test 14: 7, 9, 12, 14, 16, 21, 25, 27, 37, 46, 47, 48, 49, 50

Test 15: 18, 19, 27, 29, 31, 32, 33, 35, 36, 38, 39, 40, 41, 45, 46, 47, 48, 49, 50

Test 16: 1, 11, 13, 17, 23, 26, 29, 32, 34, 37, 38, 46, 47, 48, 49, 50

Test 17: 1, 2, 6, 9, 10, 12, 25, 29, 32, 43, 44, 45, 46, 47, 48, 49, 50

Test 18: 1, 6, 12, 18, 22, 26, 28, 30, 33, 43, 45

Test 19: 1, 3, 4, 9, 13, 15, 17, 19, 20, 23, 24, 30, 31, 33, 34, 37, 38, 40

Test 20: 1, 4, 6, 9, 10, 12, 14, 15, 16, 20, 22, 24, 31, 34, 36, 40

Obstetrics and Gynecology

Test 1: 9, 18, 29, 39, 40, 41, 42, 43, 44, 45, 46

Test 2: 2, 7, 11, 26, 30, 34, 39

Test 3: 1, 11, 21, 30, 31, 37

Test 4: 3, 9, 10, 16, 18, 21, 32

Test 5: 12, 18, 23, 27, 35, 38

Test 6: 4, 19, 21, 24, 37, 39, 40

Test 7: 11, 28, 38, 39, 40, 41, 42, 43, 44

Test 8: 2, 8, 13, 22, 26, 37, 38

Test 9: 17, 25, 26, 33, 36, 38

Test 10: 41, 42, 43, 44, 45, 46, 47, 48, 49, 50

Test 11: 1, 3, 28, 29

Test 12: 40, 41, 42, 43, 44, 45, 46

Test 13: 9, 15, 26, 30, 32, 34, 37

Test 14: 6, 39, 40, 41, 42, 43, 44, 45

Test 15: 42, 43, 44

Test 16: 12, 39, 41, 42, 43, 44, 45

Test 17: 3, 11, 18, 24, 27, 31

Test 18: 38, 39, 40, 41, 42, 46, 47, 48, 49 50

Test 19: 44, 45, 46, 47, 48, 49, 50

Test 20: 5, 8, 18, 23, 25, 28, 37

Pediatrics

Test 1: 7, 12, 14, 19, 22, 25, 28, 34

Test 2: 3, 9, 12, 19, 24, 31, 32, 35

Test 3: 2, 5, 10, 13, 15, 19, 23, 36

Test 4: 4, 7, 22, 33, 38, 40

Test 5: 6, 10, 13, 17, 29, 34, 40

Test 6: 36, 41, 42, 43, 44, 45

Test 7: 1, 17, 21, 22, 25, 26, 34

Test 8: 1, 19, 23, 24, 28, 29, 32

Test 9: 40, 41, 42, 43, 44, 45, 46, 47

Test 10: 2, 6, 11, 14, 24

Test 11: 2, 7, 8, 17, 24, 25, 39

Test 12: 3, 5, 23, 24, 31, 33 34, 39

Test 13: 3, 5, 19, 23, 24, 31, 33, 39

Test 14: 2, 8, 13, 18, 20, 24, 28, 31

Test 15: 3, 5, 9, 11, 14, 22, 25, 34, 37

Test 16: 3, 5, 7, 15, 19, 21, 28, 36

Test 17: 14, 17, 21, 23, 26, 33, 35, 37

Test 18: 2, 11, 17, 21, 24, 29, 31, 37

Test 19: 5, 7, 11, 18, 26

Test 20: 41, 42, 43, 44, 45, 46, 47, 48, 49, 50

Preventive Medicine and Public Health

Test 1: 4, 23, 38

Test 2: 17, 23, 29, 36

Test 3: 3, 25, 28

Test 4: 5, 8, 19, 30

Test 5: 41, 42, 43, 44, 45, 46, 47, 48, 49, 50

Test 6: (0)

Test 7: 2, 9, 13, 23

Test 8: 36, 48, 49, 50

Test 9: 7, 18, 35

Test 10: 4, 20, 25, 30

Test 11: 41, 42, 43, 44, 45, 46, 47, 48, 49, 50

Human Resources Management

in Canada

Canadian Eighth Edition

Human Resources Management

in Canada

Canadian Eighth Edition

Gary Dessler
Florida International University

Nina D. Cole
Brock University

Virginia L. (Gini) Sutherland
Sir Sandford Fleming College

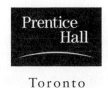

Toronto

Canadian Cataloguing in Publication Data

Dessler, Gary, 1942–
        Human resources management in Canada

Canadian 8th ed.
First–sixth eds. published under title: Human resource management in Canada.
Includes index.
ISBN 0-13-033007-8

1. Personnel management. 2. Personnel management–Canada.
I. Cole, Nina D. (Nina Dawn). II. Sutherland, Gini, (date). III. Title.

HF5549.D49 2002   658.3   C00-932774-6

0-13-033007-8

Vice President, Editorial Director: Michael Young
Acquisitions Editor: Mike Ryan
Marketing Manager: James Buchanan
Developmental Editor: Madhu Ranadive
Production Editor: Marisa D'Andrea
Copy Editor: Laurel Sparrow
Production Coordinator: Patricia Ciardullo
Page Layout: Phyllis Seto
Permissions Research: Beth McAuley
Photo Research: Alene McNeill
Art Director: Julia Hall
Interior and Cover Design: Julia Hall
Cover Art: Doug Ross

 3 4 5 6   07 06 05 04 03

Printed and bound in the United States.

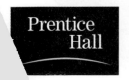

Statistics Canada information is used with the permission of the Minister of Industry, as Minister responsible for Statistics Canada. Information on the availability of the wide range of data from Statistics Canada can be obtained from Statistic Canada's Regional Offices, its World Wide Web site at http://www.statcan.ca, and its toll-free access number 1-800-263-1136.

Brief Contents

Preface   *xvii*

Part One: Human Resources Management in Perspective   1
Chapter 1: Human Resources Management: The Field and Its Environment   1
Chapter 2: The Evolving Role of HRM: From Staff Function to Strategic Partner   45
Chapter 3: The Changing Emphasis: From Legal Compliance to Valuing Diversity   74

PART TWO: Meeting Human Resources Requirements   121
Chapter 4: Designing and Analyzing Jobs   121
Chapter 5: Human Resources Planning   167
Chapter 6: Recruitment   198
Chapter 7: Selection   246

PART THREE: Developing Effective Human Resources   305
Chapter 8: Orientation and Training   305
Chapter 9: Career Development   338
Chapter 10: Managing Quality and Productivity   371
Chapter 11: Performance Appraisal   395

PART FOUR: Compensation Administration   432
Chapter 12: Establishing Pay Plans   432
Chapter 13: Pay-for-performance and Financial Incentives   474
Chapter 14: Employee Benefits and Services   505

PART FIVE: Building Effective Employee/Employer Relationships   538
Chapter 15: Fair Treatment: The Foundation of Effective Employee Relations   538
Chapter 16: The Dynamics of Labour Relations   562
Chapter 17: Collective Bargaining and Contract Administration   603
Chapter 18: Occupational Health and Safety   647

PART SIX: International Issues in Human Resources Management   686
Chapter 19: Managing Human Resources in an International Business   686

Notes   *712*

Name/Organization Index   *745*

Subject Index   *749*

Table of Contents

Preface xvii

Part One: Human Resources Management in Perspective   1

Chapter 1: Human Resources Management: The Field and Its Environment   1

Introduction to Human Resources Management   2

Information Technology and HR: HR e-Business   8

Internal Environmental Influences   12

External Environmental Influences   41

Diversity Counts: In Attaining Work/Life Balance   25

Information Technology and HR: The Time is Here for Automated Time and Attendance Systems   29

Global HRM: Canadian Government Gets a Failing Grade in Providing Family Support   32

Tomorrow's HR, Today   36

The Plan of This Book   37

The High Performance Organization: New Ways of Organizing and Managing   38

Chapter Review   38

Critical Thinking Questions   40

Application Exercises   41

Case Incident: HR Systems Inc.   42

Experiential Exercises   43

Web-based Exercises   44

e-Tutor   44

Chapter 2: The Evolving Role of HRM: From Staff Function to Strategic Partner   45

A Brief History of HRM   46

Growing Professionalism in HRM   50

The High Performance Organization: Building an Ethical Culture   54

The Current Role of HR Departments   55

Information Technology and HR: Improving Service in the e-Commerce World   58

Strategic Planning and HRM   59

The Role of the HR Department as a Strategic Partner   62

The High Performance Organization: HR as a Strategic Business Partner   63

HR Auditing   65

Information Technology and HR: High-tech Attitude Surveys   66

The Impact of Effective HRM Practices on Employee Performance and the Bottom Line   67

Chapter Review   69

Critical Thinking Questions   70

Application Exercises   71

Case Incident: Jack Nelson's Problem   71

Experiential Exercises   72

Web-based Exercises   73

Chapter 3: The Changing Emphasis: From Legal Compliance to Valuing Diversity   74

Introduction to the Legal Environment   75

Equality   76

Equal Opportunity   77

Equity   93

Diversity Counts: At TD Bank Financial Group   97

Information Technology and HR: Employment Equity Reporting   101

Impact of Equal Opportunity and Equity on HRM   106

Managing Diversity   107

Diversity Counts: In International Marketing   108

The High Performance Organization: Communicating Diversity   110

Information Technology and HR: Mentoring Online   110

Global HRM: International Rights and Pension Plan Funding   112

Chapter Review   112

Critical Thinking Questions   115

Application Exercises   115

Case Incident: Harassment   116

Experiential Exercises   117

Web-based Exercises   117

Appendix 3.1: A Guide to Screening and Selection in Employment   118

Video Case 1: Landmark Supreme Court Decision on Same-sex Benefits   120

PART TWO: Meeting Human Resources Requirements   121

Chapter 4: Designing and Analyzing Jobs   121

Organizing Work   122

Information Technology and HR: Automated Organization Charts Save Time and Money   123

Job Design   125

Diversity Counts: Older Workers Can Benefit From Ergonomic Aid   130

The Nature of Job Analysis   131

Methods of Collecting Job Analysis Information   135

Writing Job Descriptions   144

Information Technology and HR: Writing Job Descriptions Online   146

Writing Job Specifications   150

Small Business Applications: A Practical Approach   151

Job Analysis in a "Jobless" World   158

The High Performance Organization: HR Practices in a De-jobbed Company   160

Chapter Review   161

Critical Thinking Questions   163

Application Exercises   164

Case Incident: Linking Job Analysis and Pay   165

Experiential Exercises   166

Web-based Exercises   166

Chapter 5: Human Resources Planning   167

The Nature of Human Resources Planning   168

Elements of Effective HRP   173

Forecasting Future Human Resources Needs (Demand)   174

Forecasting Future Human Resources Supply   179

Information Technology and HR: Computerized Skills Inventories   183

The High Performance Organization: In Succession Planning, Being a Deputy Comes First!   185

Planning and Implementing HR Programs to Balance Supply and Demand   186

HRP Evaluation   192

Chapter Review   192

Critical Thinking Questions   194

Application Exercises   194

Case Incident: Management Trainees at Nova   195

Experiential Exercises   196

Web-based Exercise   196

Chapter 6: Recruitment   198

Introduction   199

The Recruitment Process   199

Constraints on the Recruitment Process   200

Global HRM: Bringing Home Foreign Workers With "Hot" Skills   202

Recruiting Within the Organization   205

The High Performance Organization: Effective Job Posting Enhances Commitment, Retention and Recruitment   207

Recruiting Outside the Organization   209

Information Technology and HR: Finding Interns Online   215

Small Business Applications: Using Executive Search Firms—When and Why?   219

The High Performance Organization: Innovative Recruitment Advertising   223

Information Technology and HR: Selecting an Internet Job Board   227

Small Business Applications: Online Recruiting   228

Recruiting a More Diverse Work Force   232

Diversity Counts: Helping Employees Balance Work and Family Makes
Workplaces More Attractive   233

Diversity Counts: The Benefits of a Multigenerational Work Force   234

Developing and Using Application Forms   236

Chapter Review   241

Critical Thinking Questions   242

Application Exercises   243

Case Incident: Expansion at Logans   243

Experiential Exercises   244

Web-based Exercises   244

Chapter 7: Selection   246

Introduction   247

The Selection Process   249

Constraints on the Selection Process   250

The Importance of Reliability and Validity   253

Steps in the Selection Process   255

Information Technology and HR: Screening Tools and Techniques   259

Information Technology and HR: Using Computers for Skills Assessment:
From Math and Language to Welding   266

Small Business Applications: Testing   275

Information Technology and HR: Computer-based Interviewing   281

Diversity Counts: When It Comes to Lying on Résumés   291

Small Business Applications: Reference Checking Policies   294

Information Technology and HR: Providing an RJP Online   295

The High Performance Organization: Sold on Statistical Selection   296

Chapter Review   297

Critical Thinking Questions   300

Application Exercises   300

Case Incident: The Selection Process   302

Experiential Exercises   303

Web-based Exercises   303

Video Case 2: Employers Beware!   304

PART THREE: Developing Effective Human Resources   305

Chapter 8: Orientation and Training   305

Orienting Employees   306

The High Performance Organization: Orientation and Socialization at Toyota
Canada   310

The Training Process   311

Training Needs Analysis   315

Training Techniques   318

Information Technology and HR: Launching an Online Training
Program   325

Small Business Applications: Training   326

Training for Special Purposes   327

Evaluating the Training Effort   331

Chapter Review   333

Critical Thinking Questions   334

Application Exercises   335

Case Incident: Reinventing the Wheel at Apex Door Company   336

Experiential Exercises   337

Web-based Exercises   337

Chapter 9: Career Development   338

Career Planning and Development   339

The High Performance Organization: Helping Employees to Self-actualize   339

Factors That Affect Career Choices   342

Career Development and the Responsibilities of the Manager and the Employer   346

Managing Promotions and Transfers   350

Management Development   352

Diversity Counts: Do Women Make Better Managers?   355

Using HRM to Build a Responsive Learning Organization   362

Executive Development   363

Small Business Applications: Executive Development   365

Chapter Review   366

Critical Thinking Questions   368

Application Exercises   369

Case Incident: Reality Shock   370

Experiential Exercises   370

Web-based Exercises   370

Chapter 10: Managing Quality and Productivity   371

The Importance of Quality and Productivity   372

Alternative Work Arrangements   372

Total Quality Management Programs   376

The High Performance Organization: A Transformation of Thinking!   377

Creating Team-based Organizations   384

Information Technology and HR: Virtual Teams   386

Business Process Reengineering   388

Chapter Review   390

Critical Thinking Questions   391

Application Exercises   391

Case Incident: Is the Honeymoon Over for Mazda's North American Plant?   392

Experiential Exercises   394

Web-based Exercises   394

Chapter 11: Performance Appraisal   395

The Performance Appraisal Process   396

Why Should Performance Be Appraised?   396

Defining Performance Expectations   397

The Appraisal Itself: Appraisal Methods   398

Performance Appraisal: Problems and Solutions   407

Information Technology and HR: Computerized Performance Appraisals   409

Diversity Counts: In Performance Appraisal   412

The Appraisal Interview   419

The Role of Appraisals in Managing Performance   423

Chapter Review   425

Critical Thinking Questions   427

Application Exercises   427

Case Incident: Appraising the Secretaries at Sweetwater U   428

Experiential Exercises   430

Web-based Exercises   430

Video Case 3: The Trouble with Teams   431

PART FOUR: Compensation Administration   432

Chapter 12: Establishing Pay Plans   432

Basic Aspects of Compensation at Work   433

Basic Considerations in Determining Pay Rates   434

Global HRM: Effective Rewards in China   436

Establishing Pay Rates   437

Current Trends in Compensation   456

Information Technology and HR: Computerized Job Evaluation   458

The High Performance Organization: Compensation Management
Pay for Managerial and Professional Jobs   460

Important Current Issues in Compensation Management   462

Diversity Counts: In Job Evaluation   464

Small Business Applications: Compensation Management in Smaller
Organizations   466

Chapter Review   469

Critical Thinking Questions   470

Application Exercises   471

Case Incident: Salary Inequities at Acme Manufacturing   471

Experiential Exercises   473

Web-based Exercises   473

Chapter 13: Pay-for-performance and Financial Incentives   474

Money and Motivation: Background and Trends   475

Incentives for Operations Employees   476

Incentives for Managers and Executives   479

Global HRM: Long-term Incentives for Overseas Executives   485

Incentives for Salespeople   486

Incentives for Other Professionals   488

Organization-wide Incentive Plans   490

Information Technology and HR: Technology Tackles Incentive Plan Management   491

Developing Effective Incentive Plans   495

Employee Recognition Programs   497

Chapter Review   498

Critical Thinking Questions   500

Application Exercises   500

Case Incident: Bringing the Team Concept Into Compensation—Or Not   501

Experiential Exercises   502

Web-based Exercises   504

Chapter 14: Employee Benefits and Services   505

The Changing Role of Employee Benefits   506

Government-sponsored Benefits   507

Pay for Time Not Worked   510

Insurance Benefits   514

Retirement Benefits   519

Employee Services   522

Information Technology and HR: Online EAP Counselling Services   524

Diversity Counts: What Do Young Employees Want? A Life Outside the Office   528

Flexible Benefits Programs   529

Benefits Administration   530

Small Business Applications: Benefits Administration Outsourcing for Small Employers   531

The High Performance Organization: A Benefits Program That Fosters Employee Commitment   531

Chapter Review   532

Critical Thinking Questions   533

Application Exercises   534

Case Incident: "Benefits? Who Needs Benefits?"   534

Experiential Exercises   535

Web-based Exercises   536

Video Case 4: Landmark Pay Equity Decision   537

PART FIVE: Building Effective Employee/Employer Relationships   538

Chapter 15: Fair Treatment: The Foundation of Effective Employee Relations   538

The Importance of Fair Treatment   539

Building Two-way Communication   539

Fair Treatment Programs and Employee Discipline   541

Managing Dismissals   546

Managing Separations: Layoffs and Retirements   553

The High Performance Organization: Communicating Financial Information at Marriott   556

Chapter Review   557

Critical Thinking Questions   558

Application Exercises   559

Case Incident: Job Insecurity at IBM   559

Experiential Exercises   560

Web-based Exercises   561

Chapter 16: The Dynamics of Labour Relations   562

Introduction to Labour–Management Relations   563

The Contemporary Legal Framework   564

The Labour Movement in Canada Today   569

Global HRM: Unions Protect Worker Rights Internationally   570

Information Technology and HR: Computers Help Union Leaders to Meet Changing Member Needs   577

Diversity Counts: Unions Provide Family-friendly Benefits   579

Management's Labour Relations Strategy   582

The High Performance Organization: Union–Management Cooperation Leads to Win–Win Situation   583

The Labour Relations Process   584

Union Organizing and Recognition   585

Diversity Counts: In Reasons for Unionizing   586

Information Technology and HR: Even Organizing Campaigns Are Going Online!   588

The Impact of Unionization on HRM   594

Chapter Review   595

Critical Thinking Questions   598

Application Exercises   598

Case Incident: Western College   599

Experiential Exercises   600

Web-based Exercises   600

Appendix 16.1   601

Chapter 17: Collective Bargaining and Contract Administration   603

Introduction to Collective Bargaining   604

The Collective Bargaining Process   606

Information Technology and HR: Costing for Negotiations   611

The High Performance Organization: Mutual Gains at Hercules Canada   618

Third-party Assistance and Bargaining Impasses   620

The Collective Agreement: Typical Provisions   626

Diversity Counts: In Collective Agreement Provisions   630

Introduction to Contract Administration   630

Grievance Resolution and Rights Arbitration   632

Information Technology and HR: Using Computers for Complaints/Grievance Tracking   636

Building Effective Labour–Management Relations   639

Chapter Review   640

Critical Thinking Questions   643

Application Exercises   643

Case Incident: Disciplinary Action   644

Experiential Exercises   645

Web-based Exercises   645

Chapter 18: Occupational Health and Safety   647

Why Occupational Health and Safety is Important   648

Basic Facts About Occupational Health and Safety Legislation   648

The Supervisor's Role in Safety   653

Small Business Applications: A New Occupational Health and Safety Initiative for Small Business   655

What Causes Accidents?   656

How to Prevent Accidents   659

Information Technology and HR: Health, Safety, and Disability Management Software Vendors   664

Employee Wellness Programs   664

The High Performance Organization: Healthy Workplace Keeps in Touch With Employees   665

Occupational Health Issues and Challenges   666

Diversity Counts: In Workplace Violence   680

Chapter Review   680

Critical Thinking Questions   682

Application Exercises   682

Case Incident: Introducing Ergonomics: What Went Wrong?   683

Experiential Exercises   684

Web-based Exercises   684

Video Case 5: Death of a Ballerina's Career   685

PART SIX: International Issues in Human Resources Management   686

Chapter 19: Managing Human Resources in an International Business   686

The Internationalization of Business   687

How Intercountry Differences Affect HRM   689

Improving International Assignments Through Selection   694

Diversity Counts: Sending Female Managers Abroad   698

Training and Maintaining International Employees   700

Chapter Review   707

Critical Thinking Questions   709

Application Exercises   709

Experiential Exercises   710

Web-based Exercises   710

Video Case 6: Norbert Reinhart—Employer of the Year 1999   711

Notes   712

Name/Organization Index   745

Subject Index   749

The Canadian eighth edition of *Human Resources Management in Canada* is based on two key premises: 1) that human resources are the most important asset in the majority of Canadian organizations today; and 2) that the effective management of the employment relationship is a responsibility shared by human resources (HR)/industrial relations (IR) specialists, all supervisors and managers, and increasingly, employees themselves. A strong foundation in human resources management (HRM) is important for supervisors and managers in every field and employees at every level—not just those working in HR/IR departments or aspiring to do so in the future. This book was designed to provide students specializing in HRM, those in general business or business administration programs, supervisory/managerial staff, and small business owners with a complete, comprehensive review of essential HRM concepts and techniques in a highly readable and understandable form.

As in previous editions, the Canadian eighth edition provides extensive coverage of all essential HRM topics, such as job analysis, HR planning, recruitment, selection, orientation and training, career development, compensation and benefits, performance appraisal, health and safety, and union–management relations. The High Performance Organization is introduced as an integrating theme. In The High Performance Organization boxes throughout the text, examples demonstrate the ways in which managers in firms across Canada and around the world are building better, faster, and more competitive organizations through HRM activities designed to attract and retain highly qualified employees, foster employee commitment, increase quality, and improve productivity. Ensuring fair treatment, covered in detail in Chapter 15, is emphasized throughout, as is quality management and productivity improvement, a topic explored in Chapter 10. Practical applications are discussed in the Small Business Applications boxes throughout the text, and in a feature new to this edition titled Tips for the Front Line. In addition to thorough coverage of employment legislation, legal issues are discussed throughout the book. New to this edition is a feature called Hints to Ensure Legal Compliance, in which suggestions are provided regarding ways to ensure compliance, while simultaneously increasing employee commitment and productivity.

WHAT'S NEW AND WHAT'S NOT?

Those familiar with the Canadian seventh edition will notice a number of changes:

- attractive new open design that enhances the full-colour visuals, and improves readability

- plenty of new material reflecting recent changes in the country, such as the creation of Nunavut, and emerging HR issues and trends, such as e-Business, employee leasing, video-based situational testing, micro-assessments, computerized 360-degree feedback, employee wellness programs, sick building syndrome, and international Employee Assistance Programs

- up-to-the-minute coverage of legislative changes and arbitration board, human rights tribunal, and Supreme Court decisions on issues ranging from same-sex benefits to pre-employment drug testing
- expanded coverage of such topics as human resources information systems, the uses of information technology, online recruiting, behavioural interviewing, orientation, and interest-based/mutual gains bargaining
- the introduction of the new box and features described above, as well as Research Insights, margin questions titled An Ethical Dilemma, and a number of end-of-chapter features: Critical Thinking Questions, Experiential Exercises, and Web-based Exercises
- updated text, figures, tables, boxed examples, Weblinks and video cases

The features that proved to be extremely popular in the Canadian seventh edition have been retained, such as:

- coverage of all material required to qualify for approval by the Human Resources Professionals Association of Ontario (HRPAO) and eligibility for inclusion as a recommended text in HRPAO's *Curriculum Summary*
- four leading-edge boxed features: Diversity Counts, Global HRM, Information Technology and HR, and Small Business Applications
- numerous practical examples and hints regarding applications, some based on the hands-on experience acquired by the two Canadian authors while previously employed as HR practitioners, and others based on a comprehensive literature review
- content enhancement and validation through references to research findings and the published works of many individuals, cited throughout
- the introduction of strategic HRM, key legislation affecting every aspect of HRM, and diversity issues and management early in the text, as well as a focus on these issues throughout the text
- the establishment of a link between reliability and validity and all aspects of HRM, not just selection testing
- separate chapters on managing quality and productivity and international HRM
- numerous Weblinks in the margins
- features designed to enhance learning, such as chapter outlines; learning outcomes; margin definition of key terms; chapter summaries; end-of-chapter questions, exercises, and cases; CBC video cases; and a Companion Website
- a comprehensive set of supplements for instructors

KEY FEATURES OF THE CANADIAN EIGHTH EDITION

Highlighted Themes

- **Diversity Counts** The Diversity Counts boxes describe some of the issues and challenges involved in managing the diverse work force found in Canadian organizations. Topics range from attaining work/life balance to ergonomic aids for older workers; the benefits of a multigenerational work force; gender differences in lying on resumes; reasons for unionizing and workplace violence; potential bias in performance appraisal and job evaluation; designing benefits packages to attract younger workers; and sending female managers abroad.

- **Information Technology and HR** Examples are provided throughout the book of how computers are being used, not only for storage, retrieval, and analysis of information, but for a wide range of broader applications. Topics discussed include HR e-business; automated time and attendance systems; improving service in the e-commerce world; high-tech attitude surveys; online mentoring, job descriptions, skills inventories, recruitment, counselling, and union organizing; computer-based screening tools and techniques, skills assessment, and interviewing; virtual teams; and health, safety, and disability management software.

- **The High Performance Organization** These boxes provide examples that illustrate the ways in which organizations—primarily in Canada, but not exclusively—are using effective HRM policies and practices in order to thrive in their product or service market. Topics range from new ways of organizing and managing at ABB to building an ethical culture at UPS Canada; HR practices at BP, a de-jobbed company; succession planning at Bata Ltd.; using job postings to enhance commitment, retention and recruitment at LGS; innovative recruitment advertising at UUNET; statistical selection at Toronto Hydro; orientation and socialization at Toyota Canada; benefits that foster employee commitment at FedEx Canada; communicating financial information at Marriott; mutual gains at Hercules Canada; and MDS Nordon's healthy workplace strategies.

- **Small Business Applications** Recognizing that small businesses are playing an increasingly important role in the Canadian economy, and are a major source of employment, suggestions are provided to assist those in smaller businesses with limited time and resources to implement effective HRM policies and procedures. Concrete, practical hints are included for activities ranging from writing job descriptions to using executive search firms, recruiting online, administering selection tests, checking references, setting up a training program, developing a pay plan, outsourcing benefits, and improving workplace health and safety.

- **Global HRM** Recognizing the increasing impact of globalization, topics highlighted in the Global HRM boxes range from international rights and pension plan funding to bringing home foreign workers with "hot" skills, training for international business, executive development in global companies, taking self-managed teams to Mexico, long-term incentives for overseas executives, and the role of unions in protecting human rights internationally.

NEW Highlighted Features:

- **Research Insights** Recent research findings—primarily Canadian—are highlighted in every chapter. Topics range from the impact of Generation X employees replacing aging boomers to the underutilization of women in the Canadian work force, the impact of high-involvement HR practices, what fire ants can teach humans about teamwork, current hiring and retention practices, improving the effectiveness of technology-based distance learning programs, the reliability of various job evaluation methods, the impact of open pay policies and sales commissions, reasons for unionizing, causes of workplace accidents, and factors contributing to successful foreign assignments.

- **An Ethical Dilemma** A number of questions that are designed to provoke debate and discussion on the "grey" areas of HRM appear in the margins in every chapter. Issues addressed range from dealing with functionally illiterate employees to protecting the confidentiality of employee records, accommodating employees' childcare and/or eldercare responsibilities, engaging in "headhunting" activities, denying alternative work arrangements, using the forced distribution performance appraisal method, and dealing with a supervisor who has knowingly violated the collective agreement.

- **Tips for the Front Line** Advice for front-line supervisors and managers has been included on topics ranging from how to conduct job analysis interviews and write job descriptions to how to avoid survivor sickness in downsizing situations, conduct selection interviews, set up an on-the-job training program, introduce a QC program, implement 360-degree feedback, introduce skill-based pay and gainsharing programs, reduce healthcare costs, discipline employees, retain union-free status, determine if a unionizing campaign is underway, resolve grievances, encourage workplace safety, and handle substance abuse.

- **Hints to Ensure Legal Compliance** Suggestions to help practitioners avoid legal pitfalls are provided throughout the text. Issues discussed range from introducing an employee surveillance system to ensuring a harassment-free workplace, developing legally compliant job descriptions and specifications, conducting employment interviews, avoiding negligent training charges, developing a legally compliant appraisal system, avoiding gender-bias in job evaluation, avoiding wrongful dismissal suits and charges of unfair labour practices, responding to a unionization bid, and screening out potentially violent employees.

Additional Features

- *Chapter Outlines* Each chapter begins with a chapter outline that highlights key topic areas.
- *Learning Outcomes* Specific learning goals are defined on each chapter-opening page.
- *Key Terms* Key terms appear in boldface within the text, are defined in the margins, and are listed at the end of the chapter.
- *Current Examples* Numerous real-world examples of HRM policies, procedures, and practices at a wide variety of organizations, ranging from small service providers to huge global corporations, can be found throughout the text.
- *Full-colour Figures, Tables and Photographs* Throughout each chapter, key concepts and applications are illustrated with strong, full-colour visual materials.

- *Weblinks* Helpful Internet sites are provided throughout the text and are easily identifiable by the Weblinks icon shown here.

- *End-of-Chapter Summaries* At the end of each chapter, the summary reviews key points and links the critical content.

- *End-of-Chapter Review and Discussion Questions* Each chapter contains a set of review and discussion questions.

- *Critical Thinking Questions* New to this edition are end-of-chapter questions designed to provoke critical thinking and stimulate discussion.

- *Running Case* A running case on the Carter Cleaning Company illustrates the types of HRM challenges confronted by small business owners and front-line supervisors, and is accompanied by critical thinking questions, which provide an opportunity to discuss and apply the text material.

- *Case Incident* A different case incident can be found at the end of each chapter. These cases present current HRM issues in a real-life setting, and are followed by questions designed to encourage discussion and promote the use of problem-solving skills.

- *Experiential Exercises* Each chapter now includes a number of individual and group-based experiential exercises, which provide learners with the opportunity to apply the text material and develop some hands-on skills.

- *Web-based Exercises* New to this edition, end-of-chapter web-based exercises are designed to incorporate computer-based information and research.

- *CBC Video Cases* To underscore the practical, real-world orientation of this book, a video case has been included at the end of each of the six parts of the text, based on CBC programs. They provide an additional bridge between the course material and ongoing Canadian events.

- *e-Tutor* A Companion Website has been developed to serve as a personal tutor for those using the text. Located at www.pearsoned.ca/dessler, it provides practice tests, key terms and concepts, Weblinks to related sites, news groups, CBC videos, and more.

- *Notes and References* This section, now amalgamated at the end of the text, includes references from academic and practitioner journals and books, historical information, as well as personal observations and experiences of the authors.

Supplements

Human Resources Management in Canada, Canadian eighth edition, is accompanied by a complete supplements package:

- **Instructor's Manual with Video Guide** (0-13-033008-6) This comprehensive guide contains a detailed lecture outline of each chapter, descriptions of the discussion boxes, answers to review and critical thinking questions, answers to the case questions, hints regarding the experiential and web-based exercises, and helpful video case notes.

- **Test Item File** (0-13-033009-4) The Test Item File contains more than 1500 multiple-choice, true/false, and short essay questions. Each question is rated by level of difficulty and includes a text page reference. It is available in both printed and electronic formats.

- **Pearson Education Canada Test Manager** (0-13-033000-0) This powerful computerized testing package merges the Test Item File with a state-of-the-art software package in the Windows platform, enabling instructors to create tailor-made, error-free tests quickly and easily. The Custom Test allows instructors to create an exam, administer it traditionally or online, and evaluate and track students' results—all with the click of the mouse.

- **Transparency Resource Package** (0-13-033022-1) More than 100 transparency masters highlighting key concepts featured in the text are available in printed format and electronically in PowerPoint.

- **Pearson Education Canada/CBC Video Library** (0-13-033023-X) Pearson Education Canada and the CBC have worked together to provide six segments from the CBC series *Venture* and *The National Magazine*. Designed specifically to complement the text, this case collection is an excellent tool for bringing students in contact with the world outside the classroom. These programs have extremely high production quality and have been chosen to relate directly to chapter content.

- **Companion Website** For a multitude of practice questions, experiential exercises, key terms and concepts, Weblinks to related sites, Netnews (Internet Newsgroups), Netsearch, CBC video case updates and more, instructors can check out the Human Resources Management in Canada, C/8/e, Companion Website at www.pearsoned.ca/dessler.

ACKNOWLEDGMENTS

The manuscript was reviewed at various stages of its development by a number of peers across Canada, and we wish to thank those who shared their insights and constructive criticism. Among them is Gordon Barnard, Durham College; Jane Guzar, Mohawk College; Mark Julien, University of Regina; Alex Kondra, Acadia University; Alec Lee, Camosun College; Barbara Lipton, Seneca College; Bill Kamburis, Seneca College; David McPherson, Humber College; and Don Schepens, Grant MacEwan College.

At Pearson Education Canada, we are very grateful for the support and dedicated efforts of Madhu Ranadive and Marisa D'Andrea, as well as Beth McAuley, Mike Ryan, and Laurel Sparrow.

Special thanks are extended to Susan Redhead, who proved to be an outstanding research assistant.

On a personal note, we thank our family members and friends who provided advice, moral support, and encouragement, without whom this book would never have been completed, to whom this book is dedicated.

Gary Dessler
Florida International University

Nina D. Cole
Brock University

Virginia L. (Gini) Sutherland
Sir Sandford Fleming College

Photo Credits

Chapter 1

1   Jose L. Pelaez/Stock Market
4   Andy Levin/Stock Market
24   Jose L. Pelaez/Stock Market
27   Ted Horowitz/Stock Market
37   Porter Gifford/Liaison Agency Inc.

Chapter 2

45   The Slide Farm/Al Harvey
47   The Bettmann Archive/CORBIS
55   Dick Hemingway
56   The Slide Farm/Al Harvey

Chapter 3

74   Prentice Hall Archives
81   Howell Liaon, Gamma-Liaison Inc.
88   Stacey Picks/Stock Boston
90   Mugshots/Stock Boston
109   Prentice Hall Archives

Chapter 4

121   Kevin Radford/SuperStock
123   Courtesy of Babak Varjavandi
129   Courtesy of Saturn
154   Kevin Radford/SuperStock

Chapter 5

167   Patricia Levy/Image Network Inc.
172   Alene M. McNeill
173   Courtesy of Bank of Montreal
186   Patricia Levy/Image Network Inc.

Chapter 6

198   Bob Daemmrich/Stock Boston
207   Courtesy of Celestica
224   Courtesy of UUNET
237   Bob Daemmrich/Stock Boston

Chapter 7

246   Uniphoto Picture Agency
260   SuperStock
267   © Richard T. Nowitz/CORBIS
268   John Coletti/Stock Boston
279   Uniphoto Picture Agency
289   Joe L. Peleaz/Stock Market

Chapter 8

305   Stewart Cohen/Image Network Inc.
307   Stewart Cohen/Image Network Inc.
318   Steven Rubin/J.B. Pictures Ltd./The Image Works
323   NASA/The Image Works

Chapter 9

338   The Slide Farm/Al Harvey
346   Jon Feingersh/Stock Market
356   The Slide Farm/Al Harvey
357   Courtesy of Outward Bound
360   Courtesy of Bank of Montreal

Chapter 10

371   Gabe Palmer/Stock Market
379   William Taufic/Stock Market
384   Gabe Palmer/Stock Market

Chapter 11

395   Bob Daemmrich/Bob Daemmrich Photos, Inc.
409   Uniphoto Picture Agency
414   Bob Daemmrich/Bob Daemmrich Photos, Inc.
415   Richard Pasley/Stock Boston
422   Jiang Jin/SuperStock

Chapter 12

432   Sam Sargent/Gamma Liaison
435   Vaughan Mechant/Canadian Press
457   am Sargent/Gamma Liaison

Chapter 13

474   E.I. DuPont De Nemours & Co. Inc.
480   CP Archive Photo/Canadian Press
493   © Copyright by MPL Communications Inc. Photo reproduced by permission of Canadian HR Reporter, 133 Richmond Street West, Toronto, ON M5H 3M8
497   E.I. DuPont De Nemours & Co. Inc.

Chapter 14

505   Arnold Zann/Black Star
509   Stephen Frisch/Stock Boston
517   Courtesy of Husky Injection Molding Systems, Bolton, Ontario
525   Arnold Zann/Black Star

Chapter 15

538   Tom Hanson/Canadian Press
552   Bill Truslow/Liaison Agency, Inc.
553   Tom Hanson/Canadian Press
556   Bill Wittman Photography

Chapter 16

562   John Lehman/Canadian Press
564   John Lehman/Canadian Press
581   Vancouver Sun/Ian Lindsay
588   Dick Hemingway

Chapter 17

603   The Canadian HR Reporter
613   Francisco Cruz/SuperStock
623   The Canadian HR Reporter
624   Adrian Wyld/Canadian Press
625   Paul Irish/Canadian Press

Chapter 18

647   B. Daemmrich/The Image Works
649   B. Daemmrich/The Image Works
650   Joe Carini/The Image Works
666   Frank Fisher/Gamma Liaison Inc.

Chapter 19

686   Will & Deni McIntyre/Photo Researchers Inc.
692   Owen Franken/Stock Boston
700   Will & Deni McIntyre/Photo Researchers Inc.

The Pearson Education Canada

companion Website...

Your Internet companion to the most exciting, state-of-the-art educational tools on the Web!

T he Pearson Education Canada Companion Website is easy to navigate and is organized to correspond to the chapters in this textbook. The Companion Website comprises these distinct, functional features:

Customized Online Resources

Online Interactive Study Guide

Interactivities

Communication

Table of Contents

Explore these areas in this Companion Website. Students and distance learners will discover resources for indepth study, research, and communication, empowering them in their quest for greater knowledge and maximizing their potential for success in the course.

A NEW WAY TO DELIVER EDUCATIONAL CONTENT

Course Management

Our Companion Websites provide instructors and students with the ability to access, exchange, and interact with material specially created for our individual textbooks.

- **Syllabus Manager** provides instructors with the option of creating online classes and constructing an online syllabus linked to specific modules in the Companion Website.

- **Grader** allows the student to take a test that is automatically marked by the program. The results of the test can be e-mailed to the instructor and then added to the student's record.

- **Help** includes an evaluation of the user's system and a tune-up area that makes updating browsers and plug-ins easier. This new feature will facilitate the use of our Companion Websites.

Instructor Resources

This section features modules with additional teaching material organized by chapter for instructors. Downloadable PowerPoint Presentations, Electronic Transparencies, and an Instructor's Manual are just some of the materials that may be available in this section. Where appropriate, this section will be password protected. To get a password, simply contact your Pearson Education Canada representative or call Faculty Sales and Services at 1-800-850-5813.

General Resources

This section contains information that is related to the entire book and that will be of interest to all users of the site. A Table of Contents and a Glossary are just two examples of the kind of information you may find in this section.

The General Resources section may also feature *Communication facilities* that provide a key element for distributed learning environments:

- **Message Board** – This module takes advantage of browser technology to provide the users of each Companion Website with a national newsgroup to post and reply to relevant course topics.

- **Chat Room** – This module enables instructors to lead group activities in real time. Using our chat client, instructors can display website content while students participate in the discussion.

Want some practice before an exam?

The Student Resources section contains the modules that form the core of the student learning experience in the Companion Website. The modules presented in this section may include the following:

- Learning Objectives
- Multiple-Choice Questions
- True/False Questions
- Short Answer Questions
- Internet Exercises
- Destinations
- Net Search

The question modules provide students with the ability to send answers to our grader and receive instant feedback on their progress through our Results Reporter. Coaching comments and references to the textbook may be available to ensure that students take advantage of all available resources to enhance their learning experience.

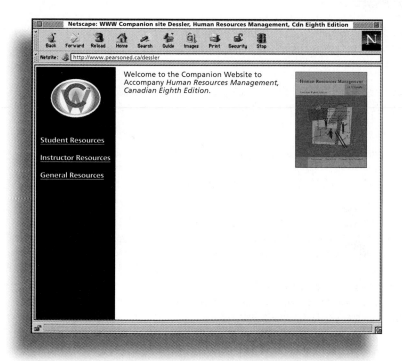

chapter 1
Student Resources
Objectives
Multiple Choice
True/False
Short Answer Questions
Internet Exercises
Destinations
Net Search
Help Syllabus
Instructor Resources
Syllabus Manager
General Resources
Welcome
Table of Contents
Glossary
Message Board
Live Chat
Feedback
Site Search

Companion Websites are currently available for:

- Mondy: Human Resource Management
- Dessler: Management
- Robbins: Organizational Behaviour

Note: Companion Website content will vary slightly from site to site depending on discipline requirements.

The Companion Website for this text can be found at:

www.pearsoned.ca/dessler

PEARSON EDUCATION CANADA

26 Prince Andrew Place
Toronto, Ontario M3C 2T8

To order:
Call: 1-800-567-3800
Fax: 1-800-263-7733

For samples:
Call: 1-800-850-5813
Fax: (416) 299-2539
E-mail:
phabinfo_pubcanada@pearsoned.com

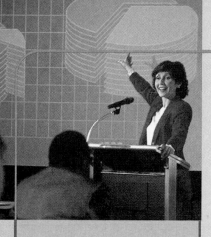

CHAPTER I

Human Resources Management:
The Field and Its Environment

CHAPTER
OUTLINE

Introduction to Human
Resources Management

Internal Environmental
Influences

External Environmental
Influences

Tomorrow's HR, Today

LEARNING OUTCOMES

After studying this chapter, you should be able to:

Define human resources management and *describe* its objectives.

Discuss the human resources management responsibilities of all managers.

Explain the role of the human resources department.

Discuss the impact of organizational culture and climate on human resources management.

Describe the external environmental factors affecting human resources management policies and practices, and *explain* their impact.

Describe the new modes of organizing and managing that have emerged and *explain* the importance of employee commitment.

Introduction to Human Resources Management

In 1994, a noted leader in the human resources (HR) field made the following observation:[1]

> Yesterday, the company with the access to the most capital or the latest technology had the best competitive advantage. Today, companies that offer products with the highest quality are the ones with a leg up on the competition. But the only thing that will uphold a company's advantage tomorrow is the calibre of people in the organization.

That predicted future is today's reality. Most managers in public- and private-sector firms of all sizes would agree that people truly are the organization's most important asset. Having competent staff on the payroll does not guarantee that a firm's human resources will be a source of competitive advantage, however. In order to remain competitive, grow, and diversify, an organization must ensure that its employees are qualified, placed in appropriate positions, properly trained, managed effectively, and committed to the firm's success. Achieving these goals is the aim of human resources management, the field that is explored in this text.

What is Human Resources Management?

human resources management (HRM)

The activities, policies, and practices involved in obtaining, developing, utilizing, evaluating, maintaining, and retaining the appropriate number and skill mix of employees to accomplish the organization's objectives.

Human resources management (HRM) refers to the management of people in organizations. It comprises the activities, policies, and practices involved in obtaining, developing, utilizing, evaluating, maintaining, and retaining the appropriate number and skill mix of employees to accomplish the organization's objectives. The goal of HRM is to maximize employees' contributions in order to achieve optimal productivity and effectiveness, while simultaneously attaining individual objectives (such as having a challenging job and obtaining recognition), and societal objectives (such as legal compliance and demonstrating social responsibility).[2]

Objectives of Human Resources Management

The objectives of HRM include:

- assisting the organization in obtaining the right number and types of employees to fulfill its strategic and operational goals
- helping to create a climate in which employees are encouraged to develop and utilize their skills to the fullest
- helping to maintain performance standards and increase productivity through effective job design; providing adequate orientation, training and development; providing performance-related feedback; and ensuring effective two-way communication
- helping to establish and maintain a harmonious employer/employee relationship
- helping to create and maintain a safe and healthy work environment
- developing programs to meet the economic, psychological, and social needs of the employees

- helping the organization to retain productive employees
- ensuring that the organization is in compliance with provincial/territorial and federal laws affecting the workplace (such as human rights, employment equity, occupational health and safety, employment standards, and labour relations legislation).

Rather than addressing organizational goals as separate and distinct from those of employees, they should be seen as compatible and mutually inclusive. A win–win situation results when this occurs. As explained by communications consultant Katie Delahaye Paine:[3]

> When you align HR with organizational strategy, you'll see growth in employee commitment, improved financial results, and find yourself better able to attract and retain the right people for your organization's business and culture.

Why is Human Resources Management Important to All Managers?

Managers at all levels must concern themselves with HRM, since they all meet their goals through the efforts of others, which requires the effective management of people. Every supervisor and manager has responsibilities related to a wide range of HRM activities. These include analyzing jobs, planning labour needs, selecting employees, orienting and training employees, managing compensation, communicating (which includes counselling and disciplining), and maintaining employee commitment. They also include ensuring fair treatment; appraising performance; ensuring employee health and safety; building and maintaining good employee/labour relations; handling complaints and grievances; and ensuring compliance with human rights, occupational health and safety, labour relations, and other legislation affecting the workplace. Regardless of field of expertise, from accounting to production control, learning about employee rights, employer responsibilities, and effective HRM practices can provide managers with knowledge that will enable them to perform more effectively.

This book is designed to provide information that will assist individuals who are currently working in an HR department or in a supervisory or managerial capacity in another department (or planning to assume such responsibilities in the future). As explained by Jim Frank, vice-president and chief economist at The Conference Board of Canada,[4]"You can see it so clearly. Some organizations in the same industry are more successful than others, and it's because they have different leadership—leadership that is able to mobilize its people around its goals and objectives."

At no time in history have effective HRM skills been more important than they are today. As we will discuss in a moment, such factors as increasing workforce diversity; rapidly changing technology; increasing government involvement in the employer–employee relationship; and globalization, have triggered an avalanche of change, one that many firms have not survived. In such an environment, the future belongs to those managers who can best manage change, but to manage change, they must have committed employees who do their jobs as if they own the company. Throughout this book, we will demonstrate that sound HRM practices and policies can play a crucial role in fostering such employee commitment and enabling organizations to better respond to change.

Society for Human Resource Management Online
www.shrm.org

Current Human Resources Management Functions

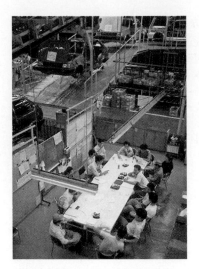

Many studies have shown that employees are more committed to their jobs when their participation is valued and encouraged. Here, assembly-line workers in a Tokyo Nissan factory participate in a worker productivity session attended by managers and supervisors.

authority
The right to make decisions, direct the work of others, and give orders.

line authority
Authorization given to managers to direct the work of those reporting to them and make decisions about operational issues.

line manager
An individual who is in charge of an aspect of operations directly linked to the organization's product(s) or service(s).

staff authority
The authority to assist, counsel, advise, or provide service to others, but not to direct or control their activities.

staff manager
The person in charge of a function or department that is not directly linked to the organization's product(s) or service(s), but rather provides assistance and support.

Except for very small businesses, most firms today have an HR department headed by an HR professional. To understand how the duties of this individual and other HR department staff relate to the HRM duties of managers throughout the rest of the organization, it is helpful to distinguish among line, staff, and functional authority.

Authority is the right to make decisions, direct the work of others, and give orders.

Line authority authorizes managers to direct the work of those reporting to them and make decisions about operational issues, and may be exercised only over employees in a manager's direct chain of command. HR professionals, for example, have line authority within the HR department and often in such service areas as the lunchroom or cafeteria.

Individuals known as **line managers** are in charge of an aspect of operations directly linked to the organization's product(s) or service(s). Hotel managers, directors of patient care, retail store managers, and managers of production and sales are generally line managers.

Staff authority, in contrast to line authority, authorizes managers to assist, counsel, advise, or provide service to others, but does not include the right to direct or control. Such authority is derived from acquired expertise and knowledge. Individuals with staff authority must rely primarily upon their ability to think strategically, their reputation, and their powers of persuasion to gain the confidence and respect of other managers. HR professionals, for example, are responsible for advising other managers on issues ranging from selection and training to grievance handling and disciplinary action, but cannot give those managers direct orders.

Managers in charge of functions or departments that are not directly linked to the organization's product(s) or service(s), but which provide assistance and support, are known as **staff managers**. HR managers, accounting managers, and managers of information technology (IT) are generally staff managers.

Functional authority involves authorization to make final decisions on issues affecting other departments or aspects of operations. The HR department is generally given functional authority for highly technical activities, such as compensation and benefits administration, and activities for which centralization enhances efficiency and effectiveness, such as recruitment. Having each department manager make decisions about pay structures, benefits, or recruitment methods could lead to inequities and excessive costs, and would be highly inefficient. The delegation of functional authority to the HR department to handle such matters ensures control (including consistent application and legal compliance), cost-efficiency, and uniformity.

Human Resources Management Responsibilities of All Managers

According to one expert, "The direct handling of people is, and always has been, an integral part of every ... manager's responsibility, from president down to the lowest-level supervisor."[5]

In small organizations, managers may carry out all of their HRM duties unassisted. As the organization grows, however, they often need the assistance, specialized knowledge, and advice of a separate human resources staff.[6]

functional authority
Authorization to make final decisions on issues affecting other departments or aspects of operations. The HR department is generally given functional authority for highly technical activities, such as compensation and benefits administration, and activities for which centralization enhances efficiency and effectiveness, such as recruitment.

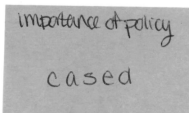

policy
A predetermined guide to thinking, established to provide direction in decision making.

procedure
A prescribed sequence of steps to be followed when implementing organizational policies.

Organization size and complexity are generally major factors in senior management's decision to establish an HR department. As an organization grows, managing human resources effectively and ensuring legal compliance become more of a burden. Once department managers and first-line supervisors find that HRM activities interfere with their other responsibilities, the benefits of delegating some of their HRM tasks to a separate HR department are generally seen to exceed the costs of establishing such an entity.

The Role of the Human Resources Department

Once an HR department has been created, it is the unit that has overall responsibility for HRM programs and activities. The primary role of the HR department is to ensure that the organization's human resources are utilized effectively and managed in compliance with company policies and procedures, government legislation, and, in unionized settings, collective agreement(s). To effectively utilize the HR department's assistance and services, all managers should be familiar with its role.

HR department staff members are involved in five distinct types of activities: formulating policies and procedures, offering advice, providing services, monitoring to ensure compliance, and serving as consultant and change agent.

Formulating Policies and Procedures

The head of the HR department usually plays a leadership role in initiating and formulating HR policies and procedures that are consistent with overall organizational objectives. These must also be compatible with current economic conditions, collective bargaining trends, and applicable employment legislation. Often, though, the actual formulation of HR policies and procedures for approval by senior management is a cooperative endeavour among managers, nonmanagerial employees, and HR department staff. A **policy** is a predetermined guide to thinking, established to provide direction in decision making. Policies are extremely important because they define the organization's position on given issues; communicate management's expectations of employees; articulate acceptable/unacceptable behaviour; ensure consistency in the treatment of employees and continuity and predictability in the course of action; and serve as standards against which performance can be measured. As illustrated in **Figure 1.1**, HR **procedures** specify a prescribed sequence of steps to be followed when implementing HR policies.

To maximize effectiveness, HR policies and procedures should be put into writing; they are often compiled in a policy manual or made available online so that they are readily accessible. This helps to ensure that the same information is communicated to all employees, and that there is consistency in employee treatment. In addition, it means that some questions and concerns can be resolved without HR departmental staff assistance.

Offering Advice

In order to cope with increasingly complex HR issues and the ever-changing work environment, managers at all levels frequently turn to the HR department staff for expert advice and counsel. Members of the HR department are expected to be completely familiar with employment legislation, HR policies and procedures, collective agreements, past practices, and the outcome of recent arbi-

FIGURE **I.I** Sample HR Policy and Procedure

Country Care **ACCESS CENTRE**	Date: May 29, 2000	Human Resource Policy
	Title: Absenteeism	
Approved by: Senior Management	References:	

Objective:

The employer recognizes that employees may be absent from work for various reasons, which may be planned, unplanned, paid or unpaid. Guidelines for the administration of these types of absence are as follows.

Unpaid Leaves of Absence

The intent of Unpaid Leaves of Absence is to provide employees with the time off to deal with personal matters that are not specifically addressed by the provisions of paid leaves of absence as defined by the collective agreements. *NOTE: There should be no expectation that Unpaid Leaves of Absence are an extension of normal vacation entitlements.*

Each request is considered on its own merit taking into account such factors as:

- The nature of the requested absence
- The effect that the employee's absence will have on daily operations
- The frequency of such requests

1.0 Unpaid Leaves of Absence of More Than One Half (1/2) Day:

    1.01 Where the Unpaid Leave of Absence request is for personal non-emergency time off, vacation and any compensation/lieu time is to be used prior to the use of Unpaid Leave of Absence; this includes vacation/compensation time that has been scheduled for future use. *NOTE: Other staff who have already scheduled vacation time will receive preference over requests for Leaves of Absence where such requests overlap.*

    1.02 Other than in cases of personal emergency, requests for Unpaid Leaves of Absence in excess of one half (1/2) day must be submitted at least two (2) weeks in advance. *NOTE: In case of emergency, or where circumstances beyond the control of the employee make such advance notice impossible, the employee's supervisor may waive the notice period.*

    1.03 Requests for Unpaid Leaves of Absence of three (3) days or less are directed to the employee's supervisor for decision.

    1.04 Requests for Unpaid Leaves of Absence in excess of three (3) days should be in the form of a letter. Such written request will be reviewed and approved by the supervisor.

    1.05 The provision of relief staffing during Unpaid Leaves of Absence will be at the discretion of the supervisor.

2.0 Leaves of Absence of One Half (1/2) Day or Less (Paid or Unpaid):

    2.01 Leaves of Absence of one half (1/2) day or less may include such things as professional appointments and personal emergencies. For these situations, the employee should seek permission from the supervisor to use medical leave, compensating time or flex-time. If flex-time is not viable and there is no paid time available for use, Unpaid Leave of Absence may be discussed with the supervisor.

    2.02 For Leaves of Absence for professional appointments or other absences where the time required is known in advance, employees are encouraged to book times so that minimal interruption to the normal work day occurs.

    2.03 The intent is to manage leaves as described in 2.01 on an informal basis between the employee and the supervisor.

tration hearings and court decisions, so that they can provide sound guidance and suggested solutions.

When assisting managers throughout the firm, the HR department staff members must keep their **employee advocacy** role in mind. This means balancing the department's primary obligation to senior management with the need to ensure that: (1) managers understand how they are expected to treat employees, (2) employees have mechanisms to contest practices that they perceive to be unfair, and (3) employees' interests are fairly represented when providing guidance and/or advice.[7]

Providing Services

The HR department generally provides services in the following areas on an ongoing basis: maintenance of HR records; recruitment, selection, orientation, training and development; compensation and benefits administration; employee counselling; and labour relations.

Monitoring to Ensure Compliance

The HR department staff members are generally responsible for monitoring to ensure compliance with established HR policies and procedures. They may analyze data pertaining to absenteeism and turnover or accident rates, for example, to identify problems with policy implementation or failures to comply with specified procedures.

In addition, the HR department staff members play a major role in ensuring compliance with employment legislation. For example, they are generally responsible for collecting and analyzing recruitment, selection, and promotion data to monitor compliance with human rights and employment equity legislation. They also assess salary and benefits data to monitor compliance with employment standards and pay equity requirements, and examine accident investigation and grievance reports to monitor compliance with health and safety and labour relations legislation.

Serving as Consultant and Change Agent

In most firms, HR department staff members serve as in-house consultants to the managers of other departments. Sometimes, HR department staff will recommend using outside consultants for assistance in solving HR issues or handling specialized assignments, such as executive recruitment and job evaluation, or suggest that certain functions or activities be outsourced.

Outsourcing, the practice of contracting with outside vendors to handle specified functions on a permanent basis, has emerged as a worldwide business megatrend. According to the Outsourcing Institute, the 1997 global outsourcing market totalled roughly $223 billion, rising to an estimated $753.5 billion in 2001.[8] While using outside experts to provide counselling services has been common for many years, more recently, the outsourcing of specific HR functions and payroll has become popular as a strategy to enable company staff to focus on core competencies and/or as a cost-savings measure. In 1999, for example, 58 percent of Canadian companies participating in one survey reported outsourcing employee training, 70 percent outsourced some of their benefits functions, and 40 percent outsourced their recruitment efforts.[9] A 1996 study revealed that the thousands of Canadian businesses outsourcing their payroll functions

---

employee advocacy
The role of the HR department staff that involves ensuring that managers understand how they are expected to treat employees, employees have mechanisms to contest practices that they perceive to be unfair, and employees' interests are fairly represented when providing guidance and/or advice.

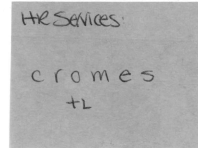
HR Services:

cromes
+L

HR Network (HRNET)
www.hronline.com/forums/index.html

outsourcing
The practice of contracting with outside vendors to handle specified functions on a permanent basis.

CFT Training and Human Resources
www.cfthr.com

were saving upwards of 50 percent of their payroll costs.[10] Today, as revealed in the following research insight, the scope of what is being outsourced is broadening, as are the kinds of outsourcing relationships that are being developed.[11]

Research Insight

In a recent research study involving 300 large global companies (including 26 Canadian organizations), 73 percent of the Canadian participants indicated that they had outsourced at least one activity or process, and 95 percent of these were somewhat or very satisfied with their outsourcing to date. About half of the respondents stated that the importance of outsourcing had increased over the previous three years. The most commonly outsourced activities (and those most likely to be outsourced in the near future) were identified as: benefits administration; payroll processing; logistics; real estate management; and internal auditing. This study also revealed that, while 63 percent reported achieving at least the expected cost savings, organizations are starting to view outsourcing strategically, as a broad management strategy rather than just as a cost-reduction tool. The major reasons for outsourcing were identified as: (1) ensuring a focus on core competencies, (2) enhancing profitability and shareholder value, and (3) avoiding the investment in technology required to enhance efficiency. Related to the latter is the trend toward a significant investment by service providers, particularly in the IT infrastructure required to support service delivery.[12]

e-business
The use of the Internet to manage everyday business processes electronically, from supply chain to delivery. Included is the use of e-mail, Web sites, and e-commerce activities.

e-commerce
Any transaction or purchase using electronic means, including the Internet transfer of funds, use of debit/credit cards, and Electronic Data Interchange.

The rapid emergence of **e-business**, defined as the use of the Internet to manage everyday business processes electronically, from supply chain to delivery,[13] is having a dramatic impact on the outsourcing environment[14]—even in the HR field, as explained in the Information Technology and HR box. e-Business includes the use of e-mail, Web sites, and e-commerce activities. **e-Commerce** involves any transaction or purchase using electronic means, and includes the Internet transfer of funds, use of debit/credit cards, and Electronic Data Interchange.[15]

INFORMATION TECHNOLOGY AND HR

HR e-Business

Everyone is going "e" these days it seems, including HR outsourcing. While only in the early stages, it is possible that e-HR—if handled well—will ultimately result in reduced administrative burdens for HR practitioners, as well as increased business possibilities for technical-minded HR consultants. Ken Duff, president of Ottawa-based HR-Dept.Com, converted his 12-year-old HR consulting company to an online-based one in 1999. He felt that it was the best way to handle his growing roster of clients, many of whom wanted a representative of the firm on-site all the time, which had become physically impossible. Now, he and the four HR consultants who assist him provide a full slate of HR services over the Internet and telephone, and can be "virtually" on-site all of the time.

HR-Dept.Com handles HR administrative functions for its client firms, which range from small start-up firms that have no HR person to medium-sized companies, thus enabling the HR practitioner or front-line managers to focus on strategic business issues. Three levels of service are available: Basic, Advantage and Premium. For a one-time $3000 fee, HR-Dept.Com creates and supports for the client a secure, customized Web site that can be accessed by managers for more information and by employees to obtain answers to HR inquiries. Ongoing costs range from $16 000 per year for Basic-level to $32 000 for Premium-level service.

Proponents of e-HR claim that it is the way of the future for small- to medium-sized companies, because it is an inexpensive and efficient way to help firms become more strategic, avoid legal pitfalls, and acquire an edge in recruitment.

Source: Based on Lesley Young, "HR e-Business: A New Form of Outsourcing," *Canadian HR Reporter* 13, no. 9 (May 8, 2000), pp. 1, 6.

HR-Dept.Com
www.hr-dept.com

proactive
Anticipating problems and taking corrective action before a problem occurs.

reactive
Responding to an already-existing problem (such as "putting out fires").

In addition to serving as consultants, HR specialists are expected to be "change agents" who provide senior managers with "up-to-date information on current trends and new methods of solving problems"[16] to help the organization increase its efficiency and effectiveness. By constantly monitoring the internal and external environments, HR specialists can help the organization to be proactive when appropriate, rather than always being reactive. Being **proactive** means that HRM problems are anticipated and corrective action begins before the problem occurs, as compared to being **reactive**, which means responding to an already-existing problem. Implementing an employment equity program on a voluntary basis in light of the changing composition of the work force is an example of a proactive strategy. Awaiting legislative requirements prior to implementation of such a program is an example of reactive HRM.

Structure of the Human Resources Department

Figure 1.2 illustrates the typical structure of the HR function in a medium-sized organization (employing 200 to 400 workers). As indicated, the HR manager usually reports to the chief executive officer (CEO), and plays a generalist role. Support staff members typically perform a wide variety of activities, including maintaining HR records, assisting with recruitment and selection, and ensuring legal compliance.

As demands on the department grow, it increases in importance and complexity. **Figure 1.3** illustrates the subdepartments and hierarchy of jobs within a typical, large-sized manufacturing firm, structured by areas of specialization. When the HR department head plays a major role in the organization's strategic planning and related processes, and the HR department makes a major con-

FIGURE 1.2 Typical Structure of the Human Resources Function in a Medium-sized Organization

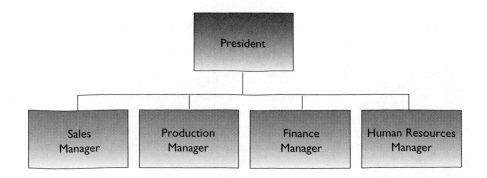

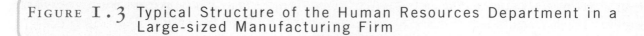

FIGURE I.3 Typical Structure of the Human Resources Department in a Large-sized Manufacturing Firm

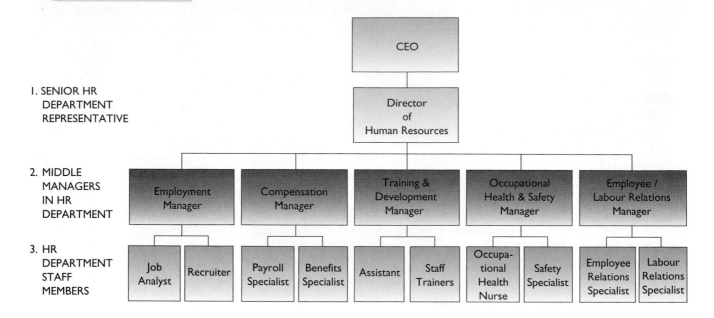

tribution to the firm, the title "director of HR" (or labour relations in a unionized setting) is often used. Those reporting to the department head typically include the following:

- employment manager (responsible for HR planning, recruitment, selection, and performance appraisals)
- compensation manager (responsible for base pay, incentives, and benefits administration)
- training and development manager (responsible for orientation, training, development, and career planning)
- occupational health and safety manager, and
- employee / labour relations manager (responsible for communications, counselling, contract administration and collective bargaining activities).

Activity managers may be supported by an assortment of specialists, assistants, and clerical staff. In large firms, the specialists actually perform such activities as recruitment and training. Community college and university graduates often start their HRM careers in specialist positions.

An Ethical Dilemma

Supervisor Jonas wants to hire Employee A. Based on reference checking results, you, the HR manager, know that Employee B would be a much more suitable hire. How would you handle this situation?

Human Resources Management: A Cooperative Effort

Regardless of the size of the HR department, in practice, good HRM is a joint, cooperative effort, with HR specialists and other managers working together. As indicated in **Table 1.1**, in some areas, such as pre-employment testing and wage and salary administration, the HR department plays the major role. In others, such as interviewing and handling disciplinary action, the duties are split more evenly with individuals in other departments.

TABLE 1.1

Division of Responsibilities for HR Activities

Activity	Responsibility for the Activity is Assigned to:		
	HR Dept. Only	HR & Other Dept(s)	Other Dept(s) Only
Employment and recruiting			
Employment interviews	31%	65%	3%
Recruiting (other than college/university recruiting)	70	29	1
Temporary labour coordination	67	28	4
Pre-employment testing	87	11	2
College/university recruiting	76	21	2
Training and development			
Orientation of new employees	61	37	1
Supervisory training/management development	45	48	7
Performance appraisal, management	36	52	12
Performance appraisal, nonmanagement	33	55	12
Skills training, nonmanagement	24	55	21
Tuition aid/scholarships	77	17	6
Career planning/development	46	49	5
Productivity/quality enhancement programs	12	55	33
Compensation			
Wage/salary administration	77	20	3
Job descriptions	61	38	1
Job evaluation	67	29	4
Payroll administration	29	29	42
Job analysis	70	29	1
Executive compensation	52	27	22
Incentive pay plans	44	45	11
Benefits			
Vacation/leave policies and administration	78	22	1
Insurance benefits administration	86	10	4
Employment Insurance	82	13	5
Pension/retirement plan administration	76	16	9
Flexible spending account administration	83	10	7
Cafeteria benefits plan administration	85	9	6
Profit sharing plan administration	57	27	16
Stock plan administration	45	28	27
Employee services			
Recreation/social programs	41%	45%	14%
Employee assistance plan/counselling	83	12	5
Relocation services	76	18	6
Preretirement counselling/retirement planning	85	9	6
Outplacement services	88	8	3
Employee and community relations			
Disciplinary procedures	44	55	2
Complaint procedures	57	41	2
Exit interviews	86	13	1
Award/recognition programs	67	30	3
Human rights compliance/employment equity programs	87	11	1
Employee communications/publications	41	46	13
Community relations/contribution programs	29	43	28
Suggestion systems	53	37	9
Attitude surveys	73	23	4
Labour relations	59	37	4

>>

HR records

HR recordkeeping	86	14	—
Promotion/transfer/separation processing	72	27	1
HRMS	68	29	3
Health and safety			
Workers' compensation administration	74	17	9
Safety training	31	42	27
Safety inspections/OHSA compliance	29	40	31
Health/wellness program	77	17	6
Strategic planning			
HR forecasting/planning	63	34	3
Organization development	37	56	7
Mergers and acquisitions	42	47	11
International HR administration	59	33	9

Source: Adapted from "SHRM-BNA Survey No. 63: Human Resource Activities, Budgets & Staffs, 1997-1998," *BNA Bulletin to Management*, pp.2–3.

Contemporary Challenges in Human Resources Management

Internal and external environmental influences play a major role in HRM. Organizational climate and culture, for example, help to shape HR policies and practices, which, in turn, have an impact on the quality of candidates that a firm can attract, as well as its ability to retain desired workers. The economic environment, labour market conditions, and unions also play a role in determining the quality and variety of employees that can be attracted and retained. There are external challenges that are dramatically changing the environment of HRM, however, and requiring it to play an ever more crucial role in organizations. These challenges include demographic trends and increasing work-force diversity, trends in technology, increasing government involvement in the employer–employee relationship, globalization, and changes in the nature of jobs and work. After briefly describing the ongoing internal and external influences, we will focus on the external challenges that are having the most significant impact on HRM in Canada today.

INTERNAL ENVIRONMENTAL INFLUENCES

How a firm deals with the following two internal environmental influences has a major impact on its ability to meet its objectives.

Organizational Culture

organizational culture
The core values, beliefs, and assumptions that are widely shared by members of an organization.

Organizational culture consists of the core values, beliefs, and assumptions that are widely shared by members of an organization. It serves a variety of purposes:

- communicating what the organization "believes in" and "stands for"
- providing employees with a sense of direction and expected behaviour (norms)
- shaping employees' attitudes about themselves, the organization, and their roles
- creating a sense of identity, orderliness, and consistency
- fostering employee loyalty and commitment.

Culture is often conveyed through an organization's mission statement, as well as through stories, myths, symbols, and ceremonies:[17]

New employees at Hewlett-Packard (HP) are told the story of how Dave Packard and Bill Hewlett started the global giant more than 60 years ago in a small backyard garage, which is now a state historical landmark in the heart of Silicon Valley and was a focal point of a major corporate brand campaign. The Rules of the Garage, depicted in Figure 1.4, are one-line principles that explain how the spirit of invention, contribution, and collaboration embodied in the founders can be demonstrated by employees and the firm in order to stay dynamic in the high-tech world.

All managers with HR responsibilities play an important role in creating and maintaining the type of organizational culture desired. Genuine concern and caring about employees can be conveyed by thorough orientation and training programs, promotion-from-within policies, strategies encouraging communication flow in all directions, providing unique benefits such as free vacations and an on-site fitness centre (as at HP Canada)[18] or offering free hotel accommodation to employees and their families (as at Four Seasons Hotels and Resorts),[19] and having an **employee assistance program** (EAP), a topic to which we'll return in Chapter 14. In organizations in which customers or clients are truly valued, employees who provide exemplary service are recognized and rewarded, and there is follow-up to ensure customer/client satisfaction.

Having a positive culture earns critical acclaim, and has a positive impact on both retention and recruitment. Firms such as 3M, HP Canada, Four Seasons Hotels and Resorts, and Bank of Montreal have gained a reputation, not only for the quality of their products and services, but also for positive relationships with their employees and customers/clients. HP Canada, for example, has an extremely low turnover rate (in the range of 5.5 to 7.5 percent) and rarely has

employee assistance program (EAP)

A company-sponsored program to help employees cope with personal problems that are interfering with or have the potential to interfere with their job performance, as well as issues affecting their well-being and/or that of their families.

FIGURE 1.4 Hewlett-Packard Principles: Rules of the Garage

Believe you can change the world.
Work quickly, keep the tools unlocked, work whenever.
Know when to work alone and when to work together.
Share—tools, ideas. Trust your colleagues.
No politics. No bureaucracy. (These are
ridiculous in a garage.)
The customer defines a job well done.
Radical ideas are not bad ideas.
Invent different ways of working.
Make a contribution every day. If it doesn't contribute,
it doesn't leave the garage.
Believe that together we can do anything.
Invent.

Source: Hewlett-Packard: Rules of the Garage, as reproduced in David Brown, "Case Study—Hewlett-Packard: Telling Stories to Attract and Retain," *Canadian HR Reporter* 13, no. 7 (April 10, 2000), p. 9. Reproduced with permission of Hewlett-Packard.

to advertise job openings due to a deluge of résumés on hand.[20] According to Vice-president of Human Resources John Cross, "It's the environment that makes people want to work for HP. We want a culture that allows people to bond with the company."[21]

Organizational Climate

organizational climate
The prevailing atmosphere that exists in an organization and its impact on employees.

Organizational climate refers to the prevailing atmosphere that exists in an organization and its impact on employees. Organizations have personalities, just like people. They can be friendly or unfriendly, open or secretive, rigid or flexible, innovative or stagnant. The major factors influencing the climate are management's leadership style, HR policies and practices, and amount and style of communication. The type of climate that exists is generally reflected in the level of employee motivation, job satisfaction, performance, and productivity, and thus has a direct impact on organizational profits and/or ongoing viability.

HR department staff members play a key role in helping managers throughout the firm to establish and maintain a positive organizational climate. They can help to develop policies and practices, for example, that encourage a spirit of teamwork and build employee commitment, which can have very positive consequences:[22]

> Unlike many firms that chose to cut staff to stay afloat during the 1990s, Teknion Furniture Systems, a Canadian designer/producer of high-end office furniture successfully competing with the U.S. giants like Steelcase, has not had a layoff in its 17-year history. Alternatives to layoffs are always examined because managers at the firm realize that layoffs result in a lack of trust between employees and management—trust that takes years to develop. The firm's no-layoff policy has had a positive impact on product quality, employee satisfaction and commitment, and customer service. With a growth rate of 46 percent during 1999, the results speak for themselves.

When organizations fail to make adjustments in their climate to keep up with environmental changes, difficulties are often experienced. The bureaucratic climate at IBM, characterized by centralized decision making, hierarchy of command, job security, and a strict promote-from-within policy, has been identified as a key factor in the firm's difficulties in maintaining a competitive position on both domestic and foreign fronts in the early 1990s. Under the leadership of Chief Executive Officer (CEO) Louis Gerstner, the climate was totally revamped. Unnecessary bureaucracy was eliminated and the firm was infused with **intrapreneurs**. The HR department, for example, was restructured into a more autonomous organization—a separate company known as Workforce Solutions (WFS). The results were excellent: delivery of HR services at a much lower cost, enhanced commitment to HR, greater flexibility and responsiveness to customer needs, streamlined HR processes, and the introduction of innovative HR programs.[23]

intrapreneur
An employee who is an innovator because he or she has been given the freedom to create new products, services, and/or production methods.

EXTERNAL ENVIRONMENTAL INFLUENCES

The external environmental factors described on the following pages have a direct or indirect influence on HRM. To be effective, HR managers must monitor the environment on an ongoing basis; assess the impact of any changes; and be proactive in implementing policies and programs to deal with such challenges.

Economic Environment

The economic environment has a major impact on business in general and the management of human resources in particular. Economic conditions affect supply and demand for products and services, which, in turn, have a dramatic impact on the **labour force** by affecting the number and types of employees required, as well as an employer's ability to pay wages and provide benefits. When the economy is healthy, companies often hire more workers as demand for products and services increases. Consequently, unemployment rates fall, there is more competition for qualified employees, and training and retention strategies increase in importance.[24] Conversely, during a downturn, some firms reduce pay and benefits in order to retain workers. Other employers are forced to downsize, by offering attractive early retirement and early leave programs or by laying off and terminating employees. Unemployment rates rise, and employers are often overwhelmed with applicants when vacancies are advertised.

As illustrated in **Figure 1.5,** although **unemployment rates** have fluctuated over the past 50 years, there was an upward trend until the last few years of the 1990s, at which point employment growth accelerated and the unemployment rate decreased significantly. As of June 2000, the seasonally adjusted labour force **participation rate** was 65.7 percent, and the unemployment rate was 6.6 percent.[25]

As illustrated in **Figure 1.6, productivity** refers to the ratio of an organization's outputs (goods and services) to its inputs (people, capital, energy, and materials).[26] To improve productivity, managers must find ways to produce more outputs with current input levels or to use fewer resources to produce current output levels.

In most organizations today, productivity improvement is essential for long-term success. Through productivity gains, managers can reduce costs, con-

labour force

Those who are employed and those actively seeking work.

unemployment rate

The percentage of individuals in the labour force who are currently unemployed.

participation rate

The percentage of adults in the total population who are in the labour force.

productivity

The ratio of an organization's outputs (goods and services) to its inputs (people, capital, energy, and materials).

FIGURE **1.5** Canadian Unemployment Rates (1946–1999)

Note: Data from 1976 on have been rebased to the 1996 Census of Population

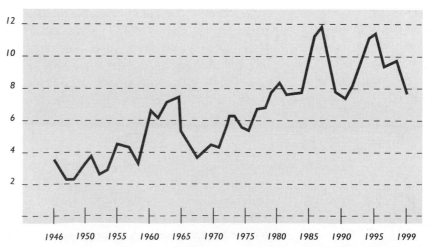

Unemployment rate (%)

Source: Reproduced from Susan Crompton and Michael Vickers, "One Hundred Years of the Labour Force," in Statistics Canada, *Canadian Social Trends,* Catalogue No. 11-008 (Summer 2000) p.11.

FIGURE I.6 Productivity Ratio

$$\text{Productivity} = \frac{\text{Outputs (Goods and Services)}}{\text{Inputs (People, Capital, Energy, Materials)}}$$

serve scarce resources, and increase profits. This leads to a win–win situation, since higher profits often result in better compensation and improved working conditions, thereby enhancing the employees' quality of work life and their motivation to further improve productivity.

Recent statistics reveal some good news and some bad. While labour productivity in Canada surged in 1999, growing at a rate of almost three times the pace of 1998,[27] the poor performance of Canadian companies—especially those in the manufacturing sector—in terms of innovation (including research and development and employee training), resulted in a relatively low productivity growth rate in comparison to that of Sweden, Germany, Japan and the U.S.[28]

Canada's relatively low productivity growth rate and high labour costs are of grave concern, since competition with foreign companies has become increasingly important. The result of the North American Free Trade Agreement (NAFTA), created to establish free trade between Canada, the United States, and Mexico, combined with the continuing liberalization of trade on a global basis and increasing deregulation in many industrialized countries, is that Canada's economic success increasingly depends on the ability of Canadian employers to meet international quality and productivity standards and become more cost-competitive. This applies to firms selling products and services in the domestic market, in which foreign competition is increasingly a factor, as well as those with international markets.

Labour Market Conditions

labour market
The geographic area from which an organization recruits employees and where individuals seek employment.

The **labour market** is the geographic area from which an organization recruits employees and where individuals seek employment. In other words, it is the area in which the forces of supply and demand interact. The labour market is often different for various employee groups within an organization. While clerical and technical employees are generally recruited locally, the labour market for senior managers and highly specialized employees is often national or even international in scope.

One measure of an organization's effectiveness is its ability to compete successfully for high-calibre human resources. Many factors motivate candidates to seek employment with a particular organization, including type of business/industry, reputation, opportunities for advancement, compensation, job security, and working conditions. In recent years, for example, lower compensation and higher income tax rates have been cited as causes of an alleged "brain drain"—the loss of highly educated workers from Canada to the U.S. Not all experts agree, however, that this phenomenon actually exists.[29]

Location and climate and other aspects of a firm's physical surroundings, such as housing, commuting, and living costs, can help or hinder a firm's ability to attract and retain employees. In large cities such as Toronto and Vancouver, experts claim that "the growing congestion of highways and transit systems poses a genuine threat to the city's economic and social growth."[30]

According to a Toronto-based executive search firm consultant, for example, it is often difficult to lure people away from centres where they don't have to put up with big-city gridlock, such as Ottawa and Kitchener-Waterloo, to accept jobs in Toronto.[31]

Recent population shifts to the west coast and small towns and rural areas can be attributed, at least in part, to the desire of many individuals to work and live in what they perceive to be a more desirable physical environment. Such shifts alter the demand for and supply of individuals in local labour markets, a factor that firms must always take into account when deciding where to establish a new venture, expand, or downsize.

Because the labour market is not controlled or influenced by any one factor, it is unstructured and often unpredictable. Nevertheless, organizations must constantly monitor and track trends affecting supply and demand of human resources. By doing so, they can gather information about the prevailing pay rates for employees with particular talents or skills, and estimate how difficult it is likely to be to attract and recruit staff. Labour market conditions should also be monitored to determine present and emerging trends (such as the changing composition of the labour force) as well as changing values and expectations, so that policies and programs can be adapted and/or designed in order to recognize and take advantage of these trends.

Labour Unions

Canada WorkinfoNET
www.workinfonet.ca

labour union
An officially recognized association of employees, practising a similar trade or employed in the same company or industry, who have joined together to present a united front and collective voice in dealing with management.

A **labour union** is an officially recognized association of employees, practising a similar trade or employed in the same company or industry, who have joined together to present a united front and collective voice in dealing with management, with the aim of securing and furthering the social and economic interests and well-being of their membership. Although both an internal and external challenge, we have listed unions as an external factor because they become an additional party in the relationship between the company and employees. Once a union has been certified or recognized to represent a specific group of employees, the union negotiates terms and conditions of employment with management, rather than individual employees doing so. The company is required by law to recognize the union and bargain with it in good faith.

In Canada, unions remain a powerful influence. Although union membership dropped slightly in 1999, 32.2 percent of employees were covered by a collective agreement.[32] This is quite different from the situation in the U.S., where union membership has decreased dramatically in recent years. Today, organized labour's share of the work force in the U.S. is about 13.9 percent of all non-agricultural paid workers.[33]

Labour unions affect organizations in several ways. Management has less discretion and flexibility in implementing and administering HR policies, procedures, and practices when dealing with unionized employees, since a negotiated collective agreement governs most terms and conditions of employment, including wages and benefits, working conditions, and job security. Often, organizations with a mix of unionized and non-unionized employees institute a policy (whether officially or unofficially) to ensure that similar or even slightly better terms and conditions of employment are provided to non-unionized staff to encourage them to retain their non-union status.

Labour unions also influence the HR policies and practices in non-unionized organizations wishing to remain union-free. Such organizations monitor bargaining activities in their community and industry, and ensure that their employees are provided with terms and conditions of employment equal to or better than those being negotiated by unions.

When some or all of an organization's employees are unionized, the HR department is responsible for helping to develop sound HR policies and practices that will promote good labour–management relations, and create and maintain a harmonious working environment. Knowledge of collective bargaining, contract administration, and pertinent labour relations legislation becomes imperative.

Demographic Trends and Increasing Work-force Diversity

demographics

The characteristics of the work force, which include age, sex, marital status, and education level.

diversity

Any attribute that humans are likely to use to tell themselves, "that person is different from me," and thus includes such factors as race, gender, age, values, and cultural norms.

Demographics refers to the characteristics of the work force, which include age, sex, marital status, and education level.[34] Demographic changes occur slowly and are well measured, which means that they are known in advance. As will be discussed further in Chapter 3, the fact that Canada's labour force is becoming increasingly diverse is one of the major challenges confronting HR managers today. **Diversity** refers to "... any attribute that humans are likely to use to tell themselves, 'that person is different from me,'" and thus includes such factors as race, gender, age, values, and cultural norms.[35]

Population Growth   The single most important factor governing the size and composition of the labour force is population growth. As of July 2000, there were 24 million Canadians 15 years of age and older, of whom 15.7 million were in the labour force.[36] Since the population growth has slowed to less than one percent per year, the average age of the work force is changing rather dramatically, the implications of which will be discussed shortly.

Canada admits more immigrants per capita than any other country, which has significant implications for the labour force, as does the fact that there has been a dramatic shift in immigration patterns. Prior to 1966, at least 90 percent of the immigrants who came to Canada were from Europe.[37] As highlighted in **Figure 1.7**, by June of 1999, that figure had dropped to 22 percent.

Currently, the fastest growing groups in the Canadian work force are women, visible minorities, Aboriginal people, and persons with disabilities. We will discuss each of these groups on the following pages, along with some of the challenges and opportunities presented by the increasing availability of members of these four groups.

baby boomers

Individuals born between 1946 and 1965.

Age   The **baby boomers**, born between 1946 and 1965, began crowding into the labour market in the late 1960s. The sheer number of "boomers" helped to expand the economy and made it easier for HR departments to focus on issues such as cost containment, since recruitment and selection, while important, were not the most critical problems. During the 1990s, individuals in this "population bulge" experienced a great deal of competition for advancement. This challenged managers to find new strategies for forging career paths, such as lateral moves, to keep this group motivated and satisfied. The oldest of the baby boomers are now in their mid-fifties. As can be seen in **Figure 1.8**, since life expectancies have increased and fertility rates have declined, the average age of the population is increasing substantially. According to Statistics Canada, between 2001 and 2016, there will be dramatic growth in the 55–59, 60–64,

FIGURE I.7 Immigrants to Canada by Country of Last Residence

July 1, 1998 to
June 30, 1999

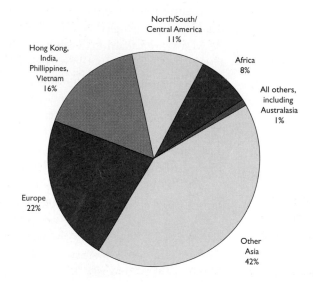

Source: "Immigrants to Canada by Country of Last Residence, July 1, 1998 to June 30, 1999," created from Statistics Canada's Website, <http://www.statcan/english/Pgdb/People/Population/demo8.htm> July 6, 2000.

65–69 age groups of 60.5, 74.8, and 67.5 percent, respectively. In contrast, the youth population, aged 15 to 24, will increase by only 0.3 percent. In fact, the 15 to 19 age group will actually decrease by seven percent.[38] Since some baby boomers have already taken advantage of generous early retirement programs and many more will be retiring over the 25 years, pension plan and social security benefits issues are starting to present a very serious concern for employers and governments, given the smaller labour force available to support the retirees. While those 65 and over currently represent about 12.4 percent of the total population, this figure will increase to 21.4 percent by 2026.[39] At present, there are approximately five active workers to support each retiree—a ratio projected to be reduced to 3.12 over the next 25 years.[40] Early retirement opportunities may soon become a thing of the past and increasing consideration given

FIGURE I.8 Population Projections for Canada

Percent Distribution of Population by Age Group
(Medium-growth Projection, Based on 1999 Population Estimates)

	0–14	15–64	65+	Mean Age
2001	18.8%	68.5%	12.7%	37.7
2006	17.1%	69.5%	13.3%	39.0
2011	15.7%	69.8%	14.5%	40.3
2016	15.2%	68.3%	16.5%	41.5
2021	15.0%	66.2%	18.8%	42.5
2026	14.8%	63.8%	21.4%	43.5

Source: "Population Projections for Canada," created from Statistics Canada's Website, www.statcan.ca/english/Pgbd/People/Population/demo23a.htm, demo23b.htm, demo23c.htm, and Statistics Canada's CANSIM Database, Matrix No. 6900, July 6, 2000.

to the abolishment of mandatory retirement at any age, a move supported by the Canadian Human Rights Commission.[41] There has also been some discussion about raising the retirement age to 67, as is now the case in the U.S. According to a recent survey, however, doing so does not have the support of the Canadian general public.[42]

Many organizations with a primary interest in the younger age group, such as retail establishments and fast-food chains, have already started to feel the impact of the fact that the population from which they have traditionally gained customers and part-time workers is starting to shrink dramatically. Some employers have undertaken initiatives to attract older workers, especially those who have taken early retirement, by offering job sharing and expanding the number of part-time hours available. Ontario school boards, for example, have been trying to entice retired teachers to return to work on a part-time basis as supply teachers, including many who took advantage of the lowered early retirement requirements introduced in April of 1998.[43] McDonald's Restaurants of Canada is another organization that is actively recruiting seniors, as well as directing advertising efforts to appeal to the senior market. Managers there take great pride in the fact that they now have employees of all ages working side by side.[44]

HR specialists must remember that many HR policies, benefits plans, and reward systems that attract and motivate employees in one age group may not appeal to those in another due to differing values and priorities.

HR Online
www.hr2000.com

Research Insight

Generation X (Nexus generation)
Individuals born between 1966 and 1980.

According to a recent survey involving in-depth interviews with senior executives from 88 major Canadian private- and public-sector companies, as **Generation X** (also known as **Nexus generation**) employees replace aging boomers, flexible work arrangements, continuous skill development and a balance between work and personal life are becoming increasingly important. Other research reveals that those in Generation X have a different work ethic than those in the baby boom generation. They are not averse to hard work, but place a premium on personal time and value a life-friendly work culture, want to be valued immediately for the skills they bring to the workplace, and like to be active participants in decision making. They view command- and authority-based cultures with disdain, and believe that security comes from transferability of skills rather than corporate loyalty.[45]

The message to employers is that having workers of diverse ages may create a need to bridge the generation gap. Young managers may have difficulty gaining the respect of those reporting to them who are older than they are, or in exerting their authority. In addition, because of their differing values, employees may have difficulty understanding and communicating with those from another generation. It has been predicted that Generation X employees—having experienced the world before and during the technological revolution—will play an increasingly significant role as a link between the baby boomers and the young people just entering the world of work, **the Net Generation** (also known as **Nexters**).[46] While successfully integrating employees of all ages may provide some challenges, organizations doing so benefit greatly from the combination of skills that a multigenerational work force offers.

Net Generation (Nexters)
Individuals born since 1980.

Sandwich Generation
A term referring to individuals who have responsibilities for rearing young dependants as well as assisting elderly relatives who are no longer capable of functioning totally independently.

The aging of the population has had another impact. Many middle-aged employees are caught in the **Sandwich Generation**, with responsibilities for rearing young dependants as well as assisting elderly relatives who are no longer capable of functioning totally independently. According to a recent Conference Board of Canada study, the number of "sandwiched" employees increased from 9.5 to 15 percent between 1989 and 1999, and will continue to grow. The study also found that those with both child- and eldercare responsibilities are much more likely to leave their jobs because of work/personal life conflicts.[47] Although some employers, such as the Royal Bank,[48] have been proactive in assisting their "sandwiched" employees, only about 10 percent of Canadian businesses have programs specifically designed to assist workers providing elder-care.[49] Recognizing that many employers will not institute voluntary initiatives and that caring for aging loved ones is likely to eclipse childcare as the pressing issue over the next 25 years, a Senate subcommittee has recommended a legis-lated solution—paid leave for palliative care.[50]

Education   The level of education of the Canadian labour force is increasing at a significant rate. In 1995, for example, an estimated 85 percent of Canadians aged 22 to 24 had completed high school.[51] In addition, more Canadians are pursuing higher education, through a variety of institutions ranging from universities and colleges/*CÉGEPs* to trade schools, private-sector organizations, and professional associations. In 1996, about one in five Canadians aged 15 to 24 pursued post-secondary studies, compared with about one in seven in 1986,[52] and more than nine million adults in the labour force had completed a college diploma or university degree, as compared with just under seven million five years previously.[53] Other trends in secondary and post-secondary education include growth in the number of cooperative-education programs, designed to enable students to gain work experience while still attending school, and of distance-education opportunities, which mesh Internet technology with the fun-damental need to continue learning. In 1997, for example, New Brunswick's TeleEducation NB launched TeleCampus on the World Wide Web; it is one of the world's first virtual universities, at which students can enroll in courses, pay their tuition, and complete their studies online.[54]

Today, the number of Canadians involved in adult education and training activities rivals the number of students enrolled in the entire elementary, second-ary and post-secondary education system,[55] a trend that many firms encourage through tuition-assistance programs. Some organizations go even further to pro-mote educational opportunities, such as hosting Master's Degree programs on-site.

Given the higher expectations of the better-educated labour force, managers are expected to try to ensure that the talents and capabilities of employees are fully uti-lized and that opportunities are provided for career growth. In today's economic cli-mate, doing so is not always possible. Many college and university graduates find themselves working in jobs that do not fully utilize their skills and knowledge. In fact, a 1994 International Adult Literacy Survey (IALS) found that one-quarter of Canadian employees do not use their skills at their jobs. At that time, those with a skills surplus not being used outnumbered those with a skill deficit by two to one.[56] Improving the quality of work life is therefore more important than ever.

The good news is that many Canadians are highly educated, and very few Canadians are illiterate in the sense of not being able to read. The bad news is that a startlingly high proportion (43 percent) have only marginal **literacy** skills,[57] defined as the ability to understand and use printed and written docu-ments in daily activities to achieve goals and to develop knowledge and poten-tial.[58] A frightening reality is that inadequate reading and writing skills have replaced lack of experience as the major reason for rejecting entry-level candi-

literacy

The ability to understand and use printed and written documents in daily activities to achieve goals and to develop knowledge and potential.

functionally illiterate
Unable to read, write, calculate, or solve problems at a level required for independent functioning or the performance of routine technical tasks.

dates.[59] While IALS found that almost three out of five Canadians between the ages of 16 and 65 are equipped to deal with the printed materials that they encounter in their daily lives, about one in six working-age Canadians is **functionally illiterate**,[60] unable to read, write, calculate, or solve problems at a level required for independent functioning or the performance of routine technical tasks.[61] Since many of these individuals are currently employed and will be in the labour market for a long time to come, functional illiteracy is exacting a toll, not only on individual social and economic opportunities but also on organizations' accident rates and productivity levels, thus affecting their ability to compete in the global economy.

Syncrude Canada Ltd. is one of a growing number of organizations that provide in-house essential skills (literacy) programs to supplement its workplace- or industry-specific training courses. Although such programs are aimed at refreshing and improving basic reading, writing, math and problem-solving skills, they also improve listening, oral communication, teamwork, leadership, and computer skills, among other things.[62]

A related problem confronting organizations is technological illiteracy. A few firms have been proactive in addressing this issue. For example, Cisco Systems Canada Co. has committed $25 million to various educational initiatives nationwide, including the Networking Academy Program (NAP), a global program—offered in 52 countries and seven languages—designed to provide secondary and post-secondary students with the skills needed to participate in the Internet economy. NAP teaches students how to build and maintain computer networks, and promotes IT as a viable career option. Cisco Canada provides ongoing financial support for NAP to the 81 participating schools across Canada.[63]

AN ETHICAL DILEMMA

The maintenance department supervisor has just come to you, the HR manager, voicing concern about the safety of two of her reporting employees whom she recently discovered are functionally illiterate. What are your responsibilities to these employees, if any?

Visible and Ethnic Minorities The proportion of visible and ethnic minorities entering the Canadian labour market is growing, in jobs ranging from general labour to technical, professional, and skilled trades. In 1996, about 3.2 million Canadians were visible-minority group members,[64] constituting 11.2 percent of the population, up from 9.2 percent in 1991 and 6.3 percent in 1986. This increase is largely the result of immigration. More than three-quarters of those who came to Canada during the 1990s were members of a visible minority group.[65] The proportion of immigrants with a mother tongue other than English or French grew from 11 percent in 1986 to nearly 17 percent in 1996.[66] The largest visible minority group in 1996 was Chinese, accounting for slightly more than 25 percent of the total visible minority population, followed by South Asians (21 percent) and Blacks (18 percent).[67] It is currently projected that the number of visible-minority group members living in Canada will increase to approximately seven million by 2016, about 19 percent of the total population.[68]

Ethnic diversity is also increasing. At the time of Confederation (1867), approximately 60 percent of Canada's population was British and 30 percent French. Although the largest ethnic groups are still those with British or French backgrounds, neither group represents a majority of the population. Currently, more than 100 different ethnic groups are represented among Canadian residents.[69]

HR specialists must ensure that policies and programs are developed in their organizations to accommodate and celebrate the diverse cultural characteristics of visible and ethnic minority employees, something that requires much more than ensuring compliance with human rights legislation.

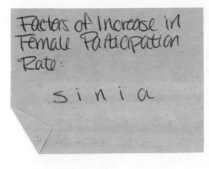

employment rate

The percentage of adults in the total population who are currently employed.

Women The growing presence of women has been one of the dominant trends in Canada's labour force since the 1950s.[70] As of 1999, there were 7.2 million women 15 years and over in the labour force, representing 45.7 percent of the total. That year, women's participation rate was 58.9 percent, while that of men was 72.5 percent.[71] Factors contributing to the dramatic increase in female participation rate include smaller family size, increased divorce rate, the need and desire for dual family incomes, increased educational level, and the availability of more-flexible working hours and part-time jobs.

The **employment rate** for women has also continued to climb. As shown in **Figure 1.9**, between 1946 and the summer of 2000, the employment rate for adult women tripled, while that for men fell by one-fifth.[72] During the 1990s, the unemployment rate for women fell below that of men and stayed there. In 1999, for example, the unemployment rate for women was 7.3 percent, while for men it was 7.8 percent. This trend reflects the fact that women have moved into occupations in which the unemployment rate is low, while men tend to be clustered in jobs in which the risk of unemployment is much higher.[73] There is still strong evidence that women are underutilized in the Canadian work force, however.

Research Insight

A 1998 study revealed that women hold just 12 percent of the corporate-officer posts at Canada's 560 largest corporations. A similar situation was revealed in a survey of top U.S. companies, where women fill 11.9 percent of such posts. In comparing the results, one major difference was unveiled, however. Canada has more than twice as many firms with no women at the corporate officer level. Further up the ranks in top Canadian firms, the numbers are even slimmer, with women filling just 3.4 percent of the positions with "clout," such as chief operating officer, executive vice-president, or chief executive officer. While 12 Canadian companies are led by women, when the subsidiaries of foreign-owned firms, private companies and Crown corporations are removed from this list, only three remain.[74]

FIGURE **1.9** Employment Rates of Canadian Men and Women (1946–1999)

Note: Data from 1976 on have been rebased to the 1996 Census of Population

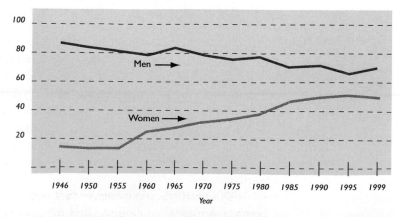

Source: Reproduced from Susan Crompton and Michael Vickers, "Employment Rates of Canadian Men and Women (1946-1999)," in Statistics Canada, *Canadian Social Trends,* Catalogue No. 11-008, (Summer 2000), p.11.

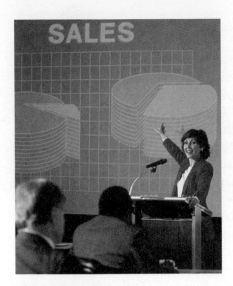

While more women are moving into management positions, there is still a 'glass ceiling' in Canadian firms that needs to be addressed.

A 1997 study revealed that women are slightly better represented at the managerial/administrative level in Canadian businesses and the professions. At that time, women made up 43 percent of all managers and administrators, up from 29 percent in 1982.[75]

Of particular significance to employers is the increasing number of women in the work force with dependent children. Between 1976 and 1998, participation rates for mothers with children under age three doubled from 32 percent to 64 percent.[76] Many organizations are making a determined effort to accommodate working women and shared parenting responsibilities, and offer one or more of the following family-friendly benefits: paid leave banks, childcare information and referral assistance, childcare subsidies, on-site daycare, leave for school functions, emergency childcare support, and flexible work programs (job sharing, a compressed workweek, a shorter workweek, a shorter workday, and/or telecommuting). Other organizations offer more comprehensive work/life programs, designed to assist employees to attain a healthier lifestyle as well as to cope with all of their non-work responsibilities (including parenting). Such programs generally include flexible work programs and some of the other family-friendly benefits listed, as well as health and fitness programs, an employee assistance plan, a wellness program, and/or eldercare.[77] As explained in the Diversity Counts box, the Royal Bank Financial Group has found that offering a work/life program can benefit the organization as well as the employees involved. Evidence of the possible benefits of such programs comes from other sources as well as the reports of individual firms. A 1999 survey of 2000 Canadian men and women revealed that management's recognition of the need for work/life balance is the most powerful driver of work-force commitment, followed by opportunities for personal growth, the organization's commitment to satisfying its customers' needs, and competitive pay.[78] In another survey, 91 percent of the participating employers indicated that work/life benefits are a strategic retention tool. Apparently, employees agree: in one company's survey of its top performers, work/life balance was one of the most frequently cited reasons for choosing to stay with the firm.[79]

Although the number of firms offering family-friendly benefits and work/life programs is on the rise, proper implementation is required to reap positive results. While 52 percent of respondents in a 1999 survey reported having some sort of work/life program (up from 33 percent in 1993), a Health Canada study released that same year concluded that Canadian organizations are not providing employees with the support necessary to strike a healthy balance between work and home. More than a third of workers were found to be experiencing a high level of work/life conflict; a third reported frequent depressed moods; and a quarter indicated that they felt "burned out" from their jobs. The study concluded that most companies have not embraced the changes that lead to substantive results. Identified factors having a negative impact on program success include lack of employee access, hesitancy on the part of employees to admit to needing help, unwillingness to use the program due to fear that doing so would be perceived to indicate a lack of commitment, an unsupportive culture, and lack of supervisory support.[80]

Francophones   Although truly a cultural mosaic (multilingual and multiracial), Canada is officially bilingual. It is the only major industrialized country with two official languages. There are large French-speaking populations in the provinces of Ontario and New Brunswick, and Quebec is predominantly French-speaking.

DIVERSITY COUNTS

In Attaining Work/Life Balance

Royal Bank Financial Group (RBFG) was one of the first Canadian organizations to recognize that acknowledging that employees have a life outside of work is critical in fostering employee commitment and attracting and retaining top talent, factors that have a direct impact on organizational efficiency. With that in mind, a Flexible Work Arrangement (FWA) program was introduced in the early 1990s. Thirty percent of employees (more than 10 000 men and women) now take advantage of the program. In recent RBFG studies, 81 percent of FWA users reported that they had become more effective in managing work and family life,

and most also reported reduced stress, more energy, and fewer work absences. The organization has also reaped some sizable benefits. In addition to better attendance, improved customer service has been noted, and an improvement in or constant level of job performance was reported by 99 percent of the managers of FWA users surveyed.

Source: David Brown, "Flex-Time Solutions in Practice," *Canadian HR Reporter* 12, no. 17 (October 4, 1999), p. 2; and Joyce Hampton, "A Balancing Between Work and Life," *Guide to Employee Benefits, Supplement to Canadian HR Reporter* 12, no. 12 (June 14, 1999), pp. G1-G2.

AN ETHICAL DILEMMA

Since not all employees require assistance in balancing work and family responsibilities, how would you justify your belief that the firm should introduce family-friendly benefits?

Organizations operating in these provinces, particularly in Quebec, must ensure that their policies, procedures, and practices conform to the requirements of relevant employment legislation, as well as meeting the expectations of all of their employees. Furthermore, although organizations functioning in French are found predominantly in Quebec and parts of New Brunswick, many firms in both the private and public sectors must be able to serve their clientele in both French and English.

Aboriginal Peoples Between 1996 and 2006, the number of First Peoples (North American Indians, Inuit, and Métis) in the prime working and family-rearing age group (35 to 54) is expected to increase 41 percent, which will exacerbate their current situation unless drastic measures are taken.[81] First Peoples are still facing considerable difficulty in obtaining jobs and advancing in the workplace. The 1999 federal Human Rights Commission annual report indicated that while the representation of First Peoples continued to increase in the federally regulated public sector in recent years (reaching 2.9 percent as of March 31, 1999), federally regulated private-sector firms hired a smaller proportion of this group for the fourth year in a row. First Peoples' high share of terminations, which stood at 1.5 percent in 1998, compounds these difficulties.[82]

Persons with Disabilities Despite the fact that human rights legislation in every Canadian jurisdiction prohibits discrimination against individuals with disabilities, Canadians with disabilities continue to confront physical barriers to equality every day. Inaccessibility is still the rule, not the exception. As of 1998, only 48 percent of Canadians with disabilities between the ages of 15 and 64 had either full- or part-time jobs, compared to 73 percent of Canadians without disabilities. Moreover, 54 percent of persons with disabilities had annual incomes of $15 000 or less.[83] Given the fact that baby boomers born between 1946 and 1965 will add 1.4 million to the population of working age Canadians with some sort of disability by 2010,[84] these statistics are rather alarming.

Even though studies show that there are no performance differences in terms of productivity, attendance, and average tenure between employees who classify themselves as having a disability and those who do not, persons with disabilities continue on average to experience high rates of unemployment and underemployment, and lower pay.

Research Insight

According to a recent Royal Bank of Canada study:

- people with disabilities have employment rates about 30 full percentage points below those without a disability
- men with a severe disability who secure full-time employment earn almost 24 percent less than their counterparts without a disability.[85]

Even in organizations covered by the federal Employment Equity Act, little progress has been made. While persons with disabilities make up 6.5 percent of all Canadian workers, they account for only 2.3 percent of employees in the federally regulated private sector, virtually unchanged over the past 12 years. Their representation in the federal public sector rose to 4.6 percent in 1999, a slight improvement from 3.9 percent in 1997.[86]

Overall Impact of Increasing Diversity Managers must be extremely aware that related to the work-force diversity described above are significant value differences about the overall importance of work, what aspects or characteristics of a job are most important, tolerance of discipline in terms of hours and pace of work, attitudes toward authority, and definition of loyalty. Employees increasingly expect to exercise more freedom from management control, and are more demanding and questioning. More people are seeking jobs that are attuned to their personal values and provide the opportunity for them to bring their personalities to work with them,[87] as well as flexible work arrangements and other programs that will enable them to balance their work and personal lives.[88] Policies and practices must be adapted to embrace the diversity of the dominant values represented in an organization's work force.

Technology

It is mainly through technological innovation that firms develop new products and services and/or improve existing ones in order to remain competitive, and gain the productivity and quality needed for competitive advantage.

Manufacturing advances, such as robotics and computer-aided design/computer-aided manufacturing (CAD/CAM), have eliminated many blue-collar jobs, replacing them with fewer but more highly skilled jobs. When robots were introduced in the automobile industry, for instance, there was a major decrease in the demand for welders and painters, but a new demand for technicians who could program, install, and service automated equipment.[89] Due to computer technology, similar changes have been occurring in the nature of office work. Optical scanners, computerized x-ray scanners, and Magnetic Resonance Imagery (MRI) are technological advances that have caused major occupational changes in the medical field over the past few decades, and such advances are being made every day. Currently, for example, a few doctors are attempting to revolutionize heart surgery using computer assistance and robotic arms.[90] The overall impact of the technological changes affecting almost every field is that labour-intensive blue-collar and clerical jobs have been decreasing, while technical, managerial, and professional

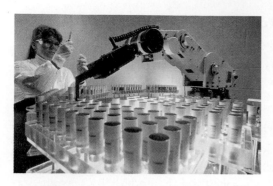

Robotics is revolutionizing work in many fields. Such technology requires highly trained and committed employees.

AN ETHICAL DILEMMA

How much responsibility does a firm have toward employees whose skills will soon become obsolete due to changing technology?

HR Technology
www.avantech.ca

jobs are on the increase. This shift in employment opportunities has many implications for organizations: jobs and organization structures are being redesigned; new incentive and compensation plans are being instituted; revised job descriptions are being written; and new programs are being instituted for employee selection, evaluation, and training/retraining—all with the help of HR specialists.

Unfortunately, the training of the Canadian labour force has not kept pace with the rate of technological change and innovation. Consequently, there is a scarcity of skills in certain fields. For example, 95 percent of the 126 firms participating in a recent Conference Board of Canada survey indicated that they are experiencing shortages in non-entry level technical jobs. Recruiting to fill such positions is taking more than four months, on average.[91]

Many Canadian firms, such as Nortel Networks, inevitably have to look outside of Canada to fill their high-tech openings, which is rather disturbing given the fact that there are currently about 1.1 million Canadians seeking employment.[92] Nortel has a history of recruiting experts from around the world to train and nurture Canadian high-tech graduates, because it has been the firm's experience that few schools in the country can keep up with the frenzied pace of technological change, with many lagging about three to five years behind.[93]

While much of the impact of information technology has been positive, it has also led to some organizational problems. For many employees, it has created anxiety, tension, resentment, and alienation. Unions have consistently expressed concerns about job displacement and health hazards, such as those related to video display terminals. All of these issues must be addressed through effective HRM practices such as information sharing, counselling, ergonomic refitting, job redesign, and training.

Information technology has also hastened what experts call the "fall of hierarchy," or promotion of egalitarianism. Power and authority are spread more evenly among all employees. For example, with "distributed computing," every employee with a personal computer on his or her desk can tap into the firm's computer network and obtain needed information. Expecting employees to make more decisions has implications for selection, training, and compensation.

Questions concerning data control, accuracy, right to privacy, and ethics are at the core of a growing controversy brought about by the new information technologies. Sophisticated computerized control systems are used to monitor employee speed, accuracy, and efficiency in some firms, including Bell Canada. More and more firms are also monitoring employee e-mail, voice mail, telephone conversations, and computer usage, and some now monitor employee behaviour using video surveillance.[94] Reasons for such monitoring include eliminating time wastage, deterring abuse of company resources, protecting network security, preventing misappropriation of company resources, ensuring compliance with health and safety standards and regulations and other legislation, and monitoring employee behaviour and performance. Employers considering monitoring employees should be aware that doing so may present both practical and legal problems:

- such monitoring may have counterproductive results such as increased job stress, decreased morale and productivity, lowered employee self-esteem, and decreased trust in and respect for the employer
- setting up and maintaining a monitoring system may involve significant economic costs

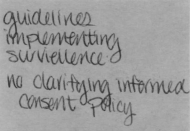

guidelines implementing surveillance·

no clarifying informed consent policy

Legal Compliance

- surveillance of employees in the workplace raises the controversial legal issue of employee privacy rights.

When introducing surveillance systems, the following guidelines should be kept in mind:[95]

1. Employees must be informed prior to the implementation of a monitoring system.

2. A policy that clearly stipulates exactly what employees can and cannot do with work resources and time should be developed; employee input is recommended to ensure that employees understand the underlying reasons and to gain acceptance.

3. Video surveillance should be used only if there are no suitable alternatives. If it is considered necessary, it should be reasonable and limited in its intrusions into employee privacy.

4. Once a monitoring system has been implemented, new employees should be required to consent to such monitoring as a term of employment.

5. Clarifying those aspects of employment in which employees should not have any expectation of privacy can help to protect employers from legal action on the part of disgruntled employees.

Human Resources Information Systems Changing technology has also had major implications for HR departments. Over the past few decades, many firms introduced a **Human Resources Information System (HRIS)** to store detailed information on employees, HR policies and procedures, government laws and regulations, collective agreements, etc. HRIS computer applications include: salary and benefits administration; tracking statistics on absenteeism, grievances, and health and safety; collecting data for government statistical reporting and employment equity purposes; advertising jobs and recruiting candidates; and communicating with employees. In a 1993 survey, to which individuals at 502 organizations from across Canada responded, computer utilization ranged from 96.3 percent in payroll management to 12.1 percent in career planning.[96]

In the Information Technology and HR boxes throughout this text, we will describe how computers are now being used not only for storage, retrieval and analysis of information but for broader applications, including basic report production, long-range forecasting and strategic planning, and evaluation of HR policies and practices. The Information Technology and HR box that follows, for example, describes the types of reports that can be generated by automated time and attendance systems. It also explains how such systems can decrease time lost to comparatively non-productive work like data entry and employee scheduling, thereby providing time for HR department employees and managers throughout the firm to focus on more strategic issues.

Today, many Canadian firms, such as Suncor, Inco and Scotiabank,[97] are utilizing computer technology even more extensively by introducing a **Human Resources Management System (HRMS)**, defined as an information management system accessible to staff at all levels, designed to ensure that the organization's human resources are recruited, selected, developed, employed, deployed, and supported effectively.[98] Functional applications include succession planning, pension plan projections and eligibility monitoring, interactive employee retirement training, and more. Self-service applications for employees

Human Resources Information System (HRIS)

A computerized system used to collect, record, store, analyze, and retrieve data pertaining to an organization's human resources.

Human Resources Management System (HRMS)

An information management system accessible to staff at all levels, designed to ensure that the organization's human resources are recruited, selected, developed, employed, deployed, and supported effectively.

INFORMATION TECHNOLOGY AND HR

The Time is Here for Automated Time and Attendance Systems

To be strategic players in the organization, HR department employees must have information at their fingertips. Time and attendance systems provide vast amounts of HR data that can be used to create valuable management reports, ranging from payroll information to absenteeism, money transaction, general employee information, actual hours worked vs. budgeted hours, and employee activity reports. Data can be collected using punch cards, keypads, bar-coded cards, badges with magnetic strips that employees swipe through a reader, or a biometric reader that uses measurements of each employee's hand to allow him/her to enter information into the system.

Time and attendance software systems can also operate with interactive voice response (IVR). These can be set up to work through the Internet, on a regular company computer network, across telephone lines, or on all three. A primary use of an IVR-operated time and attendance system is the efficient scheduling of staff, one of the most important functions of the HR department. Today's sophisticated time and attendance software systems are omniscient—they know where people are, what they want, what they can and cannot do, and who can and who cannot be trusted to come in when they say they will. Such software can be programmed to incorporate dozens—even hundreds—of possible scenarios. Scheduling basics such as vacation time, overtime and budgets can be taken into account, as well as tracking functions such as who has signed up to work but not shown up. A key advantage is that such a system operates 24 hours per day, and can therefore handle last-minute scheduling changes.

An IVR-operated time and attendance system can be invaluable in complex settings, such as school boards, which have: employees who need to be replaced from time to time (such as part-time teachers); employees who may have to be replaced at the last minute (such as full-time faculty members); and employees who are never replaced (such as the principal). At Edmonton's Public School Board, for example, a computer-driven telephone system has automated teacher absence reporting, and handles 600 to 800 placements per day. Using such a system, replacement workers can be contacted based on a number of different programmed criteria. Such criteria might involve random calls, or calls in alphabetical order, by seniority or according to the top 10 preferred substitutes. Key advantages include the fact that the likelihood of several schools calling the same person to cover on a particular day can be eliminated, while the likelihood of a school obtaining the preferred substitute is increased (provided he or she is available, of course). Such software can assume a personal touch, if so desired. An example would be permitting a teacher calling in sick to leave a recorded message for his or her substitute regarding scheduled activities, topics to be covered, etc. The system can also be programmed so that when the principal calls in sick no replacement is contacted, whereas when the head caretaker phones in, the system calls the secondary caretaker to advise that he or she will be assuming the leadership role that day.

Another setting in which an IVR system can be invaluable is one that is volume-driven, such as a hospital. To schedule staff, hospital unit heads normally discuss any scheduling discrepancies and assign workers according to their expertise and the unit's needs, something that can take hours of valuable (and expensive) time. Because no one group of people can possibly be aware of all of the hospital's scheduling needs, one department may end up sending people home on paid leave while another pays people overtime to fill in. A scheduling system knows who is currently working, each person's areas of expertise, and who is needed where. Because an automated system involves dialing in using a specific telephone and PIN number, paperwork is eliminated, as is the need for expensive and bulky equipment such as time clocks. Another key advantage of both IVR systems and biometric collection devices is that employee misuse is eliminated, as happens when one employee "punches in" for a tardy or absent colleague.

Source: Joyce Hampton, "Put Up Your Hand," *Guide to HR Technology, Supplement to Canadian HR Reporter* 12, no. 18 (October 18, 1999), p. G11; and Ian Turnbull and Joyce Hampton, "The Time is Here for Automated IVR Time and Attendance Systems," *Canadian HR Reporter* 12, no. 20 (November 29, 1999), pp. 22 & 31.

and managers ensure that information reaches those who need it, with one-time data entry, less maintenance, and improved quality and accuracy.[99]

Government

Various laws enacted by governments have had and will continue to have a dramatic impact on the employer–employee relationship in Canada. In one recent survey, 70 percent of the HR specialists responding cited changing regulatory requirements as a major factor altering their work environment.[100]

The legal framework for employment includes: constitutional law, particularly the Charter of Rights and Freedoms; acts of parliament; **common law**, which is the accumulation of judicial precedents that do not derive from specific pieces of legislation; and **contract law**, which governs collective agreements and individual employment contracts. Such laws impose specific requirements and constraints on management policies, procedures, and practices.

Some of the employment-related legislation is aimed at prohibiting discrimination in various aspects and terms and conditions of employment, such as human rights, employment equity, and pay equity. Other laws require employers to meet certain obligations, such as occupational health and safety, employment standards, and labour relations. Still others make various payments mandatory, such as Workers' Compensation, Employment Insurance, and the Canada/Quebec Pension Plans.

Accompanying each employment-related law are **regulations**, legally binding rules that are developed by the special regulatory bodies created by the government in each jurisdiction, such as human rights commissions and ministries of labour. Instead of the courts, it is these regulatory bodies that aid in the interpretation of the legislation, evaluate complaints, and enforce compliance.

All of the laws mentioned above and their regulations, which will be discussed in detail later in this book, have important implications for all managers, since they must:

- ensure currency. Because the decisions of courts and quasi-judicial bodies (such as human rights tribunals and labour relations boards) affect interpretation, and legislation itself changes frequently, keeping abreast of legislative developments is a major ongoing responsibility. Often, the HR department staff members play a major role in helping other managers to remain current by circulating reading material or holding seminars

- develop and administer legally compliant policies and practices to avoid losing government contracts, charges filed by affected employees or regulatory bodies, fines, and/or bad publicity

- try to ensure that compliance does not interfere with the efficient and effective accomplishment of their other responsibilities. This means finding ways to comply with regulatory requirements with as little cost and disruption as possible. For example, the Workplace Hazardous Materials Information System legislation (which will be discussed in Chapter 18) requires that all employees handling hazardous substances (which includes those using liquid paper correction fluid!) receive training. Many firms have developed manuals, videotapes, and self-administered quizzes, such that employees can study independently at home or at work during off-peak times, and submit their completed quizzes for evaluation and verification of training completion.

One of the factors that make the laws affecting employment in Canada so challenging is the different jurisdictions involved. Employment Insurance and the Canada Pension Plan are federal laws that apply to all employers and employees in Canada, with one exception: the Quebec Pension Plan applies to employers and employees in the province of Quebec. Other legislation varies from one jurisdiction to another. The Canada Labour Code and Canadian Human Rights Act (federal legislation) apply only to those sectors of the economy regulated by the federal government, which represents about 10 percent of the Canadian work force, including federal government departments and agencies, federal Crown corporations, chartered banks, airlines, national railways, the Canadian armed forces, shipping companies and ports, the insurance and communications industries, and certain interprovincial and international operations. Each province and territory has its own human rights, employment standards, labour relations, health and safety, and workers' compensation legislation. While there is some commonality across jurisdictions, there is also considerable variation. Minimum wage, overtime pay requirements, vacation entitlement, and grounds protected under human rights legislation, for example, vary from one province/territory to another. Furthermore, some jurisdictions have pay and employment equity legislation; others do not. Since virtually every aspect of HRM is affected by legal and/or judicial influences, legislative issues will be discussed in almost every chapter of this text.

Globalization

globalization
The tendency of firms to extend their sales or manufacturing to new markets abroad.

Globalization refers to the tendency of firms to extend their sales or manufacturing to new markets abroad. For businesses everywhere, the rate of globalization in the past few years has been nothing short of phenomenal.

While about 86 percent of Canada's exports still go to the U.S.,[101] Canada currently has approximately 200 international trading partners.[102] As one international business expert put it, "The bottom line is that the growing integration of the world economy into a single, huge marketplace is increasing the intensity of competition in a wide range of manufacturing and service industries."[103]

Production is becoming globalized, too, as firms around the world put manufacturing facilities where they will be most advantageous. For example, when Nortel Networks Corp. decided to invest another U.S. $400 million in fibre-optical networking, plans were made to build a new facility in Ottawa and expand existing facilities in the U.K. and Northern Ireland.[104]

multinational corporation
A firm that conducts a large part of business outside the country in which it is headquartered and that locates a significant percentage of its physical facilities and human resources in other countries.

There are increasing numbers of **multinational corporations**—firms that conduct a large part of business outside the country in which they are headquartered and that locate a significant percentage of their physical facilities and human resources in other countries. Many organizations are locating new plants in areas where wages and other operating costs are lower. For example, Hewlett Packard's computers are assembled in Mexico, and 3M—the manufacturer of Scotch tape, chemicals, and electrical accessories—has located one of its newest plants in India.[105]

While cheaper labour is one reason for transferring operations abroad, another is to tap into what *Fortune* magazine calls "a vast new supply of skilled labour around the world."[106] Many multinational firms set up manufacturing plants abroad, not only to establish beachheads in promising markets, but also to utilize that country's professionals and engineers. For example, Asea Brown Boveri (a $30-billion-a-year Swiss/Swedish builder of transportation and electric

GLOBAL HRM

Canadian Government Gets a Failing Grade in Providing Family Support

According to a recent report, Europeans are better able to attain a work/life balance than Canadians are because their governments provide more family support. Ottawa-based researchers found that the governments in The Netherlands, Germany, France, Norway and Sweden play a key role in supporting families by providing such benefits as parents' allowances, childcare, tax concessions, lengthy parental leaves, flexible hours, pension income for stay-at-home parents, and income supports. The governments in Canada, the U.S., and the U.K., on the other hand, generally leave it up to parents to figure out how to balance their work and home responsibilities.

Government policy on such matters has major implications for employers. According to a Health Canada report released in the spring of 1999, Canadians who feel stressed due to inability to effectively balance their work and personal lives are costing their employers at least $2.7 billion per year and the health-care system an estimated $425 million. In 1996, 19.8 million workdays were missed due to work/family conflict, and 40 percent of working Canadians reported high levels of such conflict (up from 35.6 percent in 1991). Canadians are not alone in losing the "struggle to juggle" their time. In the U.S., personal illness, family issues and personal needs account for 62 percent of unscheduled employee absences.

Source: Based on Angie Gallop, "Workaholism & The Work–Family Conflict," *HR Professional* 16, no. 5 (October/November 1999), pp. 30–32; Joey Goodings, "European Governments More Supportive of Work/Life Balance," *Canadian HR Reporter* 12, no. 5 (March 8, 1999), p. 2; and Dianne Dyck, "Make Your Workplace Family Friendly," *Guide to Employee Benefits, Supplement to Canadian HR Reporter* 12, no. 22 (December 13, 1999), p. G5.

generation systems) already has 25 000 new employees in former Communist countries and has thus shifted many jobs from Western to Eastern Europe.

This globalization of markets and manufacturing has vastly increased international competition. Throughout the world, organizations that formerly competed only with local or national firms—from airlines to automobile makers to banks—are now facing an onslaught of foreign competitors. From boosting the productivity of a global labour force to formulating selection, training, and compensation policies for expatriate employees, managing globalization and its effects on competitiveness will thus continue to be a major HR challenge in the years to come.

Trends in the Nature of Jobs and Work

Major changes have been occurring in the nature of jobs and work, in part as a response to a number of the environmental challenges already discussed.

telecommuting

The use of microcomputers, networks, and other communications technology (such as fax machines) to perform in the home work that is traditionally done in the workplace.

Telecommuting   **Telecommuting**, which will be described in more detail in Chapter 10, is the use of microcomputers, networks, and other communications

technology (such as fax machines) to perform in the home work that is traditionally done in the workplace. According to Statistics Canada, there are currently 1.5 million Canadian telecommuters (also known as teleworkers). While it is true that not all jobs are suited to telecommuting, a study released in the fall of 1998 found that: half of all employees think that their jobs are at least partially teleworkable; 43 percent would quit their jobs if another employer offered them an equivalent job allowing telework; and one-third would choose telework over a 10-percent raise. Canadian firms with telecommuting policies include the Royal Bank, the Bank of Montreal, Bell Canada, Digital Equipment of Canada Ltd., the federal government, and IBM Canada. At IBM Canada's facility in Markham, Ontario, for example, three-quarters of the staff has the ability to work on a mobile or flexible basis.[107]

contingent employees
Workers who do not have regular full-time or part-time employment status.

Use of Contingent Employees   Many firms are using more **contingent employees**—defined as workers who do not have regular full-time or part-time employment status—to handle vacation and leave coverage, peak-period demands, extra workload, and specialized tasks or assignments. Included are contract workers, seasonal workers, casual and non-regular part-time employees, temporary employees, independent contractors (freelancers), consultants, and leased employees.[108] Contingent workers currently account for about 12 percent of all jobs in Canada, a figure that is expected to reach 25 percent by 2010.[109]

While temporary employees obtained though such agencies as Manpower and Kelly Services have been a popular type of contingent employee for many years, there are a couple of relatively new contingency arrangements: freelancers and leased employees. *Freelancers* are employees who work directly for the employer through independent contract arrangements. They are often contracted to provide specialized services one or two days a week on a permanent basis. *Leased employees* are typically former company employees, now on the payroll of a leasing firm, who work for the company on an as-needed basis, often for extended periods of time.

The use of contingent workers is not restricted to clerical jobs. Many come from the executive suite or middle management—specialists in their fields—including marketing and advertising executives, HR professionals, project managers, accountants, writers, graphic designers, and lawyers.[110] In fact, it is estimated that professionals currently comprise about 20 percent of the total contingent work force.[111]

Part-time Employees   There are more regular part-time employees in Canada than ever before. These are individuals who work fewer hours than full-time core employees, typically during peak periods (such as evenings and weekends in retail stores and restaurants). Approximately 33 percent of all employed women work part-time: two-thirds of them by preference, and the other one-third because they were unable to obtain full-time employment.[112] The fact that part-time workers are often paid less than their full-time counterparts—and may not have benefits coverage—has raised some major equity concerns.

small business
A firm with fewer than 50 employees, generally characterized by individual or small-group ownership, owner involvement in the management of the company, and operations restricted to a particular geographical area (although customers may be geographically dispersed).

Small Businesses   **Small businesses**, classified as firms with fewer than 50 employees, whether sole proprietorships, partnerships or corporations, are a large and increasingly important part of the Canadian economy. Generally characterized by individual or small-group ownership, owner involvement in the management of the company, and operations restricted to a particular geographical area (although customers may be geographically dispersed), small businesses accounted for 57 percent of total job growth in 1997, and 32 percent of all jobs.[113]

Small businesses are typically run by **entrepreneurs** who are willing to accept the personal financial risks involved, knowing that they will benefit directly from the success of their enterprise. Many large corporations began as a small-business venture, including Apple Computer and Hewlett Packard, both of which started out in garages.

Unfortunately, not all small-business owners enjoy such success. The risk of failure is high. In fact, according to a recent edition of CBC's "National Magazine" (October 8, 1996), more than one-half of new business ventures fail during the first year. In 1997, 48 percent of all job loss was in this sector.[114]

A Service Society As can be seen in **Figure 1.10**, employment trends in Canada have been experiencing dramatic change. The **primary sector**, which includes agriculture, fishing and trapping, forestry, and mining, now represents only 2.8 percent of jobs. While the **secondary sector** (manufacturing and construction) grew from 1960 to 1985, between 1985 and the late 1990s employment in those industries dropped by more than 20 percent. In common with trends in Western Europe and the U.S., the sector of the Canadian economy accounting for the greatest growth in recent decades is the **tertiary or service sector**, which includes public administration, personal and business services, finance, trade, public utilities, and transportation/communications. In 1998, 86.1 percent of Canadian jobs were in this sector.[115]

While much of this growth is attributable to rapid technological change (initially in the form of automation and more recently in improvements in IT), part is due to an increase in outsourcing of particular activities by primary- and secondary-sector firms to decrease costs and increase efficiency. Subcontracted functions range from building maintenance to provision of security, cafeteria management and laundry services to payroll and training and development.

Since all jobs in this sector involve the provision of service, often in person but increasingly through the design, installation, and maintenance of service-providing technologies (such as automated banking machines and cable television), effectively managing and motivating human resources is critical. Although there are some lesser-skilled jobs (in housekeeping and food services, for example), many service-sector jobs demand **knowledge workers**, employees who transform information into a product or service, whose responsibilities include planning, problem solving, and decision making.

Knowledge Work and Human Capital Management expert Peter Drucker has said that "the foundation of an organization is not money or capital or technology—it's knowledge and education (**human capital**). By 2005, knowledge workers will be the single largest group in the labour force."[116] He is not alone in this belief. Many experts believe that the distinguishing characteristic of companies today and tomorrow is this growing emphasis on human capital. Jobs today in all sectors demand a level of expertise far beyond that required of most workers 20 or 30 years ago, which means that human capital is quickly replacing machines as the basis for most firms' success.

Furthermore, it is not unusual for more than one-quarter of sales to come from products less than five years old. As a result, "innovating—creating new products, new services, and new ways of turning out goods more cheaply—has become the most urgent concern of corporations everywhere."[117]

entrepreneur
An individual who starts, organizes, manages, and assumes responsibility for a business or other enterprise.

primary sector
Agriculture, fishing and trapping, forestry, and mining.

secondary sector
Manufacturing and construction.

tertiary or service sector
Public administration, personal and business services, finance, trade, public utilities, and transportation/ communications.

Comcheq Payroll Services
www.comcheq.ca

knowledge worker
An employee who transforms information into a product or service, whose responsibilities include planning, problem solving, and decision making.

human capital
The knowledge, education, training, skills, and expertise of a firm's workers.

FIGURE I.IO Employment Trends

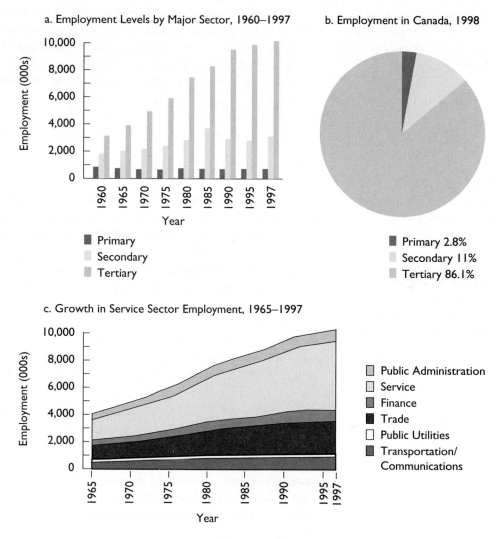

a. Employment Levels by Major Sector, 1960–1997

b. Employment in Canada, 1998

■ Primary
Secondary
Tertiary

■ Primary 2.8%
Secondary 11%
Tertiary 86.1%

c. Growth in Service Sector Employment, 1965–1997

Public Administration
Service
Finance
Trade
Public Utilities
Transportation/
Communications

Source: Reproduced from Statistics Canada's Website, www.statcan.ca/english/Pgbd/People/Labour/labor10b.htm. July 10, 2000.

For managers, the challenge of fostering intellectual or human capital lies in the fact that knowledge workers must be managed differently than workers of previous generations. New HRM systems and skills are required to select and train such employees, encourage self-discipline, win employee commitment, and spark creativity. 3M is one organization that has learned how to encourage creativity and access the skills and ideas of all of its employees:[118]

At 3M, there is a corporate policy that 30 percent of its annual revenues must come from products that are less than four years old. Thus, over the years, 3M has mastered the art of motivating employees to come up with new and useful ideas. Every 3M employee must take courses on risk taking, handling change, and assuming responsibility for his or her job. Scientists and engineers are actively encouraged to form small groups to come up with new ideas and launch new products. If they can't obtain funding from the managers of their own business units, they can seek money from other business groups. If that fails, they can appeal to a panel of scientists from across the firm to obtain a "Genesis Grant," which provides up to $50 000 in funding.

3M has a long history of success with innovations that initially seemed useless but later went on to earn millions of dollars. For example, 3M executives tried to end the Thinsulate project at least five times. Innovators within 3M persisted, however, and the light, waterproof, synthetic fibre is now used in sporting goods, shoes, and car doors. In short, Thinsulate has become a wildly successful product, but it only saw the light of day because the firm offered ways for creative employees to bring it to the market.

TOMORROW'S HR, TODAY

New Management Practices

In the organizations that have successfully responded to the dramatic changes occurring in their internal and external environments, the quest to be more competitive has led to changes in how they are organized and managed. Examples of this are as follows.

*The traditional **bureaucratic structure**,* characterized by a pyramid shape and hierarchies with many levels of management, *is being replaced by new organizational forms,* generally emphasizing cross-functional teams and improved communication flow, with corresponding de-emphasis on "sticking to the chain of command" to get decisions made.[119]

Flatter organizations are the norm. Instead of firms with seven to ten or more layers of management, flat organizations with just three or four levels are starting to prevail. At Celestica Inc., a subsidiary of IBM Canada Ltd. that manufactures computer electronics, there are only two levels of management beneath President Eugene Polistuk. Management only comprises about five percent of the firm's total staffing—and that's for 1500 people and a $1.4 billion business.[120]

Since managers have more people reporting to them in flat structures, they cannot supervise their employees as closely. *Employee **empowerment*** is thus becoming more common. At 3M's plant in Brockville, Ontario, workers on the shop floor conduct the entire recruitment and selection process, from initial interviewing to testing. The six-to-eight-person teams also handle quality control, logistics, scheduling, and shipping and receiving.[121]

Experts argue in favour of *turning the typical organization upside down.* They say today's organizations should put customers/clients on top and emphasize that every move the company makes should be toward satisfying customer/client needs. To accomplish this, front-line employees—the reception-area clerks at the Holiday Inn, customer service representatives at Canada Trust, flight attendants at Air Canada, and assemblers at GM Canada—must be given the authority to respond quickly as needs arise. The main purpose of managers in such "upside down" organizations is to ensure that the front-line staff members have the resources they need to do their jobs effectively.

Boundaryless organization structures are emerging. In this type of structure, relationships (typically joint ventures) are formed with customers, suppliers, and/or competitors, to pool resources for mutual benefit or encourage cooperation in an uncertain environment. CAMI Automotive Ltd., located in Ingersoll, Ontario, is an example. A joint venture between General Motors of Canada and Suzuki Motor Corporation, its success is attributable, at least in part, to the synthesis of Japanese management and design with a Canadian work force.[122]

bureaucratic structure (bureaucracy)
A pyramid-shaped organization, characterized by a hierarchical structure and many levels of management.

empowerment
Providing workers with the skills and authority to make decisions that would traditionally be made by managers.

boundaryless organization structure
A structure in which relationships (typically joint ventures) are formed with customers, suppliers, and/or competitors, to pool resources for mutual benefit or encourage cooperation in an uncertain environment.

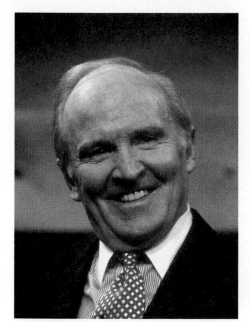

General Electric CEO Jack Welch knows the value of cultivating employee loyalty and commitment.

Work is increasingly organized around teams and processes rather than specialized functions. Over 40 percent of those responding to a recent Conference Board of Canada survey indicated that team-based activity was widespread.[123] While not all firms adopting a team-based design have introduced self-managed teams, such autonomous work groups have become more popular, and are considered a key success factor at firms ranging from Celestica to Federal Express to Xerox Canada.[124]

The bases of power are changing. According to management theorist Rosabeth Moss Kanter, position, title, and authority are no longer adequate tools for managers to rely on to get their jobs done. Instead, "success depends increasingly on tapping into sources of good ideas, figuring out whose collaboration is needed to act on those ideas, and working with both to produce results. In short, the new managerial work implies very different ways of obtaining and using power."[125] While managers in the past thought of themselves as a "manager" or "boss," today's managers increasingly think of themselves as a "facilitator" or "team leader."

Managers today must build commitment. Building adaptive, client-focussed or customer-responsive organizations means that eliciting employees' commitment and self-control is more important than ever. Jack Welch, CEO of General Electric, put it this way: "The only way I see to get more productivity is by getting people involved and excited about their jobs. You can't afford to have anyone walk through a gate of a factory or into an office who is not giving 120 percent."[126]

The following High Performance Organization box provides an example of how one firm—Asea Brown Boveri—is putting into practice changes like all of those described above.

THE PLAN OF THIS BOOK

This book is premised on two beliefs. First, we believe that HRM is the responsibility of every manager—not just those in the HR department. Throughout this book, we have therefore included practical suggestions designed to help all managers carry out their day-to-day responsibilities more effectively. The second belief is that, given the increasing need for highly competitive organizations staffed by committed employees, HR programs should be directed at helping firms to achieve this goal. Thus, we have provided numerous examples to illustrate the ways in which HR programs are helping to foster employee commitment and to make organizations better, faster, and more competitive.

This book is divided into six sections. In the remainder of Part One, we will first discuss the increasing importance of the HR function and its evolving role in strategic decision making. Then we'll present the rights of employees and obligations of managers pertaining to equal opportunity and equity, and what is involved in truly embracing and valuing diversity. In Part Two, we'll cover four critical aspects of HRM: designing and analyzing jobs, HR planning, recruitment, and selection. The focus of Part Three will be on developing effective human resources through orientation and training, career development, managing quality and productivity, and a performance appraisal. In Part Four, all aspects of compensation administration will be explored: from establishing pay plans, to the issues involved in pay-for-performance strategies and use of financial incentives, to employee benefits and services. Part Five will describe ways to build

THE HIGH PERFORMANCE ORGANIZATION

New Ways of Organizing and Managing

Zurich-based electrical equipment maker Asea Brown Boveri (ABB) provides a good example of a firm that "disorganized itself to compete in the fast-moving global market." ABB did four things to make itself super-responsive: it organized around mini-units, empowered its workers, flattened its hierarchy, and eliminated central staff. How did ABB do it?

First, within two years of taking over this $30 billion firm, Chair Percy Barnevik "de-organized" its 215 000 employees into 5000 mini-companies, each averaging only about 50 workers. For example, the ABB hydro power unit in Finland is a highly customer-focussed little business, in which employees' efforts are all centred on its local (Finnish) customers. Each of ABB's 50-person units is run by its own manager and three or four lieutenants. Such small units are very manageable: it's a lot easier to keep track of what everyone is doing when there are only 50 people than when there are 1000, let alone 5000 or 10 000.

Next, to speed up decision making, the 5000 mini-companies were empowered. The employees have the authority to make most of their own business decisions without checking first with top management. For example, if a customer has a complaint about a $50 000 machine, a mini-company employee can approve a replacement on the spot, rather than having to wait for reviews by several levels of management. Giving employees this much authority means, by the way, that ABB's 5000 businesses must be staffed, as management expert Tom Peters puts it, by "high-performance team members," highly skilled employees with the capacity and commitment to make those big decisions.

Third, ABB's 215 000-employee organization was "de-layered," leaving only three management levels (compared to the seven or eight that a company of comparable size might have). Highest is a 13-member top-management executive committee based in Zurich. Below this is a 250-member executive level that includes country managers and executives in charge of groups of businesses. The lowest level consists of the 5000 mini-company managers and their management teams.

Fourth, since decision making was pushed down to front-line ABB employees, ABB was able to eliminate most of headquarters' staff advisers. For example, when Finland's Stromberg Company was acquired, Barnevik reduced its headquarters' staff from 880 to 25. Similarly, he reduced staffing at German ABB headquarters in Mannheim from 1600 to 100.

The next effect of this reorganization, combined with superior HR systems for attracting, training, motivating and retaining employees, is responsiveness and increased competitiveness. ABB can be characterized as a lean, flat organization staffed with highly committed, empowered employees, who can respond quickly to competitors' moves and customers' needs.

Source: Tom Peters, *Liberation Management* (New York: Alfred Knopf, 1992), p. 9.

effective employee/employer relationships in both union and non-union settings, and will delve into topics such as fair treatment, the dynamics of labour relations, union organizing, collective bargaining, contract administration, and occupational health and safety. In Part Six, we'll examine international issues in HRM.

CHAPTER Review

Summary

1   Human resources management (HRM) refers to the management of people in organizations. It comprises the activities, policies, and practices involved in obtaining, developing, utilizing, evaluating, maintaining, and retaining

the appropriate number and skill mix of employees to accomplish the organization's objectives. HRM is important to all managers since they must meet their goals through the efforts of others, which requires the effective management of people.

2   Line authority authorizes managers to direct the work of those reporting to them and make decisions about production, and may be exercised only over those in a manager's direct chain of command. Line managers are in charge of an aspect of operations directly linked to the organization's products or services. Staff authority involves authorization to assist, counsel, advise, or provide service to others. Staff managers—those responsible for service departments (such as HRM and accounting)—possess such authority. Functional authority involves the right to make final decisions on issues affecting other departments. The HR department typically has functional authority for highly technical activities (such as compensation and benefits administration) and activities for which centralization enhances efficiency and effectiveness (such as recruitment).

3   Every supervisor and manager is responsible for HRM. In firms with an HR department, the role of the HR staff involves: formulating and administering policies and procedures; offering advice to managers throughout the firm; providing services in areas such as staffing, orientation, training, and labour relations; helping to ensure compliance with policies and procedures, collective agreements, and legislation; and serving as consultant and change agent.

4   The size and sophistication of the HR department and specific functional areas therein are linked to the size and complexity of the organization.

5   Internal environmental factors influencing HRM include: the organizational culture, which consists of the core values, beliefs, and assumptions that are widely shared by members of the organization; and the climate, which is the prevailing atmosphere. The climate is linked to management's leadership style, HR policies and practices, and amount and style of communication.

6   A number of external factors have an impact on HRM, including economic factors, labour market conditions, labour unions, demographic trends and increasing work-force diversity, technology, government, globalization, and trends in the nature of jobs and work.

7   In order to respond to such challenges, new modes of managing and organizing have evolved. The traditional pyramid-shaped organization is giving way to new organizational forms; flatter organizations are becoming the norm; and employees are being empowered to make more decisions. Upside-down organizations and boundaryless organization structures are becoming more common; work is increasingly organized around teams and processes; the bases of power are changing; and team leaders are replacing managers. Building employee commitment has become critical to organizational survival and success.

Key Terms

authority	common law
baby boomers	contingent employees
boundaryless organization structure	contract law
bureaucratic structure (bureaucracy)	demographics

diversity
e-business
e-commerce
employee advocacy
employee assistance program (EAP)
employment rate
empowerment
entrepreneur
functional authority
functionally illiterate
Generation X (Nexus generation)
globalization
human capital
Human Resources Information
  System (HRIS)
human resources management
  (HRM)
Human Resources Management
  System (HRMS)
intrapreneur
knowledge worker
labour force
labour market
labour union

line authority
line manager
literacy
multinational corporation
Net Generation (Nexters)
organizational climate
organizational culture
outsourcing
participation rate
policy
primary sector
proactive
procedure
productivity
reactive
regulations
Sandwich Generation
secondary sector
small business
staff authority
staff manager
telecommuting
tertiary or service sector
unemployment rate

Review and Discussion Questions

1   In your own words, define HRM and describe its objectives.
2   Differentiate among line, staff, and functional authority, and provide an example of each.
3   Describe the two major internal environmental influences on HRM and explain the impact of each.
4   Explain the ways in which labour unions influence the HR policies and practices in both unionized and non-unionized firms.
5   Describe the ways in which labour market conditions, government legislation, and globalization are affecting HRM in Canada today.
6   Explain how a Human Resources Management System (HRMS) can benefit an organization.

CRITICAL Thinking Questions

1   Explain why all managers are HR managers, and provide three examples illustrating how HRM concepts and techniques can be beneficial to all managers.
2   Explain how changing demographics and increasing work-force diversity have had an impact on the organization in which you are working or one in which you have worked.

3 A firm has requested your assistance in ensuring that their multigenerational work force functions effectively as a team. What strategies and/or programs would you recommend? Why?

4 Find a recent newspaper or journal article describing the impact of changing technology on HRM in a particular organization or sector. Briefly summarize the impact. Critically evaluate the way in which the changing technology was handled: (a) Which was the action taken: proactive or reactive? (b) Were the affected employees adequately prepared for the change? If so, how? If not, why not? (c) What steps were taken, if any, to ensure that the changing technology would reap benefits for the firm or sector?

5 Explain why employee commitment is critical in organizations today, and describe specific strategies being employed in firms in your community to build and maintain such commitment.

6 Today's managers increasingly think of themselves as "facilitator" or "team leader," rather than "manager" or "boss." Do you agree with this statement? Why or why not? Should managers today think of themselves as team leaders, rather than bosses? Why or why not?

APPLICATION *Exercises*

RUNNING CASE: Carter Cleaning Company

Introduction

The main theme of this book is that HRM is not just the job of a central HR department, but rather the responsibility of every manager. Perhaps nowhere is this more apparent than in a typical small service business. The owner/manager usually has no HR staff on whom to rely. However, the success of his or her enterprise (not to mention his or her family's peace of mind) often depends largely on the effectiveness of the processes through which employees are recruited, hired, trained, evaluated, and rewarded. Therefore, to help illustrate the HRM responsibilities of all managers and ways in which they can be handled effectively, we have included an ongoing saga—a continuing case based on a small business in southwestern Ontario. In the segment of the case at the end of each chapter, the main character—Jennifer Carter—will be confronted with HR challenges that must be resolved by applying the concepts and techniques discussed in that particular chapter.

In order to answer questions arising in the incidents at the end of subsequent chapters, the following background information is required:

Carter Cleaning Centres Jennifer Carter graduated with a degree in Business Administration from Northern University in June of 2000 and, after considering several job offers, decided to do what she had really always planned: go into business with her father, Jack.

Jack Carter opened his first laundromat in 1980 and his second in 1982. The main attraction of these coin laundry businesses to him was that they were capital- rather than labour-intensive. Once the investment in machinery was made, the laundromat could be operated with just one unskilled attendant and none of the labour problems one normally associates with being in the retail service business. The attractiveness of operating with virtually no skilled labour notwithstanding, in 1986 Jack decided to expand the services in each of his laundromats to include dry cleaning and pressing. He embarked, in other words, on a strategy of related diversification, in that he added new services that were related to and consistent with the existing coin laundry facilities. His decision was based in part on the fact that he wanted to better utilize the unused space in the rather large stores he currently had under lease, and partly because he was, as he put it, "tired of sending out the dry cleaning and pressing work that comes in from our coin laundry clients to a dry cleaner five miles away, who then takes most of what should have been our profits." To reflect the expanded line of services, he renamed his two stores "Carter Cleaning Centres." Sufficiently satisfied with their performance, he opened four more similar facilities over the next five years. Each centre had its own on-site manager and seven employees, on average, and annual revenues of about $400 000. It was this six-store chain of cleaning centres that Jennifer joined upon graduation.

Her understanding with her father was that she would serve as a troubleshooter/consultant to him, with the aims of learning the business and incorporating modern management concepts and techniques to resolve problems and facilitate growth.

Questions

1 How important is effective HRM in a small business such as Carter Cleaning Centres? Why?
2 What internal and external environmental challenges is Jennifer likely to confront? How will they affect the business?

CASE INCIDENT *HR Systems Inc.*

Lou Wally and Stan Smith founded HR Systems Inc. three years ago in Calgary, to provide three types of HR services to firms in the area.

Their first and most profitable market is small businesses. Instead of hiring a full-time person to develop employee handbooks, HR policy manuals, performance appraisal systems, job analysis questionnaires, job descriptions and specifications, compensation plans, etc., it is more cost-effective for many small firms to contract with HR Systems Inc. to do so.

The second service is the provision of an Employee Assistance Program (EAP) to participating companies for a reasonable fee.

The third service involves extensive management consulting activities, including outplacement, executive recruitment, small-business development, training and development, and problem analysis/correction/follow-up.

Lou and Stan are quite informal in their own management style. Lou is a trained psychologist and wants to have a solid working team. Stan, although telling everyone outwardly that this is what he wants, is from another school of thought. He doesn't like or trust visible minorities and believes in hierarchical management. He expects employees to be creative in their work groups but to "do as they're told or else!" The implication is that if employees don't have their noses to the grindstone—or if they disagree with his approach—they should pack up their belongings and go.

Lou and Stan fill the positions of executive vice-president and president, respectively. The company comprises approximately 20 employees and several temporary contractors. The program managers are all male. The newest hires have been females—in both professional and secretarial positions—who are paid well below the prevailing wage rates. There are no Aboriginal persons, persons with disabilities or visible minority group members, and there have been no efforts to hire any.

As stated, both Lou and Stan are informal. They believe in Friday-afternoon staff meetings that include wine, beer, and racist and dirty jokes. Some of the women in this relatively new and growing company have indicated to Lou that they feel rather uncomfortable in the staff meetings and would prefer not to attend. Stan has made it clear that attendance is mandatory.

The EAP program manager is a former salesperson who has little background or experience in the field. His performance in securing new clients is poor, and he does not appear to have an appreciation for professional confidentiality. For example, on two separate occasions he reported to managers at their firms the personal difficulties that specific employees were experiencing. Although his efforts were well intentioned (he was seeking authorization for increased services due to some extreme personal circumstances), the damage was done.

There are interpersonal problems between the various work groups and the company is rife with rumours. The employees are becoming increasingly concerned about their hard-earned credibility in a relatively small business community. Several of the professionals on staff are very angry that the owners do not practise the very management styles they are teaching and selling. Staff members are also afraid that the company might be experiencing financial problems, since cheques have been delayed and two employee paycheques bounced. This is of grave concern to several of the employees who are the sole support of their families.

Recognizing that there are a few problems in the firm, the two owners have just hired you as the HR manager, and given you responsibility for "getting things back on track."

Questions

1   Describe the organizational climate at HR Systems Inc.

2   As the new HR manager, which internal and external environmental factors would you be particularly concerned about? Why?

3   Explain the contributions that you feel you will be able to make to the organization.

4   How would you recommend that the remaining problems be addressed?

Source: Based on a case developed by Sharon Craig, while employed as a faculty member at Sir Sandford Fleming College, Peterborough, Ontario.

EXPERIENTIAL *Exercises*

1   Working individually or in groups, interview an HR department staff member at a firm in your community. Prepare a brief report—for presentation to the class or submission for critique—outlining the ways in which the HR department there handles the following five types of activities: formulating

policies and procedures, offering advice, providing services, monitoring to ensure compliance, and serving as a consultant and change agent.

2 Prepare a summary of the employment legislation affecting all employers and employees who are NOT under federal jurisdiction in your province or territory. Explain the impact of each of these laws on HRM policies and practices.

3 Prepare a brief report describing three Canadian organizations that have recently restructured or adopted a new approach to management. Explain the changes made and explain their impact.

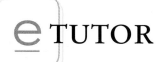

WEB-BASED *Exercises*

1 Go to the Web sites of three large Canadian organizations. Summarize the information available online about their HRM systems, policies, and procedures. Identify the major similarities across firms, and then describe the ways in which their HRM systems, policies, and procedures differ. Based on the information gleaned, how would you characterize the climate and culture at each of these organizations? Justify your response.

2 Using the Web sites of Human Resources Development Canada (**www.hrdc-drhc.ca**) and Statistics Canada (**www.statcan.ca**) as the basis of your research, identify the employment trends for two positions in each of the following fields: (a) HRM, (b) retail sales, (c) hospitality management, (d) accounting, (e) mining, and (f) manufacturing. What are the implications of these trends for those working in the positions you chose? Based on the trends identified, which fields/positions would you recommend to an individual seeking career guidance? Why?

e TUTOR

Let our Companion Web site be your personal e-Tutor! After you complete each chapter, log on to the Web site to review the material you have just read. Take practice tests that include multiple choice, true and false, fill-in-the-blanks, and essay questions! For incorrect answers, your e-Tutor will direct you to the appropriate page or section in the textbook. Check out your Companion Web site at **www.pearsoned.ca/dessler**. This site also includes key terms and concepts, Weblinks to related sites, news groups, CBC videos, and more!

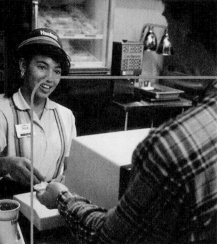

CHAPTER 2

The Evolving Role of HRM:
From Staff Function to Strategic Partner

CHAPTER
OUTLINE

A Brief History of HRM

Growing Professionalism in HRM

The Current Role of HR Departments

Strategic Planning and HRM

The Role of the HR Department as a Strategic Partner

HR Auditing

The Impact of Effective HRM Practices on Employee Performance and the Bottom Line

LEARNING OUTCOMES

After studying this chapter, you should be able to:

Describe the evolution of HRM.

Discuss the growing professionalism of HRM, and *explain* the importance of ethics and social responsibility.

Describe the current role of HR departments.

Explain the nature of strategic planning and *discuss* the role of the HR department as a strategic partner.

Describe the importance of HR auditing and *discuss* the strategies and techniques used.

Discuss the impact of effective HRM practices on employee performance and the bottom line.

A Brief History of HRM

As a result of all of the challenges discussed in Chapter 1, HRM has changed dramatically over time and has assumed an increasingly important role. The demands on HR department staff members and expectations regarding the types of assistance they should provide have increased correspondingly. As will be explained in this chapter, the emerging role of the HR department as a strategic partner has been an evolutionary process.

HR practices have been shaped by society's prevailing beliefs and attitudes about workers and their rights. **Table 2.1** outlines the three distinct stages in the

TABLE 2.1

Theories of Management

Scientific Management Model	Human Relations Model	Human Resources Model
Assumptions	**Assumptions**	**Assumptions**
1. Work is inherently distasteful to most people.	1. People want to feel useful and important.	1. Work is not inherently distasteful. People want to contribute to meaningful goals that they have helped to establish.
2. What workers do is less important than what they earn for doing it.	2. People desire to belong and to be recognized as individuals.	2. Most people can exercise far more creative, responsible self-direction and self-control than their present job demands.
3. Few want or can handle work that requires creativity, self-direction, or self-control.	3. These needs are more important than money in motivating people to work.	
Policies	**Policies**	**Policies**
1. A manager's basic task is to closely supervise and control employees.	1. A manager's basic task is to make each worker feel useful and important.	1. A manager's basic task is to make use of "untapped" human resources.
2 A manager must break tasks down into simple, repetitive, easily learned operations.	2. A manager should keep employees informed and listen to their objections to his/her plans.	2. A manager must create an environment in which all members may contribute to the limits of their ability.
3. A manager must establish detailed work routines and procedures and enforce these firmly but fairly.	3. A manager should allow employees to exercise some self-control on routine matters.	3. A manager must encourage full participation on important matters, continually broadening employees' self-direction and control.

>>

Expectations	Expectations	Expectations
1. People can tolerate work if the pay is decent and the boss is fair.	1. Sharing information with employees and involving them in routine decisions will satisfy their basic needs to belong and to feel important.	1. Expanding employee influence, self-direction, and self-control will lead to direct improvements in operating efficiency.
2. If tasks are simple enough and people are closely controlled, they will produce up to standard.	2. Satisfying these needs will improve morale and reduce resistance to formal authority—employees will "willingly cooperate."	2. Work satisfaction may improve as a "by-product" of employees making full use of their resources.

Source: Abridged and adapted from Raymond E. Miles, *Theories of Management,* (McGraw-Hill: New York, 1975). Reprinted with permission of Raymond E. Miles, Professor Emeritus and former Dean, Haas School of Business, University of California, Berkeley.

general evolution of management thinking about workers, each of which had a different focus: scientific management, human relations, and human resources.[1]

Scientific Management: Concern for Production

scientific management

The process of "scientifically" analyzing manufacturing processes, reducing production costs, and compensating employees based on their performance levels.

Frederick Taylor was the driving force behind **scientific management**, the process of "scientifically" analyzing manufacturing processes, reducing production costs, and compensating employees based on their performance.[2] The scientific management movement had a significant impact on management practices and employee–management relations in the late 1800s and early 1900s. Taylor emphasized systematic job design, task simplification, performance-based pay, selection of workers with the skills required to become superior performers, and fit between person and job. He also stressed the need for cooperation, which was achieved through the use of scientific methods, rules, and procedures that were binding on both workers and managers.

Based on his underlying assumptions about workers and the appropriate role of managers (explained in Table 2.1), he advocated achieving operational efficiency through work simplification and paying workers a piece rate, with extra pay for pieces produced in excess of the daily standard. It was his belief that such incentives would lead to higher wages for workers, increased profits for the organization, and workplace harmony.

Scientific management, which helped to shape the view that money was the primary motivator for workers, was widely accepted. It should be noted, though, that not all management theorists of Taylor's era accepted his viewpoints. An exception was Mary Parker Follet, a writer ahead of her time, who advocated: self-management; cross-functional cooperation; empowerment; and managers as leaders, not dictators.[3]

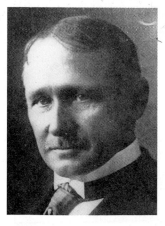

Frederick Taylor (1856–1915), the father of scientific management.

human relations movement

A management philosophy based on the belief that the attitudes and feelings of workers are important and deserve more attention.

The Human Relations Movement: Concern for People

The primary aim of the **human relations movement**, which emerged in the 1920s and '30s but was not fully embraced until the '40s, was to consider jobs from

Hawthorne Studies
A series of experiments conducted at the Hawthorne Works of the Western Electric Company between 1924 and 1933 that examined factors influencing worker morale and productivity, the conclusions of which had a significant impact on management practices.

an employee's perspective. Advocates of this model believed that worker attitudes and feelings were important and deserved more attention; they criticized managers who treated workers as machines.

This management philosophy was based on the results of the Hawthorne Studies, one of the first cooperative industry/university research efforts, conducted by Elton Mayo, Fritz J. Roethlisberger, and W. J. Dickson. These were a series of experiments conducted at the Hawthorne Works of the Western Electric Company between 1924 and 1933 that examined factors influencing worker morale and productivity. The conclusions had a significant and far-reaching impact on management practices.

The researchers discovered that the effect of the social environment is equal to or greater than that of the physical environment. They learned that workers' feelings and morale are greatly influenced by such factors as working conditions, the supervisor's leadership style, and management's philosophy regarding workers. Treating workers with dignity and respect was found to lead to higher job satisfaction and productivity levels. Economic incentives were found to be of secondary importance to workers.

The researchers also discovered that workers spontaneously form groups, establish group norms, and control productivity through social pressure. For example, those producing in excess of the group's standards were called "rate busters" by their coworkers; those whose output was unacceptably low were labelled "chisellers"; and those who complained to a superior were called "squealers." Solid evidence was found that peer pressure influences workers' behaviour.[4]

In the many firms embracing the human relations approach, working conditions improved substantially. Based on the beliefs about workers and the appropriate role of managers highlighted in Table 2.1, managerial approaches to worker motivation had a strong social emphasis. To overcome low morale, feelings of alienation, and prevailing poor performance, managers focussed on establishing better channels of communication, allowing employees to exercise more self-direction, and treating employees with consideration.

This movement came under severe criticism for overcompensating for the impersonal and dehumanizing effects of scientific management by failing to recognize the importance of structure, standards, procedures, and work rules in controlling employees' behaviour and guiding their conduct to achieve organizational goals. It was also criticized for oversimplifying the concept of employee motivation and failing to recognize individual differences in beliefs, values, needs, expectations, interests, and abilities.

The Human Resources Movement: Concern for People and Productivity

human resources movement
A management philosophy focussing on concern for people and productivity.

HRM is currently based on the theoretical assumptions of the **human resources movement**, which are listed in Table 2.1. Arriving at this joint focus on people and productivity involved four evolutionary phases.[5]

Phase One

In the early 1900s, HRM—or personnel administration, as it was then called—played a very subservient or nonexistent role. When a personnel department did exist, it was generally held in low esteem, and located at the bottom of the organization chart. At the time, there were very few laws regulating working conditions and the employee/employer relationship. Organizations focussed on maximizing productivity and increasing profits; the human element was generally considered unimportant. During this era, personnel administrators: assumed responsibility for hiring and firing, a duty formerly looked after by first-line supervisors; ran the payroll department; and administered benefits. Their job consisted largely of ensuring that procedures were followed. As technology in such areas as testing and interviewing began to emerge, personnel departments began to play an expanded role in employee selection, training, and promotion.

Phase Two

As the scientific management movement gained momentum, operational efficiency increased. However, since wages generally fell behind productivity growth, workers began to distrust management, and many turned to unions for support. The increase in unionizing activities dramatically changed the role of personnel departments. Personnel managers were expected to develop policies and practices that would enable the firm to retain non-union status, if possible; and if not, to serve as the primary contact for union representatives. The depression of the 1930s also had an important influence. Following the depression, workers sought government intervention to provide some form of financial protection in the case of job loss, and to recognize their rights to form and join unions. Various legislation was enacted, including a minimum wage act, an unemployment insurance program, and protection of workers' rights to belong to unions. Legal compliance was subsequently added to the responsibilities of personnel managers.

During the 1940s and 1950s, personnel managers were also involved in dealing with the impact of the human relations movement. Orientation, performance appraisal, and employee relations responsibilities were added to their portfolio. As a result of their expanding role, the importance of personnel departments began to increase.

Phase Three

The third major phase in personnel management was a direct result of government legislation passed during the 1960s, 1970s, and 1980s that affected employees' human rights, wages and benefits, working conditions, and health and safety. The role of personnel departments expanded dramatically. Effective employment policies and practices increased in importance because of societal, governmental, and organizational challenges and objectives, and because of the penalties for failure to meet them. Personnel departments continued to provide expertise in areas such as recruitment, screening, and training, but in an expanded capacity. During the latter part of this era, the term "human resources management" emerged. This change represented a shift in emphasis—from maintenance and administration to corporate contribution, proactive management, and initiation of change.[6]

Phase Four

The fourth phase of HRM is ongoing. Most managers today believe that workers are motivated primarily by the nature and scope of the job, social influences, the nature of the compensation and incentive systems, organizational culture and climate, management's supervisory style, and individual needs and values. It is widely recognized that employees do not all seek the same rewards and that most sincerely want to make a contribution. To harness this drive and determination, organizations must develop strategies to maximize employee performance, and potential, such that the goals and aims of both management and employees are achieved. In today's flattened, downsized, and responsive organizations, highly trained and committed employees—not machines—are often a firm's best competitive advantage. The role of HR departments has thus shifted from protector and screener to planner and change agent.

GROWING PROFESSIONALISM IN HRM

Today, senior HR practitioners must concern themselves with all aspects of HRM and their impact on organizational performance and society as a whole. Practitioners must be professionals in terms of both performance and qualifications.

Every **profession** has four major characteristics, all of which are exhibited by HRM:

- the existence of a common body of knowledge, developed through research and experimentation, that is widely communicated through professional literature and exchanged at conferences, seminars, and workshops sponsored by the professional associations
- requirements and procedures for certification of members
- performance standards established by members of the profession rather than by outsiders (self-regulation)
- a code of ethics by which members must abide.

Professional Associations and Certification

In 1990, the Personnel Association of Ontario (PAO)—now the Human Resources Professionals Association of Ontario (HRPAO)—was granted the legal right to award the Certified Human Resources Professional (CHRP) designation through an act of the provincial legislature—the first professional designation for HR practitioners in North America. HRPAO now has 28 chapters across Ontario[7] and more than 10 000 members.[8]

Nearly every province has an association of HR practitioners, with similar broad objectives:

- providing opportunities for information exchange, and cooperation in meeting and solving common problems
- assisting in the provision of HR training and skills updating
- serving as a voice for HR practitioners, especially in response to proposed legislation and legislative reforms.

The Canadian Council of Human Resources Associations (CCHRA) is the national body through which 10 provincial and specialist HR associations are affiliated. The organization, which currently represents the interests of more than 18 000 professionals across Canada, originated in 1992 and was formally established in 1996. One of its first accomplishments was member associations' adoption of a resolution to recognize the equivalency of provincial HR designations, such that those receiving the CHRP designation in one jurisdiction would be eligible for recognition of their professional status in all member provinces. CCHRA's mission is to:

[Handwritten margin note:] Profession 4 Major Characteristics exhibited by HRM: common requirement performance code

procedures for certification of members, self-regulation, and a code of ethics by which members must abide.

AN ETHICAL DILEMMA

Suppose that you, an HR professional, have just discovered that a colleague in the HR department, who is a good friend, has been "leaking" confidential information about employees. How would you handle this situation?

Human Resource Professionals Association of Ontario

www.hrpao.org

Canadian Council of HR Associations

www.chrpcanada.com

- establish national core standards for the HR profession
- foster communications among participating associations
- be the recognized resource on equivalency for HR qualifications across Canada, and
- provide a national and international collective voice on HR issues.[9]

The **International Personnel Management Association (IPMA)** – Canada, formerly CPPMA, is the national association for public-sector and quasi public-sector HR professionals.[10] A number of associations represent HR professionals specializing in specific areas such as HRP, compensation, training and development, recruitment and selection, and HRMS.

The combined interests of HR professionals in Canada, Mexico and the United States are represented by the **North American Human Resource Management Association (NAHRMA)**, which was founded on April 5, 1997 at a formal ceremony during the annual conference of the Institute for International Human Resources (IIHR), a division of the Society for Human Resource Management (SHRM)—the U.S. national body.[11] Global linkages are provided through the World Federation of Personnel Management Associations (WFPMA). Founded in 1976, its membership now represents close to 50 national HR associations and nearly 400 000 HR professionals worldwide.[12]

Every profession requires member **certification**, which is recognition for having met certain professional standards. For HR practitioners, the certification criteria vary between provinces, but generally include three requirements: membership in good standing and agreement to abide by the association's code of ethics; work experience in the field at a professional/supervisory level for a specified period of time; and completion of an approved program of study.

Many colleges and universities have created undergraduate, post-diploma, and graduate programs with specializations in HRM. HR specialists may take the courses required to meet the educational component of their professional designation through educational institutions or, in some instances, through night classes offered by the provincial association. Although HR associations in each province establish their own educational requirements, there is considerable similarity among programs offered. As an example, Ontario's academic requirements are shown in **Figure 2.1.**

Some provincial HR associations require proof of ongoing education to qualify for recertification. For senior practitioners, there is an alternative route to attainment of the CHRP designation in some jurisdictions. In Ontario, for example, it is possible for individuals assessed and accepted as senior practitioners with more than 10 years' experience at a managerial/professional level to attain the CHRP designation by writing and passing the Comprehensive Provincial Exam. The minimum eight-course requirement is waived.[13]

Ethics

The professionalization of HRM has created the need for a uniform code of ethics. **Ethics** is the discipline dealing with what is good or bad, and right or wrong, and with moral duty and obligation.

Professional associations devise codes of ethics to promote and maintain the highest possible standards of personal and professional conduct among members and assist them in handling ethical dilemmas. Agreement to abide by the

International Personnel Management Association
www.ipma-hr.org

North American Human Resource Management Association
www.shrm.org/nahrma/intro.htm

Society for HR Management
www.shrm.org

World Federation of Personnel Management Associations (WFPMA)
www.wfpma.com

certification
Recognition for having met certain professional standards.

ethics
The discipline dealing with what is good or bad, and right or wrong, and with moral duty and obligation.

FIGURE **2.1** Human Resources Professionals Association of Ontario (HRPAO) Academic Requirements

To fulfill the academic requirement for the CHRP designation, a candidate must:

1. Become a member of HRPAO; and
2. Complete all four of the Tier I compulsory subjects; and four of the seven Tier II specialty subjects; and
3. Pass the Comprehensive Provincial Examination (CPE).

Tier I—Compulsory Subjects
1. Human Resources Management
2. Organizational Behaviour
3. Finance and Accounting
4. Labour Economics

Tier II—Specialized Subjects
1. Compensation
2. Training and Development
3. Labour Relations
4. Occupational Health & Safety
5. Human Resources Planning
6. Human Resources Research and Information Systems (HRRIS)
7. Designated Elective Course (DEC)—a student may apply for ONE DEC credit.

Source: Based on HRPAO, "CHRP Academic Requirements," *Human Resources Professionals Association of Ontario.* www.hrpao.org (Summer 2000). Reproduced with permission.

Ethics Resource Centre
www.ethics.org

code of ethics is one of the requirements of maintaining professional status. The Code of Ethics of HRPAO is shown in **Figure 2.2**.

HR professionals are not only concerned with monitoring their own ethics. More and more Canadian firms are stressing ethical conduct in all aspects of business. Many, recognizing that employees and managers throughout the firm confront ethical dilemmas daily (such as those described in the margins throughout the text), have established a code of ethics to govern corporate relations with employees, clients/customers, and the public. Since what is ethical or unethical is generally open to debate, except in a few very clear-cut cases (such as willful misrepresentation), most codes do not tell employees what they should do. Rather, they provide a guide to help employees discover the best course of action by themselves.[14] Having a code is not enough, however. According to one noted ethics expert, "The ethical code of conduct is only the first step in the development of an ethical culture."[15] Integrating ethics in the workplace requires specific initiatives aligned with management policies, reporting structures, and reward and promotion systems.[16] Increasingly, HR departments are being given a greater role in communicating the organization's values and standards, providing ethics training, and monitoring to ensure compliance with the code of ethics. Some organizations have such a commitment to ethics that they have a full-time ethics officer.

Research Insight

A recent survey of CEOs at 154 Canadian firms found that:

- 86 percent have a code of ethics outlining their values and principles
- 72 percent have some type of program or initiative to promote ethical values and practices

FIGURE 2.2 Code of Ethics—Human Resources Professionals Association of Ontario (HRPAO)

Members of HRPAO strive for growth as human resources professionals and commit to the principles of the Code of Ethics to the best of their ability. Human resources professionals shall:

- continue professional growth in human resources management, in support and promotion of the goals, objectives and by-laws of the Association;
- not knowingly violate or cause to be violated, any legislated act, regulation or by-law that relates to the management of human resources;
- demonstrate commitment to such values as respect for human dignity and human rights, and promote human development in the workplace, within the profession and society as a whole;
- treat information obtained in the course of business as confidential, and avoid, or disclose, any conflict of interest that might influence personal actions or judgments;
- refrain from inappropriately using their position to secure special privileges, gain or benefit for themselves, their employers or the Association;
- acknowledge an obligation to the employer community to encourage and foster generally accepted codes of moral behaviour; and,
- practise respect and regard for other professional associations.

Source: "HRPAO Code of Ethics." *Human Resources Professionals Association of Ontario.* www.hrpao.org (Summer 2000). Reproduced with permission.

AN ETHICAL DILEMMA

How should a supervisor handle an otherwise effective employee who has just violated an important company safety regulation?

AN ETHICAL DILEMMA

Can or should an employee reveal information about a troubled coworker that was disclosed in confidence, and if so, under what circumstances?

- 41 percent have senior-level managers whose role specifically includes implementation, monitoring or assurance of ethics initiatives
- 39 percent provide some form of ethics training, but 10 percent limit their training to the application of the code of ethics
- 20 percent have a confidential reporting mechanism, such as a telephone hotline.

Thus, although the majority of firms surveyed now have a code of ethics, given the failure of many of them to implement the other initiatives required for program success, it is unlikely that an ethical culture has been attained in most of these firms.[17] A lack of ethical conduct is still quite prevalent. In fact, 57 percent of respondents in another recent survey indicated that their firm had been affected by such fraudulent activities as inflated expense reports, secret commissions, and personal use of company supplies over the previous year, and almost three-quarters identified employees as the main perpetrators. High costs are associated with such dishonesty: the average loss reported was $958 927, a drop from $1.3 million the year before![18]

The most prevalent ethical issues confronting Canadian firms today pertain to security of information (23 percent), employee and client privacy (17 percent), environment issues (14 percent), governance (13 percent), and conflicts of interest (12 percent).[19]

The major reasons for the failure of ethics programs to achieve the desired results are lack of effective leadership and inadequate training. In a study involving 1175 Canadian employees, less than one-half of the respondents stated that their CEOs and other senior managers enact the firm's ethical values in their day-to-day behaviour, and 18 percent reported that profit always trumps ethics when the two conflict.[20] Programs also fail when employees believe that they

AN ETHICAL
DILEMMA

Does expecting an employee
to over-bill clients amount to
constructive dismissal if he
or she objects to doing so?

AN ETHICAL
DILEMMA

In court litigation, costs are
typically awarded to the successful party. Assume that
you are the successful party,
and that the other party
acted unethically during the
investigation and hearing.
Should you be awarded
additional money?

exist for the purposes of: protecting top management from blame; preventing, detecting and punishing violations of law and regulation; and/or improving the company's image.[21]

Huge payoffs are associated with properly implemented ethics programs, including:

- increased confidence among stakeholders, such as clients, partners and employees
- greater client/customer and employee loyalty
- decreased vulnerability to crimes committed against the public and legal liability issues, such as those described in the margin
- reduced absenteeism
- increased employee productivity
- reduced losses due to internal theft, and
- increased profits and public trust.[22]

As explained in the High Performance Organization box, United Parcel Service (UPS) Canada is an organization that has recognized the benefits of

THE HIGH PERFORMANCE ORGANIZATION

Building an Ethical Culture

UPS is a step ahead of most corporations in implementing an ethics policy and trying to build an ethical culture. It has had an ethics policy for more than 70 years, and its old-fashioned, upright image has gone a long way in attracting the right type of employees and reinforcing ethical behaviour at work. According to Dave Cole, vice-president of HR at UPS Canada, however, while the company's commitment to ethics makes the process smoother, training is the key to making the ethics policy work.

Ethics training at UPS is carried out by senior managers, in part to show management's commitment to employees. The importance of proper ethical conduct is also reinforced through recurrent training. To determine how closely aligned employees' beliefs are with the company ethics policy, a "glass vault" exercise is used pre- and post-program implementation. This involves employees brainstorming their beliefs on core values, principles and traits of the organization. The multimedia training at UPS, developed with the help of outside trainers, managers, and employees, also includes:

- case studies
- practical ethical-dilemma class exercises and debriefing sessions

- business conduct and compliance tests, and
- an exercise in which training participants craft a personal action plan to apply the learning to their own jobs.

UPS does not rely on training alone to ensure an ethical work force. Prospective employees are screened for integrity and honesty, and are given a copy of the firm's *Business Code of Conduct* for review prior to deciding to join the company. The code clearly outlines the expected behaviour and the disciplinary action that will be taken against offenders, with penalties up to and including discharge. As Cole explains, "We want our employees to know from day one of employment that we are expecting them to preserve our legacy of honesty, integrity and ethical behaviour by meeting the high standards we set for ourselves." Numerous resources are also made available to provide additional information about the ethics policy and keep ethics in the spotlight, including a video, posters, a handbook, and a Web site.

Source: Lesley Young, "Ethics Training is the Key," *Canadian HR Reporter* 12, no. 12 (June 14, 1999), p. 2. Copyright Carswell, Thomson Professional Publishing. Reprinted by permission of *Canadian HR Reporter*, Carswell, One Corporate Plaza, 2075 Kennedy Road, Toronto M1T 3V4.

establishing an ethical culture, as well as the role of effective leadership and training in helping to ingrain ethical values.

In recent years, the concept of **social responsibility** has frequently been discussed as a complement to ethics. A company that exercises social responsibility attempts to balance its commitments—not only to its investors, but also to its employees and customers, other businesses, and the community or communities in which it operates. The Body Shop, an early and often-cited example of a socially responsible firm, proves that businesses can balance profits and principles. Despite taking a stand on anti-animal testing, human rights protection, and environmental conservation (the three main criteria against which all activities are measured), the firm's annual retail sales amount to more than $1.4 billion worldwide. Ingredients for the firm's cosmetics products are community traded, which means that the producers get a fair price for their goods and can use the income to improve their own quality of life and that of their communities. CEO Anita Roddick summed up the firm's attitude toward socially responsible global trading as follows: "By putting our money where our heart is, refusing to buy the products which exploit, and forming powerful strategic alliances, we will mold the world into a kinder, more loving shape."[23]

In an effort to enhance corporate accountability and responsibility, The Body Shop now conducts **social audits**, as do other firms known for being socially responsible (such as Ben & Jerry's and Toronto's Metro Credit Union). Such audits, also known as **responsibility audits**, involve independent reviews of a firm's social and environmental performance. They provide investors and consumers with external verification of a company's social responsibility claims.[24]

social responsibility
The implied, enforced, or felt obligation of managers, acting in their official capacities, to serve or protect the interests of groups other than themselves.

social audits (responsibility audits)
Independent reviews of a firm's social and environmental performance to provide external verification of a firm's claims of social responsibility.

THE CURRENT ROLE OF HR DEPARTMENTS

Improving Productivity

As mentioned in Chapter 1, productivity improvement is crucial in today's globally competitive environment. Organizations known for product and service quality strongly believe that employees are the key to their reputation, and that proper attention to employees improves both quality and productivity. According to Jack Welch, CEO at GE, for example, his biggest achievement is the people he hires and cultivates. "This place runs by its great people . . . the biggest accomplishment I've had is to find people. An army of them. They are all better than most. They are big hitters, and they seem to thrive here."[25]

Research Insight

The results of a recent survey commissioned by William M. Mercer Ltd. indicate that GE's CEO is not alone in recognizing the critical role played by the firm's human resources. Of the 307 CEOs polled, who were randomly selected from a list of Canada's 1200 largest corporations and other high-growth companies, 70 percent indicated that retaining key employees is a major priority. Attracting key employees was cited as a high priority by 58 percent of them.[26]

With worldwide retail sales of more than $1.4 billion, The Body Shop is an example of a company that successfully combines profits with principles.

A review of management practices in such companies as GE, FedEx Canada,[27] and 3M Canada[28] indicates that top-level commitment, employee involvement, and a conscious strategy to encourage innovation are critical for productivity improvement. All of these require the presence of an enlightened and proactive HR department.

The HR department staff members play a pivotal role in lowering labour costs, the single largest operating expense in many organizations, particularly in the service sector. Doing so might involve introducing strategies to reduce turnover, absenteeism, and/or the rate of incidence of occupational illnesses and injuries. It could also mean adopting more effective recruitment, selection, and/or training programs. At one international tire manufacturing firm, for example, adopting a behaviour-based interview strategy (which will be described in Chapter 7) as the basis for selection of entry-level engineers resulted in savings of $500 000 in three years. These savings were due to lower turnover, lower training costs, and improved capabilities of the engineering staff because of a better fit.[29]

For many firms, instituting tough headcount controls is a key strategy in reducing labour costs. The HR department generally plays the central role in planning and implementing corporate downsizings, such as those affecting many private-sector firms as well as hospitals, school boards and government organizations across the country in recent years. HR staff members typically provide assistance and support to the employees affected, and take steps to maintain the morale and performance of those remaining.

Increasing Responsiveness

Making the enterprise more responsive to product/service innovations and technological change is the basic aim of many of the management strategies listed at the end of Chapter 1. Flattening the pyramid, empowering employees, and organizing around teams are designed to facilitate communication and make it easier for decisions to be made, so that the organization can respond quickly to its customers' needs and competitors' challenges. The HR department staff members play a crucial role in accomplishing these objectives. In the High Performance Organization boxes throughout the book, numerous examples are provided of ways in which HR practices can help to boost a firm's responsiveness.

Improving Service

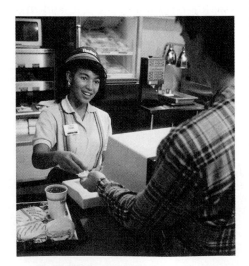

Employees in fast-food establishments are taught how to provide courteous, efficient customer service.

Employee behaviour is particularly important in firms providing in-person service, such as banks and retail establishments. If a customer is confronted by a customer-service representative or salesperson who is tactless or unprepared to discuss the pros and cons of the different products or services or, even worse, who is downright discourteous, all other efforts to attract this customer will have been wasted. Many such organizations have little to differentiate them from their competitors except superior service, and that makes them uniquely dependent on their employees' attitudes and motivation—and thus on effective HRM. As noted by Kevin Scott, senior manager of Human Resources at the Bank of Montreal, "In the financial-services sector just about everything that's new can be copied by competitors pretty quickly. What distinguishes a company is the 'people' business aspects. People are the critical differentiating component ...."[30]

Research Insight

A recent study of service firms highlights the HRM–service link. The researchers found that progressive HR practices—such as facilitating employees' career progress and developing orientation/training programs for new employees—improved employees' customer-service skills, as well as the overall quality of that service from the customers' point of view.[31]

The underlying philosophy can be summed up in the words of Fred Smith, the chairperson and founder of Federal Express, as "people—service—profits." In other words, if progressive HR practices are used to build employee commitment and morale, employees will provide excellent service, which, in turn, will generate profits. This philosophy is becoming even more relevant in today's high-tech world. In fact, as explained in the following Information Technology and HR box, the advent of e-commerce means that customer-service skills are more critical than ever before.

Helping to Build Employee Commitment

Intense global competition and the need for more responsiveness put a premium on employee commitment. As Jon Slangerup, vice-president and general manager of Federal Express Canada Ltd., explains:[32]

> It's a matter of discretionary effort—having employees do things above and beyond the call of duty every single day. To me, that is the difference between a great company and a good one.

Building employee commitment requires the joint efforts of HR department staff and managers throughout the firm. For example, two-way communication fosters commitment, and firms like Federal Express Canada Ltd. have for a long time had programs in place that guarantee two-way communication and fair treatment of all employee grievances and disciplinary matters.[33]

High-commitment firms also tend to engage in *actualizing practices*, which aim to ensure that employees fully use their skills and gifts at work and become all that they can be. HR practices are crucial here, for instance, in establishing career-oriented performance-appraisal procedures and open job-posting and job-transfer practices. Convincing employees that the company and all of its managers care about them is important, too. For this reason, high-commitment firms like Federal Express have adopted a no-layoff policy to give employees the security to go the extra mile. They are also very careful about whom they promote into management positions. All aspiring FedEx supervisors must take the firm's multistep leadership evaluation program to determine if they have the desired values and skills. Several assessments by superiors and peers are involved, as well as a project supervised by the employee's immediate superior. "It's tough," explains Slangerup. "From beginning to end, it takes from six to twelve months. We're looking for leadership ability and other skills. We want our managers to be coaches and mentors."[34]

Research Insight

There is research support for the commitment-building strategies used at FedEx. According to the latest *WorkCanada* survey, the single biggest factor affecting workplace commitment is "people awareness"—recruiting and retention procedures, valuing diversity, providing job security for good work, recognizing the need to balance work and family responsibilities, and preparing people to work in a changing environment. Job environment; being informed about business goals, strategies and results; equitable compensation; and having managers who see themselves as guides and "energizers" also have a major impact. Practices found to increase worker loyalty include providing competitive benefits, reward and recognition programs for good performance, letting employees know about reward programs, conducting employee surveys, and using self-directed teams.[35]

Many firms have recognized the link between reward and recognition programs and employee commitment and discretionary efforts. HR departments often assume a leadership role in developing such programs, as occurred at Cyanamid Crop Protection:[36]

INFORMATION TECHNOLOGY AND HR
Improving Service in the e-Commerce World

The firms that are jockeying for position in a competitive global marketplace crowded with Web site offerings are quick to recognize the Internet's potential for sales and marketing, but often ignore the customer-service side of the e-commerce frontier, something to which many Internet shoppers can attest.

Providing online service may involve a different skill set than providing in-person assistance, something that must be considered when recruiting and selecting employees. Even if an employee is suited to the job at hand, the impersonal nature of online interactions may lessen an employee's feeling of personal responsibility for a customer's care unless the employee is properly trained,.

Poor service may also result if customer service is introduced after going online, rather than being seen as a key aspect of e-commerce and planned from the outset. Even if introduced at the planning stages, customer-service initiatives may fail if a firm fails to involve customer-service and HR representatives in site design.

Perhaps more often, organizations simply miss out on the opportunity to revamp customer service when going online: they simply adopt the new technology without reviewing the processes that they intend to automate. If a firm's customer-care department is weak to begin with, the Internet will highlight this weakness, rather than leading to improved service.

Compounding the lack of forethought, inappropriate selection decisions, and/or inadequate training is the fact that Internet users, as a group, tend to be rather unforgiving if displeased with the service provided. There are typically a lot of options around the world from which to select—only a mouse click away—so most firms don't have a captive audience. When a retailer disappoints an in-person customer on one occasion, an opportunity to lure him or her back may present itself the next time that the customer is in the mall. Disappointing someone over the Internet, however, may mean never having another opportunity to interact with that person!

Customer service means connecting with people. The impersonal aspect of e-mail should not be a barrier to this; it all depends on the system that is implemented. From a customer's perspective, there is a huge difference between a service representative who sends a response into cyberspace and lets it land where it may and an individual who follows up a request with a personalized e-mail response or a telephone call.

The resources and vision that organizations apply to e-commerce must extend to e-customer care. HR department staff can provide valuable assistance in this regard.

Source: John Hobel, "Some Things Never Change," *Canadian HR Reporter* 13, no. 5 (March 13, 2000), p. 4.

According to Carolyn Cullen, director of HR at the firm, it's the thought that counts, not the reward. Employees receive sincere, spontaneous recognition through a formal day-to-day recognition program, which supplements the annual performance and long-term service award programs. Employees can recognize a coworker for outstanding performance in one of five categories: leadership, teamwork, customer service, innovation, and quality. Doing so involves choosing from a variety of $25 gift certificates for such stores as Canadian Tire and Chapters, or purchasing a gift of their own choice, valued at $25, and presenting it, accompanied by a personal thank-you card. The general manager also extends his personal congratulations, and the names of recipients are published in the quarterly company newsletter. The program, which is based on the input of a diverse employee group, is designed to reinforce the company's values, focus efforts on the company's goals, and act as a performance incentive.

Developing and Implementing Corporate Strategy

strategy

The company's plan for how it will balance its internal strengths and weaknesses with external opportunities and threats in order to maintain a competitive advantage.

Perhaps the most striking change in the role of the HR department is its growing importance in developing and implementing strategy. Traditionally, **strategy**—the company's plan for how it will balance its internal strengths and weaknesses with external opportunities and threats in order to maintain a competitive advantage—was formulated without HR department input. The CEO and senior management team would decide to enter new markets, drop product lines, or embark on a five-year cost-cutting plan, and then more or less leave the HR implications of the plan (hiring new workers, terminating employees, and arranging for outplacement services, etc.) to be carried out by the HR department staff.

Today, things are very different. Strategies increasingly depend on strengthening organizational responsiveness and building committed work teams, and these put the HR department in a central role. In the words of one senior HR practitioner,[37]

> The critical success differentiator today is people. "Best practices" and technology are available to anyone. Financing and customers will go to those companies whose people are fastest into the market with better ideas and better coordination. Our role is to make that possible.

Thus, it is increasingly common to involve HR department staff in the earliest stages of developing and implementing the firm's strategic plan, rather than simply letting them react to it. More and more firms have come to realize that HR professionals are of greatest benefit to a firm when they become strategic partners, responsible for leading organizational change initiatives, developing business strategies in cooperation with operational managers, and building effective HR strategies.[38] In the words of the senior vice-president of Aon Consulting, "I don't think [HR] has ever been as critical as it is now."[39] To explain why these changes are occurring, we next turn to an examination of strategic planning and a discussion of the strategic role of the HR department.

Strategic Planning and HRM

The Nature of Strategic Planning

Managers engage in three levels of strategic decision making in an organization,[40] as illustrated in **Figure 2.3**. Many companies consist of several different businesses. For example, Pepsi, Frito-Lay, and Pizza Hut are all part of PepsiCo.

FIGURE 2.3 Relationships Among Strategies in Multiple-business Firms

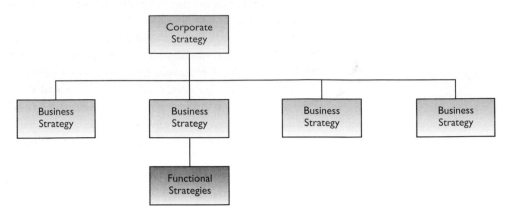

Source: James M. Higgins and Julian W. Vincze, *Strategic Management Text and Cases*, 5th ed. (Fort Worth: The Dryden Press, 1991), p. 263.

corporate-level strategy

Decisions about the portfolio of businesses that, in total, will comprise the organization, and the ways in which these will relate to each other.

business-level/ competitive strategy

Identification of how each of the firm's businesses will build and strengthen the organization's long-term competitive position in the marketplace.

functional strategy

Identification of the basic courses of action to be pursued by each department or functional area to help the business attain its competitive goals.

strategic planning

The corporate-level, organization-wide strategic planning process.

Such companies need a **corporate-level strategy** to identify the portfolio of businesses that, in total, will comprise the organization and the ways in which these will relate to each other.

At the next level down, each of these businesses, such as Pizza Hut, is guided by a **business-level/competitive strategy**, which identifies how it will build and strengthen its long-term competitive position in the marketplace.[41] Such a strategy, for instance, identifies how Pizza Hut will compete with Domino's, or Wal-Mart will compete with Zellers.

In turn, each business consists of various departments, such as manufacturing, sales, and HRM, each of which has a **functional strategy** identifying the basic courses of action to be pursued to help the business attain its competitive goals.

While companies have three types of strategies, the term **strategic planning** is usually reserved for the corporate-level planning process, which applies organization-wide. Specifically, the strategic plan outlines the overall organizational purposes and goals and how they are to be achieved, given the external opportunities and threats and internal strengths and weaknesses. Deciding whether to expand into a superstore or continue to operate small local gourmet markets is a typical strategic planning issue, as is whether to cut costs by amalgamating hospital units and reducing beds or eliminating certain departments and/or services altogether.

For example, one goal when IBM bought the Lotus software firm was the acquisition of the Lotus Notes networking programs. Sensing the opportunities and threats presented by the Internet's growing popularity and recognizing the firm's relative lack of expertise in networking software, one component of IBM's strategic plan—developed under the direction of Chairperson Louis Gerstner—was the decision to diversify by buying Lotus.

In all organizations, the three levels of strategic decision making should be interrelated and mutually supportive. For example, at the corporate level, IBM's acquisition of Lotus represented an attempt to reposition the giant corporation to compete more effectively in the business of networking computers. Having decided to acquire Lotus, Gerstner and the senior management team then had to make a business-level strategic decision regarding how to organize IBM's networking business and compete with other firms making similar products. Jim Manzi, the head of Lotus, proposed the merger of Lotus with IBM's other software divisions under his direction; this decision was rejected. Gerstner and the senior management team decided to keep Lotus and its Lotus Notes software separate, and let Manzi leave the firm.

These corporate and business-level strategic decisions, in turn, have shaped and will continue to shape IBM's functional strategies. For example, IBM's move into networking has production implications, since it may require phasing out several hardware manufacturing facilities and consolidating the firm's network program design facilities in fewer locations. Similarly, IBM's marketing and sales efforts will no doubt increasingly have to be organized around a networking sales effort. The HR department will also have to accomplish its share: there will be facilities to be closed, new ones to be staffed, and network program designers to be recruited and hired.[42]

Building Competitive Advantage

Every organization tries to achieve a **competitive advantage**, defined as any factors that allow it to differentiate its product or service from those of its competitors to increase market share.[43]

There are several strategies that can be used to achieve competitive advantage. **Cost leadership**, which means aiming to become the low-cost supplier of a product or service, is one. For example, Wal-Mart is a typical industry cost leader, due to its unique satellite-based distribution system, ability to track products from supplier to consumer more effectively than its competitors, and keeping store location costs to a minimum by choosing sites outside of the main business core.

Differentiation is a second competitive strategy. This involves seeking to be unique along dimensions that are widely valued by purchasers of the product or service.[44] Thus, Volvo stresses the safety of its cars, Canadian Tire and Petro-Canada their Canadian identity, President's Choice its reasonably priced and high-value grocery products, and Mercedes Benz the reliability and quality of its vehicles. Like Mercedes Benz, organizations can usually charge a premium price if they successfully stake out their claim to be substantially different from their competitors in some enviable way.

The aim of the **focus strategy** is to serve a narrow target market better than other firms that are competing more broadly. Achieving this objective may involve using differentiation (such as finding better ways to meet the needs of the target market), a cost-leadership strategy with this particular market, or both. An example of a firm adopting this approach is Telus, which has targeted the small- to mid-size telecommunications market in eastern Canada.[45]

Human Resources as a Competitive Advantage

In today's intensely competitive and globalized marketplace, maintaining a competitive advantage by becoming a cost leader and/or differentiator puts a heavy premium on having a highly committed and competent work force. Many experts emphasize the strategic role that committed employees play in helping organizations to achieve competitive advantage. As one puts it:[46]

> In a growing number of organizations, human resources are now viewed as a source of competitive advantage. There is a greater recognition that distinctive competencies

competitive advantage

Any factors that allow an organization to differentiate its product or service from those of its competitors to increase market share.

cost leadership strategy

The competitive strategy that aims at becoming the low-cost supplier of a product or service.

differentiation strategy

The competitive strategy that involves seeking to be unique along dimensions that are widely valued by purchasers of the product or service.

focus strategy

A strategy aimed at serving a narrow target market better than other firms that are competing more broadly, which may involve the use of differentiation, cost leadership, or both.

are obtained through highly developed employee skills, distinctive organizational cultures, management processes, and systems. This is in contrast to the traditional emphasis on transferable resources such as equipment .... Increasingly, it is being recognized that competitive advantage can be obtained with a high-quality work force that enables organizations to compete on the basis of market responsiveness, product and service quality, differentiated products, and technological innovation.

An example of an organization that has recognized the importance of its human resources as a source of competitive advantage is The Loyalty Group, the company that operates the "AIR MILES" program. Founded in 1991, it has grown from seven employees to more than 700:[47]

> President John Scullion perceives the real value of the company to lie in its intangible assets—the ability and willingness of the employees. Thus, the development of employees is a central aspect of the company's business strategy. A commitment has been made to invest three percent of revenue into employee development, and training budgets have been established at the business unit level, in HR and for the call centre. Training initiatives are aimed at the development of the core strategies required to grow the business, and performance management and compensation are both tied to employee development. Known as a firm that values and develops its employees, the company can attract and retain the best.

Strategic Human Resources Management

strategic human resources management
The linking of HRM with strategic goals and objectives in order to improve business performance and develop (an) organizational culture that fosters innovation and flexibility.

HR strategies
The specific HR actions that the company plans to pursue to achieve its competitive strategy.

The fact that employees are central to achieving competitive advantage has led to the emergence of the field known as **strategic human resources management**,[48] defined as "... the linking of HRM with strategic goals and objectives in order to improve business performance and develop (an) organizational culture that fosters innovation and flexibility ...."[49] To be effective as a strategic partner, the HR department needs a sophisticated HRMS, as described in Chapter 1.

The term "strategic HR" recognizes the HR department's partnership role in the strategic planning process, while the term "**HR strategies**" refers to the specific HR actions that the company uses to achieve its aims.[50] One of the primary objectives at Federal Express Canada Ltd. is differentiation through superior customer service. To achieve this goal, the company's overall HR strategy is aimed at building a committed work force. The specific components of the HR strategy at the firm include building healthy two-way communication, a rigorous selection process, extensive training, guaranteeing fair treatment and employee security to the greatest extent possible, and instituting various promotion-from-within activities.[51]

HR strategies that fit a cost-leadership orientation emphasize efficient, low-cost production and reinforce adherence to highly structured procedures. These include specific job descriptions, job-specific training, careful selection to ensure that employees have the necessary technical qualifications and skills, and a performance appraisal system that weeds out low performers.

THE ROLE OF THE HR DEPARTMENT AS A STRATEGIC PARTNER

The long history of staff (advisory) authority has left HR departments with a somewhat impoverished reputation. In fact, some people still view HR departments as strictly operational and believe that HR activities are not strategic at all.[52] According to this line of reasoning, HR activities simply "involve putting out small fires—ensuring that: people are paid on the right day; the job advertisement meets the newspaper deadline; a suitable supervisor is recruited for the night shift by the time it goes ahead; and the same manager remembers to observe due process before sacking the new rep who didn't work out."[53]

A more sophisticated (but perhaps no more accurate) view of HR departments is that their role is simply to "fit" HR practices to the company's strategy. In this view, top management crafts a corporate strategy—such as buying Lotus—and the HR department staff members are told to create the HR programs required to successfully implement that corporate strategy.[54] As two strategic planning experts have argued, "the human resources management system must be tailored to the demands of business strategy."[55] Their idea here is that "for any particular organizational strategy, there is purportedly a matching HR strategy."[56]

A third view is that the HR department is an equal partner in the strategic planning process. In order to forge the organization's work force into a competitive advantage, the proponents of this viewpoint believe that the HR department staff members must be equal partners in both formulation and implementation of the firm's organization-wide and competitive strategies.[57] Canadian Imperial Bank of Commerce (CIBC) is one firm in which the HR department is viewed as a strategic business partner. How this came about and what this means is explained in the High Performance Organization box that follows.

THE HIGH PERFORMANCE ORGANIZATION

HR as a Strategic Business Partner

Canadian Imperial Bank of Commerce (CIBC) has evolved into a six-business-unit structure, and the HR department evolved right along with it. The drivers contributing to HR becoming a strategic partner were cost containment pressures, customer-satisfaction focus, customer-loyalty concerns, and a focus on employee retention and well-being.

HR went from a very decentralized structure with a lot of duplication to a client-service model, which sees HR functioning very much as a consulting service with the business units as its "clients." In each business unit, there is one HR leader who reports directly to the business head, along with a team of HR consultants who act as the primary contact for all HR services. A central HR services department, providing specialized HR services, exists outside the business-unit structure and can be drawn upon as needed.

The model is successful for several reasons. It:

- provides senior HR professionals with an in-depth understanding of the business
- builds strong relationships between HR professionals and business unit managers
- provides senior executives with a confidential advisor
- provides the HR consultants with the ability to leverage the skills and ideas of others, since they are part of a larger consulting practice
- ensures appropriate strategic HR support
- reinforces the bottom-line focus, and
- enables HR processes to be better aligned and integrated with the business.

Source: "HRPAO News: HR As a Strategic Business Partner," *HR Professional* 17, no. 1 (February/March 2000), p. 56. © *HR Professional.* Reprinted by permission of the HR Professional, Suite 1902, 2 Bloor Street West, Toronto M4W 3E2.

Role in Formulating Strategy

Formulating a company's overall strategic plan requires identifying, analyzing, and balancing two sets of forces: the organization's external opportunities and threats on the one hand, and its internal strengths and weaknesses on the other.

environmental scanning

Identifying and analyzing external opportunities and threats that may be crucial to the organization's success.

This is where strategic HRM comes in. First, HR department staff can play a role in what strategic planners call environmental scanning, which involves identifying and analyzing external opportunities and threats that may be crucial to the organization's success. For example, in 1995, the Royal Bank realized that its front-line managers needed to assume more HR responsibilities in order for the company to continue to be successful in its highly competitive, service-oriented market. The decision was thus made to adopt a shared-services model.[58]

Now, Royal has a unique ISO-certified HR centre in Mississauga, staffed by about 75 HR practitioners who are responsible for HR for Royal's 60 000 employees. They handle about 3000 telephone calls per day, providing advice to front-line mangers across the country. Duplication of services has been eliminated; HR advice is delivered efficiently and effectively; and managers can rely on a centre of diverse knowledge and expertise, rather than the advice of a single HR expert. Representatives of some of Canada's largest companies have been stopping by the centre to examine the advantages of Royal's shared-service arrangements and to discuss how they could implement this model. While the reduced cost of HR is appealing, what really draws interest is the increased efficiency.

HR managers can also supply *competitive intelligence* that may be useful as the company formulates its strategic plans. Details regarding a successful incentive plan being used by a competitor, employee opinion survey data eliciting information about customer complaints, and information about pending legislative changes are examples. Furthermore, according to one expert, as a human resources specialist:[59]

From public information and legitimate recruiting and interview activities, you ought to be able to construct organization charts, staffing levels, and group missions for the various organizational components of each of your major competitors. Your knowledge of how brands are sorted among sales divisions and who reports to whom can give important clues as to a competitor's strategic priorities. You may even know the track record and characteristic behaviour of the executives.

The HR department also participates in the strategy formulation process by supplying information regarding the company's internal strengths and weaknesses. Once weaknesses have been identified, corrective action can be planned and taken. Take Canadian Pacific Hotels (CP), for example:[60]

CP's business strategy is focused on providing "four-star hotels with five-star service." While this has led to significant investments in property acquisition and capital equipment, HR professionals at CP recognized the need to make a parallel investment in their human assets to provide employees with the requisite skills. Leadership 2000 and Service Plus 2000 were launched; these are development programs that reinforce the delivery of exceptional guest satisfaction and foster the management/supervisory skills desired. Subsequently, a problem with the existing performance-management program was identified: it did little to reinforce the learning once employees were back on the job. Thus, a new performance-management program called REACH was introduced, based on the core competencies emphasized during training.

Some firms even build their strategies around an HR-based competitive advantage. For example, in the process of automating its factories, farm-equipment manufacturer John Deere developed a work force that was exceptionally talented and expert in factory automation. This, in turn, prompted the firm to establish a new technology division to offer automation services to other companies.[61]

Role in Executing Strategy

Strategy execution has traditionally been the "bread and butter" of HR's strategy role. For example, the competitive strategy at Federal Express involves differentiating itself from its competitors by offering superior customer service and guaranteed on-time deliveries. Since basically the same technologies are available to UPS, Purolator, and other competitors, it's the work force at FedEx—its human resources—that provides its crucial competitive advantage. This puts a premium on the firm's HR processes, as discussed earlier, and on the firm's ability to create a highly committed, competent, and customer-oriented work force.[62]

HR departments support strategy implementation in numerous other ways. For example, HR staff members are heavily involved in the execution of most firms' downsizing and restructuring strategies through establishing training and retraining programs, arranging for outplacement services, instituting pay-for-performance plans, and helping to redesign jobs. HR staff members also play a critical role in strategies to increase organizational effectiveness through better employee–management relations.

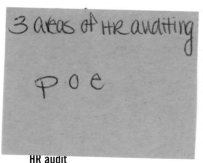

HR audit

An evaluation of the firm's HR activities and the HR department's effectiveness as a strategic partner.

Just as financial audits are conducted, periodic and systematic evaluations or audits should be conducted to assess how effectively the firm is managing its human resources.[63] Since the entire HR system should be audited, supervisors and managers throughout the organization must be involved, which helps to reinforce the important role that all managers play in HRM and the service and strategic roles of HR department staff members.

Comprehensive HR audits encompass three areas:

- The HR department's effectiveness as a strategic partner.
- Organizational compliance with applicable federal, provincial (or territorial), and municipal laws and regulations.
- The performance of specific HRM programs and functions.

In addition, area-specific audits may be conducted to evaluate issues of particular concern to management. Such audits may assess the culture of the organization, for example, or the existence of barriers to the advancement of specific employee groups, such as women and visible minorities.

attitude survey

A survey administered to determine employee thoughts and feelings about organizational issues, designed to obtain data about areas of effectiveness and those requiring improvement.

Employee attitude surveys are often one component of an HR audit. They provide a means of assessing how employees feel about a variety of issues and gaining insight into their perceptions of the organization's strengths and weaknesses. Topics surveyed typically include supervision, HR policies and programs, job-related factors, effectiveness of communication strategies, and overall leadership. As explained in the Information Technology and HR box that follows,

exit interview
A conversation with departing employees to learn their opinions of the employer, managers, policies, and other aspects of employment with the organization, and reason(s) for leaving.

focus group
A group of eight to twelve users of the services of the HR department, who provide in-depth feedback about the HR activities, programs, and services.

records analysis
A review of various organizational records to assess compliance with company policies and procedures, as well as relevant legislative standards; measure the effectiveness of various programs in meeting their stated objectives; and identify areas in which performance improvements are required.

field experiment
A research design that enables the comparison of an experimental and control group, under realistic conditions, to objectively assess the impact and effectiveness of HR programs and activities.

online and Interactive Voice Response systems are now being used to assist with such surveys. Regardless of the methodology used for data collection and analysis, the results provide excellent feedback about the effectiveness of HR policies and programs and help to identify areas requiring improvement. Survey results should be shared with employees, along with the specific strategies being implemented to address any concerns and/or correct any identified problems.

In addition to surveys, organizations use several other research tools to collect data. Interviews with employees and managers can provide specific and detailed information. Many firms conduct exit interviews with departing employees to identify any sources of dissatisfaction contributing to their decision to leave. Some organizations use focus groups to obtain in-depth information from a small group of employees. These involve an unstructured group discussion with an unbiased facilitator.

A records analysis is often included as part of an HR audit. For example, reports pertaining to health and safety, scrap rates, turnover and absenteeism, and grievances are often examined. Internal placement records, selection records, and employee files may also be looked at.

Also possible is a field experiment, which involves comparing an experimental group and a control group, under realistic conditions. For example, training in lifting techniques might be provided to half of the employees in a department (the experimental group) but not provided to the other half (the control group). After training, program effectiveness can be assessed by comparing the safety records of those in each group (in terms of number of back complaints or injuries). Field experiments are not widely used in HRM due to the drawbacks associated with them: those not selected may be dissatisfied or demotivated; there are ethical concerns about the possibility of a control group member experiencing a back injury during the course of the experiment; and results may be affected by environmental changes or information sharing between group members.

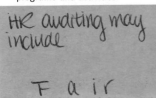

TECHNOLOGY AND HR
e Surveys

have concerns about
ormation they provide,
tive Voice Response
(IVR) systems for the administration and analysis of attitude surveys. There are three key advantages, all of which help to ensure honest, frank responses: (1) employees can respond without submitting written statements; (2) surveys can be completed away from the workplace; and (3) an independent, off-site firm receives all responses. IVR surveys also have the advantage of being accessible to all employees, even those without a computer. Respondents simply telephone a toll-free number and respond to the survey questions posed by a pre-recorded interviewer in the language spoken by the work force. Answers are conveyed using touch-tone

commands and spoken voicemail-type comments. Thus, even an employee having the most modest level of literacy can submit a useful response.

Some firms are using another high-tech alternative for the design and distribution of attitude surveys, and the collection and analysis of responses: online and Web-based solutions. Examples of available software include *Perceptor*, a Web-based system produced by Affinity Systems of Mississauga, Ontario, and *Inquisite Online*, an online survey tool available through Catapult Systems of Wakefield, Mass.

Source: Robert Boutilier, "Straight Talk," *HR Professional* 17, no. 1 (February/March 2000), pp. 38-40; and Al Doran and Ian Turnbull, "The Latest High-tech Products and Software for the HR Professional," *Guide to Technology, Supplement to Canadian HR Reporter* 13, no. 5 (March 13, 2000), p. G8.

cost–benefit analysis

A comparison of the monetary costs of a particular function with nonmonetary benefits gained, such as changes in attitudes or improvement in employee morale.

cost–effectiveness analysis

A comparison of the monetary costs and benefits of a particular initiative.

benchmarking

A continuous and systematic process for comparing some aspect of organizational performance against data from a firm considered to be superior in that particular area.

Human Resources Benchmarking Association (HRBA)

www.hrba.org

Whenever possible, audit findings should be translated into quantitative data. A cost–benefit analysis compares the monetary costs of a particular function with nonmonetary benefits gained, such as changes in attitudes or improvement in employee morale. A cost–effectiveness analysis compares the monetary costs and benefits of a particular initiative. For example, the amount spent on health and safety training might be compared to the amount saved due to reduction in equipment damage caused by unsafe practices or decreases in lost-time accidents.[64]

To be meaningful, quantifiable audit results should be compared with some accepted external measure of performance, such as industry norms or research findings. Helpful information can be obtained from Statistics Canada, Labour Canada, the Industrial Accident Prevention Association, business and industry associations, trade associations, consulting firms, and The Conference Board of Canada. Some firms, such as Xerox Canada and the Bank of Montreal, use **benchmarking**, which is a continuous and systematic process of comparing some aspect of organizational performance against data from a firm considered to be superior in that particular area. To assist with benchmarking activities and facilitate information sharing among HR professionals aimed at improving productivity, quality, and cycle time, a Human Resources Benchmarking Association (HRBA) has been formed.

The value to be derived from conducting HR audits lies in making improvements. When using a benchmarking approach, for example, survey results should be used to "peg" an organization's performance relative to that of others, identify any "performance gaps," and suggest possible corrective actions. Outstanding performers on a particular dimension can be contacted to determine how the results were achieved. Strategies for performance improvements can thus be identified and targets set to meet survey benchmarks.[65]

THE IMPACT OF EFFECTIVE HRM PRACTICES ON EMPLOYEE PERFORMANCE AND THE BOTTOM LINE

The results of systematic audits and research studies have established that sophisticated and integrated HRM practices have a positive effect on employee performance, if properly implemented and accompanied by a supportive culture and climate. In such cases, HR practices increase knowledge, skills, and abilities; improve motivation; and reduce shirking (employees avoiding work or responsibility due to laziness or selfishness). They also increase retention of productive and competent employees and have a direct and economically significant effect on organizational financial performance.

Research Insight

One study of 437 publicly traded companies demonstrated that firms that effectively manage employee performance through more sophisticated HR practices have higher profits, better cash flows, stronger stock market performance, significant productivity gains, higher sales growth per employee, and lower real growth in number of employees.[66]

Empirical studies have also established that 15 percent of the relative profit performance of an organization derives from HR strategy. Furthermore, HR systems can affect a firm's market value by $15 000 to $45 000 per employee, and HR systems can affect the probability of new-venture survival by as much as 22 percent.[67]

There is growing research evidence, however, that the presence of high-involvement HR practices alone is not sufficient to enhance organizational performance. Also required is the existence of a complementary workplace culture and climate. Studies involving more than 1200 Canadian firms and almost 800 local union leaders found that the highest performance levels are associated with high-involvement HR practices combined with a supportive work environment, characterized by participative decision making and open communication.[68]

In addition to these research findings, HR managers now have numbers to take to the boardroom to prove just how much the department can contribute to the bottom line in another form: the Human Capital Index (HCI), developed by Watson Wyatt. Based on a year-long study analyzing the HR practices at more than 400 companies, which were matched with objective financial measures, the HCI outlines 30 key HR practices and indicates, in best-case scenarios, their contributions to shareholder value. These 30 practices were then summarized in five categories: (1) recruiting excellence; (2) clear rewards and accountability; (3) collegial and flexible workplaces; (4) communications integrity; and (5) the imprudent use of resources—the negative impact of poorly implemented HR policies and practices.[69] The impact of each is shown in **Figure 2.4.**

FIGURE **2.4** HR Return on Investment

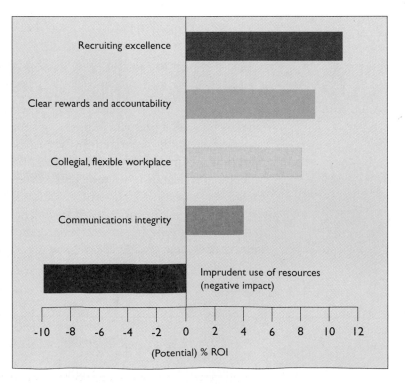

Source: Watson Wyatt, *Human Capital Index Study,* cited in David Brown, "The 30 Ways HR Adds Value to the Bottom Line," *Canadian HR Reporter* 12, no. 22 (December 13, 1999), p. 1. © Carswell, Thomson Professional Publishing. Reproduced by permission of *Canadian HR Reporter,* Carswell, One Corporate Plaza, 2075 Kennedy Road, Scarborough M1T 3V4.

CHAPTER Review

Summary

1   The historical development of HRM is linked to: scientific management, which focused on production; the human relations movement, in which the emphasis was on people; and the human resources movement, in which it was recognized that organizational success is linked to both.

2   HRM is now a recognized profession, in that it has a distinct body of knowledge, certification procedures, performance standards established through self-regulation, and a code of ethics.

3   Ethics and social responsibility are of growing importance to organizations.

4   HR departments today play an important role in: improving productivity, responsiveness, and customer service; building employee commitment; and developing and implementing corporate strategy.

5   Organizations typically formulate three types of strategies. Corporate strategies identify the mix of businesses in which the firm will engage. Business-level/competitive strategies identify how each of the firm's businesses will compete. Each function or department then has its own functional strategy, identifying how it will contribute to the business strategy.

6   There are three competitive strategies: cost-leadership, differentiation, and focus, all of which require a highly committed and competent work force.

7   Strategic HRM involves linking HRM with strategic goals and objectives to improve business performance and develop an organizational culture that fosters innovation and flexibility.

8   In more and more firms, the HR department is becoming a strategic partner, playing a role in strategy formulation and execution.

9   Just as financial audits are conducted, systematic HR audits should be conducted periodically to assess how effectively the firm is managing its human resources. Comprehensive HR audits encompass three areas: the HR department's effectiveness as a strategic partner; organizational compliance with applicable legislation; and the performance of specific HRM programs and functions.

10 Auditing techniques include attitude surveys, interviews, focus groups, records analysis, and field experiments.

11 Whenever possible, audit findings should be translated into quantitative data. A cost–benefit analysis compares the monetary costs of a particular function with nonmonetary benefits gained. A cost–effectiveness analysis compares the monetary costs and benefits of a particular initiative.

12 To be meaningful, audit results should be compared with some accepted measure of performance, such as industry norms or research findings. Benchmarking is a technique used by many firms. It involves a continuous and systematic process of comparing some aspect of organizational performance against data from a firm considered to be superior in that particular area.

13 Systematic audit results and research studies have established a link between effective HR practices, employee performance, and the bottom line, if properly implemented and accompanied by a supportive culture and climate.

Key Terms

attitude survey
benchmarking
business-level/ competitive strategy
certification
competitive advantage
corporate-level strategy
cost leadership strategy
cost–benefit analysis
cost–effectiveness analysis
differentiation strategy
environmental scanning
ethics
exit interview
field experiment
focus group
focus strategy

functional strategy
Hawthorne Studies
HR audit
HR strategies
human relations movement
human resources movement
profession
records analysis
scientific management
social audits (responsibility audits)
social responsibility
strategic human resources
  management
strategic planning
strategy

Review and Discussion Questions

1 Describe scientific management and explain its impact on organizations.

2 Explain the importance of the Hawthorne Studies.

3 Describe the forces that shaped the evolution of HRM from personnel management to strategic partner.

4 Explain why HRM is a profession.

5 Explain the role of the HR department as a strategic partner.

6 Explain why the HR system should be evaluated and describe four auditing techniques used in HRM.

CRITICAL *Thinking Questions*

1 Identify a company that is known for being both ethical and socially responsible. What types of behaviour and activities typify this organization?

2 Describe an ethical dilemma that you have confronted, explain how you handled the situation, and critique your performance. (i.e. Did you handle the situation effectively? If not, what would you do differently if you could rewrite history? If so, explain why you feel that you handled the situation appropriately.)

3   Based on inside knowledge, advertising and/or marketing, describe the corporate-level and business-level strategies of an organization with which you are familiar.

4   Briefly describe the functional strategies of the department or area in which you are currently or were most recently employed.

APPLICATION *Exercises*

RUNNING CASE: Carter Cleaning Company

Jennifer's Dilemma

One of the first problems Jennifer faces at Carter Cleaning Centres concerns the inadequacies of the firm's current HRM practices and procedures. Although she hasn't done a formal audit, she notes that there are no written policies, and the practices for recruitment, selection, and training have not been standardized.

As part of her core program of studies at university, Jennifer took several HR courses, which were recognized as credits by the Human Resources Professionals Association of Ontario (HRPAO). Because she found the HR courses quite fascinating, she chose her electives carefully to ensure that when she graduated she would have eight HRPAO credits. She wrote the Comprehensive Provincial Exam in the September after she graduated, and plans to obtain her professional designation once she acquires experience in the field.

Because of her knowledge of and interest in HRM, Jennifer would like to take over some of the HR responsibilities, but she is a little worried about "stepping on the toes" of the store managers. She knows that her father hasn't really explained her role to the Carter Cleaning employees, and she doesn't want to be seen as "taking over" or "a know-it-all."

Jennifer figures that she and her father should sit down and talk about his vision for the Centres and how she can best assist him.

Questions

1   How should Jennifer and Jack proceed?

2   Explain how a formal HR audit might assist Jennifer and Jack at this time. What systems should be audited?

3   Assuming that Jack agrees that centralization of some HR responsibilities might make sense, what should Jennifer's HR role involve? For which HR activities should the manager at each Centre remain responsible? How should these changes in roles and responsibilities be communicated to the Carter Cleaning staff?

CASE INCIDENT *Jack Nelson's Problem*

As a new member of the board of directors for a local credit union, Jack Nelson was introduced to all of the employees, starting at the home office. When he was introduced to Ruth, he was curious about her work and asked her to explain its significance and its relationship to the jobs of her coworkers. Ruth really couldn't answer his questions. She explained that she had only been working at the home office for two months. She demonstrated, however, that she knew precisely how to operate the equipment for which she was responsible, and her supervisor commented to Jack that Ruth is an excellent employee.

At one of the branch offices, the supervisor in charge spoke to Jack in confidence, telling him that something was wrong, but she didn't know what. For one thing, she explained, employee turnover was too high. No sooner had one employee been put on the job than another one resigned. With customers to see and loans to be made, she explained, she had little time to work with the new employees as they came and went.

Jack learned that all branch supervisors hire their own employees without communication with the home office or other branches. When an opening arises, the supervisor finds a suitable employee to replace the worker who quit.

After touring the 22 branches and finding similar problems in many of them, Jack wondered what action he should take. The credit union is generally regarded as a well-run institution, and has grown from 27 to 191 employees during the past eight years. The more he thought about the matter, the more puzzled he became. He couldn't quite put his finger on the problem, and didn't know whether or not to report his findings to the president.

Questions

1   What are the major problems in the home and branch offices of the credit union?

2   What do you think is causing these problems?

3   Explain how establishing an HR department could assist the firm.

4   For what specific functions should the HR department be responsible? What HR responsibilities should the other supervisors and managers have? Why?

Source: Based on Claude S. George, Jr., *Supervisor in Action*, 4th ed., (Englewood Cliffs, NJ: Prentice-Hall, 1985), pp. 307–8. Reprinted by permission.

EXPERIENTIAL *Exercises*

1   Working with a small group of classmates, contact several firms in your community to find out whether or not they have a code of ethics. If so, learn as much as possible about the specific initiatives devised to support and communicate the code. If not, find out if the firm is planning to implement such a code. If so, how does the firm intend to proceed? If not, why not?

2   Working alone or with a small group of classmates, interview an HR manager and prepare a short essay regarding his or her role in building a more responsive organization.

3   Working with a small group of classmates, contact a firm in a large metropolitan centre at which periodic HR audits are conducted. Find out which

auditing techniques are used, the frequency of audits, and how the summary data are used and communicated. Prepare a brief report and/or presentation of your findings.

WEB-BASED *Exercises*

1 Go to the Web sites of two Canadian HR associations. Compare and contrast: (a) The type of information provided on the Web site; (b) The links to other professional associations; (c) The membership requirements; (d) The services provided to members; and (e) The requirements to obtain a professional designation, if there is one available through the association.

2 Using the Web for research: (a) Identify one company that has been involved in a recent ethical scandal. Find out as much as you can about the nature of the scandal and how it was handled. (b) Identify one company that has conducted a social (responsibility) audit and find out the types of results reported. Prepare a brief report summarizing your findings.

CHAPTER 3

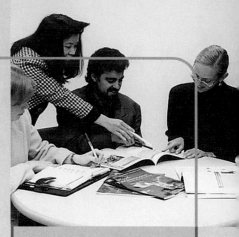

The Changing Emphasis:

From Legal Compliance to Valuing Diversity

CHAPTER OUTLINE

Introduction to the Legal Environment

Equality

Equal Opportunity

Equity

Impact of Equal Opportunity and Equity on HRM

Managing Diversity

LEARNING OUTCOMES

After studying this chapter, you should be able to:

Differentiate between "equal pay for equal work" and "equal pay for work of equal value."

Describe the impact of the Charter of Rights and Freedoms on HRM.

Discuss the grounds of discrimination prohibited under Canadian human rights legislation and *describe* the requirements pertaining to reasonable accommodation.

Discuss the types of behaviour that could constitute harassment and *describe* employers' responsibilities pertaining thereto.

Explain how the human rights legislation is enforced.

Describe the steps involved in implementing an employment equity program.

Discuss the characteristics of successful diversity management initiatives.

INTRODUCTION TO THE LEGAL ENVIRONMENT

Government of Canada
www.canada.gc.ca

As discussed in Chapter 1, government legislation and its accompanying regulations present some major challenges to managers and small-business owners. In this chapter, we will discuss the legal requirements pertaining to employee treatment in the workplace, which have evolved over the years from equality to equal opportunity to equity, primarily due to changing values and social expectations. We will also describe the ways in which some proactive organizations have moved beyond legal compliance to voluntary employment-equity initiatives, and a few have begun to truly value and capitalize on workplace diversity.

A brief overview of the legislation that will be reviewed follows.

Equality

Employment (labour) standards legislation is present in the federal jurisdiction and every province/territory. These laws establish minimum employee entitlements and set a limit on the maximum number of hours of work permitted per day or week. In most jurisdictions, they also require equality in the pay received by men and women performing similar work.

Equal Opportunity

Equal opportunity legislation makes it illegal to discriminate, even unintentionally, against various groups. Reactive in nature, since it is complaints-driven, the focus of such legislation is on the types of acts in which employers should *not* engage. Included in this category are:

1. *The Charter of Rights and Freedoms*, federal legislation that is the cornerstone of equal opportunity.
2. *Human rights legislation*, which is present in every jurisdiction. It prohibits discrimination in all aspects and terms and conditions of employment on the basis of such characteristics as race, colour, national or ethnic origin, and sex.

Equity

Equity legislation is aimed at hastening the pace of change for certain groups that, historically, have been disadvantaged in employment. Such laws fall into two categories:

1. *Employment equity laws*, which require employers to be proactive in hiring and promoting qualified individuals from four designated groups: women, visible minorities, Aboriginal people, and persons with disabilities.
2. *Pay equity legislation*, which is one component of employment equity but much narrower in focus. It is aimed at reducing the differences in pay between male-dominated and female-dominated job classes caused by the undervaluing of work traditionally performed by women.

discrimination
As used in the context of human rights in employment, a distinction, exclusion, or preference, based on one of the prohibited grounds, that has the effect of nullifying or impairing the right of a person to full and equal recognition and exercise of his or her human rights and freedoms.

Discrimination Defined

The word **discrimination** has taken on a negative connotation. When someone is accused of discrimination, it generally means that he or she is perceived to be acting in an unfair or prejudiced manner. However, definitions of the term in the *Webster's Encyclopedic Dictionary* include "choosing with care," and "good taste, discernment"; in other words, making choices based on perceived differences, which is something people do every day. Deciding which college or university to attend, for example, involves discriminating on the basis of such criteria as cost, reputation, and convenience.

What the law prohibits is unfair discrimination—making choices on the basis of perceived but inaccurate differences, to the detriment of specific individuals and/or groups. Standards pertaining to unfair discrimination have changed over time.

While discrimination is prohibited in the Charter of Rights and Freedoms and in the human rights legislation in every jurisdiction, it is not defined in any of these laws, with one exception. Section 10 of the Quebec Charter of Human Rights and Freedoms states:[1]

> Every person has a right to full and equal recognition and exercise of his human rights and freedoms, without distinction, exclusion or preference based on [specific grounds]... **Discrimination exists where such a distinction, exclusion or preference has the effect of nullifying or impairing such right**. [emphasis added]

In the discussion that follows, it will be helpful to keep this definition in mind when the term *discrimination* is used.

EQUALITY

Employment (Labour) Standards Legislation

employment (labour) standards legislation
Laws present in every Canadian jurisdiction that establish minimum employee entitlements and set a limit on the maximum number of hours of work permitted per day or week.

All employers and employees in Canada are covered by **employment (labour) standards legislation**. Those under federal jurisdiction are covered by the Canada Labour Code; the ten provinces and three territories each have an employment (or labour) standards act. These laws, which will be discussed in more detail in Chapter 12 (Establishing Pay Plans) and Chapter 14 (Employee Benefits and Services), establish minimum employee entitlements pertaining to such issues as: wages; paid holidays and vacations; leave for some mix of maternity, parenting, and adoption; bereavement leave; termination notice and overtime pay. They also set a limit on the maximum number of hours of work permitted per day or week.

Every jurisdiction in Canada has legislation incorporating the principle of equal pay for equal work. In most jurisdictions, this entitlement is found in the employment (labour) standards legislation; otherwise, it is in the human rights legislation. In the federal jurisdiction, this principle has been incorporated into the Canada Labour Code since 1971.

equal pay for equal work
The stipulation, specified in the employment (labour) standards or human rights legislation in every Canadian jurisdiction, that an employer cannot pay male and female employees differently if they are performing substantially the same work, requiring the same degree of skill, effort, and responsibility, under similar working conditions.

Equal pay for equal work specifies that an employer cannot pay male and female employees differently if they are performing substantially the same work, requiring the same degree of skill, effort, and responsibility, under similar working conditions. This principle makes it illegal, for example, for a school board to classify male employees as janitors and female employees doing virtually the same work as housekeepers and provide different wage rates based on these classifications.

Pay differences based on a valid merit or seniority system, or employee productivity are permitted; it is only sex-based discrimination that is prohibited. Enforcement is complaints-based and violators can be fined.

EQUAL OPPORTUNITY

The Charter of Rights and Freedoms

Charter of Rights and Freedoms
Federal law enacted in 1982 that guarantees fundamental freedoms to all Canadians.

The cornerstone of Canada's legislation pertaining to issues of equal opportunity is the **Charter of Rights and Freedoms,** which is part of the **Constitution Act** of 1982. The Charter applies directly only to the actions of all levels of government (federal, provincial/territorial, and municipal) and agencies under their jurisdiction. Because it takes precedence over all other laws, however, which means that all legislation must meet Charter standards, it is quite far-reaching in scope. There are two notable exceptions to this generalization. The Charter allows laws to infringe on Charter rights if they can be demonstrably justified as reasonable limits in a "free and democratic society." Since "demonstrably justified" and "reasonable" are open to interpretation, many issues challenged under the Charter eventually end up before the Supreme Court, its final interpreter. The second exception occurs when a legislative body invokes the "notwithstanding" provision, which allows the legislation to be exempted from challenge under the Charter.

The Charter provides the following fundamental rights to every Canadian:

1. Freedom of conscience and religion.
2. Freedom of thought, belief, opinion, and expression, including freedom of the press and other media of communication.
3. Freedom of peaceful assembly.
4. Freedom of association.

In addition to these fundamental freedoms, the Charter also provides democratic rights, the right to live and seek employment anywhere in Canada, legal right to due process in criminal proceedings, equality rights, minority language education rights, Canadian multicultural heritage rights, and First People's rights.[2]

When the Charter became law, it was expected by various interest groups to have significant implications for labour–management relations. In actual fact, the overall impact of the Charter on the labour relations (LR) scene has not been as extensive as predicted, in part due to the long period of time that cases take to reach the Supreme Court. As will be explained next, however, the Charter has had some effects on both HRM and LR.

Supreme Court of Canada
www.scc-csc.gc.ca

Charter Content of Particular Interest to Managers and Small-business Owners

Section Two of the Charter guarantees freedom of association, which is a central concept in LR. Under this section, unions have challenged whether this guarantees that every person should have the right to bargain collectively, strike, and picket.

equality rights
Section 15 of the Charter of Rights and Freedoms, which guarantees the right to equal protection and equal benefit of the law without discrimination.

The **equality rights** section of the Charter (Section 15) became law on April 17, 1985. In its first paragraph, it guarantees the right to:[3]

equal protection and benefit of the law without discrimination, and, in particular, without discrimination based on race, national or ethnic origin, colour, religion, sex, age, or mental or physical disability.

As anticipated, this section has resulted in many legal challenges.

Examples of Charter Applications

A number of significant Charter challenges are described briefly below.

The Right to Bargain Collectively and Strike   A long-awaited decision was issued by the Supreme Court on April 9, 1987 pertaining to the impact of the Charter on federal and provincial collective bargaining legislation.

In a four–two split decision, the Supreme Court ruled that Section Two of the Charter does not guarantee the right to bargain collectively or to strike, a judgment that was a great disappointment to the union movement. The court affirmed that Section Two protects the freedom to establish, belong to, and maintain an association, and to participate in its lawful activities without penalty or reprisal. However, the ability to bargain collectively and the right to strike were determined to be legal rights created and regulated by the various parliaments, rather than fundamental freedoms. Based on this ruling, governments can pass legislation requiring striking workers to return to work and settle outstanding bargaining issues through final and binding arbitration, generally in the case of "undue public hardship" (as when teachers go on strike). A government can also restrict unions' ability to negotiate wage increases through wage restraint legislation, and can deny certain types of workers the right to strike (such as hospital employees) and require instead that they use compulsory arbitration to settle outstanding bargaining issues.

The Right to Picket   Also a disappointment to the union movement was the Supreme Court ruling that the Charter does not protect picketing rights. Thus, employees working in settings such as malls can be denied the right to picket, and employers can impose reasonable limitations on picketing activities, including obtaining a court injunction limiting the number of picketers.

Use of Union Dues   On June 27, 1991, the union movement won a historic legal victory pertaining to LR legislation,[4] the legality of which was challenged by a community-college faculty member from northern Ontario. In a unanimous decision, the Supreme Court of Canada upheld the legality of the Rand formula, which provides for the automatic deduction of union dues from the paycheque of every person in the bargaining unit; as well as the right of unions to spend such dues to support social and political causes and organizations.

Mandatory Retirement   The Supreme Court has upheld the legality of human rights legislation *that protects only individuals of specified ages from discrimination in employment*, and therefore allows mandatory retirement at the upper age limit. In British Columbia, Ontario, and Newfoundland, for example, the upper age limit protected under the provincial human rights legislation is 65, and in Saskatchewan it is 64. The court concluded that mandatory retirement at that upper age limit, if a province chose to impose one, while discriminatory, could be justified as a reasonable limit in a "free and democratic" society.

The Supreme Court has also upheld Section 15(c) of the Canadian Human Rights Act, which excludes mandatory retirement at "the normal age" from its prohibition on age discrimination. Therefore, federal employment policies requiring that individuals retire at "the normal age" are not discriminatory.

It should be noted that these rulings do not limit the right of governments to prohibit mandatory retirement should they choose to do so. Mandatory retirement has been abolished in all Canadian provinces and territories, other than those listed above. The federal government has also abolished mandatory retirement for civil servants.

Human Rights Legislation

Every employer in Canada is affected by human rights legislation, which prohibits intentional and unintentional discrimination in its dealings with the public and in its policies pertaining to all aspects and terms and conditions of employment.

Impact

Most employment laws and regulations are limited in scope, in that they have an impact on only one or two HRM activities. For example, employment (labour) standards legislation primarily affects compensation and benefits administration, and has virtually no effect on other aspects of HRM, such as recruitment and selection, training, performance appraisal or LR.

That is not true of human rights legislation, which is extremely broad in scope. It affects virtually every aspect of HRM, including HR planning, recruitment and selection, training, LR, performance appraisal, and compensation. The ways in which employees should be treated on the job every day and the climate in which they work are also addressed. For this reason, it is critical that all supervisors and managers be thoroughly familiar with the human rights legislation, and their legal obligations and responsibilities specified therein.

Overview

human rights legislation
A family of federal and provincial/territorial laws that have a common objective: providing equal opportunity for members of protected groups in a number of areas, including accommodation, contracts, provision of goods and services, and employment.

Human rights legislation is a family of federal and provincial/territorial laws designed to provide equal opportunity to members of protected groups in a number of areas, including accommodation, contracts, provision of goods and services, and employment. Our focus is on the provisions related to employment. To review individual provincial and territorial human rights laws would be confusing because of the many but generally minor differences among them, often only in terminology (for example, some provinces use the term "creed," others "religion"). As indicated in **Figure 3.1**, the protected grounds are similar across jurisdictions and the provincial/territorial laws are similar to the federal law in terms of scope, interpretation, and application. All jurisdictions prohibit discrimination on the grounds of race, colour, religion or creed, physical and mental disability, sex (including pregnancy and childbirth), and marital status. All prohibit age-based discrimination (although the protected age groups differ), and all jurisdictions other than British Columbia and Alberta prohibit discrimination on the basis of national or ethnic origin. Discrimination on other grounds, such as sexual orientation and criminal history, are prohibited in some jurisdictions but not all.

Human rights laws do not restrict employers' ability to reward outstanding performers or penalize those who do not meet productivity standards or comply with company rules and regulations, as long as such rewards or punishments are based on work-related criteria, rather than age, sex, or other prohibited grounds.

The following discussion will focus on the federal human rights legislation.

The Nunavut Handbook
www.nunavut.com

FIGURE 3.1 Prohibited Grounds of Discrimination in Employment by Jurisdiction

Prohibited Grounds of Discrimination	Federal	Alta.	B.C.	Man.	N.B.	Nfld.	N.S.	Ont.	P.E.I.	Que.	Sask.	N.W.T.	Yukon	Nunavut*
Race	◆	◆	◆	◆	◆	◆	◆	◆	◆	◆	◆	◆	◆	◆
Colour	◆	◆	◆	◆	◆	◆	◆	◆	◆	◆	◆	◆	◆	◆
Ethnic or national origin	◆			◆	◆	◆	◆	◆	◆	◆	◆	◆	◆	◆
Ancestry or place of origin		◆	◆	◆	◆			◆			◆	◆	◆	◆
Creed or religion	◆	◆	◆	◆	◆	◆	◆	◆	◆	◆	◆	◆	◆	◆
Sex	◆	◆	◆	◆	◆	◆	◆	◆	◆	◆	◆	◆	◆	◆
Marital status	◆	◆	◆	◆	◆	◆	◆	◆	◆	◆	◆	◆	◆	◆
Family status	◆	◆	◆	◆			◆	◆	◆	◆	◆	◆	◆	◆
Age	◆	◆ 18+	◆ 19–65	◆		◆ 19–65	◆	◆ 18–65	◆	◆	◆ 18–64	◆	◆	◆
Mental & physical disability	◆	◆	◆	◆	◆	◆	◆	◆	◆	◆	◆	◆	◆	◆
Pardoned offence	◆		◆					◆		◆		◆		◆
Record of criminal conviction			◆						◆	◆			◆	
Sexual orientation	◆	◆	◆	◆	◆	◆	◆	◆	◆	◆	◆		◆	
Language								◆		◆			◆	

*Note: The legislation providing human rights protection and equal pay for equal work in Nunavut is titled the Fair Practices Act.

Source: Based on Canadian Human Rights Commission, *Prohibited Grounds of Discrimination in Canada* (December 1998), www.chrc.ccdp.ca/publications/prohibit-motifs.asp; and e-mail correspondence from Bill Riddell in Nunavut (July 24, 2000) <billr@nunanet.com>.

The Canadian Human Rights Act

Canadian Human Rights Act
Federal legislation prohibiting discrimination on a number of grounds, which applies to federal government agencies and crown corporations and to businesses and industries under federal jurisdiction.

The **Canadian Human Rights Act** is the human rights legislation that applies to businesses and industries under federal jurisdiction. Amended several times since it went into effect in March 1978, it currently specifies that:[5]

> All individuals should have an equal opportunity to make for themselves the lives that they are able and wish to have, consistent with their duties and obligations as members of society, without being hindered in or prevented from doing so by discriminatory practices based on race, national or ethnic origin, colour, religion, age, sex, sexual orientation, marital status, family status, disability or conviction for an offence for which a pardon has been granted.

Types of Discrimination Prohibited

intentional discrimination
Deliberately using criteria such as race, religion, sex, or other prohibited grounds when making employment decisions.

Intentional Discrimination Except in specific circumstances that will be described later, **intentional discrimination** is prohibited. An employer cannot discriminate *directly* by deliberately refusing to hire, train, or promote an individual, for example, on any of the prohibited grounds. It is important to realize

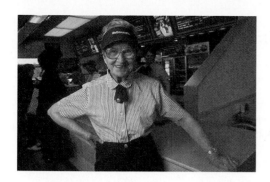

It is illegal in every jurisdiction in Canada to discriminate on the basis of age.

that deliberate discrimination is not necessarily overt. In fact, overt (blatant) discrimination is quite rare today. Subtle direct discrimination can be difficult to prove. For example, if a 60-year-old applicant is not selected for a job and is told that there was a better-qualified candidate, it is often difficult for the rejected job-seeker to determine if someone else truly did more closely match the firm's specifications or if the employer discriminated on the basis of age.

An employer is also prohibited from intentional discrimination in the form of *differential or unequal treatment.* No individuals or groups may be treated differently in any aspects or terms and conditions of employment based on any of the prohibited grounds. For example, it is illegal for an employer to request that only female applicants for a factory job demonstrate their lifting skills, or to insist that any candidates with a physical disability undergo a pre-employment medical, unless all applicants are being asked to do so.

It is also illegal for an employer to engage in intentional discrimination *indirectly*, through another party. This means that an employer may not ask someone else to discriminate on his or her behalf. For example, an employer cannot request that an employment agency refer only male candidates for consideration as management trainees, or instruct supervisors that women of childbearing age are to be excluded from consideration for promotions.

Discrimination because of association is another possible type of intentional discrimination listed specifically as a prohibited ground in six Canadian jurisdictions. It involves the denial of rights because of friendship or other relationship with a protected group member. An example would be the refusal of a firm to promote a highly qualified white male into senior management on the basis of the assumption that his wife, who was recently diagnosed with multiple sclerosis, will require too much of his time and attention, and that her needs may restrict his willingness to travel on company business.

Unintentional Discrimination

Unintentional discrimination (also known as **constructive** or **systemic discrimination**) is the most difficult to detect and combat. Typically, it is embedded in policies and practices that, although appearing neutral on the surface and being implemented impartially, have adverse impact on specific groups of people for reasons that are not job related or required for the safe and efficient operation of the business. Examples are shown in **Figure 3.2**.

Examples of Human Rights Legislation Applications

In order to clarify how the human rights legislation is applied, and the types of discrimination prohibited, a few examples follow.

Race and Colour   Discrimination on the basis of race and colour is illegal in every Canadian jurisdiction. Because these grounds are closely linked, it is often difficult to determine whether the discrimination was based on one or both. When Health Canada was found to be guilty of such discrimination by a three-person Canadian Human Rights Commission (CHRC) tribunal in March 1997, the story made news headlines:[6]

> Health Canada was found guilty of systemic discrimination for failing to promote visible minority employees to management positions. Evidence cited in the tribunal's 60-

unintentional/constructive/ systemic discrimination

Discrimination that is embedded in policies and practices that appear neutral on the surface, and are implemented impartially, but have adverse impact on specific groups of people for reasons that are not job related or required for the safe and efficient operation of the business.

FIGURE 3.2 Examples of Systemic Discrimination

- minimum height and weight requirements, such as formerly existed for the Canadian armed forces and many police forces, which screened out disproportionate numbers of women and Canadians of Asian origin, who tend to be shorter in stature
- internal hiring policies or word-of-mouth hiring in workplaces that have not embraced diversity
- limited accessibility of buildings and facilities, which poses a barrier to persons with mobility limitations
- culturally biased or non-job-related employment tests, which discriminate against specific groups
- job evaluation systems that undervalue jobs traditionally held by women
- promotions based exclusively on seniority and experience in firms that have historically been dominated by white males
- lack of explicit anti-harassment guidelines, or an organizational climate in which certain groups feel unwelcome and uncomfortable.

Source: Based on material provided by the Ontario Women's Directorate and the Canadian Human Rights Commission.

Urban Alliance on Race Relations
www.interlog.com/~uarr

page report included the fact that senior managers: considered persons of colour to be culturally different and did not consider them to be suitable for managerial positions; failed to inform them about management training opportunities or to invite them to apply for openings in such programs; and overlooked them for temporary management assignments. Since there was an adequate number of qualified visible minority candidates (16 in the management "feeder group"), the fact that only four had been selected by 1995 was attributed to the adverse impact of these employment practices. The department was given six months to begin correcting the problem and five years to complete the task, and was ordered to provide the CHRC with progress reports.

Age Age has been coming under increasing scrutiny as a criterion in employment decisions. While employers sometimes believe that specifying a minimum or maximum age is justifiable for certain jobs or types of work, there is very little evidence to support the position that age can legitimately be used to predict a person's ability to perform:[7]

A 37-year-old man filed a complaint when he was refused employment at Greyhound Lines of Canada Ltd. on the basis of age. The company, which only hired as drivers individuals between the ages of 24 and 35, justified its position based on the argument that new drivers get the least-favourable routes and must be young enough to cope with the related stress. The Tribunal ruled that there was insufficient evidence to conclude that the inability to cope with stress is related to age.

An important feature of the human rights legislation is that it supersedes the terms of any employment contract or collective agreement:[8]

In the collective agreement between an employer and the Brotherhood of Railway, Airline, and Steamship Clerks, age was used to rank on the seniority list employees hired on the same day. In her complaint against the union, Susan Tanel alleged that the policy resulted in her being denied upgrading from part-time to full-time work on the basis of age. She received compensation in settlement of her complaint. The union and employer, recognizing that their policy was an example of systemic discrimination and that age is not an appropriate measure of difference in seniority between two employees with equal length of service, no longer apply this or any other age-based seniority policy.

Sex   The Canadian Human Rights Act prohibits discrimination in employment policies and practices on the basis of sex. It is illegal for an employer to allow an individual's sex to influence its recruitment, selection, promotion, training, transfer, or termination policies and practices. Unless there is a justifiable job-related reason, it is also illegal to have separate policies for men and women (for example, specifying that certain jobs are to be performed by men only). Furthermore, employers cannot use or promote tests, standards, and/or other criteria that are biased or discriminate against one sex (or other protected group member), even if unintentionally, unless the employer can prove that such requirements are justifiable:[9]

> A woman received $3500 for lost wages and general damages in settlement of her complaint that a company's height requirement discriminated against women. She was refused an interview for a job as a bus driver because she did not meet the minimum height requirement of 173 cm (5 feet 8 inches). The case was settled, after conciliation. The company agreed to discontinue its practice of specifying a minimum height for drivers' positions, and has subsequently hired several women shorter than 173 cm. As part of the settlement, the company agreed that the CHRC would monitor its driver application records for one year.

In its 1989 decision against Canada Safeway Ltd., the Supreme Court of Canada clarified that discrimination on the basis of the fact that a woman is or could become pregnant is a form of sex discrimination and is therefore illegal. Prior to that time, it was fairly common to have short-term disability or weekly indemnity insurance plans that excluded pregnancy and related illnesses from coverage. Although the Supreme Court acknowledged that pregnancy is neither a sickness nor an accident, they ruled that it is a valid health-related reason for absence from work, and therefore cannot be excluded from benefit plan coverage or be treated differently from any other health-related absence:[10]

> Three women complained that their employer, Canada Safeway Ltd., discriminated against them on the basis of sex because, although the company provided insurance benefits to employees absent from work for medical reasons, pregnancy was excluded. The company argued that, on the basis of an earlier Supreme Court decision, although pregnant persons were treated differently from non-pregnant persons, this was not sex discrimination because not all women are or become pregnant. The Court rejected this argument and held that since only women become pregnant, a denial of health benefits to "pregnant people" is tantamount to denying those benefits to women. The Court also noted that for too long society [had] allowed employment practices to impose all of the costs of childbirth upon women.

Marital Status   Discrimination on the basis of marital status is also illegal:[11]

> An airline pilot complained to the CHRC when he lost his job. He claimed that he was released because he was married and the airline found it more convenient to employ single pilots. When the Human Rights Tribunal substantiated his claim, the company was ordered to pay him $24 487 in lost earnings and general damages.

Family Status

Only two Canadian jurisdictions do not prohibit discrimination on the basis of family status, defined in a number of jurisdictions as being in a parent-and-child relationship. The precedent-setting federal human rights commission case dealing with this ground involved the Canada Employment and Immigration Commission (CEIC)—now known as Human Resources Development Canada (HRDC):[12]

A complaint was filed by Ina Lang alleging that CEIC denied her application for funding under the Challenge '86 program because the individual whom she wished to hire to assist her in her childcare business was her daughter. A tribunal found that CEIC had discriminated on the basis of family status, and awarded Ms. Lang $1000 for hurt feelings. Although the CEIC appealed the decision, the Federal Court of Appeal upheld the tribunal's decision.

Pardoned Convicts

The federal legislation prohibits discrimination on the basis of conviction of a federal offence for which a pardon has been granted. Applications for pardon may not be submitted until a specified number of years (generally five) following release, parole, or completion of a sentence, and are investigated thoroughly by the RCMP, who verify that applicants have earned the right to have their records "expunged." The purpose is to ensure that individuals who have reformed their ways do not have past indiscretions held against them forever:[13]

A man convicted and pardoned for a drug-related offence applied for a job as a counsellor at a community correctional centre. He had extensive experience working with ex-inmates and the provincial commission on dependency, and was rated as the best candidate for the position. Correctional Services rejected him on the basis of his criminal record, however, arguing that even though he had received a pardon, he still represented a security risk. He appealed to the CHRC. Following the Commission's investigation, Correctional Services decided that the applicant's criminal record would not, in fact, inhibit his ability to meet the job requirements and, satisfied that he was suitable, offered him the position.

As indicated in CHRC's *Guide to Screening and Selection in Employment*, included as **Appendix 3.1**, employers cannot ask about arrest records. That makes sense, given that being arrested is not necessarily an indication of any wrongdoing. Employers in Ontario, Quebec, British Columbia, Nunavut, and the Northwest Territories, and those under federal jurisdiction elsewhere, cannot ask about conviction records, in general. If information about any criminal record is legitimately needed for employment purposes, the question that can be asked is: "Have you ever been convicted of a criminal offence for which a pardon has not been granted?" In British Columbia, Quebec, Prince Edward Island, and the Yukon, record of criminal conviction is a prohibited ground of discrimination, which means that even this question would be illegal. In all Canadian jurisdictions, it is permissible to ask if an applicant is eligible for bonding, if being bondable is a job requirement. (Bonding involves the firm taking out an insurance policy to cover any losses caused by employee dishonesty.)

Physical and Mental Disability

The Canadian Human Rights Act prohibits discrimination in employment policies and practices against an individual on the basis of physical or mental disability, unless accommodation would be impossible (e.g., a person who is blind cannot be employed as a truck driver or bus driver) or accommodating the individual's disability would cause the employer "undue hardship." Employers are not permitted to impose rigid physical standards for specific jobs unless they can prove that such standards are truly necessary. Those that cannot be justified may be deemed to constitute systemic discrimination. A good example is the height and weight requirements that were formerly specified by the Canadian armed forces. As this recent B.C. case illustrates, assuming that being physically fit is a legitimate job requirement is no longer permissible:[14]

> Dion Rogal was working as a security guard in Regina when he saw a help-wanted ad for carnival work in the Vancouver area. He telephoned Grace Dalgliesh, who told him that she was with West Coast Amusements and that the job, paying $1400 per month plus room and board, involved setting up and taking down rides, as well as dealing with the public. When Rogal informed Dalgliesh that he was 6'1" and 350 pounds, she replied that this was not a problem and that a West Coast uniform would fit him. Thus, Rogal accepted the job and gave his current employer two weeks' notice. During the notice period, he contacted Dalgliesh twice more to confirm their arrangements.
>
> When Rogal arrived in Vancouver, he was introduced to Grace's husband Bert, who actually managed the rides. Unbeknownst to Rogal at the time, Bert was actually an independent contractor for West Coast, running his own rides at their carnivals. Bert told Rogal that the job was for six months and confirmed the compensation arrangements. The next day, however, when he met Rogal for coffee, he told Rogal that he was "too big and too heavy" for the carnival's "fast-paced lifestyle." He stated that there were no uniforms big enough for Rogal, and handed him $179 to take the bus back to Regina.
>
> At the B.C. Human Rights Council Tribunal hearing, Rogal testified that, in firing him, Dalgliesh had "ripped his heart out" and left him with "below zero" confidence, such that he could not find employment for about six weeks thereafter. At the current time, he was working at a gas station for $5.50 per hour. Also introduced as evidence was a report by U.B.C. psychologist Mark Schaller that outlined studies "to the effect that people in North America generally have negative attitudes toward overweight individuals." Arbitrator Barbara Humphreys ruled that Dalgliesh discriminated against Rogal because of a perceived disability. There was no evidence, she noted, that size was a bona fide occupational requirement (defined on p. 86), or that Dalgliesh could not have accommodated Rogal. Since Dalgliesh did not actually work for West Coast, the firm was not held liable. She ordered Mr. Dalgliesh to pay Rogal $3500 for injury to his "dignity, feelings and self-respect" and $7750 as compensation for lost wages and expenses.

To ensure that the actual physical demands of the job are identified rather than assumed demands, some employers conduct physical demands analyses, which are described in Chapter 4. When such an analysis is distributed to each applicant, as a supplement to the job description, candidates can readily identify any job requirements that might pose a problem for them, so that accommodation strategies can be discussed.

Employers are also expected to accommodate the needs of individuals with mental disabilities, as this Quebec example illustrates:[15]

> A Quebec insurance company was ordered to pay $15 500 for failing to accommodate an employee with depression. The agent, referred to by a Quebec human rights tribunal as Ms. Grenier, was absent from work for nine months due to depression. Thereafter, on the advice of her doctor, she asked if she could work three days a week for two months, prior to returning to full-time employment. The company refused. The tribunal criticized *Assurances Générales des Caisses Désjardins* for not acknowledging Grenier's depression as a mental disability and dismissing it as a "short-term" problem.

The Canadian Council on Rehabilitation and Work
www.workink.com

Integrated Network of Disability Information and Education
www.indie.ca

Sexual Orientation

Since May of 1996, the Canadian Human Rights Act has prohibited discrimination on the basis of sexual orientation (whether an individual is heterosexual, homosexual, or bisexual). In 1998, the Supreme Court of Canada read sexual orientation into the Alberta legislation. Based on that decision, sexual orientation is now a prohibited ground of discrimination in all jurisdictions except the North West Territories and Nunavut:[16]

> In *Vriend v. Alberta*, the Supreme Court of Canada held that Alberta's Individual's Rights Protection Act violated the equality provision of the Canadian Charter of Rights and Freedoms because it did not include sexual orientation as a prohibited ground of discrimination, and ordered that the words "sexual orientation" be read into the statute.

Bolstered by the Supreme Court's decision in *Vriend,* the Ontario Court of Appeal dismantled another barrier to equal rights for gay men and lesbians in the workplace in its decision in *Rosenberg v. Canada*. In the past, federal income tax rules served as a stumbling block to equal pension benefits for homosexual employees, since the Income Tax Act only permitted private pension plans to be registered with Revenue Canada if survivor benefits were restricted to spouses of the opposite sex. In a unanimous decision, the Court of Appeal held that the definition of "spouse" in the Income Tax Act violated the equality provisions of the Charter and had to be expanded to include same-sex couples.[17]

The May 1999 Supreme Court ruling in *M v. H* (featured in the Video Case at the end of Part 1) made it clear that any legislation in which the definition of spouse did not include same-sex couples would be declared unconstitutional, if challenged under the Charter.

> The Supreme Court of Canada held that the definition of spouse in the support obligation provisions of the Ontario Family Law Act violated the Charter because it provided for benefits entitlement to opposite-sex partners only, and the provincial legislature was ordered to amend the Act within six months.

Since that time, a number of jurisdictions have introduced legislation to amend all required statutes to extend the same rights to gay spouses as are provided to those in common-law heterosexual relationships. An example is Bill C-23, The Modernization of Benefits and Obligations Act, federal legislation that received first reading on February 11, 2000. With a projected effective date of January 1, 2001, Bill C-23 was designed to amend 68 federal statutes, including the Canada Pension Plan, Employment Insurance, Old Age Security, Income Tax, and Pension Benefits Standards Acts and a series of statutory federal public service plans. It introduced a new definition of "common-law partners" to include both opposite-sex and same-sex couples who have cohabited for at least one year.[18]

Specific Human Rights Legislation Issues

Bona Fide Occupational Requirements

bona fide occupational requirement (BFOR)
A justifiable reason for discrimination based on business necessity (that is, required for the safe and efficient operation of the organization) or a requirement that can be clearly defended as intrinsically required by the tasks an employee is expected to perform.

Employers are permitted to discriminate if employment preferences are based on a **bona fide occupational requirement (BFOR)**, defined as a justifiable reason for discrimination based on business necessity (i.e., required for the safe and efficient operation of the organization) or a requirement that can be clearly defended as intrinsically required by the tasks that an employee is expected to perform. There are some settings in which a BFOR exception to human rights protection is fairly obvious. For example, if a boutique handling ladies' apparel requires its salespersons to model the merchandise, sex is clearly a BFOR. When casting in the theatre, there may be specific roles that justify using age, sex, or national origin as a recruitment and selection criterion.

The issue of BFORs gets more complicated in situations in which the occupational requirement is less obvious; the onus of proof is then placed on the employer. There are a number of instances in which BFORs have been established. For example, adherence to the tenets of the Roman Catholic Church has been deemed a BFOR when selecting faculty to teach in a Roman Catholic school.[19] The Royal Canadian Mounted Police has a requirement that guards be of the same sex as prisoners being guarded, which was also ruled to be a BFOR.[20] However, sex has often not been allowed as a BFOR in what, on the surface, might seem to be reasonable circumstances, such as a male-dominated worksite or a workplace lacking a women's washroom.[21] A 1982 Supreme Court of Canada decision established that mandatory retirement at age 60 for firefighters in Etobicoke, Ontario was not a BFOR, even though honestly imposed, because there was insufficient evidence that reaching that age impaired ability to perform adequately.[22] In another case, the CHRC ruled that visual acuity standards established by VIA Rail were not a BFOR because VIA was unable to justify the objectivity of such standards.[23] Another example of a situation in which company standards were not deemed to represent a BFOR follows:[24]

> A man, who was tested without his hearing aid, was refused a technician's job because he failed the hearing test administered by the firm. Although he asserted that he could hear well with his hearing aid and could certainly perform the job, the company's medical advisors claimed that the job required normal hearing. After conciliation, the company agreed that the applicant was correct and that normal hearing was not a BFOR. The man was hired as a technician and paid damages of $750.

Reasonable Accommodation

reasonable accommodation

The adjustment of employment policies and practices that an employer may be expected to make so that no individual is denied benefits, disadvantaged in employment, or prevented from carrying out the essential components of a job because of grounds prohibited in human rights legislation.

undue hardship

The point to which employers are expected to accommodate under human rights legislative requirements.

Employers who believe there is a BFOR for denying employment or assignment to a specific job may encounter the legal principle of **reasonable accommodation**, which requires the adjustment of employment policies and practices so that no individual is denied benefits, disadvantaged in employment, or prevented from carrying out the essential components of a job on the basis of prohibited grounds of discrimination. This may involve making adjustments to meet needs based on the group to which an individual belongs, such as scheduling adjustments to accommodate religious beliefs, or on an individual employee basis, such as work station redesign to enable an individual with a physical disability to perform a particular task.

Employers are expected to accommodate to the point of **undue hardship**, a term for which there is no definitive definition. Generally, however, to claim undue hardship, employers must present evidence that the financial cost of the accommodation (even with outside sources of funding) or health and safety risks to the individual concerned or other employees would make accommodation impossible. Factors that cannot be taken into consideration include business inconvenience, customer preference, or disruption to a collective agreement.[25]

Failure to make every reasonable effort to accommodate employees is a violation of the Act:[26]

> After becoming a member of the Worldwide Church of God, the complainant—who worked for the Central Alberta Dairy Pool at a milk-processing plant—requested unpaid leave for a particular Monday to observe a church holy day. Because Mondays were especially busy days at the plant, his request was refused. When he failed to report for work, he was fired.

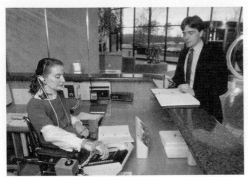

Persons with disabilities are now employed in a wide range of fields and occupations. An example is Nancy Thibeault, the telephone operator and receptionist at PAC Corporation.

The Job Accommodation Network of Canada

http://janweb.icdi.wvu.edu

IBM Canada Web site—Accommodating Persons with Disabilities

www.austin.ibm.com/sns/guidelines.htm

harassment

A wide range of behaviour that a reasonable person ought to know is unwelcome, as well as actions and activities that were once tolerated, ignored, and considered horseplay or innocent flirtation, provided that the individual who feels that he or she is being harassed makes it clear that such behaviour is unwelcome and inappropriate and asks that it be discontinued.

The Supreme Court of Canada (1990) ruled that the employer had discriminated on the basis of religion in failing to accommodate to the point of undue hardship. The court found that since Dairy Pool could cope with employee absences on Mondays due to illness, it could also accommodate a single instance of absence due to religious reasons.

In accommodating unionized employees, the employer and union have a joint (but not equal) responsibility. According to the Supreme Court of Canada (*Renaud*, 1992), there are two situations in which a union has a duty to accommodate.

The first situation is one in which the union participated in the formulation of a work rule that has a discriminatory effect on a complainant (that is, there is a provision in the collective agreement that has an adverse impact). In such case, the union shares a joint responsibility. Employers must make every effort to accommodate an employee within the parameters of a collective agreement. However, the union can become involved before the employer has exhausted all options that would not involve amendments to the union contract. The union must be involved in situations in which the proposed accommodation would have an impact on the contract or bargaining unit employee rights. While the employer is expected to initiate the accommodation process, refusal by the union to consent to reasonable accommodation measures in this type of situation would expose both parties to liability as co-discriminators.

The second situation in which the union has a duty to accommodate is one in which the lack of union support would impede the employer's reasonable efforts to accommodate an employee, even though the union did not participate in the formulation or application of the specific rule or practice that is the source of discrimination.[27]

In some situations, duty to accommodate may be related to testing standards. Employers requiring a high standard of fitness, for example, may face problems developing fair tests. If standards are set too low, people's lives may be endangered; too high a standard may mean losing otherwise highly qualified people—particularly women—to an arbitrary standard. For example, the Supreme Court ruled that the physical fitness testing being used to screen B.C. forest firefighters was illegal, since it failed to accommodate the physiological differences between men and women. (See Chapter 7 for details.)[28]

Harassment Federal legislation and that in Ontario, Quebec, and the Yukon prohibits harassment on all proscribed grounds. In a number of other jurisdictions, only sexual harassment is expressly banned. **Harassment** includes a wide range of behaviour that a reasonable person ought to know is unwelcome; however, it also encompasses actions and activities that were once tolerated, ignored, and considered horseplay or innocent flirtation, provided that the individual who feels that he or she is being harassed makes it clear that such behaviour is unwelcome and inappropriate and asks that it be discontinued. Examples of the types of behaviour that may constitute harassment are included in **Figure 3.3**. In the case of blatantly inappropriate actions, such as physical assault, one incident may constitute harassment. Generally, however, harassment involves a series of incidents. Protection against harassment extends to incidents occurring at or away from the workplace, during or outside normal working hours, provided such incidents are employment-related.[29] An employer is also responsible for dealing with employee harassment by clients or customers once it has been reported.

FIGURE 3.3 Examples of Behaviours That May Constitute Harassment

- physical assault
- unnecessary physical contact, such as patting, pinching, touching, or punching
- verbal abuse or threats
- unwelcome invitations or requests, whether subtle or explicit, and intimidation
- unwelcome remarks, jokes, innuendos, or taunting about a person's body, attire, age, marital status, ethnic or national origin, religion, etc.
- leering or other gestures
- displaying pornographic, racist, or other offensive or derogatory pictures
- practical jokes that cause awkwardness or embarrassment
- condescension or paternalism that undermines self-respect.

Source: Based on material provided by the Ontario Women's Directorate and the Canadian Human Rights Commission.

Example of Harassment on the Basis of Ethnic Origin

A federal department employee filed a complaint with the CHRC after she was harassed because of her Italian origin. Several coworkers directed toward her derogatory remarks about Italians and called her names. She complained to her supervisor, who failed to investigate her allegations, merely telling her that such behaviour went on in the office and that she was being overemotional. The commission concluded that the complainant was being harassed. The department agreed to pay the employee $1200 as compensation for hurt feelings. A memorandum was circulated to all employees reminding them that discriminatory remarks about a person's ethnic origin are a form of harassment and would not be tolerated.[30]

Employer Responsibility   In 1987 (*Robichaud v. Treasury Board*), the Supreme Court of Canada made it clear that employers and managers have a responsibility to provide a safe and healthy working environment. If harassment is occurring, of which they are aware or ought to have been aware, they can be charged as well as the alleged harasser.[31] To reduce liability, employers should establish sound corporate harassment policies, communicate such policies to all employees, enforce the policies in a fair and consistent manner, and take an active role in maintaining a working environment that is free of harassment.

Sexual Harassment   The type of harassment that has attracted the most attention in the workplace is **sexual harassment**. According to one noted scholar, sexual harassment can be divided into two categories: sexual coercion and sexual annoyance.[32]

Sexual coercion involves harassment of a sexual nature that results in some direct consequence to the worker's employment status or some gain in or loss of tangible job benefits. Typically, this involves a supervisor using control over employment, pay, performance appraisal results, or promotion, to attempt to coerce an employee to grant sexual favours. If the worker agrees to the request, tangible job benefits follow; if the worker refuses, job benefits are denied.

Sexual annoyance is sexually related conduct that is hostile, intimidating, or offensive to the employee, but has no direct link to tangible job benefits or loss thereof. Rather, a "poisoned" work environment is created for the employee, the

sexual harassment
Harassment on the basis of gender or sexual attractiveness or unattractiveness.

sexual coercion
Harassment of a sexual nature that results in some direct consequence to the worker's employment status or some gain in or loss of tangible job benefits.

sexual annoyance
Sexually-related conduct that is hostile, intimidating, or offensive to the employee, but has no direct link to tangible job benefits or loss thereof.

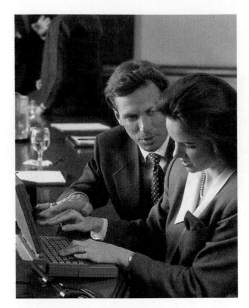

A poisoned work environment may exist even if no direct threats or promises are made.

tolerance of which effectively becomes a term or condition of employment. The following case provides an illustration of this type of harassment, as well as the consequences of management's failure to take corrective action:[33]

A woman who put up with 14 years of sexual harassment before quitting her job was awarded nearly $50 000 in damages by an Ontario Human Rights Board of Inquiry. The woman, who worked as a bookkeeper at Levac Supply Ltd., shared a general office area with the office manager, with whom she initially got along very well. After a few months, he became less friendly and began making noises and comments aimed at her, implying that she was working slowly or incompetently. He also began to make personal comments about her size, referring to her and other female employees as "fridge sisters," and making snide comments behind her back. Particularly demeaning to the woman involved were the comments "swish, swish" and "waddle, waddle" when she was wearing nylons. She sometimes yelled at him to "get off her back," but his behaviour continued. While he admitted to "bugging" and "teasing" her, he stated that he had done it simply to "get more productivity" out of her, and that he hadn't realized his comments were upsetting her. The board, however, found that monitoring her productivity was not his job and that his "digs" drove her to tears at times, a fact of which he was well aware. The complainant stated that she had complained about three or four times a year to the head of company operations about the harassment, but no one tried to remedy the situation. The board ruled that the comments—especially the ones which the woman found particularly offensive—implied sexual unattractiveness and, as such, constituted harassment because of sex (gender). The manager was found to have engaged in repeated verbal conduct of a sexual nature, which created an offensive working environment for the victim. Since the head of operations did nothing to stop the harassment, he, the office manager, and the company were ordered to pay her a total of $48 273 in damages.

Harassment Policies   An amendment to the Canada Labour Code in 1985 made it mandatory for all organizations operating under federal jurisdiction to develop and implement sexual harassment policies. Many organizations under provincial/territorial or municipal jurisdiction or receiving government funding have a similar legal obligation. Increasingly, however, organizations are developing policies to deal with harassment, whether or not they are required by law to do so.

Complying with the legal obligation to provide a "poison-free" workplace and exercise due diligence after a complaint is lodged does not necessarily require severe discipline in every case. In fact, imposing unduly harsh discipline (in view of the specific circumstances) can lead to a wrongful or constructive dismissal lawsuit.[34] A few guidelines to ensure a harassment-free workplace follow:[35]

> **Hints to Ensure Legal Compliance**

1. Develop a harassment policy that prohibits harassment on all grounds specified in the applicable human rights legislation (as in the example included as **Figure 3.4**).

2. Develop a harassment procedure that: provides several persons with whom complaints can be filed; guarantees confidentiality to the greatest extent possible; outlines the investigation process and sets time limits for each step; specifies that no record of the complaint will be placed in the HR file of the individual voicing the complaint unless he or she is proven to have filed a false charge with malicious intent; states that no record of a harassment charge will be placed in the file of the accused unless harassment is proven; and provides a range of possible penalties. Termination of employment

FIGURE 3.4 Policy for a Harassment-free Work Environment

MUTUAL RESPECT POLICY AT UNION GAS

POLICY FOR A HARASSMENT-FREE WORK ENVIRONMENT

We believe that everyone has the inherent right to work in an environment characterized by mutual respect, and we are committed to ensuring a workplace that is free from harassment.

Union Gas will treat any complaint of harassment as a serious matter. Any complaint of harassment will be investigated in a confidential manner and, where substantiated, individuals will be subject to appropriate corrective action, or disciplinary measures, up to and including dismissal.

All management and union executives have a responsibility under this policy to promote a harassment-free work environment and to ensure any complaints they receive are addressed.

Source: Excerpted from Union Gas Limited's Mutual Respect Policy, as cited in Ministry of Citizenship, Culture and Recreation, *Equal Opportunity in Ontario* (Toronto: Queen's Printer, 1999), p. 17. © Queen's Printer for Ontario, 1999. Reprinted with permission.

should be included as an option if harassment is proven or if an individual is found guilty of filing a false harassment charge with malicious intent.

3. Provide training regarding the types of behaviour that may constitute harassment and the specifics of the company policy and procedure.

4. Require each employee to sign and return a document indicating that he or she has received harassment training, is now aware of the types of behaviour that may constitute harassment, and is familiar with the company harassment policy and procedure.

5. Conduct a thorough, unbiased investigation whenever a complaint is filed. Do not assume that the alleged harasser is guilty. Provide the accused with details regarding the complaint and ample opportunity for him or her to respond to each allegation or to have someone respond on his or her behalf.

6. When harassment is proven, before deciding upon an appropriate course of action consider all relevant factors, such as the complainant's wishes, the nature and frequency of the conduct, the position and length of service of the harasser, and the potential adverse effects on the corporate culture, client/customer relations, viability of the business, etc. Options include counselling, a verbal or written apology, a verbal or written warning, a transfer or demotion, a suspension for a period ranging from one day to several months, and termination of employment.

7. Consider the same range of possible options when determining an appropriate course of action to deal with an individual found guilty of filing a false accusation with malicious intent.

8. Offer harassment victims access to counselling and support through the firm's Employee Assistance Program.

9. Monitor the workplace, both to ensure that any harassment that is occurring is being reported and to prevent a poisoned work environment from developing.

10. Remember that harassment comes in many forms. Don't forget to monitor e-mails as well as letters/memoranda, posters/calendars, verbal comments and behaviour.

Court decisions have upheld harassment as just cause for dismissal when circumstances warrant. For example, the discharge of an employee who sexually harassed his secretary (causing her to file a complaint with the Human Rights Commission) was upheld,[36] as was the discharge of a manager who was found guilty of sexually harassing a coworker (even though no complaint was filed with a Human Rights Commission).[37] Employers should be aware, however, that to justify dismissal for harassment, courts expect firms to have a harassment policy and to conduct an appropriate investigation when allegations are made. Otherwise, such dismissals may be overturned.[38]

Special Programs

Section 16(1) of the Canadian Human Rights Act legalizes employment equity initiatives, which are special programs developed by employers to remedy past discrimination and/or prevent future discrimination:[39]

> It is not a discriminatory practice for a person to adopt or carry out a special program, plan, or arrangement designed to prevent disadvantages that are likely to be suffered by, or to eliminate or reduce disadvantages that are suffered by, any group of individuals when those disadvantages would be based on or related to the prohibited grounds of discrimination, by improving opportunities respecting goods, services, facilities, accommodation, or employment in relation to that group.

Similar wording is found in the human rights legislation in most Canadian jurisdictions.

Employer Retaliation

It is a criminal offence to retaliate against someone exercising rights under human rights legislation. Whether filing charges, testifying, or participating in a human rights action in another way, individuals are protected. Thus, it is against the law for a supervisor to attempt to "get even" with an employee who has testified in a case by disciplining or demoting him/her.

Enforcement

Canadian Human Rights Commission (CHRC)
The body responsible for the implementation and enforcement of the Canadian Human Rights Act.

Canadian Human Rights Commission

www.chrc-ccdp.ca

As you may have deduced from the case examples on the previous pages, the **Canadian Human Rights Commission (CHRC)** is the body responsible for enforcing the Canadian Human Rights Act. Appointed by the Governor-in-Council, the members of CHRC include a chief commissioner, a deputy chief commissioner, full-time members appointed for a term of not more than seven years; and three to six part-time members, appointed for a maximum term of three years.

The CHRC deals with complaints concerning discriminatory practices covered by the Act, and also has the power to issue guidelines regarding its interpretation. Any individual or group may file a complaint with the CHRC, given that they have reasonable grounds to believe they have been discriminated against. The CHRC may refuse to accept the complaint for the following reasons:[40]

- there is another law that would better deal with the matter
- the matter is outside of the Commission's authority or jurisdiction

Canadian Human Rights Tribunal
www.chrt-tcdp.gc.ca

Alberta Human Rights and
Citizenship Commission
www.albertahumanrights.ab.ca

British Columbia Human Rights
Commission
www.bchrc.gov.bc.ca

Manitoba Human Rights
Commission
www.gov.mb.ca/hrc

New Brunswick Human Rights
Commission
www.gov.nb.ca/hrc-
cdp/e/index.htm

Newfoundland Human Rights
Commission
www.gov.nf.ca/hrc

Nova Scotia Human Rights
Commission
www.gov.ns.ca/humanrights

Ontario Human Rights Commission
www.ohrc.on.ca

Prince Edward Island Human
Rights Commission
www.isn.net/peihrc

Québec Commission des droits de
la personne et des droits de la
jeunesse
www.cdpdj.qc.ca

Saskatchewan Human Rights
Commission
www.gov.sk.ca/shrc

Yukon Human Rights Commission
www.yhrc.yk.ca

- the complaint seems trivial, vexatious or to have been filed in bad faith
- the complainant waited more than six months after the last incident on which the complaint is based to sign a complaint. (The CHRC can deal with a complaint filed beyond this time limit *if* it is satisfied that the delay was incurred in good faith *and* no substantial prejudice will result to any person because of the delay.)

Once the CHRC accepts the legitimacy of a written complaint, it assumes responsibility for pursuing the investigation and defending the decision reached. The steps involved in the enforcement procedure are outlined in **Figure 3.5**. It should be noted that all costs are borne by the CHRC, not by the complainant, which makes the process accessible to all employees, regardless of financial means. The CHRC itself can initiate a complaint if it has reasonable grounds to assume that a party is engaging in a discriminatory practice.

Remedies for Violations

If discrimination is found, a number of remedies can be imposed. The most common is compensation for lost wages. Other financial remedies include compensation for general damages, complainant expenses, and pain and humiliation. The violator is generally asked to restore the rights, opportunities, and privileges denied the victim, such as employment or promotion. A written letter of apology may be required. If a pattern of discrimination is detected, the employer will be ordered to cease such practices and may be required to attend a training session or hold regular human rights workshops, and may even be ordered to develop and implement an employment equity program.

Anyone obstructing an investigation or tribunal, failing to comply with the terms of a settlement, or reducing wages in order to eliminate a discriminatory practice can be found guilty of an offence punishable by a fine and/or jail sentence. The fines range from up to $5000 for an individual to $50 000 for an employer or employee organization.[41]

Provincial/Territorial Human Rights Enforcement Procedures

Each province and territory has its own human rights commission (HRC) or equivalent, with regulations and procedures similar to those of the CHRC. A person believing that he or she has been discriminated against can contact an officer, who will conduct an investigation and attempt to arrive at a settlement that satisfies everyone involved. While most cases are settled at this stage, if an agreement cannot be reached the case is presented to the HRC or equivalent. The members study the evidence and then submit a report to the minister responsible for administering the legislation, who may subsequently decide to appoint a board of inquiry, which has powers similar to those of the federal tribunal. Failing to comply with the decision of the board of inquiry can result in prosecution in a provincial/territorial court of law, resulting in a fine, the maximum amount of which varies by jurisdiction. Any provincial/territorial court decision pertaining to an issue that has implications for the nation as a whole can ultimately be appealed to the Supreme Court of Canada.

EQUITY

The Charter of Rights and Freedoms and human rights legislation focus on prohibiting various kinds of discrimination, thereby attempting to create a level playing field in the employment relationship. However, over time it became

FIGURE 3.5 The CHRC Enforcement Process

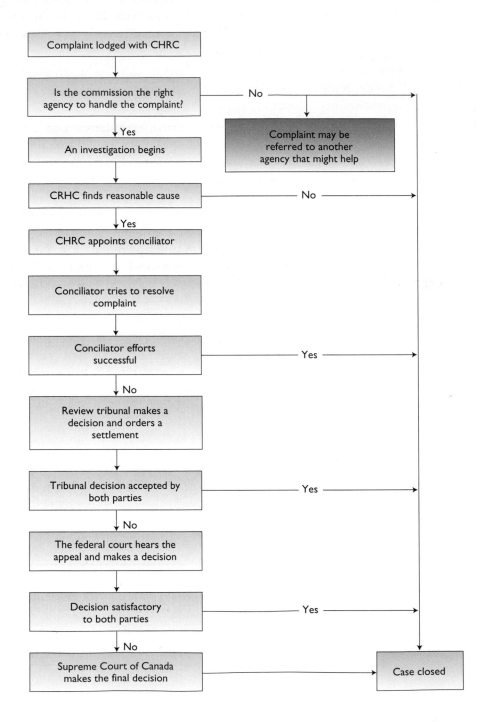

obvious that there were certain groups for whom this complaints-based, reactive approach was insufficient. Investigation revealed that four identifiable groups—women, Aboriginal people, persons with disabilities, and visible minorities—had been subjected to pervasive patterns of differential treatment by employers, as evidenced by lower pay on average, occupational segregation, higher rates of unemployment, underemployment, and concentration in low-status jobs with little potential for career growth.

occupational segregation

The existence of certain occupations that have traditionally been male dominated and others that have been female dominated.

glass ceiling

An invisible barrier, caused by attitudinal or organizational bias, which limits the advancement opportunities of qualified designated group members.

For example, historically, 60 percent of all women worked in 20 of 500 possible occupational classifications. This is known as **occupational segregation.** Advancement of women and other designated group members into senior management positions has been hindered by the existence of a **glass ceiling**, an "invisible" barrier caused by attitudinal or organizational bias, which limits the advancement opportunities of qualified individuals.

Research Insight

Several recent studies have confirmed that the glass ceiling is still intact. For example, an extensive Conference Board of Canada survey of CEOs, female executives and HR professionals found that while women make up almost half of the Canadian work force, they are still underrepresented on executive teams, comprising just 20 percent of the private sector's top jobs (defined as vice-president or higher) and 40 percent of such jobs in the public sector.[42] The study also found that there is a tremendous difference between the perceptions of CEOs and female executives. For example, while 69 percent of female executives indicated that not being taken seriously at work is more of a problem for women than for men, only 42 percent of CEOs felt that this was the case. Many of the CEOs believe that there had been a glass ceiling but now that it has been talked about and exposed, it doesn't exist anymore.[43]

underutilization

Having a smaller proportion of designated group members in particular jobs, occupations, departments, or levels of the organization than is found in the labour market.

The results of another recent study, involving 560 of Canada's largest companies and conducted by Catalyst (a nonprofit group that works for the advancement of women in business), are highlighted in **Figures 3.6 and 3.7**. In these firms, there is concrete evidence of **underutilization** of female employees. Women make up only 12 percent of corporate officers, and 7.5 percent of board

FIGURE **3.6** Snapshot: Women in Canadian Corporate Leadership Positions in Canada's 560 Largest Firms

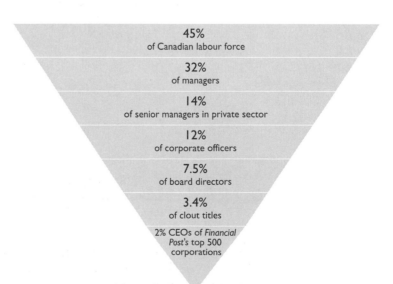

45%
of Canadian labour force

32%
of managers

14%
of senior managers in private sector

12%
of corporate officers

7.5%
of board directors

3.4%
of clout titles

2% CEOs of *Financial Post's* top 500 corporations

Source: Catalyst Census of Women Corporate Officers of Canada, in "Few Women Sitting in Top Posts," *Canadian HR Reporter* 13, no. 6 (March 27, 2000), p. 7. © Carswell, Thomson Professional Publishing. Reprinted with permission of *Canadian HR Reporter*, Carswell, One Corporate Plaza, 2075 Kennedy Road, Scarborough M1T 3V4.

FIGURE 3.7 Representation of Women Among Corporate Officers in Canada's 560 Largest Firms

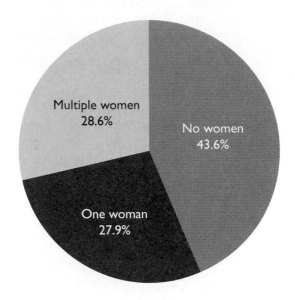

Source: Catalyst Census of Women Corporate Officers of Canada, in "Few Women Sitting in Top Posts," *Canadian HR Reporter* 13, no. 6 (March 27, 2000), p. 7. © Carswell, Thomson Professional Publishing. Reprinted by permission of *Canadian HR Reporter,* Carswell, One Corporate Plaza, 2075 Kennedy Road, Scarborough M1T 3V4.

concentration

Having a higher proportion of designated group members in specific jobs, occupations, departments, or levels of the organization than is found in the labour market.

Aboriginal Links: Canada & U.S.
www.bloorstreet.com/300block/aborcan.htm

directors; almost 44 percent of Canadian firms have no women in corporate officer positions. In this study, engineering firms fared most poorly, with women making up only 5.2 percent of all officers. Financial institutions had the highest female representation, at 17.9 percent.[44] Given these findings, it is not surprising that a Canadian financial institution, featured in the Diversity Counts box, was one of three companies awarded a 1999 Catalyst Award for outstanding initiatives to advance women into leadership roles in the workplace.

In most companies, there has tended to be a **concentration** of women in certain professions, which have been undervalued and underpaid. In 1999, 70 percent of women were working in such traditionally female-dominated occupations as teaching, nursing and other health-related occupations, clerical or administrative positions, and sales and service occupations—down from 74 percent in 1987. Women continue to be underrepresented in engineering, natural sciences and mathematics, a trend unlikely to change in the near future since women are still underrepresented in university programs in these fields.[45]

The number of young Aboriginal workers increased dramatically during the 1990s; in western Canada they account for a large portion of labour market growth. Many Aboriginal workers are concentrated in low-paying, unstable employment, especially in urban centres.

As of 1998, only 48 percent of Canadians with disabilities between the ages of 15 and 64 had either full- or part-time jobs, compared to 73 percent of Canadians without disabilities. Moreover, 54 percent of persons with disabilities had annual incomes of $15 000 or less.[46] Persons with disabilities face attitudinal barriers, physical demands unrelated to actual job requirements, and inadequate access to the technical and human support systems that would make it possible for them to obtain productive employment.

DIVERSITY COUNTS

At TD Bank Financial Group

The TD Bank Financial Group won a 1999 Catalyst Award for its program *Advancing Together,* a multiple-tier initiative that fosters career development, succession planning, respect, and flexibility for women. One strategy of the TD program involves identifying high-potential women and helping them to plan career paths, fill educational or skills gaps, and increase their visibility to senior executives.

The results verify the program's success: the number of female executive officers—individuals in positions ranging from associate vice-presidents to CEOs—more than doubled between 1994 and 1998, from eight percent to 17.8 percent.

Source: Based on "TD Bank Awarded for Program," *Canadian HR Reporter* 12, no. 3 (February 8, 1999), p. 12.

underemployment

Being employed in a job that does not fully utilize one's knowledge, skills and abilities (KSAs).

Canadian Information Centre for International Credentials

www.cicic.ca

In 1996, about 3.2 million Canadians were visible minority group members,[47] constituting 11.2 percent of the population, up from 9.2 percent in 1991 and 6.3 percent in 1986. This increase is largely the result of immigration. More than three-quarters of those who came to Canada during the 1990s were members of a visible minority group.[48] According to recent Statistics Canada findings, males aged 25 to 44 who emigrated to Canada between 1986 and 1996 were twice as likely to hold university degrees as Canadian-born males in the same age bracket (36 percent compared to 18 percent), but only 73 percent of university-educated male immigrants held jobs in 1996, compared to 92 percent of men born in Canada. A greater proportion of new immigrants ended up in sales and services jobs, and a large percentage ended up in part-time or part-year work. While women's general employment rate rose by eight percentage points to 73 percent during the same decade, immigrant women's employment dropped seven percentage points to 51 percent. Many immigrants obtain employment in jobs that do not take full advantage of their skills and qualifications; this is known as **underemployment**. Systemic barriers that have a negative impact on employment opportunities for visible minorities range from culturally biased aptitude tests, to language-skills demands in excess of job requirements, to lack of recognition of credentials gained elsewhere.[49] Recognizing how difficult it is for employers to assess educational equivalencies, various governments, professional bodies, and educational institutions have established assessment centres.

After realizing that simply levelling the playing field would not correct these patterns, a number of jurisdictions passed two categories of legislation, which will be explored next:

1. *Employment equity,* aimed at identifying and eliminating systemic barriers to employment opportunities that adversely affect these four groups.
2. *Pay equity,* which focuses on mechanisms to redress the imbalance in pay between male-dominated and female-dominated job classes resulting from the undervaluing of work traditionally performed by women.

Employment Equity

In 1983, the federal government appointed a royal commission, chaired by Judge Rosalie Abella, to review the employment practices of federal crown and government-owned operations. Its report, tabled in 1984, made recommendations about how the four traditionally disadvantaged groups identified above could be brought into the mainstream of Canada's labour force. The commission recommended that legislation be enacted to cover all federally-regulated employers, that provincial/territorial governments be urged to pass similar legislation, and that the term "employment equity" be used to distinguish Canada's approach from that taken toward "affirmative action" in the U.S. Affirmative action had, by then, become associated with quotas (described later in this chapter), a divisive political issue.[50]

Employment Equity Act

Employment Equity Act

Federal legislation, proclaimed in August of 1987, the intent of which is to remove employment barriers and promote equality for the members of four designated groups: women, visible minorities, Aboriginal people, and persons with disabilities.

Federal Employment Equity Act
http://info.load-otea.hrdc-drhc.gc.ca/~weeweb/lege.htm

The federal **Employment Equity Act** was proclaimed in August of 1987 and amended in 1995. The intent of this legislation is to remove employment barriers and promote equality for the members of the four designated groups. It requires federally-regulated employers with more than 100 employees to develop on a yearly basis a plan containing specific goals to achieve better representation of the designated group members at all levels of the organization, and timetables for goal implementation. Those covered are also required to submit an annual report to HRDC, describing their progress in meeting the goals specified in the plan, indicating the representation of designated group members by occupational groups and salary ranges, and providing information on those hired, promoted, and terminated. These reports are forwarded to the CHRC by HRDC and are available to the public. Employers are required to retain each plan and all records used to prepare their annual reports for a period of at least three years. Those failing to comply may be investigated by the CHRC and, if necessary, prosecuted under the Canadian Human Rights Act. In addition, the CHRC has the authority to monitor for compliance through the use of random audits.[51]

Federal Contractors Program

Federal Contractors Program

A provision of the Employment Equity Act that requires firms with 100 or more employees wishing to bid on federal contracts of $200 000 or more to certify their commitment to employment equity in writing and to implement an employment equity program.

A large number of employers under provincial/territorial jurisdiction are subject to federal employment equity requirements under the **Federal Contractors Program**. A provision of the Employment Equity Act, it requires firms with 100 or more employees wishing to bid on federal contracts of $200 000 or more to certify in writing their commitment to employment equity and to implement an employment equity program as a condition of the bid. These companies are subject to random on-site compliance reviews. If such a review reveals that an employer has failed to implement an employment equity program, sanctions are applied, including exclusion of the employer from future government contracts.[52]

Employment Equity Programs

Mandatory equity programs are virtually nonexistent in provincial and territorial jurisdictions. Quebec has a contract compliance program. A far-reaching, proactive employment equity law enacted in Ontario under an NDP government, which received proclamation on September 1, 1994, was subsequently repealed by the Progressive Conservative government during the fall of 1995. All provincially regulated employers were covered, except: broader public-sector employers with fewer than 10 employees; private-sector employers with fewer than 50 employees; and police forces covered by the Police Services Act.

Voluntary employment equity programs are legalized under the human rights legislation in most Canadian jurisdictions. Provincial/territorial human rights commissions often provide assistance to employers wishing to implement such initiatives.

Alliance for Employment Equity
www.web.net/~allforee

employment equity program
A detailed plan designed to identify and correct existing discrimination, redress past discrimination, and achieve a balanced representation of designated group members in the organization.

Many employers not legally required to implement an employment equity program, such as Sir Sandford Fleming College in Peterborough, Ontario, have done so voluntarily, believing that it makes good business sense. From a practical point of view, employers seldom benefit by excluding people who belong to a particular group, such as women or visible minorities, since that limits the labour pool from which to select employees. Being perceived to be discriminatory can also lead to negative public relations for a firm, consumer boycotts, and/or government intervention.

The Implementation of Employment Equity

An **employment equity program** is designed to identify and correct existing discrimination, redress past discrimination, and achieve a balanced representation of designated group members in the organization. As such, it is much more than a formal document prepared by an HR specialist; it is a major change-management exercise. Successful implementation requires that employment equity be incorporated in the organization's strategic planning process.[53] Different groups within an organization should be involved in the implementation process, including senior management, HR specialists, all other managers and supervisors, and union/nonunion employee representatives. A deliberately structured process is involved, which is tailored to suit the unique needs of the firm. The process includes six main steps, each of which will now be described.

Step One: Obtaining Senior-management Commitment and Support
Senior management's total commitment to employment equity is essential to a program's success. This commitment should be made explicit in the organization's policy statement and supporting documentation; however, senior management must also show visible support throughout the process, and assume overall responsibility and accountability for program results.

Written Policy A written policy, endorsed by senior management and strategically posted throughout the organization or distributed to every employee, is an essential first step. Sir Sandford Fleming College's employment equity policy, shown in **Figure 3.8**, illustrates how such a policy statement can convey

FIGURE **3.8** Sample Employment Equity Policy

SIR SANDFORD FLEMING COLLEGE POLICY MANUAL	
Policy No. 3-310	Approved by: Board of Governors
Page No. 1 of 1	Supersedes: _____
Date Approved: _____	
Subject: Employment Equity	
The College has as its goals the hiring, promotion, and professional development of all employees in order to achieve an equitable distribution of women, men, racial and cultural minorities, Aboriginal Peoples, and persons with disabilities throughout the institution, and to eliminate barriers to full and equal participation.	

Source: Sir Sandford Fleming College, Peterborough, Ontario. Used with permission.

senior management's approval of and commitment to the program's development and successful implementation.

Since employees at all levels often have concerns about the implications of employment equity, the policy statement should be supplemented by various communication initiatives. All employees need to know the rationale for the program, types of activities that might be involved, implications for present and future employees, and the names of contact persons. Employees must be assured that information obtained for employment equity purposes will be treated confidentially, published only as aggregate data, and not used for anything else.

Assignment of Staff Responsibility An organization should appoint a senior official to whom overall responsibility and authority for program design and implementation is assigned. Since this individual must have the status and authority necessary to gain the trust and cooperation of managers, supervisors, employees, and union representatives, many firms ensure that he or she has direct access to the chief executive officer. At Sir Sandford Fleming College, for example, this responsibility is assigned to the executive director of human and organizational development, who reports to the president.

In order for a program to be successful, however, every department manager and supervisor must be assigned accountability and responsibility for program results, since they are the ones who hire, train, interact with on a daily basis, and evaluate employees. One way to accomplish this is to require each supervisor and manager to establish employment equity goals and timetables for his or her area of responsibility, and to measure progress in meeting these targets as part of the performance appraisal process.

Many organizations have found that the best way to build commitment is to form an employment equity committee, with representatives from all departments and levels. Such committees are generally responsible for reviewing policies and practices, making recommendations, and reporting on issues. Ultimate authority usually rests with senior management, however.

Employers covered by the Employment Equity Act are legally obligated to consult with designated employee representatives or, in unionized settings, the bargaining agent(s). Employee involvement from the beginning helps to build commitment and support.

Communication Internal communication strategies should be developed that are appropriate for the organization. These might include periodic information sessions, workshops, small-group or departmental discussions, poster displays, videos, brochures, newsletters, and memoranda from union officials. Once in place, the employment equity program should be explained at new-employee orientation sessions and in the organization's employee handbook.

Organizations committed to employment equity often wish to communicate this fact externally, as well, in their promotional material, annual report, and recruitment advertising.

stock data

Data that provide a snapshot of the organization at a particular point in time, in terms of how many designated group members are employed, in what occupations, and at what levels and salaries.

Step Two: Data Collection and Analysis
The development of an internal work-force profile is necessary in order to compare internal representation with external work-force availability data, set reasonable goals, and measure progress. Such profiles must be based on both stock and flow data. **Stock data** provide a snapshot of the organization at a particular point in time, in terms of how many designated group members are employed, in what occupa-

flow data

Data tracking designated group members by employment transactions and outcomes.

tions, and at what levels and salaries. **Flow data** track designated group members by employment transactions and outcomes. This involves determining how many designated group members apply for jobs with the firm, are interviewed, hired, given opportunities for training, promoted, and terminated.

While most information necessary for employment equity planning—such as gender, occupation and career history within the firm, and pay—is available from HR and payroll files, to obtain data pertaining to the distribution of designated group members, a self-identification process is generally used. Under the Employment Equity Act, employers may collect such data, as long as employees voluntarily agree to be identified or identify themselves as designated group members, and the data are only used for employment equity planning and reporting purposes.

Prior to administering a self-identification questionnaire, a climate of trust is essential. Since individuals may fear that self-identification will lead to future discriminatory treatment, a guarantee of confidentiality and an explanation of the importance of the information and ways in which it will be used is critical. To ensure a high rate of self-identification and meet legal obligations, questionnaires should include:

Hints to Ensure Legal Compliance

- an explanation of the organization's employment equity policy, the purpose of the employment equity program, and the need for the information requested
- a guarantee that the information supplied will be kept confidential and only used for employment equity purposes
- self-identification categories, with brief definitions and examples
- space for comments and suggestions
- an indication that the form has been reviewed by the relevant human rights commission, and approved by the bargaining agent(s), where applicable
- the name of the contact person(s) for clarification or further explanation.

Once the self-identification forms have been collected, the data must be organized according to four-digit National Occupational Classification (NOC) groupings, which involves classifying all of the organization's jobs in accordance with the NOC manual developed by Statistics Canada. Once jobs have been classified, a work-force profile can be compiled.

As explained in the Information Technology and HR box, software is now available to assist employers in complying with federal requirements. Numerous other software packages have been developed for employment equity data storage and reporting purposes.

Data must also be collected on the number of designated group members available in the labour markets from which the organization recruits. As discussed in Chapter 1, these may be quite different for various employee groups within the

INFORMATION TECHNOLOGY AND HR

Employment Equity Reporting

The Employment Equity Computerized Reporting System is a stand-alone system that is technically well-supported, user-friendly, and tailored to comply with the federal government's reporting requirements. The software and technical support are free, as is the Federal Contractor Program Computer Software.

Source: Linda Gutri, "Training for Equity," *Human Resources Professional* 9, no. 2 (February 1993), p. 14.

firm. While clerical and technical personnel are often recruited locally, the search for managerial and professional employees may be national or international in scope. External labour force availability data may be obtained from Statistics Canada, HRDC, women's directorates, professional associations, and agencies providing specialized assistance to various designated group members.

The comparison of the internal work-force profile with external work-force availability is called a **utilization analysis**. This type of comparison is necessary in order to determine the degree of underutilization and concentration of designated group members in specific occupations or at particular organizational levels.

Step Three: Employment Systems Review

It is also essential that the organization undertake a comprehensive **employment systems review**. Corporate policies and procedures manuals, collective agreements, and informal practices all have to be examined, to determine their impact on designated group members so that existing intentional or systemic barriers can be eliminated. Typically, employment systems that require review include:

- job classifications and descriptions
- recruitment and selection processes
- performance appraisal systems
- training and development programs
- transfer and promotion procedures
- compensation policies and practices
- discipline and termination procedures
- access to assistance, benefits, and facilities.

To assist in identifying systemic barriers, the following questions should be asked about every system under review:[54]

- Is it job related?
- Is it valid? (Is it directly related to job performance?)
- Is it applied consistently?
- Does it have an adverse impact on designated group members?
- Is it a business necessity? (Is it necessary for the safe and efficient operation of the business?)
- Does it conform to human rights legislation?

Step Four: Plan Development

Once the work-force profile and systems reviews have been completed, the employment equity plan can be prepared.

Goals and Timetables Goals and timetables are the core of an employment equity program, since they help to ensure that changes in representation become a reality. Goals, ranging from short- to long-term in duration, should be flexible and tied to reasonable timetables. *Goals are not **quotas**.*[55] First of all, they are not imposed on the organization. Secondly, they are estimates of the results that experts in the firm have established based on knowledge of the workplace and its employees, the availability of individuals with the KSAs required by the firm in the external labour force, and the special measures that are planned.

Quantitative goals should be set, specifying the number or percentage of qualified designated group members to be hired, trained, or promoted into each

---

utilization analysis

The comparison of the internal work-force profile with external work-force availability.

employment systems review

A thorough examination of corporate policies and procedures, collective agreements, and informal practices, to determine their impact on designated group members so that existing intentional or systemic barriers can be eliminated.

quotas

Set goals and timetables for the hiring and promotion of members of each of the designated groups, often externally imposed by government or a regulatory body, a strategy associated with affirmative action in the United States.

occupational group within a specified period of time. Qualitative goals, referred to as special measures, should also be included.

Special Measures   Three types of special measures should be implemented:

1. **Positive measures** are initiatives designed to accelerate the entry, development, and promotion of designated group members, aimed at overcoming the residual effects of past discrimination. Examples include special training programs or mentoring opportunities to assist designated group members in breaking the glass ceiling, and targeted recruitment. Positive measures are intended to hasten fair representation of the designated group members within a workplace.

2. **Accommodation measures** are strategies to assist designated group members to carry out their essential job duties. These might include job redesign; reassignment of a few job duties; adjusting a work schedule; upgrading facilities; or providing technical, human, or financial support services.

3. **Supportive measures** are strategies that enable all employees to achieve a better work/life balance. A tuition advance or reimbursement program is one example. Some firms make the upgrading of skills and knowledge even more accessible by providing allowances for texts and supplies and/or childcare expenses. Flexible schedules are another example. They accommodate employees: with parenting and eldercare responsibilities; who are taking part-time courses and need to take an occasional day course to complete their degree or diploma requirements; and who prefer to work long hours early in the week so that they can spend Friday afternoons skiing or on the golf course! In northern Canada, some firms have adopted innovative work schedules so that their First Peoples employees can take part in traditional fishing and hunting activities.

positive measures
Initiatives designed to accelerate the entry, development, and promotion of designated group members, aimed at overcoming the residual effects of past discrimination.

accommodation measures
Strategies to assist designated group members.

supportive measures
Strategies that enable all employees to achieve better balance between work and other responsibilities.

Step Five: Implementation   Implementation is the process that transforms goals and timetables and special measures into reality. Implementation strategies will be different in every firm, due to each organization's unique culture and climate. The success of plan implementation is dependent on such factors as senior management commitment, effectiveness of the selected communication strategies, and commitment of lower-level managers and the employment equity committee members. Other factors include the amount of acceptance gained for the special measures planned, and whether or not sufficient human and financial resources have been allocated. Those with overall responsibility and accountability for the plan guide the implementation process.

Step Six: Monitoring, Evaluating, and Revising   An effective employment equity program requires a control system so that progress and success, or lack thereof, can be evaluated. Through program monitoring, employers can assess the overall success of equity initiatives aimed at achieving a representative work force and respond to changes in the internal and/or external environment. The monitoring process may involve activities such as a review of flow data on job applications, selection decisions, training, promotions, and terminations. It may also include personal interviews with managers and selected designated group members; committee review of management progress reports; a review of managerial performance appraisal ratings on employment equity initiatives; and examination of statistical summaries of projected versus actual goal attainment.

Periodic reports should be issued (perhaps quarterly) to update all employees regarding progress and inform them about upcoming special projects or results of completed projects. Outstanding achievements should be given special recognition; this heightens the visibility of the programs and helps to build employee acceptance and management commitment. Annual progress reports should be produced and shared with all employees.

Benefits of Employment Equity

Employment equity makes good business sense, since it contributes to the bottom line. National Grocers is one organization that recognized this fact years ago. As Robert Rocon, director of employment equity at the firm, stated in 1995:[56]

> Regardless of any legislative requirement, [employment equity] is a good business decision for us. When you consider the changing face of Canada, it just makes good business sense to reflect the customers that you serve.

One of the benefits derived from implementing employment equity is being able to attract and keep the best-qualified employees, which results in greater access to a broader base of skills. Other benefits include higher employee morale due to special measures employed, such as flexible work schedules or job sharing; and improved corporate image in the community.[57]

Impact of Employment Equity

According to the Canadian Human Rights Commission 1999 annual report, employment equity can make a difference:[58]

> The representation of women in the federally regulated private sector improved, rising from 40.1 percent in 1987 to 44.3 percent in 1998. Although this was slightly below their availability estimate of almost 46.4 percent, it still represents a substantial increase. Women's representation in the public sector increased by over 9.5 percent between 1987 and 1999, reaching 51.5 percent by March 31, 1999, indicating substantial progress overall, and representation higher than their availability rate. In both private and public federal sectors, however, women continued to be underrepresented in senior management positions across all sectors, and are overrepresented in part-time and temporary positions.

> Visible minority group members also made some progress in representation in the federal private sector, which more than doubled from 4.9 percent in 1987 to 9.9 percent in 1998. They did not fare as well in the federal public sector, however. As of March 31, 1999, their representation stood at 5.9 percent, far short of their 10.3 percent availability. Furthermore, in both sectors, they remain concentrated in specific occupational groups and underrepresented in others, such as senior management.

> Unfortunately, Aboriginal people and persons with disabilities did not fare as well as either women or visible minorities. While the representation of First Peoples continued to increase in the federally regulated public sector in recent years, reaching 2.9 percent as of March 31, 1999, federally regulated private-sector firms hired a smaller proportion of this group for the fourth year in a row. These difficulties are compounded by their high share of terminations, which stood at 1.5 percent in 1998. While persons with disabilities make up 6.5 percent of all Canadian workers, they accounted for only 2.3 percent of employees in the federally regulated private sector as of March 31, 1999, virtually unchanged since 1987. Their representation in the federal public sector rose to 4.6 percent in 1999, a slight improvement from 3.9 percent in 1997.

Pay Equity

A study released by Statistics Canada in September 2000 confirmed that the overall wage gap between men and women remains substantial: women employed full-time, year-round make 73 percent of what men take home. This chronic gap is in part due to the fact that men still aren't assuming an equal share of responsibility at home. As a result, women are more likely to be absent from work, work part-time or in other nonstandard arrangements and work shorter weeks than men.[59]

Research Insight

While the lack of shared responsibility at home may account for some of the difference in wages, according to a 1999 Statistics Canada study, the remaining portion of this wage differential cannot be attributed to differences in work experience, education, major field of study, occupation or industry of employment. The researchers concluded that "much of the wage gap still remains a puzzle, leaving at least half of the discrepancy unaccounted for."[60]

Pay equity legislation is aimed at reducing the "unaccounted for" portion of the wage differential.

pay equity

Providing equal pay to male-dominated job classes and female-dominated job classes of equal value to the employer.

Pay equity, also known as equal pay for work of equal or comparable value, is designed to augment the "equal pay for equal work" legislation mentioned at the beginning of this chapter. In some jurisdictions, such as Ontario, pay equity is covered under separate legislation. For employers under federal jurisdiction, however, pay equity was incorporated into the human rights legislation through an amendment to the Act in 1978. The federal jurisdiction, Quebec, and Ontario have the most comprehensive pay equity legislation, covering virtually all public- and private-sector employers. In Quebec, for example, a pay equity law has been in effect since November 27, 1997, covering all enterprises with 10 or more employees, with requirements that vary according to employee numbers.[61] Ontario's legislation is quite similar. A number of other jurisdictions have laws that are restricted to the public sector.

As will be explained in detail in Chapter 12, pay equity requires an employer to provide equal pay to male-dominated job classes and female-dominated job classes of equal value, on the basis of skill, effort, responsibility, and working conditions, which may require comparing jobs that are quite different, such as nurses and firefighters. The focus is on eliminating the historical income gap between male-dominated and female-dominated jobs attributable to the undervaluing of work traditionally performed by women.

The federal pay equity legislation applies to all organizations under federal jurisdiction, regardless of size. It involves a complaint-based system, which means that action is taken once a complaint has been filed by an individual, a group of employees, or a bargaining agent.[62] An example is a complaint launched by some clerical workers in 1985, in which they claimed they were being discriminated against by being paid less than their male colleagues for work of equal value. This case, which involved the Public Service Alliance of Canada and the Treasury Board, was finally resolved in 1999, following a battle that extended over a period of almost 15 years. The government ended up agreeing to pay more than $3.6 billion to about 230 000 current and former clerks, secretaries, data processors, educational support workers, health services staff, and librarians. It was determined that these individuals, mostly women, were entitled to equity payments averaging $30 000 each, representing back pay plus interest from 1985 to July 1988.[63]

IMPACT OF EQUAL OPPORTUNITY AND EQUITY ON HRM

Functional Impact

The equal opportunity and equity legislation has an impact on virtually every HR function. Human rights legislation applies to all aspects and terms and conditions of employment. Pay equity affects job evaluation and compensation administration, and employment equity systems reviews involve an examination of all policies, procedures, and practices in the workplace. Implementing required changes necessitates much more than document revision. Understanding, acceptance, and commitment are essential, which means that education and communication must be given high priority.

Reverse Discrimination

reverse discrimination
Giving preference to designated group members to the extent that nonmembers believe they are being discriminated against.

When organizations decide to adopt a "quota" approach to employment equity, as the Ontario College of Art did in 1990 (at which time a decision was made to hire only women for a 10-year period in order to correct a grave imbalance in the ratio of male to female faculty members),[64] or when a specific numerical goal is imposed to overcome past discrimination, as in the case of Canadian National Railways (CN),[65] the employer may be accused of **reverse discrimination**. This involves giving preference to designated group members to the extent that nonmembers believe they are being discriminated against.

> In August of 1984, a federal human rights tribunal issued its first decision in Canadian history with regard to a mandatory employment equity program. CN was ordered to hire women for one in four nontraditional or blue-collar jobs in its St. Lawrence region until they held 13 percent of such jobs, the proportion of women in blue-collar jobs in industry in general. At the time, women represented approximately four percent of CN's blue-collar employees. CN was also required to implement a series of special measures, ranging from changing advertising techniques for available jobs to abandoning certain mechanical aptitude tests that had an adverse impact on female applicants. This decision was upheld by the Supreme Court of Canada when appealed by CN.

AN ETHICAL DILEMMA

"Employment equity sometimes leads to reverse discrimination, which is legal, as long as it fulfills the spirit of the law." Is this ethical?

Charges of reverse discrimination place HR managers in a difficult position. On the one hand, they are responsible for eliminating concentration and underutilization resulting from past discriminatory practices. On the other hand, they must also deal with those who feel disadvantaged because of special measures for designated group members. While preferential treatment may be deemed by many to be unfair, the federal and provincial/territorial human rights legislation in Canada specifies that employment equity (special) programs that fulfill the spirit of the law are not discriminatory.

It is possible to avoid the entire issue of reverse discrimination if the approach taken to employment equity is not one of quotas, the adoption of which has given affirmative action such a mixed reaction in the United States. Canadian legislation does not require quotas; rather, it specifies that organizations are to establish reasonable goals and timetables, based on external labour force availability data. In fact, Section 33 of the federal Employment Equity Act explicitly provides that neither the CHRC nor the Tribunal may "impose a quota on an employer"; nor can either require the public service "to hire or promote persons without basing the hiring or promotion on selection according to merit."[66] When goals are seen as targets, not quotas, the end result is that a better-qualified candidate who is not a protected group member is never denied an employment-related opportunity. On the contrary, when there are two *equally qualified candidates, based on nondiscriminatory job specifications and selection criteria*, preference will be given to the designated group member. The term "equally qualified" needs to be explained, since it does not necessarily imply identical educational qualifications or years of work experience, but rather possessing the qualifications required to perform the job. Thus, if a job requires two years of previous related experience, the candidate with four years of related experience is no more qualified than the individual with two.

Managerial Decision Making

In firms that have not done a good job of educating front-line supervisors and other managers, and/or have failed to build responsibility for employment equity program results into their performance appraisals, HR department specialists may have a final say in hiring, transfer and promotion decisions in order to achieve the plan objectives. Losing the authority to make such decisions is demoralizing to the individuals concerned, and has a detrimental impact on the quality of the work environment, and should thus be avoided.

A characteristic of successful employment and pay equity programs is commitment on the part of all managers across the organization. Achieving such commitment requires extensive education and training.

The Role of the HR Department

The HR department is generally assigned overall responsibility for legal compliance with human rights legislation and employment equity program results—whether voluntary or legally required—as well as pay equity plan implementation. It is the HR department staff members who are expected to keep up-to-date with changing regulations, court decisions, and emerging legal developments, and who generally take a leadership role in acquiring information, establishing communication and training strategies, developing programs to ensure company compliance, and filing government reports. However, supervisors and managers throughout the firm should be assigned responsibility and held accountable for: compliance with human rights legislation; collecting accurate information about jobs for pay equity purposes; establishing employment equity goals and timetables, and attaining measurable results within their work area or department.

MANAGING DIVERSITY

Although many people perceive "management of diversity" to be another term for employment equity, the two are very distinct. Managing diversity goes far beyond legal compliance or even implementing an employment equity plan voluntarily.

diversity management
Activities designed to integrate all members of an organization's multicultural work force and use their diversity to enhance the firm's effectiveness.

Diversity management is broader and more inclusive in scope, and involves a set of activities designed to integrate all members of an organization's multicultural work force and use their diversity to enhance the firm's effectiveness.

As discussed in Chapter 1, the ethnocultural profile of Canada has been changing since the 1960s, and will continue to change dramatically over the next 20 years. Canada has seen continued immigration from many lands during the last four decades. Managers at organizations ranging from McDonald's to Holiday Inn, and Bell Canada to Levi Strauss, are learning not only to understand their kaleidoscopic work force but also to manage in diverse work environments. While there are ethical and social responsibility issues involved in embracing diversity, there are more pragmatic reasons for doing so:

1. It makes economic sense. According to a Carleton University researcher, for example, by 2001, the spending power of Canada's visible minorities will be $311 billion.[67]

2. Employees with different ethnic backgrounds often also possess foreign-language skills, knowledge of different cultures and business practices, and may even have established trade links in other nations, which can lead to competitive advantage.

3. Having a work force representative of the firm's clientele is of value both morally and economically. As expressed by Dominic D'Alessandro, president and CEO at Manulife Financial:

    Given that we operate in a global marketplace, it is to be expected that our work force would mirror our customer base. Not only does this allow us to better understand our customer needs, but it also helps us to be a more creative, responsive organization. Through a diverse work force, we generate creative ideas—ideas about products and services for our diverse markets, ideas for solutions to business problems, and ideas about future directions. Our diversity will help us achieve improved performance.[68]

    A dramatic example of how a more diverse work force can help the firm to identify differences in customer needs or preferences that might otherwise be overlooked is provided by Levi Strauss, at which the Dockers line of casual pants, now worth more than $1 billion a year, has been credited to ideas obtained from Argentinean employees.[69]

4. Visible minorities can help to increase an organization's competitiveness and international savvy in the global business arena. Specifically, cultural diversity can help fine-tune product design, marketing, and ultimately customer satisfaction.[70] A dramatic example is provided in the Diversity Counts box.

Ministry of Citizenship, Culture and Recreation (Ontario) Gateway to Diversity Web Site

www.equalopportunity.on.ca

DIVERSITY COUNTS

In International Marketing

According to Santiago Rodriguez, director of multicultural programs at Apple Computers (based in Cupertino, California), the firm "might have offended 1.7 billion potential consumers in the growing computer markets of India and the Middle East, had it marketed a piece of seemingly harmless audio software called a 'Moof'." Quickly pulled off the market, the Moof was a phonetic combination of a "moo" and a "woof." The "cow–dog" utterance might have been offensive to both Hindus (to whom cows are sacred), and Muslims (to whom dogs are filthy creatures).

Source: Jana Schilder, "The Rainbow Connection," *Human Resources Professional* 11, no. 3 (April 1994), pp. 13-4.

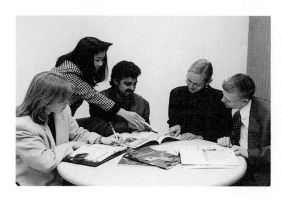

More and more firms are recognizing the benefits of employee diversity.

Although embracing employee diversity offers opportunities to enhance organizational effectiveness, transforming an organizational culture presents a set of challenges that must be handled properly. Diversity initiatives should be undertaken slowly, since they involve a complex change process. Resistance to change may have to be overcome, along with stereotyped beliefs or prejudices, and employee resentment. The aim is to ensure group cohesiveness, effective communication, retention of outstanding performers, and maximum opportunity for all employees.

Organizations that have been most successful in managing diversity tend to share the following seven characteristics:

1. Top Management Commitment

As with any major change initiative, unless there is commitment from the top, it is unlikely that other management staff will become champions of diversity. It is no coincidence that organizations that have established themselves as leaders in diversity management, such as the Bank of Montreal and Warner-Lambert Canada, Inc., have had senior-level commitment over an extended period of time.[71]

2. Diversity Training Programs

Diversity training programs are designed to provide awareness of diversity issues and to educate employees about specific gender and cultural differences and appropriate ways to handle them. Supervisors must be taught strategies to effectively manage and motivate a diverse group of employees. Often, it is appropriate to bring in an outside consulting firm with the requisite expertise to provide the training, at least initially. To be successful, diversity training must be ongoing, not a one-day workshop. Elements of diversity must be incorporated into all core training programs, based on the needs of specific business units or employee groups.[72]

3. Inclusive and Representative Communications

Organizations wishing to incorporate the value of diversity into their corporate culture must ensure that all of their internal communications and external publications convey this message. Inclusive language, such as gender-neutral terms and broad representation in terms of age, gender, race, etc. in company publications are strategies used. An example of an organization that has succeeded in this regard is Scotiabank, featured in the High Performance Organization box.

4. Activities to Celebrate Diversity

Diversity must also be celebrated in organizational activities. During the convocation ceremonies at Sir Sandford Fleming College in Peterborough, Ontario, for example, a traditional First Nations' blessing and tribute play a prominent role.

5. Support Groups or Mentoring Programs

An aim of diversity programs is to ensure that employees encounter a warm organizational climate, not one that is insensitive to their culture or background. To ensure that no one experiences feelings of alienation, isolation, or tokenism, support groups have been established in some firms to provide a nurturing climate and a means for employees who share the same background to find one another.

Other firms, such as Rogers Group, have established a mentoring program. At Rogers, the team-based mentoring program began as a six-month pilot in Toronto in mid-1999, and has since spread out to Rogers operations in the East

THE HIGH PERFORMANCE ORGANIZATION

Communicating Diversity

In 1999, Scotiabank won the communicating diversity award from the International Association of Business Communicators for its "Valuing People: Valuing Diversity" video. According to Director of Diversity Earl Miller, the project arose from Scotiabank's desire to communicate a more powerful diversity statement. He attributes the project's success to the cooperation of line managers in making a strong business case for diversity:

Our diversity program helps broaden our recruitment pool and in so doing boosts productivity and encourages teamwork. It also helps us improve our competitiveness as the employer of choice, and allows us to more effectively tap into international markets, as well as diverse communities within Canada.

The video also addresses the concern of line managers and other employees that diversity programs will increase their workload by pointing out that diversity simply provides a different way of doing things the company is already doing. As Miller explains,

Our bank has a long tradition of donations and sponsorships. Through our diversity program we have expanded our focus to include Aboriginal, Asian, West Indian and other groups. In this way, we are expanding our perspective and building our brand among a wider range of communities.

Recognizing that all videos have a limited shelf life, Scotiabank has extended the diversity initiative to include continuing education and training. The program is also now being broadened to include Scotiabank's domestic subsidiaries and foreign branches.

Source: Doug Burn, "What Have You Done for Me Lately?" pp. 13-19. Copyright Human Resources Professionals Association of Ontario, Suite 1902, 2 Bloor Street West, Toronto M4W 3E2. Reprinted by permission of the author.

and West. Not all mentoring programs follow the same path. As explained in the Information Technology and HR box, as the Internet becomes more accepted in everyday organizational life, mentors and protégés may never actually meet face-to-face.

Many organizations with mentoring programs have also established links with school boards, colleges or community organizations. At Rogers, for example, another ongoing component of the diversity strategy is participation in a Goodwill program, through which call-centre training is provided to youths and people with disabilities who, because of long-term unemployment, are not eligible for employment insurance. After two and one-half years of participation, Rogers had fully employed 20 graduates of the Goodwill program, all of whom

INFORMATION TECHNOLOGY AND HR

Mentoring Online

At the Alberta Women's Science Network is a relatively new program that electronically connects a pool of mentors with a pool of young women (typically recent university graduates) who want mentors in the science field. It's almost like having an electronic pen pal. The mentors help their protégés as they continue on in science and provide advice, assistance, and support. The mentors, all of whom are unpaid volunteers, generally assume the role because they have had a wonderful past experience with a mentor and wish to return the favour.

Source: Kira Vermond, "Making Mentoring Work," *HR Professional* 16, no. 3 (June/July 1999), pp. 19-22.

were still at the firm and performing at an above-average standard at the time a follow-up survey was conducted.[73]

6. Diversity Audits   To assess the effectiveness of an organization's diversity initiatives, **diversity audits** should be conducted. Recommended evaluation criteria include:[74]

- representation, which involves an assessment of the type of employees and their representation, and focusses on demographic and socioeconomic features. Surveys are helpful in identifying these types of data
- competency, which requires determining the diversity KSAs of employees. Self-assessments may be involved, as well as feedback from managers, peers, reporting employees, customers, etc.
- progress, which is an assessment of organizational movement from an initial state of little or no diversity commitment and infrastructure to an ideal state in which diversity is integrated into the fabric of the firm. This may involve a subjective approach (questions about how employees perceive key corporate functions such as recruitment and processes such as policy development) and objective measures (such as budgets and staff time)
- results, which requires measuring the extent to which diversity management strategies are perceived to have succeeded in promoting diversity or corporate objectives (and other subjective criteria), as well as in increasing such objective criteria as increased morale, productivity, and/or market share and decreasing turnover and absenteeism.

7. Management Responsibility and Accountability   As with employment equity, diversity management initiatives will not receive high priority unless supervisors and managers are held accountable and results are part of their formal assessment. Having managers throughout the firm committed to diversity is a major factor in program success. At Scotiabank, for example, the cooperation of line managers in making a strong business case for diversity is cited as the key reason for the success of the firm's diversity initiatives.

Managing Diversity in International Businesses

An increasing number of organizations are having to ensure that the rights of all of their employees around the world are respected, and that operations outside of Canada meet acceptable labour and human rights standards. To ensure legal compliance in all jurisdictions, companies with international operations should:[75]

- adopt a corporate code of conduct that includes labour standards and human rights issues
- ensure that the code applies internationally, as well as domestically
- provide adequate enforcement mechanisms, including external auditing
- train the key implementers, those advising and assisting implementers, and those responsible for enforcement
- educate the local work force about their rights ... workers cannot exercise rights of which they are unaware.

Taking a stand on international human rights and labour standards requires more than a code of conduct, however. It also requires ensuring that the prac-

---

diversity audit
An audit to assess the effectiveness of an organization's diversity initiatives.

Diversity Central
www.diversitycentral.com

**Hints to Ensure
Legal Compliance**

tices of the company's international clients or customers are both legal and ethical and that the firm is not inadvertently supporting less-than-desirable practices in any country around the world through even more indirect means, such as pension plan investments. As described in the Global HRM box that follows, labour standards, human rights, and ethics have become key concerns pertaining to pension plan funding.

GLOBAL HRM

International Rights and Pension Plan Funding

Increasingly, firms are having to think about the ethical and legal stance of the companies being supported by their pension plan holdings. If members don't approve of pension plan investments, they may put pressure on the employer to put their money in more ethically friendly funds. For example, in January of 2000, the largest pension fund in the U.S. unloaded its stock in Talisman Energy Inc., following reports of civilian human rights abuses in Sudan, where Talisman, a Calgary oil company, has operations. Despite the fact that Talisman had been defending itself against the accusation that its economic activity was propping up Sudan's oppressive regime, TIAA-CREF, a college teachers' fund, became the third U.S. institutional investor to withdraw its interests in Talisman.

A few months previously, the Ontario Teachers Federation indicated that it would lobby its pension fund administrators, the Ontario Teachers Pension Plan Board, to divest its $184-million stake in the company if proof of abuses was found.

Source: Peter Brewster, "Who is Paying for Your Workers' Retirement?" *Guide to Pensions & Benefits, Supplement to Canadian HR Reporter* 13, no. 11 (June 15, 2000), p. G1; and "When Members Don't Like Your Investments," *Canadian HR Reporter* 13, no. 1 (January 17, 2000), p. 9.

CHAPTER REVIEW

Summary

1 Employment (labour) standards laws, which establish minimum employee entitlements and set a limit on the maximum number of hours of work permitted per day or week, exist in every jurisdiction.

2 The principle of equal pay for equal work has been incorporated into the employment (labour) standards or human rights legislation in every jurisdiction. This specifies that an employer cannot pay male and female employees differently if they are performing substantially the same work, requiring the same degree of skill, effort, and responsibility, under similar working conditions.

3 The Charter of Rights and Freedoms is the cornerstone of Canada's legislation pertaining to equal opportunity. Although the Charter only applies directly to

the actions of all levels of government and agencies under their jurisdiction, because it takes precedence over all other laws it is quite far-reaching in scope. The Supreme Court is its ultimate interpreter. Charter rulings that have had major implications for HRM pertain to the right to bargain collectively and to strike, the right to picket, use of union dues, and mandatory retirement.

4   Every employer in Canada is affected by human rights legislation, which is a family of federal and provincial/territorial laws that prohibit intentional and unintentional discrimination in all aspects and terms and conditions of employment. All jurisdictions prohibit discrimination on the grounds of race, colour, religion or creed, physical and mental disability, sex (including pregnancy and childbirth), and marital status. All prohibit age-based discrimination (although the protected age groups differ), and all jurisdictions other than British Columbia and Alberta prohibit discrimination on the basis of national or ethnic origin. Discrimination on other grounds, such as sexual orientation and criminal history, are prohibited in some jurisdictions, but not all.

5   Employers are permitted to discriminate if employment preferences are based on bona fide occupational requirements (BFORs). In situations in which occupational requirements are not obvious, the onus of proof is on the employer.

6   Employers are required to make reasonable accommodations to the point of undue hardship. In unionized settings, the union and employer have a joint (but not equal) responsibility for accommodation.

7   Harassment includes a wide range of behaviour that a reasonable person ought to know is unwelcome. However, it also encompasses actions and activities that were once tolerated, ignored, and considered horseplay or innocent flirtation, provided the individual who feels that he or she is being harassed makes it clear that such behaviour is unwelcome and inappropriate, and asks that it be discontinued. Employers and managers have a responsibility to provide a safe and healthy working environment. If harassment is occurring, of which they are aware, or ought to have been aware, they can be charged, as well as the alleged harasser.

8   The type of harassment that has attracted the most attention in the workplace is sexual harassment, which can be divided into two categories: sexual coercion and sexual annoyance. All employers under federal jurisdiction are required by law to develop and implement sexual harassment policies. Many organizations are adopting harassment policies that encompass all of the prohibited grounds of discrimination.

9   There is a human rights commission in each jurisdiction with the authority to receive and investigate complaints, determine their validity, try to achieve a settlement between the parties and, if unsuccessful, proceed to a board of inquiry or tribunal for resolution. If the allegation is substantiated, there is a wide range of remedies, including compensation for lost wages, general damages, complainant expenses, and pain and humiliation.

10 Federal legislation pertaining to equity includes the Employment Equity Act and Federal Contractors Program. Voluntary employment equity programs are legalized under the human rights legislation in every Canadian jurisdiction.

11 The steps involved in implementing an employment equity program include: obtaining senior management commitment and support, data collection and analysis, an employment systems review, plan development,

plan implementation, and a follow-up process encompassing evaluation, monitoring, and revision.

12 Pay equity, also known as equal pay for work of equal or comparable value, requires an employer to provide equal pay to male-dominated and female-dominated job classes of equal value, based on an assessment of skill, effort, responsibility, and working conditions. Its focus is on eliminating the historical income gap attributable to the undervaluing of work traditionally performed by women.

13 Reverse discrimination is an issue that employers can avoid if they establish reasonable goals and timetables, not quotas.

14 Diversity management, which is much broader and more inclusive than employment equity, involves a set of activities designed to integrate all members of a firm's multicultural work force and use their diversity to enhance organizational effectiveness. Characteristics of successful diversity management programs include top management commitment, diversity training, inclusive and representative communication, activities to celebrate diversity, support groups or mentoring programs, diversity audits, and management responsibility and accountability.

Key Terms

accommodation measures
bona fide occupational requirement (BFOR)
Canadian Human Rights Act
Canadian Human Rights Commission (CHRC)
Charter of Rights and Freedoms
concentration
discrimination
diversity audit
diversity management
employment (labour) standards legislation
Employment Equity Act
employment equity program
employment systems review
equal pay for equal work
equality rights
Federal Contractors Program
flow data
glass ceiling

harassment
human rights legislation
intentional discrimination
occupational segregation
pay equity
positive measures
quotas
reasonable accommodation
reverse discrimination
sexual annoyance
sexual coercion
sexual harassment
stock data
supportive measures
underemployment
underutilization
undue hardship
unintentional/constructive/systemic discrimination
utilization analysis

Review and Discussion Questions

1 Describe the impact of the Charter of Rights and Freedoms on HRM.

2 Differentiate between the following types of discrimination, and provide one example of each: direct, differential treatment, indirect, because of association, and systemic.

3   Discuss the human rights requirements pertaining to reasonable accommodation, and provide five examples of workplace accommodation measures.

4   Explain employers' and managers' responsibilities pertaining to harassment.

5   Define "sexual harassment" and describe five types of behaviour that could constitute such harassment.

6   Outline the steps involved in the human rights complaint process and describe four possible remedies for violations.

7   Explain how diversity management differs from employment equity and describe the characteristics of successful diversity management initiatives.

CRITICAL *Thinking Questions*

1   Briefly describe 10 grounds of discrimination prohibited under Canadian human rights legislation, and provide an example of each that illustrates the types of activities in which an employer cannot legally engage.

2   A front-line supervisor has just informed you, the HR manager, that there are certain machine shop jobs for which he feels minimum height and weight requirements are BFORs. You disagree. How would you handle this situation?

3   A reporting employee who has been off for two months with a stress-related ailment has just contacted you, indicating that she would like to return to work next week but won't be able to work full-time for another month or so. How would you handle this?

4   Assume that you are the HR manager in a company that has decided to implement employment equity. Describe and justify each of the steps that you would take to ensure successful program implementation.

5   Differentiate between "equal pay for equal work" and "equal pay for work of equal value," and provide a specific example that illustrates the application of each.

6   Explain the difference between goals and quotas and discuss the ways in which employers can avoid the issue of reverse discrimination.

7   Describe how you would be affected by equal opportunity and equity legislation: (a) as a front-line supervisor or small-business owner and (b) as a member of the HR department.

APPLICATION *Exercises*

RUNNING CASE: Carter Cleaning Company

Discrimination?

One of the areas about which Jennifer is particularly concerned is legal compliance. She has noted that very little attention has been paid to equality, equal opportunity, and equity issues. Virtually all hiring is handled by the centre managers, three of whom are white males and three of whom are white females. None of the managers has received any training on human rights legislative requirements or the types of questions that can and cannot be asked at job interviews. During recent meetings with the managers, Jennifer learned that it is not uncommon for female applicants to be asked questions regarding child-care arrangements and visible minority candidates to be asked about their language skills. White males are not questioned about either of these issues.

Based on discussions with her father, Jennifer has deduced that the rather laid-back attitude toward equality, equal opportunity, and equity stems from her father's lack of sophistication regarding legislative requirements, as well as the fact that, as he put it, "Virtually all of our workers are women or visible minorities, anyway, so no one can come in here and accuse us of being discriminatory, can they?"

Jennifer wasn't quite sure what to say in response, so decided to mull her father's question over. Before she had time to give it much thought, however, she was faced with complaints from three employees requiring her immediate attention. Two women employed at one of the centres told her, in confidence, that their manager was making unwelcome sexual advances toward them, and one claimed that he had threatened to fire her unless she "socialized" with him after hours. On a fact-finding trip to another centre, a 63-year-old employee stated that although he had almost 40 years' experience in the business, he was being paid less than women half his age who were doing the very same job.

Jennifer has now written down five questions that she needs to consider.

Questions

1   Is it true, as her father has claimed, that they can't be accused of being discriminatory because they hire mostly women and visible minorities?

2   How should she and her father address the charges of sexual harassment? If the manager is guilty, what should they do?

3   Does the 63-year-old have a complaint for which he can file a charge? Under which legislation? How should his pay issue be addressed?

4   Aside from the two issues that require her immediate attention, what other HRM matters should she address to ensure that the centres are in compliance with the (Ontario) provincial legislation pertaining to equality and equity?

5   Given current demographic trends, should the centres be thinking beyond legal compliance? If so, how?

CASE INCIDENT   *Harassment*

Maria was hired two months ago to supervise the compensation area of the HR department, which you manage. She seems to have been accepted by her peers and reporting employees but you have noticed that, for the past three weeks, she has been the last to arrive at staff meetings and always sits as far as possible from Bob, another supervisor.

Yesterday afternoon, you had a very upsetting conversation with her. She claimed that for more than a month Bob has been repeatedly asking her to go out with him and that her constant refusals seem to be making the situation worse. Bob has accused her of being unfriendly and suggested that she thinks she is too good for him. She said that he has never touched her but that he discusses how "sexy" she looks with the other men in the department, who seem embarrassed by the whole situation. Maria also said that Bob's advances are escalating the more she refuses him and that his behaviour is interfering with her job performance to such an extent that she is thinking of resigning.

With Maria's consent, you have just spoken to Bob, who denied her allegations vehemently and believably.

Questions

1   How would you proceed in dealing with this situation?

2   What are your responsibilities to Maria and Bob?

3   If Maria is telling the truth, are you or Bob legally liable in any way? If so, under what conditions?

4   How would you resolve this matter?

Source: Based on a case provided in *Equity Works Best*, a publication of the Ontario Women's Directorate.

EXPERIENTIAL *Exercises*

1   Working in teams of six, role-play an investigation of the harassment claim described in the above case. One member of each team is to be assigned the role of Maria, another the role of Bob, and a third the role of the HR manager. The three remaining team members are to assume the roles of other HR department staff. For the purpose of this role-play, assume that Bob has made comments about how "sexy" Maria is and has asked her out, but claims that he didn't realize his behaviour was bothering Maria.

2   As the assembly department supervisor, you are responsible for hiring assemblers, supervising them, and appraising their performance. Prepare a report outlining the steps you take to ensure legal compliance when performing each of these duties.

3   Working with a small group of classmates, contact the HR manager at a company in your community that has an employment equity or diversity management program. Prepare a brief report summarizing its key features.

WEB-BASED *Exercises*

1   Visit the Web site of the Canadian Human Rights Commission (**www.chrc-ccdp.ca**). Summarize two recent cases decided in favour of employers and two decided in favour of employees. Explain the implications of these decisions for managers and small-business owners.

2   Go to the Web sites of two provincial/territorial human rights commissions. Compare and contrast: (a) The prohibited grounds of discrimination in each jurisdiction; (b) The types and volume of cases handled over the past year; and (c) The position of each on retirement age and same-sex benefits.

A Guide to Screening and Selection in Employment

Subject	Avoid Asking	Preferred	Comment
Name	about name change: whether it was changed by court order, marriage, or other reason maiden name		ask after selection if needed to check on previously held jobs or educational credentials
Address	for addresses outside Canada	ask place and duration of current or recent address	
Age	for birth certificates, baptismal records, or about age in general	ask applicants whether they are eligible to work under Canadian laws regarding age restrictions	if precise age required for benefits plans or other legitimate purposes, it can be determined after selection
Sex	males or females to fill in different applications about pregnancy, child-bearing plans, or child-care arrangements	ask applicant if the attendance requirements can be met	during the interview or after selection, the applicant, for purposes of courtesy, may be asked which of Mr, Mrs, Miss, Ms is preferred
Marital Status	whether the applicant is single, married, divorced, engaged, separated, widowed, or living common law whether an applicant's spouse may be transferred about spouse's employment	if transfer or travel is part of the job, the applicant can be asked if he or she can meet these requirements ask whether there are any circumstances that might prevent completion of a minimum service commitment	information on dependants can be determined after selection if necessary
Family Status	number of children or dependants about child care arrangements	if the applicant would be able to work the required hours and, where applicable, overtime	contacts for emergencies and/or details on dependants can be determined after selection
National or Ethnic Origin	about birthplace, nationality of ancestors, spouse, or other relatives whether born in Canada for proof of citizenship	since those who are entitled to work in Canada must be citizens, permanent residents, or holders of valid work permits, applicants can be asked if they are legally entitled to work in Canada	documentation of eligibility to work (papers, visas, etc.) can be requested after selection
Military Service	about military service in other countries	inquiry about Canadian military service where employment preference is given to veterans by law	
Language	mother tongue where language skills obtained	ask if applicant understands, reads, writes, or speaks languages required for the job	testing or scoring applicants for language proficiency is not permitted unless job related
Race or Colour	any inquiry into race or colour, including colour of eyes, skin, or hair		
Photographs	for photo to be attached to applications or sent to interviewer before interview		photos for security passes or company files can be taken after selection

Subject	Avoid Asking	Preferred	Comment
Religion	about religious affiliation, church membership, frequency of church attendance if applicant will work a specific religious holiday for references from clergy or religious leader	explain the required work shift, asking if such a schedule poses problems for the applicant	reasonable accommodation of an employee's religious beliefs is the employer's duty
Height and Weight			no inquiry unless there is evidence they are genuine occupational requirements
Disability	for list of all disabilities, limitations, or health problems whether applicant drinks or uses drugs whether applicant has ever received psychiatric care or been hospitalized for emotional problems whether applicant has received workers' compensation	ask if applicant has any condition that could affect ability to do the job ask if applicant has a condition that should be considered in selection	a disability is only relevant to job ability if it: – threatens the safety or property of others – prevents the applicant from safe and adequate job performance even when reasonable efforts are made to accommodate the disability
Medical Information	if currently under physician's care name of family doctor if receiving counselling or therapy		medical exams should be conducted after selection and only if an employee's condition is related to job duties offers of employment can be made conditional on successful completion of a medical exam
Pardoned Conviction	whether an applicant has ever been convicted if an applicant has ever been arrested whether an applicant has a criminal record	if bonding is a job requirement, ask whether the applicant is eligible	inquiries about criminal record or convictions are discouraged unless related to job duties
Sexual Orientation	any inquiry about the applicant's sexual orientation		contacts for emergencies and/or details on dependents can be determined after selection
References			the same restrictions that apply to questions asked of applicants apply when asking for employment references

Source: Canadian Human Rights Commission, *A Guide to Screening and Selection in Employment,* (Ottawa: Canadian Human Rights Commission, 1999). Reproduced with permission of the Minister of Public Works and Government Services Canada.

1

Landmark Supreme Court Decision on Same-sex Benefits

What is a spouse? Traditionally, it has meant a husband or wife, someone you married or lived with common law. Certainly it has meant a person of the opposite sex. That changed on Thursday, May 20, 1999, due to a landmark Supreme Court of Canada decision in *M v. H*. Ontario's Family Law Act was ruled to be unconstitutional, and the province was given six months to amend the Act to include same-sex couples.

Viewers have an opportunity to learn about the personal implications of this ruling for Kelly, who has been honouring the memory of her same-sex partner, Robin, and awaiting the day when her long-term relationship with Robin would be recognized with the official status of "spouse." On October 21, 1993, Robin was killed in a bike accident, and Kelly found that she had no rights to compensation as Robin's spouse under Ontario law. For her and her friends, the Supreme Court ruling felt vindicating, and was a cause for celebration.

While legal experts Brenda Cossman, a University of Toronto professor, and Ted Morton, a professor at the University of Calgary, agree that this decision will have far-reaching implications for provincial/territorial and federal statutes, they have very differing views about its legitimacy. According to Morton, sexual orientation was purposefully left out of Section 15 of the Charter, and was only added by the courts in 1995. He feels strongly that the *M v. H* ruling reflects the personal thoughts of nine Supreme Court judges, not what is in the Charter. Cossman feels that the judges' decision reflects changing public opinion about gay and lesbian rights. While acknowledging that the vast majority of Canadians may still be a little uncomfortable with the idea of gay marriage, she states that most Canadians now believe that same-sex couples should not be discriminated against and should be entitled to the same benefits and obligations as unmarried heterosexual couples. Cossman and Morton agree that the ruling will give legislatures across the country a "push" to amend the definition of spouse in all relevant statutes.

Questions

1 In your own words, describe the significance of the *M v. H* decision.

2 As highlighted in the video, reactions were varied. a) Why was the ruling a cause for celebration among gay rights activists? b) Why was Ted Morton opposed to the decision? c) Why did Brenda Cossman support the ruling?

3 What is the relationship between the *Vriend* ruling (see Chapter 3) and the one in *M v. H*?

4 What are the HRM implications of the legislative changes resulting from the *M v. H* ruling?

Video Resource: CBC, *National Magazine*, "Same Sex," May 20, 1999.

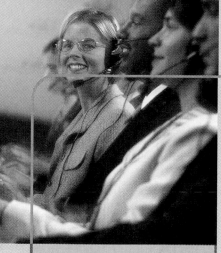

CHAPTER 4

Designing and Analyzing Jobs

CHAPTER
OUTLINE

Organizing Work

Job Design

The Nature of Job Analysis

Methods of Collecting Job Analysis Information

Writing Job Descriptions

Writing Job Specifications

Job Analysis in a "Jobless" World

LEARNING OUTCOMES

After studying this chapter, you should be able to:

Develop an organization chart.

Describe the industrial engineering, behavioural, and human engineering considerations involved in job design.

Explain the importance of job analysis information.

Describe the basic methods of collecting job analysis information and *explain* the appropriate use of each.

Analyze jobs.

Develop job descriptions and job specifications.

Explain the value of a physical demands analysis and statistically derived job specifications.

Discuss current trends in the nature of jobs and job descriptions.

ORGANIZING WORK

organizational structure

The formal relationships among jobs in an organization.

organization chart

A "snapshot" of the firm at a particular point in time, depicting the organization's structure in chart form.

An organization consists of one or more employees, who perform various tasks. The relationships between people and tasks must be structured in such a way that the organization can achieve its goals in an efficient and effective manner.

Organizational structure refers to the formal relationships among jobs in an organization. An **organization chart** is often used to depict the structure. As illustrated in **Figure 4.1**, such a chart indicates the types of departments established, the title of each manager's job, and by means of connecting lines, clarifies the chain of command and shows who is accountable to whom. An organization chart presents a "snapshot" of the firm at a particular point in time, but does not provide details about actual communication patterns, degree of supervision, amount of power and authority, or specific duties and responsibilities. As explained in the Information Technology and HR box, firms can now use high-end software to ensure that such charts are kept current and are readily accessible to all employees.

FIGURE 4.1 A Sample Organization Chart

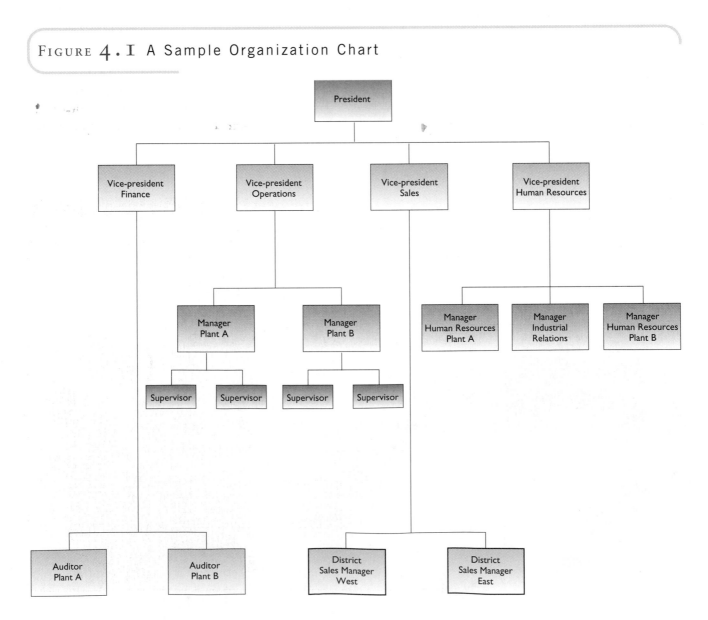

INFORMATION TECHNOLOGY AND HR
Automated Organization Charts Save Time and Money

A relatively new option in HR software is the automated organization chart. The tangible benefit of having such charts is the cost savings involved: the costs of creating, printing and distributing organization charts are eliminated and lumped into the one-time software purchase cost. A note of caution is in order, however. In order to realize such savings, the product must cost nothing to maintain, yet provide the functionality that is needed. If someone in IT or HR needs to spend a few days designing and producing each chart, then the automated solution is not living up to its potential.

Having information that can be accessed and updated easily can also lead to a number of intangible benefits. An up-to-date chart enables employees to spend less time looking for the right person and more time getting things done. In addition, automated solutions can be kept on the company intranet, thus making detailed information easier to collect and distribute. Having accurate information regarding employee headcounts at every level of the firm, as well as the number and types of employees managed by specific individuals, can also assist managers in making better decisions regarding how to structure and manage their departments.

Source: Babak Varjavandi, "Automated Org. Charts Save Time, Money," *Guide to HR Technology, Supplement to Canadian HR Reporter* 13, no. 5 (March 13, 2000), p. G4.

Designing an organization involves choosing a structure that is appropriate, given the company's strategic goals. There are three basic types of organizational structure, as depicted in **Figure 4.2**: bureaucratic, flat, and boundaryless.

Automated organization charts can be updated easily and made highly accessible to employees.

Example of Online Organization Chart
www.IntranetOrgChart.com

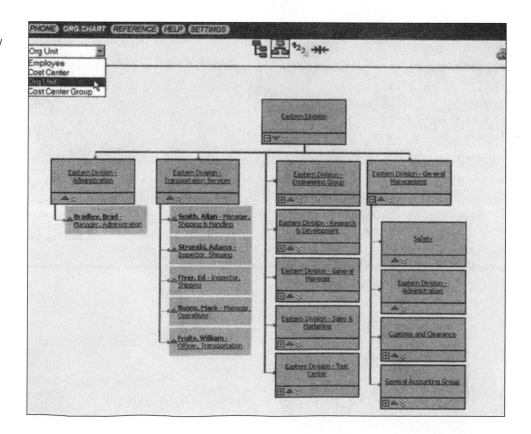

FIGURE 4.2 Bureaucratic, Flat, and Boundaryless Organizational Structures

Structure   **Characteristics**

BUREAUCRATIC

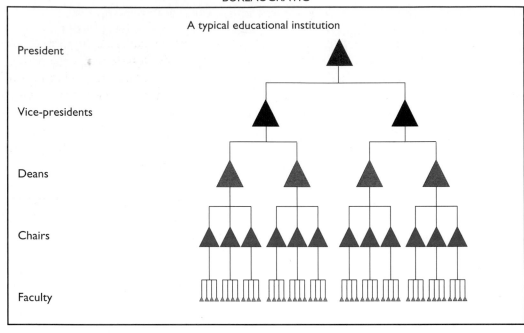

A typical educational institution

President

Vice-presidents

Deans

Chairs

Faculty

- Top-down management approach
- Many levels, and hierarchical communication channels and career paths
- Highly specialized jobs with narrowly defined job descriptions
- Focus on independent performance

FLAT

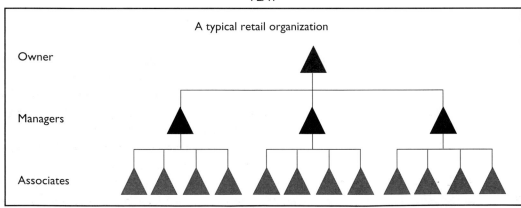

A typical retail organization

Owner

Managers

Associates

- Decentralized management approach
- Few levels and multi-directional communication
- Broadly defined jobs with general job descriptions
- Emphasis on teams and on customer service

BOUNDARYLESS

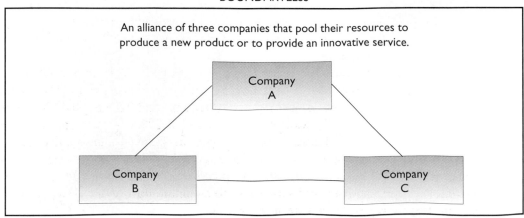

An alliance of three companies that pool their resources to produce a new product or to provide an innovative service.

Company A

Company B

Company C

- Joint ventures with customers, suppliers, and/or competitors
- Emphasis on teams whose members may cross organizational boundaries

As discussed briefly in Chapter 1 and as will be explained in more detail later in this chapter, bureaucratic designs are becoming less common; flat structures are increasingly the norm; and boundaryless organizations have started to evolve.

JOB DESIGN

job design

The process of systematically organizing work into tasks that are required to perform a specific job.

In any organization, work has to be divided into manageable units and ultimately into jobs that can be performed by employees. Job design is the process of systematically organizing work into tasks that are required to perform a specific job. An organization's strategy and structure influence the ways in which jobs are designed. In bureaucratic organizations, for example, since there is a hierarchical division of labour, jobs are generally highly specialized. In addition to organizational objectives and structure, however, effective job design also takes into consideration human and technological factors.

job

A group of related activities and duties, held by a single employee or a number of incumbents.

A job consists of a group of related activities and duties. Ideally, the duties of a job should be clear and distinct from those of other jobs, and involve natural units of work that are similar and related. This helps to minimize conflict and enhance employee performance. A job may be held by a single employee or may have a number of incumbents. The collection of tasks and responsibilities performed by one person is known as a position. To clarify, in a department with one supervisor, one clerk, forty assemblers, and three tow-motor operators, there are forty-five positions and four jobs.

position

The collection of tasks and responsibilities performed by one person.

Specialization and Industrial Engineering Considerations

The term "job" as it is known today is largely an outgrowth of the efficiency demands of the industrial revolution. As the substitution of machine power for people power became more widespread, experts such as Adam Smith, Charles Babbage, and Frederick Winslow Taylor (the father of scientific management) wrote glowingly about the positive correlation between (1) job specialization, and (2) productivity and efficiency.[1] The popularity of specialized, short-cycle jobs soared—at least among management experts and managers.

work simplification

An approach to job design that involves assigning most of the administrative aspects of work (such as planning and organizing) to supervisors and managers, while giving lower-level employees narrowly defined tasks to perform according to methods established and specified by management.

Work simplification evolved from scientific management theory. It is based on the premise that work can be broken down into clearly defined, highly specialized, repetitive tasks to maximize efficiency. This approach to job design involves assigning most of the administrative aspects of work (such as planning and organizing) to supervisors and managers, while giving lower-level employees narrowly defined tasks to perform according to methods established and specified by management.

While work simplification can increase operating efficiency in a stable environment, and may be very appropriate in settings employing individuals with mental disabilities or those lacking in education and training (as in some third-world operations), it is not effective in a changing environment in which customers/clients demand custom-designed products and/or high-quality services, or one in which employees want challenging work. Moreover, among educated employees, simplified jobs often lead to lower satisfaction, higher rates of absenteeism and turnover, and sometimes to a demand for premium pay to compensate for the repetitive nature of the work.

industrial engineering

A field of study concerned with analyzing work methods; making work cycles more efficient by modifying, combining, rearranging, or eliminating tasks; and establishing time standards.

Another important contribution of scientific management was the study of work. Industrial engineering, which evolved with this movement, is concerned with analyzing work methods and establishing time standards to improve efficiency. Industrial engineers systematically identify, analyze, and time the elements of each job's work cycle and determine which, if any, elements can be modified, combined, rearranged, or eliminated to reduce the time needed to complete the cycle.

To establish time standards, industrial engineers measure and record the time required to complete each element in the work cycle, using a stopwatch or work sampling techniques, and then combine these times to determine the total. Adjustments are then made to compensate for differences in skill level, breaks, and interruptions due to such factors as machine maintenance or breakdown. The adjusted time becomes the time standard for that particular work cycle, which serves as an objective basis for evaluating and improving employee performance and determining incentive pay.

Since jobs are created primarily to enable an organization to achieve its objectives, industrial engineering cannot be ignored as a disciplined and objective approach to job design. However, too much emphasis on the concerns of industrial engineering—improving efficiency and simplifying work methods—may result in human considerations being neglected or downplayed. What may be improvements in job design and efficiency from an engineering standpoint can sometimes prove to be physiologically or psychologically unsound. For example, an assembly line with its simplified and repetitive tasks embodies the principles of industrial engineering, but may lead to repetitive strain injuries and high turnover and low satisfaction due to the lack of psychological fulfillment. Thus, to be effective, job design must also provide for the satisfaction of human psychological and physiological needs.

Behavioural Considerations

By the mid-1900s, reacting to what they viewed as the "dehumanizing" aspects of pigeonholing workers into highly repetitive and specialized jobs and other problems associated with overspecialization, various management theorists proposed ways of broadening the numbers of activities in which employees engaged. Job enlargement involves assigning workers additional tasks at the same level of responsibility to increase the number of tasks they have to perform. Thus, if the work was assembling chairs, the worker who previously only bolted the seat to the legs might take on the additional tasks of assembling the legs and attaching the back, as well. Also known as horizontal loading, job enlargement reduces monotony and fatigue by expanding the job cycle and drawing on a wider range of employee skills. Another technique to relieve monotony and employee boredom is **job rotation**. This involves systematically moving employees from one job to another. Although the jobs themselves don't change, workers experience more task variety, motivation, and productivity. The company gains by having more versatile, multiskilled employees who can cover for one another efficiently.

More recently, psychologist Frederick Herzberg argued that the best way to motivate workers is to build opportunities for challenge and achievement into jobs through job enrichment.[2] This is defined as any effort that makes an employee's job more rewarding or satisfying by adding more meaningful tasks and duties. Also known as vertical loading, job enrichment involves increasing autonomy and responsibility by allowing employees to assume a greater role in the decision-making process and become more involved in planning, organizing, directing, and controlling their own work.

job enlargement (horizontal loading)

A technique to relieve monotony and boredom that involves assigning workers additional tasks at the same level of responsibility to increase the number of tasks they have to perform.

job rotation

Another technique to relieve monotony and employee boredom, which involves systematically moving employees from one job to another.

job enrichment (vertical loading)

Any effort that makes an employee's job more rewarding or satisfying by adding more meaningful tasks and duties.

Enriching jobs can be accomplished through such activities as:

- increasing the level of difficulty and responsibility of the job
- assigning workers more authority and control over outcomes
- providing feedback about individual or unit job performance directly to employees
- adding new tasks requiring training, thereby providing an opportunity for growth
- assigning individuals specific tasks or responsibility for performing a whole job rather than only parts of it.

Job design studies explored a new field when behavioural scientists focussed on identifying various job dimensions that would simultaneously improve the efficiency of organizations and satisfaction of employees. One of the best-known theories evolving from such research is one advanced by Richard Hackman and Greg Oldham.[3] Their job characteristics model proposes that employee motivation and satisfaction are directly linked to five core characteristics:[4]

1. Skill variety. The degree to which the job requires a person to do different tasks and involves the use of a number of different talents, skills, and abilities.
2. Task identity. The degree to which the job requires completion of a whole and identifiable piece of work, that is, doing a job from beginning to end, with a visible outcome.
3. Task significance. The degree to which the job has a substantial impact on the lives and work of others—both inside and outside the organization.
4. Autonomy. The amount of freedom, independence, and discretion the employee has in terms of scheduling work and determining procedures.
5. Feedback. The degree to which the job provides the employee with clear and direct information about job outcomes and effectiveness of his or her performance.

These core job characteristics create the conditions that enable workers to experience three critical psychological states that are related to a number of beneficial work outcomes:[5]

1. Experienced meaningfulness. The extent to which the employee experiences the work as important, valuable, and worthwhile.
2. Experienced responsibility. The degree to which the employee feels personally responsible or accountable for the outcome of the work.
3. Knowledge of results. The degree to which the employee understands, on a regular basis, how effectively he or she is performing.

As illustrated in **Figure 4.3**: skill variety, task identity, and task significance are all linked to experienced meaningfulness; autonomy is related to experienced responsibility; and feedback provides knowledge of results.

A job with characteristics that allow an employee to experience all three critical states provides internal rewards that sustain motivation. The benefits to the employer include high-quality performance, higher employee satisfaction, and lower absenteeism and turnover.

As is no doubt quite apparent, the suggestions of Herzberg, Hackman and Oldham regarding job design and redesign strategies are quite similar. The benefits of job enrichment also include increased motivation, job satisfaction, and performance.

FIGURE 4.3 The Job Characteristics Model

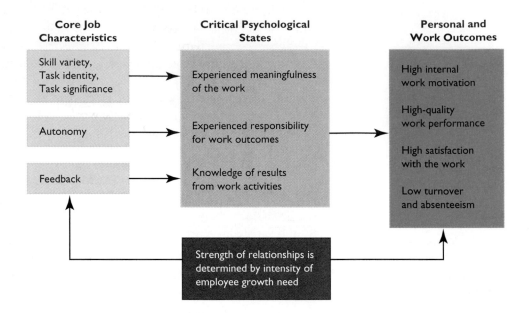

Job enrichment and the inclusion of the five core dimensions in jobs is not, however, a panacea. Job enrichment programs are more successful in some jobs and settings than in others. Moreover, not all employees want additional responsibility and challenge. Hackman and Oldham stress that the strength of the linkage among job characteristics, psychological states, and work outcomes is determined by the intensity of an individual employee's need for growth.[6] Some people prefer routine jobs and may resist job redesign efforts. In addition, job redesign efforts almost always fail when employees lack the physical or mental skills, abilities, or education needed to perform the job. Furthermore, neither approach will correct job dissatisfaction problems related to inequitable compensation, inadequate benefits, or lack of job security. Unions have sometimes resisted job enrichment, fearing that management will expect workers to take on more responsibility and challenge without additional compensation. Managers, fearing a loss of authority and control or worried about possible elimination of supervisory jobs, have also been sources of resistance.

Team-based Job Designs

team-based job designs
Job designs that focus on giving a team, rather than an individual, a whole and meaningful piece of work to do, and empowering team members to decide among themselves how to accomplish the work.

team
A small group of people, with complementary skills, who work toward common goals for which they hold joint responsibility and accountability.

A logical outgrowth of job enrichment and the job characteristics model has been the increasing use of **team-based job designs**, which focus on giving a **team**, rather than an individual, a whole and meaningful piece of work to do. Team members are empowered to decide among themselves how to accomplish the work.[7] Often they are cross-trained, and then rotated to perform different tasks. Team-based designs are best suited to flat and boundaryless organization structures.

Research Insight

Colonies of fire ants, named for their painful sting, are being studied by researchers at the University of Massachusetts, because of their capacity to work efficiently in small teams without visible leadership. The hope is that some of the findings can be applied to human teamwork. According to Abhijit Deshmukh, assistant professor of industrial engineering, there may be lessons for humans, such as letting shop teams react to immediate needs rather than relying on managers' schedules.[8]

General Motors, Saturn Division, is an extremely high-profile operation that has mastered the use of team-based job design. Initiated as a completely new venture within GM, the Saturn car assembly process involves self-managed teams with five to fifteen members. Each team reviews and hires new members, manages its own budget, schedules its work, and makes decisions regarding production and quality concerns.[9]

Human Engineering Considerations

Over time, it became apparent that in addition to considering psychological needs, effective job design must also take physiological needs and health and safety issues into account. **Human engineering** (or **ergonomics**) seeks to integrate and accommodate the physical needs of workers into the design of jobs. It aims to adapt the entire job system—the work, environment, machines, equipment, and processes—to match human characteristics. Doing so results in eliminating or minimizing product defects, damage to equipment, and worker injuries or illnesses caused by poor work design.

In addition to designing jobs and equipment with the aim of minimizing negative physiological effects for all workers, human engineering can aid in meeting the unique requirements of individuals with special needs and adapting jobs for older workers, a topic that is discussed in the Diversity Counts box.

Research Insight

It is important to note that the human engineering considerations involved in the design of jobs, workstations, and office space is important to all employees, not just older workers or those with special needs. A recent study conducted by the American Society of Interior Designers, involving interviews with 623 full-time employees and 27 HR executives and recruiters, revealed that a majority of employees rank design issues second only to compensation as a reason to accept

AN ETHICAL DILEMMA

If an organization restructures and adopts a team-based design, how should employees who can't work effectively in teams be dealt with?

human engineering (ergonomics)
An interdisciplinary approach that seeks to integrate and accommodate the physical needs of workers into the design of jobs. It aims to adapt the entire job system—the work, environment, machines, equipment, and processes—to match human characteristics.

At Saturn's auto factory, team members with complementary skills work toward common goals for which they hold joint responsibility and accountability.

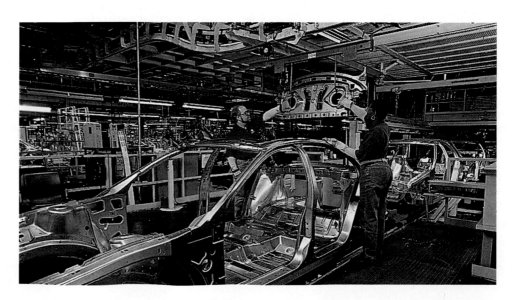

DIVERSITY COUNTS

Older Workers Can Benefit From Ergonomic Aid

More and more employees today have grey hair, stiff backs, and bifocals—a trend that will continue into the future, given Canada's current demographics.

While aging is a relatively individual process that not only affects people at different rates but also varies by body part or function, a number of changes are fairly common:

Muscular strength—Maximum strength occurs between 25 and 30 years of age. However, the rate of decline in strength appears to be a function of exercise and lifestyle. That is, an active 65-year-old may have 90 percent of his or her maximum strength, whereas a less-fit 40-year-old might have only 80 percent.

Hand function—As people age, their hands undergo a variety of changes, including a decrease in grip strength and endurance, finger and thumb strength, dexterity, precision, coordination, joint mobility, and sensitivity.

Cardiovascular capacity—The ability of the heart and lungs to supply blood to the working muscles—in order to perform light to moderate physically exhausting work—is not grossly age-dependent up to age 65, although capacity for hard, exhausting work is strongly age-dependent, with maximum capacity between ages 20 and 25.

Vision—Visual capabilities that are affected by aging include the ability to see fine detail sharply (acuity), focus on near and far objects (accommodation), distinguish between light and dark (sensitivity), discriminate certain colours, and judge distance and depth (stereopsis).

Hearing—Hearing loss with age is caused by a combination of the normal aging process, exposure to noise throughout life, and other factors. It influences ability to detect faint sounds and deal with background noise and multiple sources of noise. Detecting, understanding, and responding to speech sounds, as well as certain frequencies, becomes difficult. The need to listen and detect sounds becomes more demanding and is more tiring and prone to error.

The key for employers dealing with the effects of their aging work force is ensuring that jobs that require physical activity are designed with ergonomic principles in mind. Physical demands, such as manual materials-handling (lifting, pushing, pulling, and carrying), and upper-limb movements (reaching, grasping, pinching, and fingering), should be performed using good working postures, and as little force and repetition as possible. Items such as mechanical assists for lifting (scissor lift tables, tilters, vacuum lifts) and for assembly (screwguns and adjustable tables) are therefore becoming more essential.

As a result of diminished visual capabilities, performance of employees on assembly and inspection tasks may be greatly reduced. Visual capabilities should influence the lighting levels that are chosen and size of characters for controls and displays. The impact of aging on vision and hearing also needs to be considered when dealing with information processing and workplace communication issues.

As Canadian employers fight for competitiveness, the issues of workers' compensation, lost time due to injury, and the need to provide modified work programs top the list of challenges that must be met. Failure to incorporate ergonomic principles into the design of jobs has resulted in almost one-half of all lost-time injuries being caused by repetitive motion or overexertion. With the effects that aging has on the human body, these rates can only be expected to increase if ergonomics is not considered.

Source: Glenn Harrington, "Older Workers Need Ergonomic Aid," *Canadian HR Reporter* 10, no. 20 (November 17, 1997), p. 20.

or leave jobs. Besides wanting privacy, employees indicated a desire for access to needed equipment and people, and high-quality workspace lighting and air flow.[10]

Ergonomics has also become a collective bargaining issue. Based on the results of a joint study conducted by researchers at McMaster University and the Canadian Auto Workers Union (CAW), the CAW has determined that its members want to influence the intensity of their work and the design of their jobs, and they want the union to act on their behalf to ensure that these things occur. The CAW is therefore seeking improved job conditions for its members at the bargaining table. The aim is to create workstations that maximize comfort while allowing production standards to be met. For starters, the union wants workers to have a greater say when plants and lines are retooled or when new pieces of equipment are introduced. The union also wants to set "best practice" standards for comparable facilities and ensure that these standards are met.[11]

THE NATURE OF JOB ANALYSIS

Job Analysis Defined

job analysis

The procedure for determining the tasks, duties and responsibilities of each job, and the human attributes (in terms of knowledge skills, and abilities) required to perform it.

job description

A list of the duties, responsibilities, reporting relationships, and working conditions of a job—one product of a job analysis.

job specification

A list of the "human requirements," that is, the requisite knowledge, skills, and abilities (KSAs) needed to perform the job—another product of a job analysis.

Once jobs have been designed or redesigned, an employer's performance-related expectations need to be defined and communicated. This is best accomplished through job analysis, a process by which information about jobs is systematically gathered and organized. **Job analysis** is the procedure firms use to determine the tasks, duties, and responsibilities of each job, and the human attributes (in terms of knowledge, skills, and abilities) required to perform it. In contrast to job design, which reflects subjective opinions about the ideal requirements of a job, job analysis is concerned with objective and verifiable information about the actual requirements. Once this information has been gathered, it is used for developing **job descriptions** (what the job entails) and **job specifications** (what the human requirements are).[12]

Uses of Job Analysis Information

Job analysis is sometimes called the cornerstone of HRM. As illustrated in **Figure 4.4**, the information gathered, evaluated, and summarized through job analysis is the basis for a number of interrelated HRM activities. Having accurate information about jobs and their human requirements—which has been gathered in a gender-neutral, bias-free manner—is essential for legal compliance in each of these areas, as explained below.

Human Resources Planning

Knowing the actual requirements of jobs is essential in order to plan future staffing needs. As will be explained in the next chapter, when this information is combined with knowledge about the skills and qualifications of current employees, it is possible to determine which jobs can be filled internally and which will require external recruitment. Job analysis information is also extremely helpful in assessing how a firm's employment equity goals can be met most effectively.

Recruitment and Selection

The job description and job specification information should be used to decide what sort of person to recruit and hire. Identifying bona fide occupational

FIGURE **4.4** Uses of Job Analysis Information

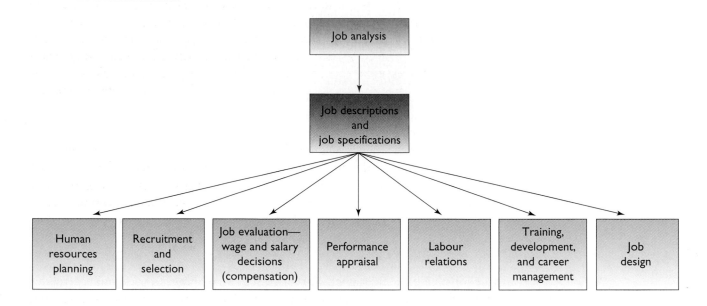

requirements, and ensuring that all activities related to recruitment and selection (such as advertising, screening, and testing) are based on such requirements, is necessary for legal compliance in all Canadian jurisdictions, something that was reinforced in a recent Federal Court of Appeal ruling:[13]

> When the Department of Employment and Immigration (now the Ministry of Citizenship and Immigration) advertised for immigration settlement counsellors, five qualifications were listed, one of which was knowledge of relevant legislation, of the branch and of issues concerning immigrant or refugee settlement. During its written and oral testing, however, the department decided to weight these knowledge requirements at only 10 percent, and three of the five candidates subsequently selected failed the knowledge requirement altogether. Two individuals who passed the knowledge requirement but were not hired launched a complaint. The Federal Court of Appeal ruled that the department "erred in law in not requiring that candidates succeed on each of the advertised qualifications of this position ... "a selection board cannot change the advertised qualifications by eliminating one or more of them: to do so is unfair to those who might otherwise have applied but failed to do so because they recognized that they did not have all of the advertised qualifications."

Job Analysis
www.ipmaac.org/link-ja.html

Compensation

Job analysis information is also essential for determining the relative value of and appropriate compensation for each job. Job evaluation should be based on the required skills, physical and mental demands, responsibilities, and working conditions—all assessed through job analysis. The relative value of jobs is one of the key factors used to determine appropriate compensation and justify pay differences if challenged under human rights or pay equity legislation. Information about the actual job duties is also necessary to determine whether a job should be classified as exempt or nonexempt for overtime pay and maximum hours purposes, as specified in employment standards legislation.

Performance Appraisal

To be legally defensible, the criteria used to assess employee performance must be directly related to the duties and responsibilities identified through job analysis. The standards used must also be justifiable. For many jobs involving routine tasks, especially those of a quantifiable nature, performance standards are determined through job analysis. For more complex jobs, performance standards are often jointly established by employees and their supervisors. To be realistic and achievable, such standards should be based on actual job requirements, as identified through job analysis.

Labour Relations

In unionized environments, the job descriptions developed from the job analysis information are generally subject to union approval prior to finalization. Such union-approved job descriptions then become the basis for classifying jobs, and bargaining over wages, performance criteria, and working conditions. Once approved, significant changes to job descriptions may have to be negotiated.

Training, Development, and Career Management

By comparing the knowledge, skills, and abilities (KSAs) that employees bring to the job with those that are identified by job analysis, managers can determine the gaps. Training programs can then be designed to bridge these gaps. Having accurate information about jobs also means that employees can prepare for future advancement by identifying gaps between their current KSAs and those specified for the jobs to which they aspire.

Job Design

Job analysis is useful for ensuring that all of the duties having to be done have actually been assigned, and identifying areas of overlap. Also, having an accurate description of each job sometimes leads to the identification of unnecessary requirements, areas of conflict or dissatisfaction, and/or health and safety concerns that can be eliminated through job redesign. Such redesign may increase morale and productivity and ensure compliance with human rights and occupational health and safety legislation.

Steps in Job Analysis

The six steps involved in analyzing jobs are as follows.

Step 1 Identify the use to which the information will be put, since this will determine the types of data that should be collected and the techniques used. Some data-collection techniques—such as interviewing the employee and asking what the job entails and what his or her responsibilities are—are good for writing job descriptions and selecting employees for the job. Other job analysis techniques (like the position analysis questionnaire, described later) do not provide qualitative information for job descriptions, but rather numerical ratings for each job; these can be used to compare jobs to one another for compensation purposes.

process chart

A diagram showing the flow of inputs to and outputs from the job under study.

Step 2 Review relevant background information such as organization charts, process charts, and job descriptions.[14] As explained earlier, organization charts show how the job in question relates to other jobs and where it fits in the overall organization. A **process chart** provides a more detailed understanding of the workflow than is obtainable from the organization chart alone. In its simplest form, a process chart (like the one in **Figure 4.5**) shows the flow of inputs to and outputs from the job under study. (In Figure 4.5, the inventory control clerk is expected to receive inventory from suppliers, take requests for inventory from the two plant managers, provide requested inventory to these managers, and give information to these managers on the status of in-stock inventories.) Finally, the existing job description, if there is one, can provide a starting point for building the revised one.

Step 3   Select the representative positions and jobs to be analyzed. This is necessary when there are many incumbents in a single job and when a number of similar jobs are to be analyzed, since it would be too time-consuming to analyze every position and job.

Step 4   Next, analyze the jobs by collecting data on job activities, required employee behaviours, working conditions, and human traits and abilities needed to perform the job, using one or more of the job analysis techniques explained later in this chapter.

Step 5   Review the information with job incumbents. The job analysis information should be verified with the worker(s) performing the job and with the immediate supervisor. This will help to confirm that the information is factually correct and complete. By providing an opportunity for review and modification, if necessary, this step can also help gain the employees' acceptance of the job analysis data, as well as the documents derived from this data and subsequent decisions reached.

Job Analysis
http://harvey.psyc.vt.edu/ja.html

FIGURE 4.5 Process Chart for Analyzing a Job's Workflow

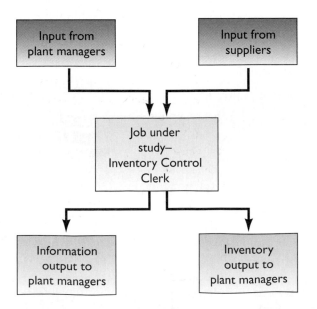

Source: Richard I. Henderson, *Compensation Management: Rewarding Performance*, 2nd ed., copyright 1985, p. 158. Reprinted by permission of Prentice-Hall, Englewood Cliffs, NJ.

Step 6 Develop a job description and job specification. A job description and a job specification are the two concrete products of the job analysis. As explained earlier, the job description is a written statement that describes the activities and responsibilities of the job, as well as important features of the job (such as working conditions and safety hazards). The job specification summarizes the personal qualities, traits, skills, and background required. While there may be a separate document describing the human qualifications, job descriptions and specifications are often combined in a single document, generally titled "Job Description."

METHODS OF COLLECTING JOB ANALYSIS INFORMATION

Various techniques are used for collecting information about the duties, responsibilities, and requirements of the job; the most important ones will be discussed in this section. In practice, when the information is being used for multiple purposes, ranging from developing recruitment criteria to compensation decisions, several techniques may be used in combination.

Who Collects the Job Information?

Collecting job analysis data usually involves a joint effort by an HR specialist, the incumbent, and the jobholder's supervisor. The HR specialist (an HR manager, job analyst, or consultant) might observe and analyze the work being done and then develop a job description and specification. The supervisor and incumbent generally also get involved, perhaps by filling out questionnaires. The supervisor and incumbent typically review and verify the job analyst's conclusions regarding the job's duties, responsibilities, and requirements.

The Interview

Three types of interviews are used to collect job analysis data: individual interviews with each employee; group interviews with employees having the same job; and supervisory interviews with one or more supervisors who are thoroughly knowledgeable about the job being analyzed. The group interview is used when a large number of employees are performing similar or identical work, and it can be a quick and inexpensive way of learning about the job. As a rule, the immediate supervisor attends the group session; if not, the supervisor should be interviewed separately to get that person's perspective on the duties and responsibilities of the job.

Whichever interview method is used, the interviewee should fully understand the reason for the interview, since there's a tendency for such interviews to be misconstrued as "efficiency evaluations." When they are, interviewees may not be willing to accurately describe their jobs or those of their reporting employees.

The interview is probably the most widely used method for determining the duties and responsibilities of a job. Its wide use reflects its advantages, which are discussed in Table 4.1 on page 140, along with the disadvantages of this technique.

Typical Questions

Some typical interview questions include:

1. What is the major purpose of the job?

2. What are the major duties? What percentage of time is spent on each?

3. What are the major responsibilities?

4. What types of equipment, machinery, and/or tools are used?

5. What are the education, experience, skill, and (where applicable) certification and licensing requirements?

6. What are the basic accountabilities or performance standards that typify the work?

7. What are the job's physical demands? What are its emotional and mental demands?

8. In what physical location(s) is the work performed? What working conditions are involved?

9. What are the health and safety conditions? To what hazard(s) is there exposure, if any?

Most fruitful interviews follow a structured or checklist format. A job analysis questionnaire like the one presented in **Figure 4.6** may be used to interview job incumbents or may be filled out by them. It includes a series of detailed questions regarding such matters as: the general purpose of the job; responsibilities and duties; education, experience, and skills required; physical and mental demands; and working conditions. A list like this can also be used by a job analyst who collects information by personally observing the work being done or by administering it as a questionnaire, two methods that will be explained shortly.[15]

Interview Guidelines
When conducting a job analysis interview, supervisors and job analysts should keep several things in mind:

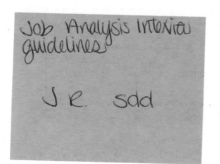

Job Analysis Interview guidelines

J.R. sdd

1. The job analyst and supervisor should work together to identify the employees who know the job best, as well as those who might be expected to be the most objective in describing their duties and responsibilities.

2. Rapport should be established quickly with the interviewee, by using the individual's name, speaking in easily understood language, briefly reviewing the purpose of the interview (job analysis, not performance appraisal), and explaining how the person came to be chosen.

3. A structured guide or checklist that lists questions and provides spaces for answers should be used. This ensures that crucial questions are identified ahead of time, so that complete and accurate information is gathered, and that all interviewers (if there is more than one) glean the same types of data, thereby helping to ensure comparability of results. However, leeway should also be permitted by including some open-ended questions like, "Was there anything that we didn't cover with our questions?"

4. When duties are not performed in a regular manner—for instance, when the incumbent doesn't perform the same tasks or jobs over and over again many times a day—the incumbent should be asked to list his or her duties *in order of importance* and *frequency of occurrence*. This will ensure that crucial activities that occur infrequently—like a nurse's occasional emergency room duties—aren't overlooked.

5. The data should be reviewed and verified by both the interviewee and his or her immediate supervisor.

FIGURE 4.6 Job Analysis Questionnaire

JOB QUESTIONNAIRE
KANE MANUFACTURING COMPANY

NAME _____   JOB TITLE _____

DEPARTMENT _____   JOB NUMBER _____

SUPERVISOR'S NAME _____   SUPERVISOR'S TITLE _____

1. *SUMMARY OF DUTIES:* State briefly, in your own words, your main duties. If you are responsible for filling out reports/records, also complete Section 8.

2. *SPECIAL QUALIFICATIONS:* List any licences, permits, certifications, etc. required to perform duties assigned to your position.

3. *EQUIPMENT:* List any equipment, machines, or tools (e.g., computer, calculator, motor vehicles, lathes, fork lifts, drill presses, etc.) you normally operate as a part of your position's duties.

    EQUIPMENT   *AVERAGE NO. HOURS PER WEEK*

4. *REGULAR DUTIES:* In general terms, describe duties you regularly perform. Please list these duties in descending order of importance and percent of time spent on them per month. List as many duties as possible and attach additional sheets, if necessary.

5. *CONTACTS:* Does your job require any contacts with other department members, other departments, outside companies, or agencies? If yes, please define the duties requiring contacts and *how often.*

6. *SUPERVISION:* Does your position have supervisory responsibilities? ( ) Yes ( ) No If yes, please fill out a *Supplemental Position Description Questionnaire for Supervisors* and attach it to this form. If you have responsibility for the work of others but do not directly supervise them, please explain.

7. *DECISION MAKING:* Please explain the decisions you make while performing the regular duties of your job.

\>>

(a) What would be the probable result of your making (i) poor judgment(s) or decision(s), or (ii) improper actions?

_____

_____

8. *RESPONSIBILITY   FOR RECORDS* : List the reports and files you are required to prepare or maintain. State, in general, for whom each report is intended.

(a)   *REPORT*   *INTENDED FOR*

_____

_____

_____

(b)   *FILES MAINTAINED*

_____

_____

9. *FREQUENCY OF SUPERVISION:* How frequently must you confer with your supervisor or other employees in making decisions or in determining the proper course of action to be taken?

( ) Frequently   ( ) Occasionally   ( ) Seldom   ( ) Never

10. *WORKING CONDITIONS*: Please describe the conditions under which you work—inside, outside, air-conditioned area, etc. Be sure to list any disagreeable or unusual working conditions.

_____

11. *JOB REQUIREMENTS*: Please indicate the minimum requirements you believe are necessary to perform satisfactorily in your position.

(a) Education:
Minimum schooling _____
Number of years _____
Specialization or major _____

(b) Experience:
Type _____
Number of years _____

(c) Special training:

        TYPE   *NUMBER OF YEARS*

_____

_____

(d) Special Skills:
Keyboarding: _____ w.p.m.   Shorthand _____ w.p.m.
Other: _____

12. *ADDITIONAL INFORMATION*: Please provide additional information, not included in any of the previous items, which you feel would be important in a description of your position.

_____

_____

_____

EMPLOYEE'S SIGNATURE _____   DATE: _____

Source: Based on Douglas Bartley, *Job Evaluation: Wage and Salary Administration* (Reading, MA: Addison-Wesley Publishing Company, 1981), pp. 101-3.

Job Analysis
www.acl.lanl.gov

Questionnaires

Having employees fill out questionnaires to describe their job-related duties and responsibilities is another good method of obtaining job analysis information.

The major decision involved is determining how structured the questionnaire should be and what questions to include. Some questionnaires involve structured checklists. Each employee is presented with an inventory of perhaps hundreds of specific duties or tasks (such as "change and splice wire"), and is asked to indicate whether or not he or she performs each and, if so, how much time is normally spent on it. At the other extreme, the questionnaire can be open-ended and simply ask the employee to describe the major duties of his or her job. In practice, a typical job analysis questionnaire often falls between the two extremes. As illustrated in Figure 4.6, there are often several open-ended questions (such as "state your main job duties"), as well as a number of structured questions (concerning, for instance, job requirements).

Whether structured, unstructured or a combination of the two, questionnaires have advantages and disadvantages, which are summarized in Table 4.1 on page 140.

Observation

Direct observation is especially useful when jobs consist mainly of observable physical activities. Jobs like those of janitor, assembly-line worker, and accounting clerk are examples. On the other hand, observation is usually not appropriate when the job entails a lot of unmeasurable mental activity (lawyer, design engineer). Nor is it useful if the employee engages in important activities that might occur only occasionally, such as year-end reports.

Direct observation and interviewing are often used together. One approach is to observe the worker on the job during a complete work cycle. (The cycle is the time that it takes to complete the job; it could be a minute for an assembly-line worker or an hour, a day, or longer for complex jobs.) All of the observed job activities are noted. Then, after as much information as possible is accumulated, the incumbent is interviewed, asked to clarify points not understood, and explain what additional activities he or she performs that weren't observed. Another approach is to observe and interview simultaneously, while the jobholder performs his or her tasks.

Participant Diary/Log

diary/log
Daily listings made by employees of every activity in which they engage, along with the time each activity takes.

Another technique involves asking employees to keep a **diary/log** or a list of what they do during the day. Each employee records every activity in which he or she is involved (along with the time) in a log. This can produce a very complete picture of the job, especially when supplemented with subsequent interviews with the employee and his or her supervisor. The employee might, of course, try to exaggerate some activities and underplay others. However, the detailed, chronological nature of the log tends to minimize this problem.

Advantages and Disadvantages of the Conventional Data Collection Methods

Interviews, questionnaires, observation, and participant diaries are known as the conventional data collection methods, since they are all qualitative in nature.

They are the most popular methods for gathering job analysis data, and provide realistic information about what job incumbents actually do and the qualification and skills required. Associated with each are certain advantages and disadvantages, as summarized in **Table 4.1** below. By combining two or more conventional techniques, some of the disadvantages can be overcome.

Quantitative Job Analysis Techniques

Although most employers use interviews, questionnaires, observations, and/or diaries/logs for collecting job analysis data, there are many times when these narrative approaches are not appropriate. For example, when the aim is to assign a quantitative value to each job so that jobs can be compared for pay purposes, a more quantitative job analysis approach may be best. The position analysis questionnaire and functional job analysis are two popular quantitative methods.

Position Analysis Questionnaire

position analysis questionnaire (PAQ)

A questionnaire used to collect quantifiable data concerning the duties and responsibilities of various jobs.

The **position analysis questionnaire (PAQ)** is a very structured job analysis questionnaire.[16] The PAQ itself is filled in by a job analyst, who should already be acquainted with the particular job to be analyzed. The PAQ contains 194 items, each of which represents a basic element that may or may not play an important role in the job. The job analyst decides whether each item plays a role on the job and, if so, to what extent. In **Figure 4.7**, for example, "written materials" received a rating of four, indicating that materials such as books, reports, and office notes play a considerable role in this job.

The advantage of the PAQ is that it provides a quantitative score or profile of the job in terms of how that job rates on five basic dimensions: (1) having

TABLE 4.1

A Summary of Conventional Data Collection Methods for Job Analysis and the Advantages/Disadvantages of Each

Method	Variations	Brief Description	Advantages	Disadvantages
Observation	Structured	• Watch people go about their work; record frequency of behaviours or nature of performance on forms prepared in advance	• Third-party observer has more credibility than job incumbents, who may have reasons for distorting information	• Observation can influence behaviour of job incumbents
	Unstructured	• Watch people go about their work; describe behaviours/tasks performed	• Focuses more on reality than on perceptions	• Meaningless for jobs requiring mental effort (in that case, use information processing method)
	Combination	• Part of the form is prepared in advance and is structured; part is unstructured		• Not useful for jobs with a long job cycle

>>

Questionnaire	Structured	• Ask job incumbents/supervisors about work performed using fixed responses	• Relatively inexpensive • Structured questionnaires lend themselves easily to computer analyses • Good method when employees are widely scattered or when data must be collected from a large number of employes	• Developing and testing a questionnaire can be time-consuming and costly • Depends on communication skills of respondents • Does not allow for probing • Tends to focus on perceptions of the job
	Unstructured	• Ask job incumbents/supervisors to write essays to describe work performed		
	Combination	• Part of the questionnaire is structured; part is unstructured		
Diary/Log	Structured	• Ask people to record their activities over several days or weeks in a booklet with time increments provided	• Highly detailed informaton can be collected over the entire job cycle • Quite appropriate for jobs with a long job cycle	• Requires the job incumbent's participation and cooperation • Tends to focus on perceptions of the job
	Unstructured	• Ask people to indicate in a booklet over how long a period they work on a task or activity		
	Combination	• Part of the diary is structured; part is unstructured		
Individual Interview	Structured	• Read questions and/or fixed response choices to job incumbent and supervisor; must be face to face	• Provides an opportunity to explain the need for and functions of job analysis • Relatively quick and simple way to collect data • More flexible than surveys • Allows for probing to extract information and provides the interviewee with an opportunity to express views and/or vent frustrations that might otherwise go unnoticed • Activities and behaviours may be reported that would be missed during observation	• Depends heavily on rapport between interviewer and respondent • May suffer from validity/reliability problems • Information may be distorted due to outright falsification or honest misunderstanding
	Unstructured	• Ask questions and/or provide general response choices to job incumbent and supervisor; must be face to face		
	Combination	• Part of the interview is structured; part is unstructured		
Group Interview	Structured	• Same as structured individual interviews except that more than one job incumbent/ supervisor is interviewed	• Groups tend to do better than individuals with open-ended problem solving • Reliability/validity are likely to be higher than with individuals because group members cross check each other	• Cost more because more people are taken away from their jobs to participate • Like individual interviews, tends to focus on perceptions of the job
	Unstructured	• Same as unstructured individual interviews except that more than one job incumbent/supervisor is interviewed		
	Combination	• Same as combination individual interview except more than one job incumbent/supervisor is interviewed		

Source: Adapted from William J. Rothwell and H.C. Kazanas, *Strategic Human Resource Planning and Management,* © 1989, pp. 66–68. Reprinted by permission of Prentice-Hall, Inc., Englewood Cliffs, New Jersey.

FIGURE 4.7 Portions of a Completed Page from the Position Analysis Questionnaire

Note: The 194 PAQ elements are grouped into six dimensions. This exhibits 11 of the "information input" questions or elements. Other PAQ pages contain questions regarding mental processes, work output, relationships with others, job context, and other job characteristics.

INFORMATION INPUT

1 INFORMATION INPUT

1.1 Sources of Job Information

Rate each of the following items in terms of the extent to which it is used by the worker as a source of information in performing the job.

	Extent of Use (U)
NA	Does not apply
1	Nominal/very infrequent
2	Occasional
3	Moderate
4	Considerable
5	Very substantial

1.1.1 Visual Sources of Job Information

1 | 4 Written materials (books, reports, office notes, articles, job instructions, signs, etc.)

2 | 2 Quantitative materials (materials that deal with quantities or amounts, such as graphs, accounts, specifications, tables of numbers, etc.)

3 | 1 Pictorial materials (pictures or picturelike materials used as *sources* of information, for example, drawings, blueprints, diagrams, maps, tracings, photographic films, x-ray films, TV pictures, etc.)

4 | 1 Patterns/related devices (templates, stencils, patterns, etc., used as *sources* of information when *observed* during use; do *not* include here materials described in item 3 above)

5 | 2 Visual displays (dials, gauges, signal lights, radarscopes, speedometers, clocks, etc.)

6 | 5 Measuring devices (rulers, calipers, tire pressure gauges, scales, thickness gauges, pipettes, thermometers, protractors, etc., used to obtain visual information about physical measurements; do *not* include here devices described in item 5 above)

7 | 4 Mechanical devices (tools, equipment, machinery, and other mechanical devices that are *sources* of information when *observed* during use or operation)

8 | 3 Materials in process (parts, materials, objects, etc., that are *sources* of information when being modified, worked on, or otherwise processed, such as bread dough being mixed, workpiece being turned in a lathe, fabric being cut, shoe being resoled, etc.)

9 | 4 Materials *not* in process (parts, materials, objects, etc., not in the process of being changed or modified, that are *sources* of information when being inspected, handled, packaged, distributed, or selected, etc., such as items or materials in inventory, storage, or distribution channels, items being inspected, etc.)

10 | 3 Features of nature (landscapes, fields, geological samples, vegetation, cloud formations, and other features of nature that are observed or inspected to provide information)

11 | 2 Man-made features of environment (structures, buildings, dams, highways, bridges, docks, railroads, and other "man-made" or altered aspects of the indoor or outdoor environment that are *observed* or *inspected* to provide job information; do not consider equipment, machines, etc., that an individual uses in the work, as covered by item 7)

Source: E.J. McCormick, P.R. Jeanneret, and R.D. Mecham, *Position Analysis Questionnaire*. Copyright 1989 by Purdue Research Foundation, West Lafayette, IN. Reprinted with permission.

decision-making/communication/social responsibilities, (2) performing skilled activities, (3) being physically active, (4) operating vehicles/equipment, and (5) processing information. Since it allows the assignment of a quantitative score to each job, based on these five dimensions, the PAQ's real strength is in classifying jobs. Results can be used to compare jobs to one another;[17] this information can then be used to determine appropriate pay levels.[18]

Functional Job Analysis

functional job analysis (FJA)
A quantitative method for classifying jobs based on types and amounts of responsibility for data, people, and things, as well as the extent to which instructions, reasoning, judgment, and verbal facility are necessary for performing assigned tasks. Performance standards and training requirements are also identified.

Functional job analysis (FJA) rates the job not only on responsibilities pertaining to data, people, and things, but also on the following dimensions: the extent to which specific *instructions, reasoning,* and *judgment* are required to perform the task; the *mathematical ability* required; and the *verbal and language facilities* involved. This quantitative technique also identifies *performance standards and training requirements.* Thus, FJA allows the analyst to answer the question, "To do this task and meet these standards, what training does the worker require?"[19]

Figure 4.8 illustrates a completed functional job analysis summary sheet. In this case, the job is that of grader (a type of heavy-equipment operator employed in road building).

FIGURE 4.8 Functional Job Analysis Task Statement

TASK CODE: GR-08

WORKER FUNCTION AND ORIENTATION						WORKER INSTRUCTIONS	GENERAL EDUCATIONAL DEVELOPMENT		
THINGS	%	DATA	%	PEOPLE	%		REASONING	MATH	LANGUAGE
3	65	3	25	1	10	3	2	1	3

GOAL:
Operates Grader–Output Basic

OBJECTIVE:
Backfilling, scarifying, windrowing, cutting firebreak, maintaining haul road, snow removal

TASK: Operates grader manipulating controls to travel forward/back, turn, raise/lower blade, position wheels and blade at correct angles; follows work order, drawing on knowledge and experience, monitoring the performance of the equipment and adapting to the changing situation, constantly alert to the presence and safety of other workers/equipment, in order to perform routine grader tasks such as backfilling, haul road maintenance, snow removal.

(To Perform This Task)

PERFORMANCE STANDARDS	TRAINING CONTENT

DESCRIPTIVE:
— Operates equipment properly.
— Is alert and attentive.

NUMERICAL:
— All work meets work order requirements.
— No accidents/damage due to improper operating techniques.

FUNCTIONAL:
— How to operate grader.
— How to do routine grader tasks, such as backfilling, scarifying, windrowing, cutting firebreak, maintaining road, snow removal.

SPECIFIC:
— Knowledge of specific grader.
— Knowledge of work requirements.
— Knowledge of specific job site (i.e., layout, soil condition, environment).

(To These Standards) ——————— ▷*(Worker Needs This Training)*

Source: Howard Olson, Sidney A. Fine, David C. Myers, and Margarette C. Jennings, "The Use of Functional Job Analysis in Establishing Performance for Heavy Equipment Operators," *Personnel Psychology*, Summer 1981, p. 354.

The *National Occupational Classification* and Job Analysis

National Occupational Classification (NOC)

A reference tool for writing job descriptions and job specifications. Compiled by the federal government, it contains comprehensive, standardized descriptions of about 25 000 occupations and the requirements for each.

The *National Occupational Classification (NOC)*, the product of systematic, field-based research by the former Occupational and Career Information Branch of Human Resources Development Canada (HRDC),[20] is an excellent source of standardized information. It contains comprehensive descriptions of approximately 25 000 occupations and the requirements for each. To illustrate the types of information included, the *NOC* listing for Specialists in Human Resources is shown in **Figure 4.9.**

Published in 1993, the *NOC* represented a new structure for analyzing and understanding the labour market, reflecting occupational changes that had occurred over the previous decade. It replaced the *Canadian Classification and Dictionary of Occupations (CCDO)* and the closely related *Standard Occupational Classification (SOC)* system devised by Statistics Canada. The *NOC* and its counselling component, the *Career Handbook* (published in 1996), both focus on occupations rather than jobs. An occupation is defined as a collection of jobs that share some or all of a set of main duties. The list of examples of job titles within each of the 522 Unit Groups in the *NOC* provides a frame of reference for the boundaries of that occupational group. The jobs within each group are characterized by similar skills.[21]

occupation

A collection of jobs that share some or all of a set of main duties.

To provide a complete representation of work in the Canadian economy, the *NOC* classifies occupations in Major Groups based on two key dimensions—skill level and skill type. The Major Groups, which are identified by two-digit numbers, are then broken down further into Minor Groups, with a third digit added, and Unit Groups, at which level a fourth digit is added. Within these three levels of classification, a Unit Group provides the actual profile of an occupation.[22] For example:

- Major Group 31—Professional Occupations in Health
- Minor Group 314—Professional Occupations in Therapy and Assessment
- Unit Group 3142—Physiotherapists

These code numbers facilitate the exchange of statistical information about jobs, and are useful for vocational counselling and charting career paths. Since the *NOC* Major Group codes are now being used for employment equity reporting purposes, many companies formerly using *CCDO* and *SOC* codes have switched to *NOC* codes.

One of the benefits of the former *CCDO* and the current *NOC* is that they have helped to promote a greater degree of uniformity in job titles and descriptions used by employers across Canada. This has facilitated the exchange of information about salaries and benefits for compensation administration purposes, and about labour supply and demand for human resources planning.

Standardized job descriptions also facilitate the movement of workers from areas experiencing high unemployment to those in which there are more job opportunities.

WRITING JOB DESCRIPTIONS

A job description is a written statement of *what* the jobholder actually does, *how* he or she does it, and *under what conditions* the job is performed.

FIGURE 4.9 *NOC* Job Description for Specialists in Human Resources

Specialists in Human Resources develop, implement, and evaluate human resources and labour relations policies, programs, and procedures and advise managers and employees on personnel matters. Specialists in Human Resources are employed throughout the private and public sectors, or may be self-employed.

Examples of titles classified in this unit group

Business Agent, Labour Union
Classification Officer
Classification Specialist
Compensation Research Analyst
Conciliator
Consultant, Human Resources
Employee Relations Officer

Employment Equity Officer
Human Resources Research Officer
Job Analyst
Labour Relations Officer
Mediator
Union Representative
Wage Analyst .

Main duties

Specialists in Human Resources perform some or all of the following duties:

- Develop, implement, and evaluate personnel and labour relations policies, programs, and procedures
- Advise managers and employees on the interpretation of personnel policies, benefit programs, and collective agreements
- Negotiate collective agreements on behalf of employers or workers, and mediate labour disputes and grievances
- Research and prepare occupational classifications, job descriptions, and salary scales
- Administer benefit, employment equity and affirmative action programs, and maintain related record systems
- Coordinate employee performance and appraisal programs
- Research employee benefit and health and safety practices and recommend changes or modifications to existing policies.

Employment requirements

- A university degree or college diploma in a field related to personnel management, such as business administration, industrial relations, commerce, or psychology

or

Completion of a professional development program in personnel administration is required.

- Some experience in a clerical or administrative position related to personnel administration may be required.

Additional information

- Progression to management positions is possible with experience.

Classified elsewhere

- *Human Resources Managers (0112)*
- *Personnel and Recruitment Officers (1223)*
- *Personnel Clerks (1442)*
- *Professional Occupations in Business Services to Management (1122)*
- Training officers and instructors (in 4131 *College and Other Vocational Instructors*)

Source: Human Resources Development Canada, *National Occupational Classification*, Cat. No. MP 53-25/1–1992-E (Ottawa: Ministry of Supply and Services, 1992). Reproduced with permission of the Minister of Public Works and Government Services Canada, 2001.

INFORMATION TECHNOLOGY AND HR

Writing Job Descriptions Online

Thanks to the Internet, assistance in writing job descriptions may be just a few keystrokes away. For example, *Workforce* has a Web site called Post-A-Job (**www.workforceonline.com/postajob/**) that employers can use to post job openings on the Internet. To aid those posting jobs, the site has a page called "Write Your Job Descriptions Online." Following it leads to a site called Descriptions Now! Direct, at **www.jobdescription.com**. Once there, for a fee, one can choose the job title of interest, pull up the relevant job description, and then fine-tune it, if so desired.

No standard format is used in writing job descriptions, but most include the following types of information: job identification, job summary, relationships, duties and responsibilities, authority of incumbent, performance standards, and working conditions. We will describe what is likely to be found under each of these headings shortly. As mentioned previously, job specifications (human qualifications) may also be included, as in the example presented in Figure 4.10 on page 147.

When writing job descriptions for the first time or updating them to keep them current, the *NOC* and its accompanying *Career Handbook* can be extremely helpful. As explained in the Information Technology and HR box, online assistance is also available.

The description in **Figure 4.10**—in this case for a marketing manager—provides an example. As can be seen, the description is quite comprehensive and includes such essential elements as identification, summary, and duties and responsibilities, as well as the human qualifications for the job.

Job Identification

As in Figure 4.10, the job identification section generally contains several types of information. The *job title* specifies the title of the job, such as marketing manager, recruiter, or inventory control clerk. The *department* or *location* is also indicated, along with the title of the immediate supervisor—in this case under the heading *reports to*. The *job status* section permits quick identification of eligibility for overtime pay. The *date* refers to the date the job description was actually written, and *prepared by* identifies the person who wrote it. There is also an indication of *who approved* the description and the *approval date*.

Many job descriptions also include a *job code*, which permits easy referencing. While some firms devise their own coding systems based on wage classification, for example, many use *NOC* codes to facilitate external comparison and employment equity reporting. Information regarding the job's salary and/or pay scale is sometimes found in the identification section, as well. If so, the grade or level of the job in the wage or salary classification system is indicated under a heading such as *grade/level*, and job evaluation points may also be shown. Some firms include a *pay range* section, in which the specific pay or pay range of the job is provided. Since pay rates change, however, many firms omit this information. Providing the grade or level facilitates cross-referencing to the collective agreement or salary grid, so that pay information can be easily obtained.

FIGURE 4.10 Sample Job Description

OLEC CORP.
Job Description

Job Title:	Marketing Manager
Department:	Marketing
Reports To:	President
ESA Status:	Non Exempt
Prepared By:	Michael George
Prepared Date:	April 1, 2000
Approved By:	Ian Alexander
Approved Date:	April 15, 2000

SUMMARY

Plans, directs, and coordinates the marketing of the organization's products and/or services by performing the following duties personally or through reporting supervisors.

ESSENTIAL DUTIES AND RESPONSIBILITIES include the following.

Establishes marketing goals to ensure share of market and profitability of products and/or services.

Develops and executes marketing plans and programs, both short and long range, to ensure the profit growth and expansion of company products and/or services.

Researches, analyzes, and monitors financial, technological, and demographic factors so that market opportunities may be capitalized on and the effects of competitive activity may be minimized.

Plans and oversees the organization's advertising and promotion acitivities including print, electronic, and direct mail outlets.

Communicates with outside advertising agencies on ongoing campaigns.

Works with writers and artists and oversees copywriting, design, layout, pasteup, and production of promotional materials.

Develops and recommends pricing strategy for the organization that will result in the greatest share of the market over the long run.

Achieves satisfactory profit/loss ratio and share of market performance in relation to pre-set standards and to general and specific trends within the industry and the economy.

Ensures effective control of marketing results and that corrective action takes place to be certain that the achievement of marketing objectives are within designated budgets.

Evaluates market reactions to advertising programs, merchandising policy, and product packaging and formulation to ensure the timely adjustment of marketing strategy and plans to meet changing market and competitive conditions.

Recommends changes in basic structure and organization of marketing group to ensure the effective fulfillment of objectives assigned to it and provide the flexibility to move swiftly in relation to marketing problems and opportunities.

Conducts marketing surveys on current and new product concepts.

Prepares marketing activity reports.

SUPERVISORY RESPONSIBILITIES

Manages three supervisors who supervise a total of five employees in the Marketing Department. Is responsible for the overall direction, coordination, and evaluation of this unit. Also directly supervises two non-supervisory employees. Carries out supervisory responsibilities in accordance with the organization's policies and applicable laws. Responsibilites include: interviewing, hiring, and training employees; planning, assigning, and directing work; appraising performance; rewarding and disciplining employees; addressing complaints and resolving problems.

QUALIFICATIONS

To perform this job successfully, an individual must be able to perform each essential duty satisfactorily. The requirements listed below are representative of the knowledge, skill, and/or ability required. Reasonable accommodations may be made to enable individuals to perform the essential functions.

EDUCATION and/or EXPERIENCE

Master's degree (M.A.) or equivalent; or four to ten years related experience and/or training; or equivalent combination of education and experience.

LANGUAGE SKILLS

Ability to read, analyze, and interpret common scientific and technical journals, financial reports, and legal documents. Ability to respond to common inquiries or complaints from customers, regulatory agencies, or members of the business community. Ability to write speeches and articles for publication that conform to prescribed style and format. Ability to efffectively present information to top management, public groups, and/or boards of directors.

MATHEMATICAL SKILLS

Ability to apply advanced mathematical concepts such as exponents, logarithms, quadratic equations, and permutations. Ability to apply mathematical operations to such tasks as frequency distribution, determination of test reliability and validity, analysis of variance, correlation techniques, sampling theory, and factor analysis.

REASONING ABILITY

Ability to define problems, collect data, establish facts, and draw valid conclusions. Ability to interpret an extensive variety of technical instructions in mathematical or diagram form.

Source: Descriptions Now! Direct at **www.jobdescription.com**.

Job Summary

The *job summary* should describe the general nature of the job, listing only its major functions or activities. Thus (as in Figure 4.10), the marketing manager "plans, directs, and coordinates the marketing of the organization's products and/or services." For the job of materials manager, the summary might state that she or he "purchases economically, regulates deliveries of, stores, and distributes all material necessary on the production line," while that for a mailroom supervisor might indicate that she or he "receives, sorts, and delivers all incoming mail properly, and he or she handles all outgoing mail including the accurate and timely posting of such mail."[23]

Relationships

There is sometimes a relationships section (not in Figure 4.10), which indicates the jobholder's relationships with others inside and outside the organization. The relationships section on the job description of an HR manager, for example, might look like this:[24]

- *Reports to:* vice-president of employee relations
- *Supervises:* HR specialist, test administrator, labour relations specialist, and one secretary
- *Works with*: all department managers and senior management team members
- *Contacts outside the company:* employment agencies, executive recruiting firms, union representatives, Human Resources Development Canada (HRDC), and various vendors.

Duties and Responsibilities

This section presents a detailed list of the job's major duties and responsibilities. As in Figure 4.10, each of the job's major duties should be listed separately, and described, in a few sentences. In the figure, for instance, the duties of the marketing manager include establishing marketing goals to ensure share of market and profitability, and developing and recommending pricing strategy. Typical duties of other jobs might include maintaining balanced and controlled inventories, making accurate postings to accounts payable, maintaining favourable purchase price variances, and repairing production line tools and equipment.

The *NOC* may be a helpful reference tool when itemizing a job's duties and responsibilities. As shown in Figure 4.9, for example, according to the *NOC*, a specialist in human resources might be expected to: "develop, implement, and evaluate personnel and labour relations policies, programs and procedures"; "advise managers and employees on the interpretation of personnel policies, benefit programs, and collective agreements"; and "research and prepare occupational classifications, job descriptions, and salary scales."

Most experts state unequivocally that "one item frequently found that should *never* be included in a job description is a 'cop-out clause' like 'other duties, as assigned.'"[25] since this leaves open the nature of the job and the people needed to staff it, and can be subject to abuse.

While the duties and responsibilities should be described in sufficient detail that training requirements and performance appraisal criteria can be identified, and the qualifications outlined in the job specification can be justified, it is gen-

Work Keys
www.freeyellow.com/members/
holleman/legal.html

erally possible to make it clear that the incumbent may be asked to perform additional related duties, without resorting to such a "cop-out clause." If not, including a statement such as, "The duties and responsibilities outlined above are representative, but not all-inclusive," may meet the firm's need for flexibility without sacrificing the quality and usefulness of the job description.

Authority

This section of a job description should define the limits of the jobholder's authority, including his or her decision-making authority, direct supervision of other employees, and budgetary limitations. For example, the jobholder might have authority to approve purchase requests up to $5000, grant time off or leaves of absence, discipline department employees, recommend salary increases, and interview and hire new employees.[26]

Performance Standards

Some job descriptions also contain a performance standards section, which indicates the standards the employee is expected to achieve in each of the job description's main duties and responsibilities.

Setting standards is never an easy matter. Most managers soon learn, however, that just telling employees to "do their best" doesn't provide enough guidance to ensure top performance. One straightforward way of setting standards is to finish the statement: "I will be completely satisfied with your work when ...." This sentence, if completed for each duty listed in the job description, should result in a usable set of performance standards.[27] Some examples would include the following:

Duty: Accurately Posting Accounts Payable

- All invoices received are posted within the same working day.
- All invoices are routed to the proper department managers for approval no later than the day following receipt.
- No more than three posting errors per month occur on average.
- Posting ledger is balanced by the end of the third working day of each month.

Duty: Meeting Daily Production Schedule

- Work group produces no less than 426 units per working day.
- No more than two percent of units are rejected at the next workstation, on average.
- Work is completed with no more than five percent overtime per week, on average.

Working Conditions and Physical Environment

The job description should also list the general working conditions involved in the job. This section generally includes information about noise level, temperature, lighting, degree of privacy, frequency of interruptions, hours of work, amount of travel, and hazards to which the incumbent may be exposed.

Job Description Guidelines

Some helpful guidelines to assist those writing job descriptions include:[28]

1. *Be clear*. Portray the job so well that the duties are clear without reference to other job descriptions.

2. *Indicate scope of authority*. Indicate the scope and nature of the work by using phrases such as "for the department" or "as requested by the manager." Include all important relationships.

3. *Be specific*. Select the most specific words to show (1) the kind of work, (2) the degree of complexity, (3) the degree of skill required, (4) the extent to which problems are standardized, (5) the extent of the worker's responsibility for each phase of the work, and (6) the degree and type of accountability. Use action words such as *analyze, gather, assemble, plan, devise, infer, deliver, transmit, maintain, supervise,* and *recommend*. Positions at the lower levels of the organization generally have the most detailed explanations of duties and tasks, while higher-level positions tend to have broader responsibility statements.

4. *Be brief*. Use short, accurate statements, since they usually best accomplish the purpose.

5. *Recheck*. Finally, to check whether the description fulfills the basic requirements, ask, "Will a new employee understand the job if he or she reads the job description?"

Writing Job Descriptions that Comply with Human Rights Legislation

As explained in Chapter 3, human rights legislation requires employers to ensure that there is no discrimination on any of the prohibited grounds in any aspect or terms and conditions of employment. To ensure that job descriptions comply with this legislation, a few key points should be kept in mind:

- job descriptions are NOT legally required, but are highly advisable
- essential job duties should be clearly identified in the job description. Indicating the percentage of time spent on each duty and/or listing duties in order of importance are strategies used to differentiate between essential and nonessential tasks and responsibilities
- when assessing suitability for employment, training program enrolment, and transfers or promotions, and when appraising performance, the only criteria examined should be KSAs required for the essential duties of the job
- even when an employee cannot perform one or more of the essential duties due to reasons related to a prohibited ground, such as a physical disability or religion, reasonable accommodation to the point of undue hardship is required.

WRITING JOB SPECIFICATIONS

Writing the job specification involves examining the duties and responsibilities and answering the question, "What human traits and experience are required to do this job?" Both skill and effort factors should be considered, as well as the human implications of the working conditions. Much of this information can be gleaned from the job analysis questionnaire. The job specification clarifies what

SMALL BUSINESS APPLICATIONS

A Practical Approach

Without their own job analysts or (in many cases) their own HR managers, many small-business owners face two hurdles when conducting job analyses and writing job descriptions. First (given their need to concentrate on other pressing matters), they often need a more streamlined approach than those provided by questionnaires like the one shown in Figure 4.6. Second, there is always the reasonable fear that in writing up their job descriptions they will inadvertently overlook duties that should be assigned to employees or assign duties to employees that are usually not associated with such positions. What they need here is an encyclopedia that includes all of the possible positions that they might encounter, with a detailed listing of the duties normally assigned to these positions. Such an "encyclopedia" exists—the *National Occupational Classification (NOC)* mentioned earlier. *The practical approach to job analysis for small-business owners presented next is built around this invaluable reference tool.*

Step 1. Decide on a plan.

Developing at least the broad outlines of a corporate plan is the first step. What is revenue expected to be next year, and in the next few years? What products/services will be emphasized? What areas or departments in the company will likely have to be expanded, reduced, or consolidated, given the firm's overall plan? What kinds of new positions will be needed in order to accomplish the strategic plans?

Step 2. Develop an organization chart.

Given the plan, the next step should be to develop an organization chart for the firm. A chart should be drawn showing who reports to the owner or CEO and who reports to each of the other managers and supervisors in the firm. Drawing up the organization chart of the present structure comes first. Then, depending upon how far in advance planning is being done, a chart can be produced that shows how the organization should look in the immediate future (say, in two months), as well as two or three other charts showing how the organization is likely to evolve over the next two or three years.

Step 3. Use a job analysis/description questionnaire.

Next, a job analysis questionnaire can be used to determine what the job entails. One of the more comprehensive job analysis questionnaires (see Figure 4.6, for instance) may be useful for collecting job analysis data. A simpler and often satisfactory alternative is to use the job description questionnaire presented in Figure 4.11. The information called for should be filled in (using the procedure outlined later) and the supervisors or the employees themselves should be asked to list their job duties (on the bottom of the page), breaking them into daily duties, periodic duties, and duties performed at irregular intervals. A sample of how one of these duties should be described (Figure 4.12) can be distributed to supervisors and/or employees.

Step 4. Obtain a copy of the *National Occupational Classification (NOC)* for reference.

Next, standardized examples of the job descriptions needed should be obtained from the *NOC*. A copy can be found in the reference section of the library in most major centres or purchased through the Ministry of Supply and Services in Ottawa.

Step 5. Choose appropriate definitions and copy them for reference.
For each department, the *NOC* job titles and job descriptions that are believed to be appropriate for the enterprise should be chosen and copied for future reference.

Step 6. Put appropriate *NOC* summaries on the top of the job description form.
Next, the corresponding *NOC* code(s) and *NOC* definition(s) should be written under the appropriate headings on the Job Description Questionnaire in Figure 4.11. Particularly when (as is usually the case) only one or two *NOC* definitions apply to the job description being written, the *NOC* definition will provide a firm foundation for the one being created. It will provide a standardized list and constant reminder of the specific duties that should be included. Including the *NOC* codes and definitions will also facilitate conversations with the local human resource centre, should this source be used to help find employees for open positions.

Step 7. Complete the job description.
An appropriate job summary for the job under consideration can then be written. Next, the job analysis information obtained in Step Three, together with the information gathered from the *NOC*, can be used to create a complete listing of the tasks and duties of each of the jobs. The working conditions section can be completed once all of the tasks and duties have been specified.

kind of person to recruit and for which qualities that person should be tested. Often—as in Figure 4.10—it is presented as part of the job description.[29]

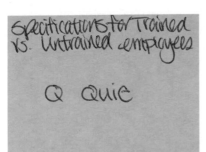

Hints to Ensure Legal Compliance

Specifications for Trained versus Untrained Employees

Writing job specifications for trained employees might seem relatively straightforward. For example, the specifications for an intermediate-level programming position, accountant, or HR manager tend to focus primarily on length of previous experience required, educational qualifications, and specialized skills or training needed. Once again, however, complying with human rights legislation means keeping a few pointers in mind:

- all listed qualifications must be justifiable, based on the current job duties and responsibilities
- unjustifiably high educational and/or lengthy experience requirements can lead to systemic discrimination. For that reason, many employers are no longer indicating that a degree or diploma is mandatory; rather, they specify that the position calls for a university degree in a specific area, a college diploma in that area, or an equivalent combination of education and work experience
- the qualifications of the current incumbent should not be confused with the minimum requirements, since he or she might be under- or overqualified. To avoid overstating or understating qualifications, it is helpful to ask the

FIGURE 4.11 Job Description Questionnaire

**Background Data
for Job Description**

Job Title _____   Department _____

Job Number _____   Written by _____

Today's Date _____   Applicable NOC Code(s) _____

I. Applicable NOC Definition(s):

II. Job Summary:
(Summarize the more important or regularly performed tasks)

III. Reports to:

IV. Supervises: _____

V. Job Duties: _____
(Briefly describe, for each duty, what employee does and, if possible, how employee does it. Show in parentheses at end of each duty the approximate percentage of time devoted to it.)

   A. Daily Duties:

   B. Periodic Duties:
   (Indicate whether weekly, monthly, quarterly, etc.)

   C. Duties Performed at Irregular Intervals:

VI. Working Conditions:

---

question, "What minimum qualifications would be required if this job were being filled in the immediate future?"

- for entry-level jobs, identifying the actual physical and mental demands is critical. Because on-the-job training will be provided, the emphasis tends to be on physical traits, personality, and/or sensory skills, instead of education and/or experience. The goal is to identify those personal traits—the human requirements—that are valid predictors of job success. For example, if the job requires detailed manipulation on a circuit-board assembly line, finger dexterity is extremely important, and is something for which

FIGURE 4.12 Examples of Background Data

Example of Job Title: Customer Service Clerk

Example of Job Summary: Answers inquiries and gives directions to customers, authorizes cashing of customers' cheques, records and returns lost charge cards, sorts and reviews new credit applications, and works at the customer-service desk.

Example of One Job Duty: Authorizes cashing of cheques: authorizes cashing of personal or payroll cheques (up to a specified amount) by customers desiring to make payment by cheque. Requests identification, such as driver's licence, from customers, and examines cheque to verify date, amount, signature, and endorsement. Initials cheque and sends customer to cashier.

---

physical demands analysis
Identification of the senses used, and type, frequency, and amount of physical effort involved in the job.

candidates should be tested. A physical demands analysis—which identifies the senses used, and type, frequency, and amount of physical effort involved in the job—is often used to supplement the job specification. A sample form is included as **Figure 4.13** on page 155. Having such detailed information is particularly beneficial when determining accommodation requirements

- as will be explained next, identifying the human requirements for a job can be accomplished through a judgmental approach or statistical analysis. Basing job specifications on statistical analysis is more legally defensible.

Job Specifications Based on Judgment

The judgmental approach is based on the educated guesses of job incumbents, supervisors, and HR managers. The usual procedure to obtain the required information is to ask questions on the job analysis questionnaire such as, "What does it take in terms of education, knowledge, training, and the like to do this job?"

The job specifications for already trained candidates, such as the call centre operators shown here, should clearly indicate which skills, like computer literacy, are job requirements.

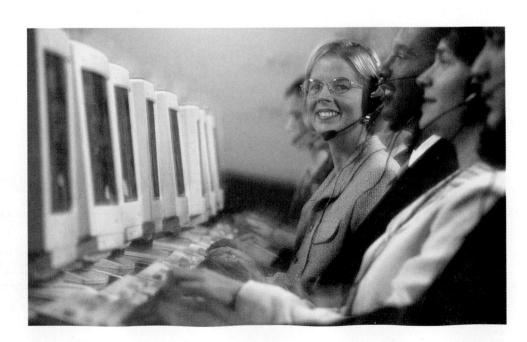

FIGURE **4.13** Physical Demands Analysis Form

Physical Demands Analysis

Physical Demands		Weight: Check if performed	Weight: Maximum (usual)	*Frequency: 0 Never	1 Seldom	2 Minor	3 Required	4 Major	Comments
Strength	Lifting								
	Carrying								
	Pushing								
	Pulling								
	Fine finger movements								
	Handling								
	Gripping								
	Reaching — Above shoulder								
	Reaching — Below shoulder								
	Foot action — One foot								
	Foot action — Two feet								
Mobility	Throwing								
	Sitting								
	Standing								
	Walking								
	Running								
	Climbing								
	Bending/stooping								
	Crouching								
	Kneeling								
	Crawling								
	Twisting								
	Balancing								
Sensory/perceptual	Hearing — Conversation								
	Hearing — Other sounds								
	Vision — Far								
	Vision — Near								
	Vision — Colour								
	Vision — Depth								
	Perception — Spatial								
	Perception — Form								
	Feeling								
	Reading								
	Writing								

Human Rights Considerations**
Essential Duties

Non-essential Duties

**Review duties before interview.
  Discuss reasonable accommodation at interview.

***Frequency** (The frequency of maximum weight should be shown without brackets and the frequency of usual weight, within brackets)
0–Not performed
1–Seldom performed
2–Minor daily activity, Less than one hour
3–Frequent repetition, for one to three hours daily
4–Major job demand, maximum ability required.
  Frequent Repetition for more than three hours daily.

Source: Developed by the Ontario Ministry of Labour. © Queen's Printer for Ontario, 1991. Reprinted with permission.

When developing job specifications, the *NOC* and *Career Handbook* can provide helpful reference information. Both include the judgments of job analysts and vocational counsellors regarding the education and/or training requirements of all of the occupations included. In addition to the types of information provided in the *NOC* (see Figure 4.9), the *Career Handbook* lists desired aptitudes and interests; and the vision, colour discrimination, hearing, body position, limb coordination, and strength demands.[30]

Job Specifications Based on Statistical Analysis

Basing job specifications on statistical analysis is more difficult than using a judgment approach. Basically, the aim is to statistically determine the relationship between (1) some predictor or human trait such as verbal or written communication skills, keyboarding speed, or finger dexterity and (2) some indicator or criterion of job effectiveness (such as performance, as rated by the supervisor). The procedure has five steps: (1) analyze the job and decide how to measure job performance; (2) select personal traits like finger dexterity that are believed to predict successful performance; (3) test job candidates for these traits; (4) measure these candidates' subsequent job performance; and (5) statistically analyze the relationship between the human trait (finger dexterity) and job performance. The objective is to determine whether there is a correlation between them, which means that the former predicts the latter. In this way, the human requirements for performing the job can be statistically ascertained.

Personality-related Job Requirements

The Personality-related Position Requirements Form (PPRF) is a new survey instrument designed to assist managers in identifying potential personality-related traits that may be important in a job. Identifying personality dimensions is difficult using most job analysis techniques, since they tend to be much better suited to unearthing human aptitudes and skills—like manual dexterity. The PPRF uses questionnaire items to assess the relevance of such basic personality dimensions as agreeableness, conscientiousness, and emotional stability to the job under study by asking whether specific items—such as "adapt(s) easily to changes in work procedures"—are "not required," "helpful," or "essential." The relevance of these personality traits can then be assessed through statistical analysis.[31]

As mentioned briefly above, statistical analysis is more legally defensible than the judgmental approach. Human rights legislation forbids using traits that could lead to discrimination on a prohibited ground in any employment decisions, *unless the employer can prove that there is a bona fide occupational requirement*. A statistical validation study provides such proof.

Completing the Job Specification Form

Once the required human characteristics have been determined, whether using statistical analysis or a judgmental approach, a job specification form should be completed.

To illustrate the types of information and amount of detail that should be provided in a well-written job specification, a sample has been included as **Figure 4.14.**

FIGURE 4.14 Municipal Trust Job Specification

Job Specification

Job Title: Customer Service Representative   Job Code: CSR.1002173
Location: Main Branch   Job Grade: CSR Level 1
Supervisor's Title: Assistant Manager   Status: Nonexempt
Author: Renée Cousineau   Date: October 06, 2000

JOB SUMMARY:

The incumbent is required to provide courteous, prompt, and efficient customer service in order to achieve a high level of customer satisfaction; identify, resolve, or refer customer banking and account maintenance needs, including the sale of bank products/services to the appropriate trained personnel; carefully handle and balance all cash and related on-line computer entries, in accordance with established Bank Security procedures; and facilitate branch work flow by assisting others with cash counts and preparing customer statements.

SKILL FACTORS:

Education
High School Diploma or an equivalent combination of education and experience. Must have some background in mathematics and accounting. Data entry/keyboarding skills are also required.

Experience
No prior experience is necessary. In-house training will be provided. Working knowledge of the physical handling/counting of cash and procedures for balancing cash and accounting entries would be an asset.

Nature of Communication Skills Required
Excellent oral communication skills are required. The incumbent must be able to communicate courteously and effectively. Excellent interpersonal skills are also mandatory. All functions must be handled with tact and diplomacy.

Customer service delivery involves almost constant contact with the public. External employment-related contacts may include government officials, local business employers and employees, social assistance recipients, and visitors to the community.

EFFORT FACTORS:

Physical Demands
The incumbent is required to stand during the majority of working hours, and spends extended periods in front of a computer monitor. Transferring coins to and from the vault involves a moderate degree of bending, lifting, and carrying.

Mental Demands
Handling customer service functions requires extended periods of mental attention. Entering customer transaction data on the online computer system and handling cash transactions requires concentrated visual attention.

Customer profile information is confidential, which requires moderate discretion.

There is a moderate level of complexity involved in this job. Duties are governed by formal policies and procedures, but dealings with the public require some independent judgment. A supervisor is available at all times to provide consultation and/or authorization.

The consequences of errors are serious, in terms of customer satisfaction and confidence in the bank and its services. Customer Service Representatives are required to balance with 100 percent accuracy at least 80 percent of the days in each month. There is a $30.00 allowance given daily, after which errors are counted against the employee. Employees who do not meet the monthly accuracy standard are subject to disciplinary action.

WORKING CONDITIONS:
The working environment makes few demands on the jobholder. (The incumbent works in a well-lit, well-ventilated, smoke-free, temperature-controlled modern office.) Customer service delivery functions may involve exposure to occasional unpleasant situations and can cause a moderate degree of stress. The incumbent may be scheduled to work on Saturdays and will be required to work overtime on occasion.

APPROVAL SIGNATURES:

_____   _____
Incumbent   Supervisor

CURRENT DATE: _____   LAST REVIEW DATE: _____

Source: Based on a job specification developed by Renée (Cousineau) Hall while a student in Compensation Administration at Sir Sandford Fleming College in the fall semester of 1994. Used with permission.

Job Analysis in a "Jobless" World

Over the past few years, the concept of *a job* has been changing quite dramatically. As one observer recently put it:[32]

> The modern world is on the verge of another huge leap in creativity and productivity, but the job is not going to be part of tomorrow's economic reality. There still is and will always be enormous amounts of work to do, but it is not going to be contained in the familiar envelopes we call jobs. In fact, many organizations are today well along the path toward being "de-jobbed."

Why Companies Are Becoming De-jobbed: The Need for Responsiveness

De-jobbing is ultimately a product of the rapid changes taking place in business today. Organizations need to grapple with a number of revolutionary forces: accelerating product and technological change, globalized competition, deregulation, political instability, demographic changes, and trends toward a service society and the information age. Forces like these have dramatically increased the need for firms to be responsive, flexible, and capable of competing in a global marketplace.

The organizational techniques firms have used to foster responsiveness have helped to blur the meaning of *job* as a set of well-defined and clearly delineated set of responsibilities. Here is a sampling of how these techniques have contributed to this blurring.

Flatter Organizations

Human Resource Consultants
www.hrcjobs.com

Instead of pyramid-shaped organizations with seven or more management layers, flat organizations with just three or four levels are becoming more prevalent. Many firms (including ABB and Celestica Inc., as described in Chapter 1) have already cut their management layers from a dozen to six or fewer. As the remaining managers are left with more people reporting to them, they can supervise them less, so every employee's job ends up involving greater breadth and depth of responsibilities.

Work Teams

Over the past decade, work has become increasingly organized around teams and processes rather than around specialized functions. While over 40 percent of those responding to a 1994 Conference Board of Canada survey indicated that team-based activity was widespread,[33] 1997 research indicated that 47 percent of Fortune 1000 firms used teams to some extent and that 60 percent planned to increase the use of teams.[34] Many organizations, such as London Life,[35] FedEx, and Xerox Canada,[36] have introduced self-managed teams. In these organizations, employees' jobs change daily; the effort to avoid having employees view their job as a limited and specific set of responsibilities is thus intentional.

In many firms, the widespread use of teams and similar structural mechanisms means that the boundaries that typically separate organizational functions (like sales and production) and hierarchical levels are reduced and made more permeable. In such firms, responsiveness is fostered by encouraging employees to rid themselves of the "it's not my job" attitude that typically creates walls between one employee area and another. Instead, the focus is on defining the job at hand in terms of the overall best interests of the organization, thereby further de-jobbing the company.

The Boundaryless Organization

As mentioned briefly in Chapter 1, boundaryless organization structures are emerging. In this type of structure, relationships (typically joint ventures) are formed with customers, suppliers, and/or competitors, to pool resources for mutual benefit or encourage cooperation in an uncertain environment. As in team-based organizations, barriers are broken down—in this case between the organization and its suppliers, customers, or competitors—and teams are emphasized. The teams may, however, include employees representing each of the companies involved in the joint venture. In such structures, jobs are defined in very general terms, since the emphasis is on the overall best interests of the organizations involved.

Reengineering

Reengineering is defined as "the fundamental rethinking and radical redesign of business processes to achieve dramatic improvements in critical, contemporary measures of performance, such as cost, quality, service, and speed."[37] In their book, *Reengineering the Corporation*, Michael Hammer and James Champy argue that the principles that shaped the structure and management of business for hundreds of years—like highly specialized divisions of work—should be retired. Instead, the firm should emphasize combining tasks into integrated, unspecialized processes that are then carried out by committed employees.

Reengineering is achieved in several ways. Specialized jobs are combined into one so that formerly distinct jobs are integrated and compressed into enlarged, enriched ones.[38] A necessary correlate of combining jobs is that workers make more decisions, since each person's responsibilities are generally broader and deeper after reengineering; supervisory checks and controls are reduced; and, indeed, committed employees largely control their own efforts. Finally, workers become collectively responsible for overall results rather than being individually responsible for just their own tasks. As a result, their jobs change dramatically. "They share joint responsibility with their team members for performing the whole process, not just a small piece of it. They not only use a broader range of skills from day to day, they have to be thinking of a far greater picture."[39] Most importantly, "while not every member of the team will be doing exactly the same work ... the lines between [the workers' jobs] blur." To that extent, reengineering also contributes to de-jobbing the enterprise.

The Future of Job Descriptions

Most firms today continue to utilize job descriptions and to rely on jobs as traditionally defined. However, it is clear that more and more firms are moving toward new organizational configurations, ones built around jobs that are broad and that may change every day. As one writer has said, "In such a situation, people no longer take their cues from a job description or a supervisor's instructions. Signals come from the changing demands of the project. Workers learn to focus their individual efforts and collective resources on the work that

reengineering
The fundamental rethinking and radical redesign of business processes to achieve dramatic improvement in contemporary measures of performance.

AN ETHICAL
DILEMMA
In view of the fact that job descriptions are not required by law and that some organizations have found them no longer relevant, would abolishing job descriptions raise any moral or legal concerns?

needs doing, changing as that changes. Managers lose their 'jobs,' too ...."[40] The High Performance Organization feature that follows describes some practical HR implications.

THE HIGH PERFORMANCE ORGANIZATION

HR Practices in a De-jobbed Company

Because job descriptions are (deservedly) so well ingrained in the way that most companies operate, it's unlikely that most firms could (or should) do without them, at least for now. For the growing number of firms that are shifting to HR systems that don't use job descriptions, however, what replaces them?

In one firm—British Petroleum's exploration division—the need for flatter organizations and empowered employees inspired management to replace job descriptions with matrices listing skills and skill levels.[1] Senior management wanted to shift employees' attention from a job description/"that's not my job" mentality to one that would motivate employees to obtain the new skills they needed to accomplish their broader responsibilities.

The solution was a skills matrix like that shown in **Figure 4.15**. Skills matrices were created for various jobs within two classes of employees: those on a management track, and those whose aims lay elsewhere (such as to stay in engineering). For each job or job family (such as drilling manager), a matrix was prepared. As in Figure 4.15, it identified (1) the basic skills needed for that job and (2) the minimum level of each skill required for that job or job family.

Such a matrix shifts employees' focus. The emphasis is no longer on a job description's listing of specific job duties. Instead the focus is on developing the new skills needed for the employees' broader, empowered, and often relatively undefined responsibilities.

The skills matrix approach has prompted other HR changes in BP's exploration division. For example, the matrices provide a constant reminder of

what skills employees must improve, and the firm's new skill-based pay plan awards raises based on skills improvement. Similarly, performance appraisals now focus more on employee skills, and training emphasizes developing broad skills like leadership and planning—ones that are applicable across a wide range of responsibilities and jobs.

Broader HR issues are also involved when firms de-job. For one thing, "... [firms] must find people who can work well without the cue system of job descriptions."[2] This puts a premium on hiring people with the skills and values to handle empowered jobs. As two reengineering experts put it:

For multidimensional and changing jobs, companies don't need people to fill a slot, because the slot will be only roughly defined. Companies need people who can figure out what the job takes and do it, people who can create the slot that fits them. Moreover, the slot will keep changing.[3]

There's also a shift from training to education: in other words, from teaching employees the "how" of the job to increasing their insight and understanding regarding its "why." In a rapidly changing industrial environment, the demands for flexibility and responsiveness mean that it's impossible to hire people "... who already know everything they're ever going to need to know...."[4] Here, continuing education over the course of the employees' organizational career becomes the norm.

[1] Milan Moravec and Robert Tucker, "Job Descriptions for the 21st Century," *Personnel Journal* (June 1992), pp. 37–44.
[2] William Bridges, "The End of the Job," Fortune (September 19, 1994), p. 68.
[3] Michael Hammer and James Champy, *Reengineering the Corporation* (New York: Harper Business, 1993), p. 72.
[4] Hammer and Champy, Reengineering, p. 72.

FIGURE 4.15 The Skills Matrix for One Job at BP

The skills matrix appears as a grid. Included but not shown are descriptors for each level of each skill, beginning at the bottom (A) with the lowest level, and increasing with the highest level at the top. For instance, under technical expertise, level A might read, "Is acquiring basic knowledge and has awareness of the key skills," while level H might read, "Conducts and/or supervises complex tasks requiring advanced knowledge of key skills or a thorough working knowledge of a range of key skills." The darker boxes indicate the minimum level of skill required for the job.

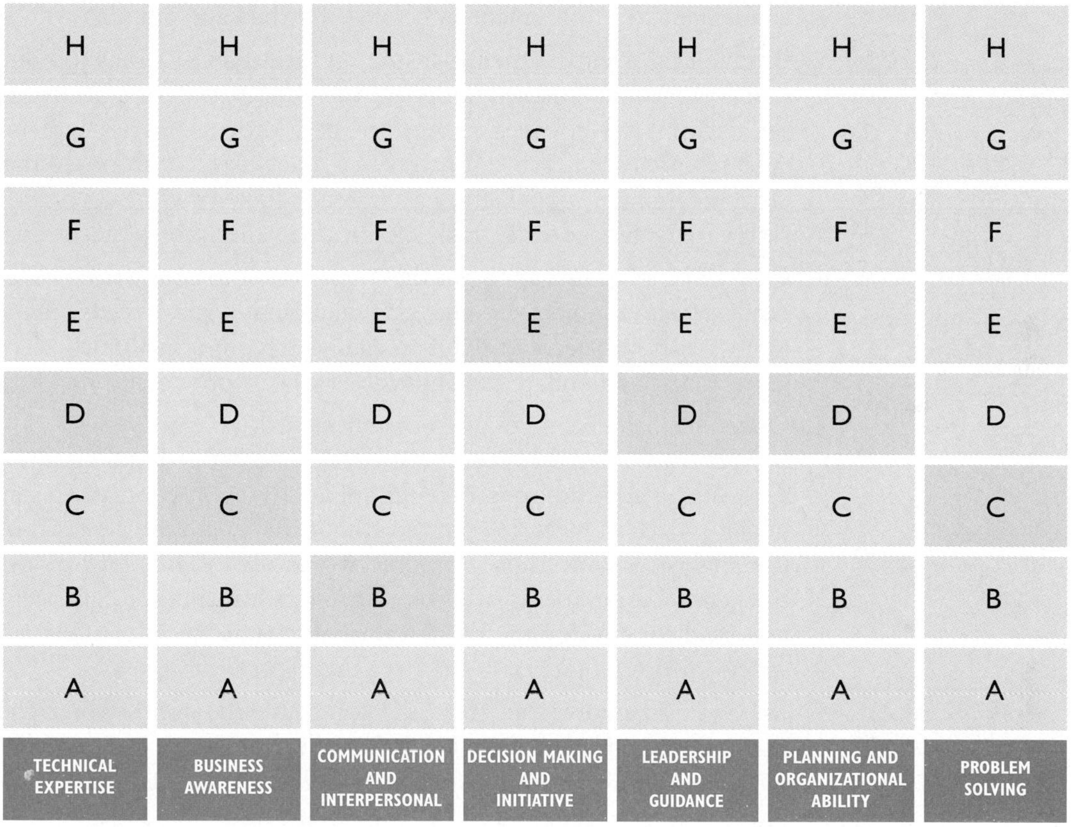

TECHNICAL EXPERTISE	BUSINESS AWARENESS	COMMUNICATION AND INTERPERSONAL	DECISION MAKING AND INITIATIVE	LEADERSHIP AND GUIDANCE	PLANNING AND ORGANIZATIONAL ABILITY	PROBLEM SOLVING
H	H	H	H	H	H	H
G	G	G	G	G	G	G
F	F	F	F	F	F	F
E	E	E	E	E	E	E
D	D	D	D	D	D	D
C	C	C	C	C	C	C
B	B	B	B	B	B	B
A	A	A	A	A	A	A

CHAPTER Review

Summary

1   Organizational structure refers to the formal relationships among jobs in an organization, and is often depicted in an organization chart. Firms can now use high-end software to ensure that such charts are kept current and are readily accessible to all employees. There are three basic types of organizational structures: bureaucratic, flat, and boundaryless.

2   In any organization, work has to be divided into manageable units and ultimately into jobs that can be performed by employees. The process of organizing work into tasks that are required to perform a specific job is known as job design.

3   The term *job* as it is known today is largely an outgrowth of the efficiency demands of the industrial revolution, which led to work simplification. Industrial engineering, which also evolved at this time, is concerned with: analyzing work methods; making work cycles more efficient by modifying, combining, rearranging, or eliminating tasks; and establishing time standards.

4   By the mid-1900s, job enlargement and job rotation evolved as popular strategies to overcome dehumanization and other problems associated with overspecialization. More recently, job enrichment—based on the premise that the best way to motivate workers is to build opportunities for challenge and achievement into jobs—has become popular.

5   Behavioural scientists then focussed on identifying various job dimensions that would simultaneously improve the efficiency of organizations and job satisfaction of employees. One of the best-known theories evolving from such research is the job characteristics model, which proposed that employee motivation and satisfaction are directly linked to five core characteristics: skill variety, task identity, task significance, autonomy, and feedback.

6   Over time, it became apparent that, in addition to considering psychological needs, effective job design must also take physiological needs and health and safety issues into account. Human engineering, or ergonomics, seeks to integrate and accommodate the physical needs of workers into the design of jobs.

7   Once jobs have been designed or redesigned, an employer's performance-related expectations need to be defined and communicated. This is best accomplished through job analysis. In contrast to job design, which reflects subjective opinions about the ideal requirements of a job, job analysis is concerned with objective and verifiable information about the actual requirements of a job. Once this information has been gathered, it is used for developing job descriptions (what the job entails) and job specifications (what the human requirements are).

8   Job analysis involves six steps: (1) determine the use to which the information will be put, (2) collect background information, (3) select the representative positions and jobs to be analyzed, (4) collect data, (5) review the information collected with the incumbents and their supervisors, and (6) develop the job descriptions and job specifications.

9   There are four conventional techniques used to gather job analysis data: interviews, questionnaires, direct observation, and participant logs. Quantitative job analysis techniques—practical when a key aim of analyzing jobs is to use the information for pay purposes—include the position analysis questionnaire (PAQ) and functional job analysis (FJA).

10   A job description is a written statement of what the jobholder actually does, how he or she does it, and under what conditions the job is performed. Typical information included is the job identification, a job summary, relationships, duties and responsibilities, authority of incumbent, performance standards, and working conditions.

11   The job specification involves examining the duties and responsibilities and answering the question, "What human traits and experience are required to do this job?" Both skill and effort factors should be considered, as well and the human implications of the working conditions. A physical demands analysis is often used to supplement the job specification.

12 De-jobbing is ultimately a product of the rapid changes taking place in business today. As firms try to speed decision making by taking steps like reengineering, individual jobs are becoming broader and much less specialized. Increasingly, firms don't want employees to feel limited by a specific set of responsibilities like those listed in a job description. As a result, more employees are de-emphasizing detailed job descriptions and often substituting brief job summaries, perhaps combined with summaries of the skills required for the position.

Key Terms

diary/log
functional job analysis (FJA)
human engineering (ergonomics)
industrial engineering
job
job analysis
job description
job design
job enlargement
job enrichment
job rotation
job specification

National Occupational Classification (NOC)
occupation
organizational structure
organization chart
physical demands analysis
position
position analysis questionnaire (PAQ)
process chart
reengineering
team
team-based job design
work simplification

Review and Discussion Questions

1 Explain work simplification. In what situations is this approach to job design appropriate?

2 Differentiate between job enlargement, job rotation, and job enrichment, and provide an example of each.

3 What is involved in the human-engineering approach to job design? Why is it becoming increasingly important?

4 We discussed several methods for collecting job analysis data—questionnaires, the position analysis questionnaire, and so on. Compare and contrast these methods, explaining what each is useful for and listing the pros and cons of each.

5 While not legally required, having job descriptions is highly advisable. Why? How can firms ensure that their job specifications are legally defensible?

CRITICAL *Thinking Questions*

1 Why isn't it always desirable or appropriate to use job enrichment or include the five core dimensions when designing jobs? How would you determine how enriched an individual employee's job should be?

2 Assume that you are the job analyst at a bicycle manufacturing company in British Columbia, and have been assigned responsibility for preparing job

descriptions (including specifications) for all of the supervisory and managerial positions. One of the production managers has just indicated that he will not complete the job analysis questionnaire you have developed. (a) How would you handle this situation? (b) What arguments would you use to attempt to persuade him to change his mind? (c) If your persuasion efforts failed, how would you go about obtaining the job analysis information you need to develop the job description for his position?

3   Since the top job in a firm (such as president, executive director, or CEO) is by nature broader in scope than any of the other jobs, is there less need for a job description for the president? Why or why not?

APPLICATION *Exercises*

RUNNING CASE: Carter Cleaning Company

Job Descriptions

Based on her review of the stores, Jennifer concludes that one of the first matters that she has to attend to involves developing job descriptions for the store managers.

As Jennifer tells it, her lessons regarding job descriptions in her basic management and HR management courses were insufficient to fully convince her of the pivotal role that job descriptions play in the smooth functioning of an enterprise. However, many times during her first few weeks on the job, Jennifer finds herself asking one of the store managers why he or she is violating what Jennifer knows to be recommended company policies and procedures. Repeatedly the answers are either, "Because I didn't know it was my job," or, "Because I didn't know that was the way we were supposed to do it." Jennifer concludes that a job description, along with a set of standards and procedures that specify what is to be done and how to do it, would go a long way toward alleviating this problem.

In general, each store manager is responsible for directing all store activities in such a way that quality work is produced, customer relations and sales are maximized, and profitability is maintained through effective control of labour, supply, and energy costs. In accomplishing that general aim, each store manager's duties and responsibilities include quality control, store appearance and cleanliness, customer relations, bookkeeping and cash management, cost control and productivity, damage control, pricing, inventory control, spotting and cleaning, machine maintenance, employee safety, hazardous waste removal, HR administration, and pest control.

The questions that Jennifer has to address follow.

Questions

1   What should be the format and final form of the store manager's job description?

2   Is it practical to specify standards and procedures in the body of the job description, or should these be kept separately?

3   How should Jennifer go about collecting the information required for the standards, procedures, and job description?

CASE INCIDENT   *Linking Job Analysis and Pay*

It wasn't until the CEO's secretary, Fay Jacobs, retired that anyone in the Winnipeg Engineering Company's HR department realized how much variation there was in the compensation of the company's secretaries.

To Tina Jessup, compensation specialist, it was quite apparent why there were inconsistent standards for secretarial pay. With the advance of office-automation technology, managers' differing styles of delegation, and secretaries' varying degrees of willingness to take on increasing managerial responsibilities, the job had assumed a variety of profiles. As the jobs now existed, it was quite likely that two individuals with the same title might be performing very different jobs.

Knowing that updated job analysis information was essential, and prepared for resistance from those who might want to protect their status and pay, she decided to use an objective method to gather information about each of the secretaries' jobs. She developed a questionnaire that she planned to distribute to each member of the firm's secretarial staff and his or her manager following a brief explanatory interview. The interviews would, she hoped, give her a chance to dispel fears on the part of any of the secretaries or managers that the purpose of the analysis was to eliminate jobs, reduce salaries, or lower the grade level of positions.

Before finalizing the questionnaire, Tina shared it with a small group of secretaries in her own department. Based on their input, she made some modifications, such as adding questions about the use of office technology and its impact on the job.

The questionnaire now covered nearly every aspect of the secretarial role, from processing mail, to making travel arrangements, to editing and preparing company correspondence, budgets, and reports. The questions also captured information about how much time was spent on each activity and how much supervision each task required. Tina hoped that, in addition to establishing standards on which Winnipeg Engineering could base a more equitable pay structure, the survey would allow the HR staff members to assess training needs, examine the distribution of work, and determine accurate specifications for recruitment and selection and for the development of employment tests to be used in the future.

Just as Tina was about to begin the interviews and distribution of questionnaires, she got a telephone call from Janet Fried, vice-president of sales. Janet had heard about the upcoming analysis and was very upset. She claimed to be worried about how much time Avril, the secretary assisting her, would have to take away from her work in order to meet with Tina and fill out the questionnaire. She also expressed concern that Avril might feel that her job was threatened and start looking for a position elsewhere. Tina agreed to meet with Janet to discuss her reservations, for which Janet thanked her profusely. Just before hanging up, Janet added, "You know, Tina, I sure wouldn't want to see Avril's job rated at a lower grade level than the secretary assisting the vice-president of operations!"

Questions

1   What do you think is the real "problem" from Janet's point of view?

2   How should Tina address each of the concerns that Janet expressed?

3   What can Tina do to prepare herself for any resistance to the job analysis on the part of the secretaries themselves?

4   Given the current advances in office technology, such as sophisticated spreadsheet programs, voice-mail systems, and email, as well as the elimination of many middle-management positions through corporate downsizings, secretaries in many firms are taking on quasi-managerial responsibilities. How can Tina account in her job analyses for the degrees to which individual secretaries at Winnipeg Engineering are doing so?

EXPERIENTIAL Exercises

1   Draw an organization chart to accurately depict the structure of the organization in which you are currently employed or one with which you are thoroughly familiar. Once you have completed this task, form a group with several of your classmates. Taking turns, each member is to show his or her organization chart to the group, briefly describe the structure depicted, explain whether or not the structure seems to be appropriate to him or her, and identify several advantages and disadvantages he or she experienced working within this structure.

2   Working individually or in groups, obtain a copy of the *National Occupational Classification* and/or the *NOC Career Handbook* from your library or nearest HRDC office. Find the descriptions for any two occupations with which you have some familiarity. Compare the Employment Requirements and/or the Profile Summaries. Based on what you know about these occupations, does the material provided seem accurate? Why or why not? What changes would you recommend, if any?

3   Working individually, prepare a job description (including job specifications) for a position that you know intimately, using the job analysis questionnaire in this chapter. Once you have done so, exchange job descriptions with someone else in the class. Critique your colleague's job description and provide specific suggestions regarding any additions/deletions/revisions that you would recommend to ensure that the job description accurately reflects the job and is legally defensible.

WEB-BASED Exercises

1   Prepare an organization chart using a software application for a firm with which you are totally familiar.

2   Go to the Web sites of three large employers in your area. Check their job specifications for entry-level HR positions. Are there any commonalities across the firms? Do you feel they are justifiable and that they meet employment equity standards? If not, what changes would you recommend?

3   Using the Web for research, identify any current trends pertaining to job descriptions. For example, are job descriptions being abolished? Are job descriptions becoming more generic? Are organizations other than British Petroleum using skills matrices?

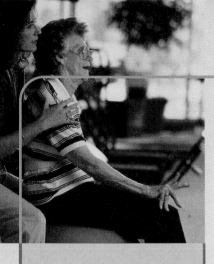

CHAPTER 5

Human Resources Planning

CHAPTER
OUTLINE

The Nature of Human
Resources Planning

Elements of Effective
HRP

Forecasting Future
Human Resources Needs
(Demand)

Forecasting Future
Human Resources
Supply

Planning and
Implementing HR
Programs to Balance
Supply and Demand

HRP Evaluation

LEARNING OUTCOMES

After studying this chapter, you should be able to:

Explain the nature of HRP and *discuss* its importance.

Describe the relationship between HRP and strategic planning and *explain* the importance of environmental scanning.

Describe various quantitative and qualitative techniques used to forecast human resources demand.

Discuss the strategies used to forecast human resources supply.

Describe the ways in which a surplus of human resources can be handled.

Explain how organizations deal with a shortage of human resources.

Describe the HRP evaluation process.

THE NATURE OF HUMAN RESOURCES PLANNING

human resources planning (HRP)
The process of reviewing human resources requirements to ensure that the organization has the required number of employees, with the necessary skills, to meet its goals.

Human Resources Planning (HRP) is the process of reviewing human resources requirements to ensure that the organization has the required number of employees with the necessary skills to meet its goals.[1] Also known as employment planning, HRP is a proactive process, which both anticipates and influences an organization's future by systematically forecasting the demand for and supply of employees under changing conditions, and developing plans and activities to satisfy these needs.[2] As illustrated in **Figure 5.1**, key steps in the HRP process include forecasting demand for labour, analyzing labour supply, and planning and implementing HR programs to balance supply and demand.

FIGURE 5.1 Human Resources Planning Model

Human Resources Planning
www.phptr.com/ptrbook/
be_0134464850.html

Step 1:   Forecast Demand for Labour

Considerations
- Organizational strategic plans
- Organizational tactical plans
- Economic conditions
- Market and competitive trends
- Government and legislative issues
- Social concerns
- Technological changes
- Demographic trends

Techniques Utilized
- Trend analysis
- Ratio analysis
- Scatter plot
- Regression analysis
- Computerized forecasting techniques
- Nominal group technique
- Delphi technique
- Managerial judgment
- Staffing tables

Step 2:   Analyze Supply

Internal Analysis
- Markov analysis
- Skills inventories
- Management inventories
- Replacement charts and development tracking
- Replacement summaries
- Succession planning

External Analysis
- General economic conditions
- Labour market conditions (national and local)
- Occupational market conditions

Step 3:   Implement Human Resources Programs to Balance Supply and Demand

Labour Shortage
- Overtime
- Hire temporary employees
- Subcontract work
- Recruitment
- Transfer
- Promotion

Labour Surplus
- Hiring freeze
- Attrition
- Buy-outs and early retirement programs
- Job sharing
- Part-time work
- Work sharing
- Reduced workweek
- Alternative jobs within the organization
- Layoffs (reverse seniority or juniority)
  - Supplemental unemployment benefits (SUBs)
- Termination
  - Severance pay
  - Outplacement assistance

FIGURE **5.2** Balancing Supply and Demand Considerations

Conditions and Possible Solutions

A. When labour demand exceeds labour supply
- Scheduling overtime hours
- Hiring temporary workers
- Subcontracting
- External recruitment
- Internal promotions and transfers
◆ *Performance management, training and retraining, and career development play a critical role.*

B. When labour supply exceeds labour demand
- Hiring freeze: reassigning current workers to job openings
- Attrition: standard employee resignation, retirement, or death
- Incentives to leave the organization: buy-outs or early retirement programs
- Job sharing
- Reducing positions to part-time
- Work sharing and reduced workweek
- Finding employees alternative jobs within the organization
- Employee layoffs
- Termination of employment
◆ *Evaluating the effectiveness of layoffs and downsizing is critical, as is managing "survivor sickness."*

C. When labour demand equals labour supply
- Vacancies are filled internally through transfers or promotions, or externally by hiring new employees
◆ *Performance management, training, and career development are critical in achieving balance.*

A fundamental HRP decision when demand exceeds supply is whether projected positions will be filled internally or externally. In other words, should the anticipated openings be filled by current employees or is the situation such that some or all vacancies must or should be filled by recruiting outside candidates? Another critical issue is what to do when the labour supply exceeds the anticipated demand. As illustrated in **Figure 5.2**, there are many alternative solutions.

The Importance of HRP

An important benefit of HRP is that it provides a framework for the coordination and integration of HRM policies and practices related to staffing and development activities, since they affect the requirements for and supply of human resources. Effective HRP helps an organization to:

- achieve its goals and objectives
- plan and coordinate recruitment, selection, training, career planning, and other staffing and development activities more effectively
- achieve economies in hiring new workers
- make major labour market demands more successfully
- anticipate and avoid shortages and surpluses of human resources

- control and/or reduce labour costs
- utilize employees' capabilities more effectively, thereby increasing performance and productivity, and reducing dissatisfaction and turnover
- establish employment equity goals and timetables that are realistic and attainable.

Lack of or inadequate human resources planning within an organization can result in:

- significant costs—both tangible and intangible. For example, unstaffed vacant positions can lead to costly inefficiencies, particularly when lengthy training is needed for new hires to reach acceptable performance standards. Requiring employees to work extra hours to perform the duties of such vacant positions or to compensate for understaffing can lead to lower productivity, fatigue, stress-related illnesses, and accidents, as well as incurring overtime premium costs. There are also costs associated with overstaffing. For example, if large numbers of employees are being laid off, extended notice periods are required in many jurisdictions, as well as severance pay
- situations in which one department is laying off employees, while another is hiring individuals with similar skills, which can have a devastating impact on morale and productivity
- inability to develop effective training, development, and career planning programs
- turnover—if employees are not qualified when vacancies arise and are therefore denied opportunities for lateral moves or promotions, turnover is the inevitable result, especially among high performers
- difficulties in meeting employment equity goals, or inappropriate staffing decisions, such as hiring or promoting underqualified target group members simply to meet established goals and timetables. This can result in poor performance or even termination and replacement, as well as costs that cannot be measured in dollars alone—perpetuation of prejudices and/or stereotypes, the undermining of employee self-confidence and self-respect associated with inadequate performance, and backlash from other employees
- inability to accomplish short-term operational plans and/or long-range strategic plans.

The Relationship Between HRP and Strategic Planning

As explained in Chapter 2, strategic planning involves making fundamental decisions about the very nature of business. Through strategic planning, organizations set major objectives and develop comprehensive plans for achieving them. Among other things, long-range strategic plans may result in: revised organizational goals; new business acquisitions; divestiture of current product lines, services or subsidiaries; new management approaches; and/or revisions to organizational structure and design. Short-range, tactical (or operational) plans deal with current operations and ways of meeting present challenges and maximizing existing opportunities. Purchasing a new software package to handle payroll more efficiently, training employees to reduce the number of back injuries, and recalling a defective product are examples.

Human Resources Planning
(HRD—L)
www.hronline.com/forums/index.
html

**AN ETHICAL
DILEMMA**

Is it wrong to hire and/or promote underqualified target group members simply to meet established employment equity goals and timetables?

Canadian Human Resource
Planners
www.chrp.ca

Whether strategic or operational, plans are made and carried out by people. Thus, determining whether or not people will be available is a critical element of both strategic and operational planning processes. For example, plans to enter new businesses, build new plants, or reduce the level of activities all influence the number and types of positions to be filled. At the same time, decisions regarding how positions will be filled must be integrated with other aspects of the firm's HR plans, for instance, those pertaining to training current and new employees, appraising performance, and terminating, transferring, or promoting staff members. In the words of a noted HRP expert, "Today, virtually all business issues have people implications; all human resource(s) issues have business implications."[3]

While production, financial, and marketing plans have long been recognized as important cornerstones in the strategic planning process, more and more firms are coming to the realization that HR plans are another essential component,[4] and that HRP and strategic planning become effective when there is a reciprocal and interdependent relationship between them.[5]

IBM is a recognized leader in the integration of HRP and strategic planning. Within IBM's manufacturing and product development businesses, the corporation's HR department develops a five-year HR strategic plan and a two-year tactical plan based on tentative business goals, formulated after an external environmental analysis and internal analysis of the company's strengths and weaknesses. The importance attributed to the HR department's role in the strategic planning process is highlighted by the fact that no major business decisions are approved until the vice-president of HR concurs with the business plan.[6] Other organizations that have long recognized the importance of integrating HRP and strategic planning include Intel and Xerox;[7] Saskatchewan Wheat Pool (the largest cooperative in Canada);[8] and Canadian Imperial Bank of Commerce.[9]

Failure to integrate HRP and strategic planning can have very serious consequences.

In early 1999, Ontario Health Minister Elizabeth Witmer announced that the government would spend an extra $375 million to hire more than 10 000 nurses in the province—after years of massive cutbacks, and spending more than $400 million on the severance packages of nurses it had laid off the year before; the B.C. government made a commitment to hire 1000 more nurses; the Alberta government indicated in its latest budget that more money would be allocated to hiring nurses; the Saskatchewan government promised to address its nursing shortage; and the Manitoba government announced $7 million to recruit more nurses. As Kathleen Connors, president of the National Federation of Nurses' Unions, said at the time, "I don't know where they're going to find the nurses, quite frankly. There is a national nursing shortage."[10] In early 2000, the provincial government in Newfoundland and Labrador decided to offer a $3000 cash incentive to fourth-year nursing students who would commit to working in the province for one year. It is feared, though, that unless workload concerns—largely resulting from staffing shortfalls—are addressed, graduates will take the incentive, work their year and leave. Despite the fact that the Canadian Nurses Association (CNA) warned governments in 1998 that an aging work force, greater emphasis on home care, and an inability to attract and retain nurses could leave the system short 113 000 nurses by 2011—a prediction now believed to be too low—a recent nationwide CNA report shows that low wages, poor working conditions and a shortage of full-time work are driving nurses out of the

Canadian Career Partners
www.career-partners.com

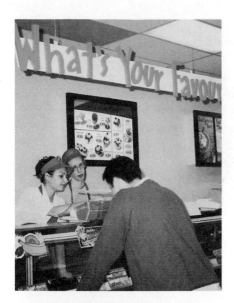

In their HR planning, employers like Baskin Robbins and others include close monitoring of trends such as the availability of entry-level labour.

quasi-public sector
Publicly supported organizations, such as health-care providers and educational institutions.

public sector
Government organizations.

profession (20 percent of new nurses), and south of the border (10 percent). Obviously there is a need for a long-term nationwide HR plan for nurses.[11] In the words of the president of the CNA, "In the past, the approach has been piecemeal. We need a national dialogue and a coordinated approach."[12]

The Importance of Environmental Scanning

As alluded to in the previous IBM example, environmental scanning is a critical component of HRP and strategic planning processes, since the most successful organizations are prepared for changes before they occur. The external environmental factors most frequently monitored include:

- Economic conditions (general, regional and local).
- Market and competitive trends.
- Government and legislative issues, such as new or revised laws and the decisions of courts and quasi-judicial bodies.
- Social concerns related to health care, childcare, and educational priorities.
- Technological changes.
- Demographic trends.

As mentioned in Chapter 1, economic conditions affect supply and demand for products and services, which in turn affect the number and types of employees required. Over the past decade, for example, many private-sector firms have restructured or downsized. Downsizing used to be relatively rare in the quasi-public and public sectors. However, due to government cost-cutting strategies, this changed in recent years. For example, as indicated in the previous discussion, nurses across the country were laid off in significant numbers during the early to mid-1990s. In February of 1995, the federal government announced plans to reduce its massive overspending by laying off 45 000 employees over the following three years.[13] Staffing cuts have affected employees at all levels and with all types of skills. Doing more with fewer employees cannot be seen as simply a temporary solution to the recession of the 1990s. Evidence that the era of downsizing is not yet over comes from numerous sources.

Research Insight

Despite the fact that tales of merger mania dominate the headlines, a *WorkCanada* survey conducted by Watson Wyatt in early 2000 revealed that more organizations underwent downsizing than grew in 1999. Only eight percent of the 1604 Canadian employees surveyed said they experienced no change in the previous year. The highlights of this study are shown in **Figure 5.3**.[14]

More recently, 79 percent of 300 Canadian business and government organization representatives responding to a Drake Beam Morin-Canada survey reported that they would begin major change or restructuring efforts over the following six months.[15]

Probably the most significant environmental factor in HRP in Canada today relates to the dramatic changes in labour-force composition. A few trends of importance include the following:

- as of July 2000, there were 16.4 million Canadians in the labour force, and population growth had slowed to less than one percent per year[16]

FIGURE 5.3 Types of Organization Change Experienced in 1999

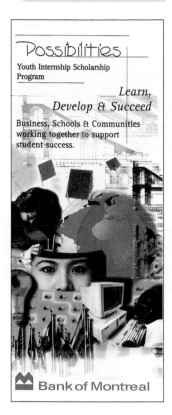

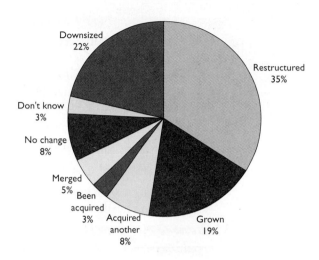

Source: Work Canada survey conducted by Watson Wyatt, reported in Lesley Young, "Employees Shaken by Downsizing Tremors," *Canadian HR Reporter* 13, no. 11 (June 5, 2000), p. 3. © Carswell, Thomson Professional Publishing. Reproduced by permission of *Canadian HR Reporter*, Carswell, One Corporate Plaza, 2075 Kennedy Road, Scarborough M1T 3V4.

The Bank of Montreal has taken numerous steps to achieve a more representative work force, including establishing a "Possibilities Foundation."

Bank of Montreal
www.bmo.com

- currently, the fastest growing groups in the Canadian work force are women, visible minorities, Aboriginal people, and persons with disabilities
- between 2001 and 2016, the number of Canadians between 55 and 69 years of age will increase dramatically. In contrast, the youth population, aged 15 to 24, will increase by only 0.3 percent. In fact, the 15 to 19 age group will actually decrease by seven percent.[17]

As discussed in Chapter 1, increasing diversity, the aging work force, and the shortage of young workers all have major implications for such HR activities as recruitment, selection, training, and compensation. Effective HRP involves monitoring such trends, anticipating their impact, and devising strategies to deal with them. The Bank of Montreal, recognizing the importance of fit between employees and customers, has incorporated equal opportunity in its strategic plan, and established an $8-million Possibilities Foundation for visible minority, Aboriginal, and disabled high-school students moving on to post-secondary education. Visible minorities, who represent 9.1 percent of the total Canadian work force, now account for more than 16.1 percent of the bank's work force.[18]

ELEMENTS OF EFFECTIVE HRP

Once the human resources implications of the organization's strategic plans have been analyzed, there are four subsequent processes involved in HRP, which will be discussed next.

1. Forecasting future human resources needs (demand).
2. Forecasting availability of internal and external candidates (supply).
3. Planning and implementing HR programs to balance supply and demand.
4. Monitoring and evaluating the results.

FORECASTING FUTURE HUMAN RESOURCES NEEDS (DEMAND)

A key component of HRP is forecasting the number and type of people needed to meet organizational objectives. Managers should consider several factors when forecasting such requirements.[19] From a practical point of view, the demand for the organization's product or service is paramount.[20] Thus, in a manufacturing firm, sales are projected first. Then, the volume of production required to meet these sales requirements is determined. Finally, the staff needed to maintain this volume of output is estimated. In addition to this "basic requirement" for staff, several other factors should be considered, including:

1. *Projected turnover* as a result of resignations or terminations.
2. *Quality and nature of employees* in relation to what management sees as the changing needs of the organization.
3. *Decisions to upgrade* the quality of products or services *or enter into new markets,* which might change the required employee skill mix.
4. *Planned technological and administrative changes aimed at increasing productivity and reducing employee headcount,* such as the installation of new equipment or introduction of a financial incentive plan.
5. The *financial resources* available to each department. For example, a budget increase may enable managers to pay higher wages and/or hire more people. Conversely, a budget crunch might result in wage freezes and/or layoffs.

In large organizations, needs forecasting is primarily quantitative in nature and is the responsibility of highly trained specialists. Quantitative techniques for determining human resources requirements include trend analysis, ratio analysis, scatter plot analysis, regression analysis, and computerized forecasting. Qualitative approaches to forecasting range from sophisticated analytical models to informal expert opinions about future needs,[21] such as a manager deciding that the cost of overtime in his or her department is beginning to outweigh that involved in hiring an additional staff member, and making plans to amend his or her staff complement during the next budget year.

Quantitative Approaches

Trend Analysis

trend analysis
Study of a firm's past employment levels over a period of years to predict future needs.

Trend analysis involves studying the firm's employment levels over the last five years or so to predict future needs. For example, the number of employees in the firm at the end of each of the last five years—or perhaps the number in each subgroup (such as sales, production, and administration)—might be computed. The purpose is to identify employment trends that might continue into the future.

Trend analysis is valuable as an initial estimate only, since employment levels rarely depend solely on the passage of time. Other factors (like changes in sales volume and productivity) will also affect future staffing needs.

Ratio Analysis

ratio analysis
A forecasting technique for determining future staff needs by using ratios between some causal factor (such as sales volume) and number of employees needed.

Another approach, ratio analysis, involves making forecasts based on the ratio between (1) some causal factor (such as sales volume) and (2) number of employees required (for instance, number of salespeople). For example, suppose a salesperson traditionally generates $500 000 in sales and that plans call for increasing the firm's sales by $3 million next year. Then, if the sales revenue–salespeople ratio remains the same, six new salespeople would be required (each of whom produces an extra $500 000 in sales).

Ratio analysis can also be used to help forecast other employee requirements. For example, a salesperson–secretary ratio could be computed to determine how many new secretaries will be needed to support the extra sales staff.

Like trend analysis, ratio analysis assumes that productivity remains about the same—for instance, that each salesperson can't be motivated to produce much more than $500 000 in sales. If sales productivity were to increase or decrease, then the ratio of sales to salespeople would change. A forecast based on historical ratios would then no longer be accurate.

The Scatter Plot

scatter plot

A graphical method used to help identify the relationship between two variables.

A scatter plot is another option. Scatter plots can be used to determine whether two factors—a measure of business activity and staffing levels—are related. If they are, then if the measure of business activity is forecast, HR requirements can also be estimated.

An example to illustrate follows.[22] Legislative changes to the health-care system require that two 500-bed Regina hospitals be amalgamated. Both previously had responsibility for acute, chronic, and long-term care. The government's plan is for one facility to specialize in acute care, while the other assumes responsibility for chronic and long-term care. In general, providing acute care requires staffing with registered nurses (RNs), while chronic and long-term care facilities can be staffed primarily with registered practical nurses (RPNs).

By the end of the calendar year, 200 beds at Hospital *A* must be converted from chronic and long-term care beds to facilities for acute patients. At the same time, Hospital *A*'s 200 chronic and long-term patients must be transferred to Hospital *B*. In a joint meeting, the directors of nursing and HR decide that a good starting point in the planning process would be to calculate the relationship between hospital size (in terms of number of acute beds) and the number of RNs required. After placing telephone calls to their counterparts at eight hospitals in larger centres across Alberta and Saskatchewan, they obtain the following information:

Size of Hospital *(Number of Acute Beds)*	*Number of* *Registered Nurses*
200	240
300	260
400	470
500	500
600	620
700	660
800	820
900	860

In order to determine how many RNs would be needed, they use the data obtained to draw the scatter plot shown in **Figure 5.4**, in which hospital size is shown on the horizontal axis and number of RNs is shown on the vertical axis. If the two factors are related, then the points will tend to fall along a straight line, as they do in this case. Carefully drawing a line that minimizes the distances

FIGURE 5.4 Determining the Relationship Between Hospital Size and Number of Nurses

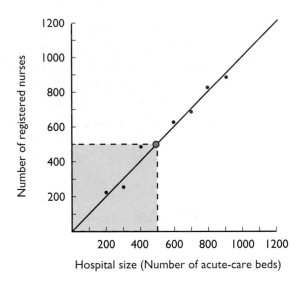

between the line and each of the plotted points permits an estimate of the number of nurses required for hospitals of various sizes. Thus, since Hospital *A* will now have 500 acute-care beds, the estimated number of RNs needed is 500.

Regression Analysis

regression analysis

A statistical technique involving the use of a mathematical formula to project future demands based on an established relationship between an organization's employment level (dependent variable) and some measurable factor of output (independent variable).

Regression analysis is a more sophisticated statistical technique to determine the "best-fit" line. It involves the use of a mathematical formula to project future demands based on an established relationship between an organization's employment level (dependent variable) and some measurable factor of output (independent variable) such as revenue, sales, or production level. When there are several dependent and/or independent variables, multiple regression analysis is used.

Computerized Forecasting Techniques

Many employers involved in quantitative forecasting use computers and software packages.[23] Typical data needed include direct labour hours to produce one unit of product (a measure of productivity) and three sales projections—minimum, maximum, and probable—for the product line in question. Based on such data, the program generates a computerized forecast of average staff levels required to meet product demands, as well as separate forecasts for direct labour (such as assembly workers), indirect labour (support staff, such as accounting clerks) and senior staff (such as managers).

computerized forecast

The determination of future staffing needs by projecting a firm's sales, volume of production, and the human resources requirements to maintain desired volume of output, using computers and software packages.

With such systems, employers can quickly translate projected productivity and sales levels into forecasts of human resources needs, and can easily check the impact of various productivity and sales levels on HR requirements.[24]

Qualitative Approaches

In contrast to quantitative approaches, which utilize statistical formulas, qualitative techniques rely solely on expert judgments. Two approaches used to gather such opinions in order to forecast human resources demand (or supply) include the nominal group and Delphi techniques.

Nominal Group Technique

nominal group technique
A decision-making technique that involves a group of experts meeting face to face. Steps include independent idea generation, clarification and open discussion, and private assessment.

The **nominal group technique** involves a group of experts (such as first-line supervisors and managers) meeting face to face. While one of its uses is human resources demand forecasting, this technique is used to deal with issues and problems ranging from identifying training needs to determining safety program incentives. The steps involved are as follows:[25]

1. Each member of the group independently writes down his or her ideas on the problem or issue (in this case, the causes of demand).

2. Going around the table, each member then presents one idea. This process continues until all ideas have been presented and recorded, typically on a flipchart or chalkboard. No discussion is permitted during this step.

3. Clarification is then sought, as necessary, followed by group discussion and evaluation.

4. Finally, each member is asked to rank the ideas. This is done independently and in silence.

Advantages of this technique include involvement of key decision makers, a future focus, and the fact that the group discussion involved in Step Three can facilitate the exchange of ideas and greater acceptance of results. Drawbacks include subjectivity and the potential for group pressure to lead to less accurate assessment than could be obtained through other means.

The Delphi Technique

Delphi technique
A judgmental forecasting method used to arrive at a group decision, typically involving outside experts as well as organizational employees. Ideas are exchanged without face-to-face interaction and feedback is provided and used to fine-tune independent judgments until a consensus is reached.

While short-term forecasting is generally handled by managers, the **Delphi technique** is useful for long-range forecasting and other strategic planning issues. It typically involves outside experts as well as company employees, based on the premise that outsiders may be able to assess changes in economic, demographic, governmental, technological, and social conditions and their potential impact more objectively. The Delphi technique involves the following steps:[26]

1. The problem is identified (in this case, the causes of demand) and each group member is requested to submit a potential solution by completing a carefully designed questionnaire. Direct face-to-face contact is not permitted.

2. After each member independently and anonymously completes the initial questionnaire, the results are compiled at a centralized location.

3. Each group member is then given a copy of the results.

4. If there are differences in opinion, each individual uses the feedback from other experts to fine-tune his or her independent assessment.

5. Steps Three and Four are repeated as often as necessary until a consensus is reached.

As with the nominal group technique, advantages include involvement of key decision makers and a future focus. The Delphi technique permits the group to critically evaluate a wider range of views, however. Drawbacks include the fact that judgments may not efficiently use objective data, the time and costs involved, and the potential difficulty in integrating diverse opinions.

Managerial Judgment

While managerial judgment is central to qualitative forecasting, it also plays a key role when using quantitative techniques. It's rare that any historical trend, ratio, or relationship will continue unchanged into the future. Judgment is thus needed to modify the forecast based on anticipated changes.

Summarizing Human Resources Requirements

staffing table

A pictorial representation of all jobs within the organization, along with the number of current incumbents and future employment requirements (monthly or yearly) for each.

The end result of the forecasting process is an estimate of short-term and long-range HR requirements. Long-range plans are, of course, general estimates of likely staffing needs, and may not include specific numbers.

Short-term plans—although still approximations—are more specific, and are often depicted in a staffing table. As illustrated in **Figure 5.5**, a staffing table is a pictorial representation of all jobs within the organization, along with the number of current incumbents and future employment requirements (monthly or yearly) for each.

FIGURE 5.5 A Sample Staffing Table

Springbrook Utilities Commission Staffing Table

Development Date: _____

Job Title	Department	Anticipated Openings											
		Total	Jan.	Feb.	Mar.	Apr.	May	June	July	Aug.	Sept.	Oct.	Nov.	Dec.
General Manager	Administration	1					1							
Director of Finance	Administration	1												1
Human Resources Officer	Administration	2	1					1						
Collection Clerk	Administration	1		1										
Groundskeeper	Maintenance	4						1	1					2
Service and Maintenance Technician	Maintenance	5	1			2					2			
Water Utility Engineer	Operations	3									2			1
Apprentice Lineperson	Operations	10	6						4					
Water Meter Technician	Operations	1												1
Engineering Technician	Operations	3			2							1		
Field Technician	Operations	8						8						
Senior Programmer/ Analyst	Systems	2				1				1				
Programmer/Operator	Systems	4		2						1			1	
Systems Operator	Systems	5					2						3	
Customer Service Representative	Sales	8	4					3				1		

FORECASTING FUTURE HUMAN RESOURCES SUPPLY

Short-term and long-range HR demand forecasts only provide half of the staffing equation by answering the question, "How many employees will we need?" The next major concern is how projected openings will be filled. There are two sources of supply:

1. Internal—present employees who can be transferred or promoted to meet anticipated needs.

2. External—people in the labour market not currently working for the organization. Included are those who are employed elsewhere, as well as those who are unemployed.

Forecasting the Supply of Internal Candidates

Before estimating how many external candidates will need to be recruited and hired, management must determine how many candidates for projected openings will likely come from within the firm. This is the purpose of forecasting the supply of internal candidates.

Estimating internal supply involves much more than simply calculating the number of employees. Some firms use the Markov analysis technique to track the pattern of employee movements through various jobs and develop a transitional probability matrix for forecasting internal supply by specific categories, such as position and gender. As illustrated in **Figure 5.6**, such an analysis shows the actual number (and percentage) of employees who remain in each job from one year to the next, as well as proportions promoted, demoted, transferred, and leaving the organization. It is these proportions (probabilities) that are used to forecast human resources supply.

In addition to such quantitative data, the skills and capabilities of current employees must be assessed, and skills inventories prepared. From this information, replacement charts and/or summaries and succession plans can be developed.

Skills Inventories

Skills inventories contain comprehensive information about the capabilities of current employees. Prepared manually or using a computerized system, data gathered for each employee include name, age, date of employment, current position, present duties and responsibilities, educational background, previous work history, skills, abilities, and interests. Information about current performance and readiness for promotion is generally included, as well. Data pertaining to managerial staff are compiled in management inventories. In addition to the information listed above, such inventories also include the number and types of employees supervised, duties of such employees, total budget managed, previous managerial duties and responsibilities, and managerial training received.

To be useful, skills and management inventories must be updated regularly. Failure to do so can lead to present employees being overlooked for job openings. Updating every two years is generally adequate if employees are encouraged to report significant qualifications changes (such as new skills learned and/or courses completed) to the HR department as they occur.

Manual Systems

Several types of manual systems are used to keep track of employees' qualifications. An example of a skills inventory and development record is shown in

Markov analysis

A method of forecasting internal labour supply that involves tracking the pattern of employee movements through various jobs and developing a transitional probability matrix.

skills inventories

Manual or computerized records summarizing employees' education, experience, interests, skills, etc., which are used to identify internal candidates eligible for transfer and/or promotion.

management inventories

Manual or computerized records summarizing the background, qualifications, interests, skills, etc. of management employees, as well as information about managerial responsibilities, duties in current and previous position(s), and management training, used to identify internal candidates eligible for transfer and/or promotion opportunities.

FIGURE 5.6 Hypothetical Markov Analysis for a Manufacturing Operation

→ 2000 1999	Plant Manager	Foreperson	Team Leaders	Production Worker	Exit
Plant Manager (*n* = 5)	80% 4				20% 1
Foreperson (*n* = 35)	8% 3	82% 28			10% 4
Team Leader (*n* = 110)		11% 12	70% 77	7% 8	12% 13
Production Worker (*n* = 861)			6% 52	72% 620	22% 189
Projected Supply	7	40	129	628	

Percentages represent transitions (previous year's actuals).
Actual numbers of employees are shown as whole numbers in each block
(projections for 2000 based on current staffing).

Figure 5.7. Such a form may be completed by each employee or filled in by a member of the HR department following a face-to-face interview. Once the information has been compiled and recorded, it can be used to determine which current employees are available for and interested in transfer or promotion.

Replacement Charts

replacement charts

Visual representations of who will replace whom in the event of a job opening. Likely internal candidates are listed, along with their age, present performance rating, and promotability status.

Replacement charts are a visual representation of who will replace whom in the event of a job opening, and are typically used to keep track of potential internal candidates for the firm's most important positions. As can be seen in **Figure 5.8**, such charts typically indicate age and replacement status of potential internal candidates. While age cannot be used as a criterion in making selection or promotion decisions, such information is necessary to project retirement dates, plan lateral moves, etc. Replacement status consists of two variables:

1. present performance—gleaned from performance appraisals
2. future promotability—based on information provided by the employee about future career aspirations and a subjective assessment by the employee's immediate supervisors of likelihood of future success.

To provide a more objective estimate of future potential, this information may be supplemented by results of psychological tests, interviews with HR specialists, and/or a visit to an assessment centre (which is explained in Chapter 7).

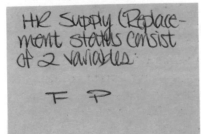

FIGURE 5.7 Skills Inventory Form Appropriate for Manual Storage and Retrieval

HUMAN RESOURCES SKILLS INVENTORY AND DEVELOPMENT RECORD			Date: month, year
Department	Area or sub-department	Branch or section	Location

Human Resources Skills Inventory and Development Record form

Replacement Summaries

While **replacement charts** provide an excellent quick reference tool, they contain very little information. For that reason, many firms prefer to use **replacement summaries.** Such summaries list likely replacements for each position and their relative strengths and weaknesses, as well as information about current position, performance, promotability, age, and experience. These additional data can be extremely helpful to decision makers, although caution must be taken to ensure that there is no discrimination on the basis of age, sex, etc.

FIGURE 5.8 Management Replacement Chart

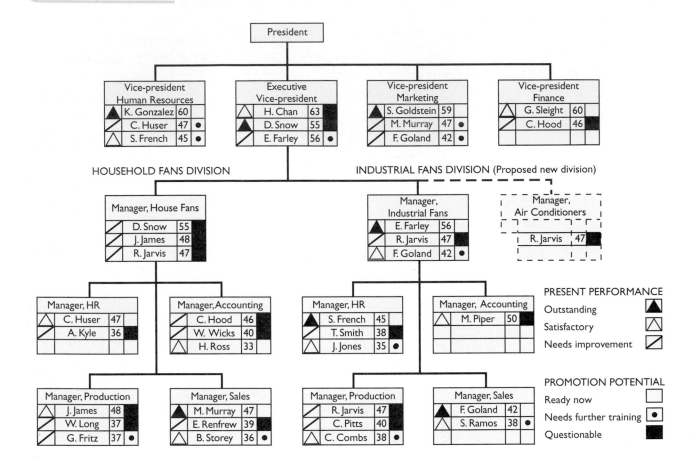

Computerized Information Systems

Skills inventories on hundreds or thousands of employees cannot be adequately maintained manually. Many firms—including DuPont Canada and Hewlett Packard (Canada)—computerize this information, and packaged systems are available for accomplishing this task.[27]

In one such system, employees fill out a 12-page booklet in which they describe their background and experience. This information is then transferred to the firm's HRMS. When a manager needs a position filled, he or she simply enters the job specifications (such as skill and/or experience requirements). After scanning its bank of possible candidates, the computer generates a printout of qualified candidates.

A computerized skills inventory should include the following types of information:

- work experience codes: the individual's present, previous, and desired jobs in coded format

- product or service knowledge: level of familiarity with the employer's product lines or services as an indication of where the person might be transferred or promoted

- industry experience: amount and type of industry experience, which may be relevant for certain positions

- formal education: the name of each post-secondary educational program completed, the field of study, and degree, diploma or certificate granted

- training courses: a brief description of company-sponsored courses taken or conducted by the employee, as well as courses taken through outside providers, such as the Canadian Institute of Management

- language skills: degree of proficiency in languages other than English and/or French

- relocation limitations: relocation limitations, if any, and/or preferred locales

- career interests: an indication of what the employee would like to be doing for the employer in the future; priority of choices; and whether the employee's main qualification for that work is experience, knowledge, or interest—all in coded format

- performance appraisal ratings: current data regarding the employee's achievement on each dimension appraised, along with a summary of the employee's strengths and deficiencies.[28]

Skills are often included in these types of data banks. Including "training courses completed" only shows what the employee is trained to do, not what he or she has actually done. Including specific skills, such as "remove boiler casings and doors," along with number of times performed, date last performed, and time spent, enables firms to use the computer to identify which employees are competent to accomplish the task at hand. Skill level can also be included, perhaps ranging from 1 (can lead or instruct others), to 2 (can perform the job with minimum supervision), 3 (has some experience; can assist experienced workers), and 4 (has not had opportunity to work on this job).[29] The role of computerized skills inventories and benefits associated with them are discussed in more detail in the Information Technology and HR box.

Succession Planning

Forecasting the availability of inside candidates is particularly important in succession planning. In a nutshell, succession planning refers to the plans a company makes to fill its most important executive positions. In the days when companies were hierarchical and employees tended to remain with the firm for years, executive succession was often straightforward: staff climbed the ladder one rung at a time, and it wasn't unusual for someone to start on the shop floor and end up in the president's office. While that kind of ascent is still possible, employee turnover and flatter structures mean that the lines of succession are no

The Expertise Center
www.expertcenter.com

succession planning

The process of ensuring a suitable supply of successors for current and future senior or key jobs, so that careers of individuals can be effectively planned and managed.

INFORMATION TECHNOLOGY AND HR

Computerized Skills Inventories

Using **SkillView.net**, a skills inventory program available via the Internet from SkillView Technologies, employees can receive a comprehensive printout analyzing their skills gaps (if any) and recommendations on how to address deficiencies. It is an interactive application, which allows users to rate their skills for their current job, obtain immediate online advice about how to fill any gaps, and rate their skills in other jobs if so desired. Group-based summary reports are available to managers who need to analyze employee skills gaps.

Source: "Bridging the Gap," Marketplace, *HR Professional* 16, no. 2 (April/May 1999), p. 44.

SkillView Technologies
www.skillview.com

longer so direct.[30] Thus, today, the succession planning process often involves a series of fairly complicated and integrated steps, as illustrated in the High Performance Organization box. For example, potential successors for top positions might be routed through the top jobs at several key divisions, as well as overseas, and sent through a university graduate-level, advanced management program. As a result, the comprehensive definition of succession planning shown in the margin is more applicable today.[31]

Since succession planning requires balancing the organization's top-management needs with the potential and career aspirations of available candidates, it includes these activities:

- analysis of the demand for managers and professionals by company level, function, and skill
- audit of existing executives and projection of likely future supply from internal and external sources
- planning of individual career paths based on objective estimates of future needs, performance appraisal data, and assessments of potential
- career counselling
- accelerated promotions, with development targeted against future business needs
- performance-related training and development to prepare individuals for future roles, as well as current responsibilities
- planned strategic recruitment, aimed at obtaining people with the potential to meet future needs, as well as filling current openings
- the actual activities by which openings are filled.[32]

It should be noted that replacement charts, replacement summaries, and succession plans are considered to be highly confidential in most organizations.

Forecasting the Supply of External (Outside) Candidates

It is not possible to fill all future openings with current employees. External sources of supply must be considered when entry-level jobs need to be filled or when there are no qualified internal replacements.

Employer growth is primarily responsible for the number of entry-level openings. While there are some higher-level jobs that require such unique talents and skills that they are impossible to fill internally, and some jobs are vacated unexpectedly, a key factor in determining the number of positions that must be filled externally is the effectiveness of the organization's training and development and career planning initiatives. If employees are not encouraged to expand their capabilities, they may not be ready to fill vacancies as they arise, and external sources must be tapped.

To project the supply of outside candidates, employers assess general economic conditions, national labour market conditions, local labour market conditions, and occupational market conditions.

General Economic Conditions

The first step is to forecast general economic conditions and the expected unemployment rate. The national unemployment rate provides the HR managers

The High Performance Organization

In Succession Planning, Being a Deputy Comes First!

Bata Ltd., a multinational shoe company with more than 55 000 employees worldwide, provides a great deal of in-house and external development, and relies on a highly structured system to groom future executives, a system that was recently overhauled to address a concern about an impending shortage of leadership talent. At Bata, every senior position has three high-potential employees—at different stages of development—being groomed for succession. While the process at Bata is more sophisticated than some, many large global companies have similar succession planning programs to safeguard the success of the firm. Such plans are neither a commitment nor a promise: the company agrees to provide opportunities for further development and expects employee dedication in return.

At Bata, a succession-planning chart provides a snapshot of the company superstructure at each of the 67 subsidiaries. For every senior position, there is a box with the names of the incumbent and three potential successors. The first is considered to be ready to step into the role immediately; the second is deemed to require two years to prepare for the position; and the third is expected to be management material in five years. Individual career plans are then prepared for those employees on the succession chart—about 200 individuals around the world. Such plans identify expected highest position and the date

on which that position should be attained, programs and training completed, areas still requiring improvement, and scheduled development programs.

Employees who are not on the chart can work to earn a spot thereon. At least once a year, candidates go through a formal review process (individual progress assessments) with their managers to assess how they are doing and determine what training they should pursue. Once functional training needs have been identified, candidates are taught best practices—both internal and external, and then "deputized." This involves being assigned to a position (usually replacing someone on holiday or attending an executive development session) for a trial period of two months or so, which provides an opportunity for the development of any deficient skills.

Like many firms today, Bata is cognizant of the need for new blood. Very aware of the impact of rapid change, demographics, and globalization, the company doesn't just want managers who look and think and talk like those before them. Instead, Bata is are looking for people who will constantly seek opportunities to improve ways of doing business, who are open to divergent opinions, and who are willing to go abroad.

Source: David Brown, "You Have to Be Deputy Before You Become Sheriff," *Canadian HR Reporter* 13, no. 3 (February 14, 2000), p. 9.

with an estimate of how difficult it is likely to be to acquire new employees in the immediate future. In general terms, the lower the rate of unemployment, the smaller the labour supply and the more difficult it will be to recruit. It is important to note, though, that even when unemployment rates are high, some positions will still be difficult to fill, since unemployment rates vary by occupation and also by geographic location (one city or province to another).

National Labour Market Conditions

Demographic trends have a significant impact on national labour market conditions. Fortunately for HR planners, these trends are well measured and projected, and there is a wealth of information available from government and private sources.[33]

Statistics Canada, for example, publishes annual, monthly, quarterly and occasional reports on labour force conditions. In addition to census data and population projections by sex and province, data is provided on labour income

Statistics Canada
www.statcan.ca

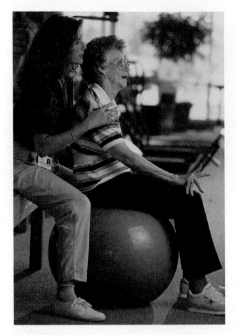

Physiotherapy is a skills-shortage occupation: the demand for physiotherapists exceeds the supply.

and total labour force projections based on geographic area, occupation, and demographics. Such information may have significant implications for organizations:

When CAMI Automotive Inc., a joint venture of Suzuki and General Motors, began operation in 1988, a corporate decision was made to include people with disabilities in CAMI's outreach recruitment, since there was recognition that this designated group represents a vast source of untapped potential.[34] (As of 1998, only 48 percent of Canadians with disabilities between the ages of 15 and 54 had either full- or part-time jobs, compared to 73 percent of Canadians without disabilities. Moreover, 54 percent of persons with disabilities had annual incomes of $15 000 or less.)[35]

Local Labour Market Conditions

Local labour markets are affected by many conditions, including community growth rates and attitudes. If growth is frowned upon or businesses receive little support, present employers may move elsewhere, and individuals losing their jobs may be forced to relocate. In communities experiencing such population declines, it is often impossible to attract new business, since potential employers fear future local HR supply shortages. The end result is that there are fewer and fewer jobs and more and more people leaving the local labour market—a vicious downward spiral. Conversely, one reason growing cities are attractive to employers is the promise of large future labour markets.

Chambers of Commerce and provincial/local development and planning agencies can be excellent sources of local labour market information.

Occupational Market Conditions

In addition to looking at the overall labour market, organizations also generally want to forecast the availability of potential candidates in specific occupations (engineers, drill press operators, accountants, and so on) for which they will be recruiting. In recent years, for example, there has been an undersupply of IT specialists, physiotherapists, and physicians in many parts of the country.

Forecasts for various occupations are available from a number of sources. For example, Human Resources Development Canada (HRDC) publishes both short-term and long-term labour force projections. as well as a publication projecting domestic occupational requirements (demand) and supply, nationally and provincially, for periods of up to 10 years. This report is useful for determining whether any projected imbalances will be self-correcting or will require specific intervention on the part of governments and/or private-sector organizations. The computerized supplement to this report integrates the impact of technological change on occupational composition.[36]

Human Resources Development Canada
www.hrdc-drhc.gc.ca

PLANNING AND IMPLEMENTING HR PROGRAMS TO BALANCE SUPPLY AND DEMAND

Once the supply and demand of human resources have been estimated, program planning and implementation commence. To successfully fill positions internally, organizations must manage performance and careers. Performance is managed

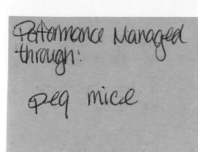

Performance Managed through:

peq mice

through: effective job design and quality of working life initiatives; establishing performance standards and goals, coaching, measuring and evaluating; and implementing a suitable reward structure (compensation and benefits).

To manage careers effectively, policies and systems must be established for recruitment, selection and placement (including transfer, promotion, retirement, and termination), and training and development. Policies and systems are also required for job analysis, individual employee assessment, replacement and succession planning, and career tracking, as well as career planning and development.[37]

Specific strategies must be formulated to balance supply and demand considerations. As was illustrated in Figure 5.2, there are three possible scenarios:

- labour supply exceeds demand (surplus)
- labour demand exceeds supply (shortage)
- expected demand matches supply.

Labour Surplus

A labour surplus exists when the internal supply of employees exceeds the organization's demand. Most employers respond initially by instituting a **hiring freeze**, which means that openings are filled by reassigning current employees, and no outsiders are hired unless authorization is granted by the CEO due to extenuating circumstances. The surplus is slowly reduced through **attrition**, which is the normal separation of employees due to resignation, retirement, or death. Because attrition is initiated by the employee, rather than the organization, it leads to the fewest problems. As people leave voluntarily, the vacancies created are not filled, and the staffing level decreases gradually without having to separate anyone involuntarily. In addition to the time that it takes, a major drawback of this approach is that the firm has no control over who stays and who leaves. Thus, valuable high performers may leave, while less-needed or lower-performing employees stay. Other potential problems include remaining employees being overburdened with work or lacking necessary skills, resulting in decreased or inferior performance and stagnation due to the lack of new skills and ideas.

Some organizations attempt to accelerate attrition by offering incentives to employees to leave, such as **buyout and early retirement programs**. Staffing levels are reduced and internal job openings created by offering attractive buyout (also known as early leave) packages or the opportunity to retire on full pension, with an attractive benefits package, at a relatively early age (often as young as 50 or 55). To be successful, buyouts must be handled very carefully. Selection criteria should be established, to ensure that key people who cannot be easily replaced do not leave the firm. A drawback of buyouts and early retirement packages is that they often require a great deal of money up-front. The New Brunswick government's early retirement program for civil servants, offered to 1700 of the 10 000 employees in January 2000, for example, will incur an increase in pension liability of at least $60 million, a cost that will be added to the province's net debt. Originally the pension liability was expected to increase by about $50 million. However, more than 1300 employees chose to accept the offer, rather than the projected 1000.[38] Care must also be taken to ensure that early retirement is voluntary, since forced early retirement is a contravention of human rights legislation, the consequences of which can be extremely costly. In

hiring freeze

A common initial response to an employee surplus. Openings are filled by reassigning current employees, and no outsiders are hired.

attrition

The normal separation of employees from an organization due to resignation, retirement, or death.

buyout and early retirement programs

Strategies used to accelerate attrition, which involve offering attractive buyout (early leave) packages or the opportunity to retire on full pension, with an attractive benefits package.

Options for Job Surplus: When large heavy beals just attack randomly.

job sharing
A strategy that involves dividing the duties of a single position between two or more employees.

work sharing
A layoff-avoidance strategy introduced by the federal government in 1977, by which employees worked three or four days a week and received unemployment insurance (now called employment insurance) on their non-work day(s).

reduced workweek
A layoff-avoidance strategy involving employees working fewer hours and receiving less pay.

layoff
The temporary withdrawal of employment to workers for economic or business reasons; another strategy used to correct an employee surplus.

reverse seniority
The employees hired most recently are the first to be laid off and the last to be recalled.

juniority clause
A provision in the collective agreement that senior workers (those with the greatest length of service) must be offered layoff first. If they accept, they are laid off and collect employment insurance (and organizational benefits), while junior employees retain their jobs.

a precedent-setting Ontario case, an older worker forced to accept early retirement was awarded $250 000 plus benefits.[39]

Another strategy used to deal with an employee surplus involves reducing total number of work hours. Job sharing involves dividing the duties of a single position between two or more employees.[40] Reducing full-time positions to *part-time work* is sometimes more effective, especially if there are peak demand periods. Creating a job-share position and/or offering part-time employment can be win–win strategies, since layoffs can be avoided. Although the employees involved work fewer hours and thus have less pay, they are still employed, and may enjoy having more free time at their disposal. The organization benefits by retaining good employees.

In 1977, the federal government introduced a work-sharing scheme, a layoff-avoidance strategy that involved employees working three or four days a week and receiving unemployment insurance (now called employment insurance—EI) on their non-workday(s).[41] Armco (now Armtec), a manufacturer of prefabricated steel buildings in Guelph, Ontario, was one organization that used work sharing to avoid layoffs and save jobs.

Similar to work sharing, but without a formal arrangement with government regarding EI benefits, is a reduced workweek. Employees simply work fewer hours and receive less pay. The organization retains a skilled work force, lessens the financial and emotional impact of a full layoff, and yet manages to reduce production costs. The only potential drawback is that it is sometimes difficult to predict in advance, with any degree of accuracy, how many hours of work should be scheduled each week.

Some organizations with progressive HR policies are able to find *alternative jobs within the organization* for surplus and displaced employees. For example, when Dylex closed its Town and Country stores, more than 500 of the 600 redundant employees in Ontario were placed in other Dylex chain stores.[42]

Another strategy for correcting an employee surplus is a layoff, the temporary withdrawal of employment to workers for economic or business reasons. Layoffs may be short in duration, as when plants close for brief periods to adjust inventory levels or retool for a new product line, but can last for months or even years if caused by a major change in business cycle. Layoffs are not pleasant for either managers or workers, but are sometimes needed if attrition will take too long or be insufficient to reduce numbers to the required level.

In unionized settings, layoffs are typically handled on the basis of reverse seniority—the employees hired most recently are the first to be laid off and the last to be recalled. The rights of employees during layoffs and the conditions and obligations pertaining to recall are clearly specified in the collective agreement. It is common for re-employment (recall) rights of laid-off employees to be preserved for periods of up to one or two years, provided they do not refuse to return to work if recalled sooner.

When a layoff is expected to be brief, as is common in the automotive industry when plants shut down for several weeks to change tooling for a new model, juniority may be used instead. If there is a juniority clause in the collective agreement, senior workers (those with the greatest length of service) must be offered layoff first. If they accept, they are laid off and collect EI (and organizational benefits), while junior employees retain their jobs. Long-service employees are often quite willing to accept a short-term layoff, since they can have time off for other pursuits, while their take-home pay remains virtually the same (EI cheques don't involve payroll deductions for benefits, union dues, etc.) and they can use the time off to pursue other interests. When layoffs are expected to be lengthy or are of unknown duration, long-service employees generally decline to exercise their juniority rights, since EI can only be collected for a limited period of time. In such situations, the employees who are lower on the seniority list are laid off.

In non-union settings, the ability of employees to change jobs and learn new skills, in addition to performance and competencies, is often given more weight than seniority in layoff decisions.

A key advantage of seniority and juniority clauses is objectivity. Using length of service as the basis for layoff and recall decisions is perceived by many to be most fair, since judgment of ability is subjective and favouritism may come into play. Employees themselves can calculate the probability of layoff and recall. There are drawbacks to using seniority as the governing factor, however. Less-competent employees receive the same rewards and security as those who are more competent. Talent and effort are ignored. When layoffs occur in reverse seniority order, the payroll is also higher, since those with the most seniority tend to earn more. Also, there is often a disproportionate impact on designated group members, since they are generally more recent hires.

To ease the financial burden of layoffs, some organizations offer **supplemental unemployment benefits (SUBs)**, which increase income levels closer to what an employee would receive if on the job. SUB programs are generally negotiated through collective bargaining. Benefits are payable until the pool of funds set aside has been exhausted.

When employees are no longer required, the employment relationship may be severed. **Termination** is a broad term that encompasses permanent separation from the organization for any reason. Since "termination" is often associated with discharge (being fired as a form of disciplinary action), some firms prefer to use the term "permanent layoff" when employees must be separated for economic or business reasons. In situations in which employment is terminated involuntarily, employees with acceptable or better performance ratings are often offered severance pay and outplacement assistance.

Severance pay is a lump-sum payment that is given to employees who are being permanently separated. While legally required in certain situations, such as mass layoffs (as will be explained in Chapter 15), severance pay is expected when employees are being terminated through no fault of their own. In addition to pay, severance packages often include benefits continuation for a specified period of time. In determining the appropriate package, employers should take salary, years of service, the employee's age and his or her likelihood of obtaining another job into consideration. To avoid costly court battles, many employers make reference to "ballpark," "reasonable range," or "reasonable offer" court decisions.[43]

Executives may be protected by a *golden parachute clause* in their contract of employment, a guarantee by the employer to pay specified compensation and benefits in the case of employee termination due to downsizing or restructuring.

Outplacement assistance may be provided to lessen the impact of termination. Generally offered by an outside agency, such programs are designed to assist affected employees in finding employment elsewhere. Typical aids provided include counselling; job-search skills training; use of office space, secretarial services, a computer, photocopier, and fax machine; and access to long-distance telephone calls. Sometimes letters are sent to other employers or placed in publications such as the *HR Professional* outlining the qualifications of displaced

supplemental unemployment benefits (SUBs)
A top-up to employment insurance, generally negotiated through collective bargaining, to increase income levels closer to what an employee would receive if on the job.

termination
A broad term that encompasses permanent separation from the organization for any reason.

severance pay
A lump-sum payment that is given to employees who are being permanently separated.

outplacement assistance
A program designed to assist terminated employees in finding employment elsewhere.

HR on the Net
www.njhrpg.org/fhomeres.htm

employees and a contact number. Such efforts not only assist the employees affected, but also indicate to the remaining employees and the public that the firm is truly interested in and committed to its human resources.

Re-evaluating Restructuring

While restructuring initiatives ranging from layoffs to mergers and acquisitions have certainly been prevalent in Canadian firms in recent years, in many instances, the consequences have not been as positive as anticipated.

Research Insight

In a study involving a sample of almost 500 major unionized and non-unionized Canadian organizations ranging in size from less than 200 to 1000 or more employees, employers whose firms had undergone work-force reductions reported significant expenditure cuts, a decline in the firm's reputation, difficulty in accomplishing work, a decline in financial performance, pressure on managers to focus on short-term profit or budget goals, a less favourable employee perception of top management, more vocal special interest groups, present employee concern about job security, difficulty in retaining top performers, and increased stress among managers. Permanent work-force reductions were also found to be associated with significantly lower overall employee satisfaction rates; noticeably poorer employer–employee relations (including higher rates of grievances and absenteeism), and more conflict within the organization; and moderately poorer economic performance, including somewhat lower productivity, product/service quality, market share, product/service innovation, and profitability.[44]

As those firms discovered—and which has been revealed in numerous studies— a high cost associated with downsizing is **survivor sickness,** a range of emotions that can include feelings of betrayal or violation, guilt, and detachment. The remaining employees, anxious about the next round of terminations, often suffer stress symptoms including depression, proneness to errors, and reduced performance. Despite the fact that survivor sickness is a well-publicized phenomenon, the *WorkCanada* survey described earlier found that firms tend to do a better job of handling acquisitions, growth, or mergers than they do of handling downsizing.[45] Given that fact, the results of another recent study are truly frightening: almost one in three mergers and acquisitions fails to achieve its business goals because of mishandled people issues and the inability to garner employee buy-in![46]

To avoid survivor sickness in downsizing situations, supervisors should:[47]

survivor sickness

A range of negative emotions experienced by employees remaining after a major restructuring initiative, which can include feelings of betrayal or violation, guilt and detachment; and result in stress symptoms, including depression, proneness to errors, and reduced productivity.

- get the process right by providing abundant, honest communication
- provide assistance to those being laid off
- treat victims and survivors with dignity and respect
- allow remaining employees to grieve and deal with repressed feelings and emotions
- increase their accessibility
- help survivors to recapture their sense of control and self-esteem
- use ceremonies, such as special meetings or small-group sessions, to provide people with a chance to acknowledge the changes and their reactions to them

Tips for the Front Line

An Ethical Dilemma

How much time, effort and money should firms devote to helping "surviving" employees deal with downsizing? mergers and acquisitions?

- reshape the systems to lessen dependency-creating processes by: eliminating rewards and recognition based on length of service; blurring differences between permanent, temporary and contract workers; and encouraging employees to think of themselves as self-employed entrepreneurs.

Labour Shortage

A labour shortage exists when the internal supply of human resources cannot fulfill the organization's needs. Scheduling overtime hours is often the initial response. Another short-term solution is to hire temporary employees. Employers may also subcontract work (if not prohibited by the collective agreement) on a temporary or permanent basis.

As vacancies are created within the firm, opportunities are generally provided for employee transfers and promotions, which necessitate performance management, training (and retraining), and career development. Internal movement does not eliminate a shortage, so recruitment will be required. Hopefully, though, resultant vacancies will be for entry-level jobs, which can be filled more easily externally.

A transfer involves lateral movement—from one job to another that is relatively equal in pay, responsibility, and/or organizational level. Such a move can lead to more effective utilization of human resources; broaden an employee's knowledge, skills and perspectives, in preparation for future promotional opportunities; result in additional technical or interpersonal challenges that lead to improved motivation and/or satisfaction; or offer some variety, which may also increase employee motivation and/or satisfaction.

A promotion involves the movement of an employee from one job to another that is higher in pay, responsibility, and/or organizational level. Such a move may be based on merit, seniority, or a combination of both.

A merit-based promotion is awarded in recognition of an employee's outstanding performance in his or her current job, or an assessment of his or her future potential. Such promotions should be based on an objective measure of performance and not personal biases, since decisions based on favouritism result in incompetent people in higher-level, more demanding positions, and resentment among those not selected. Another potential problem associated with promotions based on merit is the Peter Principle, which states that, in a hierarchy, people tend to rise to their level of incompetence.[48] This principle recognizes that being good in one job does not guarantee that one will be good in a higher-level position. An employee who is outstanding technically may make a very poor manager, for example, due to a lack of "people" or "team" skills.

In unionized settings, seniority may be the governing factor in promotion and transfer decisions, or the deciding factor in the event of a tie in candidates' skills and abilities. Unions often prefer seniority to be the deciding factor, since length of service is a matter of record and is therefore totally objective. The drawback is that because all workers are not equally capable, the individual who is transferred or promoted may not be the most competent.

transfer

Movement of an employee from one job to another that is relatively equal in pay, responsibility, and/or organizational level.

promotion

Movement of an employee from one job to another that is higher in pay, responsibility, and/or organizational level, usually based on merit, seniority, or a combination of both.

Peter Principle

The idea that in a hierarchy, people tend to rise to their level of incompetence, a potential problem with merit-based promotions.

Labour Supply Matches Labour Demand

When there is a match between expected supply and demand, organizations replace employees who leave the firm with individuals transferred or promoted from inside or hired from outside. As in shortage situations, performance management, training, and career development play a crucial role.

HRP Evaluation

HRP evaluation
An annual assessment to determine the effectiveness of HRP in meeting management's expectations, which involves determining whether or not goals were reached and reasons for failure, and identifying areas in need of change.

HR planning should be assessed on an annual basis with an **HRP evaluation** to determine its effectiveness in meeting management's expectations. Since HRP links an organization's HRM activities with its strategic goals and objectives, the strength and adequacy of these linkages should be assessed.[49] Whether or not goals were reached, reasons for failure should be determined and areas in need of change should be identified.

Specific criteria often assessed include:

- actual staffing levels versus established staffing requirements
- the ratio of internal placements to external hiring
- actual internal mobility flow (movement of employees within the organization) versus career development plans
- internal mobility flow versus turnover
- employment equity achievements as compared to established goals and timetables.

Chapter Review

Summary

1 Human Resources Planning (HRP) is the process of reviewing HR requirements to ensure that the organization has the required number of employees with the necessary skills to meet its goals.

2 Whether strategic or operational, plans are made and carried out by people. Thus, determining whether or not people will be available is a critical element of both strategic and operational planning processes. HRP and strategic planning become effective when there is a reciprocal and interdependent relationship between them.

3 Environmental scanning is a critical component of the HRP and strategic planning processes. The external environmental factors most frequently monitored include: economic conditions; market and competitive trends; government and legislative issues; social concerns related to health care, childcare, and educational priorities; technological changes; and demographic trends.

4 Once the HR implications of the organization's strategic plans have been analyzed, there are four subsequent processes involved in HRP: forecasting future human resources needs (demand); forecasting availability of internal and external candidates (supply); planning and implementing HR programs to balance supply and demand; and monitoring and evaluating the results.

5 The end result of the forecasting process is an estimate of short-term and long-range HR requirements. Long-range plans are general statements of

probable needs. Short-term plans, although still approximations, are more specific, and are often depicted in a staffing table.

6   Once the supply and demand have been estimated, program planning and implementation commence. Organizations must manage performance and careers and formulate specific strategies to balance supply and demand considerations.

7   Strategies to deal with a labour surplus include: the implementation of a hiring freeze and downsizing through attrition; speeding up attrition through attractive buyout (early leave) and early retirement programs; reducing hours through job sharing, part-time hours, work sharing or reduced workweeks; finding alternative jobs within the organization for displaced workers; laying off workers on the basis of reverse seniority or juniority; and terminating employment.

8   Scheduling overtime is often the initial response to a human resources shortage. Another short-term solution is to hire temporary employees. Employers may also subcontract work (if not prohibited by the collective agreement) on a temporary or permanent basis. As vacancies are created within an organization, opportunities are generally provided for employee transfers and promotions.

9   When there is a match between expected supply and demand, organizations replace employees who leave the firm with individuals transferred or promoted from inside or hired from outside.

10   HR planning should be assessed on an annual basis to determine its effectiveness in meeting management's expectations. Whether or not goals were reached and reasons for failure should be determined, and areas in need of change identified.

Key Terms

attrition	ratio analysis
buyout and early retirement programs	reduced workweek
computerized forecast	regression analysis
Delphi technique	replacement charts
hiring freeze	replacement summaries
human resources planning (HRP)	reverse seniority
HRP evaluation	scatter plot
job sharing	severance pay
juniority clause	skills inventories
layoff	staffing table
management inventories	succession planning
Markov analysis	supplemental unemployment benefits (SUBs)
nominal group technique	
outplacement assistance	survivor sickness
Peter Principle	termination
promotion	transfer
public sector	trend analysis
quasi-public sector	work sharing

Review and Discussion Questions

1 Explain the nature of human resources planning (HRP) and describe the costs associated with lack of or inadequate HRP.

2 Describe the relationship between HRP and strategic planning.

3 Differentiate between replacement charts and replacement summaries, and explain why replacement summaries are generally preferred.

4 Discuss various layoff-avoidance strategies that can be used to reduce a surplus of human resources.

5 Differentiate between the reverse seniority and juniority approaches to lay-offs and explain the advantages and disadvantages of each.

6 Differentiate between the seniority and merit-based approaches to promotion and describe the advantages and disadvantages associated with each.

CRITICAL *Thinking Questions*

1 In this chapter, we discussed a number of quantitative and qualitative techniques for forecasting human resources demand. Working in groups, identify which strategies would be most appropriate for (a) various sized companies, (b) industries undergoing rapid change, and (c) businesses/industries in which there are seasonal variations in HR requirements.

2 Suppose that it has just been projected that, due to a number of technological innovations, your firm will need 20 percent fewer clerical employees within the next five years. What actions would you take to try to retain your high-performing clerical staff members?

3 Suppose that you are the HR manager at a firm at which a hiring freeze has just been declared. The plan is to downsize through attrition. What steps would you take to ensure that you reap the advantages of this strategy, while minimizing the disadvantages?

APPLICATION *Exercises*

RUNNING CASE: Carter Cleaning Company

To Plan or Not to Plan?

One aspect of HRM that Jennifer studied at university was HR planning. Her professor in the course emphasized its importance, especially for large organizations. While Carter Cleaning is certainly not large at this time—with only six centres, each staffed by its own on-site manager and seven employees, on average—she wonders if HRP might help to resolve some of their current problems.

At this point, there is only an informal succession plan—both Jennifer and her father are counting on the fact that Jennifer will take over the firm when her father decides to retire.

Carter Cleaning is heavily dependent on its managers—three white males and three white females—and skilled cleaner-spotters and pressers. Employees generally have no more than a high-school education (often less). The market for skilled staff is very competitive. Over a typical weekend, literally dozens of want ads for experienced pressers or cleaner-spotters can be found in area newspapers. Paid little more than minimum wage, people in these jobs tend to move around a great deal. Virtually all of the incumbents in these positions at the centres are women and/or visible minorities. Turnover (as in the stores of many of Carter Cleaning's competitors) sometimes approaches 400 percent.

Jennifer is pondering the following questions:

Questions

1 In what ways might HRP benefit Carter Cleaning?
2 Should they decide to proceed with HRP, what steps should Jennifer and her father take?
3 What HRP techniques would be appropriate for them to use?
4 What other issues would have to be addressed to make HRP worthwhile?

CASE INCIDENT *Management Trainees at Nova*

It's that time of year again at Nova! Each year, Carl Adams, recruitment officer at head office of the retail chain, visits colleges and universities across Canada to recruit graduates for sales, marketing, human resources, and purchasing management-trainee positions for its 26 locations.

In order to predict the number of management trainees required, HRP is done each year, based on the budget and forecasted sales. The previous year's plan is also reviewed. There has been virtually no change in the HR plan over the past 10 years.

Natalie Gordon, vice-president of human resources, is feeling rather concerned about what happened last year and wondering how to ensure that it doesn't happen again. Based on the HR plan, 50 new management trainees were hired. Unfortunately, six months after they started, the company experienced a drastic drop in sales due to a downturn in the economy, combined with increased foreign competition. Half of the recently hired management trainees had to be laid off.

Carl, who started at Nova as a management trainee when he completed the Business Administration–Human Resources Management program at Central Community College, has just returned from an on-campus recruitment campaign, which happened to be at his old alma mater, and reported that his experience was not as pleasant as usual. One of the candidates that he interviewed knew someone who had been hired and laid off last year, and indicated that she was rather worried about considering a position with the firm in light of that fact, despite Nova's excellent reputation for promotion from within and overall stability. (Nova, which currently employs more than 8000 people in its head office and retail stores across the country, has been in business for more than 70 years.)

Carl has just finished telling Natalie how embarrassed he was by this candidate's probing questions about job security and how uncomfortable he felt. He ended up simply reassuring the candidate that such a situation could never happen again. Natalie is now wondering how to make Carl's reassurance a reality.

Questions

1 What are the consequences of poor HRP at Nova?
2 What problems do you see with Nova's present HRP process?
3 What should Natalie do to more accurately forecast the demand for management trainees for the coming year before Carl does any more on-campus recruiting?

EXPERIENTIAL *Exercises*

1 Develop a realistic, hypothetical staffing table for a department or organization with which you are familiar.

2 Contact the HR manager at a firm in your area and find out whether or not the firm uses any of the following: (a) skills/management inventories, (b) replacement charts or summaries and (c) a succession plan. Prepare a brief summary of the information gleaned. Once you have completed these tasks, form a group with several of your classmates. Share your findings with the group members. Were there similarities across firms? Did company size seem to make a difference in terms of strategies used for forecasting the supply of internal candidates? Can you identify any other factors that seem to play a role in the choice of forecasting techniques used?

3 This assignment requires working within teams of five or six. Half of the teams are to assume the role of management team-members at a firm that is about to undergo major downsizing. The other half of the teams are to assume the roles of employees—some of whom will be affected and others of whom will remain. Each management team is to be paired up with an employee team, and assigned responsibility for preparing a realistic simulation. Managers should work toward the goal of minimizing the negative impact on those who will be affected as well as those who will be remaining. Individuals in employee roles are asked to try to envision what their thoughts and feelings would be (if they have never actually been in this situation, that is) and to portray them as realistically as possible.

WEB-BASED *Exercise*

1 Visit the Web sites of Statistics Canada (**www.statcan.ca**) and Human Resources Development Canada (**www.hrdc-drhc.gc.ca**) and answer the following questions: (a) What is the current unemployment rate in your province or territory? How does the unemployment rate in your province or territory compare to the overall Canadian unemployment rate? (b) In which occupations are there currently skills shortages across Canada? Are there any provincial/territorial differences in this regard? (c) Which occupa-

tions are in high demand in your province or territory? (d) Select two occupations. Compare the supply and demand for these occupations across four provinces or territories. Summarize your findings and be prepared to be called upon to present them to the class as a whole or a small group of classmates.

CHAPTER 6

Recruitment

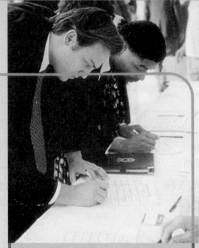

CHAPTER
OUTLINE

Introduction

The Recruitment Process

Constraints on the
Recruitment Process

Recruiting Within the
Organization

Recruiting Outside the
Organization

Recruiting a More
Diverse Work Force

Developing and Using
Application Forms

LEARNING OUTCOMES

After studying this chapter, you should be able to:

Define recruitment and *describe* its purposes.

Explain the recruitment process.

Describe the constraints on recruitment.

Describe the role of job posting, human resources records, and skills inventories in promotion from within.

Describe the methods used for external recruitment and *explain* the appropriate use of each.

Discuss strategies for recruiting a more diverse work force.

Explain the importance of application forms and *design* a legally compliant application form.

INTRODUCTION

recruitment
The process of searching for and attracting an adequate number of qualified candidates, from whom the organization may select the most appropriate to staff its job requirements.

Recruitment is the process of searching for and attracting an adequate number of qualified candidates, from whom the organization may select the most appropriate to staff its job requirements. The process begins when the need to fill a position is identified and ends with the receipt of résumés and/or completed application forms.

The Purposes of Recruitment

According to one expert, recruitment of the right people is a key ingredient of corporate health and well-being.[1] Because the quality of a firm's human resources depends to a great extent upon the quality of its recruits, recruitment is a critical HR function. Its purposes are to:

- ensure that an adequate pool of applicants is generated at minimum possible cost
- eliminate (or at least minimize) unqualified or poorly qualified candidates, thus improving the success rate of the selection process[2]
- find and attract individuals who not only meet the job requirements, but are also suited to the organization's unique culture and climate
- help the firm to meet its employment equity goals by attracting a diverse applicant pool.

The Role of the HR Department in the Recruitment Process

recruiter
A specialist in recruitment, whose job it is to find and attract capable candidates

As was mentioned in Chapter 1, in firms with an HR department, functional authority for recruitment is generally delegated to HR staff members. In large organizations, in which recruiting is done on an almost continuous basis, the HR team typically includes specialists, known as **recruiters**, whose job it is to find and attract qualified applicants.

THE RECRUITMENT PROCESS

As illustrated in **Figure 6.1**, there is a number of steps in the recruitment process:

1. Job openings are identified through HR planning or manager request. HR plans play a vital role in the identification process, because they indicate present and future openings and specify which should be filled internally and which externally. Openings do arise unexpectedly, however, in which case the immediate supervisor may have to complete a **human resources requisition form** or a business plan to obtain authorization to proceed with recruitment and selection.

human resources requisition form
A form that must be completed to obtain authorization for recruitment, outlining the position, job specifications, reason for the opening, and date required.

2. The job requirements are determined. This involves reviewing the job description and the job specification and updating them, if necessary. Manager comments may also prove helpful in identifying requirements, particularly pertaining to personality and fit.

FIGURE **6.1** The Recruitment Process

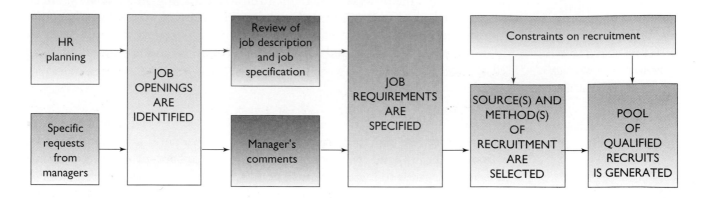

3. Appropriate recruiting source(s) and method(s) are chosen. There is no single, best, recruiting technique, and the most appropriate for any given position depends on a number of factors, which will be discussed next.

4. A pool of qualified recruits is generated.

CONSTRAINTS ON THE RECRUITMENT PROCESS

To be successful in his or her search, a recruiter must be aware of the constraints affecting the process. These come from organizational policies and plans, the job specifications, recruiter preferences, inducements of competitors, and environmental factors.

Organizational Policies

Promote-from-within

Most firms have a promote-from-within policy. Collective agreements often require that jobs be posted internally for a specified period of time before external recruitment can begin, and many organizations have adopted a similar policy for their non-union positions. While this practice has numerous advantages, which will be discussed shortly, having such a policy may mean that a recruiter cannot start recruiting externally until the period is over, even if he or she is aware that there are no suitable internal candidates.

Compensation

The pay structure and benefits package can pose a constraint, since they influence the attractiveness of the job to potential applicants. Recruiters typically do not have the authority to deviate from established pay ranges, and may be further constrained by an organizational policy specifying that no one can be hired at a rate higher than the midpoint or other set level within the range.

Employment Status

Some organizations have a policy prohibiting the hiring of part-time, temporary, or contract employees, which means that only those seeking full-time positions are eligible for consideration as recruits. In other firms, there is a restriction on full-time hiring, which means that recruiters are authorized to hire on a part-time, temporary or contract basis only.

Local Hiring

Many firms with international operations hire locally whenever possible. Hiring host-country nationals (HCNs) has a number of advantages. It reduces the likelihood of charges of economic exploitation, reduces relocation expenses, and minimizes the likelihood of cultural and family adjustment problems. HCNs are also more apt to be fluent in the language and to understand and accept local customs and business practices. Moreover, in many countries, including Canada, there are legal restrictions on the right to recruit outside the country if there are qualified candidates available within.

There are some drawbacks to hiring HCNs, however. In addition to the challenge of recruiting a good performer in an unfamiliar labour market, time must be spent helping the HCN to learn and adopt the organization's corporate culture. The firm may also have to provide the technical knowledge required, such that the new employee can operate effectively as a local agent. Many organizations have found, though, that providing indoctrination and support systems for an HCN are less onerous than training and supporting a domestic manager on an expatriate assignment.[3]

AN ETHICAL DILEMMA

Are there circumstances in which it would be both ethical and prudent for firms to offer jobs to expatriates when there are qualified HCNs available?

Organizational Plans

Human Resources Plan

The HR plan provides valuable guidance to recruiters by indicating how many candidates will be required for various positions and when they will be needed, but may also pose some restrictions, since such plans specify which positions should be filled internally and which externally.

Employment Equity Plan

Whether legally required or voluntarily initiated, if there is an employment equity plan, it must be consulted, since it will specify the organization's goals and timetables pertaining to designated group members. To increase the number of qualified candidates from the designated groups, recruiters often use nontraditional (outreach) strategies, a topic that will be explored later in this chapter.

Recruitment Budget

The budget established for recruitment also poses some constraints. The costs of telephone calls, travel, advertising, etc. must be taken into consideration. Some positions can be filled very cheaply; others will require extensive advertising and considerable time and travel. Recruiters have to decide how to allocate their allotted budget dollars in the most effective manner. Careful HR planning and forethought by recruiters can minimize expenses. For example, recruiting for several job openings simultaneously can reduce the cost per recruit.

Costs have to be balanced with other considerations, however. For example, relying on three very popular and inexpensive techniques—walk-ins, write-ins, and word-of-mouth hiring, which will be described later in this chapter—can result in systemic discrimination. Also, as will be explained shortly, the ~~recruitment method~~ chosen ~~affects the quality of hires and turnover rates.~~

Job Specifications

The actual requirements of the job for which recruits are being sought pose some constraints. Skilled and specialized workers, for example, often have to be hired externally and are generally more difficult to locate and attract than unskilled or semi-skilled ones. The length of time required, scope of the search area (local, regional, national, or international), amount of compensation required to attract candidates, and recruitment campaign budget are all linked to the job specifications. As explained in the Global HRM box, filling certain high-tech positions may mean seeking recruits from around the world, something that is not easy, given Canada's strict immigration laws.

GLOBAL HRM

Bringing Home Foreign Workers With "Hot" Skills

The Canadian government has fairly strict immigration requirements. Recognizing, though, that there are skills shortages in a number of fields, both government and industry agree that bringing in foreign workers with skills that are in high demand is of economic benefit to Canada, specifically if these jobs cannot be filled by Canadians.

The Software Development Worker Pilot Project, which has now become the blueprint for an overall temporary foreign worker project, was introduced by Citizenship and Immigration Canada (CIC) in May of 1997, in conjunction with Human Resources Development Canada (HRDC), Industry Canada (IC), and the Software Human Resource Council (SHRC), a nonprofit, non-government body. In recognition of the drastic shortage of information technology (IT) professionals possessing specific skills, the aim of the project was to fast-track the entry of qualified software professionals to Canada for temporary employment with a Canadian employer, by removing HRDC's normal job validation requirement.

Seven job descriptions were published as the basis for expedited processing of applications from IT workers possessing specific skills, provided the applications were accompanied by a written job offer from a Canadian employer, along with other required documentation. The positions involved include: (1) embedded systems software engineer, (2) software products developer, (3) MIS software engineer, (4) multimedia software developer, (5) senior animation editor, (6) software developer—services, and (7) application developer.

The project was initially extended to the end of 1999 to enable CIC and HRDC to review the results and consider various ways of addressing labour market shortages in a number of high-skill occupations. It was then further extended until a sectoral agreement involving the SHRC could be concluded. Between May 1997 and January 2000, more than 100 Canadian employers and close to 3000 foreign workers took advantage of the program.

Based on findings that key foreign workers actually create employment opportunities for Canadians and support a much-needed skills transfer, on

January 21, 2000, CIC and HRDC announced a number of improvements to Canada's Temporary Foreign Worker Program for skills-shortage occupations, which range from IT professionals to blue-collar workers. These include:

- the formal introduction of sectoral agreements by councils or organizations that represent and/or advocate on behalf of the interests of defined skills groups

- the introduction of an improved computerized information exchange process in early April 2000 to speed up the processing of the applications of skilled temporary foreign workers in skills-shortage occupations

- permission for employers who require significant numbers of foreign workers to meet their HR needs, due to a proven labour market shortage, to enter into individual agreements with HRDC that provide for preapproval of job validations for a specific number of foreign workers, in exchange for a commitment to train and hire Canadian workers or undertake other labour market initiatives.

Source: Howard D. Greenberg, "Ottawa Serves Up Fast Tracking for Entry of Foreign Workers with Hot Skills," *Canadian HR Reporter* 13, no. 3 (February 14, 2000), pp. 6-7; and "Software Development Worker Pilot Project: The Achievement" *Software Human Resource Council*, www.shrc.ca/ss2b/sdwpp/achievement.html. August 22, 2000.

Software Human Resource Council (SHRC)

www.shrc.ca

Recruiter Preferences

With time and success, recruiters acquire preferences. Although such preferences can save time and enhance efficiency, they can also lead to perpetuation of past mistakes or failure to consider alternatives that might be more effective.

Using the same method repeatedly may make it difficult, if not impossible, to reach employment equity goals, and may result in a ~~pool of employee~~s who share the ~~same strengths and weaknesses~~.

Inducements of Competitors

Attracting qualified candidates requires marketing. Monetary and non-monetary inducements are used to stimulate interest. The types of inducements being offered by the competition impose a constraint, since recruiters must try to meet the prevailing standards or use alternative inducements to overcome limitations. For example, if a competitor is offering excellent pay as an inducement, and the organization has a far more modest salary range, the recruiter may try to sell: the job (interesting projects, the opportunity to use leading-edge tools); the work environment (a high level of intellectual stimulation, a collegial environment); the firm (a track record of job security, reputation as a prestigious blue-chip company); the community (good schools, a low crime rate, accessible cultural and entertainment options); the location (along the Cabot Trail, in the heart of the Okanagan Valley); or unique benefits (a generous educational subsidy plan, flextime, childcare facilities). The types of inducements offered today range from computers and Internet access at home for a nominal fee to signing bonuses and stock options.[4]

There is a caution to be noted in the use of inducements, however. The Supreme Court of Canada decision in *Queen v. Cognos* (1993) makes it clear that employers must take extreme care in describing the nature and existence of an employment opportunity to prospective employees. Representations made must be accurate, not misleading, or the firm can be charged with negligent misrepresentation:[5]

> Douglas Queen, a Calgary accountant who moved to Ottawa for a job at Cognos Inc., a computer software company, was awarded $67 244 in a wrongful hiring suit. When he was recruited, Mr. Queen was not informed that the financing for the project for which he was being enticed to move to Ottawa had not been finalized. Shortly after being hired, the funding fell through and the responsibilities he thought he would be assuming evaporated.

Environmental Factors

As described in detail in Chapter 1, external environmental conditions impose a major constraint on many aspects of employment. Changes in the labour market, unemployment rate, economy and legislation, and the recruiting activities of labour-market competitors all affect a recruiter's efforts. Although an environmental scan is an important component of HRP, the economic climate may change after the firm has finalized its HR plan. Thus, recruiters should check several measures to ensure that the assumptions on which the plan was based are valid at the time of search:

Leading Economic Indicators

Each month, Statistics Canada announces the direction of the leading economic indicators. If these indices signal a sudden downturn or upturn in the economy, it may be necessary to modify recruiting plans.

Want-ads Index

Statistics Canada monitors and reports as an index the volume of want ads in major metropolitan newspapers. An upward trend in this index, such as that experienced over the past three years,[6] reflects a high degree of competition for recruits sought nationally, such as professionals and managers. To monitor the amount of competition for workers recruited locally or regionally, such as clerical and production employees, recruiters may wish to monitor changes in want-ad volume in local and regional newspapers and create their own indices. Generally, the more competition there is, the more vigorous and extensive the recruitment campaign must be. A drop in level of competition may narrow the scope of the area of search or make less-costly recruitment methods viable.

Actual Activity versus Predicted Activity

Most organizations produce monthly reports in which actual levels of activity (such as sales volume or number of patients admitted) are compared with projections. Variations between what was predicted, as reflected in the HR plan, and what is actually occurring may necessitate modifications to recruiting plans.

Recruiting Sources

There are two sources of recruits: the pools of workers internal and external to the company. Although recruiting often brings employment agencies and classified ads to mind, current employees are generally the largest source of recruits.

Research Insight

In a recent survey involving 718 Canadian firms, internal advertising or posting and a database search of internal candidates were reported as being "very useful" recruitment methods for salaried positions at all levels.[7] Another recent study of 100 executives in Canada's largest companies revealed that firms are more likely to promote from within these days than they were three years ago. Sixty-two percent of the respondents indicated they are more likely to promote from within, while only 19 percent said they are less likely to do so.[8]

RECRUITING WITHIN THE ORGANIZATION

Filling open positions with inside candidates has several advantages:

* employees see that competence is rewarded, thus enhancing commitment, morale and performance
* having already been with the firm for some time, insiders may be more committed to the company's goals and less likely to leave
* managers are provided with a longer-term perspective when making business decisions
* it is generally safer to promote from within, since the firm is likely to have a more accurate assessment of the person's skills and performance level than would otherwise be the case
* inside candidates require less orientation than outsiders.

Promotion from within also has a number of drawbacks, however:

* employees who apply for jobs and don't get them may become discontented. Informing unsuccessful applicants as to why they were rejected and what remedial action they might take to be more successful in the future is thus essential[9]
* managers may be required to post all job openings and interview all inside candidates, even when they already know whom they wish to hire, thus wasting considerable time and creating false hope on the part of those employees not genuinely being considered
* employees may be less satisfied and accepting of a boss appointed from within their own ranks than they would a newcomer
* it is sometimes difficult for a newly chosen leader to adjust to no longer being "one of the gang"[10]
* there is a possibility of "inbreeding." When an entire management team has been brought up through the ranks, there may be a tendency to make decisions "by the book" and to maintain the status quo, when a new and innovative direction is needed.

AN ETHICAL
DILEMMA
Is it ethical to require a manager to post all jobs and interview all internal candidates, even if he or she has already made a decision about the individual who will be selected for the position?

Most firms recognize that to be effective, promotion from within requires using job posting, human resources records, and skills inventories. In a recent study involving 718 Canadian firms, for example, internal advertising or posting as a strategy for identifying candidates for lower-level salaried positions was identified by 64 percent of respondents as being very useful, and internal databases were rated as very useful by 53 percent. For executives, internal advertising or posting was reported by 38 percent of respondents as being very useful, and internal databases were rated as very useful by 42 percent.[11]

Job Posting

job posting

The process of notifying current employees about vacant positions.

Job posting is a process of notifying current employees about vacant positions. This may involve placing on designated bulletin boards throughout the firm a form outlining the title, duties (as listed in the job description), qualifications (taken from the job specification), hours of work, pay range, posting date, and closing date (as in **Figure 6.2**). Such bulletin boards may be enclosed in glass cases and kept locked, so that no unauthorized postings can be placed and postings cannot be removed prior to the closing date. Some firms require that interested employees submit a current résumé to the HR department; others have forms that can be completed.

FIGURE 6.2 Sample Job Posting

Renfrew County Board of Education

Job Posting Notice

Secretary

(Special Education)

This is a full-time position starting November 15, 2000.

Any employee who feels s/he is qualified and wishes to apply, in accordance with the Collective Agreement, must submit an up-to-date resume with attached cover letter to the Director, Human Resources Services, up to and including October 30, 2000.

The secretarial position is responsible for providing secretarial and clerical support services for the Special Education Administrator, Psychologist, and other professional staff and committees. Specifically, this will include setting up, word processing, duplicating, and distributing reports, handbooks, policy and procedure manuals, etc.; receiving inquiries by mail, telephone, and in person, from parents, teachers, and other staff; updating student information files; and other related clerical duties.

QUALIFICATIONS: secretarial, clerical training and/or experience; excellent written and oral communication skills; good organizational skills; high ethical standards; and the ability to take initiative.

HOURS:	9:00 a.m. to 5:00 p.m. (40 hrs/week)
DATE POSTED:	October 15, 2000
DATE CLOSED:	October 30, 2000

A detailed job description is available from the Human Resources Department.

DEDICATED TO EMPLOYMENT EQUITY; QUALIFIED DESIGNATED GROUP MEMBERS ARE ENCOURAGED TO APPLY

Source: Lorann Martinell. Reproduced with permission.

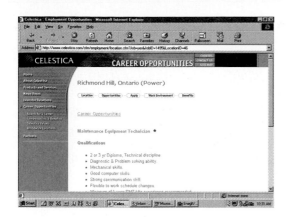

Posting jobs on the company's intranet can be an effective way of spreading the word about job opportunities to existing employees.

Not all firms use bulletin boards. Some post jobs in employee publications, have special-announcement handouts, or send out notices by mail. Others, such as DuPont Canada, now have computerized job-posting systems, such that information about vacancies can be found on the company's intranet or is accessible 24 hours a day by calling a specific telephone number.

As mentioned earlier, many collective agreements require that all vacant jobs in the bargaining unit be posted for a specified number of days, and stipulate that only bargaining unit members can initially be considered. This helps to ensure that the bargaining unit members receive fair consideration when opportunities for lateral moves or promotions arise within the local. Many firms have job-posting policies covering their non-union employees as well. An example is presented in **Figure 6.3**. Included therein are important guiding principles for such policies, such as the fact that all permanent employees are eligible to apply for positions under the policy and that all employees in all locations will be advised about job openings.

As illustrated in **Figure 6.4**, there are advantages and disadvantages to using job postings to facilitate the transfer and promotion of qualified internal candidates. As highlighted in the High Performance Organization box, an effective job-posting policy can increase commitment and retention, and linking job postings to career development not only increases retention, but also provides an edge in recruiting external candidates.

Human Resources Records

Human resources records are often consulted to ensure that qualified individuals are notified, in person, of vacant positions. An examination of employee files, including résumés and application forms, may uncover: employees who are working in jobs below their education or skill levels; people who already have the requisite KSAs; or persons with the potential to move into the vacant position if given some additional training.

THE HIGH PERFORMANCE ORGANIZATION

Effective Job Posting Enhances Commitment, Retention and Recruitment

Recognizing the critical link between employee development and ability to qualify for transfers and promotions, LGS—an international IT consulting firm—launched the Career Managers program to enhance the firm's promote-from-within policy. The program's sole focus is to support employees' career aspirations and provide them with client assignments and training that will support their desired career path. Since the introduction of Career Managers, voluntary turnover has dropped from 25 percent to 12 percent. Linking job posting and career development has not only enhanced commitment and retention; it has also given the firm an edge in recruitment. In fact, because of the firm's focus on career growth, people have declined multiple other job offers in order to join LGS—something that is not surprising given the aspirations and values of workers today (described in Chapter 1).

Source: Based on Sue Nador, "Breaking Down Retention Barriers by Building Up Internal Opportunities," *Canadian HR Reporter* 12, no. 9 (May 3, 1999), p. 11.

FIGURE 6.3 One Firm's Job Posting Policy

ELIGIBILITY

- All permanent employees who have completed their probationary period are eligible to use the open position listing policy in order to request consideration for a position that would constitute a growth opportunity.
- Employees who have been promoted or transferred, or who have changed jobs for any reason, must wait a six-month period before applying for a different position.

POLICY

- A list of open positions will be communicated to all employees in all facilities. Notices will include information on job title, salary grade, department, supervisor's name and title, location, brief description of the job content, qualifications, and instructions concerning whether or not candidates will be expected to demonstrate their skills during the interview process.
- Basic job qualifications and experience needed to fill the job will be listed on the sheet. Employees should consult with the human resources department if there are questions concerning the promotional opportunities associated with the job.
- Open position lists will remain on bulletin boards for five working days.
- Forms for use in requesting consideration for an open position may be obtained from the human resources department.
- The human resources department will review requests to substantiate the employee's qualifications for the position.
- The hiring manager will review requests for employees inside the company before going outside the company to fill the position.
- It is the responsibility of the employees to notify their managers of their intent to interview for an open position.
- The hiring manager makes the final decision when filling the position; however, the guidelines for filling any open position are based on the employees' ability, qualifications, experience, background, and the skills they possess that will allow them to carry out the job successfully. It is the responsibility of the hiring manager to notify the previous manager of the intent to hire the employee.
- Employees who are aware of a pending opening, and who will be on vacation when the opening occurs, may leave a request with the human resources department for consideration.
- It is the manager's responsibility to ensure that the human resources department has notified all internal applicants that they did or did not get the job before general announcement by the manager of the person who did get the job.
- "Blanket" applications will not be accepted. Employees should apply each time a position they are interested in becomes available.
- Since preselection often occurs, employees should be planning for their career growth by scheduling time with potential managers before posting, to become acquainted with them, and to secure developmental information to be used in acquiring appropriate skills for future consideration.
- There are occasions when jobs will not be listed. Two such examples might be (1) when a job can be filled best by natural progression or is a logical career path for an employee, and (2) when a job is created to provide a development opportunity for a specific high-performance employee.
- In keeping with this policy, managers are encouraged to work with employees in career development in order to assist them in pursuing upward movement in a particular career path or job ladder.

Source: From *Human Resource Director's Handbook,* by Mary F. Cook ©1984. Used by permission of the publisher, Prentice-Hall, Inc., Englewood Cliffs, NJ.

FIGURE 6.4 Advantages and Disadvantages of Job Posting

Advantages

- Provides every qualified employee with a chance for a transfer or promotion
- Reduces the likelihood of special deals and favouritism
- Demonstrates the organization's commitment to career growth and development
- Communicates to employees the organization's policies and guidelines regarding promotions and transfers
- Provides equal opportunity to all qualified employees

Disadvantages

- Unsuccessful job candidates may become demotivated, demoralized, discontented, and unhappy if feedback is not communicated in a timely and sensitive manner
- Tensions may rise if it appears that a qualified internal candidate was passed over for an equally qualified or less qualified external candidate
- The decision about which candidate to select may be more difficult if there are two or more equally qualified candidates

Skills Inventories

Skills inventories, described in Chapter 5, are an even better reference tool. While such inventories may be used instead of job postings, they are more often used as a supplement. Whether computerized or manual, referring to such inventories ensures that qualified internal candidates are identified and considered for transfer or promotion when opportunities arise.

Limitations of Recruiting from Within

It is rarely possible to fill all non-entry-level jobs with current employees. Middle- and upper-level jobs may be vacated unexpectedly, with no internal replacements yet qualified or ready for transfer or promotion; or may require such specialized training and experience that there are no potential internal replacements.

In many firms with a policy of promoting from within, potential external candidates are also considered, to prevent the inbreeding problem described previously. Hiring someone from outside may be preferable in order to acquire the latest knowledge and expertise or gain new ideas and revitalize the department or organization.[12]

RECRUITING OUTSIDE THE ORGANIZATION

Unless there is a work-force reduction, even in firms with a promote-from-within policy, a replacement from outside must eventually be found to fill the job left vacant once all eligible employees have been given the opportunity for transfer and/or promotion. In addition, most entry-level positions must be filled by external candidates. The advantages of external recruitment include:

- generation of a larger pool of qualified candidates, which may have a positive impact on the quality of the selection decision (as will be explained in Chapter 7)

- availability of a more diverse applicant pool, which can assist in meeting employment equity goals and timetables
- acquisition of skills or knowledge not currently available within the organization and/or new ideas and creative problem-solving techniques
- elimination of rivalry and competition caused by employees jockeying for transfers and promotions, which can hinder interpersonal and interdepartmental cooperation
- potential cost savings resulting from hiring individuals who already have the skills, rather than providing extensive training.

Planning External Recruitment

When choosing external recruitment method(s), in addition to the constraints mentioned earlier, there are several factors that should be taken into consideration: the type of job, the relationship between the method chosen and quality of hire, the yield ratio, and the amount of lead time.

Type of Job

The type of job to be filled has a major impact on the recruitment method selected. This fact is clearly illustrated by the results of a comprehensive study of the recruiting practices of 718 Canadian firms, representing diverse sectors, industries, and businesses. Sixty-nine percent of the respondents indicated that they normally rely on professional search firms for recruiting executive-level employees. Fifty-four percent indicated that they relied on such firms for recruiting managers/supervisors, 50 percent for recruiting professional/technical employees, and 41 percent for recruiting other salaried employees. In contrast, local newspaper advertising was rated as very useful for recruiting executives by 40 percent of respondents, for recruiting manager/supervisors by 47 percent, for recruiting professional/technical employees by 48 percent, and for recruiting other salaried employees by 54 percent.[13]

Another recent study highlights the types of jobs for which online recruitment is effective. According to a survey conducted by *CareerMosaic*, the Web is becoming an appropriate recruitment tool for jobs ranging from writer to teacher, nurse, HR professional, and executive. While computer and engineering jobs are still widely sought online, the two most popular searches during the first six months of 1999 were for management and sales positions.[14]

Relationship of Method Chosen and Quality of Hire

Several studies have suggested that the recruitment methods chosen can affect subsequent tenure and job performance.[15] In general, applicants who find employment as walk-ins or through referral by a current employee tend to remain with the organization longer and be higher-quality performers than those recruited through advertising and employment agencies.

Research Insight

Highlights of the results of a study comparing four external recruiting methods follow. The four methods were convention/journal advertising, newspaper advertising, college/university placement offices, and self-initiated walk-ins.

They were assessed in terms of: employee effectiveness, measured by quality of performance and dependability; absenteeism; satisfaction with supervision; and job involvement.[16]

- Quality and dependability. Applicants who made contact based on their own initiative or in response to convention or professional journal advertising were superior to those recruited through educational institution placement offices and newspaper advertising.
- Absenteeism. Those recruited through newspaper ads missed almost twice as many days as did those recruited using any of the other methods.
- Job involvement and satisfaction with supervision. Recruits obtained through college/university placement offices reported significantly lower levels of both job involvement and satisfaction with supervision than did employees recruited in other ways.

As mentioned previously, the results of such research must be weighed against employment equity and cost considerations.

Yield Ratios

yield ratio
The percentage of applicants that proceed to the next stage of the selection process.

Yield ratios help to indicate which recruitment methods are the most effective at producing qualified job candidates. A **yield ratio** is the percentage of applicants that proceed to the next stage of the selection process.

A recruiting yield pyramid, such as that shown in **Figure 6.5**, can be devised for each method, by calculating the yield ratio for each step in the selection process. The firm in this example typically hires 50 entry-level accountants each year through on-campus recruitment at colleges and universities. The firm has calculated that using this method leads to a ratio of offers made to actual new hires of two to one (about half of the candidates to whom offers are made accept). The firm also knows that the ratio of candidates interviewed to offers made is three to two, while the ratio of candidates invited for interviews to candidates actually interviewed is generally four to three. Finally, the firm knows that the ratio between leads generated and candidates selected for interviews is six to one. In other words, of six leads generated through college/university recruiting efforts, one applicant is invited to attend an interview. Given these ratios, the firm knows that, using this particular recruitment method, 1200 leads must be generated in order to hire 50 new accountants.

FIGURE 6.5 Recruiting Yield Pyramid

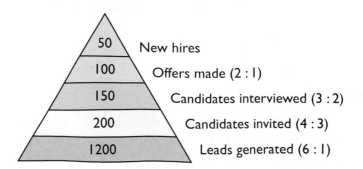

By calculating and comparing yield pyramids for each recruiting method, it is possible to determine which method results in the most new hires for each type of job.

Amount of Lead Time

time-lapse data

The average number of days from when the company initiates a recruitment method to when the successful candidate begins work.

The average number of days from when the company initiates a recruitment method to when the successful candidate begins to work is called time-lapse data. Similar to yield ratios, data should be collected for each step in the process.

Let's assume that the accounting company in the above example found the following: six days elapsed between submission of application forms and résumés to invitation for an interview; five days then passed from invitation to actual interview; five days from interview to job offer; six days from job offer to acceptance; and 23 days from acceptance of job offer to commencement of work. These data indicate that, using on-campus recruiting, the firm must initiate recruitment efforts at least 45 days prior to the anticipated job opening date.

Calculating time-lapse data for each recruitment method means that the amount of lead time available can be taken into account when deciding which strategy or strategies would be most appropriate.

External Recruitment Methods

Walk-ins and Write-ins

Individuals who go to organizations in person to apply for jobs without referral or invitation are called walk-ins. Relying on walk-ins is a popular and inexpensive recruitment method used primarily for entry-level and unskilled positions. When walk-ins drop off a résumé, they are often asked to complete an application form. These applications and résumés are then screened, and those considered suitable are kept on file for a period of three to six months and reviewed when a relevant vacancy arises for which external candidates are being considered.

People who submit unsolicited résumés to organizations via mail, e-mail, Web, or fax are known as write-ins. Relying on unsolicited résumés is a valuable and inexpensive recruitment method used primarily for managerial, clerical, professional, sales, and technical positions. In many firms, there is a practice of acknowledging the interest of write-in applicants by sending a brief thank-you note. The résumés of write-ins are generally screened by a member of the HR department. If an applicant is considered suitable, his or her résumé is retained on file for a period of three to six months or passed on to the relevant department manager if there is an immediate or upcoming opening for which he or she is qualified.

Some organizations are using computer databases to store the information found on the résumés and application forms of walk-in and write-in candidates. Whether the original document is paper-based or submitted via e-mail, Web, or fax, it can be scanned and stored on databases for fast, easy access using a few key words.[17]

Employee Referrals

Some organizations encourage applications from friends and relatives of current employees by mounting an employee referral campaign. Openings are announced in the company's newsletter or posted on a bulletin board or the intranet, along with a request for referrals. Cash awards or prizes may be offered for referrals that culminate in a new hire. At Nortel Networks, for example, at which 48 percent of new hires are the result of internal referrals, any employee whose referral is hired receives U.S. $2000.[18] Platform Computing Corp. is another organization committed to this recruitment method. A workload-management software firm, which grew from 10 employees in 1994 to more than 200 in 1999, Platform Computing pays employees a $1000 bonus for every referral hired. The results are amazing: 113 of the current employees were hired through the referral program.[19] Because there are no advertising or agency fees involved, paying bonuses such as these still represents a low recruiting cost. Other advantages include: the fact that employees with hard-to-find job skills may know others in their field; the recruits obtained tend to have a positive, yet realistic impression of the organization; and the candidates referred are of high quality (since employees are generally willing to refer only those in whom they have great confidence). It should be noted, however, that the success of such programs depends largely on the morale of employees.[20]

Employee referral programs are quite popular. Forty percent of the firms responding to one survey said they use some sort of employee referral system and hire about 15 percent of their employees in this manner. The use of cash awards (the amount of which varied with company size) for referring candidates who are hired was listed as the most common type of referral incentive. The cost per hire was uniformly low—far below the cost of an employment agency.[21]

Disadvantages associated with employee referrals include the potential of inbreeding and nepotism to cause morale problems, and dissatisfaction of employees whose referral is not hired. Perhaps the biggest drawback, however, is that this method may result in systemic discrimination in workplaces that are not diverse, since employees tend to recommend individuals who have backgrounds similar to their own in terms of race, ethnicity, religion, and so on. To avoid this potential problem, employers using referral programs should: adopt an employment equity policy; educate their employees about the purpose, importance, and value of diversity; and highlight the organization's commitment to equity in all of their job postings and referral requests.

nepotism
A preference for hiring relatives of current employees.

Educational Institutions

Recruiting at educational institutions is extremely effective when candidates require formal training but relatively little full-time work experience. High schools can provide recruits for clerical and blue-collar jobs. Universities and colleges can supply qualified applicants for positions ranging from police officer to management trainee.

Most Canadian universities and community colleges have placement centres. Organizations provide such centres with information about their job openings, which is then posted. When students see postings in which they are interested, they submit an application form and résumé to the placement centre on or before the closing date specified. The centre staff typically does not do any pre-screening; centre staff members simply submit to the employer a single package containing all applications received. The employer then selects those applicants who appear to best fit the job specifications and arranges with the centre to conduct interviews with those individuals on campus.

Each year, many companies throughout Canada visit selected educational institutions to conduct on-campus recruitment activities. Since such activities can be time-consuming and expensive, the number of universities or colleges at which each recruits tends to be limited. In a recent survey of more than 200 Canadian firms, 61 percent of the respondents planning to recruit business graduates in 2000 indicated that they would focus on no more than three colleges or universities. Twenty-one percent stated they would recruit at four to six schools. Only eight percent of respondents indicated that they conduct an international search for such graduates. Forty-five percent stated that they search nationally, and 47 percent indicated that they limit the scope of their search to the region in which they are situated.[22]

Most high schools, colleges, and universities have counselling centres that provide job-search assistance to students through activities such as skills assessment testing and workshops on résumé preparation and interview strategies. Sometimes they arrange for on-site job fairs, at which employers set up displays outlining the types of job opportunities available. The largest such job fair in Canada is held at Wilfrid Laurier University each February. Bringing together the three post-secondary institutions in Kitchener–Waterloo (University of Waterloo, Wilfrid Laurier University, and Conestoga College) and the University of Guelph, the fair attracts 175 to 200 companies and 2500 to 3000 students.[23]

Cooperative education (co-op) and field placement programs have become increasingly popular in Canada. These programs require students to spend a specified period of time working in organizations as an integral part of their academic program, thereby gaining some hands-on skills in an actual work setting. Co-op programs are now offered in some high schools, as well as in colleges and universities. Woodstock General Hospital (in Woodstock, Ontario) has for more than 15 years provided co-op opportunities in departments ranging from Physiotherapy to Medical Records for students from Fanshawe College, Huron Park Secondary School, and Woodstock Collegiate Institute. Nortel Networks hires more than 3000 North American university co-op students each year. Placement sites vary, but most Canadian co-op students work in Ottawa, Toronto, Calgary, or Montreal.[24]

Summer internship programs are part of the recruitment strategy at organizations such as Celestica in Toronto and Shell Canada in Calgary. College and/or university students are hired to complete summer projects between their second-last and final year of study. Their performance is assessed, and those who are judged to be superior are offered permanent positions following graduation.

Other firms, such as the Ministry of Natural Resources in Peterborough, Ontario, offer internship opportunities to graduates, thereby enabling them to acquire hands-on skills to supplement their education. As with student internships, outstanding performers are often offered full-time employment at the end of the program. It is now possible for firms to recruit graduate interns online through Career Edge, described in the Information Technology and HR box.

Internship, co-op, and field placement programs can produce a win–win result. The employer is provided with an excellent opportunity to assess the skills and abilities of a potential employee, without incurring any significant costs, while benefiting from the current knowledge and enthusiasm of bright, talented individuals. Because co-op and field placement students and student/graduate interns have been exposed to the organization and its expectations, they are, if hired, less likely to leave shortly after hire than recruits with no previous exposure to the firm.[25] Recognizing these benefits has made such programs a major recruitment method in many organizations. Most of the col-

Campus WorkLink (The National
Graduate Register)

ngr.schoolnet.ca

INFORMATION TECHNOLOGY AND HR

Finding Interns Online

Career Edge is a national, nonprofit, private-sector organization committed to helping university, college, and high-school graduates gain essential career-related experience through internships. The aim is to help overcome the youth unemployment/underemployment problem: there are currently more than 600 000 graduates in Canada who are unemployed or underemployed, and the youth unemployment rate is just over 12 percent—almost double that of adults. Recognizing the existence of such trends, a group of more than 70 of Canada's largest companies launched Career Edge in October of 1996. Charter members include the Toronto-Dominion Bank, The Boston Consulting Group of Canada Limited, Noranda Inc., PanCanadian Petroleum Limited, Nortel and Bell Canada.

Career Edge uses the Internet as its sole means of bringing companies and youth together. Interested organizations register with Career Edge and, once approved, are invited to provide information about their internship positions on the Career Edge Web site. Prospective interns visit the site, view available positions, and apply directly to the company. Host organization staff then reviews the applications and selects the intern(s).

Interns become employees of Career Edge. Host organizations pay $18 500 ($18 900 in British Columbia, Manitoba and Quebec), plus applicable taxes, of which $16 200 goes to the intern and the balance to payroll taxes, medicare and workers' compensation, and administrative costs. No government funding is involved.

Host organizations provide on-the-job training, coaching from an experienced employee, and networking opportunities. By completing a six-, nine-, or twelve-month paid internship, participating graduates gain the skills and experience they need to become more marketable. Host organizations benefit by gaining fresh ideas from bright, committed graduates. The program is definitely a success. As of August 2000, 4493 interns had been placed and there were 269 participating organizations.

Source: Career Edge, "About Our Program, Career Edge Potential Hosts—The Private Sector Response, Career Edge Potential Hosts—The Youth Unemployment Problem, and Career Edge Potential Hosts—How the Program Works," Career Edge Web Site: www.careeredge.org, extracted August 23, 2000.

Career Edge
www.careeredge.org

lege and university graduates who end up working at Nortel, for example, have done previous internships or co-op work terms. In fact, Nortel is Canada's largest employer of co-op students and student interns, welcoming about 2000 each year.[26] Another organization that is sold on graduate internship programs is Deltaware Systems of Charlottetown, P.E.I., which participated in the Software Human Resource Council's (SHRC's) national youth software internship program for small to medium-sized companies (up to 200 employees) in the IT industry in 1999, and subsequently hired intern Lisa Bruce on a full-time basis.[27]

Funding university chairs is an additional industry/educational institution cooperative venture, which supplements traditional recruitment methods. Dofasco Inc. of Hamilton, Ontario funds chairs in advanced steel processing at the University of British Columbia (UBC) and at McMaster University in Hamilton. Angiotech Pharmaceuticals Inc. of Vancouver sponsors a chair at UBC's Faculty of Pharmaceutical Sciences, as well as academic laboratories at other universities. Although funding chairs is very costly, both firms believe that the expense is quite justified, since the chairs act as a breeding ground for future employees.[28] According to William Hunter, chair and CEO at Angiotech, "Grad students working on these projects learn the field that's the core part of our business, and then when they graduate we're one of the most obvious choices to work for." The familiarization process works both ways. He adds, "Invariably they've worked with myself or our chief scientific officer, and if you've worked with a person for three years while they're doing their Ph.D. you have a pretty good idea of how they think and their potential."[29]

Human Resources Development Canada (HRDC)

HRDC fulfills its mission, which is to enable Canadians to participate fully in the workplace and the community, through four types of programs: Employment Insurance income benefits, human resources investment, income security, and labour. These programs are delivered by a network of more than 300 Human Resource Centres across the country, call centres, kiosks, and Web sites.

Through its various human resources investment programs, HRDC helps unemployed individuals to find suitable jobs and employers to locate qualified candidates to meet their needs. There is no cost to either party. Employers can call and place job postings with HRDC, which are then accessed by job seekers via telephone, using the Employment Telemessage system, or online. In addition, HRDC now operates the Electronic Labour Exchange (ELE). This computer-based system matches employer job specifications with job-seeker profiles.

While used primarily to obtain blue-collar, unskilled, and clerical employees, because there is a National Job Bank that provides a Canada-wide listing of job orders, HRDC can sometimes help employers locate highly skilled workers who happen to be living in an area of high unemployment and are willing to relocate.

HRDC also manages the Employment Insurance program, and offers a variety of other services ranging from providing labour market information to assisting individuals with their job search. For example, in addition to the "Taking Charge Self-Help Series," which deals with topics ranging from job hunt preparation to starting a successful business, job seekers can access Work Search, an interactive site designed to guide users through all aspects of the work search process. Other HRDC programs include learning and literacy, special youth initiatives such as a youth resource network, a student summer program, and an Aboriginal youth network.[30] HRDC also funds numerous jobsMARKETS and jobsMARKETS for Persons With Disabilities across the country, which are free events designed to enable employers and job seekers to interact.[31] If job seekers require additional training and/or upgrading to help match their skills with available jobs, HRDC provides assistance ranging from subsidizing wages and training costs for on-the-job training to paying tuition fees and providing income assistance to those attending a community college.

Another fairly recent initiative of HRDC is ON-SITE, a program through which qualified professionals are provided to firms across Canada for periods of up to six months. Professionals are available in a number of fields, including quality management, export development, IT, occupational health and safety, and environmental or energy management. There is no obligation to hire, and while the operating costs of ON-SITE are covered by the participating employers ($2600 per placement), the wages of the ON-SITE workers are paid through

Electronic Labour Exchange
www.ele-spe.org

National Job Bank
www.jb-ge.hrdc-drhc.gc.ca/
index.html

Work Search
www.worksearch.gc.ca
The JobsMARKETS
www.jobsmarket.org

HRDC and provincial labour market development agreements. As of August 2000, more than 4000 firms across the country had utilized the program to increase their productivity and competitiveness.[32]

Private Employment Agencies

Private employment agencies, which are quite widespread throughout Canada, are often called upon to provide assistance to employers seeking intermediate- to senior-level clerical staff, and professional, technical or managerial employees. Such agencies take an employer's request for recruits and then solicit job seekers, relying primarily on advertising and walk-ins/write-ins. They serve two basic functions: expanding the applicant pool and performing preliminary interviewing and screening. To match the employer's job specifications with the abilities and interests of potential applicants, agencies may perform a range of functions, including: advertising; testing for skills, aptitudes, and interests; interviewing; and reference checking.[33] It should be noted, though, that the amount of service provided varies widely, as does the level of professionalism and the calibre of staff. While most agencies carefully screen applicants, some simply provide a stream of applicants and let the client's HR department staff do the screening. Where agency staff are paid on a commission basis, their desire to earn a commission may occasionally compromise their professionalism, and they may encourage job seekers to accept jobs for which they are neither qualified nor suited.

Generally, it is the employer who pays the agency fee. In many jurisdictions, it is illegal for private employment agencies to charge jobseekers a fee; in others permissible fees are regulated. It is common for employers to be charged a fee equal to 15 to 30 percent of the first year's salary of the individual hired through agency referral. This percentage may vary depending on the type of employee being recruited or the volume of the business generated by the client.

There are reasons for firms to use an employment agency to handle some or all of their recruiting needs. Specific situations in which an agency might be used include the following:

- the organization does not have an HR department and/or has no one with the requisite time and/or expertise
- the firm has experienced difficulty in generating a pool of qualified candidates for the position or a similar type of position in the past
- a particular opening must be filled quickly
- there is a desire to recruit a greater number of designated group members than the firm has been able to attract on its own
- the recruitment effort is aimed at reaching individuals who are currently employed and might therefore feel more comfortable answering ads placed by and dealing with an employment agency.

There are many advantages to using a professionally operated private employment agency.[34] The agency can: save the organization a great deal of time by finding, interviewing, and selecting qualified candidates for referral to the hiring manager; cut down on the number of people for the employer to interview; and help to ensure that only candidates matching the job specifications are interviewed. Agencies failing to do a proper screening job or violating human rights legislative standards earn a bad reputation among HR professionals and rapidly lose credibility.

To ensure that the agency–employer relationship is positive and to avoid any legal compliance problems, references provided by the agency should be contacted to confirm suitability and professionalism. In addition, it is recommended that organizations do the following:[35]

1. Give the agency an accurate and complete job description. The better the agency understands the job(s) to be filled, the greater the likelihood that a reasonable pool of qualified applicants will be generated.

2. Specify the tools or devices that the agency should use to screen applicants on the firm's behalf. At the very least, find out what devices the agency uses for applicant screening and ensure that they meet the firm's standards and expectations.

3. If possible, periodically review data on accepted and rejected candidates. This will serve as a check on the agency's processes and practices.

4. If feasible, develop a long-term relationship with one or two agencies. It may also be advantageous to designate one person in the HR department to serve as the liaison between the firm and agency and/or to have a specific contact at the agency coordinating the firm's recruiting needs.

Executive Search Firms

Employers retain executive search firms to seek out middle- to senior-level professional, technical, and managerial employees. Paid a fee by the employer, executive search firms are typically used to fill jobs for which the pay range exceeds $40 000 or $50 000. While the percentage of a firm's positions filled by such firms is generally small, they typically include the most critical positions. For executive positions, using a search firm may be the firm's only recruitment method.

Such firms can be very useful. They often specialize in a particular type of talent, such as executives, sales, technical, scientific or middle-management employees. They typically know and understand the marketplace, have many contacts, and are especially adept at contacting qualified candidates who are employed and not actively looking to change jobs (which is why they have been given the nickname "headhunters"). To broaden their candidate pools, the world's three largest headhunters have now set up online recruiting Web sites catering to middle-management-level employees. Smaller headhunting firms are following suit.[36] Executive search firms can keep their client organization's name confidential until late in the search process and save considerable top-management time by looking after advertising, pre-screening of what could turn out to be hundreds of applicants, and doing careful reference checking. Search firms' fees range from 25 to 50 percent of the annual salary for the position, and are often payable even if the employer terminates the search for any reason. Generally, one-third of the fee is payable as a retainer at the outset. Compared to the value of the time savings realized by the client firm's executive team, however, such a fee often turns out to be insignificant.

There are some potential pitfalls to using this recruitment method. Executive search firms cannot do an effective job if they are given inaccurate or incomplete information about the job and/or the firm. It is therefore essential for employers to explain in detail the type of candidate required—and why. A few head-

AN ETHICAL DILEMMA

Is it ethical for HR professionals to engage in "headhunting" activities themselves, rather than relying on executive search firms to do so?

hunters are more salespeople than professionals, and are more interested in persuading the employer to hire a candidate than in finding one who really meets the job specifications. Some firms have also been known to present an unpromising candidate to a client simply to make their one or two other prospects look that much better.

Some helpful hints for small-business owners considering using an executive search firm are provided in the Small Business Applications box.

Small Business Applications

Using Executive Search Firms—When and Why?

There comes a time in the life of most small businesses when it dawns on the owner that his or her managers are not capable of taking the company into the realm of expanded sales or innovative services. A decision must then be made regarding what kinds of people to hire from outside and how this hiring should take place. Should the owner decide what type of person to hire and recruit this person himself or herself, or should an outside expert be brought in to help with the search?

The heads of most large firms often don't think twice about hiring executive search firms. However, owners of small firms may hesitate before committing to a fee that could reach $20 000 to $30 000 for a $60 000 to $70 000 marketing manager. Such hesitation may be short-sighted when the options are actually reviewed.

Engaging in an executive search is not at all like looking for secretaries, supervisors, or data-entry clerks. Recruiting lower-level employees can usually be accomplished easily by contacting the local Human Resource Centre, placing ads, using relatively low-cost employment agencies, or even by placing a "help wanted" sign in the front window. However, when seeking a key executive to help run the firm, the chances are high that this person won't be found by placing ads or using most of the other traditional methods. For one thing, the person being sought is probably already employed and is not reading the want ads. Even if a potential candidate does happen to glance at the ads, unless he or she is extremely unhappy at present, there is little likelihood that the ad will spark the effort to embark on a job search.

In other words, there is a danger of ending up with lots of résumés from people who are, for one reason or another, out of work or unhappy with their work, and would also be unsuited to the job. It then falls to the small-business owner to try to find several gems among these résumés, and then to interview and assess the most promising applicants. This is hardly an attractive proposition, unless the owner happens to be an expert at interviewing and reference checking (and has little else to do).

Thus, there are two potential problems small-business owners may encounter when conducting an executive search without assistance. First, as a non-expert, the individual concerned may not even know where to begin: how to write a suitable ad, where to place an ad, where to search, whom to contact, how to screen out those who appear to be good on paper but are actually unsuitable candidates, or how to perform adequate reference checking. Second, to be done effectively, the process is generally extremely time-consuming and may divert attention from more important duties. Many business owners find that when they consider the opportunity costs involved with doing their own searches, they are not saving any money at all. For example, the time spent may cost enough in terms of lost sales calls that the company actually comes out behind financially. Often, the question is not whether the small-business owner can afford to use an executive search firm, but whether he or she can afford not to.

Advertising

Advertising is one of the most often-used recruiting methods. While commonly used media range from television and radio to professional journals, the advantages and disadvantages of which are shown in **Table 6.1**, newspaper advertising seems to be the most popular.[37]

For advertising to bring the desired results, two issues must be addressed: the media to be used, and the construction of the ad.[38] The selection of the best medium—whether it is the local newspaper, a national newspaper, or a technical journal—depends on the types of positions for which the organization is recruiting. Reaching individuals who are already employed and not actively seeking alternative employment requires a different medium than is appropriate to attract those who are unemployed.

To achieve optimum results from an advertisement, the following four-point guide, called *AIDA*, should be kept in mind as the ad is being constructed:

1. The ad should attract *attention*. The ads that stand out have borders, a company logo or picture, and effective use of empty white space. To attract attention, key positions should be advertised in display ads, not lost in the columns of classified ads.

2. The ad should develop *interest* in the job. Interest can be created by the nature of the job itself, by pointing out the range of duties and/or the amount of challenge or responsibility involved. Sometimes other aspects of the job, such as its location or working conditions, are useful in attracting interest. To ensure that the individuals attracted are qualified, the job specifications should always be included.

3. The ad should create a *desire* for the job. This may be done by capitalizing on the interesting aspects of the job itself and by pointing out any unique benefits or opportunities associated with it, such as the opportunity for career development or travel. Desire may also be created by stressing the employer's commitment to employment equity. The target audience should be kept in mind as the ad is being created.

4. The ad should instigate *action*. To prompt action, ads often include a closing date and a statement such as "Call today," "Send your résumé today by fax or e-mail," "Check out our Web site for more information," or "Go to the site of our next job fair."

If properly constructed, advertisements can be an effective instrument for recruiting, as well as for communicating the organization's corporate image to the general public. A newspaper ad incorporating the AIDA guidelines is shown in **Figure 6.6**.

TABLE 6.1

Advantages and Disadvantages of Some Major Types of Media

TYPE OF MEDIUM	ADVANTAGES	DISADVANTAGES	WHEN TO USE
Newspapers	Short deadlines. Ad size flexibility. Circulation concentrated in specific geographic area. Classified sections well organized for easy access by active job seekers.	Easy for prospects to ignore. Considerable competitive clutter. Circulation not specialized— a great number of unwanted readers must be paid for. Poor printing quality.	When it is desirable to limit recruiting to a specific area. When sufficient numbers of prospects are clustered in a specific area. When enough prospects are reading help wanted ads to fill hiring needs.
Magazines	Specialized magazines reach pin-pointed occupation categories. Ad size flexibility. High-quality printing. Prestigious editorial environment. Long life— prospects keep magazines and reread them.	Wide geographic circulation— usually cannot be used to limit recruiting to specific area. Long lead-time for ad placement.	When job is specialized. When time and geographic limitations are not of utmost importance. When involved in ongoing recruiting programs.
Radio and television	Difficult to ignore. Can reach prospects who are not actively looking for a job better than newspapers and magazines. Can be limited to specific geographic areas. Creatively flexible. Can dramatize employment story more effectively than printed ads. Little competitive recruitment clutter.	Only brief, uncomplicated messages are possible. Lack of permanence; prospect cannot refer back to it. (Repeated airings necessary to make impression.) Creation and production of commercials—particularly TV—can be time-consuming and costly. Lack of special-interest selectivity; paying for waste circulation.	In competitive situations when not enough prospects are reading printed ads. When there are are multiple job openings and there are enough prospects in specific geographic area. When a large impact is needed quickly. A "blitz" campaign can saturate an area in two weeks or less. Useful to call attention to printed ads.
"Point-of-purchase" (promotional materials at recruiting location)	Calls attention to employ- ment story at a time when prospects can take some type of immediate action. Creative flexibility.	Limited usefulness; prospects must visit a recruiting loca- tion before it can be effective.	Posters, banners, brochures, audiovisual presentations at special events such as job fairs, open houses, conventions, as part of an employee referral program, at placement offices, or whenever prospects visit organization facilities.

Source: Adapted from Bernard S. Hodes, "Planning for Recruitment Advertising: Part II," *Personnel Journal* 28, no. 5 (June 1983), p. 499. Reprinted with the permission of *Personnel Journal*, Costa Mesa, CA. All rights reserved.

want ad

A recruitment ad describing the job and its specifications, the compen- sation package, and the hiring employer. The address to which applications and/or résumés should be submitted is also provided.

blind ad

A recruitment ad in which the identity and address of the employ- er are omitted.

There are two general types of newspaper advertisements: want ads and blind ads. Want ads describe the job and its specifications, the compensation package, and the hiring employer. They also provide the address(es) to which applications and/or résumés should be submitted, often including an e-mail address and/or fax number. While the content pertaining to the job, specifications, and compensation is identical in blind ads, such ads omit the identity and address of the hiring employer. Potential candidates are instructed to forward their responses to a post office box number or a newspaper box number. While many job seekers do not like responding to blind ads, since there is always the danger of unknowingly sending a résumé to the firm at which they are currently employed, such ads do have some advantages. The opening can remain confidential (which may be necessary if the position is still staffed), telephone

FIGURE 6.6 Newspaper Recruitment Advertisement, Demonstrating AIDA Principles

You and our customers—our most valued assets!

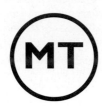

Do you have an interest in a career in banking and excellent oral communication and interpersonal skills?

If so, a front-line position in our progressive organization may provide the opportunity you are seeking to get your career on track!

Customer Service Representatives

We are recruiting individuals with a High School Diploma or an equivalent combination of education and experience, who have some background in mathematics/accounting and data entry keyboarding skills, to provide courteous, prompt, efficient customer service in order to achieve a high level of customer satisfaction. Other responsibilities include identifying, resolving or referring customer banking and account maintenance needs to appropriate trained personnel; carefully handling and balancing cash and related on-line computer entries, in accordance with established Bank Security procedures; and facilitating branch work flow by assisting others.

Although the job involves a moderate amount of discretion and complexity and the consequences of errors can be serious, NO PRIOR EXPERIENCE IS NECESSARY. In-house training will be provided.

If are have the qualifications specified above and are seeking a position that involves key customer service responsibilities and leads to various career opportunities in a bank that is committed to promotion from within, please apply in writing by March 05, 2001, citing **Competition #03/01**, to: **Human Resources Manager, Municipal Trust, 1015 14th Street N.W., Calgary, Alberta T2M 3N3. Fax: (403) 282-8367**

No agencies or telephone calls, please.
We thank all applicants; however only those selected for an interview will be contacted.

Visit our Web site at: www.municipaltrust.ca

Municipal Trust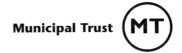

Dedicated to Employment Equity.
Qualified designated group members are encouraged to apply.

inquiries are eliminated, and it is possible to avoid some of the public relations problems associated with unsuccessful applicants.

Many factors make advertising a useful recruiting method. Employers can use advertisements to reach and attract potential job applicants from a diverse labour market in as wide or narrow a geographical area as desired. In order to meet employment equity goals and timetables, ads can be placed in publications read by designated group members, such as a minority-language newspaper or the newsletter of a nonprofit agency assisting individuals who have a particular mental or physical disability. As explained in the High Performance

THE HIGH PERFORMANCE ORGANIZATION

Innovative Recruitment Advertising

In 1999, UUNET, an Internet provider, demonstrated the benefits that can be reaped from a unique and aggressive recruitment advertising campaign. Recognizing that employees are the firm's strongest selling point, UUNET developed a recruitment initiative using its own staff members to attract more great people. First, a marketing campaign was launched using a series of six posters featuring close-ups of UUNET employees from its offices across Canada. These appeared at more than 135 locations across Toronto. The campaign ran for two weeks in June of 1999, and then again for four weeks in the fall. The first set of posters described the relationship between the employees' outside interests and the qualities they bring to their jobs. For example, "Nancy Worth, Systems Administrator, sailor, world traveler ...." The second set, slightly more crisply designed, hit the streets on a larger scale. The goal was to reach potential employees at the grassroots level, and at a fraction of the cost of conventional advertising.

To continue the momentum created by the posters, the company launched a relatively inexpensive aerial campaign. On a Tuesday, Thursday and Saturday in late September/early October, an airplane circled the city for two hours trailing a banner that read "COOLJOBS @ WWW.UUNET.CA."

As a result of this campaign combined with traditional recruitment activities, UUNET hired more than 60 people for its corporate headquarters in Toronto during the fourth quarter of 1999. During this same quarter, turnover was very low—averaging just two percent. The company's creative advertising campaign, which was outsourced to The Farm (a Toronto-based communication design agency), cut its recruitment costs by about 80 percent. Typically, a campaign culminating in 60 new hires, using newspaper ads and recruiters, costs a firm about $125 000. The campaign at UUNET achieved the same results for only $25 000.

Source: Susan Pahl, "Creativity Key to Attracting High-Tech Professionals," *Guide to Recruitment and Staffing, Supplement to Canadian HR Reporter* 13, no. 3 (February 14, 2000), p. G6.

Organization box, being creative and innovative in choice of media and ad construction can increase the effectiveness of a recruitment campaign.

Professional and Trade Associations

Professional and trade associations can be extremely helpful when recruiters are seeking individuals with specialized skills in fields such as IT, engineering, HR, and accounting, particularly if experience is a job requirement. Many such associations conduct ongoing placement activities on behalf of their members, and most regularly send all of their members newsletters or magazines in which organizations can place job advertisements. Such advertising may attract individuals who hadn't previously thought about changing jobs, as well as those actively seeking employment. Some professional associations have expanded the types of job search assistance provided. HRPAO, for example, now has an employment referral service called The Hire Authority. Employers can post HR job opportunities of all levels on the HRPAO Web site for a $25 charge and/or request a referral search for positions involving two or more years of experience at a nominal fee, which results in the résumés of qualified applicants being sent to them.[39]

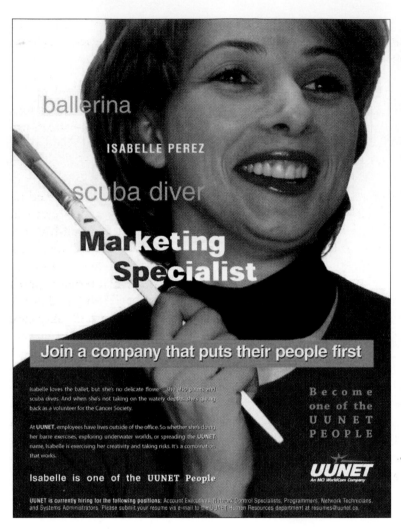

Innovative recruitment campaign at UUNET results in 60 new hires and low turnover.

Labour Organizations

Some firms, particularly in the construction industry, obtain recruits through union hiring halls. The union maintains a roster of members (typically skilled tradespeople such as carpenters, pipe fitters, welders, plumbers, and electricians), whom it sends out on assignment as requests from employers are received. Once the union members have completed their contracted work at one firm, they notify the union of their availability for another assignment.

Military Personnel

The Canadian military may also provide qualified recruits, since individuals leave the forces on a regular basis. Many have been trained in fields in which there tends to be a skills shortage, such as mechanics and pilots; others have received a university or college education, as well as military leadership training, and are potential civilian managerial employees. Thus, military establishments, such as the Royal Military College in Kingston, Ontario, may be an excellent contact for recruiters.

Reservists are also potential recruits. The Canadian Forces Liaison Council (CFLC), formed in 1992, is responsible for promoting the hiring of reservists by civilian employers, the merits of which organizations such as A&P have recognized.[40]

The Council is also trying to encourage civilian employers to give reservists time off for military training without endangering their jobs or seniority. Organizations such as Air Canada—Flight Operations in Montreal, Litton Systems of Canada in Nova Scotia,[41] and Bristol Aerospace in Winnipeg[42] have been sold on the value of such leave. To date, more than 2000 Canadian employers have signed a Statement of Support for the Reserve Force with the CFLC. More than 550 employers have sent CFLC copies of HR policies that provide reservists in their employ with time off to attend military training, and, where necessary, time off to participate in domestic and foreign military operations.[43]

Online Recruiting

Almost half of Fortune Global 500 companies now recruit online. This is a fairly new recruitment method that has caught on in a big way.[44] Online recruiting involves three possible approaches: accessing one or more Internet job boards; purchasing software to install on the company's server (such that the firm's intranet can be used for internal job postings and generating employee referrals and its Web site for external advertising); and renting recruitment software through an Application Service Provider (ASP) for the same purposes.

At Montreal-based Bombardier Aerospace, for example, the Web site doesn't just provide a mechanism for e-mailing a résumé or filling in an application. The pre-screening starts on the spot with a series of click-to-answer questions designed to determine the fit between the applicant and job specifications. Although the questions appear on Bombardier's site, the job advertisements and pre-screening questions actually reside on a server operated by California-based ASP Recruitsoft.com Inc. Bombardier became a charter Recruitsoft subscriber in November of 1999, in part because the HR department staff members could no longer cope with the more than 30 000 résumés per year being received in Montreal alone.[45] E-Cruiter.com Inc. is another firm that offers a full-featured Web-based recruiting solution. ASPs such as Recruitsoft and e-Cruiter.com "rent" recruitment software to clients on a subscription basis. Their Web-based software frees their clients from the demands of managing the internal support structure required by client-server applications. By using such Web-based applications, firms can also remain current with technology, since the ASP takes care of upgrading, while reducing IT costs, since there are no installation or maintenance expenses.[46]

Whether using a Web-based solution or client-server application, using the company's Web site for recruiting has other advantages. It tends to reduce cycle times, particularly if pre-screening is done by e-mail, and is much less costly than print-based advertising. It has been estimated that this e-cruitment strategy can reduce time-to-hire by weeks and save companies at least 30 percent on cost-per-hire. By targeting star candidates and acting immediately, firms can gain competitive advantage.[47]

Research Insight

A recently published study based on a survey of recruiters and technology specialists at 58 Canadian companies using the Internet for recruiting purposes found that 96 percent of them posted openings on their Web site, and approximately half were receiving more than 50 percent of their résumés online, via either e-mail or a résumé builder. Sixty-six percent of the respondents indicated that the Internet generated higher-calibre applicants than other recruitment methods. The majority (74 percent) also reported that hiring over the Internet was faster than traditional means. An overwhelming 82 percent stated that the Internet was cheaper than traditional advertising.[48]

Another advantage of using the firm's Web site for recruitment purposes is that company recruiters at one location can mine the candidate database and share résumés and candidate profiles with hiring managers and/or recruiters at other sites. Most software—whether rented or purchased—enables recruiters to track individual candidates through the recruitment and selection processes and permits candidates to keep their profiles up to date. Using pre-screening strategies is virtually essential, however. As the HR department staff members at Bombardier have discovered, the volume of résumés definitely does not diminish when the firm accepts them online. At Hewlett Packard, for example, more than one million online applications are received each year.[49] Another way of coping with this volume is to generate automatic replies acknowledging receipt of applications. These are an excellent public relations tool, and also help to avoid numerous follow-up e-mails and/or telephone calls.[50]

E-cruitment is one of the fastest growing sectors on the Internet, with predictions of its becoming a $1.7 billion industry by 2003, a growth from $1.5 million in 1998.[51] In fact, online recruitment is becoming so popular that there is now an association of online recruiters in Canada, known as canRecruit! Experts caution, though, that e-cruiting must be an extension of the company's overall marketing strategy, and convey the same image and atmosphere as the organization itself. Recruitment is a two-way street, and having a world-class Web site provides an opportunity to sell the company and jobs to prospective applicants. To be effective, though, such Web sites must be user-friendly.[52]

The Canadian Association of Recruiters Online
www.canRecruit.com

Research Insight

General Job Boards
Acti-Job Canada
www.actijob.com

Canadajobs.com
www.canadajobs.com

Canjobs.com
www.canjobs.com

Careerclick.com
www.careerclick.com

CareerMosaic
www.careermosaic.com

Monster Board Canada
www.monster.ca

Workopolis.com
www.workopolis.com

The Canadian Job Board Comparison
www.careerboards.com

A recent survey of college graduates showed that 94 percent of them had used corporate Web sites to gain information about potential employers, and to screen potential employers online.[53] Other research found that about 80 percent of visitors to job boards check the employer's Web site before applying for job openings.[54]

Based on this research, it is clear that a company's corporate Web site can become even more powerful if used in combination with commercial job boards, the most popular of which reported between 10 000 and 20 000 "hits" per day in early 1999.[55] There are more than 50 job boards in Canada from which to choose: some are general in nature, others are student-oriented, and still others specialize in particular types of postings ranging from acting to health care and physical therapy. With this number and variety, it's nice to know that an online product is available to assist with the selection process (it is highlighted in the Information Technology and HR Box).[56] Another component of a well-rounded e-cruiting strategy is banner advertising, which is designed to drive applicant traffic to the firm's job posting on a commercial board or on the company Web site. Such banner ads are much cheaper than more common forms of advertising. In order to ensure that e-cruiting effectively reaches passive job seekers, it is also recommended that companies register their Web site with various search engines and areas other than employment sites (since the active job seeker surfing the job boards may not be the most qualified for the jobs), and that they post jobs with newsgroups. Potential employees should also be "sourced" by searching for résumés in résumé databases, on personal home pages, and in newsgroups.[57]

With 9.5 million Canadians having Internet access and the résumés of 300 000 Canadians currently online, the Internet provides recruiters with a large audience for job postings and a vast talent pool.[58] Whether using corporate Web sites, e-cruitment service companies or job boards, having a presence on the Web is becoming more necessary if firms want the best talent working for them. E-cruitment does not replace the need for interviews, testing, and thorough reference checking, nor is it the best recruitment method for all types and levels of positions. However, it does provide an excellent supplement to the more traditional recruitment methods, and, as is highlighted in the Small Business Applications box, e-cruiting can benefit firms of all sizes.

Research Insight

According to a recent Forrester Report, recruiters plan to increase the amount spent on online recruiting by 52 percent by 2004, primarily at the expense of print advertising and search firm fees. This research found, however, that the Internet still plays a relatively small role in consumer job searches and is still far less influential than employee referrals or newspaper advertising. Also highlighted in this report is the fact that ~~online recruitment is most popular for technical and administrative jobs~~. Thirty-seven percent of online job seekers are looking for technology-related positions and 21 percent of administrative jobs. Only six percent of those seeking jobs online are interested in executive positions.[59]

Another recent study confirms that recruiters should not abandon the more traditional recruitment methods. Those surveyed reported that their greatest recruitment successes are due to old-fashioned networking and targeted "sourcing." This study also confirmed that the Internet may not be the most appropriate tool for executive searches. Less than one-third of employed executives surveyed said that they think posting their résumé on the Internet is a good idea, mainly because they can't target the specific recipient within a company. Thus, the emergence of e-cruiting has not reduced the time required to fill executive positions. Participating search firms indicated that filling such jobs still takes more than three months on average, and the HR executives surveyed said that it takes longer than that.[60]

INFORMATION TECHNOLOGY AND HR

Selecting an Internet Job Board

Criteria that should be taken into consideration when selecting an appropriate Internet job board for recruitment advertising include: industry, regional focus, the number of visitors to the site each day, the number of résumés connected with the job board, the average length of visit, and the cost per posting. The Canadian Job Board Comparison (www.careerboards.com) is an online service, available on a subscription basis, which can assist with this review process. Revised each month in order to remain current, it acts as an impartial third party in evaluating various Internet services and products. In addition to reviewing the criteria listed above, it also takes into consideration any added features that the board may offer employers, including résumé management, multiple job postings, a link to the company's corporate Web site, and whether or not new résumés will be e-mailed to the firm as they become available. It also compares added features for job seekers, such as anonymity and e-mail notification of new job openings.

Another service provided by The Canadian Job Board Comparison is the Intelligent Advisor. Recruiters can input information regarding desired regional focus and type of job, and the Advisor will reply with tables indicating which boards best meet these criteria. Links to these job boards are offered, including a link to the boards' online pricing information. Thus, checking out the recommended job board(s) is as easy as point-and-click. Intelligent Advisor also verifies the figures provided by the job boards through the boards' log files, and indicates when the board provides log-file access through a banner on the individual job board listings. In this way, the authenticity of the information provided by each board can be verified.

Source: Jennifer Clarke, "Using an Internet Job Board," *Guide to Recruitment and Staffing, Supplement to Canadian HR Reporter* 12, no. 4 (February 22, 1999), p. G7.

SMALL BUSINESS APPLICATIONS

Student Connection Program
www.scp-ebb.com

Online Recruiting

Online recruiting has helped to level the playing field for small businesses competing with large firms for talent. Ninety-one percent of the more than 5000 users surveyed by globecareers.com indicated that the availability of online recruiting sites led job hunters to consider companies that they had never before heard of and/or considered. Thus, given the importance of acquiring top talent, online recruitment is a strategy that small-business owners should seriously consider. Tips for small-business owners planning to recruit online include:

• sell the company, as well as the job

• highlight the ways in which "smaller is better"

• shortlist and screen applicants before arranging for interviews.

Small-business owners wanting to learn more about the ways in which the Internet can aid them with recruitment and many other aspects of business operations may wish to take advantage of the Student Connection Program. Initially an Industry Canada and Youth Employment Strategy program that is now sponsored by the government and five private-sector corporations, it was created to foster youth employment and provide Internet and e-commerce training to those working in small to medium-sized Canadian enterprises. Since 1996, the program has hired and trained 3100 post-secondary students and recent graduates as Student Business Advisors, who have provided on-site customized Internet training and e-commerce services to more than 64 000 businesspeople across Canada.

Sources: "Online Recruiting Boon for Small Business," *HR Professional* 17, no. 1 (February/March 2000), p. 10; and Government of Canada Publication, "Student Connection Program."

Open Houses

An increasingly popular recruitment method involves holding an open house. Common in retail firms looking to staff a new store from the ground up, open houses have also been the choice of high-tech corporations trying to draw out the much-coveted IT worker in an ultratight job market.[61] For example, Nortel hosts an open house several times a year. One event, held in June 1996, days after Nortel unveiled its Ottawa expansion plans, attracted 9000 people and resulted in the hiring of 200 applicants.[62] Similarly, when Canadian Tire hosted its first-ever open house in September of 1997, more than 1000 job seekers were attracted to its conference centre in Toronto:[63]

> Needing to hire for a wide range of positions in finance, IT, marketing, and logistics, the firm invited skilled professionals with a minimum of three years of experience to drop by. While awaiting their turn for an interview with the hiring manager in their area of expertise, applicants spent time watching a corporate video that regaled them with the firm's attributes, examining the annual report, and reading feature articles chronicling the firm's much-publicized turnaround under CEO Stephen Bachand.

The open house was merely one component of Canadian Tire's recruitment strategy; also involved were newspaper and online advertising, and participation in high-tech career fairs. An open house is an ideal recruitment method when a firm has a lot of hiring needs. Additional benefits include increased department manager commitment due to their direct involvement, and the fact that open houses tend to attract more highly qualified candidates than newspaper advertising does.[64]

Information Sessions/Job Fairs

Another recruitment method, particularly popular with high-tech firms, involves hosting information sessions in communities across the country or holding a job fair on-site. At such events, recruiters share information about the organization and job opportunities in an informal, relaxed setting with those attending. Refreshments are generally provided. Top prospects are invited to visit the firm or to return at a later date for a more in-depth assessment. The response is often overwhelming:

> When IBM extended the invitation to IT professionals with at least five years' experience to attend a one-night job fair at the firm's Markham, Ontario headquarters, 5000 people showed up. Given the fact that IBM had specified that 500 jobs paying a salary of $75 000 plus were available immediately, a large turnout was expected—in the neighbourhood of 2000 to 3000. While the larger-than-anticipated response meant that the complimentary food didn't last to the end of the evening, things went very smoothly thanks to the more than 350 IBM staff volunteers on hand to assist. Candidates were greeted as they arrived and shepherded inside, where a senior executive gave a brief presentation every half-hour describing the company, its current state, and the firm's future objectives. Attendees then stopped by the booths of those business units that interested them to learn more about the specifics of that unit and the fit between their KSAs and those required. In addition to having an opportunity to learn about the jobs available and the firm itself, meet some of the senior executives, and talk to potential co-workers, candidates identified as likely prospects based on a brief résumé perusal were pulled aside by the hiring manager for a mini-interview. Since many of the attendees brought résumés for friends, the HR department staff had more than 7000 résumés on hand by the end of the evening. Within 24 hours, 400 high-potential candidates had been selected for further interviews.[65] By mid-August, 500 of those whose résumés were received at the job fair had been interviewed, and more than 100 individuals had received job offers.[66]

Recruiting Non-permanent Staff

Fifty-seven percent of the major companies surveyed recently by The Conference Board of Canada indicated that they had increased their use of contingent workers over the past two years, and most expected to rely even more heavily on them in the future. In these firms, contingent workers are seen as a key to attaining labour flexibility and acquiring special expertise on an as-needed basis.[67] In these firms, recruiters are spending more time seeking temporary (term, seasonal, casual) and contract workers and less time recruiting permanent staff.

According to a Statistics Canada report released in September 1997, the number of Canadians whose main source of income is from contingency jobs has grown to about 11 percent or 1.3 million workers. The stereotype of contingency work being primarily clerical, manual, or service-oriented is simply not true. Twenty-nine percent of non-permanent employees are from professional and technical fields and six percent are managers and administrators.[68]

Temporary Help Agencies

Temporary help agencies, such as Kelly Services and Office Overload, exist in all major cities in Canada. These agencies specialize in providing supplemental workers, rather than recruits. Firms use temporary employees (temps) to fill in for vacationing, sick, or on-leave employees and to handle seasonal work, peak workloads, and special projects for which there are no current employees with time and/or expertise. While the term "temp" tends to bring clerical staff to mind, temps are becoming more and more common in legal work, engineering, computer programming, and other jobs requiring advanced professional training.[69] Intercom Management Resources Group is one of many new firms starting up in response to the increasing need for middle- to senior-level specialists for a specific project or term.[70] Temps are agency employees, and are reassigned to another employer when their services are no longer required.

Temps provide employers with three major benefits:

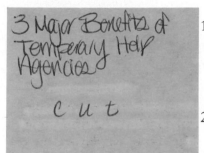

3 Major Benefits of Temporary Help Agencies

cut

1. They cost much less than permanent employees. This relates not only to the fact that temps generally receive less compensation than permanent staff and do not go on the company payroll or benefits plans, but also to savings related to the recruitment, selection, training, and severance costs associated with permanent employees.

2. If a temp performs unsatisfactorily, a substitute can be requested immediately. Generally, a suitable replacement is sent to the firm within one business day.

3. Individuals working as temps who are seeking full-time employment are often highly motivated, knowing that many firms choose full-time employees from the ranks of their top-performing temps. In such case, a fee similar to that charged by a private employment agency is paid to the temporary firm, less the amount already paid while the individual was working as a temp. Since their performance has already been assessed in the actual work setting, hiring temps as permanent employees is a relatively low-risk strategy.

Contract Workers

Contract workers, also known as consultants and freelancers, are employees who develop work relationships directly with the employer for a specific type of work or period of time.[71] Sometimes they are contracted to provide specialized services one or two days a week on a permanent basis. PPL Marketing Services—a mid-sized firm in Mississauga, Ontario with a core staff of some 80 people—uses contract workers on a regular (both project-based and permanent) basis. As projects come and go, so do the writers or production people contracted to complete the jobs. PPL also has a senior HR professional on contract, working two days a week, handling critical issues like hiring, exit interviews, and developing salary structures.[72]

Many professionals with specialized skills become contract workers. Included are marketing and advertising executives, HR professionals, project managers, accountants, writers, and graphic designers,[73] as well as lawyers, physicians, editors, and professors. Some have consciously made a decision to work for themselves; others have been unable to obtain full-time employment in their field of expertise or have found themselves out of a full-time job due to cutbacks. Thus, some wish to remain self-employed; others (such as many adjunct professors at universities and part-time college faculty members) work on a contract basis, hoping to obtain a full-time position eventually. Some firms hire former employees (such as retirees or laid-off workers) on a contract basis. Others learn about potential contract workers through word-of-mouth referrals or advertising or obtain contract employees through agencies.

Because contract workers are not part of the company head count, managers can rely on their services while honouring company staffing restrictions aimed at reducing payroll costs. Contract workers can often be relied upon to be more productive and efficient than in-house employees because they can focus on the task at hand and do not get involved in countless meetings or organizational politics. They can also provide expertise not available in-house or a fresh, outsider's perspective. The major drawback of using contract workers is that their commitment to the employer may be somewhat lower than that of permanent staff, and the demands and deadlines of their multiple clients may conflict at times.

Employee Leasing

employee leasing

An arrangement that typically involves a company transferring specific employees to the payroll of an employee leasing firm or Professional Employer Organization (PEO) in an explicit joint-employment relationship.

Employee leasing is a relatively new concept that permits firms to realize many of the advantages of contract and temporary employees, and to avoid some of the drawbacks associated with these staffing strategies. **Employee leasing arrangements typically involve a company transferring specific employees to the payroll of an employee leasing firm or Professional Employer Organization (PEO) in an explicit joint-employment relationship.** These employees then become employees of the PEO, which leases these individuals back to the client company on a permanent basis. The PEO maintains the HR files for the leased employees, handles the administration of their pay and benefits, and performs most of the other functions normally handled by a firm's HR department staff members. In return, the PEO receives a placement fee—typically five to ten percent of payroll cost.[74]

Not all leasing arrangements are based on the transfer of staff from the client organization to a PEO. Some leasing companies also hire workers themselves and then lease them out to client organizations. For example, Minacs Group, based in Pickering, Ontario, leases employees who perform such functions as data processing and marketing.[75]

Outsourcing/Subcontracting

As explained in Chapter 1, outsourcing or subcontracting is the process by which employers transfer work to another organization specializing in that type of work, which has the ability to perform it more efficiently. Outsourcing agreements may result in a long-term relationship between the employer and subcontractor, although both parties retain the ability to renew or sever the relationship at their convenience.

While data processing, security, cafeteria services, and housekeeping have been outsourced for many years, companies have recently begun to hire subcontractors to provide services that are important to the business but not within its core capabilities, including research and development, marketing research, product design, specific HR functions, and payroll. In 1999, for example, 58 percent of Canadian companies surveyed by Buck Consultants reported outsourcing employee training, 70 percent outsourced some of their benefits functions, and 40 percent outsourced their recruitment efforts.[76] A 1996 Deloitte & Touche study revealed that the thousands of Canadian businesses outsourcing their payroll functions were saving upwards of 50 percent of their payroll costs.[77]

Improving the Effectiveness of External Recruitment

Organization size is the major factor that determines who is responsible for recruitment. In large firms, there may be a number of recruiters on the HR department team. In smaller organizations, recruiting is generally handled by the HR generalist. In firms with no HR position, recruitment is the responsibility of every supervisor and manager.

The structure of the firm also has an impact on who performs the function, however. In organizations emphasizing teamwork, such as 3M's plant in Brockville, Ontario, the team members are responsible for this function.[78]

Regardless of who does the recruiting, it is imperative that those responsible have a good understanding of the job specifications and the organization's philosophy and values. Proper training in recruitment strategies and etiquette is also essential, since recruiters are often the main reason applicants select one organization over another. For example, one study showed that recruiters can have a significant impact on perceived job attractiveness, regard for the job and organization, and intention to accept a job.[79] Thus, choosing personable, enthusiastic, and competent recruiters should improve the effectiveness of an organization's recruitment program.

RECRUITING A MORE DIVERSE WORK FORCE

Recruiting a diverse work force is not just socially responsible, it's a necessity. As noted previously, the composition of Canada's work force is changing dramatically. Trends of particular significance include a decrease in the availability of young workers, a dramatic increase in the average age of employees, and an increase in the number of women, visible minorities, Aboriginal people, and persons with disabilities in the work force. The number of employees in the Sandwich Generation, trying to balance work with child- and eldercare responsibilities, is also increasing. As described in the Diversity Counts box, helping such employees to balance work and family responsibilities makes workplaces more attractive and aids in recruitment and retention.

Attracting Older Workers

Many employers, recognizing the fact that the work force is aging, are encouraging retirement-age employees to stay with the company or are actively recruiting employees who are at or beyond retirement age. There are significant benefits to hiring and retaining older employees. A 1993 study by the American Association of Retired Persons found that older workers have qualities that make them a valuable resource. These include: the highest job satisfaction of any age group; a strong sense of loyalty and organizational commitment; a strong work ethic; good people skills such as patience, empathy, and helpfulness; willingness to work in a variety of roles, including part-time; high potential for successful retraining; and a greater likelihood of staying with the firm.[80]

DIVERSITY COUNTS

Helping Employees Balance Work and Family Makes Workplaces More Attractive

According to one expert, "Top performers consistently say the number-one reason for staying with the company is the ability to balance work and life." He adds, "The danger may not even be in losing current employees, but in losing the ability to recruit new ones."[1]

Based on a Conference Board of Canada report released in June 2000, it seems that many Canadian employers have recognized the validity of these statements. Ninety-three percent of employers surveyed offered at least one type of flexible work arrangement to their employees, and most provide a range of options. Flextime and part-time hours are the most common, although the number providing telecommuting/work-at-home opportunities increased from 11 percent in 1989 to 50 percent in 1999.

However, childcare and other dependant care benefits are still limited. Fewer than half of the employers surveyed have implemented even one program to assist their employees in dealing with dependant care issues. Only slightly more than half offer any childcare benefits. The exception is the financial services industry, which has taken a lead in providing childcare and other dependant care benefits.[2]

An example is the Royal Bank, which provides a combination of access to information (including personal counselling and printed material) and Flexible Work Arrangements (FWAs) to all employees requiring such support. The increasing necessity of programs to assist employees in balancing their work–life responsibilities is highlighted by Royal Bank data: 42 percent of the 1800 employees involved in FWAs in 1998 were doing so for dependant care reasons.[3]

[1] Cited in Michael Miller, "The New Entrant to the Work/Life Balancing Act: Eldercare," *HR Professional* 16, no. 4 (August/September 1999), p. 40

[2] The Conference Board of Canada, "News Release: Employers Are Responding to Employees' Need for Work-Life Balance," The Conference Board of Canada Web site: www.conferenceboard.ca, extracted August 23, 2000.

[3] Miller, "The New Entrant to the Work/Life Balancing Act," pp. 40-1.

Studies have also shown that since older employees are less likely to get work injuries and have lower rates of turnover and absenteeism, their employers benefit from significantly reduced costs.[81]

Recruiting and attracting older workers involves any or all of the methods described earlier, but with one big difference. It generally requires a comprehensive effort before recruiting begins to make the company attractive to older workers. Specifically, organizations should:[82]

- deal with stereotypical attitudes toward older workers as vigorously as any other form of bias, through education and proactive efforts to eliminate discriminatory practices

- check HR policies, procedures, and practices to ensure that they do not discourage recruitment of seniors or encourage valuable older people to leave (for example, promoting early retirement, providing benefits only to full-time employees, and offering no flexibility in benefits or hours of work)

- develop flexible work options such as part-time positions, job sharing, shorter work weeks, consulting jobs, seasonal work, reduced hours with reduced pay, flextime, and phased retirement. At Polaroid Corp. and Aetna Insurance, for example, phased-retirement programs retain talented older workers, decrease burnout, and lower costs by prorating benefits payments over gradually reduced work hours. Many of these flexible work options are inducements that will make the workplace more attractive to a wide range of recruits

- redesign or create jobs. To accommodate older adults experiencing a decrease in dexterity and strength, manufacturing jobs may need to be redesigned, for example. At Xerox, unionized hourly workers over 55 with 15 years of service (and those over 50 with 20 years of service) can bid on jobs at lower stress and lower pay levels if they so desire.[83] In offices, brighter lighting, firm chairs, and ergonomic workstations may be required to lessen physical stress and fatigue

- invest in training, retraining, career development, and reward systems suitable for workers of all ages

- offer flexible benefits plans. Being able to pick and choose among benefits options can be attractive to all employees. Older employees may have different preferences, such as longer vacations or continued accrual of pension credits.

Attracting Younger Employees

As explained in the Diversity Counts box, many firms are recognizing the benefits of a multigenerational work force, and are not only trying to attract older workers, but are taking steps to address the pending shortage of younger employees. A program designed to assist employers in doing so is Experience Canada (EC). It is intended for young people between the ages of 18 and 29 and offers them the opportunity to acquire work experience in their field of study, for a 24-week period, in a Canadian province/territory other than their own. Although there is no obligation to hire the young people placed in jobs through this program, who are paid and insured by EC, firms often choose to do so. An example is the Town of Markham, Ontario. Initially placed in its economic market research department for a six-month term through EC, Patrick Joly was subsequently offered a full-time position and has been promoted to business development officer.[84]

DIVERSITY COUNTS

The Benefits of a Multigenerational Work Force

People of different ages have different skills. While older employees have comparatively wider experience and wisdom, the young bring energy, enthusiasm and physical strength to their positions. According to Robert Barnard, co-author of *Chips and Pop: Decoding the Nexus Generation*, "The really successful organizations are the ones that figure out how to balance the different kinds of experience within the company."[1] Mary Ann Drummond, vice-president of human resources at McDonald's Restaurants of Canada Ltd. (one of the largest employers of youth in the country and an active recruiter of seniors), agrees with Barnard's viewpoint. She feels that it is critical for organizations in the service industry to have employees who mirror their customer base. It has been her experience that each member of their multi-age teams brings a particular strength, which leads to synergy, respect, and team-building.

[1] Cited in Sarah B. Hood, "Generational Diversity in the Workplace," *HR Professional* 17, no. 3 (June/July 2000), p. 20.

Source: Hood, "Generational Diversity in the Workplace," pp. 18-20.

Recruiting Designated Group Members

Many of the prescriptions that apply to recruiting older workers, described earlier, also apply to the recruitment of members of the employment equity-designated groups—women, visible minorities, Aboriginal people, and persons with disabilities. In other words, employers have to formulate comprehensive plans for attracting such candidates, including overcoming stereotypes and biases; reevaluating HR policies and practices; developing flexible work options; redesigning jobs; investing in training, retraining, and career development; and offering flexible benefits.

Most of the recruitment methods discussed previously can be used to attract designated group members, provided that the employer's commitment to equity and diversity is made clear to all involved in the recruitment process—whether it is employees asked for referrals or private employment agencies. This can also be stressed in all recruitment advertising. Alternative publications—ones targeted to the designated groups—should be considered for advertising, and linkages can be formed with organizations and agencies (both for-profit and nonprofit) interested in or specializing in assisting designated group members. Specific examples follow:

- the Canadian Council for Aboriginal Business runs an employment agency called Aboriginal Choice Placement Services for clerical, technical, and engineering positions

- a national Aboriginal Apprenticeship campaign was launched by the Canadian Labour Force Development Board in 1999[85]

- the Bank of Montreal, which is committed to both education and employment equity, has established an $8 million Possibilities Foundation, aimed at visible minority, Aboriginal, and disabled high-school students moving on to post-secondary education. Selected students are eligible for summer employment and a $1000 scholarship. Partners in the program include the Halifax Regional School Board, the National Council of Black Educators of Canada, the Black Educators Association, the Canadian Council on Rehabilitation and Work, and the Micmac Native Friendship Centre.[86]

There are two recent publications (produced by a joint effort of Ontario businesses, community service agencies, and government) aimed at ensuring that persons with disabilities are integrated into the workplace. Both are available through the Centre for Management of Community Services, a nonprofit agency that participated in the project. *Opportunity Knocks* is a how-to guide for community agencies to assist them in convincing employers to hire people with disabilities. *It's a Smart Move* targets the corporate sector, and dispels many of the common myths associated with hiring people with disabilities. These include fears that hiring such employees causes Workers' Compensation premiums to rise and that it's impossible to interview candidates with disabilities without violating human rights legislation. Both publications include case studies of organizations committed to adding persons with disabilities to their work force, such as Canada Trust, McDonald's, CAMI Automotive, Wal-Mart, the Bank of Montreal, and A&P Canada. According to the firms interviewed for the employer profiles, there are many advantages to hiring individuals with disabilities, including:[87]

- access to a broader pool of job candidates

- enhanced corporate image

- a more reliable work force
- lower staff turnover
- a work force better prepared to deal with customers or clients with disabilities
- improved staff morale
- better customer service.

DEVELOPING AND USING APPLICATION FORMS

The Purposes of Application Forms

application form

A form completed by applicants for employment designed to collect information about education, prior work record, and job-related skills in a uniform and standardized manner.

Once the organization has a pool of qualified applicants, the selection process can begin. For most employers, completion of an **application form** is the last step in the recruitment process. An application form provides an efficient means of collecting verifiable historical data from each candidate in a standardized format; it usually includes information about education, prior work history, and other job-related skills.

A completed application form can provide the recruiter with four types of data:[88]

1. Information on substantive matters, such as whether the applicant has the education and experience to do the job.

2. A brief overview of the applicant's career progress and growth, traits that are especially important for management candidates.

3. An indication of the applicant's dependability and stability. (Caution is required when examining work history, though. Numerous job changes may be the result of contract jobs or layoffs at the candidate's previous places of employment, rather than a reflection of his or her lack of commitment and/or ability.)

4. Information that can be used to predict whether or not the candidate will succeed on the job. (As will be explained shortly, not all application forms provide predictor data.)

In practice, most organizations need several application forms. For technical and managerial positions, for example, the form may require detailed information about the applicant's education, previous responsibilities, and so on. The form for factory workers might require much briefer responses to questions about education and work history, focusing instead on the types of equipment and tools the applicant has used.

Reasons for Application Forms

Even when detailed résumés have been submitted, most firms also request that a standardized company application form be completed. There are many reasons for this practice:[89]

- candidate comparison is facilitated because information is collected in a uniform manner
- the information that the company requires is requested; it is not simply left to the candidate to include that which he or she wishes to reveal. By asking

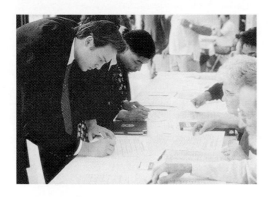

Most firms require that a standardized company application form be completed, even if a résumé has been submitted.

for work history in reverse chronological order and insisting that dates be provided, for example, gaps in work history may be revealed that are concealed on the candidate's résumé

- candidates are typically asked to complete an application form while on the company premises, which means that the application form is more likely to be a sample of the candidate's own work. (It is not uncommon for job applicants to get help—even paid professional assistance—with their résumés. In fact, obtaining assistance is getting easier and more affordable every day. Some Web sites, such as Monster.ca, now offer online résumé building options.)[90]

- the way in which an application form is completed reveals information about the candidate's ability to organize his or her thoughts, as well as spelling and grammar skills. This can be extremely important for certain positions, such as a secretary, HR manager, or management trainee

- application forms typically ask the candidate to provide written authorization for reference checking. A photocopy of this section can be faxed or mailed to individuals being asked for references, if so requested. (Many employers today will not give out any reference information until such written authorization has been received.)

- candidates are asked to sign and date their application form, acknowledging that the information provided is true and accurate, to the best of their knowledge. Beside that affirmation, there is typically a statement about the consequences of lying, such as, "I understand that a false statement may disqualify me from employment, or cause my dismissal." This protects the company somewhat from candidates who falsify their credentials

- many application forms today have a section regarding designated group member status, which candidates are asked, but not required, to complete. An example is provided in **Figure 6.7**. As indicated, the data collected are used for employment equity tracking purposes.

Human Rights Legislation and Application Forms

As explained in Chapter 3, human rights legislation in every Canadian jurisdiction prohibits discrimination on the grounds of race, religion or creed, colour, marital status, sex, and physical disability. Age-based discrimination is also prohibited, although the protected age groups differ, and most jurisdictions prohibit discrimination on the basis of mental disability. There are other prohibited grounds, which vary by jurisdiction. Application forms cannot ask questions that would *directly* or *indirectly* classify candidates on the basis of any of the prohibited grounds. Employers with operations in a number of provinces have to ensure that their application forms comply with the human rights code provisions in each.

Thus, candidates should not be asked to supply any of the following on an application form:

- information that could lead to direct, intentional discrimination such as age, gender, sexual orientation, marital status, maiden name, date of birth, place of origin, number of dependants, etc.

Hints to Ensure Legal Compliance

FIGURE 6.7 Self-identification for Employment Equity Purposes

Completion of this section of the application form is considered OPTIONAL and VOLUNTARY.

We are committed to employment equity and outreach recruitment. For purposes of employment equity tracking, we ask that applicants provide us with the following information. All answers will be considered confidential and used only for employment equity data-collection purposes. Eligibility as an applicant will not be affected: All of our selection decisions are based on merit.

Please check the appropriate box(es):

Are you:

❑ Male   ❑ Female

❑ White (Caucasian)

❑ A visible minority (Black, Chinese, South Asian, etc.)

❑ Aboriginal (Canadian Indian, Inuit, Métis)

❑ A person with a physical or mental disability (including learning disabilities)

Please note: This application form has been reviewed and approved by the provincial Human Rights Commission.

- an indication of whether he or she would prefer to be addressed as Mr./Mrs./Miss/Ms.
- his or her social insurance number
- a photograph
- information pertaining to citizenship
- information about height and weight (unless this is a bona fide job requirement)
- an indication of his or her mother tongue or how any language skills possessed were acquired
- the name, address, and dates of educational institutions attended
- information about illnesses, disabilities, or workers' compensation claims
- accommodation requirements, if any
- information about military service, in general
- information pertaining to arrests and/or criminal record
- his or her religious affiliation or ability to work on specific religious holidays
- references from relatives or members of the clergy.

If there are illegal questions on an application form, an unsuccessful candidate may challenge the legality of the entire recruitment and selection processes. In such case, the burden of proof is on the employer. Thus, taking human rights legislative requirements into consideration when designing application forms is imperative. *The Guide to Screening and Selection in Employment* in the Appendix to Chapter 3 provides helpful hints. Specific guidelines regarding questions that can and cannot be asked on application forms are available through the human rights commissions in each jurisdiction. **Figure 6.8,** a sam-

AN ETHICAL DILEMMA

There is a job that you really want. However, the application form that you have been asked to complete has a number of illegal questions, including date of birth, marital status, number of dependants, and religious affiliation. How would you handle this?

FIGURE 6.8 Sample Application Form

APPLICATION FOR EMPLOYMENT

Position being applied for	Date available to begin work

PERSONAL DATA

Last name   Given name(s)

Address	Street	Apt. No.	Home Telephone Number
City	Province	Postal Code	Business Telephone Number

Are you legally eligible to work in Canada?   ☐ Yes   ☐ No

Are you 18 years or more and less than 65 years of age?   ☐ Yes   ☐ No

Are you willing to relocate in Ontario? ☐ Yes ☐ No	Preferred location

To determine your qualification for employment, please provide (below and on the reverse) information related to your academic and other achievements including volunteer work, as well as employment history.
Additional information may be attached on a separate sheet.

EDUCATION

SECONDARY SCHOOL ■	BUSINESS, TRADE OR SECONDARY SCHOOL ■
Highest grade or level completed	Name of course Length of course
Type of certificate or diploma obtained	Licence, certificate or diploma awarded? ☐ Yes ☐ No

COMMUNITY COLLEGE ■	UNIVERSITY ■
Name of program Length of program	Length of course Degree awarded ☐ Pass ☐ Yes ☐ No ☐ Honours
Diploma received ☐ Yes ☐ No	Major subject
Other courses, workshops, seminars	Licences, certificates, degrees

Work-related skills

Describe any of your work-related skills, experience, or training that relate to the position being applied for.

Source: Application for employment from the Ontario Human Rights Commission, *Employment Application Forms, Interviews,* (1992). Reproduced with permission of the Ontario Human Rights Commission.

ple application form developed by the Ontario Human Rights Commission, illustrates the types of information that can legally be requested. As indicated therein, employers have the right to elicit detailed information about educational qualifications, employment history, and job-related skills—all of the data required to compare the qualifications of each candidate with the job specifications. Figure 6.7 shows a self-identification that prospective employees may fill out voluntarily on an optional basis.

Using Application Forms to Predict Job Performance

Some firms use application forms to predict which candidates will be successful and which will not, in much the same way that employers use tests for screening.

One approach involves designing a weighted application blank (WAB). Statistical studies are conducted to find the relationship between (1) responses on the application form and (2) measures of success on the job. A scoring system is subsequently developed by weighting the different possible responses to those particular items. By scoring an applicant's response to each of those questions and then totalling the scores obtained, a composite score can be calculated for each applicant. It should be noted that the scoring system is not shown on the application form. Thus, there is no difference in appearance between a WAB and a regular application form.

weighted application blank (WAB)
A job application form on which applicant responses have been weighted based on their statistical relationship to measures of job success.

Research Insight

As an example, the goal of one study, conducted at a large insurance company, was to determine whether there was a relationship between application form responses and turnover. At the time, the company was experiencing a 48-percent turnover rate among its clerical staff. (In other words, for every two employees hired at the same time, there was about a 50–50 chance that one of them would leave the firm within 12 months.) The researcher obtained the application forms of about 160 clerical employees from the company's HR files and divided them into two categories: long-tenure and short-tenure employees. After performing various statistical analyses, it became quite apparent that certain responses on the application form were highly related to job tenure. An application form weighted on the basis of this information enabled the firm to predict which applicants would be more likely to stay.[91]

Although studies have shown that WABs can be highly valid predictors, and they can be developed fairly easily, such forms are used by relatively few organizations.

Another type of application form that can be used to predict performance is a biographical information blank (BIB), also known as a biodata form. Like the WAB, it is a self-report instrument. However, all questions are in multiple-choice format, and the issues covered are much broader in scope than on a WAB. Essentially, it is a more detailed version of an application form, focussing on biographical data found to be predictive of job success. Candidates respond to a series of questions about their background, experiences, and preferences, including willingness to travel and leisure activities. Because biographical questions rarely have right or wrong answers, BIBs are difficult to fake. As with a WAB, responses are scored.

The development of a BIB requires that the items that are valid predictors of job success be identified and that weights be established for different responses

biographical information blank (BIB)
A detailed job application form requesting biographical data found to be predictive of success on the job, pertaining to background, experiences, and preferences. As with a WAB, responses are scored.

to these items. By totalling the scores for each item, it is possible to obtain a composite score for each applicant. BIBs have ~~moderate validi~~ty in predicting job performance.[92]

CHAPTER *Review*

Summary

1   Recruitment is the process of searching for and attracting an adequate number of qualified candidates, from whom the organization may select the most appropriate to staff its job requirements.

2   There is a number of steps in the recruitment process. First, job openings are identified through HR planning or manager request. The job description and job specification are then reviewed to determine the job requirements. Next, appropriate recruiting source(s) and method(s) are chosen. Using these strategies, a pool of qualified candidates is generated.

3   In order to be successful, a recruiter must be aware of the constraints affecting the recruitment process. These come from organizational policies and plans, the job requirements, recruiter habits, inducements of competitors, and environmental conditions.

4   There are two sources of recruits: the pools of workers internal and external to the company. Although recruiting often brings employment agencies and classified ads to mind, current employees are generally the largest source of recruits. To be effective, promotion from within requires using job posting, HR records, and skills inventories.

5   Unless there is a work-force reduction, even in firms with a promote-from-within policy, a replacement from outside must eventually be found to fill the job(s) left vacant once all eligible employees have been given the opportunity for transfer and/or promotion. In addition, most entry-level positions must be filled by external candidates.

6   When choosing external recruitment method(s) there is a number of factors that should be taken into consideration: the type of job, the relationship between method chosen and quality of hire, the yield ratio, and the amount of lead time.

7   External recruitment methods include walk-ins/write-ins, employee referrals, educational institutions, HRDC, private employment agencies, executive search firms, advertising, professional and trade associations, labour organizations, military personnel, online recruiting, hosting an open house, and holding information sessions/job fairs.

8   Strategies for obtaining non-permanent staff include using temporary help agencies, hiring contract workers, leasing employees, and outsourcing/subcontracting.

9   Recruiting a diverse work force is not just socially responsible, it's a necessity. To do so means formulating comprehensive plans to attract a diverse group of candidates, including: overcoming stereotypes and biases; reevaluating HR policies and practices; developing flexible work options; redesign-

ing jobs; investing in training, retraining and career development; and offering flexible benefits.

10 For most employers, completion of a standardized company application form is the last step in the recruitment process. Application forms cannot ask questions that would directly or indirectly classify candidates on the basis of any of the grounds prohibited in human rights legislation. Some firms design weighted application blanks and/or biographical information blanks, and use them to predict which candidates will be successful and which will not.

Key Terms

application form	recruiter
biographical information blank (BIB)	recruitment
blind ad	time-lapse data
employee leasing	want ad
human resources requisition form	weighted application blank (WAB)
job posting	yield ratio
nepotism	

Review and Discussion Questions

1 Describe the constraints on recruitment.

2 Discuss the advantages and disadvantages of recruiting within the organization.

3 Describe the role of job posting, HR records, and skills inventories in promotion from within.

4 List the advantages of external recruitment.

5 Explain why the type of job, the relationship between the method chosen and quality of hire, the yield ratio, and the amount of lead time should be taken into consideration when selecting external recruitment methods.

6 Under what circumstances should a blind ad be used?

7 Even when detailed résumés have been submitted, most firms also request that a standardized company application form be completed. Why?

CRITICAL *Thinking Questions*

1 Describe the external recruitment methods that would be appropriate for each of the following: factory worker, management trainee, senior engineer with twelve years of experience, senior secretary, Certified Management Accountant, accounts payable clerk, HR manager, junior buyer, and company president. Explain your choices.

2 Describe a position for which you would recommend using a professional search firm and explain the reasons for your recommendation.

3   Compare and contrast the advantages and disadvantages of temporary help agencies, contract employees, leased employees, and outsourcing and describe a specific situation in which you feel each would be the most appropriate strategy for recruiting non-permanent employees.

4   As the newly hired HR recruiter, you have been told that the firm wishes to diversify its work force. Explain the strategies you would use to ensure that this goal is met.

APPLICATION *Exercises*

RUNNING CASE: Carter Cleaning Company

Getting Better Applicants

If you were to ask Jennifer and her father what they considered to be their major challenge in running the six cleaning centres, their answer would be immediate and brief: hiring good people. To attract their management staff as well as skilled cleaner-spotters and pressers, they rely primarily on newspaper advertising and word of mouth. Putting a "help wanted" sign in the front window of the centre with the job opening has generally led to lots of applications but few hires, since most of the applicants lacked the required skills.

There is no promotion-from-within policy. As mentioned previously, virtually all of the employees at the centres, other than the managers, are women and/or visible minorities. Turnover among the experienced pressers and cleaner-spotters sometimes approaches 400 percent.

Jennifer recently spent some time discussing the benefits of HRP with her father and is now focusing on more effective recruitment strategies. Specifically, she is pondering the following questions.

Questions

1   How could a promote-from-within policy benefit Carter Cleaning? What would be necessary to make such a policy effective?

2   What other external recruitment methods should she and her father consider? Why?

3   How could a more diverse group of applicants be attracted?

CASE INCIDENT *Expansion at Logans*

Business has been so good at the Logans Department Store outlet in the outskirts of Halifax that management has decided to expand it to include a bakery and deli, a cosmetic department, and a sporting goods department. No other outlets have a bakery and deli, but several have small cosmetics and sporting goods departments. The chain has a reputation for high-quality merchandise and personal attention to customers, standards that new hires will be expected to meet.

Management has estimated that the new departments, scheduled to begin operations in 12 months, will require 15 new employees. Projected staffing for the bakery and deli includes one baker, one butcher, two customer-service representatives, and one manager. The projected HR requirements for the cosmetics and sporting goods departments are four customer-service representatives and one manager each. These estimates have been based on anticipated customer demand for the new products and services and on the level of service the firm wishes to maintain (i.e. customer-service representative to customer ratio).

Although there is a corporate promote-from-within policy for supervisory and management-level positions, the uniqueness of the new departments makes it unlikely that qualified applicants can be found internally.

Kim Vu has worked as an HR specialist at Logans corporate offices in downtown Halifax for the past two years. Although she has recruited for a number of positions, she has never previously been asked to conduct a recruitment campaign of this magnitude. She has a challenge ahead of her now, though, since her boss, Vice-president of HR Bea Tjoveld, has asked her to prepare a recruiting plan and budget for staffing the expansion.

Questions

1 Assume that you are Kim. Prepare a recruiting plan and budget to meet the projected staffing needs. Your plan should outline your recommended recruiting sources and methods for each of the positions, accompanied by reasons for each of your recommendations. Your plan should also include cost and lead-time estimates.

2 After you have prepared your plan, assume a scenario in which there is a marked downturn in the economy. How might this affect your recruiting plan?

EXPERIENTIAL *Exercises*

1 Working individually or in groups, examine the classified and display ads appearing in the help-wanted section of a recent newspaper. Using the AIDA guidelines presented in this chapter, analyze their effectiveness.

2 Working individually or in small groups, design an application form that meets human rights legislative requirements.

WEB-BASED *Exercises*

1 Before coming to class, visit the HRDC Web site (**www.hrdc.drhc.gc.ca**). Come to class prepared to discuss the following questions: (a) What programs and services are available to link employers and potential employees? How does each work? (b) To what extent would HRDC be helpful if you were responsible for recruiting technical, managerial, or professional employees? Why? (c) What other programs and services are offered?

2   Compare and contrast the Internet recruiting sites of two employers of your choice. Prepare a brief report outlining: (a) the features of each site; (b) strengths and weaknesses of each site; (c) your opinion regarding which site is more "job seeker friendly" and why; (d) your opinion on which site is more successful in assisting the firm to recruit a good-sized pool of qualified applicants and why.

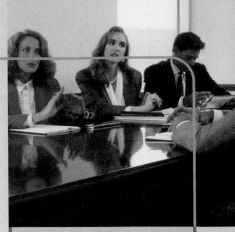

CHAPTER 7

Selection

CHAPTER OUTLINE

Introduction

The Selection Process

Constraints on the Selection Process

The Importance of Reliability and Validity

Steps in the Selection Process

LEARNING OUTCOMES

After studying this chapter, you should be able to:

Define selection and *discuss* its purpose and importance.

Describe the constraints on the selection process.

Define reliability and validity and *explain* their importance.

Describe at least four types of testing used in selection and *discuss* the legal and ethical concerns related to medical examinations and drug testing.

Describe the major types of selection interviews and the problems that can undermine their effectiveness.

Design and *conduct* an effective interview.

Explain the importance of reference checking, *describe* strategies to make such checking effective, and *discuss* the legal issues involved.

Describe the supervisor's role in selection.

Explain how firms evaluate the selection process.

INTRODUCTION

selection
The process of choosing individuals with the relevant qualifications to fill existing or projected job openings.

Selection is the process of choosing individuals with the relevant qualifications to fill existing or projected job openings. Whether considering current employees for a transfer or promotion, or outside candidates for a first-time position with the firm, information about the applicants must be collected and evaluated. Each step in the selection process, from preliminary reception and initial screening to the hiring decision, is performed under legal, organizational, and environmental constraints that protect the interests of both applicant and organization.[1]

multiple-hurdle strategy
An approach to selection involving a series of successive steps or hurdles. Only candidates clearing the hurdle are permitted to move on to the next step.

Most firms use a sequential selection system involving a series of successive steps—a **multiple-hurdle strategy**. Only candidates clearing the "hurdle" (typically pre-screening, testing, interviewing, and background/reference checking) are permitted to move on to the next step. Clearing the hurdle requires meeting or exceeding the minimum requirements established for each screening technique. At each step, some applicants are eliminated. Thus, only candidates who have cleared all of the previous hurdles remain in contention for the position at the time that the hiring decision is being made.

Purpose and Importance of Selection

The purpose of selection is to find the "best" candidate for the job—an individual who possesses the required KSAs and personality, who will perform well, embrace the corporate mission and values, and fit the organizational culture. The importance of fit is being recognized by more and more firms. In fact, in a recent survey of 200 Canadian companies, fit with organizational culture was identified as the second most important hiring criterion for business graduates, surpassed only by relevant areas of study.[2]

Proper selection is important for three key reasons: (1) its impact on company performance, (2) the costs involved, and (3) its legal implications.

Company Performance

While proper selection was important during the years when the Canadian economy was predominantly production oriented, it is even more vital now that the major part of the nation's gross national product is based on the provision of services. More and more managers have come to the realization that the quality of the company's human resources is often the single most important factor in determining whether the firm is going to survive, be successful in reaching the objectives specified in its strategic plan, and realize a satisfactory return on its investment. In fact, after increasing profits, the top priority of 300 CEOs participating in a recent survey was attracting and retaining key employees.[3]

Cost

In recent years, the cost of recruitment and selection has risen substantially. For example, one expert estimates that the cost of hiring is approximately two to three times an individual's salary.[4] Costs do not end, of course, with the selection decision. Even if an internal candidate is chosen, that person will require orientation and training. Often, the cost of training surpasses that of hiring.

Since labour costs make up such a big percentage of overhead expenses in many Canadian organizations (up to 80 or 85 percent in service-sector firms, such as hospitals), there are also tremendous costs associated with inappropriate selection decisions.

Much emphasis has been placed on effective training and development and various motivational techniques as means of ensuring that employees make a worthwhile contribution. However, if the wrong employee is selected initially, no training program or motivational strategy—no matter how well conceived and designed—is likely to compensate adequately or offset the original hiring error.

The high cost of training and development makes it all the more critical that the selection process receive careful attention, such that subsequent training and development efforts will "fall on fertile soil." Furthermore, a good selection process for vacancies being filled by external applicants will ensure that qualified, promotable employees are brought into the firm.

When an unsuccessful employee must be terminated while on probation, or quits during this time, the recruitment and selection process must begin all over again, and the successor must be properly oriented and trained. These "visible" costs vary widely from job to job, and firm to firm, but there are always costs involved, even for the lowest-level, lowest-paid positions. The "hidden" costs are frequently even higher, including: the low quality of work performed by the unsuccessful/unhappy employee while on the job; internal disorganization and disruption the employee may have caused; and customer/client ill will or alienation that may have been generated.

More often than not, really unsatisfactory applicants are screened out. Those that somehow "slip through" usually reveal their deficiencies and shortcomings early and are terminated during the probationary period. This is not the case, however, with the marginal (or borderline) employee, someone who really is not capable enough to be considered truly satisfactory, and never makes a worthwhile contribution to the firm. Virtually all organizations have some marginal employees. In retrospect, these people probably should never have been hired in the first place.

Once marginal employees are on the payroll, it becomes exceedingly difficult to terminate their employment. When they were first hired, their deficiencies and shortcomings may not have been readily appreciable; after all, most people are on their best behaviour while on probation. Typically, it is only after they have been on the job for a while that their limitations become apparent.

Frequently, marginal employees are hired when the firm is in the midst of expansion, especially if there is no formalized selection process. Under the pressure of the moment, they are not properly screened out. Sometimes an interviewer even realizes that a particular applicant does not really meet all of the critical requirements, but does not have the written policy backing (or authority) to insist that selection standards not be compromised. The interviewer may truly believe that with time and training the applicant will develop into a better employee than he or she appears to be at present. In reality, this hope is rarely fulfilled. If anything, the marginal applicant usually turns out to be even less satisfactory an employee than expected.

Using a sequential selection system and adopting policies and procedures requiring strict adherence to selection standards can help to ensure that unsuitable applicants do not "slip through" and that marginal employees never end up on the company's payroll.[5] Such improvements to the firm's selection process also reduce total recruitment and selection costs by an estimated 20 to 40 percent.[6]

marginal employee

Someone who really is not capable enough to be considered truly satisfactory, and never makes a worthwhile contribution to the firm.

Many organizations are now focussing on teamwork skills, for example. In such firms, the entire team may be involved in the selection process. At 3M's plant in Brockville, Ontario, workers on the shop floor, who work closely together in teams of six or eight, are responsible for choosing new team members. They have been trained to assess applicants in three ways. First, they determine whether recruits have the desired values; next, they conduct some basic paper-and-pencil testing of problem-solving skills; and finally, teamwork skills are assessed through group exercises.[9] Recognizing that how people get along with each other will have a major impact on the success of plant operations, 3M has the workers decide whom they can best work with, right from the start.

Selection Budget

Since the selection process is not an end, but a means through which firms obtain employees, a selection budget is established, within which HR staff members must work. If there were no budget limitations, they could refine selection procedures. The benefits of such refinements, however, might be outweighed by the negative impact on organizational effectiveness of unnecessarily high selection expenses.

Employment Equity Plan

If there is an employment equity plan, whether legally required or voluntarily initiated, it must be taken into consideration when planning the selection process. This is because selection is one of the major HR activities by which the goals and timetables established by the firm and specified in their employment equity plan can be reached.

The Job Requirements

As explained in Chapter 4, it is through job analysis that the duties, responsibilities, and human requirements for each job are identified. By defining bona fide occupational requirements through job analysis and basing selection criteria on these requirements, firms can create a legally defensible hiring system.[10]

The skills required, mental and physical demands, responsibilities, and working conditions should provide the basis for the information obtained from the applicant and his or her previous employers and other references, as well as for any employment tests administered. Individuals hired after thorough screening against carefully developed selection criteria (based directly on the job description and job specification) learn their jobs readily, are productive, and generally adjust to their jobs with a minimum of difficulty. As a result, both the individual and organization benefit.

Supply Challenges

Although it is desirable to have a large pool of qualified recruits from which to choose, that is not always possible. In fields in which there is a supply shortage, such as physiotherapy, middle and senior management, and Information Technology,[11] there is often a very small selection ratio. A **selection ratio** is the relationship between the number of applicants hired and the total number of

selection ratio
The ratio of the number of applicants hired to the total number of applicants.

applicants available, calculated by dividing the number of applicants hired by the total number of applicants.

A small selection ratio, such as 1:2, means that there are very few applicants from which to select, and may also mean low-quality recruits. If this is the case, it is generally better to start the recruitment process over again, even if it means a hiring delay, rather than taking the risk of hiring an employee who will be a marginal performer at best.

Ethics

An Ethical
Dilemma

As the company recruiter, how would you handle a request from the CEO that you hire her son for a summer job, knowing that, given current hiring constraints, the sons and daughters of other employees will not be able to obtain such positions?

Since members of the HR department have a major impact on the hiring decision, it is important that they have a strong sense of professional ethics.[12] Being offered gifts from a private employment agency wanting the firm's business or being pressured to hire an underqualified designated group member are examples of ethical dilemmas that those involved in the selection process may encounter.

Ethical standards pertaining to privacy and confidentiality are also important. The applicant's right to privacy must be balanced against the organization's right to know.

Legislative Requirements

As mentioned earlier, all steps in the selection process must meet human rights and employment equity legislative standards (where applicable). Organizations must ensure that their selection criteria and screening techniques are justifiable, based on the job requirements, and that none leads to discrimination—whether intentional or systemic.

Legal compliance concerns also require that employers exercise due diligence in employee screening and reference checking. Suggested guidelines for avoiding negative legal consequences, such as human rights complaints, liability for negligent hiring, and unjust discharge suits, include:[13]

Hints to Ensure
Legal Compliance

1. Ensuring that all selection criteria and strategies are based on the job description and job specification. Doing so will enable the employer, if charged under human rights legislation, to prove that a protected group member was denied employment on the basis of legitimate and bona fide grounds.

2. Adequately assessing the applicant's ability to meet performance standards or expectations. If an applicant passes a test given to evaluate his or her abilities in a particular area, is subsequently hired based in part on the test results, and is later discharged due to inadequate skills in that area, the employer would be found liable in a wrongful discharge suit. It is the employer's responsibility to ensure that the candidate possesses the necessary KSAs to fulfill the job requirements.

3. Carefully scrutinizing all information supplied on application forms and résumés. To avoid negligent hiring charges, unexplained gaps in employment history should be explored. Any discrepancies between the information provided on paper and that gleaned during the interview process should also be thoroughly investigated. In unjust discharge cases, courts may decide in an employee's favour if the employer had objective informa-

tion that contradicted the applicant's misrepresentations or embellishments, and ignored it or failed to act upon it.

4. Obtaining written authorization for reference checking from prospective employees, and checking references very carefully. Where justified, based on the job requirements, permission should also be obtained to check credit history, driving record, and/or criminal record. The results of such checking may lead to candidate rejection if the individual's history indicates unsuitability for the job in question. (This requires delicate balancing of the candidate's legal rights—discussed in Chapter 3—and the fear of negligent hiring.)

5. Saving all records and information obtained about the applicant during each stage of the selection process. Having such records, which make it clear that there were bona fide reasons for candidate rejection, is essential for defence against charges of discrimination under human rights or employment equity legislation. Having records that prove that due diligence was exercised in assessing applicant suitability is necessary in order to defend against charges of wrongful hiring.

6. Rejecting applicants who make false statements on their application forms or résumés. Doing so enables firms to avoid dishonest employees who may have something serious to hide, which could lead to a charge of negligent hiring. Most wrongful dismissal cases involving applicant misrepresentation have been decided in the employer's favour because the misrepresentation resulted in gross incompetence, breach of trust (that is, dishonesty), or both; except in cases in which the employer received both accurate and embellished information, and had objective data that should have enabled him or her to distinguish between the two.

Two critical issues related to legal compliance are reliability and validity, which will be discussed next.

The Importance of Reliability and Validity

Reliability

reliability

The degree to which interviews, tests, and other selection procedures yield comparable data over a period of time; in other words, the degree of dependability, consistency, or stability of the measures used.

The degree to which interviews, tests, and other selection procedures yield comparable data over a period of time is known as **reliability**. Reliability is thus concerned with the degree of dependability, consistency, or stability of the measures used.[14] For example, if a group of interviewers selects three candidates as their top choices today that are not those they chose yesterday, their judgments are obviously not reliable. Similarly, a test that results in widely variable scores when it (or an equivalent version of the test) is administered on different occasions to the same individual is unreliable.[15]

Reliability also refers to the extent to which two or more methods (such as tests and reference checking) yield the same results or are consistent, as well as the extent to which there is agreement between two or more raters (inter-rater reliability).

When dealing with tests, another measure of reliability that is taken into account is internal consistency. For example, suppose that there were 10 items on a vocational interest test, all of which were supposed to measure, in one way or another, the person's interest in working outdoors. To assess internal reliability, the degree to which responses to those 10 items vary together would be statistically analyzed. (That is one reason why tests often include questions that appear rather repetitive.)

There are at least four sources of unreliability:

1. The selection instrument might do a poor job of sampling. For example, one version of a college course test might focus on specific chapters more than the supposedly equivalent version does. Similarly, interview questions may be worded in such a way that they do not do a good job of measuring what they were supposed to, such as knowledge about a particular subject.

2. Errors may result from chance response tendencies. For example, a test may be so hard or so boring that the candidate gives up and starts answering questions at random.

3. The conditions under which the instrument is administered might cause errors. An interview room with construction noise outside may unnerve a candidate, for example, resulting in a far different performance than if the interview had been conducted in a quiet setting.

4. There could be changes within the applicant. Interview performance after a sleepless night is typically far different from that when a candidate is well rested, for example.

Validity

validity
The accuracy with which a predictor measures what it is supposed to measure.

Validity refers to the accuracy with which a predictor measures what it is supposed to measure. In the context of selection, validity is an indicator of the extent to which data from a selection technique, such as a test or interview, are related to or predictive of subsequent performance on the job.[16] Selection procedures must, above all, be valid. Without proof of validity, there is no logical or legally permissible reason to continue using the technique to screen job applicants.

To ensure that the selection techniques being used are valid, validation studies should be conducted. There are three distinct types of validity: criterion-related, content, and construct. Since construct validity is not frequently used in selection, we will focus on the former two.

Criterion-related Validity

criterion-related validity
The extent to which a selection tool predicts or significantly correlates with important elements of work behaviour.

The extent to which a selection tool predicts or significantly correlates with important elements of work behaviour is known as **criterion-related validity**. Demonstrating criterion-related validity requires proving that those who do well on a test or in an interview, for example, also do well on the job, and that individuals who do poorly on the test or in the interview receive low job-performance ratings.[17]

Content Validity

content validity
The extent to which a selection instrument, such as a test, adequately samples the knowledge and skills needed to perform the job.

When a selection instrument, such as a test, adequately samples the knowledge and skills needed to perform the job, **content validity** is assumed to exist. The closer the content of the selection instrument is to actual samples of work or work behaviour, the greater the content validity.[18] For example, asking a candidate for a secretarial position to demonstrate word processing skills, as required on the job, has high content validity.

Ensuring content validity sounds easier that it is in practice. Demonstrating that the tasks a person performs in an interview or a test situation are, in fact, a comprehensive and random sample of the tasks performed on the job and that the conditions under which they are performed resemble the work situation is not always easy. Nevertheless, content validity is the most direct and least complicated type of validity to assess.

Construct Validity

The extent to which a selection tool measures a theoretical construct or trait deemed necessary to perform the job successfully is known as **construct validity**. Intelligence, verbal skills, analytical ability, and leadership skills are all examples of constructs. Measuring construct validity requires demonstrating that the psychological trait or attribute is related to satisfactory job performance, as well as showing that the test or other selection tool used accurately measures the psychological trait or attribute.[19]

Regardless of the method used, cross-validation is essential. **Cross-validation** is the process of verifying the results obtained from a validation study by administering a test or test battery to a different sample drawn from the same population.

Experts also recommend assessing **differential validity**—using separate validation studies to confirm that the selection tool accurately predicts the performance of all possible employee subgroups. Otherwise, a procedure may be a valid predictor of job success for one group (such as white male applicants), but not for all candidates, thereby leading to systemic discrimination. As may be recalled from Chapter 3, the issue of differential validity played a significant role in the 1987 landmark decision of the Supreme Court of Canada, upholding a federal human rights tribunal ruling. CN Rail was ordered to cease using the Bennet Mechanical Comprehension Test as a selection tool for entry-level blue-collar jobs in its St. Lawrence region because the test had an adverse impact on female applicants.[20]

The overall effectiveness of a selection program depends on the validity of its components. **Table 7.1** summarizes the results of one study of the validity of various selection tools. Tests with high face validity (that appear valid)—such as tests of actual performance, including work sampling, peer evaluations, and assessment centres—rated highest. Indirect evaluations, such as psychological tests or academic performance, rated lower.

construct validity
The extent to which a selection tool measures a theoretical construct or trait deemed necessary to perform the job successfully.

cross-validation
The process of verifying the results obtained from a validation study by administering a test or test battery to a different sample drawn from the same population.

differential validity
Confirmation that the selection tool accurately predicts the performance of all possible employee subgroups, including white males, women, visible minorities, persons with disabilities, and Aboriginal Peoples.

Research Insight

Tests with high face validity may also be more acceptable to candidates. In a recent study involving 259 college students from France and the U.S., face validity was found to be the most important determinant of students' reactions to various selection techniques. Tests high in face validity, such as interviews and work sampling, were viewed much more favourably than those low in face validity, such as graphology. Other strong predictors of favourable reactions included beliefs that the employer had the right to obtain information using that particular technique and the extent to which the procedure is widely used in industry.[21]

STEPS IN THE SELECTION PROCESS

In order to gain as reliable and valid a picture as possible of each applicant's potential for success on the job, organizations typically rely on a number of

TABLE 7.1

Validity of Various Selection Devices

PREDICTOR	VALIDITY
Cognitive Ability and Special Aptitude	Moderate
Personality	Low
Interest	Low
Physical Ability	Moderate–High
Biographical Information	Moderate
Interviews	Low
Work Samples	High
Seniority	Low
Peer Evaluations	High
Reference Checks	Low
Academic Performance	Low
Self-Assessments	Moderate
Assessment Centres	High

Source: Neal Schmitt and Raymond Noe, "Personal Selection and Equal Employment Opportunity," in *International Review of Industrial and Organizational Psychology*, eds. Cary L. Cooper and Ivan T. Robertson. Copyright 1986 by John Wiley & Sons, Ltd. Reproduced by permission of John Wiley & Sons Limited.

sources of information. As mentioned earlier, the number of steps in the selection process and their sequence varies not only with the organization, but also with recruiting source and method. Reference checking with former employers is not generally a step in the selection of an internal candidate for transfer or promotion, for example. Private employment agencies and executive search firms perform screening, and often do testing and reference checking. Thus, when using either of these recruiting methods, the company's selection process may only involve three steps: a supervisory interview, a realistic job preview, and making the final hiring decision.

As illustrated in **Figure 7.2**, after applicants have been pre-screened, the most common selection strategies revealed in a recent study involving 718 Canadian firms include reference checks with previous employers and one-on-one interviews, while the least frequent are handwriting analysis and videoconference interviews.[22]

The type and level of job also make a difference. For example, while 58 percent of those responding to a recent survey of 202 Canadian organizations indicated that they use letters of reference for at least some jobs, as illustrated in **Figure 7.3**, such letters are requested least frequently for blue-collar jobs and most frequently for white-collar professional positions.[23]

Each of the steps commonly involved in the selection process, as identified in Figure 7.1, will now be described.

Step One: Applicant Reception

The selection process is a two-way street: organizations select employees, and applicants select employers. How initial reception is handled affects an applicant's opinion of the employer.

In many firms, initial contact is made directly with the HR department, either in person or in writing, or by the exchange of some basic information

FIGURE 7.2 Selection Strategies for Pre-screened Candidates

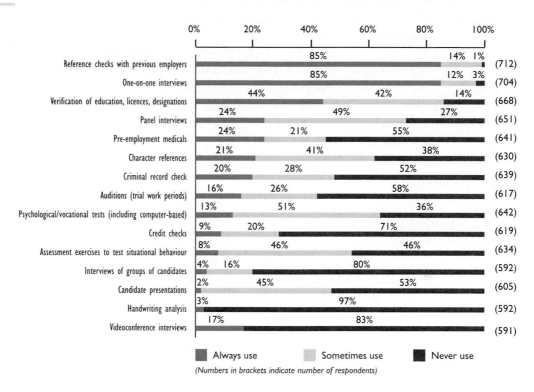

	0%	20%	40%	60%	80%	100%	
Reference checks with previous employers			85%			14% 1%	(712)
One-on-one interviews			85%			12% 3%	(704)
Verification of education, licences, designations		44%		42%		14%	(668)
Panel interviews	24%		49%		27%		(651)
Pre-employment medicals	24%	21%		55%			(641)
Character references	21%		41%		38%		(630)
Criminal record check	20%	28%		52%			(639)
Auditions (trial work periods)	16%	26%		58%			(617)
Psychological/vocational tests (including computer-based)	13%		51%		36%		(642)
Credit checks	9%	20%		71%			(619)
Assessment exercises to test situational behaviour	8%	46%		46%			(634)
Interviews of groups of candidates	4%	16%		80%			(592)
Candidate presentations	2%	45%		53%			(605)
Handwriting analysis	3%		97%				(592)
Videoconference interviews	17%		83%				(591)

■ Always use   ■ Sometimes use   ■ Never use

(Numbers in brackets indicate number of respondents)

Source: Murray Axmith & Associates Ltd., *Survey 2000: Canadian Hiring, Retention and Dismissal Practices*, (Toronto: Murray Axmith & Associates Ltd.) p. 13. Reprinted by permission.

FIGURE 7.3 Letters of Reference as a Selection Strategy

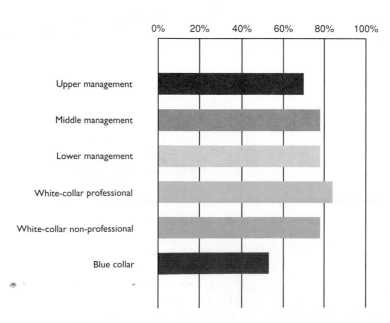

Source: Sean A. Way and James W. Thacker, "Selection Practices: Where are Canadian Organizations?" *HR Professional* 16, no. 5 (October/November 1999), p. 33. Reprinted by permission of Professer James W. Thacker.

through the receptionist, such as nature of jobs available, pay rates, and hours of work. In such organizations, candidates are typically required to complete an application form as part of the preliminary reception process.

An applicant appearing in person may be granted a preliminary interview as a matter of good public relations, especially if there is an opening for which he or she may be qualified. Such a "courtesy interview" is very brief, but enables a member of the HR department to confirm whether or not the candidate has the "must have" selection criteria and to screen out candidates who are unsuitable or undesirable.

Candidates who apply in writing may be sent a letter of acknowledgment. If such candidates have desirable qualifications, an application form may be enclosed, with the request that it be completed and returned. Some applicants may self-select themselves out of the process at this stage if they realize that they are unqualified or decide that they have no desire to work for the firm based on some of the information relayed or the treatment received.

In some Canadian firms, most individuals interested in work are now making their initial contact online or using an interactive voice response (IVR) system, rather than by mail or in person. In such cases, preliminary reception and initial applicant screening may occur simultaneously.

Step Two: Initial Applicant Screening

Initial applicant screening is generally performed by members of the HR department. Application forms and résumés are reviewed. Those candidates not meeting the "must have" selection criteria are eliminated first. Then, the remaining applications are examined and those candidates who most closely match the remaining job specifications are identified and given further consideration.

As explained in the Information Technology and HR box, an increasing number of firms are taking advantage of IVR screening, applicant-tracking systems, skills-management software, and/or Web-based applications to speed up the initial screening process and make it far less labour intensive.

Step Three: Selection Testing

Selection testing is a common screening device used by organizations for both hiring and promotion purposes. The tests assess specific job-related skills, as well as general intelligence, personality characteristics, mental abilities, interests, and preferences. Tests may involve a demonstration of skills, a simulation, or a written exercise. Testing techniques provide efficient, standardized procedures for screening large numbers of applicants. The use of valid tests can significantly assist in the selection of the most qualified candidate, and increase output substantially. According to researcher Stephen Cronshaw, for example, the utility for a single year of testing Canadian Armed Forces' clerical applicants was $50 million.[24]

The use of tests to assist with hiring and/or promotion decisions has been increasing. In a recent study involving 202 Canadian firms, two-thirds of the respondents indicated that they use at least one type of testing method in their selection process, to supplement interview results.[25] **Table 7.2** indicates the types of testing methods used.

In general, testing is more prevalent in larger organizations. This reflects their greater need for efficient, standardized procedures to screen large numbers of applicants, as well as their ability to finance testing programs.

Microsoft Online Résumé Building and Pre-screening
www.microsoft.com/jobs/

Cisco Online Résumé Building and Pre-screening
www.cisco.com/jobs/

INFORMATION TECHNOLOGY AND HR
Screening Tools and Techniques

IVR is a telephone-based system ideal for situations involving the screening of many hundreds or even thousands of applicants. Candidates access the system by calling a designated telephone number and then, using the touch-tone pad, respond to the job-related questions posed. By asking questions that gauge each applicant's fit with the job specifications, an IVR system can help the HR department staff members to quickly identify those who are qualified and screen out those who are not, thereby eliminating the time typically spent sorting through stacks of résumés and/or application forms.

Alternatively, some firms are starting to take advantage of applicant-tracking systems, which can scan each résumé—whether received by mail, fax or e-mail—and search for key words that will indicate whether or not the applicant has the requisite KSAs. Such systems sort candidates into two categories: those that are worthy of further consideration and those that are not. The résumés of individuals considered suitable for future consideration are added to the firm's database.

Another option involves the use of skills-management software. As résumés are received for an advertised position, high-potential candidates are provided with a computer-generated skills ques-

tionnaire, designed to elicit information about their level of proficiency in the relevant skills. The consistency provided by the firm's skill definitions and rating scale form the basis for meaningful analysis. When the questionnaire is completed, returned, and keyed into the skills application, it becomes that applicant's skills profile. Merely requesting applicants to explicitly state their abilities in defined skills acts as a screening tool, since candidates who know that they do not have the appropriate skill set and/or those who have something to hide typically do not bother returning the questionnaire.

Going one step further, some experts predict that 10 years from now, paper-based résumés will be a distant memory. Already, high-tech firms such as Microsoft and Cisco have developed Web sites that not only construct résumés for applicants but also screen them based on a series of job-related questions.

Source: Michael Callans, "Using Technology to Hire the Best," *Canadian HR Reporter* 12, no. 14 (August 9, 1999); Hank Reihl, "Skills-Based Management—A More Effective Tool for Hiring Technical People," *Guide to Recruitment & Staffing, Supplement to Canadian HR Reporter*, 12, no. 4 (February 22, 1999), p. G10; and Al Doran, "Paper Résumés Out, Electronic Résumé Creation In," *Canadian HR Reporter*, 12, no. 3 (February 8, 1999), p. 9.

Fundamental Guidelines to Effective Testing

The Canadian Psychological Association has developed and published comprehensive testing standards, covering such areas as test instrumentation, test use and administration, scoring, and reporting.[26]

TABLE 7.2

Selection Testing Methods Used in Canadian Firms (n = 133)

Paper & Pencil Tests			Rapid Screening		Behavioural		
Personality	Aptitude	Other	WAB	BIB	Assessment Centre	Work Sampling	Others
25%	36%	23%	3%	6%	12%	29%	7%

Source: Adapted from Sean A. Way and James W. Thacker, "Selection Practices: Where are Canadian Organizations?" *HR Professional* 16, no. 5 (October/November 1999), p. 34. Reprinted by permission of Professor James W. Thacker.

Selection testing involves many different varieties of tests that purport to measure such diverse attributes of candidates as job performance and honesty. It is important, therefore, that firms do a great deal of planning, analysis, and experimentation in order to ensure that the tests they use best satisfy their needs. Basic guidelines[27] for setting up a testing program include:[28]

Hints to Ensure Legal Compliance

1. Use tests as supplements to other techniques, such as interviews and background checks. Tests are not infallible. Even in the best of cases, the test score usually accounts for only about 25 percent of the variation in the measure of performance. In addition, tests are often better at telling which candidates will fail than which will succeed.

2. Validate the tests in the organization. Both legal requirements and good testing practice demand in-house validation. The fact that the same tests have been proven valid in similar organizations is not sufficient.

3. Analyze all current hiring and promotion standards. Questions should be asked, such as: "What proportion of Aboriginal or visible minority applicants are being rejected at each stage of the hiring process?" and "Why are we using this standard—what does it mean in terms of actual behaviour on the job?" The burden of proof is always on the organization to show that the predictor (such as intelligence) is related to success or failure on the job.

4. Keep accurate records of why each applicant was rejected, using objective, fact-based statements. A general note such as "not sufficiently well qualified" will not meet Human Right Commission standards, should a rejection decision be questioned at a later date.

5. Begin a validation program if the firm either does not currently use tests or uses tests that have not been validated. A predictive validation study is preferable. This requires administering a test to applicants, hiring the applicants without referring to the test scores, and at a later date correlating test scores with the employees' performance on the job.

6. Use a certified psychologist. The development, validation, and use of selection standards (including tests) generally require the assistance of a qualified psychologist.

7. Provide appropriate testing conditions. Tests should be administered in a private, quiet, well-lit, and well-ventilated setting, and all applicants must take tests under the same conditions.

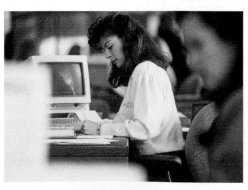

To assess the traits on which job success depends, many firms, such as those that rely on computer literacy, administer a skills assessment test before hiring.

Individual Rights of Test Takers and Test Security

Under the Canadian Psychological Association's Standards, test takers have the right to expect that:[29]

- results will be treated as highly confidential and used only with their informed consent

- results will be shared only with those having a legitimate need for the information, who are either qualified to interpret the scores or who have been provided with sufficient information to ensure their appropriate interpretation

- tests are equally fair to all test takers in the sense of being equally familiar, which requires security measures, such that no one taking a test has any prior information concerning the questions or answers.

Types of Tests

A number of the tests commonly used in selection can conveniently be classified according to whether they measure cognitive (thinking) abilities, motor and physical abilities, personality and interests, or achievement.[30] Other potential testing strategies include work sampling, management assessment centres, video-based situational testing, micro-assessments, the miniature job training and evaluation approach, graphology, medical examination, and drug testing.

Tests of Cognitive Abilities

Included in this category are tests of general reasoning ability (intelligence), tests of emotional intelligence, and tests of specific thinking skills like memory and inductive reasoning.

intelligence (IQ) tests
Tests that measure general intellectual abilities, such as verbal comprehension, inductive reasoning, memory, numerical ability, speed of perception, spatial visualization, and word fluency.

Intelligence Tests
Intelligence (IQ) tests are tests of general intellectual abilities. They measure not a single "intelligence" trait, but rather a number of abilities including memory, vocabulary, verbal fluency, and numerical ability.

Originally, IQ (intelligence quotient) was literally a quotient: a child's mental age (as measured by the intelligence test), divided by his or her chronological age, multiplied by 100. Thus, if an eight-year-old child answered questions as a 10-year-old might, his or her IQ would be 10 divided by 8, times 100, or 125.

For adults, of course, the notion of mental age divided by chronological age would not make sense. For example, we would not necessarily expect a 30-year-old to be more intelligent than a 25-year-old. Therefore, an adult's IQ score is actually a *derived* score, reflecting the extent to which the person is above or below the "average" adult's intelligence score.

Intelligence is often measured with individually administered tests, such as the Stanford-Binet Test or the Wechsler Test. Other IQ tests, such as the Wonderlic, can be administered to groups of people.

emotional intelligence (EI) tests
Tests that measure ability to monitor one's own emotions and the emotions of others and use that knowledge to guide thoughts and actions.

Emotional Intelligence Tests
Emotional intelligence (EI) tests measure ability to monitor one's own emotions and the emotions of others and use that knowledge to guide thoughts and actions. Someone with a high emotional quotient (EQ) is self-aware, can control his or her impulses, motivates him or herself, and demonstrates empathy and social awareness.

While some circles are hailing EI as the next great wave, others argue that EI is not new at all, but is made up of a number of factors that have been published in the academic literature for years. Many people believe that EQ, which can be modified through conscious effort and practice, is actually a more important determinant of success than having a high IQ. This is reflected in the fact that the EQ-i (Emotional Quotient Inventory) is now used in more than 600 organizations around the world, ranging from businesses to counselling centres to the U.S. armed forces.[31]

aptitude tests
Tests that measure an individual's aptitude or potential to perform a job, provided he or she is given proper training.

Specific Cognitive Abilities
There are also measures of specific thinking skills, such as inductive and deductive reasoning, verbal comprehension, memory, and numerical ability.

Tests in this category are often called **aptitude tests**, since they purport to measure the applicant's aptitudes for the job in question, that is, the applicant's potential to perform the job once given proper training. An example is the test of mechanical comprehension illustrated in **Figure 7.4**. It tests the applicant's understanding of basic mechanical principles. It may therefore reflect a person's aptitude for jobs—like that of machinist or engineer—that require mechanical comprehension. Other tests of mechanical aptitude include the Mechanical Reasoning Test and the SRA Test of Mechanical Aptitude.

Multidimensional aptitude tests commonly used in applicant selection include the General Aptitude Test Battery (GATB), the Employee Aptitude Survey (EAS), the Flanagan Aptitude Classification Test (FACT), and the Differential Aptitude Test (DAT). Some firms are now administering and scoring aptitude tests online. At Microsoft, for example, after completing the online aptitude test, visitors to the site are provided with a list of recommended jobs.

Microsoft Online Aptitude Testing
www.microsoft.com/skills2000

Tests of Motor and Physical Abilities

There are many *motor abilities* that a firm might want to measure. These include finger dexterity, manual dexterity, speed of arm movement, and reaction time. The Crawford Small Parts Dexterity Test, as illustrated in **Figure 7.5**, is an example. It measures the speed and accuracy of simple judgment, as well as the speed of finger, hand, and arm movements. Other tests include the Stromberg Dexterity Test, the Minnesota Rate of Manipulation Test, and the Purdue Peg Board.

Tests of physical abilities—such as static strength (lifting weights), dynamic strength (like pull-ups), body coordination (as in jumping rope), and

---

FIGURE **7.4** Two Problems from the Test of Mechanical Comprehension

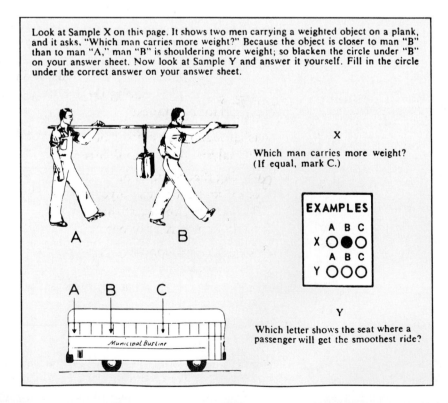

Source: Reproduced by permission. Copyright 1967, 1969 by The Psychological Corporation, New York, NY. All rights reserved. Author's note: 1969 is latest copyright on this test, which is still the main one used for this purpose.

FIGURE 7.5 Crawford Small Parts Dexterity Test

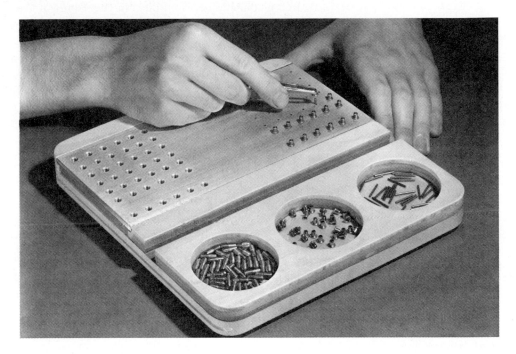

Source: The Psychological Corporation.

stamina[32]—may also be required.[33] For example, some firms are now using Functional Abilities Evaluations (FAE) to assist with placement decisions. An FAE, which measures a whole series of physical abilities—ranging from lifting, to pulling and pushing, sitting, squatting, climbing, and carrying—is particularly useful for positions with a multitude of physical demands, such as firefighter and police officer.[34] Ensuring that physical abilities tests do not violate human rights legislation requires:

Hints to Ensure Legal Compliance

- basing such tests on bona fide, essential job duties, as identified through job analysis. A physical demands analysis can be particularly helpful

- ensuring that the tests duplicate the actual physical requirements of the job. For example, if an employee will be required to lift parts that weigh up to 20 kilograms, applicants may be asked to demonstrate their ability to lift 20-kilogram parts, but not parts weighing 30, 40, or 50 kilograms

- developing and imposing such tests honestly and in good faith. For example, candidates cannot be asked to demonstrate the aerobic equivalence of a marathon runner if the fitness level required to perform the job is that of a couch potato

- ensuring that those administering the tests are properly trained and that the tests are administered in a consistent manner

- ensuring that testing standards are related to job performance in an objective sense. In other words, firms must be able to demonstrate that the standards are necessary to assure the efficient and economical performance of the job without endangering the employee, fellow employees, and/or the general public.[35] If standards have an adverse impact on protected group members, inability to justify them on these grounds can lead to charges of systemic discrimination:[36]

In a unanimous decision, the Supreme Court of Canada restored Tawney Meiorin's position as a firefighter with the B.C. Ministry of Forests, ruling that the physical fitness test being used by the province, although developed in good faith, failed to properly take into account the differing physiology of males and females. After three years on the job, Meiorin was permanently laid off when she took 49.4 seconds too long to complete a 2.5-kilometre run (a component of the newly introduced physical testing program), despite the fact that she passed all of the other physical tests. In reaching a decision, the court took into account the fact that 65 to 70 percent of men taking the test were able to pass it on their first attempt, but only 35 percent of the female applicants did so. The Ministry was also unable to prove that inability to run the race in the specified time would pose a serious safety risk to Ms. Meiorin, her fellow employees, or the public at large.

Measuring Personality and Interests

A person's mental and physical abilities are seldom sufficient to explain his or her job performance. Other factors such as the person's motivation and interpersonal skills are important too. Personality and interests inventories are sometimes used as predictors of such intangibles.

personality tests

Instruments used to measure basic aspects of personality, such as introversion, stability, motivation, neurotic tendency, self-confidence, self-sufficiency, and sociability.

Personality tests can measure basic aspects of an applicant's personality, such as introversion, stability, and motivation. Many of these tests are projective. An ambiguous stimulus (like an ink blot or clouded picture) is presented to the test taker, and he or she is asked to interpret or react to it. Since the pictures are ambiguous, the person's interpretation must come from within—he or she supposedly *projects* into the picture his or her own emotional attitudes about life. Thus, a security-oriented person might describe the woman in **Figure 7.6** as "my mother worrying about what I will do if I lose my job." Examples of personality tests (more properly called personality inventories) include the Thematic Apperception Test, the Guilford-Zimmerman Temperament Survey, and the Minnesota Multiphasic Personality Inventory. The Guilford-Zimmerman survey measures personality traits such as emotional stability versus moodiness, and friendliness versus criticalness. The Minnesota Multiphasic Personality Inventory taps traits like hypochondria and paranoia.

Personality tests—particularly the projective type—are the most difficult tests to evaluate and use. An expert must analyze the test taker's interpretations and reactions and infer from them his or her personality. The usefulness of such tests for selection then assumes that it is possible to find a relationship between a measurable personality trait (such as introversion) and success on the job.[37]

Research Insight

The difficulties notwithstanding, recent studies confirm that personality tests can help companies to hire more effective workers. For example, industrial psychologists often talk in terms of the "Big Five" personality dimensions as they apply to employment testing: *extroversion, emotional stability, agreeableness, conscientiousness, and openness to experience.*[38] One study focussed on the extent to which these dimensions predicted performance (in terms of job and training proficiency, for example) for professionals, police officers, managers, sales workers, and skilled/semiskilled workers. Conscientiousness showed a consistent relation-

FIGURE 7.6 Sample Picture from Thematic Apperception Test

How do you interpret this picture?

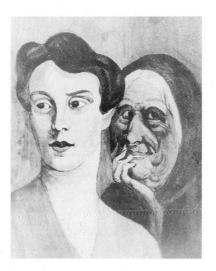

interest inventories

Tests that compare a candidate's interests with those of people in various occupations.

achievement tests

Tests used to measure knowledge and/or proficiency acquired through education, training, or experience.

ship with all performance criteria for every occupation. Extroversion was a valid predictor of performance for managers and sales employees—the two occupations involving the most social interaction. Both openness to experience and extroversion predicted training proficiency for all occupations.[39] Another study involving a sample of 89 university employees concluded that absenteeism was inversely related to extroversion and conscientiousness.[40]

A third study confirms the potential usefulness of personality tests for selection, while underscoring the importance of job analysis. The researchers concluded that the predictive power of a personality test can be quite high.[41] However, they also found that the full potential of personality testing in selection will be realized only when careful job analysis becomes the "standard practice for determining which traits are relevant to predicting performance on a given job ..."[42] In summary, personality tests can help employers to predict which candidates will succeed on the job and which will not. However, the job analysis and validation study must be carefully executed.

Interest inventories compare a candidate's interests with those of people in various occupations. Thus, a person taking the Strong-Campbell Inventory would receive a report comparing his or her interests to those of people already in occupations such as accountant, engineer, manager, or medical technologist.

Interest inventories have many uses. One is career planning, since people generally do better in jobs involving activities in which they have an interest. Another is selection. If the firm can select people whose interests are roughly the same as those of high-performing incumbents in the jobs for which it is hiring, the new employees are more likely to be successful.[43]

Achievement Tests

An achievement test is basically a measure of what a person has learned. Most of the tests taken in school are achievement tests. They measure knowledge and/or proficiency in areas such as economics, marketing, or HRM.

Achievement tests are also widely used in selection. For example, the Purdue Test for Machinists and Machine Operators tests the job knowledge of experi-

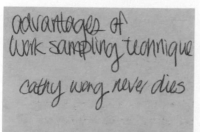

enced machinists with questions like "What is meant by 'tolerance'?" Other tests are available for electricians, welders, carpenters, and so forth. In addition to job knowledge, achievement tests measure the applicant's abilities; a keyboarding test is one example. The use of computers for achievement testing is discussed in the Information Technology and HR box.

Work Sampling for Employee Selection

work samples

Actual job tasks used in testing applicants' performance.

Work samples and simulations like assessment centres can be considered tests. However, they differ from most of the tests that we have discussed because they focus on measuring job performance directly.[44] Personality and interest inventories, on the other hand, aim to predict job performance by measuring traits such as extroversion or interests.

work sampling technique

A testing method based on measuring performance on a actual basic job tasks.a

The work sampling technique, which measures how a candidate actually performs some of the job's basic tasks,[45] has a number of advantages:

- since actual on-the-job tasks are being measured, it is harder for an applicant to fake answers
- the clear link between the work sample and actual job requirements makes such testing more legally defensible
- there is virtually no chance of such testing being viewed as an invasion of privacy, since it does not delve into the applicant's personality or psyche
- well-designed work samples are high in validity.

Information Technology and HR

Using Computers for Skills Assessment: From Math and Language to Welding

When a candidate claims to be a Grade-12 graduate, does this mean that his or her math and reading comprehension skills are currently at a Grade-12 level? Not necessarily! Basic skills-testing software, such as the Wonderlic Basic Skills Test (WBST), can help firms to measure an individual's math and reading skills accurately, so that competency level in those key areas can be assessed. Thus, such software can help firms to:

- establish appropriate minimum hiring standards, using the actual skill levels of current, successful incumbents as a benchmark
- make hiring, transfer, and promotion decisions more objectively through basic skills assessment
- identify which applicants and current employees could benefit most from math and language training
- determine the effectiveness of the firm's basic skills training programs.

Computerized testing is now available for a wide range of skills. For example, Industrial Edge is software designed to assist in the selection of applicants for industrial and manufacturing jobs. The validated tests cover everything from shop math and blueprint reading to CNC machining and welding. Another example is Pre.valuate, software that companies can access on the Internet. Available skills assessment programs evaluate skills ranging from clerical ability to proficiency with technical programming languages.

Source: "Measuring Math and Language Skills," *Guide to HR Technology, Supplement to Canadian HR Reporter* 12, no. 18 (October 18, 1999), p. G9; Al Doran and Ian Turnbull, "The Latest High-Tech Products and Software for the HR Professional: Testing," *Guide to HR Technology, Supplement to Canadian HR Reporter* 13, no. 5 (March 13, 2000), p. G9; and Michelle Griffith, "Marketplace: Testing 1-2-3, Testing 1-2-3," *HR Professional* 16, no. 2 (April/May 1999), p. 44.

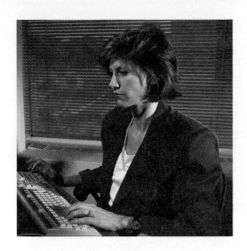

Interactive employment tests administered on the computer are becoming popular as screening devices at many firms.

The basic procedure[46] involved in developing and validating a work sampling test is illustrated in the following example:

In developing a work sampling test for maintenance mechanics, experts first list all of the possible tasks that jobholders would be required to perform. Then, by listing the frequency of performance and relative importance of each task, key tasks are identified. Thus, four crucial tasks might be: installing pulleys and belts, disassembling and installing a gear box, installing and aligning a motor, and pressing a bushing into a sprocket.

Next, the steps required to complete each of the crucial tasks are identified. Since some techniques for completing each step are better than others, the experts assign varying weights to different possible approaches. This is illustrated in **Figure 7.7**, which shows one of the steps required for installing pulleys and belts: "checks key before installing." The different possible approaches for completing this step include checking the key against (1) the shaft, (2) the pulley, or (3) neither; each possible approach has been assigned a weight (as shown on the right of the figure).

As each applicant performs the crucial tasks, his or her work is monitored by the test administrator, who completes a checklist like the one in Figure 7.7 to record the approach taken.

Finally, the work sampling test is validated by determining the relationship between the applicants' scores on the work samples and their actual performance on the job. Then, once it is shown that the work sample is a valid predictor of job success, the employer can begin using it for selection.

Management Assessment Centres

management assessment centre
A strategy used to assess candidates' management potential using a combination of realistic exercises, management games, objective testing, presentations, and interviews.

In a two- to three-day **management assessment centre,** the management potential of 10 or 12 candidates is assessed by expert appraisers who observe them performing realistic management tasks. The centre may be a plain conference room, but it is often a special room with a one-way mirror to facilitate unobtrusive observations. Examples of the types of activities and exercises involved include:

1. *An in-basket exercise.* Each candidate is faced with an accumulation of reports, memos, messages from incoming phone calls, letters, and other materials collected in the in-basket of the simulated job that he or she is to take over, and is required to take appropriate action. For example, he or she must write letters, return phone calls, and prepare meeting agendas. The trained evaluators then review the results.

FIGURE 7.7 Example of a Work Sampling Question

This is one step in installing pulleys and belts.

CHECKS KEY BEFORE INSTALLING AGAINST:		
_____ shaft	score	3
_____ pulley	score	3
_____ neither	score	1

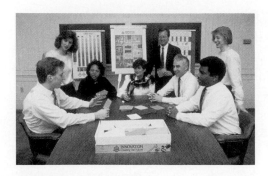

A management game or simulation is a typical component in a management assessment centre.

2. *A leaderless group discussion.* A leaderless group is given a discussion question and told to arrive at a group decision. The raters evaluate each candidate's interpersonal skills, acceptance by the group, leadership ability, and individual influence.

3. *Management games.* Participants engage in realistic problem solving, usually as members of two or more simulated companies that are competing in the marketplace. Decisions might have to be made about such issues as how to advertise and manufacture and how much inventory to keep in stock.

4. *Individual presentations.* During oral presentations on an assigned topic, each participant's communication skills and persuasiveness are evaluated.

5. *Objective tests.* Candidates may be asked to complete paper-and-pencil or computer-based personality, aptitude, interest and/or achievement tests.

6. *An interview.* Most centres also require an interview between at least one of the expert assessors and each participant to evaluate interests, background, past performance, and motivation.

Research Insight

A recent U.S. survey found that: (1) assessment centres are most commonly used for selection, promotion, and development purposes; (2) supervisory recommendations play a key role in participant selection; (3) line managers generally serve as assessors; and (4) ratings are typically reached through a consensus process.[47]

Studies indicate that assessment centres that sample realistic job behaviour can be effective as selection tools.[48] Yet, studies also raise an important question regarding one of the main disadvantages of this strategy—its high costs.[49] While one study suggests that this approach is financially efficient, another concluded that a review of participants' HR files can predict which individuals will succeed as well as an assessment centre evaluation can.[50] In another study, a combination of the assessment centre results and an evaluation of the candidate's records was found to be a better predictor than the assessment centre alone.[51]

Video-based Situational Testing

situational tests

Tests in which candidates are presented with hypothetical situations representative of the job for which they are applying and are evaluated on their responses.

In situational tests, candidates are presented with hypothetical situations representative of the job for which they are applying and are evaluated on their responses.[52] Several of the assessment centre exercises described previously are examples.

Video-based situational testing is growing in popularity. In a typical test, a number of realistic video scenarios are presented, and each is followed by a multiple-choice question with several possible courses of action, from which candidates are asked to select the "best" response, in their opinion.[53] While the evidence is somewhat mixed, the results of several recent studies suggest that video-based situational tests can be useful for employee selection.[54]

Micro-assessments

micro-assessment

A series of verbal, paper-based or computer-based questions and exercises that a candidate is required to complete, covering the range of activities required on the job for which he or she is applying.

An entirely performance-based testing strategy that focusses on individual performance is a micro-assessment. In a micro-assessment, each applicant completes a series of verbal, paper-based or computer-based questions and exercises that cover the range of activities required on the job for which he or she is applying. In addition to technical exercises, participants are required to solve a set of work-related problems that demonstrate their ability to perform well within the confines of a certain department or corporate culture. Exercises are simple to develop because they are taken directly from the job. Such assessments, which take one to three hours to complete, are generally used to identify the strengths, weaknesses, work habits, and organizational, personal and cultural fit of short-listed candidates. If only the top three performers are subsequently interviewed, such assessments can eliminate 60 to 75 percent of interviews, thereby resulting in significant cost and time savings. Other key advantages include the fact that such assessments can be:[55]

- used for any level of position in organizations of all sizes
- completed by more than one applicant at the same time
- used for both internal and external applicants, thereby levelling the playing field and helping to eliminate bias
- completed and submitted electronically by applicants down the hall, across the country, and/or on the other side of the world
- sent out at the end of the hiring party's work day, completed and returned by a prearranged time (documented by the receiving fax or e-mail), and evaluated the following morning
- easily scored within 15 minutes or so.

The Miniature Job Training and Evaluation Approach

In this performance-based approach, candidates are trained to do a representative sample of the tasks involved in the job for which they are applying and their performance is subsequently evaluated. The underlying premise is that a person who can demonstrate the ability to learn and perform a few of the required tasks will be able to learn and perform the entire job.

Advantages include the fact that it is "content relevant" and may be more acceptable and fair to some applicants (such as those for whom English or French is a second language) than the usual paper-and-pencil tests. The key disadvantage relates to its emphasis on individual instruction during training, which makes it a relatively expensive screening device.[56]

The Polygraph and Honesty Testing

polygraph (lie detector)
A device that measures physiological changes associated with stress, such as increased perspiration, blood pressure, and heart rate.

A few firms use the **polygraph** (or **"lie detector"**) for honesty testing. This is a device that measures physiological changes like increased perspiration caused by the emotional stress that accompanies lying. An applicant or current employee has painlessly attached to his or her body electrodes that transmit physiological data to the machine. The person is then asked a series of neutral questions by the polygraph expert, such as confirming his or her name and address. Once the person's emotional reaction to giving truthful answers to neutral questions has been ascertained, questions are asked such as, "Have you ever stolen anything without paying for it?" and "Have you ever been convicted of a crime for which a pardon has not been granted?" In theory, the expert can then accurately determine whether or not the applicant is lying.

There are good arguments against the use of polygraphs:

- estimates about their ability to distinguish between who is lying and who is not range from about 70 to 90 percent. Some emotional people may

Aspentree Software
www.aspentree.com

honesty tests

Psychological tests that measure an individual's attitude toward honest versus dishonest behaviours or lack of candour.

demonstrate the changes in perspiration, breathing, blood pressure, and pulse rate normally associated with lying, even when telling the truth; while others, accomplished actors, for example, may be able to tell a lie with no discernable physiological changes. Because of their questionable accuracy, polygraphs are not legally permissible as a selection tool in some Canadian jurisdictions, such as Ontario

- the experience can be demeaning and embarrassing.

Thus, even in jurisdictions in which administering polygraphs is legal, employers often choose less offensive and more accurate means to assess applicant honesty.

Paper-and-pencil honesty tests are psychological tests designed to predict job applicants' proneness to dishonesty and other forms of counterproductivity.[57] Most measure attitudes regarding things like tolerance of others who steal, acceptance of rationalizations for theft, and admission of theft-related activities. An example is the Phase II profile, owned by Wackenhut Corporation of Coral Gables, Florida. Similar tests are published by London House, Incorporated, and Stanton Corporation.[58]

While several psychologists initially raised concerns about the validity of many of the paper-and-pencil honesty tests on the market,[59] several recent studies supported the validity of honesty testing as a selection technique.

Research Insight

One study focussed on 111 employees hired by a major retail convenience store chain to work as counter persons in their stores or gas station outlets. "Shrinkage" was estimated to equal three percent of sales, and internal theft was believed to account for much of this. The researchers found that scores on an honesty test successfully predicted actual theft, as measured by termination for theft.[60]

A recent large-scale review of the use of such tests for measuring honesty, integrity, conscientiousness, dependability, trustworthiness, and reliability concluded that the "pattern of findings" regarding the usefulness of such tests "continues to be consistently positive."[61]

Despite these findings, there are several reasons to be cautious about honesty testing:

1. As noted earlier, doubt has been expressed regarding the validity of many (or most) paper-and-pencil honesty-testing instruments.

2. On purely humanitarian grounds, it can be argued that a rejection (let alone an incorrect rejection) for dishonesty carries more stigma than does being rejected for, say, poor mechanical comprehension or even poor sociability. While it is true that others may never know why a candidate was rejected, the subject, having just taken and "failed" what was likely fairly obviously an honesty test, may leave the premises feeling that his or her treatment was less than proper.

3. Test questions pose serious invasion-of-privacy issues, delving as they do into areas such as how the applicant feels about stealing, or whether he or she has ever stolen anything.

It is for these reasons that honesty testing is not legally permissible in many Canadian jurisdictions. Even where legally permissible, until more widespread evaluations are done, such tests should never be used as the sole selection strategy, but rather as a supplement to other techniques, such as interviewing and reference checking.

Graphology

graphology

The use of handwriting analysis to assess an applicant's basic personality traits.

The use of **graphology** (handwriting analysis), based on the assumption that the writer's basic personality traits will be expressed in his or her handwriting,[62] has some resemblance to projective personality tests. In graphology, the handwriting analyst studies an applicant's handwriting and signature in order to discover the person's needs, desires, and psychological makeup.[63] According to the graphologist, the writing in **Figure 7.8** exemplifies "uneven pressure, poor rhythm, and uneven baselines." The variation of light and dark lines shows a "lack of control" and is "one strong indicator of the writer's inner disturbance."

While it is true that the classified sections of international periodicals like *The Economist* run ads from graphologists offering to aid employers in selection, and that an estimated 500 Canadian companies were using handwriting analysis to assess job applicants in the early 1990s,[64] many scientists doubt its predictive validity for job performance and occupational success. The use of graphology in selection decisions is also viewed with considerable skepticism by applicants.[65]

Physical Examination

There are three main reasons why firms may include a medical examination as a step in the selection process:

1. To determine that the applicant *qualifies for the physical requirements* of the position and, if not, to document any *accommodation requirements*.

2. To establish a *record and baseline* of the applicant's health for the purpose of future insurance or compensation claims.

3. To *reduce absenteeism and accidents* by enabling the applicant and physician to identify any health- or safety-related issues or concerns that need to be addressed, including communicable diseases of which the applicant may have been unaware.

In large firms, the physician and occupational health nurse on staff look after medical testing. Smaller employers retain the services of consulting physicians to perform such exams, which are paid for by the employer. Regardless of size of

---

FIGURE 7.8 Handwriting Exhibit Used by Graphologist

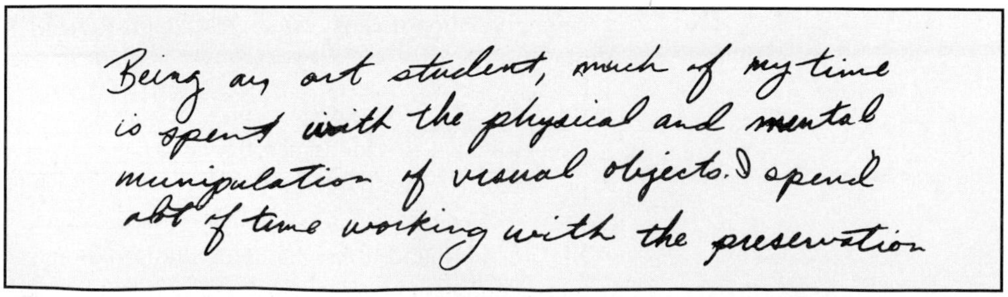

Source: Reproduced with permission from Kathryn Sackhein, *Handwriting Analysis and the Employee Selection Process* (New York: Quorum Books, 1990), p. 45.

firm, if medical testing is a step in the selection process, certain guidelines must be kept in mind:

- a medical exam is only permitted after a written offer of employment has been extended (except in the case of bona fide occupational requirements, as in food handlers)
- if used, medical exams must be required of all applicants for the job in question
- a person with a disability cannot be rejected for a job if he or she is otherwise qualified and could perform the job duties with reasonable accommodation
- while an interviewer may ask a candidate if he or she has any disability-related needs that would require accommodation, the focus must be on the type of accommodation that the employer might be expected to provide
- companies have no right to request information regarding the nature of a candidate's disability, either from the applicant or the physician performing the medical examination. The physician should only be asked to indicate, in writing, whether or not the applicant is capable of performing the essential job duties and, if not, what type of accommodation might be required
- all medical information should be retained by the examining physician, never placed in employees' HR files.

Drug Testing

The purpose of pre-employment drug testing, which is usually based on urinalysis, is to avoid hiring employees who would pose unnecessary risks to themselves or others, have an attendance problem, and/or perform below expectations.

The legal issues surrounding such testing are somewhat complex. Under human rights legislation, as with any other type of medical examination, pre-employment drug testing is only permitted after a written job offer has been extended. Based on the decision in a protracted case involving the Toronto-Dominion Bank, it seems that employers in Canada cannot use blanket drug testing, even if the results are handled in a non-punitive manner. Drug testing is only permissible if the firm can demonstrate a bona fide occupational requirement.[66]

A lower-court decision several years ago pertaining to the drug-testing policy at the Toronto-Dominion Bank (TD) affirmed the legality of blanket drug testing, as long as test results were handled appropriately. At TD, potential employees were not denied employment nor were current employees dismissed due to drug dependence. Instead, every possible opportunity was provided for rehabilitation. Dismissal was the recourse only when a habitual substance abuser refused to participate in a rehabilitation program or such a program was of no avail. Casual users faced similar disciplinary action if they tested positive on three or more occasions and continued to use drugs.

On July 23, 1998, however, TD's policy was declared discriminatory by a Federal Court of Appeal. One issue of concern was the lack of job-related rationale for the program, since the bank could not prove that drugs had actually contributed to substandard employee performance and/or theft. In addition, Justice F. Joseph McDonald found that the rehabilitation policy failed to satisfy the reasonable accommodation standard. According to McDonald, retesting is only justifiable if an employee's post-treatment performance remains inadequate, and cannot be routinely required.

There is an additional human rights issue pertaining to drugs and drug testing that employers must keep in mind: addiction to drugs or alcohol is considered to be a disability, which must be accommodated to the point of undue hardship. Thus, to deny or terminate employment to an individual with an addiction problem—whether unveiled through drug testing or on-the-job performance-related concerns—would be construed as discrimination on the basis of disability, unless undue hardship can be proven.

What complicates the legal situation even further are employers' obligations under health and safety legislation and in preventing negligent hiring.[67] Certainly, employers can legally discipline employees for being impaired on the job, with sanctions up to and including discharge. Where there is a bona fide occupational requirement, as in safety-sensitive positions, pre-employment and routine drug testing have been accepted by human rights commissions for a number of years. If an applicant refuses, he or she can be denied employment; a current employee refusing to undergo such testing can be dismissed. For example:[68]

> An arbitrator upheld Canadian Pacific's decision to discharge a train conductor who refused to submit to a drug test. The individual concerned had been charged by the police with cultivation of marijuana and had a previous conviction for possession. The arbitrator ruled that the employer "was charged with the safe operation of a railroad" and had "a particular obligation to ensure that those employees responsible for the movement of trains perform their duties unimpaired by the effect of drugs."

Legality notwithstanding, there is widespread opposition to drug testing in the workplace. The Canadian Civil Liberties Association has taken the stance that "no person should be required to share urine with a stranger" as a condition of employment.[69] Invasion of privacy concerns and questionable accuracy are at the root of this controversy.

- urine sampling is considered by many to be an invasion of privacy, as well as degrading and intrusive. While the human rights commissions have adopted the position that, to protect individual privacy, test samples should be analyzed only for the purpose intended,[70] there is nothing to prevent an unscrupulous employer from performing other analyses, such as pregnancy tests for female candidates

- while breathalyzers and blood tests for alcohol (like those given by police officers on the roadside to drivers suspected of being inebriated) do correlate closely with impairment levels, urine and blood tests for other drugs only indicate whether drug residues are present: they cannot measure impairment, habituation, or addiction[71]

- because drug tests cannot indicate whether the individual is impaired at the time that the sample is provided, only the use of a substance during preceding days or weeks, or the use of drugs during leisure hours may be identified through workplace drug testing, and yet have little or no relevance to the individual's job[72]

- as with polygraphs, drug tests are not infallible. Some less-expensive tests have been known to generate both false negative and false positive results. For example, popular over-the-counter pain pills such as Advil and Nuprin can produce positive results for marijuana; and some illegal substances do not register on commonly used tests. In response to criticism about the highly personal nature of urine analysis, and concerns about the accuracy of results, some employers have turned to hair follicle testing.[73]

In conclusion, an employer's decision to use drug testing for pre-employment or monitoring purposes involves a delicate balancing of individual right to privacy against risk of liability.[74] Because such tests do not yield data about current impairment or usage level, and may be inaccurate, even an employer's pursuit of a healthy, unimpaired work force and safe working environment do not seem to justify drug testing. The good news is that relatively simple tests that demonstrate the extent of impairment are being developed for manual dexterity and hand–eye coordination, as well as tasks of an intellectual nature.[75] It is hoped that such tests will not only be far more effective in identifying impaired conditions than drug testing, but will also be far less invasive and controversial.

Step Four: The Selection Interview

The interview is one of the most common and popular devices used for selecting job applicants. In fact, it was the only selection method being used by 100 percent of the respondents in a recent survey of 202 Canadian firms.[76] Whether candidates are interviewed prior to or following testing varies greatly. The selection interview, which involves a process of two-way communication between the interviewee(s) and the interviewer(s), can be defined as "... a procedure designed to predict future job performance on the basis of applicants' oral responses to oral inquiries."[77]

Interviews are considered to be one of the most important aspects of the selection process, and generally have a major impact on both applicants and interviewers. Interviews significantly influence applicants' views about the job and organization, enable employers to fill in any gaps in the information provided on application forms and résumés, and supplement the results of any tests administered. They may also reveal entirely new types of information.

A major reason for the popularity of selection interviews is that they meet a number of objectives of both interviewer and interviewee. Interviewer objectives include:[78]

- assessing applicants' qualifications
- observing relevant aspects of applicants' behaviour, such as verbal communication skills, degree of self-confidence, and interpersonal skills
- gathering information about applicants that will help to predict future performance (such as how well they will perform and how long they are likely to remain in the organization)
- providing candidates with information about the job and expected duties and responsibilities
- promoting the organization and highlighting its attractiveness
- determining how well the applicants would fit into the organization.

Typical objectives of job applicants include:[79]

- presenting a positive image of themselves
- selling their skills and marketing their positive attributes to the interviewer(s)
- gathering information about the job and the organization so that they can make an informed decision about the job, career opportunities in the firm, and the work environment.

selection interview
A procedure designed to predict future job performance on the basis of applicants' oral responses to oral inquiries.

SMALL BUSINESS APPLICATIONS

Testing

Just because a company is small does not mean that it should not engage in selection testing. Quite the opposite is true: hiring one or two mistakes may not be a big problem for a very large firm, but it could cause chaos in a small operation.

A number of tests are so easy to administer that they are particularly good for smaller firms. One is the Wonderlic Personnel Test. This easy-to-use test measures general cognitive ability. Given in the form of a four-page booklet, it takes less than 15 minutes to administer. The instructions are read to the candidate and then the time taken to work through the 50 problems on the two inside sheets is measured. The person's test is then scored by totalling the number of correct answers. The person's score can next be compared to the minimum scores recommended for various occupations (**Figure 7.9**) to determine whether the person achieved the minimally acceptable score for the type of job in question.

FIGURE **7.9** Minimum Scores on Wonderlic Personnel Test for Various Occupations

Position	No. of Questions Answered Correctly in 12 minutes
Chemist	31
Electrical Engineer	30
General Manager	30
Administrator	29
Computer Programmer	29
Claims Adjuster	28
Librarian	27
Management Trainee	27
News Writer	26
Office Worker	24
Salesperson	24
Cashier	24
Secretary	24
Drafter	23
Bank Teller	22
Order Clerk	22
Foreperson	22
General Clerk	21
Police Officer	21
Receptionist	21
Typist	21
Unskilled Labourer	20
Mechanic's Helper	19
Maintenance Person	18
Security Guard	17
Nurse's Aide	17
Assembler	16
Packer	15
Warehouse Person	15

See the tables presented in this manual, "Test Scores by Position Applied For" and "Minimum Occupational Scores for The Wonderlic Personnel Test," for additional data on established scores.

Source: Based on Wonderlic Personnel Test Manual (Northfield, IL: E.F. Wonderlic & Associates, Inc., 1998), p. 14.

A test like this can help to identify people who are not up to the tasks required, however, care must be taken to avoid misuse. In the past, for instance, unnecessarily high cutoff scores were required by some employers for certain jobs, a tactic that, in effect, unfairly discriminated against some designated group members. Similarly, it would probably be neither fair nor wise to choose between two candidates who both exceeded the minimum score for a job by choosing the one with the higher score, since people of lower ability but higher motivation will often outperform those with higher ability but less motivation. Therefore, tests like the Wonderlic are only useful as supplements to a comprehensive screening program. The Wonderlic is available to employers, business owners, and HR managers with or without previous training in selection testing.[1]

The Predictive Index is another example of a test that is used by large companies, but is equally valuable for small ones because of its ease of administration and interpretation. The index measures personality traits, drives, and behaviours that are work-related—in particular, dominance (ranging from submissive to arrogant), extroversion (ranging from withdrawn to gregarious), patience (ranging from volatile to lethargic), and attention to detail (ranging from sloppy to perfectionistic). The Predictive Index test is a two-sided sheet on which candidates or current employees check off the words that best describe them (such as "helpful" or "persistent"). The test is then easily scored with the use of a scoring template.

The Predictive Index provides valuable information about the candidate. For example, a candidate rating toward the careless end of the range would not be suitable for a job involving painstaking attention to detail, whereas, for an exceedingly boring job, preference might be given to candidates who are patient. Each candidate taking the Predictive Index will probably have his or her own unique pattern of responses. However, the Predictive Index program includes 15 standard patterns that are typical. For example, there is the "social interest" pattern, representing a person who is generally unselfish, congenial, persuasive, patient, and fairly unassuming. This is a person who would be good with people and a good interviewer, for instance.

Computerized testing programs like those described earlier in this chapter can be especially useful for small employers. For example, rather than depending on informal tests of keyboarding and filing skills when hiring office help, a better way to proceed is to use a PC-based program like the Minnesota Clerical Assessment Battery published by Assessment Systems Corp. Since it includes a series of tests assessing keyboarding, proofreading, and filing skills, as well as knowledge of business vocabulary, business math, and clerical procedures, it is useful for evaluating candidates for such positions as secretary, clerk, bookkeeper, and filing clerk. Because it is computerized, administration and scoring are simplified and each test can be adapted to the particular position for which the individual is applying.[2]

[1] Information and tests may be obtained from E.F. Wonderlic and Associates, Inc., 820 Frontage Rd., Northfield, IL 60093. (Telephone: (312) 445-8900)

[2] Assessment Systems Corporation may be reached at 2233 University Avenue, Suite 440, St. Paul, MN 55114. (Telephone: (612) 647-9220)

Types of Interviews

Selection interviews can be classified in four ways, according to: (1) degree of structure; (2) purpose; (3) content; and (4) the way in which the interview is administered. In turn, the main types of interviews used in selection—structured, unstructured, mixed, situational, behavioural, sequential, panel, stress, computerized, and videotaped or videoconferenced—can each be classified in one or more of these four ways.

The Structure of the Interview

unstructured interview
An unstructured, conversational-style interview. The interviewer lpursues points of interest as they come up in response to questions.

First, interviews can be classified according to the degree to which they are structured. In an unstructured (or nondirective) interview, questions are asked as they come to mind. While questions may be specified in advance, they usually are not, and there is seldom a formalized guide for scoring the quality of each answer. Interviewees for the same job thus may or may not be asked the same or similar questions, and the interview's unstructured nature allows the interviewer to ask questions based on the candidate's last statements and to pursue points of interest as they develop. While extremely friendly, unstructured interviews lack reliability, and are used for selection purposes by only 17 percent of Canadian firms.[80]

structured interview
An interview following a set sequence of questions.

The interview can also be structured. In the classical structured (or directive) interview, the questions and acceptable responses are specified in advance and the responses are rated for appropriateness of content.[81] In practice, however, most structured interviews do not involve specifying and rating responses in advance. Instead, each candidate is asked a series of predetermined, job-related questions, based on the job description and specification. Such interviews are generally high in validity and reliability, and enable inexperienced supervisors or HR practitioners to conduct useful, valid interviews. On the other hand, a totally structured interview does not provide the flexibility to pursue points of interest as they develop, which may result in an interview that seems quite mechanical to all concerned.

mixed (semi-structured) interview
An interview format that combines the structured and unstructured techniques.

Between these two extremes is the mixed (semi-structured) interview, which involves a combination of preset, structured questions based on the job description and specification, and a series of preset candidate-specific, job-related questions based on information provided on the application form and/or résumé. The questions asked of all candidates facilitate candidate comparison, while the job-related, candidate-specific questions make the interview more conversational. A realistic approach that yields comparable answers and in-depth insights, the mixed interview format is extremely popular.

The Purpose of the Interview

stress interview
An interview in which the applicant is made uncomfortable by a series of often-rude questions. This technique helps to identify hypersensitive applicants and assess degree of tolerance for stress.

A stress interview is a special type of selection interview in which the applicant is made uncomfortable by a series of questions that are sometimes rude. The aim is to help identify sensitive applicants and assess degree of tolerance for stress.

The interviewer might first probe for weaknesses in the applicant's background, such as a job that the applicant left under questionable circumstances. Having identified these, the interviewer can then focus on them, hoping to get the candidate to lose his or her composure. Thus, a candidate for customer-relations manager who obligingly mentions having had four jobs in the past two years might be told that frequent job changes reflect irresponsible and immature behaviour. If the applicant then responds with a reasonable explanation of why the job changes were necessary, another topic might be pursued. On the other hand, if the formerly tranquil applicant reacts explosively with anger and disbelief, this might be taken as a symptom of low tolerance for stress.

The stress approach can help to identify hypersensitive applicants who might be expected to overreact to mild criticism with anger and abuse. On the other hand, such interviews only sample a small portion of the behaviour expected on most jobs. Because of this limited relevance, the uneven diagnostic abilities of interviewers, and the invasive and ethically questionable nature of such interviews, this interview technique is not recommended for selection purposes.

The Content of the Interview Interviews can also be classified according to the content of their questions. A situational interview is one in which the questions focus on the individual's ability to project what his or her behaviour would be in a given situation.[82] The underlying premise is that intentions predict behaviour. For example, a candidate for a supervisory position might be asked how he or she would respond to an employee coming to work late three days in a row. The interview can be both *structured and situational*, with predetermined questions requiring the candidate to project what his or her behaviour would be. In a structured situational interview, the applicant could be evaluated, say, on whether he or she would try to determine if the employee was experiencing some difficulty in getting to work on time or would simply issue a verbal or written warning to the employee.

The behavioural interview is gaining in popularity. Also known as a behaviour description interview (BDI), this technique involves describing various situations and asking interviewees how they behaved *in the past* in such situations.[83] Thus, while situational interviews ask interviewees to describe how they *would* react to a situation, the BDI asks interviewees to describe how they *did* react to situations in the past, giving specific examples.[84] The underlying assumption is that the best predictor of future performance is past performance in similar circumstances.

Finally, *psychological interviews* may be used for selection purposes. Often included in assessment centre evaluations, for example, such psychologist-conducted interviews are used to assess personality traits such as dependability.[85] Such interviews generally have a significant unstructured element.

Administering the Interview Interviews can also be classified based on how they are administered: one-on-one or by a panel of interviewers; sequentially or all at once; and computerized, audiotaped, videotaped, videoconferenced, teleconferenced, or conducted entirely in person.

Most interviews are administered *one-on-one*. For example, in one recent study, one-on-one interviews were "always used" by 85 percent of the participating employers.[86] As the name implies, this process involves one interviewer and one interviewee.

Most selection processes are sequential. In a *sequential interview* the applicant is interviewed by several persons in sequence before a selection decision is made. In an *unstructured sequential interview* each interviewer may look at the applicant from his or her own point of view, ask different questions, and form an independent opinion of the candidate. On the other hand, in a structured sequential or serialized interview, each interviewer rates the candidate on a standard evaluation form, and the ratings are compared before the hiring decision is made.[87]

A panel interview involves the candidate being interviewed simultaneously by a group (or panel) of interviewers. The panel typically comprises a represen-

---

situational interview
A series of job-related questions that focus on how the candidate would behave in a given situation.

behavioural or behaviour descriptive interview (BDI)
A series of job-related questions that focus on relevant past job-related behaviours.

serialized interview
An interview in which the applicant is interviewed sequentially by several persons who each rate the applicant on a standard form.

panel interview
An interview in which a group of interviewers questions the applicant.

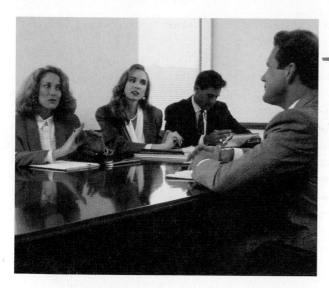

A panel interview is an efficient and cost-effective way of permitting a number of qualified persons to assess a candidate's KSAs.

tative of the HR department, the hiring manager, and potential coworkers, superiors, and/or reporting employees. Panel interviews are becoming increasingly popular. In fact, they are "always" used by 24 percent of the employers responding to a recent survey, and "sometimes used" by 49 percent of respondents.[88] The key advantages associated with this technique are as follows:

- having a number of people present, with varied backgrounds, increases the likelihood that the information provided will be heard and recorded accurately

- because of their differing perspectives and areas of expertise, interview team members may focus on different aspects of interviewee behaviour

- the finalist interviewees typically only have to attend one interview rather than two or three, thereby minimizing travel/accommodation expenses (which are often reimbursed by the interviewing employer, especially in the case of senior-level applicants), and saving a great deal of time.

- the almost inevitable duplication of questions involved in sequential interviews (unless they are carefully orchestrated) can be avoided

- the likelihood of human rights/employment equity violations is greatly reduced, since an HR department representative is present at the only interview that the top candidates attend

- each interviewer can ask and answer questions pertaining to his or her area of expertise, thereby ensuring that more in-depth information is gathered and provided

- there is less likelihood of interviewer error. Advance planning and preparation are required in order to coordinate the team, and there is a virtual guarantee that at least one member (and likely more) will have thorough knowledge of the job. Also, team members can build on strengths (such as one member's warm, personable manner) and compensate for weaknesses (such as the tendency of one interviewer to jump to conclusions, and another to do too much talking, for example)

- interviewees may actually be more comfortable with a team, especially if there is representation from both sexes and various cultural, racial, etc. groups

- despite the fact that panel interviews tend to be more thorough and often a little lengthier than single-person interviews, less time tends to be spent, overall. (In multiple interview situations, each interviewer has to take time to build rapport, discuss the job and firm, answer interviewee questions, and explain subsequent steps. In a single, panel interview, these steps occur only once.)

computerized selection interview
An interview technique involving a computer, rather than a person. A candidate's oral and/or computerized responses to computer-generated oral or written questions and/or situations are obtained and assessed.

A more stressful variant of the panel interview is the *mass interview*, which involves a panel simultaneously interviewing several candidates. The panel poses a problem to be solved and then sits back and watches which candidate takes the lead in formulating an answer.

Increasingly, interviews aren't administered by people at all but are computerized, teleconferenced, or videoconferenced. A **computerized selection interview** is one in which a job candidate's oral and/or computerized responses are

HR Software
www.peoplesoft.com

obtained in response to computerized oral or written questions and/or situations. The basic idea is to present to each applicant a series of questions (often multiple choice) regarding his or her KSAs for the job for which he or she has applied. Once the questions have been answered, they are automatically scored and the candidates are ranked, according to a predetermined weighting scale based on the relative importance of each of the selection criteria.

Computer-based interviewing can be very advantageous. Often, such interviews are used to narrow down the applicant pool, and only the two or three candidates most closely matching the job specifications are invited in for a personal interview, thereby saving considerable time and money.[89] Applicants are also reportedly more honest with computers than they would be with people, presumably because computers are not judgmental.[90] A computer can also be sneaky: If an applicant takes longer than average to answer a question like, "Can you be trusted?" he or she may be summarily screened out or later asked probing questions in that area by a human interviewer. Several of the interpersonal interview problems that we will discuss later in this chapter (such as making a snap judgment based a candidate's appearance) are also avoided with this nonpersonal interviewing approach.[91] On the other hand, the mechanical nature of computer-based interviews can leave applicants with the impression that the prospective employer is rather impersonal. A description of a relatively sophisticated, actual computer-based interview is presented in the Information Technology and HR box.

There are some other technology-based alternatives. Videotaped or audiotaped interviews involve a combination of in-person and technology-based techniques. First, a traditional face-to-face interview is conducted and taped (with the consent of the interviewee). At the completion of the interview, the candidate is assessed by the interviewer. The videotape or audiotape is then taken to the company for review by another interviewer or interviewers, including the hiring manager. Those conducting such a review assess the applicant independently, and the assessments are then pooled to arrive at a final candidate evaluation.

There are also two entirely technology-based strategies, **teleconferencing** and **videoconferencing**, which permit "real-time" interviews. Interest in such technology-based alternatives to traditional face-to-face interviews is related to: the expansion of national and international markets and satellite or off-site offices; the increasing frequency of home-based employees; increasing competition for qualified employees; and decreasing recruitment and selection budgets. All of these factors have contributed to the need for more cost-effective strategies. Alternatives that enable organizations to conduct "long-distance" interviews can save time, money, and effort. Aggressive marketing and increased demand mean that even the smallest organization can now easily access video and teleconference services at a reasonable cost.[92]

videotaped/audiotaped interview

An interview technique that involves both an in-person and technology-based component. A face-to-face interview is conducted and taped. The video or audiotape is then independently assessed by interviewers who have not met the candidate.

videoconferenced/ teleconferenced interview

An interview technique that is entirely technology-based. Using a combination of video and audio equipment, or audio equipment alone (in the case of a teleconference), interviews are conducted with candidates who are physically distant from both conference location and interviewer.

Research Insight

A 1997 study assessing videoconferenced college recruitment interviews found that while the employers involved preferred face-to-face interviews, they believed that through videoconferencing they were able to gather appropriate information to screen out less-qualified candidates. The students participating also preferred traditional interviews, but reported being comfortable with the process. Both employers and students identified access to a wider pool (of appli-